Orthopaedics for the Physical Therapist Assistant

Mark Dutton, PT

Allegheny General Hospital
Pittsburgh, Pennsylvania

Content Review
Debra A. Belcher, PT, DPT
Associate Professor, PTA Program
Sinclair Community College
Dayton, Ohio

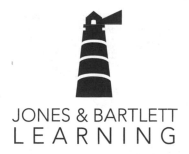

JONES & BARTLETT
LEARNING

World Headquarters
Jones & Bartlett Learning
40 Tall Pine Drive
Sudbury, MA 01776
978-443-5000
info@jblearning.com
www.jblearning.com

Jones & Bartlett Learning books and products are available through most bookstores and online booksellers. To contact Jones & Bartlett Learning directly, call 800-832-0034, fax 978-443-8000, or visit our website, www.jblearning.com.

Substantial discounts on bulk quantities of Jones & Bartlett Learning publications are available to corporations, professional associations, and other qualified organizations. For details and specific discount information, contact the special sales department at Jones & Bartlett Learning via the above contact information or send an email to specialsales@jblearning.com.

Some images in this book feature models. These models do not necessarily endorse, represent, or participate in the activities represented in the images.

The author, editor, and publisher have made every effort to provide accurate information. However, they are not responsible for errors, omissions, or for any outcomes related to the use of the contents of this book and take no responsibility for the use of the products and procedures described. Treatments and side effects described in this book may not be applicable to all people; likewise, some people may require a dose or experience a side effect that is not described herein. Drugs and medical devices are discussed that may have limited availability controlled by the Food and Drug Administration (FDA) for use only in a research study or clinical trial. Research, clinical practice, and government regulations often change the accepted standard in this field. When consideration is being given to use of any drug in the clinical setting, the health care provider or reader is responsible for determining FDA status of the drug, reading the package insert, and reviewing prescribing information for the most up-to-date recommendations on dose, precautions, and contraindications, and determining the appropriate usage for the product. This is especially important in the case of drugs that are new or seldom used.

Production Credits
Publisher: David D. Cella
Acquisitions Editor: Katey Birtcher
Associate Editor: Maro Gartside
Production Manager: Julie Champagne Bolduc
Production Editor: Jessica Steele Newfell
Marketing Manager: Grace Richards
Manufacturing and Inventory Control Supervisor: Amy Bacus
Composition: Glyph International
Cover Design: Kate Ternullo
Rights and Permissions Supervisor: Christine Myaskovsky
Assistant Photo Researcher: Elise Gilbert
Cover Image: © Patrick Hermans/ShutterStock, Inc.
Printing and Binding: Edwards Brothers Malloy
Cover Printing: Edwards Brothers Malloy

Library of Congress Cataloging-in-Publication Data
Dutton, Mark, author.
 Orthopaedics for the physical therapist assistant / Mark Dutton, PT, Allegheny General Hospital, Pittsburgh ; content review, Debra A. Belcher, PT, DPT, Associate Professor, PTA Program, Sinclair Community College.
    p. ; cm.
 Includes bibliographical references and index.
 ISBN 978-0-7637-9755-3 (paperback : alk. paper)
 1. Orthopedics. 2. Allied health personnel. 3. Musculoskeletal system—Diseases—Physical therapy. I. Title.
 [DNLM: 1. Orthopedic Procedures—methods. 2. Allied Health Personnel. 3. Musculoskeletal Diseases—therapy.
 4. Physical Therapy Modalities. 5. Wounds and Injuries—therapy. WE 190]
 RC925.5.D88 2011
 616.7—dc22
                            2010052508

6048
Printed in the United States of America
18 17 16 15   10 9 8 7 6 5 4

To my Mum, who is no longer around to do those things that Mums do best.

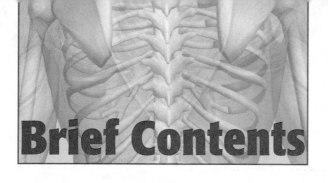

Brief Contents

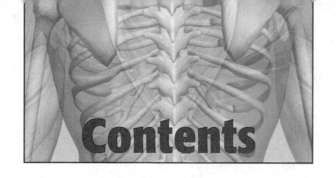

Contents

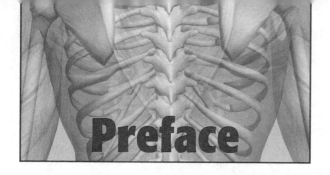

Preface

The aim of *Orthopaedics for the Physical Therapist Assistant* is to fill a void in the present literature and to be of value to the physical therapist assistant (PTA) student studying orthopaedics. The management of the patient/client is a complex process involving an intricate blend of experience, knowledge, and interpersonal skills. There is a vast amount of information available related to orthopaedics, and, with an ever-increasing demand for instant results and the continuing advances in technology, the PTA is tasked to provide an efficient level of care with other members of the healthcare team.

Although the medical profession is moving toward an increased reliance on the findings from imaging studies such as computed axial tomography (CAT) and magnetic resonance imaging (MRI), physical therapy continues to rely on the subjective and objective findings from the physical examination. For any patient interaction to be successful, an accurate diagnosis is essential, and through the move toward evidence-based testing, the accuracy of the physical therapy diagnosis continues to be enhanced.

Once established, the diagnosis must be followed by a carefully planned and specific rehabilitation program for both the affected area and its related structures. This approach must take into consideration the anatomy and biomechanics of the structure involved and the stage of healing. Each intervention must be individualized to the patient, requiring an eclectic approach, because no single approach works all of the time.

This text attempts to provide the student with the essential information regarding the anatomy and biomechanics of each major area of the body together with evidence-based guidelines for the assessment and rehabilitation of the orthopaedic patient. Therapeutic exercise is a major component of the intervention plan for orthopaedic impairments, and the exercises for each of the areas are covered in detail.

Although it would be nice to be able to give myself credit for the contents of this book, that would be a gross misrepresentation. I owe a huge debt to all those practitioners who continue to publish their findings for our benefit. I merely serve as a conduit for that information and present those techniques and principles that have worked for me as practicing clinician. I hope this book will be seen as the best available textbook, guide, review, and reference for orthopaedic students.

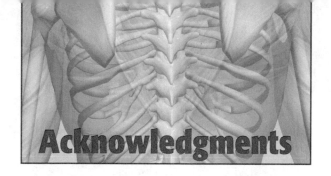

Acknowledgments

It is my firm belief that our accomplishments in life are due to a supporting cast of people who help shape, direct, and inspire. I, therefore, would like to thank the following:

- My family. Certain sacrifices to family life are always necessary when a task of this size is undertaken.
- The team at Jones & Bartlett Learning: David Cella for his confidence in this project, and Maro Gartside for her patience, guidance, and support.
- My parents for teaching me the importance of hard work and perseverance.
- Bob Davis for his excellent eye during our photo shoots and for the resulting photos.
- Leah for agreeing to be the photographic model even before she knew what it entailed.
- The staff of Human Motion Rehabilitation, Allegheny General Hospital.

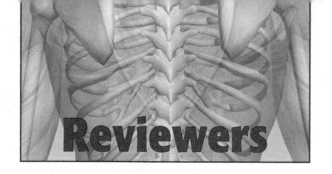
Reviewers

Denise Abrams, PT, DPT, MA
Chairperson
Physical Therapist Assistant Program
Broome Community College

Jessica M. Goodman, PT, DPT
Professor
Gateway Community College

Jacki Klaczak Kopack, PT, DPT
Director
Physical Therapist Assistant Program
Harcum College

Julianne Martin, PT, MA
Assistant Professor
Physical Therapist Assistant Program
Broome Community College

Jose M. Milan, PTA, BSc
Assistant Professor
Austin Community College

Jennifer Pitchford, PTA, BS
Instructor
Physical Therapist Assistant Program
Jefferson Community and Technical College

Laurie Schroder, PT, DPT
Program Manager
Physical Therapist Assistant Program
Daymar Institute

Verla Ubert, MA, PT, MBA
Director
Physical Therapist Assistant Program
Kennebec Valley Community College

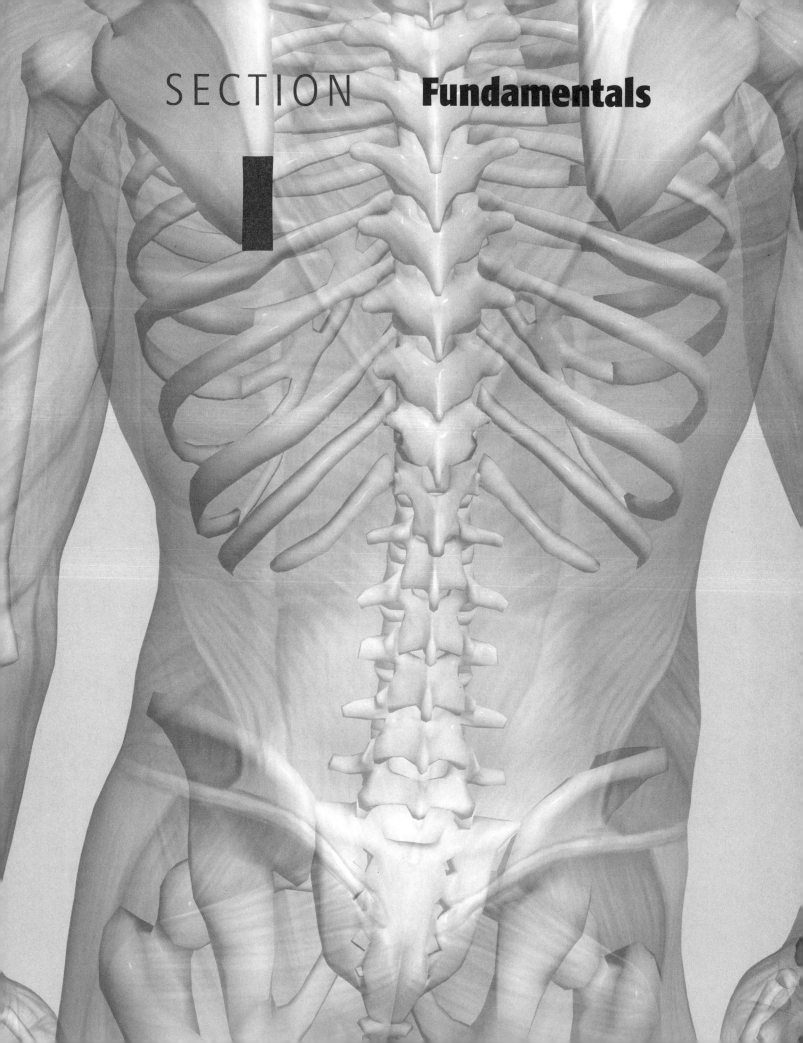

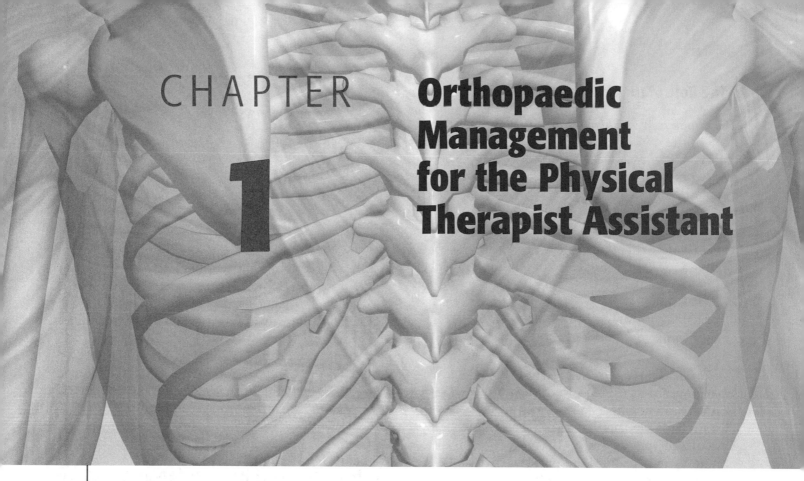

CHAPTER

1

Orthopaedic Management for the Physical Therapist Assistant

Chapter Objectives

At the completion of this chapter, the reader will be able to:

1. Describe the role of the physical therapist assistant in the orthopaedic setting.
2. List the different members of the orthopaedic rehabilitation team and describe their respective roles.
3. Describe the model of disablement used by the *Guide to Physical Therapist Practice*.
4. Recognize a medical emergency in the orthopaedic setting.
5. Understand the importance of monitoring vital signs.
6. Outline some of the common causes of edema.
7. Discuss the important concepts of an intervention.
8. Describe some of the medications used in orthopaedics and their potential impact.
9. Discuss what the SOAP note is, and the importance of accurate documentation.
10. Have a working knowledge of the types of abbreviations used in the orthopaedic setting.

Overview

The management of the orthopaedic patient involves a complex relationship between the clinician and the patient. The aim of the management process is to develop a rapport between clinician and patient while providing an efficient and effective exchange. The success of this process involves a myriad of skills. Successful clinicians demonstrate effective communication skills, clinical reasoning, critical judgment, creative decision-making, knowledge, and competence.

The Role of the Physical Therapist Assistant

The *Guide to Physical Therapist Practice* was developed by the American Physical Therapy Association (APTA) "to encourage a uniform approach to physical therapist practice and to explain to the world the nature of that practice."[1] The *Guide* is divided into two parts:

- Part 1 delineates the physical therapist's scope of practice and describes patient management by physical therapists (PTs).
- Part 2 describes each of the diagnostic preferred practice patterns of patients typically treated by PTs.

Physical therapy is defined as the care and services provided by or under the direction and supervision of a physical therapist. Physical therapists are the only professionals who provide physical therapy. Physical therapist assistants (PTAs)—under the direction and supervision of the physical therapist—are the only paraprofessionals who assist in the provision of physical therapy interventions. The *Guide for Conduct of the Physical Therapist Assistant*[2] is provided in Appendix A.

● **Key Point** The APTA House of Delegates (HOD) first authorized the training of PTAs at the 1967 Annual Conference by adopting the policy statement *Training and Utilization of the Physical Therapist Assistant.* In 1977, the Commission on Accreditation in Education (CAE), the precursor to the Commission on Accreditation in Physical Therapy Education (CAPTE), was established and recognized by the U.S. Department of Education and by the Council on Postsecondary Accreditation. The activities of the CAE included accreditation of programs for PTAs.

The role of the PTA has continued to evolve since its conception, and PTAs practice in a broad range of inpatient, outpatient, and community-based settings. According to the APTA's HOD (HOD 06-96-39 and HOD 06-00-16-27), the PTA is specifically defined as "a technically educated health care provider who assists the physical therapist in the provision of physical therapy. ... In the contemporary provision of physical therapy services, the physical therapist is considered the professional practitioner of physical therapy, while the physical therapist assistant, educated at the technical level, is considered the paraprofessional."

● **Key Point** Supervision of the PTA is governed by a number of factors including:

- APTA standards.
- Individual state and federal laws regulating practice acts, including administrative rules for practice. Supervision of the PTA may be spelled out separately from other support personnel, or the PTA may be included in language that defines supervision for all support personnel. When the state laws do not delineate supervision requirements, PTs and PTAs should rely on the APTA guidelines. State regulations always supersede the APTA guidelines.
- Specifications of entitlement programs such as Medicare.

It is the responsibility of the PT to examine the patient; evaluate the data and identify problems; determine the diagnosis, prognosis, and plan of care (POC); and implement the POC (intervention).[3] The PTA may help the PT with the initial examination, gathering specific data that the PT requests. The PT evaluates the results of data collection and makes a judgment about data value. The PTA does not interpret the results of the initial examination. The PT establishes the goals or outcomes to be accomplished by the POC and treatment plan and performs the patient's interventions. The PTA performs selected interventions as directed by the PT. The PTA must also recognize when involvement of the PT is warranted.

● **Key Point** The PTA is responsible for data collection, carrying out the PT's POC, providing proper patient supervision, communicating with the PT, recording the patient's progress or lack of progress since the initial examination and evaluation, and providing clinical observation during treatment sessions.

The PTA is frequently called upon to modify or adjust therapeutic interventions, either to progress the patient as directed by the PT or to ensure patient safety and comfort. These modifications or adjustments include, but are not limited to, any or all interventions in response to changes in a patient's signs and symptoms, range of motion (ROM), strength, endurance, function, balance, and coordination (**Table 1-1**). The PTA also may ask the PT to perform a re-examination.

● **Key Point** When performing data collection, it is important for the PTA to consider why a change in patient status has occurred. For example, when the PTA is using a goniometer to measure knee range of motion of a patient and finds that the patient is unable to perform the last 5 degrees of extension, the PTA should begin thinking about possible reasons why the patient is unable to achieve full knee extension. However, the PTA is obligated to consult with the supervising PT before making any changes outside of the POC.

TABLE 1-1

Essential Data Collection Skills for Carrying Out an Orthopaedic Plan of Care

Aerobic Capacity and Endurance
Measures standard vital signs
Recognizes and monitors responses to positional changes and activities
Observes and monitors thoracoabdominal movements and breathing patterns with activity

Anthropometrical Characteristics
Measures height, weight, length, and girth

Arousal, Mentation, and Cognition
Recognizes changes in the direction and magnitude of patient's state of arousal, mentation, and cognition

Assistive, Adaptive, Orthotic, Protective, Supportive, and Prosthetic Devices
Identifies the individual's and caregiver's ability to care for the device
Recognizes changes in skin condition while using devices and equipment
Recognizes safety factors while using the device

Gait, Locomotion, and Balance
Describes the safety, status, and progression of a patient while engaged in gait, locomotion, and balance

Integumentary Integrity
Recognizes absent or altered sensation
Recognizes normal and abnormal integumentary changes

Joint Integrity and Mobility
Recognizes normal and abnormal joint movement

Muscle Performance
Measures muscle strength by manual muscle testing
Observes the presence or absence of muscle mass
Recognizes normal and abnormal muscle length
Recognizes changes in muscle tone

Pain
Administers standardized questionnaires, graphs, behavioral scales, or visual analog scales for pain
Recognizes activities, positioning, and postures that aggravate or relieve pain or altered sensations

Posture
Describes resting posture in any position
Recognizes alignment of trunk and extremities at rest and during activities

Range of Motion
Measures functional range of motion
Measures range of motion using a goniometer

Applicable Standards
3.3.2.9. Adjusts interventions within the plan of care established by the physical therapist in response to patient clinical indications and reports this to the supervising physical therapist
3.3.2.10. Recognizes when intervention should not be provided due to changes in the patient's status and reports this to the supervising physical therapist
3.3.2.11. Reports any changes in the patient's status to the supervising physical therapist
3.3.2.12. Recognizes when the direction to perform an intervention is beyond that which is appropriate for a physical therapist assistant and initiates clarification with the physical therapist
3.3.2.13. Participates in educating patients and caregivers as directed by the supervising physical therapist
3.3.2.14. Provides patient-related instruction to patients, family members, and caregivers to achieve patient outcomes based on the plan of care established by the physical therapist
3.3.2.15. Takes appropriate action in an emergency situation
3.3.2.16. Completes thorough, accurate, logical, concise, timely, and legible documentation that follows guidelines and specific documentation formats required by state practice acts, the practice setting, and other regulatory agencies
3.3.2.17. Participates in discharge planning and follow-up as directed by the supervising physical therapist
3.3.2.18. Reads and understands the healthcare literature

Data from Accreditation Handbook: PTA Criteria, Appendix A-32.

Strong interpersonal communication between the patient, the physical therapist, and the PTA; keen observation; and sound clinical decision-making are needed for the PTA to function effectively and efficiently.

The Rehabilitation Team

The PTA is only one vital member of the rehabilitation team (**Table 1-2**).[2] The PTA is responsible and accountable to the other members of the team. However, the responsibility for the patient care is shared by the entire rehabilitation team and requires the active participation of the patient. **Table 1-3** provides the standards for the PTA's role in administering physical therapy.

● **Key Point**   The PTA should always be looking for ways to establish relationships with the other team members and to use the resources that they can provide.

Fundamental differences involving protocols and treatment approaches can exist among the members of the rehabilitation team due to different backgrounds and types of education; these can place the PTA in uncomfortable situations. For example, when transferring the patient from bed to chair, a nurse may insist that the PTA transfers the patient using a technique that the PTA considers will put the patient at increased risk. The PTA must use these scenarios as opportunities for communication, learning, and increased understanding of the other team members.

TABLE 1-2   Potential Key Members of the Orthopaedic Rehabilitation Team

Personnel	Function
Orthopaedic surgeon	A surgeon concerned with conditions involving the musculoskeletal system. Orthopaedic surgeons use both surgical and nonsurgical approaches to treat musculoskeletal trauma, sports injuries, degenerative diseases, infections, tumors, and congenital disorders.
Physiatrist	A physician specializing in physical medicine and rehabilitation, who has been certified by the American Board of Physical Medicine and Rehabilitation. The primary role of the physiatrist is to diagnose and treat patients with disabilities involving musculoskeletal, neurological, cardiovascular, or other body systems.
Primary care physician (PCP)	A practitioner, usually an internist, general practitioner, or family medicine physician, providing primary care services and managing routine healthcare needs. Most PCPs serve as gatekeepers for managed-care health organizations, providing authorization for referrals to other specialty physicians or services, including physical therapy.
Chiropractor (DC)	A doctor trained in the science, art, and philosophy of chiropractic. A chiropractic evaluation and treatment is directed at providing a structural analysis of the musculoskeletal and neurologic systems of the body. According to chiropractic doctrine, abnormal function of these two systems may affect function of other systems in the body.
Physical therapy director/ manager	The director or manager is typically a physical therapist who has demonstrated qualifications based on education and experience in the field of physical therapy and who has accepted the inherent responsibilities of the role. He or she establishes guidelines and procedures that will delineate the functions and responsibilities of all levels of physical therapy personnel in the department and the supervisory relationships inherent to the functions of the department and the health system.
	This person also ensures that the objectives of the service are efficiently and effectively achieved within the framework of the stated purpose of the organization and in accordance with safe physical therapist practice, interprets administrative policies, acts as a liaison between line staff and administration, and fosters the professional growth of the staff.
Staff physical therapist (PT)	The staff PT is responsible for the examination, evaluation, diagnosis, prognosis, and intervention of patients. He or she assists in the supervision of physical therapy personnel in the service.
Physical therapist assistant (PTA)	A PTA works under the supervision of a physical therapist. Care provided by a PTA may include teaching patients/clients exercise for mobility, strength, and coordination, and training patients for activities such as walking with crutches, canes, or walkers, and using adjunctive interventions. The PTA may modify an intervention only in accordance with changes in patient status and within the established plan of care developed by the physical therapist.

| | TABLE 1-2 | Potential Key Members of the Orthopaedic Rehabilitation Team (continued) |

Personnel	Function
PT/OT aide	Aides are support personnel who may be involved in support services directed by PTs and PTAs. They receive on-the-job training and are permitted to function only with continuous on-site supervision by a physical therapist, or in some cases, a physical therapist assistant. Their duties are limited to those methods and techniques that do not require clinical decision making or clinical problem solving by a physical therapist or a physical therapist assistant.
PT or PTA student	The PT or PTA student can perform duties commensurate with their level of education. The PT clinical instructor (CI) is responsible for all actions and duties of the affiliating student, and can supervise both physical therapy and physical therapist assistant students. (A PTA may only supervise a PTA student, not a PT student.)
Volunteer	A member of the community who is interested in assisting with rehab departmental activities. Responsibilities include taking phone messages and basic nonclinical/secretarial duties. Volunteers may not provide or set up patient treatment, transfer patients, clean whirlpools, or maintain equipment.
Occupational therapist (OT)	OTs assess functioning in activities of everyday living, including dressing, bathing, grooming, meal preparation, writing, and driving, which are essential for independent living. The minimum educational requirements for the registered occupational therapist are described in the current *Essentials and Guidelines of an Accredited Educational Program for the Occupational Therapist.*
Certified OT assistant (COTA)	An OT assistant works under the direction of an occupational therapist. He or she performs a variety of rehabilitative activities and exercises as outlined in an established treatment plan. The minimum educational requirements for the COTA are described in the current *Essentials and Guidelines of an Accredited Educational Program for the Occupational Therapy Assistant.*
Certified orthotist (CO)	A CO designs, fabricates, and fits orthoses (e.g., braces, splints, collars, corsets), prescribed by physicians, to patients with disabling conditions of the limbs and spine.
Certified prosthetist (CP)	A CP designs, fabricates, and fits prostheses for patients with partial or total absence of a limb.
Physician's assistant (PA)	A PA is a medically trained professional who can provide many of the healthcare services traditionally performed by a physician, such as taking medical histories and doing physical examinations, making a diagnosis, and prescribing and administering therapies.
Nurse practitioner (NP)	An NP is a registered nurse with additional specialized graduate-level training who can perform physical exams and diagnostic tests, counsel patients, and develop treatment programs.
Certified athletic trainer (ATC)	The certified athletic trainer is a professional specializing in athletic health care. In cooperation with the physician and other allied health personnel, the athletic trainer functions as an integral member of the athletic healthcare team in secondary schools, colleges and universities, sports medicine clinics, professional sports programs, and other athletic healthcare settings.

| | TABLE 1-3 | The PTA's Role in Administration |

Administration

Standard 3.3.2.21. Interacts with other members of the health care team in patient-care and nonpatient-care activities

Standard 3.3.2.22. Provides accurate and timely information for billing and reimbursement purposes

Standard 3.3.2.23. Describes aspects of organizational planning and operation of the physical therapy service

Standard 3.3.2.24. Participates in performance improvement activities (quality assurance)

Data from Accreditation Handbook: PTA Criteria, Appendix A-3.

Models of Disablement

A disablement model is designed to detail the functional consequences of and relationships among disease, impairment, and functional limitations (**Table 1-4**). The PTA's understanding of the process of disablement, and the factors that affect its development, is crucial to achieving the goal of restoring or improving function and reducing disability in the individual. The *Guide to Physical Therapist Practice*[3] employs terminology from the Nagi disablement model (an example of which is shown in **Table 1-5**)[4]

TABLE 1-4 Disablement Model Comparisons

The International Classification of Functioning, Disability and Health (ICFDH-I)	Nagi Disablement Model	The International Classification of Functioning, Disability and Health (ICFDH-II)
Disease The intrinsic pathology or disorder	**Pathology/Pathophysiology** Interruption of or interference with normal processes and efforts of an organism to regain normal state	**Health Condition** Dysfunction of a body function and/or structure
Impairment Loss or abnormality of psychological, physiologic, or anatomic structure or function	**Impairment** Anatomic, physiologic, mental, or emotional abnormalities or loss	**Impairment** Problems in body function or structure such as a significant deviation or loss
Disability Restriction or lack of ability to perform an activity in a normal manner	**Functional Limitation** Limitation in performance at the level of the whole organism or person	**Activity Limitation** Limitation in execution of a task or action by an individual
Handicap Disadvantage or disability that limits or prevents fulfillment of a normal role (depends on age, sex, and sociocultural factors for the person)	**Disability** Limitation in performance of socially defined roles and tasks within a sociocultural and physical environment	**Participation Restriction** Prevents fulfillment of involvement in a life situation

TABLE 1-5 Example of Nagi Disablement Model

Pathology/Pathophysiology	Impairment	Related Functional Limitation	Disability
Osteoarthritis	Loss of range of motion (ROM)	Slow, painful gait—unable to ambulate 20 feet in 9 seconds	Does not leave house
	Muscle weakness	Unable to rise from chair	
		Unable to ascend/descend 10 steps	

but also describes its framework as being consistent with other disablement models.[5] In 1980 the Executive Board of the World Health Organization (WHO) published a document for trial purposes, the *International Classification of Functioning, Disability and Health* (ICFDH-I or ICF). In 2001, a revised edition was published (ICFDH-II) that emphasized "components of health" rather than "consequences of disease" (i.e., participation rather than disability) and environmental and personal factors as important determinants of health.[6] The following defines some of the terms used in that document:

- *Impairment:* Loss or abnormality of anatomic, physiologic, or psychologic structure or function. Not all impairments are modifiable by physical therapy, and not all impairments cause activity limitations and participation restrictions.[1]
- *Primary impairment:* An impairment that can result from active pathology or disease. Examples include loss of sensation and loss of strength. Primary impairment can create secondary impairments and can lead to secondary pathology.

- *Secondary impairment:* An impairment that originates from primary impairment and pathology.[1] Examples include conditions that result from limited mobility (e.g., pressure sores, contractures, and cardiovascular deconditioning).
- *Composite impairment:* When an impairment is the result of multiple underlying causes and arises from a combination of primary or secondary impairments.[7] For example, a patient who sustained a fracture of the tibial plateau and whose knee was immobilized for several weeks is likely to exhibit a balance impairment of the involved lower extremity after the immobilization has been removed. It is important to be able to recognize functionally relevant impairments, because not all impairments are necessarily linked to functional limitations or disability.
- *Functional limitation:* A restriction of the ability to perform at the level of the whole person, a physical action, an activity, or a task in an efficient, typically expected, or competent manner.[1]

The Five Elements of Patient/Client Management

The PTA must be aware of the sequence, organization, and administration of an examination performed by the PT. This awareness increases the PTA's understanding of the rationale for decision making and the plan of care. The five elements of patient/client management are as follows:[3]

1. Examination of the patient
2. Evaluation of the data and identification of problems
3. Determination of the diagnosis
4. Determination of the prognosis and POC
5. Implementation of the POC (intervention)

An outline of the physical therapy examination for each of the joints is provided in the relevant chapters of this book. Throughout the patient's plan of care, the PTA must communicate changes in the patient's status relative to data from the initial examination and make safe and appropriate modifications to the existing program based on consultation with the supervising PT.

Examination

The examination is an ongoing process that begins with the patient referral or initial entry and continues throughout the course of the rehabilitation program.

The process of examination includes gathering information from the chart, other caregivers, the patient, the patient's family, caregivers, and friends in order to identify and define the patient's problem(s).[8] The examination consists of three components of equal importance—patient history, systems review, and tests and measures.[3] These components are closely related, in that they often occur concurrently. One further element, observation, occurs throughout.

> **● Key Point** A continual assessment by the PTA with each treatment session allows the PT to evaluate progress and modify interventions as appropriate.[3] It is not unusual for a patient to neglect to provide the PT with information pertinent to their condition during the initial examination, often because they felt it was irrelevant. If the patient provides such information to the PTA, he or she must decide whether the information warrants communication with the PT.

Patient History

The patient history involves gathering information from a review of the medical records and interviews with the patient, family members, caregiver, and other interested persons about the patient's history and current functional and health status.[9]

> **● Key Point** It is estimated that 80 percent of the information needed to explain the presenting patient problem can be provided by a thorough history.[10]

Systems Review

The systems review is a brief or limited examination that provides additional information about the patient's general health and the continuum of patient/client care throughout the lifespan. The purpose of the systems review is to:

- Help determine the anatomic and physiologic status of all systems (musculoskeletal, neurologic, cardiovascular, pulmonary, integumentary, gastrointestinal, urinary, and genitoreproductive)
- Provide information about communication skills, affect, cognition, language abilities, education needs, and learning style of the patient
- Narrow the focus of subsequent tests and measures
- Define areas that may cause complications or indicate a need for precautions during the examination and intervention processes
- Screen for physical, sexual, and psychological abuse

- Make a determination of the need for further physical therapy services based on an evaluation of the information obtained
- Identify problems that require consultation with, or referral to, another healthcare provider

Tests and Measures

The tests and measures portion of the examination involves the physical examination of the patient and provides the PT with objective data to accurately determine the degree of specific function and dysfunction.[9] A number of recognized tests and measures are commonly performed; however, not all are used every time. The physical examination may be modified by the PT based on the history and the systems review.

Numerous special tests exist for each area of the body. These tests are performed by the PT only if there is some indication that they would be helpful in confirming or implicating a particular structure or providing information as to the degree of tissue damage. For example, in the joints of the spine, special tests include directional stress tests (posterior–anterior pressures and anterior, posterior, and rotational stressing), joint quadrant testing, vascular tests, and repeated movement testing. Examples of special tests in the peripheral joints include ligament stress tests (e.g., Lachman for the anterior cruciate ligament), articular stress testing (valgus stress applied at the elbow), and rotator cuff impingement tests.

Only those special tests that have appeared in peer-reviewed literature are included in the various chapters of this book so that the PTA can have a full appreciation of their purpose and implications. It is important to remember that the interpretation of the findings from the special tests depends on the sensitivity and specificity of the test, the skill and experience of the PT, and the PT's degree of familiarity with the tests.

Evaluation

Following the history, systems review, and tests and measures, the PT makes an evaluation based on an analysis and organization of the collected data and information.[2] An evaluation is the level of judgment necessary to make sense of the findings in order to identify a relationship between the symptoms reported and the signs of disturbed function.[11] The evaluation process also may identify possible problems that require consultation with, or referral to, another provider.

Diagnosis

Diagnosis, as performed by a PT, refers to a cluster of signs and symptoms, syndromes, or categories, and is used to guide the PT in determining the most appropriate intervention strategy for each patient.[12] A physical therapy diagnosis includes a prioritization of the identified impairments, functional limitations, and disabilities.

Prognosis and Plan of Care

The prognosis, determined by the PT, is the predicted level of optimum function that the patient will attain and an identification of the barriers that may impact the achievement of optimal improvement—such as age, medication(s), socioeconomic status, comorbidities, cognitive status, nutrition, social support, medical prognosis, and environment—within a certain time frame.[2] This prediction helps guide the intensity, duration, frequency, and type of the intervention, in addition to providing justifications for the intervention. Knowledge of the severity of an injury; the age, physical status, and health status of a patient; and the healing processes of the various tissues involved are among the factors used by the PT in determining the prognosis.

The plan of care (POC), which outlines anticipated patient management, involves the setting of goals, coordination of care, progression of care, and discharge. The POC:[12]

- Is based on the examination, evaluation, diagnosis, and prognosis, including the predicted level of optimal improvement
- Includes statements that identify anticipated goals and the expected outcomes
- Describes the specific interventions to be used, and the proposed frequency and duration of the interventions that is required to reach the anticipated goals and expected outcomes
- Includes documentation that is dated and appropriately authenticated by the PT who established the plan of care
- Includes patient and family (as appropriate) goals, and a focus on patient education
- Includes plans for discharge of the patient/client, taking into consideration achievement of anticipated goals and expected outcomes, and provides for appropriate follow-up or referral

Intervention

According to the *Guide to Physical Therapist Practice*,[2] an intervention is "the purposeful and skilled interaction of the PT and the patient/client and, when appropriate, with other individuals involved in the patient/client care, using various physical therapy procedures and techniques to produce changes in the condition consistent with the diagnosis and prognosis." One of the primary purposes of rehabilitative interventions after orthopaedic injury is to improve the tolerance of a healing tissue to tension and stress, and to ensure that the tissue has the capacity to tolerate the various stresses that will be placed on it (see Chapter 4). As an example, with contractile tissues, such as the muscles, this can be accomplished through measured rest, rehabilitative exercise, high-voltage electrical stimulation, central (cardiovascular) aerobics, general conditioning, and absence from overuse.[13]

● **Key Point** Three components comprise the physical therapy intervention:[2]

1. Coordination, communication, and documentation
2. Patient/client-related instruction
3. Direct interventions

The inert structures, such as ligaments and menisci, rely more on the level of tension and force placed on them for their recovery, which stimulates the fibroblasts to produce fiber and glycosaminoglycans (see Chapter 2).[14] Thus, the intervention chosen for these structures must involve the repetitive application of modified tension in the line of stress based on the stress of daily activities or sporting activity.[14]

● **Key Point** The most successful intervention programs are those that are custom designed from a blend of clinical experience and scientific data. The level of improvement achieved is related to accurate goal setting and the attainment of those goals.

The therapeutic strategy is determined solely from the responses obtained from tissue loading and the effect that loading has on symptoms. Once these responses have been determined, the focus of the intervention is to provide for patients sound and effective self-management strategies that avoid harmful tissue loading.[15] Interventions are typically aimed at addressing short- and long-term goals, both of which are dynamic in nature, being altered as the patient's condition changes by designing strategies with which to achieve those goals (**Table 1-6**). Intervention strategies can be subdivided into active (direct) or passive (indirect), with the goal being to make the intervention as active as possible at the earliest opportunity. As part of a comprehensive intervention, the principles listed in **Table 1-7** should be applied (see also Chapter 5).

Rehabilitative Modalities

Clinicians have at their disposal a battery of physical agents and electrotherapeutic modalities for use throughout all phases of healing. The modalities used during the acute phase involve the application of cryotherapy, electrical

TABLE 1-6 Acute Intervention Goals and Strategies

Presenting Issue	Goal	Strategies and Implementation
Pain and inflammation	Increase pain-free mobility while promoting tissue repair/regeneration	Rest/ice Supports/braces Gentle ROM Modalities
Decreased strength	Increase muscle strength/endurance	Isometric exercises Concentric exercises Eccentric exercises Isokinetic exercises Stabilization exercises
Decreased range of motion (ROM)	Increase range of motion	Passive, active assisted, and active range of motion Stretching Joint mobilizations
Deconditioning	Increase aerobic capacity	Cardiovascular exercises (e.g., treadmill, upper body ergometer, elliptical)
Decreased function	Enhance function/independence	Address psychosocial factors Improve ergonomic factors Gait progression as appropriate Closed kinetic chain exercises Neuromuscular and agility drills
Poor balance	Improve balance	Eyes open—eyes closed Stable to unstable surfaces Single movements in single planes to multiple movements in multiple planes

TABLE 1-7	Intervention Principles
Control pain and inflammation	
Promote and progress healing	
Strengthen or increase flexibility	
Correct posture and movement impairment syndromes	
Analyze and integrate the entire kinetic chain	
Incorporate neuromuscular re-education	
Improve functional outcome	
Maintain or improve overall fitness	
Provide patient education and self-management	
Ensure a safe return to function	

TABLE 1-8	General Recommendations for Verbal Communication
Verbal commands	Should focus the patient's attention on specifically desired actions for intervention.
Instruction	Should remain as simple as possible and must never incorporate confusing medical terminology.
	The general sequence of events should be explained to the patient before initiating the intervention.
Questions	The patient should be asked questions before and during the intervention to establish a rapport with the patient and to provide feedback as to the status of the current intervention.
Tone of voice	The PTA should speak clearly in moderate tones and vary his or her tone of voice as required by the situation.
Sensitivity	The PTA should be sensitive to the patient/client's level of understanding and cultural background.

Data from Dreeben O: Introduction to physical therapy for physical therapist assistants. Sudbury, MA, Jones & Bartlett Learning, 2007

stimulation, pulsed ultrasound, and iontophoresis (see Chapter 7). These are generally used to decrease pain and inflammation. Modalities used during the later stages of healing include thermotherapy, phonophoresis, electrical stimulation, ultrasound, iontophoresis, and diathermy (see Chapter 7). Thermal modalities are used to promote blood flow to the healing tissues and to prepare the tissues for exercise or manual techniques.

At present, with the exception of cryotherapy, there is simply insufficient evidence to support or reject the use of various modalities.[16–18] However, the absence of evidence does not always mean that there is evidence of absence of effect, and there is always the risk of rejecting therapeutic approaches that are valid.[19]

● **Key Point** It is important for the clinician to understand the principles that relate to a particular modality so the modality is used when indicated and the maximum therapeutic benefit may be derived from its use.

At the earliest opportunity, the patient should be weaned away from these modalities, and the focus of the intervention should shift to the application of movement and the repeated and prolonged functional restoration of the involved structures.

Patient Communication

Much about becoming an effective clinician relates to an ability to communicate with the patient, the patient's family, and to the other members of the

healthcare team. Good communication involves an understanding of human behavior, effective listening, and the ability to detect subtle changes in mood, tone of voice, and body language (**Table 1-8**). The nonverbal cues such as mood and body language are especially important, because they often are performed subconsciously.

● **Key Point** Communication involves interacting with the patient using terms he or she can understand.

Communication between clinician and patient begins when the clinician first meets the patient, and continues throughout any future sessions. The introduction to the patient should be handled at eye level and in a professional yet empathetic tone. Listening with empathy involves understanding the ideas being communicated and the emotion behind the ideas. In essence, empathy is seeing another person's viewpoint, so that a deep and true understanding of what the person is experiencing can be obtained.

Patient Assessment, Progression, and Compliance

During the physical therapy visits, the PTA and the patient work together to alter the patient's perception of their functional capabilities. Discussions about intervention goals must continue throughout the rehabilitative process and must be mutually acceptable. Open-ended questions or statements, such as "Tell me how you are feeling today," are used initially to encourage the patient to provide narrative information and to decrease the opportunity for bias on the part of the clinician.[10] More specific questions, such as "How would you rate pain today on a scale of 0 to 10?" are asked as the session proceeds. The specific questions help to obtain specific responses and deter irrelevant information. The clinician should provide the patient with encouraging responses, such as a nod of the head, when the information is relevant and when needed to steer the patient into supplying necessary information. *Neutral* questions should be used whenever possible. These questions are structured to avoid leading the patient into giving a particular response. Avoid leading questions, such as "Does it hurt more when you walk?" A more neutral question would be, "What activities make your symptoms worse?" It is also important to use statements that summarize the data that have been collected; for example, "Would I be right in saying that your neck only hurts when you turn your head to the right?" Summarizing the patient's information helps clarify the purpose of the intervention, while increasing patient involvement.

Misjudgments are sometimes made with the intervention. In general, the patient's pain should not last more than a couple of hours after an intervention. Pain that lasts longer than 2 hours is usually an indication that the intensity of the intervention, rather than the intervention itself, has been inappropriate. However, remember that therapeutic exercise has the potential to cause pain, discomfort, and soreness that can last 24–48 hours after exercise.

Motivation and Compliance

Many factors can contribute to the patient's resistance to improvement. In some cases, it may be an individual factor that, when eliminated, will allow the patient to respond well. In the majority of cases, the resistance to improvement is based on the interaction of multiple factors, which must be recognized and corrected. Patient motivation and compliance are paramount in the rehabilitation program.

Motivation

Anecdotally, unmotivated patients may progress more slowly. Much literature has conceptualized or reported poor motivation in rehabilitation as secondary to patient-related factors, including depression, apathy, cognitive impairment, low self-efficacy (e.g., low confidence in one's ability to successfully rehabilitate), fatigue, and personality factors.[20]

Compliance

Compliance is vitally important and varies from patient to patient. Several factors have been outlined to improve compliance, among them:[21-23]

- Involving the patient in the intervention planning and goal setting
- Setting realistic short- and long-term goals
- Promoting high expectations regarding final outcome
- Promoting perceived benefits
- Projecting a positive attitude
- Providing clear instructions and demonstrations with appropriate feedback
- Keeping the exercises pain-free or with a low level of pain
- Encouraging patient problem solving

Patient Education

Patient/client-related instruction forms the cornerstone of every intervention and plan of care (**Table 1-9**). It is imperative that the PTA spend time educating the patient about his or her condition, so the patient can fully understand the importance of his or her role in the rehabilitation process and become an educated consumer. Educating the patient about strategies to adopt in order to prevent recurrences, and to

TABLE 1-9	The Role of the PTA in Patient Education

Education

Standard 3.3.2.19. Under the direction and supervision of the physical therapist, instructs other members of the health care team using established techniques, programs, and instructional materials commensurate with the learning characteristics of the audience

Standard 3.3.2.20. Educates others about the role of the physical therapist assistant

Data from Accreditation Handbook: PTA Criteria, Appendix A-3.

self-manage his or her condition, is also very important to ensure an interactive environment. The aim of patient education is to create independence, not dependence, and to foster an atmosphere of learning in the clinic. A detailed explanation should be given to the patient in a language that he or she can understand. This explanation should include the following:

- *The name of the structure(s) involved, and the cause of the problem:* Whenever possible, an illustration or model of the involved structure should be shown to the patient to explain principles in layperson's terms.
- *Information about the interventions that are planned, and the PT's prognosis for the problem:* An estimation of healing time is useful for the patient, so he or she does not become frustrated at a perceived lack of progress.
- *What the patient can and cannot do:* This includes the allowed use of the joint or area, and a brief description about the relevant stage of healing and the vulnerability of the various structures during the pertinent healing phase. This information makes the patient aware and more cautious when performing activities of daily living (ADLs), recreational activities, and the home exercise program. Emphasis should be placed on dispelling the myth of "no pain, no gain." Patients should be encouraged to respect pain. Also, patients often have misconceptions about when to use heat and ice, and it is the role of the clinician to clarify such issues.
- *Home exercise program:* Before instructing a patient on his or her home exercise program (HEP), the PTA should take into consideration the time that will be needed to perform the program. In addition, the level of tolerance and motivation for exercise varies among

individuals, and is based on their diagnosis and stage of healing. A short series of exercises, performed more frequently during the day, should be prescribed for patients with poor endurance or when the emphasis is functional re-education. Longer programs, performed less frequently, are aimed at building strength or endurance. Each HEP needs to be individualized to meet the patient's specific needs. The patient's HEP should start on the first day of intervention and continue through and beyond the day of discontinuation of physical therapy. At the earliest opportunity, the patient must be educated about the signs and symptoms that warrant discontinuation of an exercise and when the PT or physician should be contacted (see Section II: Therapeutic Exercise). The HEP must be modified continuously and updated and follow the guidelines in **Table 1-10**. Any prescribed exercise should be simple and instructions should include the frequency, number of repetitions, number of sets, how long to hold, the amount of exercise resistance, and the position for performing the exercise. Whenever possible, pictures of the exercises should be provided to maximize carryover.

● **Key Point** Educational materials need to be written in plain language, consistently using the same words. Sentences should be short and simple, with each item preceded by a bullet point. Instructions should be taught one step at a time using appropriate demonstrations and descriptions.

There are probably as many ways to teach as there are to learn. The PTA needs to be aware that people may have very different preferences for how, when,

TABLE 1-10	Basic Requirements for the Home Exercise Program (HEP)

The HEP should be organized, concise, and written in layperson's terms (fifth or sixth grade reading level) using a font size of 12 points or larger.

The HEP should represent an extension of the interventions.

The HEP should include uncomplicated diagrams or pictures.

Data from Dreeben O: Introduction to physical therapy for physical therapist assistants. Sudbury, MA, Jones & Bartlett Learning, 2007

where, and how often to learn. It is not within the scope of this text to discuss all of the theories on learning, but an overview of the major concepts is merited. Litzinger and Osif[25] organized individuals into four main types of learners, based on instructional strategies:

1. *Accommodators:* This type of learner relies heavily on other people for information rather than on their own analytic ability, often enjoy being active participants in their learning, and will ask many questions, such as, "What if?" and "Why not?" For example, when instructing such a patient about the precautions following a total hip replacement (see Chapter 19), the patient may ask why they are being told not to place any weight through the involved hip.

2. *Divergers:* This type is motivated to discover the relevancy of a given situation and prefers to have information presented in a detailed, systematic, and reasoned manner. For example, this type of learner prefers to have the information provided in a sequential fashion with the rationale for each stage.

3. *Assimilators:* This type is motivated to answer the question, "What is there to know?" These learners like accurate, organized delivery of information, and they tend to respect the knowledge of the expert. They are perhaps less instructor-intensive than some other types of learners and will carefully follow prescribed exercises, provided a resource person is clearly available and able to answer questions. For example, this type would respond well to clear verbal and written instructions, the rationale behind the exercises, and specific details as to how often the exercises should be performed.

4. *Convergers:* This type of learner can make decisions and apply practical ideas to solve problems. Generally, these people can organize knowledge by using hypothetical deductive reasoning. The instructions given to this type of learner should be interactive, not passive. For example, this type responds well to being asked to demonstrate an exercise rather than hearing a description.

Another frequently used way of classifying learners describes three common learning styles:

1. *Visual:* As the name suggests, the visual learner assimilates information by observation, using visual cues and information such as pictures, anatomic models, and physical demonstrations.

2. *Auditory:* Auditory learners prefer to learn by having things explained to them verbally.

3. *Tactile:* Tactile learners, who learn through touch and interaction, are the most difficult of the three groups to teach. Close supervision is required with this group until they have demonstrated to the clinician that they can perform the exercises correctly and independently. Proprioceptive neuromuscular facilitation (PNF) techniques, with the emphasis on physical and tactile cues, often work well with this group (see Chapter 6).

A patient's learning style can be identified by asking how he or she prefers to learn. Some patients will prefer a simple handout with pictures and instructions; others will prefer to see the exercises demonstrated, and then be supervised while they perform the exercises. Some may want to know why they are doing the exercises, which muscles are involved, why they are doing three sets of a particular exercise, and so on. Others will require less explanation.

> **● Key Point** When educating a patient who has a hearing impairment, the PTA should choose a quiet environment, face the patient, and speak clearly without exaggerating the pronunciation.

If in doubt as to the patient's learning style, it is recommended that each exercise first be demonstrated by the clinician, and then by the patient, both at the end of a session and at the beginning of the next session. The rationale and purpose behind each of the exercises must be given, as well as the frequency and intensity expected.

> **● Key Point** The PTA should always consider cultural diversity and pay attention to nonverbal communication such as voice volume, postures, gestures, and eye contact.

It is important that the patient view his or her rehabilitative progression with a healthy respect for pain, combined with the importance of returning to normal levels of function as early as possible. Pain is, unfortunately, a necessary component of the healing process; however, the patient needs to be educated about what constitutes healing pain in comparison to harmful pain (an increase in pain that lasts more than 2–4 hours). Clear instructions must be given to the patient on how to recognize injurious pain and how to avoid additional strain. The frequency and duration of the patient's care need to be addressed with the PT. The common practice is to see patients two to three times per week; however, this is not always necessary, particularly with well-motivated patients. It is the duty of all clinicians to make the patient's visit meaningful. Clinic visits must include a level of skilled intervention that the patient cannot receive in the home environment. Placing the patient on a hot pack and then having him or her perform a routine rehabilitation program that is not constantly being updated or modified is a waste of the patient's time, and does little to foster public confidence in the profession. Each session must have a purpose. The PTA should attempt to explain any gains or losses the patient has made since the previous session, and the possible reasons. New goals should be discussed, and any changes to the intervention plan, and their rationale, should be discussed with the PT and then the patient.

Documentation

Documentation of the assessment and intervention processes is an important part of any therapeutic regimen. Documentation in health care includes any entry made in the patient/client record. As a record of client care, documentation provides useful information for the clinician, other members of the healthcare team, and third-party payers. The APTA Board of Directors has approved a number of guidelines for physical therapy documentation that are intended to be a foundation for the development of more specific guidelines in specialty areas, while at the same time providing guidance across all practice settings. The APTA's Documentation Guidelines are outlined in Appendix B. In all instances, it is the APTA's position that the physical therapy examination, evaluation, diagnosis, prognosis, and intervention must be documented, dated, and authenticated by the PT or PTA, as appropriate.

The SOAP (Subjective, Objective, Assessment, Plan) note format has traditionally been used to document the examination and intervention process.

- *Subjective:* Information about the condition from patient or family member
- *Objective:* Measurement a clinician obtains during the physical examination
- *Assessment:* Analysis of the problem including the long- and short-term goals
- *Plan:* A specific intervention plan for the identified problem

More recently, the patient/client management format is being used by those clinicians familiar with the *Guide to Physical Therapist Practice*.[8] The

patient/client management model described in the *Guide to Physical Therapist Practice* has the following components:

- *History:* Information gathered about the patient's history.
- *Systems review:* Information gathered from performing a brief examination or screening of the patient's major systems addressed by physical therapy. Also includes information gathered about the patient's communication, affect, cognition, learning style, and education needs.
- *Tests and measures:* Results from specific tests and measures performed by the PT.
- *Diagnosis:* Includes a discussion of the relationship of the patient's functional deficits to the patient's impairments and/or disability as determined by the PT as well as a discussion of other healthcare professionals to which the PT has referred the patient or believes the patient should be referred.
- *Prognosis:* Includes the predicted level of improvement that the patient will be able to achieve according to the PT and the predicted amount of time to achieve that level of improvement. The prognosis also should include the PT's professional opinion of the patient's rehabilitation potential.
- *Plan of care:* Includes the expected outcomes (long-term goals), anticipated goals (short-term goals), and interventions, including an education plan for the patient or the patient's caregivers or significant others.

The purposes of documentation are as follows:[8]

- To document what the clinician does to manage the individual patient's case.
- To record examination findings, patient status, intervention provided, and the patient's response to treatment.
- To communicate with all other members of the healthcare team; this helps maintain consistency among the services provided and includes communication between the PT and PTA.
- To provide information to third-party payers, such as Medicare and other insurance companies, who make decisions about reimbursement based on the quality and completeness of the physical therapy note.
- To be used for quality assurance and improvement purposes and for issues such as discharge planning.

The PTA reads the initial documentation of the examination, evaluation, diagnosis, prognosis, anticipated outcomes and goals, and intervention plan, and is expected to follow the POC as outlined by the PT in the initial patient note.[8] After the patient has been seen by the PTA for a period of time (the time varies according to the policies of each facility or healthcare system and state law), the PTA must write a progress note documenting any changes in the patient's status that have occurred since the PT's initial note was written.[8] Also, after a discussion with the PT about the diagnosis and prognosis, expected outcomes, anticipated goals, and interventions, the PTA rewrites or responds to the previously written expected outcomes and documents the revised POC accordingly.[8] In many facilities (according to the policies of each facility or healthcare system and state law), the PT then cosigns the PTA's notes, indicating agreement with what is documented.[8]

Abbreviations

Medical abbreviations are used throughout the various disciplines in health care to document client status or progression. To avoid miscommunication, it is important to remember that before using abbreviations the PTA must ensure that they are approved for use by the facility. Appendix C outlines some of the more common abbreviations used by orthopaedic physical therapy professionals.

Patient Confidentiality

In the majority of situations, the patient's written authorization is required for the release of medical information. For example, authorization is required:

- For any member of the patient's family (except where a member of the family has received durable power of attorney for healthcare agencies)
- For the patient's attorney or insurance company
- For the patient's employer (unless a worker's compensation claim is involved)

General Medical Assessment

Although it is the PT's responsibility to perform the initial systems review and evaluation of general health, the PTA must be aware of and continually assess a patient for vital signs, response to care, and medical complications/emergencies. Monitoring of the vital signs can provide the PTA with important information as to the health status of the patient. The four so-called vital signs, which are standard in most medical settings, are temperature, heart rate, blood pressure, and respiratory rate. Pain is considered by many to be the fifth vital sign. Based on a patient's medical history, it may be necessary to take vital signs at every session both before and after treatment.

Temperature

Body temperature is one indication of the metabolic state of an individual; measurements provide information concerning basal metabolic state, possible presence or absence of infection, and metabolic response to exercise.[26] In most individuals there is a diurnal (occurring every day) variation in body temperature of 0.5–2 degrees, with the lowest ebb occurring during sleep. "Normal" adult body temperature is 98.6°F (37°C); however, a temperature in the range of 96.5°–99.4°F (35.8–37.4°C) is not at all uncommon. The normal temperature of infants is 98.2°F (36.8°C). The normal temperature of a child or an adolescent is the same as for adults.

Fever or pyrexia is a temperature exceeding 100°F (37.7°C).[27] At this point, physical therapy should be discontinued. *Hyperpyrexia* refers to extreme elevation of temperature (above 106°F or 41.1°C).[26] *Hypothermia* refers to an abnormally low temperature (below 95°F or 35°C).

It is worth remembering that in adults over 75 years of age and in those who are immune-compromised (e.g., transplant recipients, corticosteroid users, persons with chronic renal insufficiency, anyone taking excessive antipyretic medications), fever response may be blunted or absent.[26] Menstruating women have a well-known temperature pattern that reflects the effects of ovulation, with the temperature dropping slightly before menstruation and then dropping further 24–36 hours prior to ovulation.[27] Coincident with ovulation, the temperature rises and remains at a somewhat higher level until just before the next menses.

Both the degree of temperature change and its duration are relevant to diagnostic processes when elevated body temperature is evident. Although an increase in localized skin temperature as compared to the normal side is to be expected as part of the inflammatory process following an injury, a systemic increase in temperature, which may be a sign of illness or infection, should be communicated to the PT. The testing of skin temperature can also help the PT to differentiate between a venous and an arterial insufficiency. With venous insufficiency, an increase in skin temperature is usually noted in the area of occlusion, and the area also appears bluish in color. Pitting edema, especially around the ankles, sacrum, and hands, also may be present. However, if pitting edema is present and the skin temperature is normal, the lymphatic system may be at fault. With arterial insufficiency, a decrease in skin temperature is usually noted in the area of occlusion, and the area appears whiter. It is also extremely painful.

It is very important to be able to recognize the signs and symptoms of infection so that the PT and the patient's physician can be notified immediately. An infection may cause redness, warmth, and inflammation around the affected area and the area may become stiff, drain pus, and begin to lose range of motion.

> **● Key Point** Infection and inflammation are not to be confused:
> - *Infection:* The harmful colonization of a host by an infecting organism
> - *Inflammation:* The complex biological response of vascular tissues to harmful stimuli while initiating the healing process for the tissue (see Chapter 5)

The PTA must always exercise vigilance with proper hygiene techniques, especially with regular hand washing in between patients and the cleaning and disinfection of all treatment areas and equipment as per the policy and procedure of the facility (**Table 1-11**).

Heart Rate

In most people, the pulse is an accurate measure of heart rate. The heart rate or pulse is taken to obtain information about the resting state of the cardiovascular system and the system's response to activity or exercise and recovery.[26] It is also used to assess patency of the specific arteries palpated and the presence of any irregularities in the rhythm.[26]

> **● Key Point**
> - *Normal resting adult heart rate (HR):* 70 beats per minute (bpm) (range = 60–100); a true resting heart rate should be taken prior to the patient getting out of bed in the morning
> - *Bradycardia:* Less than 60 bpm; at <60 bpm, the supervising PT should be informed as the patient may need to be monitored carefully
> - *Tachycardia:* More than 100 bpm; at 110 bpm, the supervising PT should be informed and the patient should be monitored carefully
> - *Normal infant HR:* 120 bpm (range = 70–170)
> - *Normal child HR:* 125 bpm (range = 75–140)
> - *Normal adolescent HR:* 85 bpm (range = 50–100)

Respiratory Rate

In adults, the normal chest expansion difference between the resting position and the fully inhaled position is 2–4 cm. (It is greater for females than for males.) As per the PT's instructions, the PTA should compare measurements of both the anterior-posterior diameter and the transverse diameter during rest and at full inhalation.

> **● Key Point**
> - *Normal adult respiratory rate (RR):* 12–18 breaths/min; at 30 breaths/min the supervising PT should be informed and the patient should be monitored carefully
> - *Normal infant RR:* 30–50 breaths/min
> - *Normal child RR:* 20–40 breaths/min
> - *Normal adolescent RR:* 15–22 breaths/min

Blood Pressure

Blood pressure is a measure of vascular resistance to blood flow.[26] Blood pressure values, measured with a sphygmomanometer, are usually given in millimeters of mercury (mm Hg). The values consist of two parts:

- *Systolic pressure:* The pressure exerted on the brachial artery when the heart is contracting[26]
- *Diastolic pressure:* The pressure exerted on the brachial artery during the relaxation phase of the heart contraction[26]

> **● Key Point** The values for resting blood pressure in adults are:
> - *Normal:* Systolic blood pressure <120 mm Hg and diastolic blood pressure <80 mm Hg
> - *Prehypertension:* Systolic blood pressure 120–139 mm Hg or diastolic blood pressure 80–90 mm Hg
> - *Stage 1 hypertension:* Systolic blood pressure 140–159 mm Hg or diastolic blood pressure 90–99 mm Hg
> - *Stage 2 hypertension:* Systolic blood pressure ≥160 mm Hg or diastolic blood pressure ≥100 mm Hg
>
> The normal values for resting blood pressure in children are:
> - *Systolic:* Birth to 1 month, 60 to 90 mm Hg; up to 3 years of age, 75 to 130 mm Hg; over 3 years of age, 90 to 140 mm Hg
> - *Diastolic:* Birth to 1 month, 30 to 60 mm Hg; up to 3 years of age, 45 to 90 mm Hg; over 3 years of age, 50 to 80 mm Hg

TABLE
1-11   Standard Precautions

Handwashing

1. Wash hands after touching blood, body fluids, secretions, excretions, and contaminated items, whether or not gloves are worn.

2. Wash hands immediately after removing gloves, between patient contacts, and when otherwise indicated to reduce transmission of microorganisms.

3. Wash hands between tasks and procedures on the same patient to prevent cross-contamination of different body sites.

4. Use plain (non-antimicrobial) soap for routine handwashing.

5. An antimicrobial agent or a waterless antiseptic agent may be used for specific circumstances (hyperendemic infections), as defined by infection control.

Patient Care Equipment

1. Handle used patient care equipment soiled with blood, body fluids, secretions, or excretions in a manner that prevents skin and mucous membrane exposures, contamination of clothing, and transfer of microorganisms to other patients or environments.

2. Ensure that all equipment, including but not limited to BP equipment, weights, exercise toys, and dumbbells, is not used for the care of another patient until it has been cleaned and reprocessed appropriately.

3. Ensure that single use items are discarded properly.

Gloves

1. Wear gloves (clean, unsterile gloves are adequate) when touching blood, body fluids, secretions, excretions, and contaminated items; put on clean gloves just before touching mucous membranes and nonintact skin.

2. Change gloves between tasks and procedures on the same patient after contact with materials that may contain high concentrations of microorganisms.

3. Remove gloves promptly after use, before touching uncontaminated items and environmental surfaces, and before going on to another patient; wash hands immediately after glove removal to avoid transfer of microorganisms to other patients or environments.

Environmental Control

1. Follow hospital procedures for the routine care, cleaning and disinfection of environmental surfaces, beds, bed rails, bedside equipment, and other frequently touch surfaces.

Linen

1. Handle, transport, and process used linen soiled with blood, body fluids, secretions, and excretion in a manner that prevents skin and mucous membrane exposures and contamination of clothing, and avoids transfer of microorganisms to other patients or environments.

Adapted from Centers for Disease Control, Hospital Infection Control Practices Advisory Committee: Part II Recommendations for Isolation Precautions in Hospitals. February 1997.

Orthostatic (postural) hypotension is a form of hypotension in which a person's blood pressure drops upon standing up, particularly after resting. The decrease is typically greater than 20/10 mm Hg. The symptoms, which can include dizziness, lightheadedness, nausea, headache, blurred or dimmed vision, generalized (or extremity) numbness/tingling, and fainting, are the consequences of insufficient blood pressure and cerebral perfusion (blood supply to the brain).

● Key Point White coat hypertension (WCH), also known as the white coat effect or isolated office hypertension, is the presence of higher BP when measured in the physician's office than at other times.[28–30] Whether WCH is a benign phenomenon or carries increased cardiovascular risk is still not known.

Pain

Concomitant with most soft tissue injuries is pain, inflammation, and edema (see Chapter 5). Pain serves as a protective mechanism, allowing an individual to be aware of a situation's potential for producing tissue damage and to minimize further damage. With the exception of constant pain, the presence of pain should not always be viewed negatively by the clinician. After all, its presence helps to determine the location of the injury, and its behavior aids the clinician in determining the stage of healing and the impact it has on the patient's function; for example, whether the pain is worsening, improving, or unchanging provides information on the effectiveness of an intervention. In addition, a gradual increase in the intensity of the symptoms over time may indicate to the clinician that the condition is worsening or that the condition is nonmusculoskeletal in nature. If pain is present, the PTA's major focus should be to seek methods to help control it throughout each interaction.

● **Key Point** Remember that the location of symptoms for many musculoskeletal conditions is quite separate from the source, especially in those peripheral joints that are more proximal, such as the shoulder and the hip. The term *referred pain* is used to describe symptoms that have their origin at a site other than where the patient feels the pain. The concept of referred pain is often difficult for patients to understand, so an explanation of referred pain can enable the patient to better understand and answer questions about symptoms they might otherwise have felt irrelevant.

Pain may be constant, variable, or intermittent. Variable pain is pain that is perpetual, but that varies in intensity. Variable pain usually indicates the involvement of both a chemical and a mechanical source.

Myofacial pain syndrome (MPS) often manifests with symptoms suggestive of neurologic disorders, including diffuse pain and tenderness, headache, vertigo, visual disturbances, paresthesias, incoordination, and referred pain that often can be clarified by the musculoskeletal and neurologic examination.[31] MPS is characterized by the presence of myofascial trigger points (MTrPs).[32–36] An MTrP is a hyperirritable location, approximately 2 to 5 cm in diameter,[37] within a taut band of muscle fibers that is painful when compressed and that can give rise to characteristic referred pain, tenderness, and tightness.[38] Some confusion exists as to the difference between trigger points and tender points. Although MTrPs can occur in the same sites as the tender points of fibromyalgia, MTrPs can cause referral of pain in a distinct and characteristic area, remote from the trigger point site, not necessarily in a dermatomal distribution.[32]

The mechanical cause of constant pain is less understood than the chemical causes of pain but is thought to be the result of the deformation of collagen, which compresses or stretches the nociceptive free nerve endings, with the excessive forces being perceived as pain.[39] Thus, specific movements or positions should influence pain of a mechanical nature. Chemical, or inflammatory, pain is more constant and is less affected by movements or positions than mechanical pain. Intermittent pain is unlikely to be caused by a chemical irritant. Usually, this type of pain is caused by prolonged postures, a loose intra-articular body, or an impingement of a musculoskeletal structure.

● **Key Point** Constant pain following an injury continues until the healing process has sufficiently reduced the concentration of noxious irritants.

Unfortunately, the source of the pain is not always easy to identify, because most patients present with both mechanical and chemical pain. It is therefore important that the PTA be able to determine the following:

■ Any change in the patient's pain since their last PT visit or examination. If the perception of pain has increased since the last visit, further questioning may be needed to determine whether the increase is due to postexercise muscle soreness rather than deterioration in the patient's condition.

■ The response of the pain to any of the interventions, or direction of movement of the involved structure (e.g., does the patient complain of more pain with lumbar flexion or with extension?). Musculoskeletal conditions are typically aggravated with movement and alleviated with rest.

■ The nature and pattern of the pain. Because pain is variable in its nature, quality, and location, describing pain is often difficult for the patient.

■ The intensity of the pain. One of the simplest methods to quantify the intensity of pain is to use an 11-point (0–10) visual analog scale (VAS). The VAS is a numerically continuous scale that requires the pain level be identified by making a mark on a 100-mm line, or by circling the appropriate number in a 0–10 series.[40] The patient is asked to rate his or her present pain compared with the worst pain ever experienced, with 0 representing no pain, 1 representing minimally perceived pain, and 10 representing pain that requires immediate attention.[41]

Several tools are at the clinician's disposal to help to control pain, inflammation, and edema, including the application of electrotherapeutic and physical modalities, gentle ROM exercises, and graded manual techniques (see Chapter 6 and 7). Most episodes of pain resolve on their own, provided that the condition is not exacerbated through constant re-injury and that the injured tissue is allowed to progress through the natural stages of healing. If this natural progression does not occur, chronic pain can result. The prognosis for chronic pain syndromes is generally poor, and often requires a biopsychosocial approach. In these instances, the PTA may need to discuss with the PT resources that will aid the patient both physically and emotionally. This can include referrals for counseling, pain control, stress management, and self-help groups.

> ● **Key Point** Symptom magnification, an exaggerated subjective response to symptoms in the absence of adequate objective findings, is an increasingly common occurrence in the clinic. The patients who display this type of behavior are a difficult population to deal with. The causes of symptom magnification can be categorized into two main patient types:
>
> 1. Patients with a psychosomatic overlay and those whose symptoms have a psychogenic cause
> 2. Patients who are involved in litigation
>
> In either case, the PTA must inform the PT.

Recognizing a Medical Emergency

It is extremely important that the PTA be able to detect malfunctions of the various systems, often referred to as *red flags*, through observation and receiving subjective complaints. Any of the following should cause immediate concern for the PTA and require consultation with the supervising PT or medical personnel:[42]

- *Fatigue:* Complaints of feeling tired or run down are extremely common and therefore often only become significant if the patient reports that tiredness interferes with the ability to carry out typical daily activities and when the fatigue has lasted for 2–4 weeks or longer. Many serious illnesses can cause fatigue.

> ● **Key Point** The signs and symptoms of hyperglycemia (high blood sugar of more than 200 mg/dL) include:
>
> - Fatigue and lethargy
> - Blurred vision and dry skin
> - Extreme thirst and frequent urination
> - Dizziness and increased appetite
> - Nausea, vomiting, or abdominal pain
>
> Hyperglycemia can result in ketoacidosis and ultimately a diabetic coma. If hyperglycemia is suspected, the PTA should call for medical assistance, monitor the patient until help arrives, and inform the supervising PT. Ideally, to prevent such occurrences, the patient exercise program should be planned in conjunction with food intake, and insulin should be administered and the patient's glucose levels monitored before exercise.

- *Malaise:* A sense of uneasiness or general discomfort that is often associated with conditions that generate fever.
- *Fever/chills/sweats:* These are signs and symptoms that are most often associated with systemic illnesses such as cancer, infections, hypoglycemia, and connective tissue disorders

such as rheumatoid arthritis. To qualify as a red flag, the fever should have some longevity (2 weeks or longer).

> ● **Key Point** The signs and symptoms of hypoglycemia (low blood sugar of less than 50 mg/dL) include:
>
> - Sweating, unsteadiness, and weakness
> - Increased heart rate and lightheadedness
> - Headache, fatigue, and impaired vision
> - Clumsiness and tingling sensation in the mouth
> - Confusion, pallor, and behavior changes
>
> If the PTA suspects hypoglycemia, the patient should be provided with sugar (half a cup of orange juice, a glass of milk, or four or five candies). The supervising PT should be notified. Ideally, to prevent such occurrences, the patient exercise program should be planned in conjunction with food intake and insulin administration, and the patient's glucose levels should be monitored before exercise.

- *Unexpected weight change:* A sensitive but nonspecific finding that can be a normal physiologic response, but also may be associated with depression, cancer, or gastrointestinal disease.
- *Nausea/vomiting:* Persistent vomiting is an uncommon complaint reported to a physical therapist, because the physician will have already been contacted. However, a low-grade nausea can be caused by systemic illness or an adverse drug reaction.
- *Dizziness/lightheadedness:* Dizziness (vertigo) is a nonspecific neurologic symptom that requires a careful diagnostic workup. A report of vertigo, although potentially problematic, is not a contraindication to the continuation of the examination. Differential diagnosis includes primary central nervous system diseases, vestibular and ocular involvement, and, more rarely, metabolic disorders.[43]

> ● **Key Point** Dizziness provoked by head movements or head positions could indicate an inner ear dysfunction. Dizziness provoked by certain cervical motions, particularly extension or rotation, may indicate vertebral artery compromise.

- *Paresthesia/numbness/weakness:* Because motor and sensory axons run in the same nerves, disorders of the peripheral nerves (neuropathies) usually affect both motor and sensory functions. Peripheral neuropathies can manifest as abnormal, frequently unpleasant sensations, which are variously described by the patient as numbness, pins and needles, and tingling.[44] When these sensations occur spontaneously without an external sensory stimulus, they are called *paresthesias*. Patients with paresthesias typically demonstrate a reduction in the perception of cutaneous and proprioceptive sensations.

■ *Change in mentation/cognition:* Can be a manifestation of multiple disorders including delirium, dementia, head injury, stroke, infection, fever, and adverse drug reactions. The clinician notes whether the patient's communication level is age appropriate; whether the patient is oriented to person, place, and time; and whether his or her emotional and behavioral responses appear to be appropriate to his or her circumstances.

Medical Emergency Diagnoses

The PTA may encounter a number of diagnoses that are recognized as medical emergencies. A knowledge of these diagnoses is essential because early recognition of these conditions can have a significant impact on the prognosis.

Compartment Syndrome

Compartment syndromes, caused by compression of nerves and blood vessels within a fascial compartment, can be acute or chronic. Chronic compartment syndromes can occur when muscle hypertrophy causes compression. The acute syndrome occurs when fluid accumulation within a closed osseofascial space (compartment) causes neurovascular compression. For example, an acute compartment syndrome can be caused by the application of a tight bandage or plaster cast; a decrease in arterial flow, as in peripheral vascular disease (PVD); or an increase in venous pressure. A number of recognized acute compartment syndromes exist:

■ *Gluteal:* A tense, swollen buttock following a mechanism of severe contusion, such as a fall from a height.[45] The swelling in the buttock can result in necrosis of the gluteal muscles or sciatic neuropathy, or both.
■ *Thigh:* A pulsating, expanding swelling of the upper thigh.
■ *Forearm (Volkmann's ischemic contracture):* Severe pain of the forearm, exacerbated with passive stretch of the forearm muscles.
■ *Anterior aspect of the lower leg:* Tenderness along the proximal half of the lower leg, with swelling and tightness over the anterior compartment.
■ *Lateral aspect of the lower leg:* Tenderness along the proximal half of the lower leg,

with swelling and tightness over the lateral compartment.
■ *Posterior aspect of the lower leg:* Acute calf pain with activity that improves with rest.

● **Key Point** An acute compartment syndrome is a medical emergency and requires immediate consultation with the supervising PT. Clinical findings include:[46]

• A swollen and tense tender compartment
• Severe pain, exacerbated with passive stretch of the surrounding muscles or with exercise
• Sensory deficits in the involved area
• Motor weakness or paralysis
• Absence of related peripheral pulses

The clinical signs of compartment syndrome can be remembered using the mnemonic of the five Ps: pain, paralysis, paresthesia, pallor, and pulses. Pain, especially disproportionate pain, is often the earliest sign, but the loss of normal neurologic sensation is the most reliable sign.[47,48]

Deep Vein Thrombosis

A thrombus, or blood clot, is an obstruction of the venous or arterial system. If a thrombus is located in one of the superficial veins, it is usually self-limiting. Venous thromboembolism is a vascular disease that manifests as deep vein thrombosis (DVT) or pulmonary embolism (PE). A DVT most commonly appears in the lower extremity and is typically classified as being either proximal (affecting the popliteal and thigh veins) or distal (affecting the calf veins). Proximal DVT is the more dangerous form of lower extremity DVT because it is more likely to cause life-threatening PE.

DVT is caused by an alteration in the normal coagulation system. This alteration in the fibrinolytic system, which acts as a system of checks and balances, results in a failure to dissolve the clot. If the clot becomes dislodged, it enters into the circulatory system through which it can travel to become lodged in the lungs (PE), obstructing the pulmonary artery or branches that supply the lungs with blood. If the clot is large and completely blocks a vessel, it can cause sudden death.

Certain patients are at increased risk for DVT:[49–53]

■ Strong risk factors include fracture (e.g., pelvis, femur, tibia), hip or knee replacement, major general surgery, major trauma, or spinal cord injury. A recent study indicated that up to 60 percent of patients undergoing total hip replacement surgery may develop a DVT without preventative treatment.[54,55]

- Moderate risk factors include arthroscopic knee surgery, central venous lines, chemotherapy, congestive heart or respiratory failure, hormone replacement therapy, malignancy, oral contraceptive therapy, cerebrovascular accident, pregnancy/postpartum, previous venous thromboembolism, and thrombophilia.
- Weak risk factors include bed rest for more than 3 days, immobility due to sitting (e.g., prolonged air travel), increasing age, laparoscopic surgery, obesity, pregnancy/antepartum, and varicose veins.

> **● Key Point** Two-thirds of the fatalities resulting from DVT occur within 30 minutes of the initial symptoms.[56-58] Both DVT and PE can be symptomatic or asymptomatic. Clinical signs of a DVT have traditionally been described as including swelling of the extremity, tenderness or a feeling of cramping of the calf muscles that increases with weight bearing, vascular prominence, elevated temperature in the region of the clot, tachycardia, and inflammation and discoloration or redness of the extremity. However, a purely clinical diagnosis is fraught with a high incidence of false positives and negatives.

The traditional test used to detect a DVT was the Homan's sign—the gentle passive stretching of the ankle into full dorsiflexion. The test is considered positive if the symptoms increase when the ankle is dorsiflexed. However, a positive Homan's sign has been found to be insensitive, nonspecific, and is present in fewer than 30 percent of documented cases of DVT,[58,59] and the performance of the test may increase the risk of producing a PE. The most commonly used method to predict clinical probability, the Wells score, is a clinical prediction rule (**Table 1-12**).

Prevention is the key with DVT. Methods of prevention may be classified as pharmacologic and nonpharmacologic:

- *Pharmacologic:* Includes anticoagulant drugs such as low-dose Coumadin (warfarin), low molecular weight heparin, adjusted-dose heparin, and heparin-antithrombin III

combination; these drugs work by altering the body's normal blood-clotting process

- *Nonpharmacologic:* Attempts to counteract the effects of immobility through early mobilization, calf and foot/ankle exercises, and compression stockings

Edema

Edema is an observable swelling from fluid accumulation in the tissue spaces of the body. The swelling occurs as a result of changes in the local circulation and an inability of the lymphatic system to maintain equilibrium, which causes an accumulation of excess fluid under the skin in the interstitial spaces or compartments within the tissues that are outside of the blood vessels. Edema can be generalized or localized. Generalized edema is diffused over a larger area and most commonly occurs due to a systemic disorder (e.g., congestive heart failure, renal disease); if it occurs in the feet and legs, it is referred to as peripheral edema.

> **● Key Point** The more serious reasons for swelling include fracture, tumor, congestive heart failure, compartment syndrome, and deep vein thrombosis.

Injury or trauma to musculoskeletal tissue typically results in localized edema at the site of an injury. In general, the amount of swelling is related

TABLE 1-12	The Wells Score			
Criteria	Scoring	Traditional Interpretation	Alternate Interpretation
Clinically suspected DVT	3.0 points	Score >6.0: High probability	Score >4: PE likely; consider diagnostic imaging.
Alternative diagnosis is less likely than PE	3.0 points	Score 2.0 to 6.0: Moderate probability	
Tachycardia	1.5 points	Score <2.0: Low probability	Score 4 or less: PE unlikely; consider D-dimer to rule out PE.
Immobilization/surgery in previous 4 weeks	1.5 points		
History of DVT or PE	1.5 points		
Hemoptysis	1.0 point		
Malignancy (treatment for within 6 months, palliative)	1.0 point		

Data from Wells P, Anderson D, Rodger M, et al: Derivation of a simple clinical model to categorize patients' probability of pulmonary embolism: Increasing the model's utility with the SimpliRED D-dimer. Thromb Haemost 83(3):416-420, 2000

to the severity of the condition. Assessment of edema by a PTA involves measurement of the edematous part or extremity. The measurement can occur in one of two ways:

- *Volumetric measurement:* Involves immersing the limb into a specially designed container of fluid, a volumeter, and measuring the amount of water displaced
- *Tape measurement:* Uses a tape measure to obtain circumferential measurements using recognized landmarks of the involved region (**Table 1-13**).

Petersen et al. performed a study to determine the interrater and intrarater reliability of water volumetry and the figure-of-eight method (shown in (Figure 1-1)) on subjects with ankle joint swelling, and found high interrater reliability for both the water volumetry (intraclass correlation coefficient [ICC] = 0.99) and the figure-of-eight method (ICC = 0.98). Additionally, intrarater reliability was high (ICCs = 0.98–0.99). The authors concluded that both methods are reliable measures of ankle swelling, although they recommended the figure-of-eight method because of its ease of use, time efficiency, and cost effectiveness. However, water volumetry

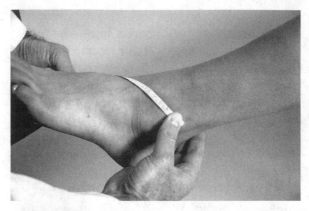

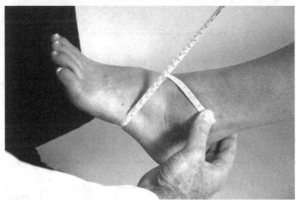

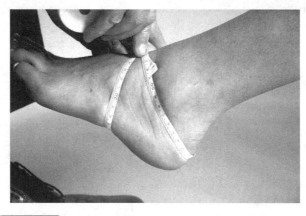

(Figure 1-1)   Figure-of-eight measurement for ankle swelling.

may be more appropriate when measuring diffuse lower extremity swelling. Edema can also be assessed based on its quality (**Table 1-14**).

Integumentary Changes

The integumentary system includes the skin, hair, and nails. Changes in the integumentary system may be manifestations of systemic disorders. Cyanosis in the nails, hands, and feet may be a sign of a central dysfunction (advanced lung disease, pulmonary edema, congenital heart disease, or low hemoglobin level) or peripheral dysfunction (pulmonary edema, or venous obstruction).[26] Palpation of the skin in

TABLE 1-13	Examples of Common Tape Measurement Methods for Edema
Body Region	**Method**
Elbow	A circumferential measurement is made 4 inches above the elbow, 2 inches above the elbow, at the elbow (from the cubital fossa around the elbow, crossing the olecranon process), 2 inches below the elbow, and 4 inches below the elbow.
Ankle	Figure-of-eight method: The clinician places a tape measure midway between the tibialis anterior tendon and lateral malleolus. The tape is then drawn medially and is placed just distal to the navicular tuberosity. The tape is then pulled across the arch and just proximal to the fifth metatarsal. The tape is then pulled across the tibialis anterior tendon and around the ankle to a point just distal to the medial malleolus, before being finally pulled across the Achilles tendon and placed just distal to the lateral malleolus and across the start of the tape.

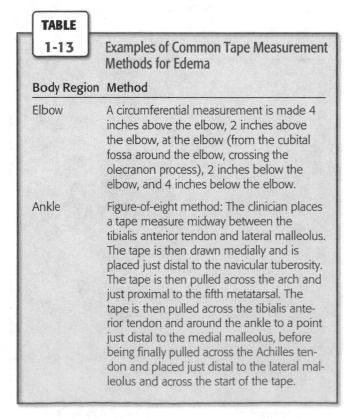

TABLE 1-14	Quality Descriptors of Edema	

Descriptor	Characteristics
Pitting	Formation of a sustained indentation when the swollen area is compressed. Can be quantified using the following scale: 1+ = slight pitting/2 mm, disappears rapidly 2+ = somewhat deeper pit/4 mm, disappears in 10–15 seconds 3+ = deep pit/6 mm, may last >1 minute; dependent extremity is swollen 4+ = very deep pit/8 mm, lasts 2–5 minutes, dependent extremity is grossly distorted
Brawny/ nonpitting	Feels tough, thick, or leathery
Dependent	The fluid shifts in response to gravity. For example, if the patient is lying down, the fluid accumulates on the side of the body in contact with the bed.

general should include assessment of temperature, texture, moistness, mobility, and turgor (degree of fluid loss or dehydration).[26] Skin mobility may be decreased in areas of edema or in scleroderma.

● Key Point Skin temperature is best felt over large areas using the back of the clinician's hand.

Viscerogenic Symptoms

Visceral symptoms can be produced by chemical damage, ischemia, or spasm of the smooth muscles. Although not evoked from all viscera, the symptoms are generally described as diffuse and poorly localized and are often accompanied by autonomic reflexes, such as nausea and vomiting. Symptoms arising from problems in the peritoneum, pleura, or pericardium differ from those of other visceral impairments because of the innervation of these structures.

● Key Point A visceral source of the symptoms should always be suspected if the symptoms are not altered with movement or position changes.

Palpatory findings of tenderness, gross abnormal masses, or abnormal pulsations are indicative of a broad range of abdominal pathologies, including tumor, obstruction, infection, and abdominal aortic aneurysm.[60] Any of these findings warrant a call to the physician.

● Key Point The clinician should always be alert for the presence of cancer. The most common signs and symptoms of cancer include:
- Unexplained weight loss
- Fever
- Constant pain
- Night pain
- Fatigue
- Changes in bowel and/or bladder function
- Unexplained skin changes

Vasculogenic Symptoms

Vasculogenic symptoms tend to result from venous congestion or arterial deprivation to the musculoskeletal areas. Vasculogenic pain may mimic a wide variety of musculoskeletal, neurologic, and arthritic disorders because this type of pain is often worsened by activity.

● Key Point Clinical evidence of arterial insufficiency includes lower calf pain with walking, extremity asymmetry, skin condition changes, skin temperature and color changes, and diminishing pulses. Venous insufficiency is characterized by leg aching, swelling, cramping, heaviness, and soreness, which are improved by walking or by elevating the legs.

The term *intermittent claudication* is used to describe activity-related discomfort associated with peripheral artery disease (PAD). Patients suffering from intermittent claudication often experience effort-related cramp in the calves, thighs, and buttocks, which disappears at rest.

● Key Point Unlike the pain from spinal stenosis, the pain from PVD is not relieved by trunk flexion or aggravated with sustained trunk extension

Pain may occur at more regular intervals as the disease process continues to its end stage—critical limb ischemia—until finally it occurs when the patient is at rest (rest pain). At this stage, rest pain is usually worse when the legs are elevated and during sleep, with the patient gaining relief by hanging the foot over the side of the bed. The development of nonhealing wounds or gangrene (tissue death) may occur at this stage. Any significant changes in the resting vascular signs and symptoms or during exercise must be reported to the PT or physician. **Table 1-15** outlines the general signs and symptoms that warrant the discontinuation of a physical therapy intervention.

TABLE 1-15	The General Signs and Symptoms that Warrant the Discontinuation of a Physical Therapy Intervention
Temperature	>100°F
Systolic BP	>240 mm Hg
Diastolic BP	>110 mm Hg
Fall in systolic BP	More than 20 mm Hg
Rise in HR	More than 220 − age
Resting HR	More than 130 bpm or less than 40 bpm
Oxygen saturation (the percentage of hemoglobin binding sites in the bloodstream occupied by oxygen)	Less than 90%. At low partial pressures of oxygen, most hemoglobin is deoxygenated. An Sao_2 (arterial oxygen saturation) value below 90% causes hypoxemia.
Blood glucose	More than 250 mg/dL

Data from Dreeben O: Introduction to physical therapy for physical therapist assistants. Sudbury, MA, Jones & Bartlett Learning, 2007

Evidence-Based Practice

Evidence-based practice (EBP) involves the integration of three key elements: best research evidence from systematic research, clinical expertise, and patient values.[61] Judging the strength of the evidence becomes an important part of the decision-making process. One of the major problems in evaluating studies is that the volume of literature makes it difficult for the busy clinician to obtain and analyze all of the evidence necessary. In addition, an understanding of how to appraise the quality of the evidence offered by clinical studies and deciding whether the results from the literature are definite enough to indicate an effect other than chance is important.[62] Judging the strength of the evidence becomes an important part of the decision-making process.

● **Key Point** Clinical prediction rules (CPRs) are tools designed to assist clinicians in decision making when caring for patients. However, although there is a growing trend toward producing more CPRs in the field of physical therapy, few reliable and valid CPRs presently exist.

The efficacy of a test or intervention is determined by clinical trials, that is, prospective studies assessing the effect and value of a test or intervention against a control in human subjects.[63] Unfortunately, many of the experimental studies that deal with physical therapy topics are not clinical trials, because there is no control to judge the efficacy of the test or intervention, and there are no tests or interventions from which to draw comparisons.[64] The best evidence comes from randomized controlled trials, systematic reviews, and evidence-based clinical practice guidelines.[65] The ideal clinical trial includes a blinded, randomized design and a control group. A hierarchy of evidence grading is outlined in **Table 1-16**, with Grade A representing the best evidence. Two terms used in the table, and throughout this text, are:

- *Sensitivity:* This represents the proportion of patients with the target disorder who test positive with the diagnostic test. A test that can correctly identify every person who has the target disorder has a sensitivity of 1.0.
- *Specificity:* This represents the proportion of the study population without the target disorder who test negative.[66] A test that can correctly identify every person who does not have the target disorder has a specificity of 1.0.

● **Key Point** A test with a very high sensitivity but low specificity, and vice versa, is of little value. The acceptable levels for each are generally set at between 50% (unacceptable test) and 100% (perfect test), with an arbitrary cut-off of about 80 percent.[66]

It may be possible to discriminate between high- and low-quality trials by asking three simple questions:[65]

- *Were subjects randomly allocated to conditions?* Random allocation implies that a nonsystematic, unpredictable procedure was used to allocate subjects to conditions.
- *Was there blinding of assessors and patients?* Blinding (the people are unaware of which subjects have been assigned to which group) of assessors and patients minimizes the risk of the placebo effect and the "Hawthorne effect," an experimental artifact that is of no clinical utility, where patients report better outcomes than they really experienced because they perceive that this is what is expected from them.[67]
- *Was there adequate follow-up?* Ideally, all subjects who enter the trial should subsequently be followed up to avoid bias. In practice this rarely happens. As a general rule, losses to follow-up of less than 10 percent avoid serious bias, but losses to follow-up of more than 20 percent cause potential for serious bias.

TABLE 1-16	A Hierarchy of Evidence Grading			
Level of Evidence Grading = A	Level of Evidence Grading = B	Level of Evidence Grading = C	Level of Evidence Grading = D	Level of Evidence Grading = E
Randomized clinical trial	Cohort study	Nonrandomized trial with concurrent or historical controls Case study Study of the sensitivity and specificity of a diagnostic test Population-based descriptive study	Cross-sectional study Case series Case report	Expert consensus Clinical experience

Laboratory Values

Although PTAs are not involved in the administration or interpretation of laboratory values, an understanding of normal lab values is essential when reviewing medical charts and other documentation. Laboratory tests can be used for screening, diagnosing, and monitoring patient health and disease. A laboratory test result is interpreted using a reference range appropriate for the age and sex of the patient; the range is the interval between and including the lower and upper reference limits. Reference ranges of the more common laboratory values are provided in Appendix D. The traditional reference range for a quantitative test is the range of values of the central 95 percent of the healthy population.[68]

Musculoskeletal Pharmacology

A drug is any substance that can be used to modify a chemical process or processes in the body, for example, to treat an illness, relieve a symptom, enhance performance or an ability, or alter states of mind. Drug therapy (**Table 1-17**) is one of the mainstays of modern treatments, and PTAs often encounter patients who are taking various medications. These medications may be administered to treat preexisting conditions that are not directly related to the condition being treated with physical therapy, but they can nonetheless have an impact on the patient's response to rehabilitation.[69] As PTAs monitor the effects of their interventions, they must also understand the effect and potential interactions of all available and reasonable resources, including

TABLE 1-17	Pharmacology Terms and Definitions
Term	**Definition**
Pharmacology	The science of studying both the mechanisms and the actions of drugs, usually in animal models of disease, to evaluate their potential therapeutic value
Pharmacy	The mixing and dispensing of drugs The monitoring of drug prescriptions for appropriateness and the monitoring of patients for adverse drug interactions
Pharmacotherapeutics	The use of chemical agents to prevent, diagnose, and cure disease
Pharmacokinetics	The study of how the body absorbs, distributes, metabolizes, and eliminates a drug
Pharmacodynamics	The study of the biochemical and physiologic effects of drugs and their mechanisms of action at the cellular or organ level
Pharmacotherapy	The treatment of a disease or condition with drugs
Pharmacogenetics	The study of how variation in human genes leads to variations in our response to drugs; helps direct therapeutics according to a person's genotype
Toxicology	A study of the negative effects of chemicals on living things, including cells, plants, animals, and humans

TABLE 1-18	Controlled Substances
Schedule	**Description**
I	These drugs are available only for research. They have a high abuse potential, leading to dependence without any acceptable medical indication. Examples include heroin, LSD, and marijuana.
II	These drugs also have a high abuse potential but also have accepted medical uses. Examples include amphetamines, morphine, and oxycodone.
III	Although these drugs have a lower abuse potential and dosing schedule than I or II, they also may be abused and can result in some physical and psychological dependence. Examples include mild to moderately strong opioids, barbiturates, and steroids.
IV	These drugs have less of an abuse potential. No more than five refills within 6 months are allowed under one prescription. Examples include opioids, benzodiazepines, and some stimulants.
V	These drugs have the lowest abuse potential and often are available without prescription. Examples include various cold and cough medicines containing codeine.

pharmacologic interventions, offered by other members of the healthcare team.

Controlled substances are drugs classified according to their potential for abuse. These drugs are regulated under the Controlled Substances Act, which classifies these compounds into schedules from I to V (**Table 1-18**).[1] A black box warning (also sometimes called a black label warning or boxed warning), named for the black border that usually surrounds the text of the warning, appears on the package insert for prescription drugs that carry a significant risk of serious or even life-threatening adverse effects. The U.S. Food and Drug Administration (FDA) can require a pharmaceutical company to place a black box warning on the labeling of a prescription drug, or in literature describing it. It is the strongest warning that the FDA requires.

Drugs are widely used in the management of infection, both acute and chronic pain, and inflammation. The following discussion emphasizes those drugs that are prescribed to control infection, pain, and/or inflammation.

> **Key Point** In the absence of data supporting a therapeutic benefit, toxicity can be associated with any drug, including herbal supplements.

Antibacterial Drugs

Bacteria are unicellular organisms that consist of a cell wall, sometimes a membrane, DNA without a nuclear envelope, and protoplasm containing metabolites and enzymes. Drugs that affect these microorganisms are called antibacterial or antibiotic drugs and are relatively specific for bacteria only. Most antibacterial drugs have five major sites of action as follows:

1. Inhibition of synthesis and/or damage to the bacterial cell wall
2. Inhibition of synthesis and/or damage to the cytoplasmic membrane
3. Modification of synthesis and/or metabolism of microbial nucleic acids
4. Inhibition or modification of microbial protein synthesis by disrupting ribosomal function
5. Inhibition or modification of microbial cell metabolism

Antibacterials/antibiotics are among the most frequently prescribed medications in modern medicine. Although there are well over 100 antibiotics, the majority come from only a few types of drugs. The main classes of antibiotics are outlined in **Table 1-19**. In orthopaedics, antibiotics are commonly used to treat general bone infections (e.g., osteomyelitis) and joint infections (e.g., septic arthritis), for preoperative surgical prophylaxis, and for fracture management with internal fixation.

> **Key Point** Despite excellent antibiotics and preventative treatments, patients who undergo a joint replacement can develop an infection, which will often require removal of the implanted joint in order to treat the infection effectively.

In general, antibacterial drugs can cause nausea, vomiting, allergic reactions, and superinfections.

> **Key Point** Healthcare professionals have been shown to be a primary source of spreading infections. These are referred to as *nosocomial infections*. Between patients, gloves worn by the PTA should be discarded, hands should be washed with soap for at least 15 to 30 seconds, or disinfective solutions should be used to minimize the spread of infection.

TABLE 1-19 Antibiotics

Type	Action	Examples	Implications for Physical Therapy
Penicillin	Bactericidal agent; acts by inhibiting cell membrane synthesis.	Penicillin and amoxicillin	Advise patients to follow prescription schedule strictly and to continue taking drugs even if clinical signs or symptoms have subsided.
Cephalosporin	Bactericidal agent; mainly used to counter staphylococcal organisms	Cephalexin (Keflex)	
Aminoglycosides	Bactericidal agent; generally effective against aerobic gram-negative bacteria (*Klebsiella, Pseudomonas, Escherichia coli*)		Adhere to drug warnings that tetracyclines and quinolones must be taken as prescribed because their use with food or antacids can render them ineffective.
Macrolide	Bacteriostatic agent; inhibits organism replication and is used to counter organisms such as *Chlamydia, Clostridium, Staphylococcus aureus*, and *Bacteroides*	Erythromycin (E-Mycin), clarithromycin (Biaxin), and azithromycin (Zithromax)	Notify supervising PT if patient exhibits an unexplained rash or abdominal discomfort.
Quinolone	Bacteriostatic agent; broadly effective against all gram-negative rods (e.g., *E. coli*, salmonella, and *Pseudomonas*)	Ciprofloxacin (Cipro), levofloxacin (Levaquin), and ofloxacin (Floxin)	Advise the patient to avoid exposure to sunlight because these drugs can cause photosensitization.
Sulfonamide	Bacteriostatic agent; prescribed for the treatment of certain urinary tract infections but also for other (non-orthopedic-related) infections	Co-trimoxazole (Bactrim) and trimethoprim (Proloprim)	
Tetracycline	Bacteriostatic agent; rarely used in the treatment of orthopedic infections	Tetracycline (Sumycin, Panmycin) and doxycycline (Vibramycin)	

Opioid Analgesics

Most of the narcotics used in medicine are referred to as opioids, because they are derived directly from opium or are synthetic opiates. Examples of these opioids include codeine, Darvon (propoxyphene hydrochloride), morphine, and Demerol (meperidine).

Nonopioid Analgesics

Cyclooxygenase (COX) is an enzyme responsible for the formation of important biological mediators called prostanoids, including prostaglandins, prostacyclin, and thromboxane. Pharmacologic inhibition of COX can provide relief from the symptoms of inflammation and pain. The main COX inhibitors are the nonsteroidal anti-inflammatory drugs (NSAIDs), including Voltaren (diclofenac), Relafen (nabumetone), Naprosyn (naproxen), Motrin (ibuprofen), Indocin (indomethacin), Feldene (piroxicam), Lodine (etodolac), Celebrex (celecoxib), and many others.

● **Key Point** Different tissues express varying levels of COX-1 and COX-2. Although both enzymes act basically in the same fashion, selective inhibition can make a difference in terms of side effects.

The NSAIDs are not selective and inhibit all types of COX. The resulting inhibition of prostaglandin and thromboxane synthesis has the effect of reducing inflammation as well as causing antipyretic, antithrombotic, and analgesic effects. The most frequent adverse effect of this class of medication is an irritation of the gastric mucosa, a direct effect of inhibition of prostaglandin synthesis, which normally has a protective role in the gastrointestinal tract.

NSAIDs also may alter kidney blood flow by interfering with the synthesis of prostaglandins in the kidneys involved in the autoregulation of blood flow and glomerular filtration.[73]

Because COX-2 is usually specific to inflamed tissue, there is much less gastric irritation associated with COX-2 inhibitors, with a decreased risk of peptic ulceration. (Currently the only COX-2 inhibitor available in the United States is celecoxib [Celebrex].) The selectivity of COX-2 does not seem to negate other side effects of NSAIDs, most notably an increased risk of renal failure, and there is evidence that indicates an increase in the risk for heart attack, thrombosis, and stroke through an increase of thromboxane unbalanced by prostacyclin (which is reduced by COX-2 inhibition).

Corticosteroids

Corticosteroids are natural anti-inflammatory hormones produced by the adrenal glands under the control of the hypothalamus. An injection of corticosteroids can be used to decrease pain at the site of inflammation, at least temporarily.

Synthetic corticosteroids (cortisone, dexamethasone) are commonly used to treat a wide range of immunological and inflammatory musculoskeletal conditions. Corticosteroids exert their anti-inflammatory effects by binding to a high-affinity intracellular cytoplasmic receptor present in all human cells.[75] As a result, these agents are capable of producing undesirable and sometimes severe systemic adverse effects that may offset clinical gains in many patients. The side effects from corticosteroids emulate those from exogenous hypercortisolism, which is similar to the clinical syndrome of Cushing's disease. These side effects include:[76]

- *Cutaneous manifestations:* Cutaneous manifestations of hypercortisolism include delayed wound healing, acanthosis nigricans (a velvety, thickened, hyperpigmented plaque that usually occurs on the neck or in the axillary region), acne, ecchymoses after minor trauma, hyperpigmentation, hirsutism, petechia, and striae.
- *Hypokalemia:* Hypokalemia is a well-recognized side effect of corticosteroid therapy and is probably related to the mineralocorticoid effect of hydrocortisone, prednisone, and prednisolone. Dexamethasone has no mineralocorticoid effect.
- *Myopathy:* There are two recognized forms of corticosteroid-induced myopathy: acute and chronic. Acute myopathy may in part be caused by hypokalemia, although corticosteroids (especially massive dosages) may have a direct effect on skeletal muscle. Both proximal and distal muscle weakness occur acutely, usually with an associated and significant elevation in serum creatinine phosphokinase, which is indicative of focal and diffuse muscle necrosis. In the more chronic form of myopathy, weakness is more insidious in onset and primarily involves proximal muscle groups.
- *Hyperglycemia:* Although it is not clear how corticosteroid use causes it, hyperglycemia, especially when combined with the immunosuppressive effect of corticosteroids, may significantly increase the risk for infection.
- *Neurological impairments:* These can include vertigo, headache, convulsions, and benign intracranial hypertension.
- *Osteoporosis:* Corticosteroids inhibit bone formation directly via inhibition of osteoblast differentiation and type I collagen synthesis and indirectly by inhibition of calcium absorption and enhancement of urinary calcium excretion.
- *Ophthalmologic side effects:* Corticosteroids increase the risk of glaucoma by increasing intraocular pressure, regardless of whether administered intranasally, topically, periocularly, or systemically.

- *Growth suppression:* Corticosteroids interfere with bone formation, nitrogen retention, and collagen formation, all of which are necessary for anabolism and growth.

> ● **Key Point** Both iontophoresis and phonophoresis can be used to deliver corticosteroids, without the potential for systemic effects.

> ● **Key Point** Pain medications and nonsteroidal anti-inflammatory drugs including corticosteroids can mask signs and symptoms, thereby affecting examination findings and increasing the potential for injury during the performance of prescribed exercises.[77] However, if the patient has a significant amount of pain, appropriate use of these medications may enhance treatment, allowing a more rapid progression than would otherwise be possible. However, as the patient improves, the need for this medication should lessen.

Muscle Relaxants

Muscle relaxants, such as Robaxin and Soma, are thought to decrease muscle tone without impairment in motor function by acting centrally to depress polysynaptic reflexes. Because muscle guarding and spasm accompanies many musculoskeletal injuries, it was originally thought that these drugs, by eliminating the spasm and guarding, would facilitate the progression of a rehabilitation program. However, other drugs with sedative properties, such as barbiturates, also depress polysynaptic reflexes, making it difficult to assess if centrally acting skeletal muscle relaxants actually are muscle relaxants as opposed to nonspecific sedatives.[78]

A description of most common drugs, their indications, and their implications to physical therapy is provided in **Table 1-20**.

TABLE 1-20	The Most Common Drugs, Their Indications, Mechanism of Action, and Implications to Physical Therapy		
Drug	**Indications**	**Mechanism of Action**	**Implications**
ACE inhibitors	Hypertension Congestive heart failure Diabetic nephropathy Migraine headaches	Inhibit ACE (angiotensin-converting enzyme), which causes less stimulation of angiotensin receptors, blood vessel dilation, and a fall in blood pressure	Advise patients to change positions and get up slowly because orthostatic hypotension may occur. Notify the physician if the patient complains of a sore throat (early warning sign of agranulocytosis).
α agonists	Nasal congestion Allergic conditions Bronchoconstriction	Stimulate α agonist receptors resulting in constriction of blood vessels (with increased peripheral resistance and increased blood pressure), and prevent urinary outflow	Some of these drugs are available OTC, and patients often assume that OTC drugs are safe. Advise older men that use of OTC α agonists can lead to urinary hesitancy or even retention in the presence of benign prostatic hyperplasia. Inquire about the use of OTC medications that contain α agonists if you notice that blood pressure has increased in a patient.
α blockers	Hypertension Benign prostatic hyperplasia	Block α agonist receptors resulting in dilation of blood vessels (with decreased peripheral resistance and decreased blood pressure), and increased urinary outflow	Advise patients to change positions and get up slowly because orthostatic hypotension may occur. Monitor patients after strenuous exercise because of risk of hypotensive episode.
Antiarrhythmic drugs	Arrhythmias/dysrhythmias	These drugs can affect the movement of electrical and muscular activity of the heart. There are four major classes: • Sodium channel blockers • β blockers • Drugs that slow the efflux of potassium • Calcium channel blockers	Advise patients to strictly adhere to the prescribed dosing, and avoid caffeine. Monitor patients for peripheral edema or dyspnea. Advise patients to change positions and get up slowly because orthostatic hypotension may occur.

(continued)

TABLE 1-20

The Most Common Drugs, Their Indications, Mechanism of Action, and Implications to Physical Therapy (continued)

Drug	Indications	Mechanism of Action	Implications
Anticholinergics	Arrhythmias Peptic ulcer and irritable bowel syndrome Urinary bladder hypermotility Asthma Parkinson's disease	Inhibit muscarinic (M) cholinergic receptors, thereby reducing the action of acetylcholine resulting in increased heart rate and contractility, dilation of bronchial muscles, and decreased gut and bladder activity	Expect some increases in heart rate in all patients, and some mental confusion in older patients. Keep the exercise environment cool because these patients have a decreased ability to sweat and lose heat.
β blockers	Angina pectoris Hypertension Arrhythmias	Bronchial constriction, blood vessel constriction, decreased heart rate, and decreased systolic blood pressure	When exercising a patient, be aware that because the heart rate will be reduced by the drug, the use of target heart rate needs to be altered accordingly.
Corticosteroids	Inflammation Adrenocortical insufficiency	Multiple metabolic effects on glucose, carbohydrate, and lipid metabolism as well as on inflammatory processes	Observe standard precautions with patients on long-term, high-dose steroid therapy due to the likelihood of a weakened immune system. Be aware of the association between osteoporosis and long-term, high-dose steroid therapy. Be aware that steroid injections can weaken ligaments and tendons. Monitor blood pressure in these patients because hypertension can be a side effect.
Nonsteroidal anti-inflammatory drugs (NSAIDs)	General inflammation Dysmenorrhea Fever Ocular inflammation	See text	Advise the patient that these drugs must be used with caution. NSAIDs may mask pain during exercises. Notify supervising PT if the patient complains about stomach problems, upper respiratory infection, muscle aching, a rash with blisters, or any indications of dermatitis.
Opioid analgesics	Moderate to severe pain Therapy for opioid dependence and withdrawal	Stimulation of opioid receptors in the CNS, which can prevent pain impulses from reaching their final destination	Analgesics may mask pain during exercises. Monitor patients for drowsiness and respiratory depression. Advise patients to change positions and get up slowly because orthostatic hypotension may occur.
Skeletal muscle relaxants	Spasticity Spasm Malignant hyperthermia/tetanus/seizures/neuralgia/cosmetic purposes (Botox)	Enhance the action of the inhibitory GABA system and reduce muscle tone Suppress polysynaptic reflex activity Suppress calcium release from the sarcoplasmic reticulum in skeletal muscles	Monitor patients who have previously used extensor spasticity to maintain balance. Monitor all patients when walking or getting up because drowsiness and muscle weakness can cause falls.

Data from Vogel W: Introduction to pharmacology, in Sueki D, Brechter J (eds): Orthopedic Rehabilitation Clinical Advisor. St Louis, MO, Mosby, 2010, pp 873–922.

Imaging Studies

For healthcare professionals involved in the primary management of neuromusculoskeletal disorders, diagnostic imaging is an essential tool. The availability of diagnostic images varies greatly depending on the practice setting. Although the interpretation of diagnostic images is always the responsibility of the radiologist, it is important for the clinician to know what importance to attach to these reports, and the strengths and weaknesses of the various techniques that image bone and soft tissues, such as muscle, fat, tendon, cartilage, and ligament. In general, imaging tests have a high sensitivity (few false negatives) but low specificity (high false-positive rate), so they are not used in isolation.

Conventional (Plain Film) Radiography

Tissues of greater density allow less penetration of the x-rays and therefore appear lighter on the film. The following structures are listed in order of descending density: metal, bone, soft tissue, water or body fluid, fat, and air. Metal structures (total joint components) are denser than bone and therefore appear as the lightest structures. In contrast, because air is the least dense material in the body, it absorbs the least amount of x-ray particles, thereby appearing as the darkest structure on the film. When studying radiographs, a systematic approach such as the mnemonic ABCS is recommended:[79]

- *A: Architecture or alignment.* The entire radiograph is scanned from top to bottom, side to side, and in each corner to check for the normal shape and alignment of each bone. The outline of each bone should be smooth and continuous. Breaks in continuity usually represent fractures. Malalignments may indicate subluxations or dislocations, or in the case of the spine, scoliosis. Malalignment in a setting of trauma must be considered traumatic rather than degenerative until proven otherwise.[80]
- *B: Bone density.* The clinician should assess both general bone density and local bone density. The cortex of the bone should appear denser than the remainder of the bone. Subchondral bone becomes sclerosed in the presence of stress in accordance with Wolff's law[81] (see Chapter 5) and increases its density. This is a radiographic hallmark of osteoarthritis.
- *C: Cartilage spaces.* Each joint should have a well-preserved joint space between the articulating surfaces. A decreased joint space typically indicates that the articular cartilage is thinned from a degenerative process such as osteoarthritis.
- *S: Soft tissue evaluation.* Trauma to soft tissues produces abnormal images resulting from effusion, bleeding, and distension.

Arthrography

Arthrography is the study of structures within an encapsulated joint using a contrast medium with or without air that is injected into the joint space. The contrast medium distends the joint capsule. This type of radiograph is called an *arthrogram*. An arthrogram outlines the soft tissue structures of a joint that would otherwise not be visible with a plain-film radiograph. This procedure is commonly performed on patients with injuries involving the shoulder or the knee.

Myelography

Myelography is the radiographic study of the spinal cord, nerve roots, dura mater, and spinal canal. The contrast medium is injected into the subarachnoid space, and a radiograph is taken. This type of radiograph is called a *myelogram*. Myelography is used frequently to diagnose intervertebral disk herniations, spinal cord compression, stenosis, nerve root injury, or tumors. The nerve root and its sleeve can be observed clearly on direct myelograms.

Diskography

Diskography is the radiographic study of the intervertebral disk. A radiopaque dye is injected into the disk space between two vertebrae. A radiograph is then taken. This type of radiograph is called a *diskogram*. An abnormal dye pattern between the intervertebral disks indicates a rupture of the disk.

Angiography

Angiography is the radiographic study of the vascular system. A water-soluble radiopaque dye is injected either intra-arterially (arteriogram) or intravenously (venogram). A rapid series of radiographs is then taken to follow the course of the contrast medium as it travels through the blood vessels. Angiography is used to help detect injury to or partial blockage of blood vessels.

Computed Tomography

A CT scanner system, also known as computerized axial tomography (CAT) and computerized transaxial tomography (CT), consists of a scanning gantry that holds the x-ray tube and detectors (moving parts), a moving table or couch for the patient, an x-ray generator, a computer processing unit, and a display console or workstation.[82] Images are obtained in the transverse (axial) plane of the patient's body by rotating the x-ray tube 360 degrees. The x-rays are absorbed in part by the patient's body. The amount of x-rays transmitted through the body is detected in the opposite side of the gantry by an array of detectors. The quality of the image is dependent on variables selected by the operator. Two parameters are used to determine image quality:[82]

- *Spatial resolution:* The ability of the system to distinguish between two closely spaced objects.
- *Contrast resolution:* The ability of the system to discriminate between two adjacent areas. The contrast resolution of CT is dramatically better than conventional radiography, providing the operator with greater soft tissue detail compared with plain films.[80]

As with plain radiographs, air appears as the darkest portion of the film, and bone appears white.

CT Myelogram (CTM)

CTM is a diagnostic tool that uses radiographic contrast media (dye) that is injected into the subarachnoid space (cerebrospinal fluid, CSF). After the dye is injected, the contrast medium serves to illuminate the spinal canal, cord, and nerve roots during imaging. The low viscosity of the water-soluble contrast permits filling of the nerve roots and better visualization.[80]

Magnetic Resonance Imaging (MRI)

Unlike CT, which depends upon multiple thin slices of radiation that are "backplotted" through Fourier transformers, MRI is the result of the interaction among magnetic fields, radiofrequency (RF) waves, and complex image reconstruction techniques. Normally, the axes of protons in the body have a random orientation. However, if the body or body part is placed within a high magnetic field, the protons align themselves parallel with or perpendicular to the direction of the magnetic field. The protons, now spinning synchronously at an angle within the magnetic field, induce a current in a nearby transmitter-receiver coil or antenna. This small nuclear signal is then recorded, amplified, measured, and localized (linked to the exact location in the body where the MRI signal is coming from), producing a high contrast, clinically useful MR image.

Radionucleotide Scanning

Radionucleotide scanning involves the introduction of bone-seeking isotopes that are administered to the patient orally or intravenously and allowed to localize to the skeleton. The photon energy emitted by the isotopes is then recorded using a gamma camera 2–4 hours later. The pathophysiologic basis of the technique is complex but depends on localized differences in blood flow, capillary permeability, and metabolic activity that accompany any injury, infection, repair process, or growth of bone tissue.[83] The most common radionuclide scanning test is the bone scan. This test is used to detect particular areas of abnormal metabolic activity within a bone. The abnormality shows up as a so-called hot spot, which is darker in appearance than normal tissue.

Summary

The role of the PTA in the orthopaedic setting continues to evolve, and the responsibilities placed on the PTA continue to increase. With this increased responsibility comes the need to be fully prepared by having a sound knowledge base from which to work from. However, what has not changed is the importance of communication among the PTA, the PT, the patient, and other members of the healthcare team.

REVIEW Questions

1. A PT asks you to perform a joint mobilization. Whether you can perform the mobilization depends upon:
   a. Ethical principles
   b. State licensure laws
   c. Departmental procedures
   d. Whether the patient has medical insurance
2. What was developed to "encourage a uniform approach to physical therapist practice and to explain to the world the nature of that practice"?
   a. State licensure laws
   b. *Guide to Physical Therapist Practice*
   c. National Physical Therapy Examination
   d. Medicare Act of 1973
3. What is the function of the Commission on Accreditation in Physical Therapy Education (CAPTE)?
   a. To design policies and procedures with regard to physical therapy
   b. To make autonomous decisions concerning the accreditation status of continuing

education programs for physical therapists and physical therapist assistants

   c. To design questions for the National Physical Therapy Examination

   d. To oversee state licensing laws

4. A loss or abnormality of anatomic, physiologic, or psychologic structure or function is a description of which category of the disablement model?

   a. Impairment

   b. Functional limitation

   c. Disability

   d. None of the above

5. Which element of patient/client management includes gathering information from the chart, other caregivers, the patient, the patient's family, caregiver, and friends in order to identify and define the patient's problem(s)?

   a. Evaluation

   b. Intervention

   c. Examination

   d. Tests and measures

6. Which component of the examination includes an analysis of posture, structural alignment or deformity, scars, crepitus, color changes, swelling, and muscle atrophy?

   a. Palpation

   b. Observation

   c. Patient history

   d. None of the above

7. Which of the elements of patient/client management attempts to identify a relationship between the symptoms reported and the signs of disturbed function?

   a. Tests and measures

   b. Patient history

   c. Examination

   d. None of the above

8. Which of the elements of patient/client management determines the predicted level of function that the patient will attain and identifies the barriers that may impact the achievement of optimal improvement—age, medication(s), socioeconomic status, comorbidities, cognitive status, nutrition, social support, and environment—within a certain time frame?

   a. Evaluation

   b. Examination

   c. Prognosis

   d. Diagnosis

9. Which of the following statements is true about the plan of care?

   a. It is based on the examination, evaluation, diagnosis, and prognosis, including the predicted level of optimal improvement.

   b. It describes the specific interventions to be used, and the proposed frequency and duration of the interventions that are required to reach the anticipated goals and expected outcomes.

   c. It includes plans for discharge of the patient/client, taking into consideration achievement of anticipated goals and expected outcomes, and provides for appropriate follow-up or referral.

   d. All of the above.

10. Which of the elements of patient/client management can be defined as "the purposeful and skilled interaction of the PTA and the patient/client and, when appropriate, other individuals involved in the patient/client care, using various physical therapy procedures and techniques to produce changes in the condition consistent with the diagnosis and prognosis."

   a. Examination

   b. Prognosis

   c. Intervention

   d. Evaluation

11. What are the four components of the traditional SOAP note?

12. True or false: Correction fluid/tape can be used to correct text when documenting in medical records.

13. True or false: A PTA may modify an intervention only in accordance with changes in patient status and within the established plan of care developed by the physical therapist.

14. Which of the following duties cannot be performed legally by a physical therapist assistant?

   a. Call a physician about a patient's status

   b. Add 3 pounds to a patient's current exercise protocol

   c. Allow a patient to increase in frequency from 2 times a week to 3 times a week

   d. Perform an ultrasound on a patient

15. A PTA is performing a chart review and discovers that lab results reveal that the patient has malignant cancer. When later treating the patient, the PTA is asked by the patient, "Did

my lab results come back?" The appropriate response for the physical therapist assistant is:
a. To inform the patient about the results and contact the social worker to assist in consultation of the family
b. To inform the patient that it would be inappropriate for you to comment on the lab results before the physician has assessed the lab results and spoken to the patient
c. To inform the patient that he or she has a malignant cancer
d. To tell the patient the results are in, but that PTAs are not allowed to comment on the results

16. You are completing documentation using a SOAP note. Where should "The patient reports wanting to return to playing soccer in 5 weeks" be placed in a SOAP note?
a. Subjective
b. Objective
c. Assessment
d. Plan

17. A physical therapist assistant checks the vital signs of a 40 year-old patient who has a history of cardiac disease. The heart rate is steady at 65 beats per minute; respiratory rate is 8 breaths per minute; blood pressure is 120/72 mm Hg; and the oral temperature is 98.6°F. The vital sign that presents the most concern at this time is the patient's:
a. Respiratory rate
b. Heart rate
c. Blood pressure
d. Temperature

18. A patient with hepatitis B receives a bleeding skin tear on the right forearm during a treatment session. To prevent transmission of the disease while cleaning up, the physical therapist assistant should:
a. Wear disposable gloves
b. Wash both hands before and after cleaning up
c. Wipe up the blood with gauze and dispose in a trash container
d. Wear a mask with a splash guard

19. You are working with a patient who begins to exhibit signs and symptoms of unresponsiveness. You should:
a. Activate emergency protocols and check for vital signs
b. Sit the patient down and monitor blood pressure and pulse rate

c. Administer chest compressions
d. Allow the patient to rest, then resume exercise activities at a lighter pace

References

1. American Physical Therapy Association: Guide to physical therapist practice. Second edition. Phys Ther 81:1–746, 2001
2. Guide to physical therapist practice. Phys Ther 81:S13–S95, 2001
3. American Physical Therapy Association: Guide to physical therapist practice: Revisions. Phys Ther 1–79, 2001
4. Nagi S: Disability concepts revisited: Implications for prevention, in Pope A, Tartov A (eds): Disability in America: Toward a National Agenda for Prevention. Washington, DC, National Academy Press, 1991, pp 309–327
5. Brandt EN, Jr., Pope AM: Enabling America: Assessing the role of rehabilitation science and engineering. Washington, DC, Institute of Medicine, National Academy Press, 1997
6. Palisano RJ, Campbell SK, Harris SR: Evidence-based decision-making in pediatric physical therapy, in Campbell SK, Vander Linden DW, Palisano RJ (eds): Physical Therapy for Children. St. Louis, Saunders, 2006, pp 3–32
7. Schenkman M, Butler RB: A model for multisystem evaluation, interpretation, and treatment of individuals with neurologic dysfunction. Phys Ther 69:538–547, 1989
8. Kettenbach G: Background information, in Kettenbach G (ed): Writing SOAP Notes with Patient/Client Management Formats (ed 3). Philadelphia, FA Davis, 2004, pp 1–5
9. O'Sullivan SB: Clinical decision-making, in O'Sullivan SB, Schmitz TJ (eds): Physical Rehabilitation (ed 5). Philadelphia, FA Davis, 2007, pp 3–24
10. Goodman CC, Snyder TK: Introduction to the interviewing process, in Goodman CC, Snyder TK (eds): Differential Diagnosis in Physical Therapy. Philadelphia, Saunders, 1990, pp 7–42
11. Grieve GP: Common Vertebral Joint Problems. New York, Churchill Livingstone, 1981
12. American Physical Therapy Association: Guide to physical therapist practice. Second edition. Phys Ther 81:9–746, 2001
13. Nirschl RP: Prevention and treatment of elbow and shoulder injuries in the tennis player. Clin Sports Med 7:289–308, 1988
14. Grimsby O, Power B: Manual therapy approach to knee ligament rehabilitation, in Ellenbecker TS (ed): Knee Ligament Rehabilitation. Philadelphia, Churchill Livingstone, 2000, pp 236–251
15. McKenzie R, May S: Introduction, in McKenzie R, May S (eds): The Human Extremities: Mechanical Diagnosis and Therapy. Waikanae, New Zealand, Spinal Publications New Zealand, 2000, pp 1–5
16. Chapman CE: Can the use of physical modalities for pain control be rationalized by the research evidence? Can J Physiol Pharmacol 69:704–712, 1991
17. Feine JS, Lund JP: An assessment of the efficacy of physical therapy and physical modalities for the control of chronic musculoskeletal pain. Pain 71:5–23, 1997

18. McMaster WC, Liddle S, Waugh TR: Laboratory evaluation of various cold therapy modalities. Am J Sports Med 6:291–294, 1978

19. Watson T: The role of electrotherapy in contemporary physiotherapy practice. Man Ther 5:132–141, 2000

20. Lenze EJ, Munin MC, Quear T, et al: The Pittsburgh Rehabilitation Participation Scale: Reliability and validity of a clinician-rated measure of participation in acute rehabilitation. Arch Phys Med Rehabil 85:380–384, 2004

21. Blanpied P: Why won't patients do their home exercise programs? J Orthop Sports Phys Ther 25:101–102, 1997

22. Chen CY, Neufeld PS, Feely CA, et al: Factors influencing compliance with home exercise programs among patients with upper extremity impairment. Am J Occup Ther 53:171–180, 1999

23. Friedrich M, Cermak T, Madebacher P: The effect of brochure use versus therapist teaching on patients performing therapeutic exercise and on changes in impairment status. Phys Ther 76:1082–1088, 1996

24. Deyo RA: Compliance with therapeutic regimens in arthritis: Issues, current status, and a future agenda. Semin Arthritis Rheum 12:233–244, 1982

25. Litzinger ME, Osif B: Accommodating diverse learning styles: Designing instruction for electronic information sources, in Shirato L (ed): What Is Good Instruction Now? Library Instruction for the 90s. Ann Arbor, MI, Pierian Press, 1993

26. Bailey MK: Physical examination procedures to screen for serious disorders of the low back and lower quarter, in Wilmarth MA (ed): Medical Screening for the Physical Therapist. Orthopaedic Section Independent Study Course 14.1.1 La Crosse, WI, Orthopaedic Section, American Physical Therapy Association, 2003, pp 1–35

27. Judge RD, Zuidema GD, Fitzgerald FT: Vital signs, in Judge RD, Zuidema GD, Fitzgerald FT (eds): Clinical Diagnosis (ed 4). Boston, Little, Brown and Company, 1982, pp 49–58

28. Huber MA, Terezhalmy GT, Moore WS: White coat hypertension. Quintessence Int 35:678–679, 2004

29. Chung I, Lip GY: White coat hypertension: Not so benign after all? J Hum Hypertens 17:807–809, 2003

30. Alves LM, Nogueira MS, Veiga EV, et al: White coat hypertension and nursing care. Can J Cardiovasc Nurs 13:29–34, 2003

31. Aronoff GM: Myofascial pain syndrome and fibromyalgia: A critical assessment and alternate view. Clin J Pain 14:74–85, 1998

32. McClaflin RR: Myofascial pain syndrome: Primary care strategies for early intervention. Postgrad Med 96:56–73, 1994

33. Travell JG, Simons DG: Myofascial Pain and Dysfunction—The Trigger Point Manual. Baltimore, MD, Williams & Wilkins, 1983

34. Fricton JR: Myofascial pain. Baillieres Clin Rheumatol 8:857–880, 1994

35. Vecchiet L, Giamberardino MA, Saggini R: Myofascial pain syndromes: Clinical and pathophysiological aspects. Clin J Pain 7:16–22, 1991 (suppl)

36. Grodin AJ, Cantu RI: Soft tissue mobilization, in Basmajian JV, Nyberg R (eds): Rational Manual Therapies. Baltimore, MD, Williams & Wilkins, 1993, pp 199–221

37. Fricton JR: Management of masticatory myofascial pain. Semin Orthod 1:229–243, 1995

38. Esenyel M, Caglar N, Aldemir T: Treatment of myofascial pain. Am J Phys Med Rehab 79:48–52, 2000

39. Bogduk N: The anatomy and physiology of nociception, in Crosbie J, McConnell J (eds): Key Issues in Physiotherapy. Oxford, Butterworth-Heinemann, 1993, pp 48–87

40. Huskisson EC: Measurement of pain. Lancet 2:127, 1974

41. Halle JS: Neuromusculoskeletal scan examination with selected related topics, in Flynn TW (ed): The Thoracic Spine and Rib Cage: Musculoskeletal Evaluation and Treatment. Boston, Butterworth-Heinemann, 1996, pp 121–146

42. Boissonnault WG: Review of systems, in Boissonnault WG (ed): Primary Care for the Physical Therapist: Examination and Triage. St Louis, MO, Elsevier Saunders, 2005, pp 87–104

43. Mohn A, di Ricco L, Magnelli A, et al: Celiac disease–associated vertigo and nystagmus. J Ped Gastroent Nutr 34:317–318, 2002

44. Rowland LP: Diseases of the motor unit, in Kandel ER, Schwartz JH, Jessell TM (eds): Principles of Neural Science (ed 4). New York, McGraw-Hill, 2000, pp 695–712

45. Owen CA: Gluteal compartment syndromes. Clin Orthop 132:57, 1978

46. Botte MJ, Gelberman RH: Acute compartment syndrome of the forearm. Hand Clin 14:391–403, 1998

47. Mars M, Hadley GP: Raised intracompartmental pressure and compartment syndromes. Injury 29:403–411, 1998

48. Matsen FA, Winquist RA, Krugmire RB: Diagnosis and management of compartment syndromes. J Bone Joint Surg 62A:286–291, 1980

49. Gorman WP, Davis KR, Donnelly R: ABC of arterial and venous disease. Swollen lower limb-1: General assessment and deep vein thrombosis. BMJ 320:1453–1456, 2000

50. Anderson FA, Wheeler HB: Natural history and epidemiology of venous thromboembolism. Orthop Rev 23:5–9, 1994

51. Anderson FA, Jr., Spencer FA: Risk factors for venous thromboembolism. Circulation 107:109–I16, 2003

52. Anderson FA, Jr., Wheeler HB: Venous thromboembolism. Risk factors and prophylaxis. Clin Chest Med 16:235–251, 1995

53. Anderson FA, Jr., Wheeler HB, Goldberg RJ, et al: The prevalence of risk factors for venous thromboembolism among hospital patients. Arch Intern Med 152:1660–1664, 1992

54. McNally MA, Mollan RAB: Total hip replacement, lower limb blood flow and venous thrombogenesis. J Bone Joint Surg 75B:640–644, 1993

55. McNally MA, Mollan RAB: The effect of active movement of the foot on venous blood flow after total hip replacement. J Bone Joint Surg 79A:1198–1201, 1997

56. Skaf E, Stein PD, Beemath A, et al: Fatal pulmonary embolism and stroke. Am J Cardiol 97:1776–1777. Epub Apr 27, 2006

57. Perrier A, Bounameaux H: Accuracy or outcome in suspected pulmonary embolism. N Engl J Med 354:2383–2385, 2006

58. McRae SJ, Ginsberg JS: Update in the diagnosis of deep-vein thrombosis and pulmonary embolism. Curr Opin Anaesthesiol 19:44–51, 2006

59. Aschwanden M, Labs KH, Engel H, et al: Acute deep vein thrombosis: Early mobilization does not increase

the frequency of pulmonary embolism. Thromb Haemost 85:42–46, 2001

60. Stowell T, Cioffredi W, Greiner A, et al: Abdominal differential diagnosis in a patient referred to a physical therapy clinic for low back pain. J Orthop Sports Phys Ther 35:755–764, 2005

61. Sackett DL, Rosenberg WM, Gray JA, et al: Evidence based medicine: What it is and what it isn't. BMJ 312: 71–72, 1996

62. Cleland J: Introduction, in Orthopedic Clinical Examination: An Evidence-Based Approach for Physical Therapists. Carlstadt, NJ, Icon Learning Systems, 2005, pp 2–23

63. Friedman LM, Furberg CD, DeMets DL: Fundamentals of Clinical Trials (ed 2). Chicago, Mosby-Year Book, 1985, pp 2, 51, 71

64. Bloch R: Methodology in clinical back pain trials. Spine 12:430–432, 1987

65. Maher CG, Herbert RD, Moseley AM, et al: Critical appraisal of randomized trials, systematic reviews of randomized trials and clinical practice guidelines, in Boyling JD, Jull GA (eds): Grieve's Modern Manual Therapy: The Vertebral Column. Philadelphia, Churchill Livingstone, 2004, pp 603–614

66. Van der Wurff P, Meyne W, Hagmeijer RHM: Clinical tests of the sacroiliac joint, a systematic methodological review. Part 2: Validity. Man Ther 5:89–96, 2000

67. Wickstrom G, Bendix T: The "Hawthorne effect"—what did the original Hawthorne studies actually show? Scand J Work Environ Health 26:363–367, 2000

68. Wall LJ: Laboratory tests and values, in Boissonnault WG (ed): Primary Care for the Physical Therapist: Examination and Triage. St Louis, Elsevier Saunders, 2005, pp 348–367

69. Ciccone CD: Basic pharmacokinetics and the potential effect of physical therapy interventions on pharmacokinetic variables. Phys Ther 75:343–351, 1995

70. Teitz CC, Garrett WE, Jr., Miniaci A, et al: Tendon problems in athletic individuals. J Bone Joint Surg 79-A:138–152, 1997

71. Pease BJ, Cortese M: Anterior knee pain: Differential diagnosis and physical therapy management, Orthopaedic Physical Therapy Home Study Course 92-1. La Crosse, WI, Orthopaedic Section, American Physical Therapy Association, 1992

72. Sperling RL: NSAIDs. Home Healthc Nurse 19:687–689, 2001

73. Clive DM, Stoff JS: Renal syndromes associated with nonsteroidal antiinflammatory drugs. N Engl J Med 310:563–572, 1984

74. Leadbetter WB: Corticosteroid injection therapy in sports injuries, in Leadbetter WB, Buckwalter JA, Gordon SL (eds): Sports-Induced Inflammation: Clinical and Basic Science Concepts. Park Ridge, IL, American Academy of Orthopaedic Surgeons, 1990, pp 527–545

75. Brattsand R, Linden M: Cytokine modulation by glucocorticoids: Mechanisms and actions in cellular studies. Aliment Pharmacol Ther 10:81–90, Discussion 1–2, 1996 (suppl 2)

76. Buchman AL: Side effects of corticosteroid therapy. J Clin Gastroent 33:289–294, 2001

77. Stetts DM: Patient examination, in Wadsworth C (ed): Current Concepts of Orthopaedic Physical Therapy—Home Study Course 11.2.2. La Crosse, WI, Orthopaedic Section, American Physical Therapy Association, 2001

78. Elenbaas JK: Centrally acting oral skeletal muscle relaxants. Am J Hosp Pharm 37:1313–1323, 1980

79. Swain JH: An introduction to radiology of the lumbar spine, in Wadsworth C (ed): Orthopedic Physical Therapy Home Study Course. La Crosse, WI, Orthopedic Section, American Physical Therapy Association, 1994

80. Iwasaki T, Zheng M: Sensory feedback mechanism underlying entrainment of central pattern generator to mechanical resonance. Biol Cybern 94:245–261. Epub Jan 10, 2006

81. Wolff J: The Law of Remodeling (Maquet P, Furlong R, trans). Berlin, Springer-Verlag, 1986 (1892)

82. Yamaguchi T: The central pattern generator for forelimb locomotion in the cat. Prog Brain Res 143:115–122, 2004

83. Norris BJ, Weaver AL, Morris LG, et al: A central pattern generator producing alternative outputs: Temporal pattern of premotor activity. J Neurophysiol 96:309–326. Epub Apr 12, 2006

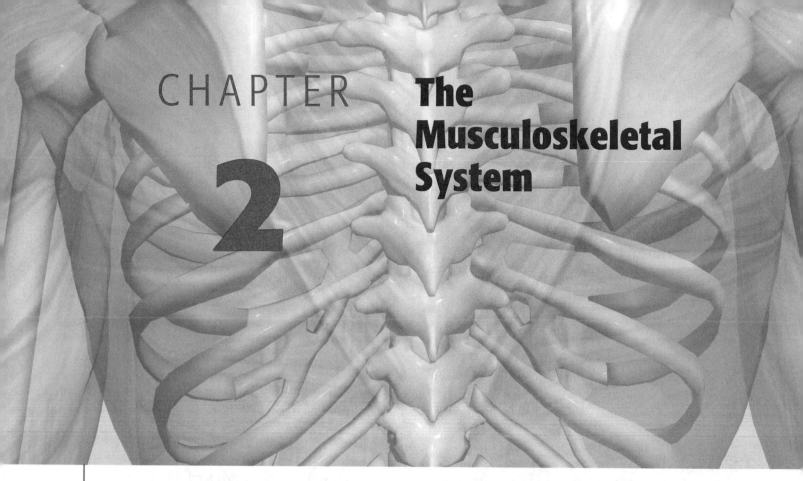

CHAPTER 2

The Musculoskeletal System

Chapter Objectives

At the completion of this chapter, the reader will be able to:

1. Describe the various structures of the musculoskeletal system.
2. Describe the types of connective tissue related to orthopaedics.
3. Outline the function of the various components of connective tissue, including collagen and elastin.
4. Describe the structural differences and similarities among fascia, tendons, and ligaments.
5. Describe the structure and function of a bone as it relates to physical therapy.
6. Outline the different types of cartilage tissue.
7. Describe the main constituents of a synovial joint.
8. Describe the main cellular components of skeletal muscle.
9. Outline the sequence of events involved in a muscle contraction.
10. Describe the major components of a musculoskeletal assessment.

Overview

A working knowledge of the musculoskeletal system forms the foundation of every orthopaedic assessment and intervention by a PTA. A basic tenet in the study of anatomy and biomechanics is that design relates to function, in that the function of a structure can often be determined by its design and vice versa. On the basis of design and function, the tissues of the body are classified into four basic kinds: epithelial, nervous, connective, and muscle tissue:[1]

- *Epithelial tissue* is found throughout the body in two forms: membranous and glandular. Membranous epithelium forms such structures as the outer layer of the skin, the inner lining of the body cavities and lumina, and the covering of visceral organs. Glandular epithelium is a specialized tissue that forms the secretory portion of glands.

- *Nervous tissue* (described in Chapter 3) helps coordinate movements via a complex motor control system of prestructured motor programs and a distributed network of reflex pathways mediated through the autonomic, peripheral, and central nervous systems.[2]
- *Connective tissue* is found throughout the body. It is divided into subtypes according to the matrix that binds the cells. Connective tissue provides structural and metabolic support to other tissues and organs of the body. It includes bone, cartilage, tendons, ligaments, fascia, and blood tissue. The properties of connective tissue are described in the next section of this chapter.
- *Muscle tissue* is responsible for the movement of circulatory materials through the body, the movement of one part of the body with respect to another, and locomotion. There are three types of muscle tissue: smooth, cardiac, and skeletal tissue. In this chapter, human skeletal muscle tissue is described.

> **● Key Point** Together, connective tissue and skeletal muscle tissue form the musculoskeletal system. The musculoskeletal system functions intimately with nervous tissue to produce coordinated movement and to provide adequate joint stabilization and feedback during sustained positions and purposeful movements, such as when climbing and dancing.

Connective Tissue

The anatomic and functional characteristics of the four types of connective tissue that predominate in the joints of the musculoskeletal system are summarized in **Table 2-1**.

The primary types of connective tissue cells are fibroblasts, which are the principal cells of connective tissue; macrophages, which function as phagocytes to clean up debris; and mast cells, which release chemicals associated with inflammation (see Chapter 5).[3] The connective tissue types are differentiated according to the extracellular matrix (ECM) that binds the cells.

Fibroblasts (Figure 2-1) produce collagen, elastin, and reticulin fibers. All connective tissues are made up of varying levels of collagen, elastin, and reticulin:

- Collagen fibers, the most common fibers in connective tissue proper, are long, straight, and unbranched. The collagens are a family of ECM proteins that play a dominant role in maintaining the structural integrity of various tissues and in providing tensile strength

Typical "connective tissue"

Collagen fiber
Elastic fiber
Fibroblast
Amorphous ground substance

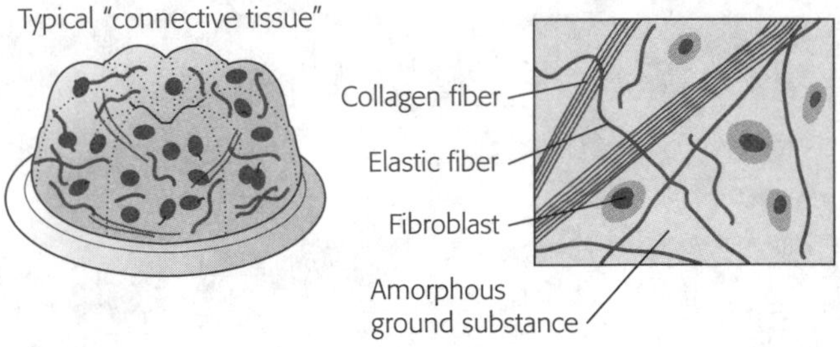

Figure 2-1 Typical connective tissue.

to tissues. The most common forms of collagen (types I–IV) are outlined in **Table 2-2**.[4]

> **● Key Point** Collagen can be visualized as being like the little strands that run through packing tape.

- Elastic fibers contain the protein elastin and are branched and wavy. Elastin is synthesized and secreted from several cell types, including chondroblasts, myofibroblasts, and mesothelial and smooth muscle cells. As its name suggests, elastin provides elastic properties to the tissues in which it is situated.[5] Elastin fibers can stretch, but they normally return to their original shape when the tension is released. The presence of elastin determines the patterns of distention and recoil in most organs, including the skin and lungs, blood vessels, and connective tissue. These characteristics can be useful in preventing injury because they allow the tissues to deform a great deal before breaking.
- Reticular fibers are the least common of the three and are thinner than collagen fibers, forming a branching, interwoven network in various organs providing structural support.

> **● Key Point** Collagen and elastin fibers are embedded within a water-saturated matrix known as *ground substance*, which is composed primarily of glycosaminoglycans, water, and solutes. These materials allow many fibers of the body to exist in a fluid-filled environment that disperses millions of repetitive forces affecting the joints throughout a lifetime.[5]

Fascia

Fascia is an example of loose connective tissue. From the functional point of view, the body fascia may be regarded as a continuous laminated sheet of connective tissue that extends without interruption from the top of the head to the tips of the toes. It surrounds and permeates every other tissue and organ of the

TABLE 2-1 Types of Connective Tissue that Form the Structure of Joints

Joint Type	Anatomic Location	Fibers	Mechanical Specialization
Dense irregular connective tissue (CT)	Composes the external fibrous layer of the joint capsule Forms ligaments, fascia, tendons, and fibrous membranes	High type I collagen fiber content; low elastin fiber content	*Ligament:* Binds bones together and restrains unwanted movement at the joints; resists tension in several directions *Tendon:* Attaches muscle to bone *Fascia:* A layer of fibrous tissue that permeates the human body and that performs a number of functions, including enveloping and isolating the muscles of the body, providing structural support and protection
Articular cartilage	Covers the ends of articulating bones in synovial joints	High type II collagen fiber content; fibers help anchor cartilage to subchondral bone and restrain the ground substance	Resists and distributes compressive forces (joint loading) and shear forces (surface sliding); very low coefficient of friction—the ratio of the force of friction between two bodies and the force pressing them together The coefficient of friction depends on the materials used; for example, ice on steel has a low coefficient of friction, whereas rubber on pavement has a high coefficient of friction
Fibrocartilage	Composes the intervertebral discs and the disc within the pubic symphysis Forms the intraarticular discs (menisci) of the tibiofemoral, sternoclavicular, acromioclavicular, and distal radioulnar joints Forms the labrum of the glenoid fossa and the acetabulum	Multidirectional bundles of type I collagen	Provides some support and stabilization to joints; primary function is to provide "shock absorption" by resisting and distributing compressive and shear forces
Bone	Forms the internal levers of the musculoskeletal system	Specialized arrangement of type I collagen to form lamellae and osteons and to provide a framework for hard mineral salts (e.g., calcium crystals)	Resists deformation; strongest resistance is applied against compressive forces due to body weight and muscle force Provides a rigid lever to transmit muscle force to move and stabilize the body

body, including nerves, vessels, tendons, aponeuroses, ligaments, capsules, and the intrinsic components of muscle.[6,7] Theoretically, injury, inflammation, disease, surgery, and excess strain can cause the fascia to scar and harden. This can cause tension not only in adjacent, pain-sensitive structures but also in other areas of the body. This is because of the complete integration of fascia with all the other systems. Myofascial release (see Chapter 6) is a form of soft tissue therapy used to treat dysfunction and accompanying pain and restriction of motion by relaxing contracted muscles, increasing circulation, increasing venous and lymphatic drainage, and stimulating the stretch reflex of muscles and overlying fascia

Tendons

Tendons (Figure 2-2), a type of dense connective tissue, are cordlike structures that attach muscle to bone.[8] Tendons are made up of densely packed parallel-oriented bundles of fibers.[9] The thickness of each tendon varies and is proportional to the size of the muscle from which it originates. Tendons deform

TABLE 2-2	Major Types of Collagen
Type	**Description/Location**
I	Thick and rough
	Designed to resist elongation
	Found in bone, skin, ligament, and tendon
II	Thinner and less stiff than type I fibers
	Provide a framework for maintaining the general shape and consistency of structures such as hyaline cartilage and nucleus pulposus
III	A small and slender fiber of collagen
	Found in extensible connective tissues such as skin, lung, and the vascular system
IV	Overall arrangement causes the collagen to form in a sheet
	Found primarily in the basement membrane (a thin sheet of fibers that underlies the epithelium, which lines the cavities and surfaces of organs, or the endothelium, which lines the interior surface of blood vessels)

less than ligaments under an applied load and are able to transmit the load from muscle to bone.[10] However, tendons transmit forces from muscle to bone and are subject to great tensile stresses.

● **Key Point** Although tendons withstand strong tensile forces well, they resist shear forces less well and provide little resistance to compression force (see Chapter 4).

As the tendon joins the muscle, it fans out into a much wider and thinner structure. The site where the muscle and tendon meet is called the *myotendinous junction (MTJ)*. Despite its viscoelastic mechanical characteristics, the MTJ is very vulnerable to tensile failure.[11,12] Indeed, the MTJ is the location of most common muscle strains caused by tensile forces in a normal muscle–tendon unit.[10,13]

● **Key Point** A tendency for a tear near the MTJ has been reported in the biceps and triceps brachii, rotator cuff muscles, flexor pollicis longus, fibularis (peroneus) longus, medial head of the gastrocnemius, rectus femoris, adductor longus, iliopsoas, pectoralis major, semimembranosus, and the entire hamstring group.[14–16]

Ligaments

Skeletal ligaments, a type of dense connective tissue, connect bones across joints (refer to Figure 2-2). The gross structure of the ligaments varies with their location (intra-articular or extra-articular, capsular) and function.[9] The orientation of the collagen fibers has a less unidirectional organization in ligaments

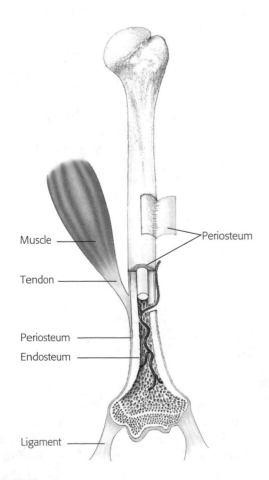

Muscle

Tendon

Periosteum

Endosteum

Ligament

Periosteum

Figure 2-2 Tendon, ligament, bone, and muscle.

than it does in tendons, but this irregular crossing pattern still provides stiffness (resistance to deformation) and makes ligaments ideal for sustaining tensile loads from several different directions.[17,18]

> **● Key Point** Ligaments have a rich sensory innervation through specialized mechanoreceptors and free nerve endings that provide information about proprioception and pain, respectively.

Ligaments contribute to the stability of joint function by preventing excessive motion,[19] acting as guides to direct motion, and providing proprioceptive information for joint function (**Table 2-3** and **Table 2-4**).[20,21]

> **● Key Point** Immobilization and disuse dramatically compromise the structural material properties of ligaments (see Chapter 5), resulting in a significant decrease in the ability of the ligament to resist strain.[9]

Bone

Bone is a highly vascular and metabolically active form of connective tissue, composed of collagen, calcium phosphate, water, amorphous proteins, and cells. There are approximately 206 bones in the body.

There are three types of bone cells:

- *Osteocytes:* Control extracellular concentrations of calcium and phosphorus. Actively involved with the maintenance of the bony matrix.
- *Osteoclasts:* Responsible for bone resorption. An increased number of osteoclasts is characteristic of diseases with increased bone turnover.
- *Osteoblasts:* Responsible for bone formation.

TABLE 2-3   Major Ligaments of the Upper Quadrant

Joint	Ligament	Function
Shoulder complex	Coracoclavicular	Fixes the clavicle to the coracoid process
	Costoclavicular	Fixes the clavicle to the costal cartilage of the first rib
	Coracohumeral	Reinforces the upper portion of the joint capsule
	Glenohumeral	Reinforces the anterior and inferior aspect of the joint capsule
	Coracoacromial	Protects the superior aspect of the joint
Elbow and forearm	Annular	Maintains the relationship between the head of the radius and the humerus and ulna
	Ulnar (medial) collateral	Provides stability against valgus (medial) stress, particularly in the range of 20–130° of flexion and extension
	Radial (lateral) collateral	Provides stability against varus (lateral) stress and functions to maintain the ulnohumeral and radiohumeral joints in a reduced position when the elbow is loaded in supination
	Interosseous membrane of the forearm	Divides the forearm into anterior and posterior compartments, serves as a site of attachment for muscles of the forearm, and transfers forces from the radius to the ulna to the humerus
Wrist	Extrinsic palmar	Provides the majority of the wrist stability
	Intrinsic	Serves as rotational restraints, binding the proximal carpal row into a unit of rotational stability
	Interosseous	Binds the carpal bones together
	Triangular fibrocartilage complex (TFCC)	Suspends the distal radius and ulnar carpus from the distal ulna
		Provides a continuous gliding surface across the entire distal face of the radius and ulna for flexion-extension and translational movements
		Provides a flexible mechanism for stable rotational movements of the radiocarpal unit around the ulnar axis
		Cushions the forces transmitted through the ulnocarpal axis
Fingers	Volar and collateral interphalangeal	Prevents displacement of the interphalangeal joints

TABLE 2-4

Major Ligaments of the Spine and Lower Quadrant

Joint	Ligament	Function
Spine	Anterior longitudinal ligament	Functions as a minor assistant in limiting anterior translation and vertical separation of the vertebral body
	Posterior longitudinal ligament	Limits hyperextension of the spine
		Resists vertebral distraction of the vertebral body
		Resists posterior shearing of the vertebral body
		Acts to limit flexion over a number of segments
		Provides some protection against intervertebral disk protrusions
	Ligamentum flavum	Resists separation of the lamina during flexion
	Interspinous	Resists shear forces and separation of the spinous processes during flexion; prevents excessive rotation
	Intratransverse	Resists side bending of the spine and helps in preventing rotation
	Iliolumbar (lower lumbar)	Resists flexion, extension, axial rotation, and side bending of L5 on S1
	Nuchal (represents the supraspinal ligaments of the lower vertebrae)	Resists cervical flexion
Sacroiliac	Sacrospinous	Resists forward tilting of the sacrum on the hip bone during weight bearing of the vertebral column
	Sacrotuberous	Resists forward tilting (nutation) of the sacrum on the hip bone during weight bearing of the vertebral column
	Interosseous	Resists anterior and inferior movement of the sacrum
	Posterior (dorsal) sacroiliac	Resists backward tilting (counternutation) of the sacrum on the hip bone during weight bearing of the vertebral column
	Anterior (ventral) sacroiliac	Consists of numerous thin bands; a capsular ligament
Hip	Ligamentum teres	Transports nutrient vessels to the femoral head
	Iliofemoral (Y ligament)	Strongest of the hip ligaments; limits hip extension
	Ischiofemoral	Limits anterior displacement of the femoral head and internal rotation of the hip
	Pubofemoral	Limits hip extension and abduction of the hip
Knee	Medial collateral	Stabilizes medial aspect of tibiofemoral joint against valgus stress
	Lateral collateral	Stabilizes lateral aspect of tibiofemoral joint against varus stress
	Anterior cruciate	Resists anterior translation of the tibia and posterior translation of the femur
	Posterior cruciate	Resists posterior translation of the tibia and anterior translation of the femur
Ankle	Medial collaterals (deltoid)	Include the tibionavicular, calcaneotibial, anterior talotibial, and posterior talotibial ligaments; provide stability between the medial malleollus, navicular, talus, and calcaneus against eversion
	Lateral collaterals	Include the anterior talofibular, calcaneofibular, talocalcaneal, posterior talocalcaneal, and posterior talofibular ligaments; static stabilizers of the lateral ankle, especially against inversion
Foot	Long plantar	Provides indirect plantar support to the calcaneocuboid joint, by limiting the amount of flattening of the lateral longitudinal arch of the foot
	Bifurcate	Supports the medial and lateral aspects of the foot when weight bearing in a plantarflexed position
	Calcaneocuboid	Provides plantar support to the calcaneocuboid joint and possibly helps to limit flattening of the lateral longitudinal arch

Bone is the most rigid of the connective tissues. Despite its rigidity, bone is a dynamic tissue that undergoes constant metabolism and remodeling. The collagen of bone is produced in the same manner as that of ligaments and tendons, but by a different cell, the osteoblast.[22]

At the gross anatomical level, each bone has a distinct morphology (**Table 2-5**) comprising both cortical bone and cancellous bone.

- Cortical (compact) bone is relatively dense and found in the outer shell of the diaphysis of long bones. The osteon, or Haversian system, is the fundamental functional unit of much compact bone.
- Cancellous (trabecular) bone is porous and is typically found within the epiphyseal and metaphyseal regions of long bones as well as throughout the interior of short bones.[11]

The function of a bone is to provide support, enhance leverage, protect vital structures, provide attachments for both tendons and ligaments, and store minerals, particularly calcium.

Blood Supply to Bone

Bone has a rich vascular supply, receiving 10–20 percent of the cardiac output. The blood supply varies with different types of bones, but blood vessels are especially rich in areas that contain red bone marrow. The long bones are supplied by the following:

- *Diaphyseal nutrient artery:* The most important supply of arterial blood to a long bone

TABLE 2-5	**General Structure of Bone**
Site	**Description**
Epiphysis	The region between the growth plate or growth plate scar and the expanded end of bone, covered by articular cartilage
	The location of secondary ossification centers during development
	Forms bone ends
Physis (also known as epiphyseal plate)	The region that separates the epiphysis from the metaphysis
	The zone of endochondral ossification in an actively growing bone or the epiphyseal scar in a fully grown bone
	Vulnerable prior to growth spurt and mechanically weak
Metaphysis	The junctional region between the growth plate and the diaphysis
	Contains abundant cancellous (trabecular) bone, which heals rapidly, but the cortical bone thins here relative to the diaphysis
	Common site for many primary bone tumors and similar lesions (osteomyelitis)
Diaphysis	Forms shaft of bone
	Large surface for muscle origin
	Composed mainly of cortical (compact) bone
	The medullary canal contains marrow and a small amount of trabecular bone

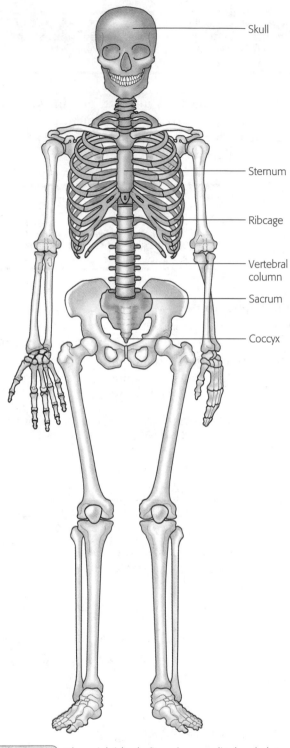

Figure 2-3 The axial (shaded) and appendicular skeleton.

Skull

Sternum

Ribcage

Vertebral column

Sacrum

Coccyx

- *Metaphyseal and epiphyseal arteries:* Supply the ends of bones
- *Periosteal arterioles:* Supply the outer layers of cortical bone

The large irregular, short, and flat bones receive a superficial blood supply from the periosteum, as well as frequently from large nutrient arteries that penetrate directly into the medullary bone.

> **● Key Point** Bone remodeling is a lifelong process that involves the replacement of old bone by new bone based on the functional demands of the mechanical loading according to Wolff's law (see Chapter 5).

Articular Cartilage

The development of bone is usually preceded by the formation of articular (hyaline) cartilage tissue, commonly called gristle. Articular cartilage is a highly organized viscoelastic material composed of cartilage cells called *chondrocytes*, water, and an ECM. The ECM contains proteoglycans, lipids, water, and dissolved electrolytes. Articular cartilage is devoid of any blood vessels, lymphatics, and nerves.[23,24] It covers the ends of long bones and, along with the synovial fluid that bathes it, provides a smooth, almost frictionless articulating surface.[25]

> **● Key Point**
> • Articular cartilage is the most abundant cartilage within the body.
> • Most of the bones of the body form first as articular cartilage and later become bone in a process called *endochondral ossification*.

Articular cartilage distributes the joint forces over a large contact area, dissipating the forces associated with the load. The normal thickness of articular cartilage is determined by the contact pressures across the joint—the higher the peak pressures, the thicker the cartilage.[9] This distribution of forces allows the articular cartilage to remain healthy and fully functional throughout decades of life.

> **● Key Point** The patella has the thickest articular cartilage in the body.

Articular cartilage may be grossly subdivided into four distinct zones with differing cellular morphology, biomechanical composition, collagen orientations, and structural properties (Figure 2-4).

Fibrocartilage

Fibrocartilage consists of a blend of white fibrous tissue and cartilaginous tissue. The white fibrous tissue provides flexibility and toughness, while the cartilage tissue provides elasticity.

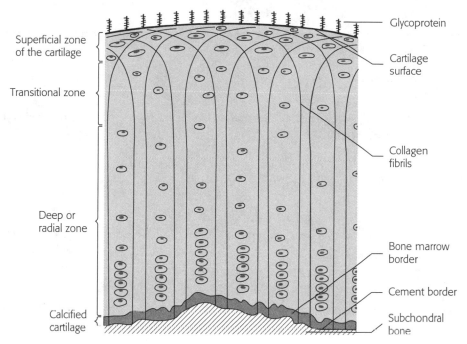

Superficial zone of the cartilage

Transitional zone

Deep or radial zone

Calcified cartilage

Glycoprotein

Cartilage surface

Collagen fibrils

Bone marrow border

Cement border

Subchondral bone

Figure 2-4 Articular layers of cartilage.

Meniscus

The meniscus is a specialized viscoelastic fibrocartilaginous structure capable of load transmission, shock absorption, stability, articular cartilage lubrication, and proprioception.[9] The collagen fibers of the menisci are arranged parallel to the peripheral border in the deeper areas, and are more radially oriented in the superficial region. The radially oriented fibers provide structural rigidity and the deep fibers resist tension. Menisci tend to be found in noncongruent joints, such as the knee. The pathology of the knee meniscus and implications for the PTA are described in Chapter 20.

Intervertebral Disc

An intervertebral disk (IVD) is located between adjacent vertebrae in the spine, and combined represent the largest avascular structure in the body.[24] In the human spinal column, the combined heights of the IVDs account for approximately 20–33 percent of the total length of the spinal column.[26] The human vertebral column is designed to provide structural stability while affording full mobility as well as protection of the spinal cord and axial neural tissues.[27] The presence of an IVD not only permits motion of the segment in any direction up to the point that the disk itself is stretched but also allows for a significant increase in the weight-bearing capabilities of the spine.[28] Vertebral disks have traditionally been described as being composed of three parts: the annulus fibrosus (AF), the vertebral end plate, and a central gelatinous mass, called the nucleus pulposus (NP).

Three main types of structural disruption are recognized: herniation, protrusion, and prolapse (see Chapter 15).

Joints

A joint represents the junction between two or more bones. Joints are regions where bones are capped and surrounded by connective tissues that hold the bones together and determine the type and degree of movement between them.[29] Joints may be classified as synovial, fibrous, or cartilaginous (**Table 2-6**).

> **● Key Point** An amphiarthrosis, a type of joint formed primarily by fibrocartilage and hyaline cartilage, plays an important role in shock absorption. An example of an amphiarthosis is the intervertebral body joints of the spine.

Every synovial joint contains at least one "mating pair" of articular surfaces—one convex and one concave. If only one pair exists, the joint is called simple; more than one pair is called compound. If a disk is present, the joint is termed complex. Synovial joints have five distinguishing

TABLE 2-6	Joint Types	
Type	**Characteristics**	**Examples**
Synovial		
Diarthrosis	Fibroelastic joint capsule, which is filled with a lubricating substance called *synovial fluid*	Hip, knee, shoulder, and elbow joints
Fibrous		
Synarthrosis (eventual fusion is termed a synostosis)	United by bone tissue, ligament, or membrane Immovable joint	Sagittal suture of the skull
Syndesmosis	Joined together by a dense fibrous membrane Very little motion	The interosseous membrane between the tibia and fibula
Gomphosis	Bony surfaces connected like a peg in a hole (the periodontal membrane is the fibrous component)	The teeth and corresponding sockets are the only gomphosis joints in the body
Cartilaginous (amphiarthrosis)		
Synchondrosis	Joined by either hyaline or fibrocartilage May ossify to a synostosis once growth is completed	The epiphyseal plates of growing bones and the articulations between the first rib and the sternum
Symphysis	Generally located at the midline of the body Two bones covered with hyaline cartilage and connected by fibrocartilage	The symphysis pubis

characteristics: joint cavity, articular cartilage, synovial fluid, synovial membrane, and a fibrous capsule (Figure 2-5). Synovial joints can be broadly classified according to structure or analogy into the following categories:[1]

- *Spheroid:* As the name suggests, a spheroid joint is a freely moving joint in which a sphere on the head of one bone fits into a rounded cavity in the other bone. Spheroid (ball and socket) joints allow motions in three planes (refer to Chapter 4). Examples of a spheroid joint surface include the heads of the femur and humerus.
- *Trochoid:* The trochoid (pivot) joint is characterized by a pivot-like process turning within a ring, or a ring on a pivot, the ring being formed partly of bone, partly of ligament. Trochoid joints permit only rotation. Examples of a trochoid joint include the proximal radioulnar joint and the atlantoaxial joint.
- *Condyloid:* The condyloid joint is characterized by an ovoid articular surface, or condyle. One bone may articulate with another by one

surface or by two, but never more than two. If two distinct surfaces are present, the joint is called condylar or bicondylar. The elliptical cavity of the joint is designed in such a manner as to permit the motions of flexion, extension, adduction, abduction, and circumduction, but no axial rotation (see Chapter 4). The wrist joint is an example of this form of articulation.
- *Ginglymoid:* A ginglymoid (hinge) is characterized by a spool-like surface and a concave surface. An example of a ginglymoid joint is the humeroulnar joint.
- *Ellipsoid:* Ellipsoid joints are similar to spheroid joints in that they allow the same type of movement, albeit to a lesser magnitude. The ellipsoid joint allows movement in two planes (flexion, extension; abduction, adduction) and is biaxial (refer to Chapter 4). Examples of this joint can be found at the radiocarpal articulation at the wrist and the metacarpophalangeal articulation in the phalanges.
- *Planar:* As its name suggests, a planar (gliding) joint is characterized by two flat

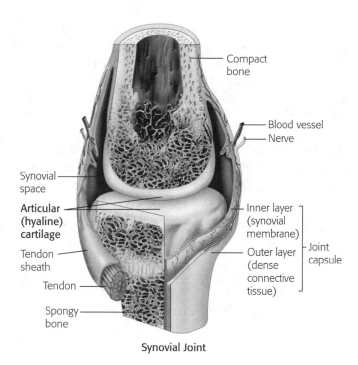

Synovial Joint

- Compact bone
- Blood vessel
- Nerve
- Synovial space
- Articular (hyaline) cartilage
- Inner layer (synovial membrane)
- Joint capsule
- Outer layer (dense connective tissue)
- Tendon sheath
- Tendon
- Spongy bone

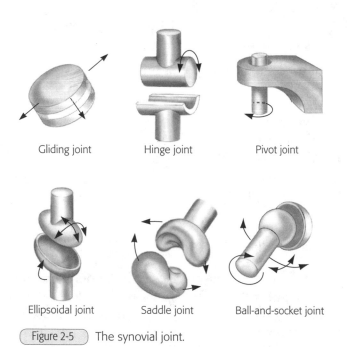

Gliding joint   Hinge joint   Pivot joint

Ellipsoidal joint   Saddle joint   Ball-and-socket joint

Figure 2-5 The synovial joint.

surfaces that slide over each other. Movement at this type of joint does not occur about an axis and is termed nonaxial. Examples of a planar joint include the intermetatarsal joints and some intercarpal joints.

■ *Sellar:* The other major type of articular surface is the sellar (saddle) joint.[2] Sellar joints are characterized by a convex surface in one cross-sectional plane and a concave surface in the plane perpendicular to it. Examples of a sellar joint include the carpometacarpal joint of the thumb, the humeroulnar joint, and the calcaneocuboid joints.

Although the above-mentioned categories give a broad description of joint structure, this classification does not sufficiently describe the articulations or the movements that occur. In reality, no joint surface is planar or resembles a true geometric form. Instead, joint surfaces are either convex in all directions or concave in all directions, that is, they resemble either the outer or inner surface of a piece of eggshell.[2] Because the curve of an eggshell varies from point to point, these articular surfaces are called *ovoid*.

Joint Receptors
All synovial joints of the body are provided with an array of corpuscular receptor endings (mechanoreceptors) and noncorpuscular receptor endings (nociceptors) imbedded in articular, muscular, and cutaneous structures with varying characteristic behaviors and distributions depending on articular tissue (**Table 2-7**).

Synovial Fluid
Articular cartilage is subject to a great variety of loading conditions (see Chapter 4); therefore, joint lubrication through synovial fluid is necessary to minimize frictional resistance between the weight-bearing surfaces. Fortunately, synovial joints are blessed with a very superior lubricating system, which permits a remarkably frictionless interaction at the joint surfaces.

> ● **Key Point** In terms of design, a synovial joint imparts very little friction at the joint surfaces. By way of a comparison, a lubricated cartilaginous interface has a coefficient of friction* of 0.002[64]; ice moving on ice has a much higher coefficient of friction of 0.03.[30]

The composition of synovial fluid is nearly the same as that of blood plasma, but with a decreased total protein content and a higher concentration of hyaluronan.[31] Indeed, synovial fluid is essentially a dialysate of plasma to which hyaluronan has been added.[32] Hyaluronan is a glycosaminoglycan

---

*Coefficient of friction is a ratio of the force needed to make a body glide across a surface compared with the weight or force holding the two surfaces in contact. The higher the coefficient, the greater the force required and the greater heat generated.

TABLE 2-7 Characteristics of Mechanoreceptors and Nociceptors

Receptor Type	Type of Stimulus and Example	Receptor Type and Location
Mechanoreceptors	Pressure	
	Movement of hair in a hair follicle	Afferent nerve fiber (base of hair follicles)
	Light pressure	Meissner's corpuscle (skin)
	Deep pressure	Pacinian corpuscle (skin)
	Touch	Merkel's touch corpuscle (skin)
Nociceptors	Pain (stretch)	Free nerve endings (wall of gastrointestinal tract, skin)
Proprioceptors	Distension	Ruffini corpuscles (skin and capsules in joints and ligaments)
	Length changes	Muscle spindles (skeletal muscles)
	Tension changes	Golgi tendon organs (between muscles and tendons)
Thermoreceptors	Temperature changes	
	Cold	Krause's end bulbs (skin)
	Heat	Ruffini corpuscles (skin and capsules in joints and ligaments)

(GAG) that is continually synthesized and released into synovial fluid by specialized synoviocytes.[33] Hyaluronan is a critical constituent component of normal synovial fluid and an important contributor to joint homeostasis.[34]

● **Key Point** Hyaluronan imparts anti-inflammatory and antinociceptive properties to normal synovial fluid and contributes to joint lubrication. It is also responsible for the viscoelastic properties of synovial fluid[31] and contributes to the lubrication of articular cartilage surfaces.[32,33]

The mechanical properties of synovial fluid permit it to act as both a cushion and a lubricant to the joint. Fluid lubrication results when a film of synovial fluid is established, and maintained, between the two surfaces as long as movement occurs.

Bursae

Closely associated with some synovial joints are flattened, saclike structures called *bursae* that are lined with a synovial membrane and filled with synovial fluid. The bursa produces small amounts of fluid,

allowing for smooth and almost frictionless motion between contiguous muscles, tendons, bones, ligaments, and skin.[35–37] A tendon sheath is a modified bursa. Bursitis is defined as inflammation of a bursa, and it occurs when the synovial fluid becomes infected by bacteria or gets irritated because of too much movement. Symptoms of bursitis include inflammation, localized tenderness, warmth, edema, erythema of the skin (if superficial), and loss of function. Any signs of a pathologic or inflamed bursa should be reported to the supervising PT. The list of bursae that may become inflamed is quite extensive:

- Subacromial (subdeltoid) bursitis
- Olecranon bursitis
- Iliopsoas bursitis
- Trochanteric bursitis
- Ischial bursitis
- Prepatellar bursitis
- Infrapatellar bursitis
- Anserine bursitis

Skeletal Muscle Tissue

Skeletal muscle tissue consists of individual muscle cells or fibers (Figure 2-6). A single muscle cell is called a *muscle fiber* or *myofiber*. Individual muscle fibers are wrapped in a connective tissue envelope called *endomysium*. Bundles of myofibers, which form a whole muscle (fasciculus), are encased in the perimysium. The perimysium is continuous with the deep fascia. Groups of fasciculi are surrounded by a connective sheath called the epimysium. An electron microscope reveals that each of the myofibers consists of thousands of *myofibrils*, which extend throughout its length (Figure 2-7). Myofibrils are composed of sarcomeres arranged in series).[38]

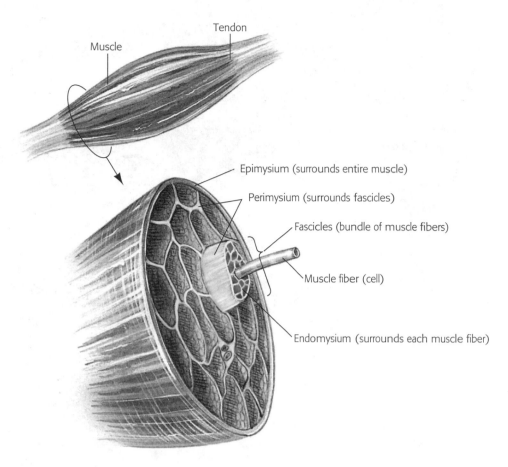

Muscle

Tendon

Epimysium (surrounds entire muscle)

Perimysium (surrounds fascicles)

Fascicles (bundle of muscle fibers)

Muscle fiber (cell)

Endomysium (surrounds each muscle fiber)

Figure 2-6 Muscle tissue.

Machinery of Movement

One of the most important roles of connective tissue is to mechanically transmit the forces generated by the skeletal muscle cells to provide movement. Each muscle cell contains many structural components called *myofilaments*, which run parallel to the myofibril axis. The myofilaments are made up of two protein filaments: actin (thin) and myosin (thick) (Figure 2-7). The most distinctive feature of skeletal muscle fibers is their striated (striped) appearance. This cross-striation is the result of an orderly arrangement within and between structures called sarcomeres and myofibrils.[39] The sarcomere is the contractile machinery of the muscle. The striations are produced by alternating dark (A) and light (I) bands that appear to span the width of the muscle fiber. The A bands are composed of myosin filaments, whereas the I bands are composed of actin

filaments. The actin filaments of the I band overlap into the A band, giving the edges of the A band a darker appearance than the central region (H band), which contains only myosin. At the center of each I band is a thin, dark Z line (Figure 2-7). A *sarcomere* represents the distance between each Z line. Each muscle fiber is limited by a cell membrane called a *sarcolemma*. The protein *dystrophin* plays an essential role in the mechanical strength and stability of the sarcolemma.[40]

When a muscle contracts, the distance between the Z lines decreases, the I band and H bands disappear, but the width of the A band remains unchanged.[39] This shortening of the sarcomeres is not produced by a shortening of the actin and myosin filaments, but by a sliding of actin filaments over the myosin filaments, which pulls the Z lines together.

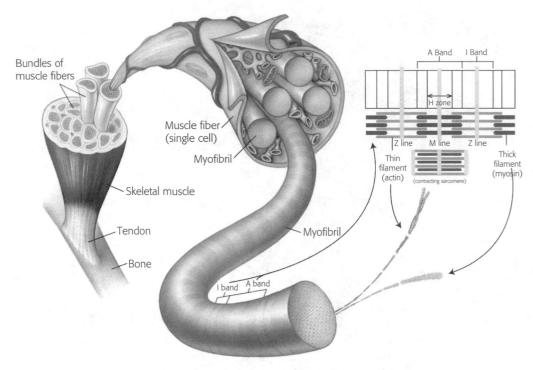

Figure 2-7 Contractile machinery.

Structures called *myosin cross-bridges* connect the actin and myosin filaments (refer to Figure 2-7). The myosin filaments contain two flexible, hinge-like regions, which allow the cross-bridges to attach and detach from the actin filament. During contraction, the cross-bridges attach and undergo power strokes, which provide the contractile force. During relaxation, the cross-bridges detach. This attaching and detaching is asynchronous, so that some are attaching while others are detaching. Thus, at each moment, some of the cross-bridges are pulling while others are releasing. The regulation of cross-bridge attachment and detachment is a function of two proteins found in the actin filaments: tropomyosin and troponin (Figure 2-8). Tropomyosin attaches directly to the actin filament, whereas troponin is attached to the tropomyosin rather than directly to the actin filament. Tropomyosin and troponin function as the switch for muscle contraction and relaxation. In a relaxed state, the tropomyosin physically blocks the cross-bridges from binding to the actin. For contraction to take place, the tropomyosin must be moved.

Each muscle fiber is innervated by a somatic motor neuron. One neuron, and the muscle fibers it innervates, constitutes a motor unit or functional unit of the muscle. Each motor neuron branches as it enters the muscle to innervate a number of muscle fibers. The area of contact between a nerve and a muscle fiber is known as the motor end plate or neuromuscular junction. The release of a chemical, acetylcholine, from the axon terminals at the neuromuscular junctions causes electrical activation of the skeletal muscle fibers. When an action potential propagates into the transverse tubule system (narrow membranous tunnels formed from and continuous with the sarcolemma), the voltage sensors on the transverse tubule membrane signal the release of Ca^{2+} from the terminal cisternae portion of the sarcoplasmic reticulum (a series of interconnected sacs and tubes that surround each myofibril).[39] The released Ca^{2+} then diffuses into the sarcomeres and binds to troponin, displacing the tropomyosin and allowing the actin to bind with the myosin cross-bridges. At the end of the contraction (the neural activity and action potentials cease), the sarcoplasmic reticulum actively accumulates Ca^{2+} and muscle relaxation occurs. The return of Ca^{2+} to the sarcoplasmic reticulum involves active transport, requiring the degradation of adenosine triphosphate (ATP) to adenosine diphosphate (ADP) (see Chapter 8).[39]

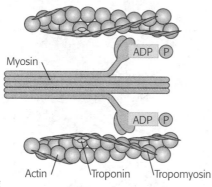
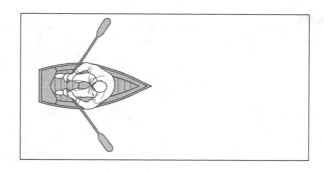

Myosin

ADP Ⓟ

ADP Ⓟ

Actin   Troponin   Tropomyosin

Resting

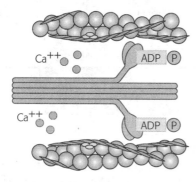
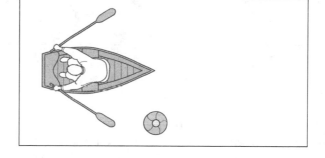

Ca++

ADP Ⓟ

Ca++

ADP Ⓟ

Figure 2-8   Troponin and tropomyosin.

● Key Point Because sarcoplasmic reticulum function is closely associated with both contraction and relaxation, changes in its ability to release or sequester Ca^{2+} markedly affect both the time course and magnitude of force output by the muscle fiber.[41]

Activation of varying numbers of motor neurons results in gradations in the strength of muscle contraction. The stronger the electrical impulse, the stronger the muscle twitch. Whenever a somatic motor neuron is activated, all of the muscle fibers that it innervates are stimulated and contract with *all-or-none* twitches. Although the muscle fibers produce all-or-none contractions, muscles are capable of a wide variety of responses, ranging from activities requiring a high level of precision to activities requiring high tension.

● Key Point The graded contractions of whole muscles occur because the number of fibers participating in the contraction varies. An increase in the force of movement is achieved by recruiting more cells into cooperative action.

When rapid successive impulses activate a muscle fiber already in tension, *summation* occurs, and tension is progressively elevated until a maximum value for that fiber is reached.[42] A fiber repetitively activated so that its maximum tension level is maintained for a time is in *tetanus*. If the state of tetanus is sustained, fatigue causes a gradual decline in the level of tension produced.

Muscle Fiber Types

The basic function of a muscle is to contract. On the basis of their contractile properties, two different types of muscle fibers have been recognized within skeletal muscle: type I (slow-twitch red oxidative) and type II (fast-twitch white glycolytic). Type II fibers can be broken down further into three distinct subsets: type II, A; type II, AB; and type II, B[43] (**Table 2-8**).

Slow-twitch fibers have a high capacity for oxygen uptake. They are, therefore, suitable for activities of long duration or endurance, including the maintenance of posture. Fast-twitch fibers have a low capacity for oxygen uptake, and are therefore suited to quick, explosive actions, including such activities as sprinting.

● Key Point In fast-twitch fibers, the sarcoplasmic reticulum embraces every individual myofibril. In slow-twitch fibers, it may contain multiple myofibrils.[44]

TABLE 2-8	Comparison of Muscle Fiber Types			
Characteristics	Type I	Type II A	Type II AB	Type II B
Diameter	Small	Intermediate	Large	Very large
Capillaries	Many	Many	Few	Few
Resistance to fatigue	High	Fairly high	Intermediate	Low
Glycogen content	Low	Intermediate	High	High
Respiration	Aerobic	Aerobic	Anaerobic	Anaerobic
Twitch rate	Slow	Fast	Fast	Fast
Major storage fuel	Triglycerides	Creatine phosphate Glycogen	Creatine phosphate Glycogen	Creatine phosphate Glycogen

Theory dictates that a muscle with a large percentage of the total cross-sectional area occupied by slow-twitch type I fibers should be more fatigue resistant than one in which the fast-twitch type II fibers predominate. The shape of a muscle determines its specific action. A number of muscle shapes are recognized:

- *Circular:* As their name suggests, these muscles appear circular in shape and are normally sphincter muscles that surround an opening such as the mouth or eyes.
- *Fusiform:* These muscles are more spindle-shaped, with the muscle belly being wider than the origin and insertion. Typically, these muscles are built to provide large ranges of motion. Examples include the biceps brachii and the psoas major.
- *Triangular (convergent):* These are muscles where the origin is wider than the point of insertion. This fiber arrangement allows for maximum force production. Examples include the gluteus medius and pectoralis major.

● Key Point
- *Origin:* The proximal attachment of a muscle, tendon, or ligament
- *Insertion:* The distal attachment of a muscle, tendon, or ligament

- *Parallel (strap):* These are normally long muscles capable of producing large movements; although they are not very strong, they have very good endurance. Examples include the sartorius and sternocleidomastoid. Some textbooks include fusiform muscles in the parallel group.
- *Rhomboidal:* These muscles are characterized by expansive proximal and distal attachments, which make them well-suited to either stabilize a joint or provide large forces. Examples include the rhomboids and gluteus maximus.
- *Pennate:* These muscles resemble the shape of a feather, with muscle fibers approaching a central tendon at an oblique angle. This diagonal orientation of the fibers maximizes the muscle's force potential and many more muscle fibers can fit into the muscle compared with a similar sized fusiform muscle. They can be divided into the following subcategories:
  - ❏ *Unipennate:* These fibers are arranged to insert in a diagonal direction onto the tendon, which allows for greater strength. Examples include the lumbricals (deep hand muscles) and the extensor digitorum longus (wrist and finger extensor).
  - ❏ *Bipennate:* These have two rows of muscle fibers, facing in opposite diagonal directions, with a central tendon, like a feather. This arrangement allows for even greater power than the unipennate but less range of motion. An example is the rectus femoris.
  - ❏ *Multipennate:* These muscles have multiple rows of diagonal fibers, with a central tendon that branches into two or more

tendons. An example is the deltoid muscle, which has three sections, anterior, posterior, and middle.

Muscle Function

Muscle groups are classified based on the following functions (Figure 2-9):

- *Agonist muscle:* An agonist muscle contracts to produce the desired movement.
- *Antagonist muscle:* The antagonist muscle typically opposes the desired movement and is responsible for returning a limb to its initial position. Antagonists ensure that the desired motion occurs in a coordinated and controlled fashion by relaxing and lengthening in a gradual manner.
- *Synergist muscle (supporters):* Synergist muscles are muscle groups that perform, or assist in performing, joint motions. Although synergists can work with the agonists, they can also oppose the agonists, as occurs in force couples.

- *Neutralizers:* These muscles help cancel out, or neutralize, extra motion from the agonists to make sure the force generated works within the desired plane of motion. An example is when the flexor carpi ulnaris and extensor carpi ulnaris neutralize the flexion/extension forces at the wrist to produce ulnar deviation.
- *Stabilizers (fixators):* These muscles provide the necessary support to help stabilize an area so that another area can be moved. For example, the trunk core stabilizers become active when the upper extremities are being used.

Stable posture results from a balance of competing forces, whereas movement occurs when competing forces are unbalanced.[46]

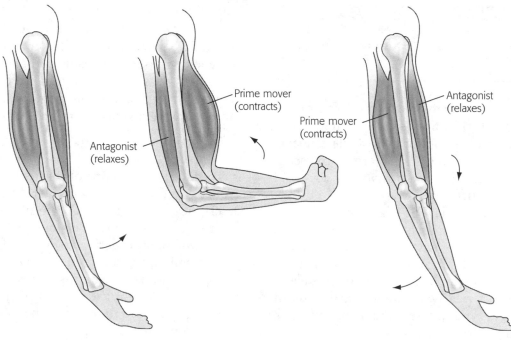

Antagonist
(relaxes)

Prime mover
(contracts)

Prime mover
(contracts)

Antagonist
(relaxes)

Figure 2-9 Agonist and antagonist muscle actions.

TABLE 2-9	Examples of Skeletal Muscles That Cross Two or More Joints
Erector spinae	
Biceps brachii	
Long head of the triceps brachii	
Hamstrings	
Iliopsoas	
Sartorius	
Rectus femoris	
Gastrocnemius	
A number of muscles crossing the wrist/finger and foot/ankle joints	

● Key Point

- Movements generated or stimulated by active muscle are referred to as *active movements*.
- Movements generated by sources other than muscular activation, such as gravity, are referred to as *active-assisted* or *passive movements*.

Most skeletal muscles span only one joint; however, some skeletal muscles cross two or more joints (**Table 2-9**). A two-joint muscle is more prone to adaptive shortening than a one-joint muscle.

● Key Point The graded contractions of whole muscles occur because the number of fibers participating in the contraction varies. The increase in the force of movement is achieved by recruiting more cells into cooperative action. The different types of muscle contractions are described in Chapter 10.

The physiologic cross-sectional area of the muscle describes its thickness—an indirect and relative measure of the amount of contractile elements available to generate force.[45] The larger a muscle's cross-sectional area, the greater its force potential (see Chapter 4). Different activities place differing demands on a muscle. For example, movement activities involve a predominance of fast-twitch fiber recruitment, whereas postural activities and those activities requiring stabilization entail more involvement of the slow-twitch fibers. In humans, most limb muscles contain a relatively equal distribution of each muscle fiber type, whereas the back and trunk demonstrate a predominance of slow-twitch fibers.

If a contraction proceeds normally there is an orderly recruitment of muscle fibers, which proceeds according to the following: slow twitch→ fast twitch→ fast twitch A→ fast twitch AB→ fast twitch B.

Although it would seem possible that physical training may cause fibers to convert from slow twitch to fast twitch or the reverse, this has not been shown to be the case.[47] However, fiber conversion from fast twitch A to fast twitch B, and vice versa, has been found to occur with training.[48] Muscle tissue is capable of significant adaptions. The various types of muscle contraction and their relationship to therapeutic exercise and impaired muscle performance are described in Chapter 10.

Assessment of Musculoskeletal Tissues

Assessment of the musculoskeletal tissues involves an examination of range of motion, flexibility, joint mobility, and strength.

● Key Point For the purpose of an orthopaedic examination, Cyriax subdivided musculoskeletal tissue into *contractile* and *inert* (noncontractile) tissues.[49]

Range of Motion

A normal joint has an available range of active, or physiologic, motion, which is limited by a physiologic barrier as tension develops within the surrounding tissues. At the physiologic barrier, there is an additional amount of passive range of motion. Beyond the available passive range of motion, the anatomic barrier is found. This barrier cannot be exceeded without disruption to the integrity of the joint. Both passive and active range of motion can be measured using a goniometer, which has been shown to have a satisfactory level of intraobserver reliability.[50–52]

Goniometry

It is not within the scope of this text to cover every aspect of goniometry, but merely to provide a description so that the PTA can fully appreciate its function in the overall assessment of a patient. The term *goniometry* is derived from two Greek words, *gonia* meaning angle and *metron* meaning measure. Thus, a goniometer is an instrument used to measure angles. Within the field of physical therapy, goniometry is used to measure the total amount of available motion at a specific joint. Goniometry can be used to measure both active and passive range of motion.

Goniometers are produced in a variety of sizes and shapes and are usually constructed of either plastic or metal. The two most common types of instruments used to measure joint angles are the bubble inclinometer and the traditional goniometer.

The bubble goniometer has a 360° rotating dial and scale with fluid indicator. The traditional goniometer consists of three parts:

1. *Body:* The body of the goniometer is designed like a protractor and may form a full or half circle. A measuring scale is located around the body. The scale can extend either from 0 to 180 degrees and 180 to 0 degrees for the half circle models, or from 0 to 360 degrees and from 360 to 0 degrees on the full circle models. The intervals on the scales can vary from 1 to 10 degrees.
2. *Stationary arm:* The stationary arm is structurally a part of the body and therefore cannot move independently of the body.
3. *Moving arm:* The moving arm is attached to the fulcrum in the center of the body by a rivet or screwlike device that allows the moving arm to move freely on the body of the device. In some instruments, the screwlike device can be tightened to fix the moving arm in a certain position or loosened to permit free movement.

The correct selection of which type of goniometer to use depends on the joint angle to be measured. The length of arms varies among instruments and can range from 3–18 inches. Extendable goniometers allow varying ranges from 9½ inches to 26 inches. The longer armed goniometers, or the bubble inclinometer, are recommended when the landmarks are further apart, such as when measuring hip, knee, elbow, and shoulder movements. Bubble inclinometers are recommended when measuring spinal motions. In the smaller joints such as the wrist and hand and foot and ankle, a traditional goniometer with a shorter arm is used.

To use the goniometer, the patient is positioned in the recommended testing position. While stabilizing the proximal joint component, the clinician gently moves the distal joint component through the available range of motion until the end feel is determined. An estimate is made of the available range of motion, and the distal joint component is returned to the starting position. The clinician palpates the relevant bony landmarks and aligns the goniometer. A record is made of the starting measurement. The goniometer is then removed and the patient moves the joint through the available range of motion. Once the joint has been moved through the available range of motion, the goniometer is replaced and realigned, and a measurement is read and recorded. A brief summary of the goniometric technique for each of the upper and lower extremity joints is provided in **Table 2-10** and **Table 2-11**.

Active Range of Motion

Active range of motion testing gives the clinician information about:

- The quantity of available physiologic motion
- The presence of muscle substitutions
- The willingness of the patient to move
- The integrity of the contractile and inert tissues
- The quality of motion
- Symptom reproduction
- The pattern of motion restriction

Active range of motion testing may be deferred if small and unguarded motions provoke intense pain because this may indicate a high degree of joint irritability.

Full and pain-free active range of motion suggests normalcy for that movement, although it is important to remember that normal *range* of motion is not synonymous with normal motion.[53] Normal motion implies that the control of motion must also be present. Single motions in the cardinal planes are usually tested first. Dynamic testing involves repeated movements in specific directions. Pain that increases after the repeated motions may indicate a retriggering of the inflammatory response, and repeated motions in the opposite direction should be explored.

> ● **Key Point** Static testing involves sustaining a position. Sustained static positions may be used to help detect postural syndromes.[54]

Combined motions, as their name suggests, use single plane motions with other motions superimposed. For example at the elbow, the single plane motion of elbow flexion is tested together with forearm supination and then forearm pronation. The active range of motion will be found to be either abnormal or normal. Abnormal motion is typically described as being reduced. It must be remembered,

**TABLE
2-10**

Goniometric Techniques for the Upper Extremity

Joint	Motion	Axis	Stationary Arm	Movable Arm	Normal Ranges (Degrees)
Shoulder	Flexion	Acromion process	Mid-axillary line of the thorax	Lateral midline of the humerus using the lateral epicondyle of the humerus for reference	0–180
	Extension	Acromion process	Mid-axillary line of the thorax	Lateral midline of the humerus using the lateral epicondyle of the humerus for reference	0–40
	Abduction	Anterior aspect of the acromion process	Parallel to the midline of the anterior aspect of the sternum	Medial midline of the humerus	0–180
	Adduction	Anterior aspect of the acromion process	Parallel to the midline of the anterior aspect of the sternum	Medial midline of the humerus	90–0
	Internal rotation	Olecranon process	Parallel or perpendicular to the floor	Ulna using the olecranon process and ulnar styloid for reference	0–80
	External rotation	Olecranon process	Parallel or perpendicular to the floor	Ulna using the olecranon process and ulnar styloid for reference	0–90
Elbow	Flexion	Lateral epicondyle of the humerus	Lateral midline of the humerus using the center of the acromion process for reference	Lateral midline of the radius using the radial head and radial styloid process for reference	0–150
	Extension	Lateral epicondyle of the humerus	Lateral midline of the humerus using the center of the acromion process for reference	Lateral midline of the radius using the radial head and radial styloid process for reference	0–5
Forearm	Pronation	Lateral to the ulnar styloid process	Parallel to the anterior midline of the humerus	Dorsal aspect of the forearm, just proximal to the styloid process of the radius and ulna	0–75
	Supination	Medial to the ulnar styloid process	Parallel to the anterior midline of the humerus	Ventral aspect of the forearm, just proximal to the styloid process of the radius and ulna	0–85
Wrist	Flexion	Lateral aspect of the wrists over the triquetrum	Lateral midline of the ulna using the olecranon and ulnar styloid process for reference	Lateral midline of the fifth metacarpal	0–80
	Extension	Lateral aspect of the wrists over the triquetrum	Lateral midline of the ulna using the olecranon and ulnar styloid process for reference	Lateral midline of the fifth metacarpal	0–60

| TABLE 2-10 | Goniometric Techniques for the Upper Extremity (continued) |

Joint	Motion	Axis	Stationary Arm	Movable Arm	Normal Ranges (Degrees)
	Radial deviation	Over the middle of the dorsal aspect of the wrist over the capitate	Dorsal midline of the forearm using the lateral epicondyle of the humerus for reference	Dorsal midline of the third metacarpal	0–20
	Ulnar deviation	Over the middle of the dorsal aspect of the wrist over the capitate	Dorsal midline of the forearm using the lateral epicondyle of the humerus for reference	Dorsal midline of the third metacarpal	0–30
Thumb	Carpometacarpal flexion	Over the palmar aspect of the first carpometacarpal joint	Ventral midline of the radius using the ventral surface of the radial head and radial styloid process for reference	Ventral midline of the first metacarpal	CMC: 45–50; MCP: 50–55; IP: 85–90
	Carpometacarpal extension	Over the palmar aspect of the first carpometacarpal joint	Ventral midline of the radius using the ventral surface of the radial head and radial styloid process for reference	Ventral midline of the first metacarpal	MCP: 0; IP: 0–5
	Carpometacarpal abduction	Over the lateral aspect of the radial styloid process	Lateral midline of the second metacarpal using the center of the second metacarpal or phalangeal joint for reference	Lateral midline of the first metacarpal using the center of the first metacarpal or phalangeal joint for reference	60–70
	Carpometacarpal adduction	Over the lateral aspect of the radial styloid process	Lateral midline of the second metacarpal using the center of the second metacarpal or phalangeal joint for reference	Lateral midline of the first metacarpal using the center of the first metacarpal or phalangeal joint for reference	30
Fingers	Metacarpophalangeal flexion	Over the dorsal aspect of the metacarpophalangeal joint	Over the dorsal midline of the metacarpal	Over the dorsal midline of the proximal phalanx	Flexion: MCP: 85–90; PIP: 100–115; DIP: 80–90
	Metacarpophalangeal extension	Over the dorsal aspect of the metacarpophalangeal joint	Over the dorsal midline of the metacarpal	Over the dorsal midline of the proximal phalanx	Extension: MCP: 30–45; PIP: 0; DIP: 20
	Metacarpophalangeal abduction	Over the dorsal aspect of the metacarpophalangeal joint	Over the dorsal midline of the metacarpal	Over the dorsal midline of the proximal phalanx	Abduction: 20–30
	Metacarpophalangeal adduction	Over the dorsal aspect of the metacarpophalangeal joint	Over the dorsal midline of the metacarpal	Over the dorsal midline of the proximal phalanx	Adduction: 0

(continued)

TABLE 2-10

Goniometric Techniques for the Upper Extremity (continued)

Joint	Motion	Axis	Stationary Arm	Movable Arm	Normal Ranges (Degrees)
Fingers	Proximal interphalangeal flexion	Over the dorsal aspect of the proximal interphalangeal joint	Over the dorsal midline of the proximal phalanx	Over the dorsal midline of the middle phalanx	
	Proximal interphalangeal extension	Over the dorsal aspect of the proximal interphalangeal joint	Over the dorsal midline of the proximal phalanx	Over the dorsal midline of the middle phalanx	
	Distal interphalangeal flexion	Over the dorsal aspect of the proximal interphalangeal joint	Over the dorsal midline of the middle phalanx	Over the dorsal midline of the distal phalanx	
	Distal interphalangeal extension	Over the dorsal aspect of the proximal interphalangeal joint	Over the dorsal midline of the middle phalanx	Over the dorsal midline of the distal phalanx	

TABLE 2-11

Goniometric Techniques for the Lower Extremity

Joint	Motion	Axis	Stationary Arm	Movable Arm	Normal Ranges (Degrees)
Hip	Flexion	Over the lateral aspect of the hip joint using the greater trochanter of the femur for reference	Lateral midline of the pelvis	Lateral midline of the femur using the lateral epicondyle for reference	0–125
	Extension	Over the lateral aspect of the hip joint using the greater trochanter of the femur for reference	Lateral midline of the pelvis	Lateral midline of the femur using the lateral epicondyle for reference	0–30
	Abduction	Over the anterior superior iliac spine (ASIS) of the extremity being measured	Aligned with an imaginary horizontal line extending from one ASIS to the other ASIS	Anterior midline of the femur using the midline of the patella for reference	0–40
	Adduction	Over the anterior superior iliac spine (ASIS) of the extremity being measured	Aligned with an imaginary horizontal line extending from one ASIS to the other ASIS	Anterior midline of the femur using the midline of the patella for reference	0–20
	Internal rotation	Anterior aspect of the patella	Perpendicular to the floor or parallel to the supporting surface	Anterior midline of the lower leg using the crest of the tibia and a point midway between the two malleoli for reference	0–40
	External rotation	Anterior aspect of the patella	Perpendicular to the floor or parallel to the supporting surface	Anterior midline of the lower leg using the crest of the tibia and a point midway between the two malleoli for reference	0–50

| TABLE 2-11 | Goniometric Techniques for the Lower Extremity (continued) |

Joint	Motion	Axis	Stationary Arm	Movable Arm	Normal Ranges (Degrees)
Knee	Flexion	Lateral epicondyle of the femur	Lateral midline of the femur using the greater trochanter for reference	Lateral midline of the fibula using the lateral malleolus and fibular head for reference	0–150
	Extension	Lateral epicondyle of the femur	Lateral midline of the femur using the greater trochanter for reference	Lateral midline of the fibula using the lateral malleolus and fibular head for reference	0–5
Ankle	Dorsiflexion	Lateral aspect of the lateral malleolus	Lateral midline of the fibula using the head of the fibula for reference	Parallel to the lateral aspect of the fifth metatarsal	0–20
	Plantarflexion	Lateral aspect of the lateral malleolus	Lateral midline of the fibula using the head of the fibula for reference	Parallel to the lateral aspect of the fifth metatarsal	0–40
	Inversion	Anterior aspect of the ankle midway between the malleoli	Anterior midline of the lower leg using the tibial tuberosity for reference	Anterior midline of the second metatarsal	0–30
	Eversion	Anterior aspect of the ankle midway between the malleoli	Anterior midline of the lower leg using the tibial tuberosity for reference	Anterior midline of the second metatarsal	0–20

though, that abnormal motion may also be excessive. Excessive motion is often missed and is erroneously classified as normal motion. To help determine whether the motion is normal or excessive, passive range of motion, in the form of passive overpressure, and the end feel is assessed by the PT.

Passive Range of Motion
If the active motions do not reproduce the patient's symptoms, or the active range of motion appears incomplete, it is important to perform gentle passive range of motion and overpressure at the end of the active range in order to fully test the motion. The passive overpressure should be applied carefully in the presence of pain. The barrier to active motion should occur earlier in the range than the barrier to passive motion. Pain that occurs at the end-range of active and passive movement is suggestive of hypermobility or instability, a capsular contraction, or scar tissue that has not been adequately remodeled.[55]

● **Key Point** If active and passive motions are limited/painful in the same direction, the injured tissue is likely inert in nature. If active and passive motions are limited/painful in the opposite direction, the injured tissue is likely contractile in nature. The exception to these generalizations occurs with tenosynovitis.

Passive range of motion testing gives the clinician information about the integrity of the contractile and inert tissues, and the *end feel*. Cyriax[49] introduced the concept of the end feel, which is the quality of resistance at end range. The end feel can indicate to the clinician the cause of the motion restriction (**Table 2-12**). If the PTA detects an abnormal end feel that was not present at the time of initial examination, the intervention must be terminated and the supervising PT must be notified immediately.

● **Key Point** An association has been demonstrated between an increase in pain and abnormal-pathological end feels compared to normal end feels.[56]

TABLE 2-12 End Feels

Type	Cause	Characteristics and Examples
Bony	Produced by bone-to-bone approximation	Abrupt and unyielding Examples: *Normal:* Elbow extension *Abnormal:* Cervical rotation (may indicate osteophyte)
Elastic/stretch	Produced by the muscle–tendon unit	Stretch with elastic recoil Examples: *Normal:* Wrist flexion with finger flexion, and ankle dorsiflexion with the knee extended *Abnormal:* Decreased dorsiflexion of the ankle with the knee flexed as compared to knee extended
Soft tissue approximation	Produced by the contact of two muscle bulks on either side of a flexing joint	A very forgiving end feel Examples: *Normal:* Knee flexion, elbow flexion *Abnormal:* Elbow flexion with an obese subject
Capsular/firm	Produced by capsule or ligaments	Various degrees of stretch without elasticity Stretch ability depends on the thickness of the tissue Examples: *Normal:* Wrist flexion (soft), elbow flexion in supination (medium), and knee extension (hard) *Abnormal:* Inappropriate stretch ability for a specific joint
Springy	Produced by the articular surface rebounding from an intra-articular meniscus or disc	A rebound sensation Examples: *Normal:* Axial compression of the cervical spine *Abnormal:* Knee flexion or extension with a displaced meniscus
Boggy	Produced by fluid (blood) within a joint	A "squishy" sensation as the joint is moved towards its end range Further forcing feels as if it will burst the joint Examples: *Normal:* None *Abnormal:* Hemarthrosis at the knee
Spasm	Produced by reflex and reactive muscle contraction	An abrupt end to movement that is unyielding With acute joint inflammation, it occurs early in the range Note: Muscle guarding is not a true end feel because it involves a co-contraction Examples: *Normal:* None *Abnormal:* Significant traumatic arthritis, recent traumatic hypermobility, grade II muscle tears
Empty	Produced solely by pain	The limitation of motion has no tissue resistance component The resistance is from the patient being unable to tolerate further motion due to severe pain Examples: *Normal:* None *Abnormal:* Acute subdeltoid bursitis, sign of the buttock

The PT bases the planned intervention and its intensity on the type of tissue resistance to movement demonstrated by the end feel and the acuteness of the condition.[49] This information may indicate whether the resistance is caused by pain, muscle, capsule ligament, disturbed mechanics of the joint, or a combination.

Recording Range of Motion
The methods of recording range of motion vary. The measurements depicted in **Tables 2-13**, **Table 2-14**, and **Table 2-15** highlight one method.

Flexibility
Flexibility is examined to determine if a particular structure, or group of structures, has sufficient extensibility to perform a desired activity. The extensibility and habitual length of connective tissue is a factor of the demands placed upon it. These demands produce changes in the viscoelastic properties and, thus, the length–tension relationship of a muscle or muscle group (see Chapter 4), resulting in an increase or decrease in the length of those structures. A loss of flexibility can be produced by:

- Restricted mobility
- Poor posture
- Tissue damage secondary to trauma
- Prolonged immobilization
- Disease
- Hypertonia (the muscle will feel hard and may stand out from those around it)

> **● Key Point** The concepts of contracture and adaptive shortening are important to understand.
>
> - A contracture is a condition of fixed high resistance to passive stretch of the tissue resulting from fibrosis or shortening of the soft tissues around the joint, including the muscles. Contractures occur after injury, surgery, or immobilization and are the result of the remodeling of dense connective tissue.
> - Adaptive shortening occurs when the length of the tissue shortens relative to its normal resting length. Immobilization of the tissue in a shortened position or a prolonged posture results in adaptive shortening.

Capsular and Noncapsular Patterns of Restriction
A capsular pattern of restriction is a limitation of pain and movement in a joint-specific ratio, which is usually present with arthritis, or following prolonged

---

TABLE 2-13   Recording Range of Motion Measurements for the Spine

Region	Normal AROM (in degrees)	Clinical Examples	
		Patient Example	Documentation Recording (in degrees)
Cervical	Extension (60) Flexion (50)	Patient extends to 30 degrees and flexes to 45 degrees	30-0-45
	Sidebend (45)	Patient bends 30 degrees to left, 40 degrees to right	30-0-40
	Rotation (80)	Patient rotates 40 degrees to the left, 50 degrees to the right	40-0-50
Thoracic	Extension (5) Flexion (45)	Patient extends to 0 degrees, flexes to 45 degrees	0-0-45
	Sidebend (45)	Bends left 45 degrees, right 20 degrees	45-0-20
	Rotation (30)	Rotates left 15 degrees, right 20 degrees	15-0-20
Lumbar	Extension (25) Flexion (60)	Extends to 25 degrees, flexes to 40 degrees	25-0-40
	Left side bend-0-Right lateral bend (25-0-25)	Ankylosis of the spine in 20 degrees left side bend	20-0
		Restricted motion from 20–30 degrees of left lateral bending	F: 30-20-0

AROM, active range of motion.
Data from American Medical Association: Guides to the Evaluation of Permanent Impairment (ed 5). Chicago, American Medical Association, 2001

TABLE 2-14 Recording Range of Motion Measurements for the Upper Extremities

Joint	Normal AROM (in degrees)	Clinical Examples	
		Patient Example	Documentation Recording (in degrees)
Shoulder	Extension (40) Flexion (180)	Patient extends left shoulder to 40 degrees, flexes to 150 degrees	Left: 40-0-150
	Abduction (180) Adduction (30)	Patient extends left shoulder to 100 degrees, adducts to 10 degrees	Left: 100-0-10
	External rotation (90) Internal rotation (80)	Patient rotates left shoulder to 90 degrees, internal rotation to 80 degrees	Left: 90-0-80
Elbow	Extension-0-Flexion (0)-0-(150)	Patient extends left elbow to 0 degrees, flexes to 150 degrees	Left: 0-0-150
		Patient hyperextends left elbow to 5 degrees, flexes to 110 degrees	Left: 5-0-110
Forearm	Supination-0-Pronation (80)-0-(80)	Left supinates to 60 degrees, pronates to 80 degrees	Left: 60-0-80
Wrist	Extension-0-Flexion (60)-0-(60)	Patient extends left wrist to 20 degrees, flexes to 50 degrees	Left: 20-0-50
Wrist	Radial deviation-0-Ulnar deviation (20)-0-(30)	Patient radial deviates left wrist to 20 degrees, ulnar deviates to 30 degrees	Left: 20-0-30

AROM, active range of motion.
Data from American Medical Association: Guides to the Evaluation of Permanent Impairment (ed 5). Chicago, American Medical Association, 2001

TABLE 2-15 Recording Range of Motion Measurements for the Lower Extremities

Joint	Normal AROM (in degrees)	Clinical Examples	
		Patient Example	Documentation Recording (in degrees)
Hip	Extension (30) Flexion (100)	Patient extends the left hip to 30 degrees, flexes to 80 degrees	Left: 30-0-80
	Abduction (40) Adduction (20)	Patient abducts the left hip to 30 degrees, adducts to 10 degrees	Left: 30-0-10
	External rotation (50) Internal rotation (40)	Patient externally rotates the left hip to 30 degrees, internally rotates to 30 degrees	Left: 30-0-30
Knee	Extension (0) Flexion (150)	Patient extends the left knee to 0 degrees, flexes to 150 degrees	Left: 0-0-150
Ankle (Talocrural)	Dorsiflexion (20) Plantarflexion (40)	Patient dorsiflexes left ankle to 10 degrees, plantarflexes to 10 degrees	Left: 10-0-10
Ankle (Subtalar)	Eversion (20) Inversion (30)	Patient everts left ankle to 20 degrees, inverts to 30 degrees	Left: 20-0-30

AROM, active range of motion.
Data from American Medical Association: Guides to the Evaluation of Permanent Impairment (ed5). Chicago, American Medical Association, 2001

<table>
<tr><th colspan="2">TABLE 2-16   Capsular Patterns of Restriction</th></tr>
</table>

Joint	Limitation of Motion (Passive Angular Motion)
Glenohumeral	External rotation > Abduction > Internal rotation (3:2:1)
Acromioclavicular	No true capsular pattern; possible loss of horizontal adduction, pain (and sometimes slight loss of end range) with each motion
Sternoclavicular	See above: acromioclavicular joint
Humeroulnar	Flexion > Extension (±4:1)
Humeroradial	No true capsular pattern; possible equal limitation of pronation and supination
Superior radioulnar	No true capsular pattern; possible equal limitation of pronation and supination with pain at end ranges
Inferior radioulnar	No true capsular pattern; possible equal limitation of pronation and supination with pain at end ranges
Wrist (carpus)	Flexion = Extension
Radiocarpal	See above: wrist (carpus)
Carpometacarpal	
Midcarpal	
First carpometacarpal	Retroposition
Carpometacarpal 2–5	Fan > Fold
Metacarpophalangeal 2-5	Flexion > Extension (±2:1)
Interphalangeal	
Proximal (PIP)	Flexion > Extension (±2:1)
Distal (DIP)	
Hip	Internal rotation > Flexion > Abduction = Extension > other motions
Tibiofemoral	Flexion > Extension (±5:1)
Superior tibiofibular	No capsular pattern: pain at end range of translatory movements
Talocrural	Plantarflexion > Dorsiflexion
Talocalcaneal (subtalar)	Varus > Valgus
Midtarsal	
Talonavicular calcaneocuboid	Inversion (plantarflexion, adduction, supination) > Dorsiflexion
First metatarsophalangeal	Extension > Flexion (±2:1)
Metatarsophalangeal 2–5	Flexion ≥ Extension
Interphalangeal 2–5	
Proximal	Flexion ≥ Extension
Distal	Flexion ≥ Extension

Data from Cyriax J: Textbook of Orthopaedic Medicine, Diagnosis of Soft Tissue Lesions (ed 8). London, Bailliere Tindall, 1982

immobilization (**Table 2-16**).[49] A noncapsular pattern of restriction is a limitation in a joint in any pattern other than a capsular one, and may indicate the presence of either a derangement, a restriction of one part of the joint capsule, or an extra-articular lesion, that obstructs joint motion.[49]

Joint Integrity and Mobility

The small motion available at joint surfaces is referred to as *accessory* or *arthrokinematic motion*. A variety of measurement scales have been proposed for judging the amount of accessory joint motion present between two joint surfaces, most of which are based on a comparison with a comparable contralateral joint using manually applied forces in a logical and precise manner.[57] Using these techniques to assess the joint glide, the PT can describe joint motion as hypomobile (restricted), normal (unrestricted but not excessive), or hypermobile (excessive).

Passive accessory mobility tests assess the accessory motions of a joint. The joint glides are tested in the loose (open) pack position of a peripheral joint (see Chapter 6) and at the end of available range in the spinal joints to avoid soft tissue tension affecting the results. The information gathered from these tests will help the PT determine the integrity of the inert structures.

Muscle Strength

Strength measures the power with which musculotendinous units act across a bone–joint lever-arm system to actively generate motion or passively resist movement against gravity and variable resistance.[58]

> **● Key Point** A measure of a person's strength is really a measurement of an individual's torque production (see Chapter 4). Specific joint positions are used when performing manual muscle testing because force production is highly dependent on muscular length and joint angle.

A number of methods can be used to measure strength including dynamometry, isokinetics, and cable tensiometry. The *Guide to Physical Therapist Practice* lists both manual muscle testing (MMT) and dynamometry as appropriate measures of muscle strength.

- Manual muscle testing evaluates the function and strength of individual muscles and muscle groups based on the effective performance of a movement in relation to the forces of gravity and manual resistance.
- Dynamometry is a method of strength testing using sophisticated strength measuring devices (e.g., hand-grip, hand-held, fixed, isokinetic dynamometry).

Manual Muscle Testing

Manual muscle testing (MMT) is traditionally used by the clinician to assess the strength of a muscle or muscle group. MMT is designed to assess a muscle or muscle group's ability to isometrically resist the force applied by the clinician. When performing strength testing, a particular muscle or muscle group is first isolated, and then an external force is applied. Resistance applied at the end of the tested range is

termed a *break test*. This method is best used solely as a screening tool. Resistance applied throughout the range is termed a *make test*. The results of the strength testing differ depending on the method used. The isometric hold (break test) shows the muscle to have a higher test grade than the resistance given throughout the range (make test).

Whichever testing method is used, resistance should be applied and released gradually to give the patient sufficient time to offer resistance. Following the manual muscle test, the muscle tested is said to be "weak" or "strong" based upon the muscle's ability to resist the externally applied force over time. If a position other than the standard position is used, it must be documented.

Interpretation of Manual Muscle Testing Results
A number of grading scales have been devised to assess muscle strength (**Table 2-17**).[59,60] Each system specifies patient testing position, clinician positioning to maximize patient stabilization and minimize substitution of agonist muscles, the force vector for clinician resistance, and a corresponding grading scheme describing the clinician's results (**Table 2-18**).[61] In the Medical Research Council scale, the grades of 0, 1, and 2 are tested in the gravity-minimized position (contraction is perpendicular to the gravitational force). All other grades are tested in the antigravity position. The Daniels and Worthingham grading system is considered by some as the most functional of the three grading systems outlined in Table 2-17 because it tests a motion that utilizes all of the agonists and synergists involved in the motion.[62] The Kendall and McCreary approach is designed to test a specific muscle rather than the motion, and it requires both selective recruitment of a muscle by the patient and a sound knowledge of anatomy and kinesiology on the part of the clinician to determine the correct alignment of the muscle fibers.[62]

> **● Key Point** Choosing a particular grading system is based on the skill level of the clinician while ensuring consistency for each patient, so that coworkers who may be re-examining the patient are using the same testing methods.
> To confirm a finding, another muscle that shares the same innervation (spinal nerve or peripheral nerve) is tested. Knowledge of both spinal nerve and peripheral nerve innervation will aid the clinician in determining which muscle to select.

All of the grading systems for manual muscle testing produce ordinal data with unequal rankings between grades, and all are innately subjective

TABLE 2-17   Comparison of MMT Grades

Medical Research Council	Daniels and Worthingham	Kendall and McCreary	Explanation
5	Normal (N)	100%	Holds test position against maximal resistance
4+	Good + (G+)		Holds test position against moderate to strong pressure
4	Good (G)	80%	Holds test position against moderate resistance
4−	Good − (G−)		Holds test position against slight to moderate pressure
3+	Fair + (F+)		Holds test position against slight resistance
3	Fair (F)	50%	Holds test position against gravity
3−	Fair− (F−)		Gradual release from test position
2+	Poor + (P+)		Moves through partial ROM against gravity *or* Moves through complete ROM gravity eliminated and holds against pressure
2	Poor (P)	20%	Able to move through full ROM gravity eliminated
2−	Poor − (P−)		Moves through partial ROM gravity eliminated
1	Trace (T)	5%	No visible movement; palpable or observable tendon prominence/flicker contraction
0	0	0%	No palpable or observable muscle contraction

Data from Frese E, Brown M, Norton B: Clinical reliability of manual muscle testing: Middle trapezius and gluteus medius muscles. Phys Ther 67:1072–1076, 1987; Daniels K, Worthingham C: Muscle Testing Techniques of Manual Examination (ed 5). Philadelphia, WB Saunders, 1986; and Kendall FP, McCreary EK, Provance PG: Muscles: Testing and Function. Baltimore, Williams & Wilkins, 1993

TABLE 2-18   Manual Muscle Testing Procedure

Explanation	It is important that the clinician provides instructions to the patient. For example, the following statements may be used: "I'm going to test the strength of one of the muscles that bends your elbow." "This is the movement pattern I want you to do. Do it first on your uninvolved side."
Patient positioning	The patient and the part to be tested should be positioned comfortably on a firm surface in the correct testing position. The correct testing position ensures that the muscle fibers to be tested are correctly aligned. The patient is properly draped so that the involved body part is exposed as necessary.
Stabilization	Stabilization, which helps to prevent substitute movements can be provided manually or through the use of an external support such as a belt. The stabilization is applied to the proximal segment using counterpressure to the resistance.
Active range of motion	The patient moves through the test movement actively against gravity. (If using the Daniels and Worthingham grading system, the clinician passively moves the patient's joint through the test movement.) The clinician palpates the muscle for activity and also notes any adaptive shortening (slight to moderate loss of motion), substitutions or trick movements (weakness or instability), or contractures (marked loss of motion). The joint is then returned to the start position. If the patient is unable to perform the muscle action against gravity, the patient is positioned in the gravity-minimized position.

(continued)

TABLE 2-18	Manual Muscle Testing Procedure (continued)
Test	The test should be completed on the uninvolved side first to ascertain normal strength before being repeated on the involved side. The patient is instructed to complete the test movement again and then hold the segment in the desired position. The clinician alerts the patient that resistance will be applied and then applies resistance in the appropriate direction and in a smooth and gradual fashion. The proper location for the application of resistance is as far distal as possible from the axis of movement on the moving segment without crossing another joint. Resistance should never cross an intervening joint unless the integrity of the joint has been assessed as normal. The resistance is applied in a direction opposite the muscle's rotary component and at right angles to the long axis of the segment (opposite the line of the pull of the muscle fibers). The test is repeated three times and the muscle strength grade is determined. Fatigue with three repetitions may be suggestive of nerve root compression.

because they rely on the subject's ability to exert the maximal contraction.

> ● **Key Point** The primary tenet of manual muscle testing is that each muscle should be tested just proximal to the next distal joint of the muscle's insertion and that the clinician must place the subject in positions that will isolate, as much as possible, the specific muscle or muscles being examined and eliminate substitution of agonist muscles.[61]

To be a valid test, strength testing must elicit a maximum contraction of the muscle being tested. Four strategies ensure this:

1. *Placing the muscle to be tested in a shortened position.* This puts the muscle in an ineffective physiologic position, and has the effect of increasing motor neuron activity.
2. *Having the patient perform an eccentric muscle contraction by using the command "Don't let me move you."* The tension at each crossbridge and the number of active cross-bridges is greater during an eccentric contraction, so the maximum eccentric muscle tension developed is greater with an eccentric contraction than with a concentric one.
3. *Breaking the contraction.* It is important to break the patient's muscle contraction in order to ensure that the patient is making a maximal effort and that the full power of the muscle is being tested.
4. *Holding the contraction for at least 5 seconds.* Weakness due to nerve palsy has a distinct fatigability. The muscle demonstrates poor endurance because it is usually able to sustain a maximum muscle contraction for only about 2–3 seconds

before complete failure occurs. This is based on the theories behind muscle recruitment wherein a normal muscle performing a maximum contraction uses only a portion of its motor units, keeping the remainder in reserve to help maintain the contraction. A palsied muscle with its fewer functioning motor units has very few, if any, in reserve. If a muscle appears to be weaker than normal, further investigation is required. The test is repeated three times. Muscle weakness resulting from disuse will be consistently weak and should not get weaker with several repeated contractions.

> ● **Key Point** Multiple studies have shown good intertester and intratester reliability with manual muscle testing and a high degree of exact consistency to within one grade using some form of the Medicine Research Council's grading sequence (0–5).[61]

Substitutions by other muscle groups during testing indicate the presence of weakness. They do not, however, tell the clinician the cause of the weakness.

> ● **Key Point** From a functional perspective, wherever possible, strength testing by the clinician should assess the function of a muscle. If a power muscle is assessed, its ability to produce power should be assessed. In contrast, an endurance muscle should be tested for its ability to sustain a contraction for a prolonged period, such as that which occurs with sustained postures.

Whenever possible, the same muscle is tested on the opposite side, using the same testing procedure, as a comparison is made.

Dynamometry

A handheld dynamometer (HHD) is a precision measurement instrument designed to obtain more discrete, objective measures of strength during MMT than can be achieved via traditional MMT. A prerequisite for quality MMT measures, and likewise HHD measures, is adequate force-generating capacity by the testers performing the measurements. When subject strength is clearly beyond a tester's capability to control, use of an HHD does not appear to be indicated. This issue is often encountered when attempting to measure plantar flexion. Aside from limitations regarding mechanical advantage and strength when using an HHD, there is also the issue of patient comfort as a potential limitation. Even though the HHD is padded, it does not and cannot conform to a given body part like a tester's hand, and a common subject complaint is tenderness over the dynamometer placement site.

Clinical Relevance of Strength Testing

According to Cyriax, pain with a contraction generally indicates an injury to the muscle or a capsular structure.[49] The PT confirms this by combining the findings from the isometric test with the findings of the passive motion and the joint distraction and compression. In addition to examining the integrity of the contractile and inert structures, strength testing may also be used to examine the integrity of the myotomes. A myotome is a muscle or group of muscles served by a single nerve root. *Key muscle* is a better, more accurate term, because the muscles tested are the most representative of the supply from a particular segment. Cyriax reasoned that if you isolate and then apply tension to a structure, you could make a conclusion as to the integrity of that structure.[49] His work also introduced the concept of tissue reactivity, which is the manner in which different stresses and movements can alter the clinical signs and symptoms. This knowledge can be used to gauge any subtle changes to the patient's condition.[67]

Pain that occurs consistently with resistance, at whatever the length of the muscle, may indicate a tear of the muscle belly. Pain with muscle testing may indicate a muscle injury, a joint injury, or a combination of both.

Pain that does not occur during the contraction, but occurs upon the release of the contraction, is thought to have an articular source, produced by the joint glide that occurs following the release of tension.

Summary

Numerous types of tissue exist throughout the body, each having specific functional capabilities; for example, upon studying the structure and function of joints, one can see that some joints are designed for mobility (e.g., glenohumeral), whereas other joints are designed for stability (e.g., elbow). Although these characteristics are helped by joint design, other factors such as ligamentous and muscular support play a role. The various types of connective tissue that are contained in fascia, tendons, ligaments, bone, and muscle give each of these structures unique characteristics based on the function they must perform. In physical therapy, injury to any of the musculoskeletal structures must be diagnosed and treated. The physical therapy diagnosis is based on an assessment that includes range of motion measurements, measurement of joint and ligament integrity, and the measurement of muscle performance.

REVIEW Questions

1. True or false: Connective tissue (CT) is found throughout the body and serves to provide structural and metabolic support for other tissues and organs of the body.
2. What are the three types of cartilage and bone tissue?
3. True or false: Fascia is an example of dense regular connective tissue.

4. True or false: A bursa is a synovial membrane–lined sac.

5. All of the following functions are true of the living skeleton except:
   a. It supports the surrounding tissues.
   b. It assists in body movement.
   c. It provides a storage area for mineral salts.
   d. It determines the individual's developing somatotype.

6. What is the type of cartilage found in synovial joints called?

7. Approximately how many bones are in the human body?

8. True or false: Hyaline and elastic cartilage has no nerve supply whereas fibrocartilage is well innervated.

9. What is the shaft of a long bone called?

10. Which area of the bone is responsible for increasing the bone length during growth?

11. What are the three types of muscle tissue?

12. Which structure separates each muscle fiber from its neighbor?

13. Which type of muscle fiber is activated during moderate-intensity, long-duration exercise?

14. What is the function of a tendon?

15. True or false: Bone is a highly vascular form of connective tissue.

16. Give four functions of bone.

17. The smallest organized unit of the contractile mechanism of skeletal muscle is the:
    a. Myofilaments
    b. Actin
    c. Myosin
    d. Sarcomere

18. All of the following are true about the epiphyseal plate except:
    a. It is formed from cartilage.
    b. It serves as the site of progressive lengthening in long bones.
    c. It is located between the epiphysis and the diaphysis.
    d. It is found in all bones.

19. Hyaline cartilage is nourished through the:
    a. Vessels from the periosteum
    b. Haversian canals
    c. Joint fluid
    d. Nutrient arteries

20. The epiphysis of a bone is located:
    a. Directly adjacent to the periosteum
    b. Directly above the diaphysis
    c. Directly below the metaphysis
    d. Directly adjacent to the joint

21. The biceps is an elbow flexor. Which of the following are considered antagonists to the biceps?
    a. Brachioradialis
    b. Supinator
    c. Triceps
    d. Supraspinatus

22. A patient who is substituting with the sartorius muscle during testing of the iliopsoas muscle for a grade 3 (fair) muscle test would demonstrate:
    a. External rotation and abduction of the hip
    b. Internal rotation and abduction of the hip
    c. Flexion of the hip and extension of the knee
    d. Extension of the hip and knee

23. Manual muscle testing of a grade 4/5 (good) strength lower trapezius muscle (for scapular depression and adduction) should be conducted with the patient prone and shoulder positioned in:
    a. 145 degrees of abduction, the forearm in neutral with the thumb pointing at the ceiling
    b. 180 degrees of abduction and fully externally rotated
    c. 90 degrees of abduction, elbow flexed to 90 degrees, and the forearm in neutral with the thumb pointing inward
    d. Neutral at the side and the shoulder and forearm internally rotated with the thumb pointing inward

24. The stationary arm of a goniometer is placed in line with the lateral midline of the trunk, the fulcrum is placed at the greater trochanter, and the movable arm is aligned with the lateral femoral condyle. What motion is being measured?
    a. Hip flexion
    b. Hip abduction
    c. Trunk lateral flexion
    d. Trunk extension

25. When assessing joint range of motion for ankle dorsiflexion and plantarflexion, the preferred goniometric technique is to align the stationary arm parallel to the midline:
    a. Of the fibula and the moving arm parallel to the fifth metatarsal, keeping the patient's knee somewhat flexed
    b. Of the fibula and the moving arm parallel to the fifth metatarsal, keeping the knee stabilized and fully extended

c. Of the tibia and the moving arm parallel to the first metatarsal, keeping the knee somewhat flexed

d. Of the tibia and the moving arm parallel to the first metatarsal, keeping the knee stabilized and fully extended

References

1. Van de Graaff KM, Fox SI: Histology, in Van de Graaff KM, Fox SI (eds): Concepts of Human Anatomy and Physiology. New York, WCB/McGraw-Hill, 1999, pp 130–158

2. Williams GR, Chmielewski T, Rudolph KS, et al: Dynamic knee stability: Current theory and implications for clinicians and scientists. J Orthop Sports Phys Ther 31:546–566, 2001

3. Prentice WE: Understanding and managing the healing process, in Prentice WE, Voight ML (eds): Techniques in Musculoskeletal Rehabilitation. New York, McGraw-Hill, 2001, pp 17–41

4. Jackson-Manfield P, Neumann DA: Structure and function of joints, in Jackson–Manfield P, Neumann DA (eds): Essentials of Kinesiology for the Physical Therapist Assistant. St. Louis, MO, Mosby Elsevier, 2009, pp 21–34

5. Starcher BC: Lung elastin and matrix. Chest 117(5):229S–234S, 2000 (suppl 1)

6. Barnes J: Myofascial Release: A Comprehensive Evaluatory and Treatment Approach. Paoli, PA, MFR Seminars, 1990

7. Smolders JJ: Myofascial pain and dysfunction syndromes, in Hammer WI (ed): Functional Soft Tissue Examination and Treatment by Manual Methods—The Extremities. Gaithersburg, MD, Aspen, 1991, pp 215–234

8. Clancy WG, Jr.: Tendon trauma and overuse injuries, in Leadbetter WB, Buckwalter JA, Gordon SL (eds): Sports-Induced Inflammation. Park Ridge, IL, American Academy of Orthopaedic Surgeons, 1990, pp 609–618

9. Vereeke West R, Fu F: Soft tissue physiology and repair, Orthopaedic Knowledge Update 8: Home Study Syllabus. Rosemont, IL, American Academy of Orthopaedic Surgeons, 2005, pp 15–27

10. Teitz CC, Garrett WE, Jr., Miniaci A, et al: Tendon problems in athletic individuals. J Bone Joint Surg 79-A:138–152, 1997

11. Reid DC: Sports Injury Assessment and Rehabilitation. New York, Churchill Livingstone, 1992

12. Garrett W, Tidball J: Myotendinous junction: Structure, function, and failure, in Woo SL-Y, Buckwalter JA (eds): Injury and Repair of the Musculoskeletal Soft Tissues. Rosemont, IL, American Academy of Orthopaedic Surgeons, 1988, pp 29–54

13. Garrett WE, Jr.: Muscle strain injuries: Clinical and basic aspects. Med Sci Sports Exerc 22:436–443, 1990

14. Garrett WE: Muscle strain injuries. Am J Sports Med 24:S2–S8, 1996

15. Safran MR, Seaber AV, Garrett WE: Warm-up and muscular injury prevention: An update. Sports Med 8:239–249, 1989

16. Huijbregts PA: Muscle injury, regeneration, and repair. J Man Manip Ther 9:9–16, 2001

17. Amiel D, Kleiner JB: Biochemistry of tendon and ligament, in Nimni ME (ed): Collagen. Boca Raton, FL, CRC Press, 1988, pp 223–251

18. Woo SL-Y, An K-N, Arnoczky SP, et al: Anatomy, biology, and biomechanics of tendon, ligament, and meniscus, in Simon S (ed): Orthopaedic Basic Science. Rosemont, IL, American Academy of Orthopaedic Surgeons, 1994, pp 45–87

19. Safran MR, Benedetti RS, Bartolozzi AR, III., et al: Lateral ankle sprains: A comprehensive review: Part 1: Etiology, pathoanatomy, histopathogenesis, and diagnosis. Med Sci Sports Exer 31:S429–S437, 1999

20. Smith RL, Brunolli J: Shoulder kinesthesia after anterior glenohumeral dislocation. Phys Ther 69:106–112, 1989

21. McGaw WT: The effect of tension on collagen remodelling by fibroblasts: A stereological ultrastructural study. Connect Tissue Res 14:229, 1986

22. Engles M: Tissue response, in Donatelli R, Wooden MJ (eds): Orthopaedic Physical Therapy (ed 3). Philadelphia, Churchill Livingstone, 2001, pp 1–24

23. Junqueira LC, Carneciro J, Kelley RO: Basic Histology. Norwalk, CT, Appleton and Lange, 1995

24. Lundon K, Bolton K: Structure and function of the lumbar intervertebral disk in health, aging, and pathological conditions. J Orthop Sports Phys Ther 31:291–306, 2001

25. Cohen NP, Foster RJ, Mow VC: Composition and dynamics of articular cartilage: Structure, function, and maintaining healthy state. J Orthop Sports Phys Ther 28:203–215, 1998

26. White AA, Punjabi MM: Clinical Biomechanics of the Spine (ed 2). Philadelphia, JB Lippincott, 1990

27. Singer KP, Boyle JJW, Fazey P: Comparative anatomy of the zygapophysial joints, in Boyling JD, Jull GA (eds): Grieve's Modern Manual Therapy: The Vertebral Column. Philadelphia, Churchill Livingstone, 2004, pp 17–29

28. Buckwalter JA: Spine update: Aging and degeneration of the human intervertebral disc. Spine 20:1307–1314, 1995

29. Junqueira LC, Carneciro J: Bone, in Junqueira LC, Carneciro J (eds): Basic Histology (ed 10). New York, McGraw-Hill, 2003, pp 141–159

30. Chaffin D, Andersson G: Occupational Biomechanics (ed 4). New York, Wiley Interscience, 2006

31. Dahl LB, Dahl IMS, Engstrom-Laurent A, et al: Concentration and molecular weight of sodium hyaluronate in synovial fluid from patients with rheumatoid arthritis and other arthropathies. Ann Rheum Dis 44:817–822, 1985

32. Namba RS, Shuster S, Tucker P, et al: Localization of hyaluronan in pseudocapsule from total hip arthroplasty. Clin Orthop Relat Res 363:158–162, 1999

33. Marshall KW: Intra-articular hyaluronan therapy. Curr Opin Rheumatol 12:468–474, 2000

34. Laurent TC, Fraser JRE: Hyaluronan. FASEB J 6:2397–2404, 1992

35. Ho G, Jr., Tice AD, Kaplan SR: Septic bursitis in the prepatellar and olecranon bursae: An analysis of 25 cases. Ann Intern Med 89:21–27, 1978

36. Buckingham RB: Bursitis and tendinitis. Compr Ther 7:52–57, 1981

37. Reilly J, Nicholas JA: The chronically inflamed bursa. Clin Sports Med 6:345–370, 1987

38. Jones D, Round D: Skeletal Muscle in Health and Disease. Manchester, England, Manchester University Press, 1990

39. Van de Graaff KM, Fox SI: Muscle tissue and muscle physiology, in Van de Graaff KM, Fox SI (eds): Concepts of Human Anatomy and Physiology. New York, WCB/McGraw-Hill, 1999, pp 280–305

40. Armstrong RB, Warren GL, Warren JA: Mechanisms of exercise-induced muscle fibre injury. Med Sci Sports Exerc 24:436–443, 1990

41. Williams JH, Klug GA: Calcium exchange hypothesis of skeletal muscle fatigue. A brief review. Muscle Nerve 18:421, 1995

42. Hall SJ: The biomechanics of human skeletal muscle, in Hall SJ (ed): Basic Biomechanics. New York, McGraw-Hill, 1999, pp 146–185

43. Brooke MH, Kaiser KK: The use and abuse of muscle histochemistry. Ann N Y Acad Sci 228:121, 1974

44. Jull GA, Janda V: Muscle and motor control in low back pain, in Twomey LT, Taylor JR (eds): Physical Therapy of the Low Back: Clinics in Physical Therapy. New York, Churchill Livingstone, 1987, pp 253–278

45. Jackson-Manfield P, Neumann DA: Structure and function of skeletal muscle, in Jackson-Manfield P, Neumann DA (eds): Essentials of Kinesiology for the Physical Therapist Assistant. St. Louis, MO, Mosby Elsevier, 2009, pp 35–49

46. Brown DA: Muscle: The ultimate force generator in the body, in Neumann DA (ed): Kinesiology of the Musculoskeletal System: Foundations for Physical Rehabilitation. St. Louis, MO, Mosby, 2002, pp 41–55

47. Fitts RH, Widrick JJ: Muscle mechanics; adaptations with exercise training. Exerc Sport Sci Rev 24:427, 1996

48. Allemeier CA, Fry AC, Johnson P, et al: Effects of spring cycle training on human skeletal muscle. J Appl Physiol 77:2385, 1994

49. Cyriax J: Textbook of Orthopaedic Medicine, Diagnosis of Soft Tissue Lesions (ed 8). London, Bailliere Tindall, 1982

50. Boone DC, Azen SP, Lin C-M, et al: Reliability of goniometric measurements. Phys Ther 58:1355–1360, 1978

51. Mayerson NH, Milano RA: Goniometric measurement reliability in physical medicine. Arch Phys Med Rehab 65:92–94, 1984

52. Riddle DL, Rothstein JM, Lamb RL: Goniometric reliability in a clinical setting: Shoulder measurements. Phys Ther 67:668–673, 1987

53. Farfan HF: The scientific basis of manipulative procedures. Clin Rheumat Dis 6:159–177, 1980

54. McKenzie RA, May S: The lumbar spine: Mechanical diagnosis and therapy (ed 2). Waikanae, New Zealand, Spinal Publications New Zealand, 2003

55. McKenzie R, May S: Physical examination, in McKenzie R, May S (eds): The Human Extremities: Mechanical Diagnosis and Therapy. Waikanae, New Zealand, Spinal Publications New Zealand, 2000, pp 105–121

56. Petersen CM, Hayes KW: Construct validity of Cyriax's selective tension examination: Association of end-feels with pain at the knee and shoulder. J Orthop Sports Phys Ther 30:512–527, 2000

57. Riddle DL: Measurement of accessory motion: Critical issues and related concepts. Phys Ther 72:865–874, 1992

58. American Medical Association: Guides to the Evaluation of Permanent Impairment (ed 5). Chicago, IL, American Medical Association, 2001

59. Sapega AA: Muscle performance evaluation in orthopedic practice. J Bone Joint Surg 72A:1562–1574, 1990

60. Janda V: Muscle Function Testing. London, Butterworths, 1983

61. Nadler SF, Rigolosi L, Kim D, et al: Sensory, motor, and reflex examination, in Malanga GA, Nadler SF (eds): Musculoskeletal Physical Examination—An Evidence-Based Approach. Philadelphia, PA, Elsevier-Mosby, 2006, pp 15–32

62. Palmer ML, Epler M: Principles of examination techniques, in Palmer ML, Epler M (eds): Clinical Assessment Procedures in Physical Therapy. Philadelphia, JB Lippincott, 1990, pp 8–36

63. Bohannon RW: Measuring knee extensor muscle strength. Am J Phys Med Rehab 80:13–18, 2001

64. Ottenbacher KJ, Branch LG, Ray L, et al: The reliability of upper- and lower-extremity strength testing in a community survey of older adults. Arch Phys Med Rehab 83:1423–1427, 2002

65. Escolar DM, Henricson EK, Mayhew J, et al: Clinical evaluator reliability for quantitative and manual muscle testing measures of strength in children. Muscle Nerve 24:787–793, 2001

66. Bohannon RW, Corrigan D: A broad range of forces is encompassed by the maximum manual muscle test grade of five. Percept Mot Skills 90(3 Pt 1):747–750, 2000

67. Tovin BJ, Greenfield BH: Impairment-based diagnosis for the shoulder girdle, in Tovin BJ, Greenfield BH (eds): Evaluation and Treatment of the Shoulder: An Integration of the Guide to Physical Therapist Practice. Philadelphia, FA Davis, 2001, pp 55–74

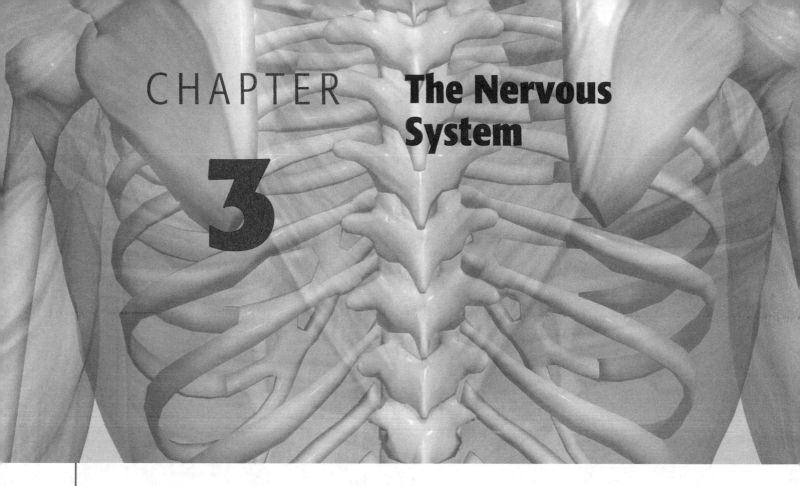

CHAPTER 3 The Nervous System

Chapter Objectives

At the completion of this chapter, the reader will be able to:

1. Describe the various components of the central and peripheral nervous systems as they relate to the orthopaedic setting.
2. Describe the anatomic and functional organization of the nervous system as it relates to the orthopaedic setting.
3. Describe the various components and distributions of the cervical, brachial, and lumbosacral plexuses.
4. Outline the various methods by which pain is transmitted.
5. Recognize the characteristics of a lesion to the central nervous system that can occur during an orthopaedic assessment.
6. List the findings and impairments associated with the more common peripheral nerve lesions.
7. Describe some of the medical interventions following a nerve injury.
8. List the categories for the various nerve injuries.
9. Outline a number of tests performed by the physical therapist related to neurologic dysfunction.

Overview

The nervous system can be divided into two anatomic divisions, the central nervous system (CNS) and peripheral nervous system (PNS), each with their own subdivisions (Figure 3-1).

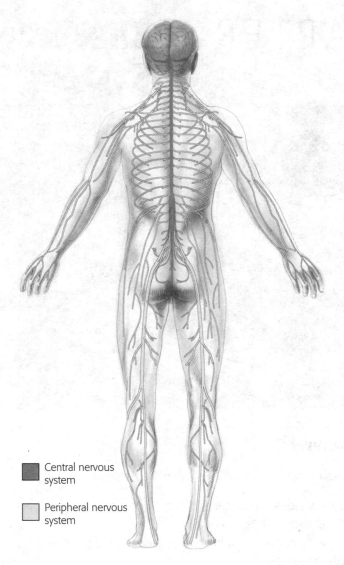

Central nervous system

Peripheral nervous system

Figure 3-1 The nervous system.

Central Nervous System

The central nervous system (CNS) is composed of the brain and the spinal cord. The brain, contained within the skull (cranium), begins its embryonic development as the cephalic end of the neural tube before rapidly growing and differentiating into three distinct swellings: the prosencephalon, the mesencephalon, and the rhombencephalon (**Table 3-1**).

The spinal cord has an external segmental organization (**Figure 3-2**). Each of the 31 pairs of spinal nerves that arise from the spinal cord has a ventral root (motor) and a dorsal root (sensory), with each root made up of one to eight rootlets, and each rootlet consisting of bundles of nerve fibers.[1] In the dorsal root of a typical spinal nerve lies a dorsal root ganglion, a swelling that contains sensory nerve cell bodies.[1]

The spinal cord provides a conduit for the two-way transmission of messages between the brain and the body. These messages may descend or ascend along pathways, or tracts, which are fiber bundles of similar groups of neurons, each with specific functions.

● Key Point Myelin is a lipid-rich membrane that coats, protects, and insulates nerves. Most of the axons of the PNS and CNS are covered by myelin, which is divided into segments about 1 millimeter long by small gaps where the myelin is absent, called *nodes of Ranvier*. As the brain sends messages through the nerves of the spinal cord, the impulses jump from node to node through a process called *salutatory conduction*.

The central gray matter of the spinal cord, which roughly resembles the letter *H*, contains two anterior (ventral) and two posterior (dorsal) horns united by gray commissure within the central canal.

Derivation and Functions of the Major Brain Structures

	Region	Structure	Description/Function
Prosencephalon (forebrain)	Telencephalon	Cerebrum	Lies in front or on top of the brainstem and is the largest and most developed of the major divisions of the brain.
			Consists of six paired lobes within two hemispheres, which are folded into many gyri (crests) and sulci (grooves), which allows the cortex to expand in surface area without taking up much greater volume.
			Controls most sensory processing, conscious and volitional movements, language and communication, learning, and memory.
		Limbic system	A set of brain structures including the hippocampus, amygdala, anterior thalamic nuclei, and limbic cortex, which support a variety of functions including emotion, behavior, long-term memory, and olfaction.
		Basal ganglia	Associated with a variety of functions, including motor control, motor learning, and action selection.
	Diencephalon	Thalamus	Functions include the relaying of sensation, spatial sense, and motor signals to the cerebral cortex, along with the regulation of consciousness, sleep, and alertness.
		Hypothalamus	Regulation of food and water intake, body temperature, and heart rate. One of the most important functions of the hypothalamus is to link the nervous system to the endocrine system via the pituitary gland.
		Pituitary gland	Considered to be the "master gland."
			Regulation of homeostasis and of various endocrine functions.
Mesencephalon (midbrain)	Mesencephalon	Superior colliculi	Visual reflexes (hand–eye coordination).
		Inferior colliculi	Auditory reflexes.
		Cerebral peduncles	Important fibers running through the cerebral peduncles include the corticospinal tract and the corticobulbar tract. This area contains many nerve tracts conveying motor information to the brain and from the brain to the rest of the body.
Rhombencephalon (hindbrain)	Metencephalon	Cerebellum	Balance/equilibrium and coordination of skeletal muscle contractions (force, direction, extent, and sequencing of movement).
		Pons	Relay center; contains nuclei (pontine nuclei).
	Myelencephalon	Medulla oblongata	Relay center; contains many nuclei; visceral autonomic center (e.g., respiration, heart rate, vasoconstriction).

Data from Van de Graaff KM, Fox SI: Central nervous system, in Van de Graaff KM, Fox SI (eds): Concepts of Human Anatomy and Physiology. New York, WCB/McGraw-Hill, 1999, pp 407–446

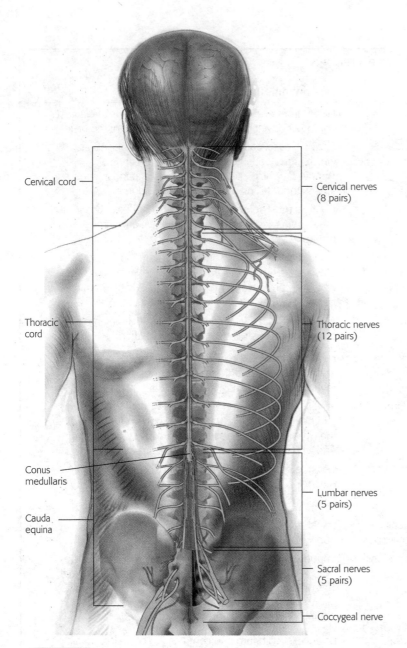

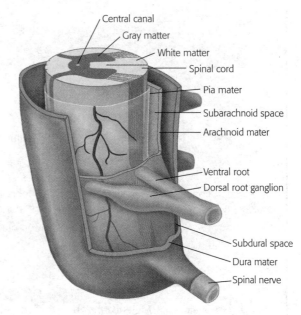

Figure 3-2 Segmental organization of the spinal cord.

Key Point *Anterior horns* contain cell bodies that give rise to motor (efferent) neurons. Gamma motor neurons connect to muscle spindles (**Box 3-1**). Alpha motor neurons connect to effect muscles. *Posterior horns* contain sensory (afferent) neurons whose nerve cell bodies are located in the dorsal root ganglia.[1]

Three membranes, or meninges, envelop the structures of the CNS: the dura mater, the arachnoid mater, and the pia mater (Figure 3-3). The meninges, and related spaces, are important for both the nutrition and protection of the spinal cord. The cerebrospinal fluid that flows through the meningeal spaces, and within the ventricles of the brain, provides a cushion for the spinal cord. The meninges also form

barriers that resist the entrance of a variety of noxious organisms.

Key Point Occasionally, spinal cord compression may occur secondary to bony encroachment from spinal stenosis, space-occupying lesions, trauma, or disease. Clinical signs and symptoms that may be associated with spinal cord compression include:

- Segmental deficits (paraparesis or quadriparesis)
- Hyperreflexia
- Extensor plantar response and other pathologic reflexes
- Loss of sphincter tone (with bowel and bladder dysfunction)
- Sensory deficits

Subacute or chronic spinal cord compression may begin with local back pain, often radiating down the distribution of a nerve root (radicular pain), and sometimes includes hyperreflexia and loss of sensation. Sensory loss may begin in the sacral segments.

Box 3-1

Muscle Spindle and Golgi Tendon Organs

Muscle Spindle

Essentially, the purpose of the muscle spindle is to compare the length of the spindle with the length of the muscle that surrounds the spindle. Within each muscle spindle are 2–12 long, slender, and specialized skeletal muscle fibers called *intrafusal fibers*. The central portion of the intrafusal fiber is devoid of actin or myosin and, thus, is incapable of contracting. As a result, these fibers are capable of putting tension on the spindle only. The intrafusal fibers are of two types: nuclear bag fibers and nuclear chain fibers.

- Nuclear bag fibers primarily serve as sensitivity meters for the changing lens of the muscle.[a,b]
- Nuclear chain fibers each contain a single row or chain of nuclei and are attached at their ends to the bag fibers.
  Whereas muscles are innervated by alpha motor neurons, muscle spindles have their own motor supply, namely gamma motor neurons.

  The muscle spindle can be stimulated in two different ways:

- By stretching the whole muscle, which stretches the mid-portion of the spindle thereby exciting the receptor
- By contracting only the end portion of the intrafusal fibers, thereby exciting the receptor (even if muscle length does not change)

Golgi Tendon Organs

Golgi tendon organs (GTOs) are relatively simple sensory receptors that that are arranged in series with the extrafusal muscle fibers and, therefore, become activated by stretch. In a normal person, the Golgi tendon organs contribute to control of muscle activity over the whole range of movement, not just at its extremes.[c] They appear to serve a protective function, while supplying tension information for complicated tension-maintaining reflexes or supplying inhibition at the appropriate moment to switch from flexion to extension movements in walking or running. They may also play a role in increasing muscle force during fatigue. Thus, during fatigue the muscle produces less force, which reduces Golgi tendon organ activity, thereby decreasing inhibition. Activity in the group Ib afferent fibers, associated with Golgi tendon organs, inhibit a process called *autogenic inhibition* (reflex inhibition of a motor unit in response to excessive tension in the muscle fibers it supplies). It was originally thought that this inhibition served only to protect the muscle from being injured when contracting against too heavy a load. Now it is thought that it occurs at the point where autogenic inhibition is great enough to overcome the stretch reflex excitation.

a. Grigg P: Peripheral neural mechanisms in proprioception. J Sport Rehabil 3:1–17, 1994
b. Swash M, Fox K: Muscle spindle innervation in man. J Anat 112:61-80, 1972
c. de Jarnette B: Sacro-occipital technique. Nebraska City, Major Bertrand de Jarnette, DC, 1972

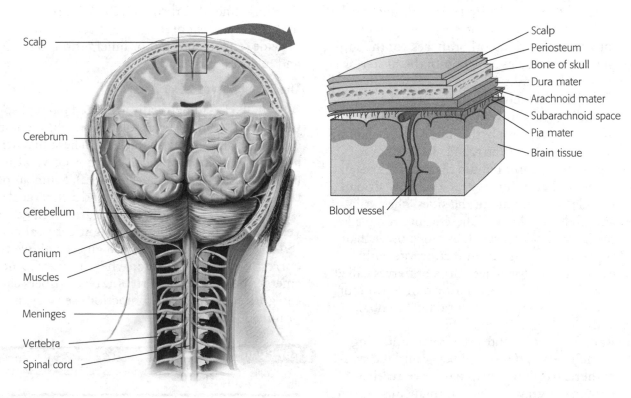

Scalp
Cerebrum
Cerebellum
Cranium
Muscles
Meninges
Vertebra
Spinal cord

Scalp
Periosteum
Bone of skull
Dura mater
Arachnoid mater
Subarachnoid space
Pia mater
Brain tissue
Blood vessel

Figure 3-3 The meninges.

Peripheral Nervous System

The peripheral nervous system (PNS) is composed of the following:

- *Cranial nerves:* The brain stem, which is literally the stalk of the brain, gives rise to 10 of the 12 pairs of cranial nerves, which provide the main motor and sensory innervation to the face and neck.
- *Spinal nerve roots:* The posterior (dorsal) and anterior (ventral) roots of the spinal nerves are located within the vertebral canal. In the region of the intervertebral foramen, the posterior (afferent) and anterior (efferent) roots come together in a common neural sheath to form a spinal nerve root, which is a mixed sensory-motor nerve. Shortly after a spinal nerve exits the intervertebral foramen, it branches into the posterior (dorsal) ramus, anterior (ventral) ramus, and rami communicantes. Each of these three structures carries both sensory and motor information.
  - The posterior (dorsal) rami branches carry visceral motor, somatic motor, and sensory information, and as a rule are smaller than their anterior counterparts. They are directed posteriorly, and, with the exceptions of those of the first cervical, the fourth and fifth sacral, and the coccygeal, divide into medial and lateral branches for the supply of the muscles and skin of the posterior part of the trunk.
  - The anterior (ventral) ramus branches, including the sinuvertebral (recurrent meningeal) nerve, supply the limbs and the anterolateral parts of the trunk. In the thoracic region these rami remain distinct from each other, and each innervates a narrow strip of muscle and skin along the sides, chest, ribs, and abdominal wall. These rami are called the intercostal nerves. In regions other than the thoracic, ventral rami converge with each other to form networks of nerves called *nerve plexuses*. The anterior rami form four main plexuses: cervical, brachial, lumbar, and sacral.
  - Rami communicantes is a communicating branch between a spinal nerve and the sympathetic trunk. Each spinal nerve receives a branch—a gray ramus communicans—from the adjacent ganglion of the sympathetic trunk. The thoracic, and the first and second lumbar nerves each contributes a branch—a white ramus communicans—to the adjoining sympathetic ganglion.
- *Dorsal root ganglia (or spinal ganglia):* A dorsal root ganglion is a nodule on a dorsal root that contains cell bodies of neurons in afferent spinal nerves.

> ● **Key Point** The recurrent meningeal or sinuvertebral nerve, a branch of the spinal nerve, passes back into the vertebral canal through the intervertebral foramen. This nerve supplies the anterior aspect of the dura mater, outer third of the annular fibers of the intervertebral discs, vertebral body, and epidural blood vessel walls, as well as the posterior longitudinal ligament.[2] The two structures capable of transmitting neuronal impulses that result in the experience of pain are the sinuvertebral nerve and the nerve root.

- The peripheral nerve trunks and their terminal branches
- The peripheral autonomic nervous system

The somatic divisions (the parts that produce voluntary action) of the peripheral nervous system consist of the cranial nerves and the spinal nerves.

The Cranial Nerves

The cranial nerves (CN) are typically described as comprising 12 pairs, which are referred to by the Roman numerals I through XII (**Table 3-2**). The cranial nerve roots enter and exit the brain stem to provide sensory and motor innervation to the head and muscles of the face.

The Spinal Nerves

A total of 31 symmetrically arranged pairs of spinal nerves exit from all levels of the vertebral column, each derived from the spinal cord. The spinal nerves are divided topographically into 8 cervical pairs (C1–C8), 12 thoracic pairs (T1–T12), 5 lumbar pairs (L1–L5), 5 sacral pairs (S1–S5), and a coccygeal pair (see Figure 3-1). Although there are seven cervical vertebrae (C1–C7), there are eight cervical nerves (C1–C8). All nerves except C8 emerge above their corresponding vertebrae, whereas the C8 nerve emerges below the C7 vertebra. Nerve fibers can be categorized according to function: sensory, motor, or mixed (**Table 3-3**).

> ● **Key Point** A dermatome is an area of skin that is mainly supplied by a single spinal nerve. Dermatomes are useful for determining the site of a nerve lesion.

TABLE 3-2	Cranial Nerves and Their Functions

Cranial Nerve	Function and Testing
I: Olfactory	The olfactory nerve is responsible for the sense of smell. The sense of smell is tested by having the patient identify familiar odors (e.g., coffee, vanilla) with each nostril.
II: Optic	The optic nerve is responsible for vision. The optic nerve is tested by examining visual acuity and confrontation.
III: Oculomotor	The somatic portion of the oculomotor nerve supplies the levator palpabrae superioris muscle; the superior, medial, and inferior rectus muscles; and the inferior oblique muscles, all of which are responsible for some eye movements. The visceral efferent portion of this nerve is responsible for papillary constriction. The nerve is tested by using eye movements and assessing pupil dilation. Cranial nerves III, IV, and VI are typically tested together.
IV: Trochlear	The trochlear nerve supplies the superior oblique muscle of the eye. This nerve is tested using eye movements.
V: Trigeminal	The trigeminal nerve supplies sensory information to the soft and hard palates, maxillary sinuses, upper teeth, upper lip, and the mucous membrane of the pharynx, and supplies motor information to the muscles of mastication, both pterygoids, the anterior belly of digastric, tensor tympani, tensor veli palatini, and mylohyoid. The sensory branches of the trigeminal nerve are tested with a pin-prick close to the mid-line of the face. The motor components are tested by asking the patient to clench his or her teeth while the clinician palpates the temporal and masseter muscles.
VI: Abducens	The abducens nerve innervates the lateral rectus muscle of the eye. This nerve is tested using eye movements.
VII: Facial	The facial nerve is composed of a sensory (intermediate) root, which conveys taste, and a motor root, the facial nerve proper, which supplies the muscles of facial expression, the platysma muscle, and the stapedius muscle of the inner ear. The clinician inspects the face at rest and in conversation with the patient, and notes any asymmetry. The patient is asked to smile. If there is asymmetry, the patient is asked to frown, or wrinkle the forehead.
VIII: Vestibulocochlear (Auditory)	The cochlear portion is concerned with the sense of hearing. The vestibular portion is part of the system of equilibrium, the vestibular system. The vestibular nerve can be tested in a number of ways depending on the objective.
IX: Glossopharyngeal	The glossopharyngeal nerve serves a number of functions. The gag reflex is used to test this nerve but is reserved for only severely affected patients.
X: Vagus	The vagus nerve contains somatic motor, visceral efferent, visceral sensory, and somatic sensory fibers. The functions of the vagus nerve are numerous. The patient is asked to open their mouth and say "aah." The clinician watches the movements of the soft palate and pharynx.
XI: (Spinal) Accessory	The cranial root is often viewed as an aberrant portion of the vagus nerve. The spinal portion of the nerve supplies the sternocleidomastoid and trapezius muscles. The patient is asked to shrug both shoulders upward against the clinician's hand and the strength of contraction is noted.
XII: Hypoglossal	The hypoglossal nerve is the motor nerve of the tongue, innervating the ipsilateral side of the tongue as well as helping to innervate the infrahyoid muscles. The patient is asked to stick out his or her tongue. The clinician looks for asymmetry, atrophy, or deviation from the midline.

Peripheral nerves are enclosed in three layers of tissue of differing character. From the inside outward, these are the:

- *Endoneurium:* Encloses the myelin sheath of a nerve fiber and serves to support capillary vessels, which form a network.

- *Perineurium:* Arranges axons into fascicles (a bundle of axons/nerve fibers).
- *Epineurium:* The outermost layer of connective tissue surrounding a peripheral nerve. It includes the blood vessels supplying the nerve. The epineurium binds fascicles into bundles.

TABLE 3-3 Nerve Fiber Types and Their Functions

Nerve Fiber Type	Function	Examples
Sensory	Carry afferents from a portion of the skin.	Lateral femoral cutaneous nerve
	Carry afferents to the skin structures. This area of distribution is called a *dermatome*, which is a well-defined segmental portion of the skin (refer to Figure 3-4), and generally follows the segmental distribution of the underlying muscle innervation.	Saphenous nerve Interdigital nerves
Motor	Carry efferents to muscles and return sensation from muscles and associated ligamentous structures. Any nerve that innervates a muscle also mediates the sensation from the joint upon which that muscle acts.	Ulnar nerve Suprascapular nerve Dorsal scapular nerve
Mixed	Combination of skin, sensory, and motor functions.	Median nerve Ulnar nerve (at the elbow as it enters the tunnel of Guyon) Common peroneal nerve Ilioinguinal nerve

Spinal nerves and peripheral nerves can be injured anywhere along their distribution, although some sites are more commonly injured than others. Peripheral nerve injuries can occur at the level of the axon (i.e., axonopathy), the motor neuron, or the dorsal root ganglion (i.e., neuronopathies). Compression and/or irritation of cervical or lumbar nerve roots can cause radiculopathy, a common cause of symptoms.

> ● **Key Point** Because motor and sensory axons run in the same nerves, disorders of the peripheral nerves (neuropathies) usually affect both motor and sensory functions distal to the lesion. Symptoms can manifest as abnormal, frequently unpleasant sensations, which are variously described by the patient as numbness, pins and needles, or tingling, but are more correctly termed *paresthesias*.

Paresthesias can occur anywhere within a dermatomal distribution, or within a peripheral nerve distribution (Figure 3-4). Central nervous system causes of paresthesia include ischemia, obstruction, compression, infection, inflammation, and degenerative conditions.

The Cervical Nerves

The eight pairs of cervical nerves are derived from cord segments between the level of the foramen magnum and the middle of the seventh cervical vertebra.[3] The C1 (suboccipital) nerve serves the muscles of the suboccipital triangle, with very few sensory fibers.[3]

The Cervical Plexus (C1–C4)

The cervical plexus (Figure 3-5) is formed from the anterior primary divisions of the first four cervical nerves (C1–C4). Nerves formed from the cervical plexus innervate the back of the head, as well as some neck muscles. The cervical plexus has two types of branches: cutaneous and muscular.

The cutaneous branch contains:

- *Lesser occipital nerve:* Innervates the lateral part of the occipital region (C2 *only*)
- *Great auricular nerve:* Innervates skin near the hollow of the auricle of the external ear and external acoustic meatus (C2–C3)
- *Transverse cervical nerve:* Innervates the anterior region of neck (C2–C3)
- *Supraclavicular nerves:* Provide sensory innervation to the suprascapular, shoulder, and upper thoracic regions (C3–C4)

The muscular branch contains:

- *Ansa cervicalis (loop formed from C1–C3):* Innervates the geniohyoid, thyrohyoid, sternothyroid, sternohyoid, and omohyoid muscles
- *Phrenic (C3–C5, primarily C4):* Contain motor, sensory, and sympathetic nerve fibers that provide the only motor supply to the diaphragm, the key breathing muscle

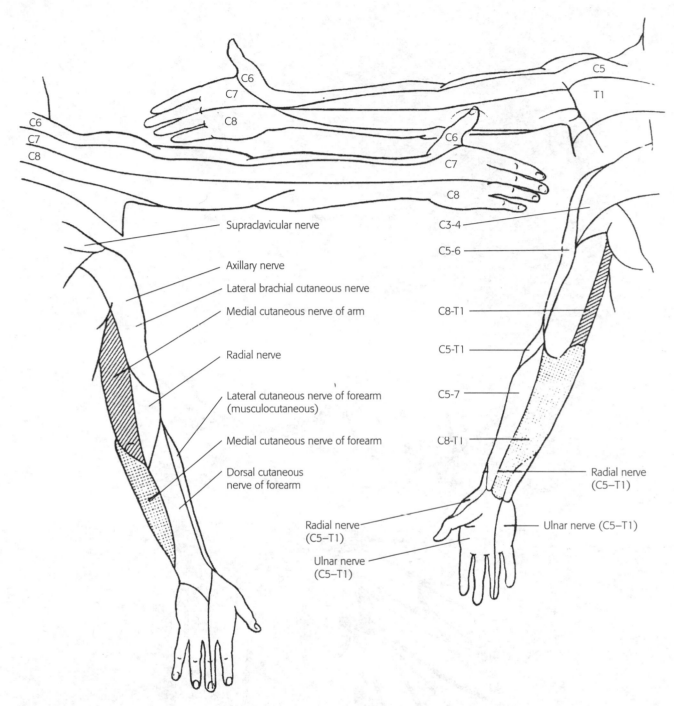

Figure 3-4   Dermatomes of the upper extremity.

Labels in figure: C6, C7, C8, C5, T1, C6, C7, C8, C3-4, C5-6, C8-T1, C5-T1, C5-7, C8-T1

Supraclavicular nerve
Axillary nerve
Lateral brachial cutaneous nerve
Medial cutaneous nerve of arm
Radial nerve
Lateral cutaneous nerve of forearm (musculocutaneous)
Medial cutaneous nerve of forearm
Dorsal cutaneous nerve of forearm
Radial nerve (C5–T1)
Ulnar nerve (C5–T1)
Radial nerve (C5–T1)
Ulnar nerve (C5–T1)

■ *Segmental branches (C1–C4):* Is a branch to the sternocleidomastoid muscle from C2 and branches to the trapezius muscles (C3–C4) via the subtrapezial plexus; smaller branches to the adjacent vertebral musculature supply the rectus capitis lateralis and rectus capitis anterior (C1), the longus capitis (C2, C4) and longus coli (C1–C4), the scalenus medius (C3, C4) and scalenus anterior (C4), and the levator scapulae (C3–C5)

The Brachial Plexus

The brachial plexus (Figure 3-6) arises from the anterior primary divisions of the fifth cervical through the first thoracic nerve roots, with occasional contributions from the fourth cervical and second thoracic roots. The C5 and C6 roots of the plexus join to form the upper trunk, the C7 root becomes the middle trunk, and the C8 and T1 roots join to form the lower trunks. Each of the trunks divides into anterior and posterior divisions, which then form cords. The

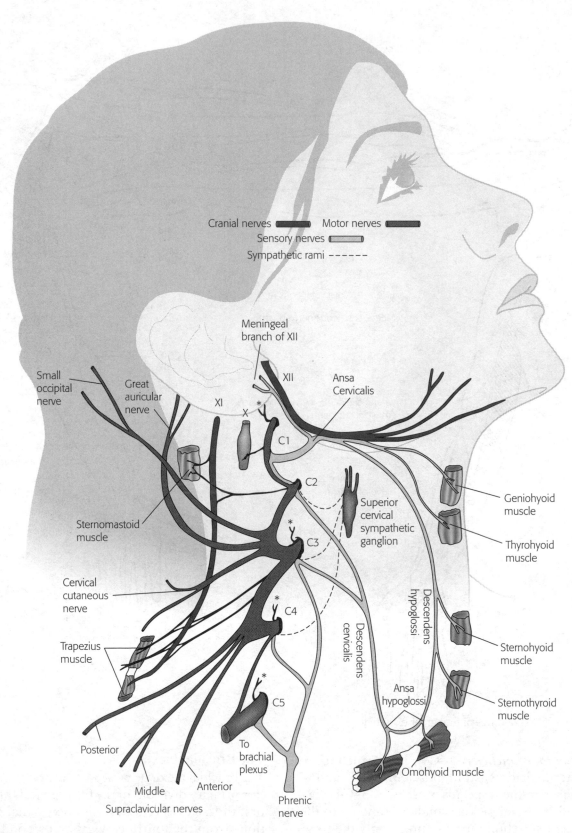

Legend:
- Cranial nerves
- Motor nerves
- Sensory nerves
- Sympathetic rami - - - - -

Labels:
- Meningeal branch of XII
- Small occipital nerve
- Great auricular nerve
- XI
- X
- XII
- Ansa Cervicalis
- C1
- Sternomastoid muscle
- C2
- Superior cervical sympathetic ganglion
- Geniohyoid muscle
- Thyrohyoid muscle
- Cervical cutaneous nerve
- C3
- Descendens hypoglossi
- Trapezius muscle
- C4
- Descendens cervicalis
- Sternohyoid muscle
- Posterior
- C5
- Ansa hypoglossi
- Sternothyroid muscle
- Middle
- Anterior
- To brachial plexus
- Omohyoid muscle
- Supraclavicular nerves
- Phrenic nerve

Figure 3-5   The cervical plexus.

*To adjacent vertebral musclature

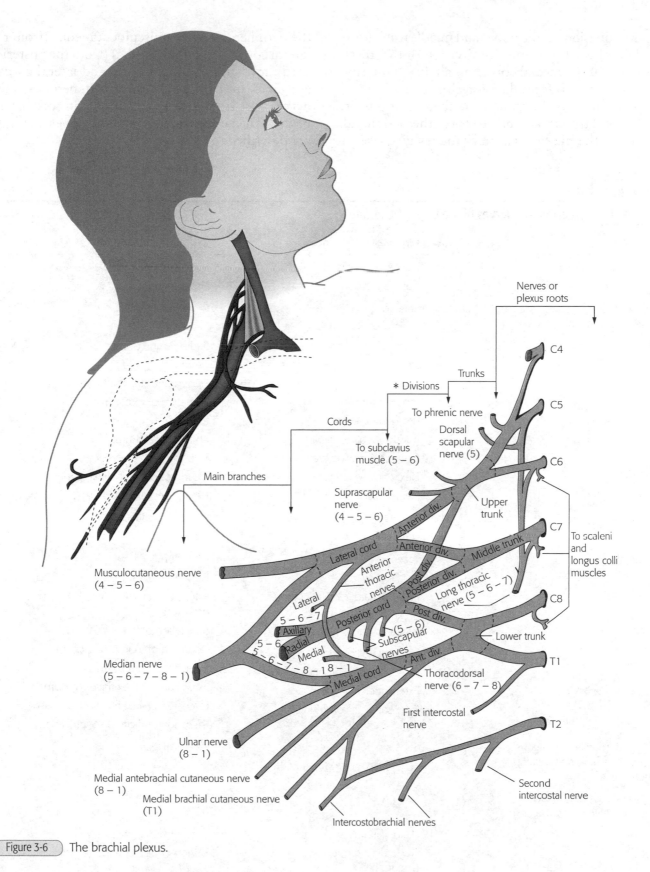

Nerves or plexus roots

C4

Trunks

C5

* Divisions

To phrenic nerve

Cords

Dorsal scapular nerve (5)

C6

To subclavius muscle (5 – 6)

Suprascapular nerve (4 – 5 – 6)

Upper trunk

Main branches

Anterior div.

C7

To scaleni and longus colli muscles

Lateral cord

Anterior div.

Middle trunk

Musculocutaneous nerve (4 – 5 – 6)

Anterior thoracic nerves

Post div.

Posterior div.

Long thoracic nerve (5 – 6 – 7)

Lateral 5 – 6 – 7

Posterior cord

Post div.

C8

Axillary 5 – 6

(5 – 6)

Lower trunk

Radial 5 – 6 – 7 – 8 – 1

Subscapular nerves

Median nerve (5 – 6 – 7 – 8 – 1)

Medial

Ant. div.

T1

Medial cord

Thoracodorsal nerve (6 – 7 – 8)

First intercostal nerve

T2

Ulnar nerve (8 – 1)

Medial antebrachial cutaneous nerve (8 – 1)

Second intercostal nerve

Medial brachial cutaneous nerve (T1)

Intercostobrachial nerves

Figure 3-6 The brachial plexus.

*Splitting of the plexus into anterior and posterior divisions is one of the most significant features in the redistribution of nerve fibers, because it is here that libers supplying the flexor and extensor groups of muscles of the upper extremity are separated. Similar splitting is noted in the lumber and sacral plexuses for the supply of muscles of the lower extremity.

anterior divisions of the upper and middle trunk form the lateral cord; the anterior division of the lower trunk forms the medial cord; and all three posterior divisions unite to form the posterior cord.

The three cords, named for their relationship to the axillary artery, split to form the peripheral nerves of the plexus. These branches give rise to the peripheral nerves: musculocutaneous (from the lateral cord), axillary and radial (from the posterior cord), median (from the medial and lateral cords), and ulnar (from the medial cord).[4] Numerous smaller nerves arise from the roots, trunks, and cords of the plexus. The peripheral nerves of the upper quadrant are described in **Table 3-4**.

TABLE 3-4   Peripheral Nerves of the Upper Quadrant

Nerves	Nerve Root	Muscles	Action
Musculocutaneous	C5–C6	Biceps, brachialis	Flexion of elbow
		Coracobrachialis	Shoulder flexion
Lateral brachial cutaneous nerve of the arm	C5–C6	Sensory	Refer to Figure 3-4
Median	C5–T1	Flexor carpi radialis	Radial flexion of wrist
		Flexor digitorum superficialis	Flexion of middle phalanges (digiti II–V)
		Flexor digitorum profundus (lateral half)	Flexion of distal phalanges (digiti II, III)
		Pronator teres	Pronation of forearm
		Pronator quadratus	Pronation of forearm
		Abductor pollicis brevis	Abduction of thumb
		Opponens pollicis brevis	Opposition of thumb
		Flexor pollicis longus	Flexion of distal phalanx of thumb
		Flexor pollicis brevis	Flexion of proximal phalanx of thumb
Axillary	C5–C6	Deltoid	Shoulder abduction
		Teres minor	
Radial	C5–T1	Triceps	Extension at elbow
		Brachioradialis	Flexion of forearm
		Extensor carpi radialis/ulnaris	Extension at wrist with radial/ulnar deviation
		Supinator	Supination of forearm
		Extensor pollicis brevis	Extension of thumb (proximal)
		Extensor pollicis longus	Extension of thumb (distal)
		Extensor indicis proprius	Extension of index finger (proximal)
		Extensor digiti V proprius	Extension of little finger (proximal)
		Extensor digiti communis	Extension of digits (II–V, proximal)
Medial (dorsal) cutaneous (antebrachial) nerve of the forearm	C6–T1	Sensory	Refer to Figure 3-4
Lateral cutaneous (antebrachial) nerve of the forearm	C5–C6	Sensory	Refer to Figure 3-4
Ulnar	C8–T1	Flexor carpi ulnaris	Ulnar flexion of wrist
		Flexor digitorum profundus (medial half)	Flexion of distal phalanges (digiti IV, V)
		Abductor digiti minimi	Abduction of digiti V
		All other intrinsics of hand	Finger abduction/adduction

The Thoracic Nerves

The thoracic posterior (dorsal) rami travel posteriorly, close to the vertebral zygapophyseal (facet) joints before dividing into medial and lateral branches. The posterior ramus contains nerves that serve the posterior portions of the trunk carrying visceral motor, somatic motor, and sensory information to and from the skin and muscles of the back. There are 12 pairs of thoracic anterior (ventral) rami, and all but the twelfth are located between the ribs, serving as intercostal nerves. All of the intercostal nerves supply the thoracic and abdominal walls, with the upper two also supplying the upper limbs. The thoracic anterior rami of T3–T6 supply only the thoracic wall, whereas the lower five rami supply both the thoracic and abdominal walls. The subcostal nerve supplies both the abdominal wall and the gluteal skin.

The Lumbar Plexus

The lumbar plexus (Figure 3-7) forms the upper part of the lumbosacral plexus. It is formed by the anterior divisions of the first four lumbar nerves (L1–L4) and from contributions of the subcostal nerve (T12), which is the last thoracic nerve (in approximately 50 percent of cases). **Table 3-5** outlines the peripheral nerves of the lumbar plexus.

The Sacral Plexus

The L4 and L5 nerves join medial to the sacral promontory, becoming the lumbosacral trunk. The lumbosacral trunk (L4, L5) descends into the pelvis, where it enters the formation of the sacral plexus (Figure 3-8). The S1–S4 nerves converge with the lumbosacral trunk in front of the piriformis muscle, forming the broad triangular band of the sacral plexus. The upper three nerves of the sacral plexus divide into two sets of branches:

- The medial branches are distributed to the multifidi muscles.
- The lateral branches become the medial cluneal nerves. The medial cluneal nerves supply the skin over the medial part of the gluteus maximus.

The lower two posterior primary divisions, with the posterior division of the coccygeal nerve, supply the skin over the coccyx.

Collateral branches from the anterior divisions extend to the quadratus femoris and gemellus inferior muscles (from L4, L5, and S1) and to the obturator internus and gemellus superior muscles (from L5 and S1, S2).

The muscles innervated by the sacral plexus are listed in **Table 3-6**.

The Sciatic Nerve

The sciatic nerve (refer to Figure 3-8) is the largest nerve in the body. It arises from the L4, L5, and S1–S3 nerve roots as a continuation of the lumbosacral plexus. The nerve is composed of the independent tibial (medial) and common fibular (peroneal) (lateral) divisions (refer to Table 3-6), which are usually united as a single nerve down to the lower portion of the thigh.

The Pudendal and Coccygeal Plexuses

The pudendal and coccygeal plexuses are the most caudal portions of the lumbosacral plexus and supply nerves to the perineal structures.

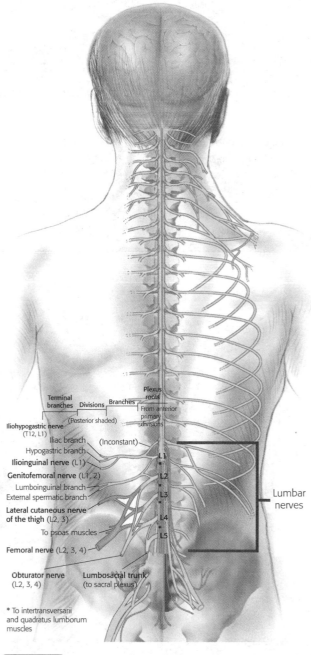

Figure 3-7   The lumbar plexus.

TABLE 3-5

Peripheral Nerves of the Lumbar Plexus

Nerves	Nerve Root	Muscles	Function
Iliohypogastric	T12, L1	Sensory	The lateral (iliac) branch supplies the skin of the upper lateral part of the thigh while the anterior (hypogastric) branch supplies the skin over the symphysis
Ilioinguinal	L1	Sensory	Supplies the skin of the upper medial part of the thigh and the root of the penis and scrotum or mons pubis and labia majora
Genitofemoral	L1, L2	Sensory	The genital branch supplies the cremasteric muscle and the skin of the scrotum or labia while the femoral branch supplies the skin of the middle upper part of the thigh and the femoral artery
Femoral	L2–L4	Iliopsoas	Flexion of hip
		Quadriceps femoris	Extension of knee
		Pectineus	
		Sartorius	
Saphenous	L3–L4	Sensory	Medial aspect of the knee, leg, and foot
Obturator	L2–L4	Adductor longus, adductor brevis, adductor magnus	Adduction of hip
Lateral cutaneous (femoral) nerve of the thigh	L2–L3	Sensory	Anterior and lateral parts of the thigh, as far as the knee
Posterior cutaneous nerve of the thigh	L2–L3	Sensory	The gluteal region, the perineum, and the back of the thigh and leg
Anterior cutaneous (femoral) nerve of the thigh	L2–L3	Sensory	Anterior aspect of the thigh, leg, and foot

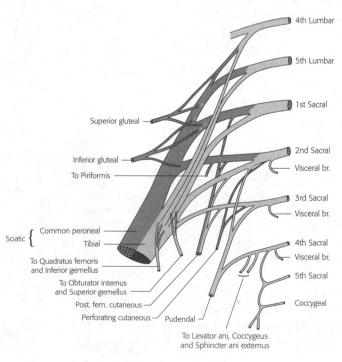

Figure 3-8　The sacral plexus.

Source: Gray H: Anatomy of the Human Body (ed 20). Philadelphia, Lea and Febiger, 1918.

TABLE 3-6	Peripheral Nerves (Motor) of the Sacral Plexus		
Nerves	**Nerve Root**	**Muscles**	**Action**
Superior gluteal	L4–S1	Gluteus medius, gluteus minimus, and tensor fasciae latae	Abduction of the hip (With the hip flexed, the gluteus medius and minimus externally rotate the thigh. With the hip extended, the gluteus medius and minimus internally rotate the thigh.)
Inferior gluteal	L5–S2	Gluteus maximus	Extension of the hip
Sciatic	(Common fibular and tibial nerves travel in a common sheath)	Biceps femoris (long head), semitendinosus, semimembranosus, and adductor magnus	Hip extension, knee flexion, and hip adduction
Common fibular	L4, L5 and S1, S2	Biceps femoris (short head), fibularis (peroneus) longus, fibularis (peroneus) brevis, tibialis anterior, extensor digitorum longus, fibularis (peroneus) tertius, extensor hallucis longus (propius), extensor digitorum brevis, and extensor hallucis brevis	Varies according to muscle
Tibial	L 4, 5 and S 1, 2, 3	Gastrocnemius, popliteus, soleus, plantaris, tibialis posterior, flexor digitorum longus, flexor hallucis longus, abductor hallucis, flexor digitorum brevis, flexor hallucis brevis, the first lumbrical, quadratus plantae, flexor digiti minimi, adductor hallucis, the interossei, three lumbricals, and abductor digiti minimi.	Varies according to muscle

Autonomic Nerves

The autonomic nervous system (ANS) is the division of the peripheral nervous system that affects heart rate, digestion, respiration rate, salivation, perspiration, diameter of the pupils, micturition (urination), and sexual arousal (Figure 3-9). The ANS has two components: sympathetic and parasympathetic, each of which is differentiated by its site of origin as well as the transmitters it releases.[5] In general, these two systems have antagonist effects on their end organs.

- *Sympathetic:* General action is to mobilize the body's resources under stress, to induce the "flight-or-fight" response. An example of an aberrant sympathetic reaction is complex regional pain syndrome, an unusual cause of paresthesias, pain, and autonomic dysfunction that can occur after minor soft tissue injuries or fractures and usually affects the distal extremities.[6]
- *Parasympathetic:* Actions can be summarized as "rest and digest." A parasympathetic imbalance can result in a decrease in pulse and breathing rates and an increase in tear and salivation production.

Transmission of Pain

The nociceptive (pain) system is normally a dormant system requiring strong, intense, potentially damaging stimulation before it becomes activated.[7] Any tissue that contains free nerve endings involved with nociception is capable of being a source of pain. Nociceptor stimulation can only occur in one of three ways:[8]

1. Mechanical deformation resulting in the application of sufficient mechanical forces to stress, deform, or damage a structure
2. Excessive heat or cold
3. The presence of chemical irritants in sufficient quantities or concentrations (bradykinin, serotonin, histamine, potassium ions, protons, prostaglandins, leukotrienes, cytokines, and growth factors)[9]

Specific peripheral nerve fibers (A-delta and C) carry information regarding the state of the body to the posterior horn of the spinal cord. Some of these fibers react only to painfully intense (noxious) stimuli, whereas others do not differentiate noxious from non-noxious stimuli.

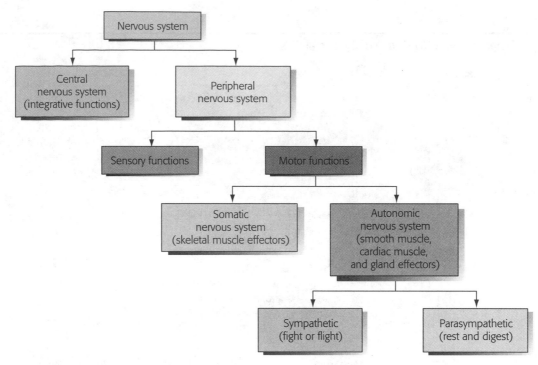

Figure 3-9 The ANS and its relation to the other components of the nervous system.

Three major mechanism are involved in the suppression of pain:

- *Gate control:* Although largely discounted in the literature, the gate control theory continues to be used clinically to explain the control of pain. The theory proposes that the large-diameter nerve fibers that carry information about touch, pressure, and vibration and the smaller nerve fibers that carry information about pain meet at two places in the posterior horn of the spinal cord: the "transmission" (T) cells and the inhibitory cells. Both the large fiber signals and the small fiber signals excite the T cells, and when the output of the T cells exceeds a critical level, pain is felt. The T cells are the gate for pain, and inhibitory cells can shut the gate.
- *Endogenous opiate control:* When sensory nerves are subjected to certain types of stimulation, enkephalin may be released from local sites within the CNS and β-endorphin may be released from the pituitary gland into the cerebrospinal fluid.[10–12] Enkephalin and β-endorphin bind to the body's opioid receptors and are considered the body's natural pain killers.
- *Central biasing:* Intense stimulation, approaching a noxious level, of the smaller C or pain fibers produces a stimulation of the descending neurons, which results in an inhibition of pain.

Over the last decade, researchers have begun to investigate the influence of pain on patterns of neuromuscular activation and control.[7] It has been suggested that the presence of pain leads to inhibition or delayed activation of muscles or muscle groups that perform key synergistic functions to limit unwanted motion.[13] This inhibition usually occurs in deep muscles—local to the involved joint—that perform a synergistic function in order to control joint stability.[14–16] It is now also becoming apparent that in addition to being influenced by pain, motor activity and emotional state can, in turn, influence pain perception.[7,17]

Clinical Implications of the Neuromuscular System

It is believed that certain programs for movement patterns are inherent in the CNS, and that these naturally develop during the maturation process of the CNS. For example, gait is an inherent motor program (see Chapter 25). Other activities require learning through successful repetition and the formation of a program within the CNS. Once this program is formed, the individual no longer has to concentrate on performing the activity, but can do so with very little cortical involvement. A patient cannot succeed in functional and recreational activities if his or her neuromuscular system is not prepared to meet the demands of the specific activities.[18] A motor program that is particularly important is that of postural stability—the ability to maintain a stable upright stance against internal and external perturbations. The key components involved in postural stability are proprioception, kinesthesia, neuromuscular control, and balance (see Chapter 11). The visual system, which involves CN II, III, IV, and VI, assists in balance control by providing input about the position of the head or the body in space. Proprioception occurs at rest, sensing the position of a limb, while kinesthesia is the perception of motion.[19,20] Reflexes are also important to motor control and motor learning.

A reflex is a subconscious, programmed unit of behavior in which a certain type of stimulus from a receptor automatically leads to the response of an effector. Reflexes can be controlled by spinal or supraspinal (brain stem) pathways. The stretch reflex (myotatic or deep tendon) is an example of a spinal reflex. The stretch reflex is a preprogrammed response by the body to a stretch stimulus in the muscle (Figure 3-10). When a muscle spindle (refer to Box 3-1) is stretched, an impulse is immediately sent to the spinal cord and a response to contract the muscle is received (Figure 3-11). Because the impulse

only has to go to the spinal cord and back, not all the way to the brain, it is a very quick impulse. It generally occurs in 1–2 milliseconds. This is designed as a protective measure for the muscles, to prevent tearing. At the same time, the stretch reflex has an inhibitory aspect to the antagonist muscles. When the stretch reflex is activated the impulse is sent from the stretched muscle spindle and the motor neuron is split so that the signal to contract can be sent to the stretched muscle, while a signal to relax can be sent to the antagonist muscles. The stretch reflex is very important in posture. It helps maintain proper posturing because a slight lean to either side causes a stretch in the spinal, hip, and leg muscles to the other side, which is quickly countered by the stretch reflex in a constant process of adjustment and maintenance.

● **Key Point** In contrast to muscle spindles, which are sensitive to changes in muscle length, Golgi tendon organs (GTO) detect and respond to changes in muscle tension that are caused by passive stretch or muscular contraction.

Lesions of the Nervous System

As with all neuromusculoskeletal structures, the nervous system is prone to injury through trauma or

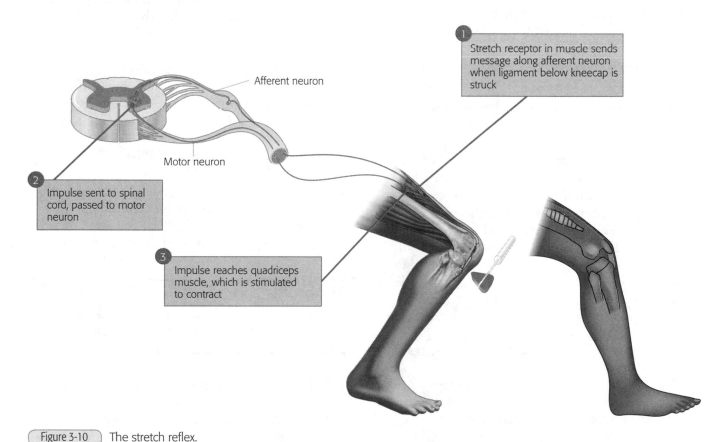

1. Stretch receptor in muscle sends message along afferent neuron when ligament below kneecap is struck

Afferent neuron

Motor neuron

2. Impulse sent to spinal cord, passed to motor neuron

3. Impulse reaches quadriceps muscle, which is stimulated to contract

Figure 3-10   The stretch reflex.

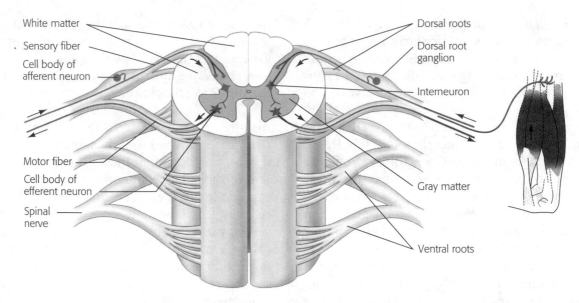

White matter
Sensory fiber
Cell body of afferent neuron
Motor fiber
Cell body of efferent neuron
Spinal nerve

Dorsal roots
Dorsal root ganglion
Interneuron
Gray matter
Ventral roots

Figure 3-11 The muscle spindle and golgi tendon organ.

disease. The resultant signs and symptoms depend on the location and extent of the injury.

Upper Motor Neuron Lesion

Upper motor neurons (UMN) are located in the white columns of the spinal cord and the cerebral hemispheres. An upper motor neuron lesion is a lesion of the neural pathway above the anterior horn cell or motor nuclei of the cranial nerves. It is important that the PTA be aware of the signs and symptoms associated with UMN lesions because they can constitute a medical emergency. A UMN lesion can be characterized by:

- *Nystagmus:* An involuntary loss of control of the conjugate movement of the eyes (about one or more axes).
- *Dysphasia:* A problem with vocabulary that results from a cerebral lesion in the speech areas of the frontal or temporal lobes.
- *Ataxia:* Often most marked in the extremities. In the lower extremities, it is characterized by the so-called drunken-sailor gait pattern, with the patient veering from one side to the other and having a tendency to fall toward the side of the lesion. Ataxia of the upper extremities is characterized by a loss of accuracy in reaching for, or placing, objects. Although ataxia can have a number of causes, it generally suggests CNS disturbance.
- *Spasticity:* A motor disorder characterized by a velocity-dependent increase (resistance increases with velocity) in tonic stretch reflexes with exaggerated tendon jerks.[21–23]

> ● **Key Point** Spasticity can occur as a result of a new or enlarged CNS lesion, a genitourinary tract dysfunction (e.g., infection, obstruction) and/or gastrointestinal disorder (e.g., bowel impaction, hemorrhoids), venous thrombosis, fracture, muscle strain, or pressure ulcers in those patients who already have a UMN lesion.

- *Vertical diplopia:* A patient report of "double vision" or seeing two images, one atop or diagonally displaced from the other.[24]
- *Dysphonia:* Presents as a hoarseness of the voice. Usually, no pain is reported. Painless dysphonia is a common symptom of a condition called Wallenberg's syndrome (difficulty with swallowing, speaking, or both, caused by interrupted blood supply to parts of the brain).[25]
- *Hemianopia:* This finding, a loss in half of the visual field, is always bilateral.
- *Ptosis:* A pathologic depression of the superior eyelid such that it covers part of the pupil.
- *Miosis:* The inability to dilate the pupil. It is one of the symptoms of Horner's syndrome.

> ● **Key Point** The symptoms of Horner's syndrome include miosis, ptosis, exophthalmos, facial reddening, and anhydrosis. If Horner's syndrome is suspected, the patient should immediately be returned or referred to a physician for further examination and not treated again until the cause is found to be relatively benign.

- *Dysarthria:* A previously undiagnosed change in articulation.
- *Aphasia:* An acquired language disorder in which there is an impairment of any language

TABLE 3-7	Types of Aphasia	

Type	Description
Nonfluent aphasia (Broca's aphasia, motor aphasia, expressive aphasia)	Speech is typically awkward, restricted, and produced with effort.
Fluent aphasia (Wernicke's aphasia, receptive aphasia)	Spontaneous speech is preserved but auditory comprehension is impaired. Despite the fluency, the speech is full of emptiness and gibberish jargon, which may include invented words known as neologisms.
Conduction aphasia	Language output is fluent, but naming and repetition are impaired. Hesitations and word-finding pauses are frequent.
Global aphasia	Marked impairment in the comprehension and production of language, with deficits in repeating, naming, understanding, and producing fluent speech.
Transcortical aphasia	Patients can repeat what they hear, but they have difficulty naming or producing spontaneous speech or understanding spoken speech.
Anomic aphasia	Patients present with fluent speech, intact or mostly intact repetition, and an inability to name things.

modality. This may include difficulty in producing or comprehending spoken or written language (**Table 3-7**).

- *Apraxia:* A disorder caused by damage to specific areas of the cerebrum, characterized by loss of the ability to execute or carry out learned purposeful movements
- *Perceptual dysfunction:* A compromised ability to attain awareness or understanding of sensory information.
- *Visual-spatial deficits:* Visual-spatial deficits manifested as poor visual recall, faulty space perceptions, poor sense of directionality, and poor comprehension of visually presented material.
- Examples include cerebrovascular accident (CVA), spinal cord injury (SCI), traumatic brain injury (TBI), and Parkinson's.

Lower Motor Neuron Lesion

A lower motor neuron (LMN) lesion affects nerve fibers traveling from the anterior horn of the spinal cord to the relevant muscle(s). The characteristics of an LMN lesion include muscle weakness or paralysis with atrophy and hypotonus, diminished or absent deep tendon reflex of the areas served by a spinal nerve root or a peripheral nerve, and absence of pathologic signs or reflexes. These lesions can be the result of direct trauma, toxins, infections, ischemia, compression, or from a congenital or acquired nervous system pathology. Examples of LMN pathology include:

- Guillain-Barré syndrome

- Cauda equina syndrome
- Bell's palsy

Peripheral Nerve Entrapment Syndromes

The majority of peripheral nerve entrapments result from chronic injury to the nerve layers along their various routes; the compression usually is between ligamentous, muscular, or bony surfaces. Although peripheral nerve entrapments are more common in the upper extremities, particularly in the forearm and wrist, they also occur in the lower extremities. The consequences of nerve compression are ischemia and disruption of the nerve fiber (**Table 3-8** and **Table 3-9**).

Neurovascular Healing

Neuriums (the nerve coverings) provide a framework for support of the nerve; they facilitate sliding of the nerve and provide a protective barrier. The area surrounding nerves is drained by the body's lymphatic system, and the nerve itself has a blood and nerve barrier to prevent foreign substances from invading the nerve. However, there is no lymphatic system inside the blood–nerve barrier, resulting in poor drainage. Due to the presence of mast cells in the epineurium, there is a potential for nerve repair, but because neurons are incapable of dividing and migrating, regeneration occurs only through existing neurons. Nerve growth is dependent upon several factors including the health of tissue, the state of the nerve and nerve sheath, and the region of the injury. On average, nerves regenerate at a rate of 1 to 3 millimeters per day.

Cord and Nerve	Level of Injury	Motor Loss	Cutaneous Loss
Posterior cord: Radial nerve (C5–T1)	Plexus: proximal to axillary nerve	All muscles innervated by radial nerve All muscles innervated by axillary nerve	Throughout the radial and axillary distribution
	Axilla (brachio-axillary angle)	Triceps (medial and lateral heads), anconeus	Posterior brachial cutaneous
	Spiral groove	All muscles innervated by radial nerve except medial head of triceps	Posterior antebrachial cutaneous
	Proximal to lateral epicondyle	Brachialis, brachioradialis, ECRL, ECRB	None
	Arcade of Frohse	Supinator, all muscles innervated by the posterior interosseous nerve	Superficial radial (Wartenberg's syndrome)
Posterior cord: Axillary nerve (C5–C6)	Axilla (quadrangular space)	Teres minor, deltoid	Lateral arm
Medial and lateral cord: Median nerve (C5–T1)	Plexus (proximal to the joining of the medial and lateral cords): thoracic outlet syndrome	All muscles innervated by the median, musculocutaneous, and ulnar nerves	Throughout the median, musculocutaneous, and ulnar distributions
	Ligament of Struthers: proximal to medial epicondyle	Pronator teres	None
	Cubital fossa exit: between the two heads of the pronator teres	Pronator teres, FCR, FDS, PL, lumbricales I and II	None
	Forearm	Anterior interosseous: FDP (I and II), FPL, PQ	Palmar branch: radial half of thumb
		Median muscular branch: thenar muscles (APB, FPB, OP), lumbricales I and II	Digital branch: Dorsal tips of thumb, index, and middle fingers, and radial half of ring finger
Lateral: Musculo-cutaneous nerve (C5–C7)	Coracobrachialis	Coracobrachialis Biceps Brachialis	None
	Elbow	None	Lateral antebrachial cutaneous nerve: lateral forearm
Medial: Ulnar nerve (C8–T1)	Cubital tunnel	FCU, FDP, adductor pollicis, lumbricales, and interossei	Dorsal and palmar aspects on the ulnar side of the hand
	Between the two heads of the FCU	FDP, FCU	None
	Proximal to wrist	Deep branch: all hand muscles innervated by the ulnar nerve Superficial branch: palmaris brevis	Dorsal cutaneous: medial aspect of ring and little fingers, dorsum of hand Dorsal digital: DIP aspect of little finger, PIP aspect of ring and middle fingers Palmar cutaneous: medial third of palm
	Guyon canal	Muscles of the hypothenar eminence (hand of benediction), interossei	Ulnar aspect of the hand

ECRL, extensor carpi radialis longus; ECRB, extensor carpi radialis brevis; FCR, flexor carpi radialis; FDS, flexor digitorum superficialis; PL, palmaris longus; FDP, flexor digitorum profundus; FPL, flexor pollicis longus; PQ, pronator quadratus; APB, abductor pollicis brevis; FPB, flexor pollicis brevis; OP, opponens pollicis; FCU, flexor carpi ulnaris; DIP, distal interphalangeal; PIP, proximal interphalangeal.

TABLE
3-9

Peripheral Nerve Entrapment Syndromes of the Lower Extremity

Nerve Involved	Mechanism/Entrapment Site
Iliohypogastric nerve	Rarely injured in isolation.
	The most common causes of injury are surgical procedures
	Sports injuries such as trauma or muscle tears of the lower abdominal muscles also may result in injury to the nerve
	Occurs on rare occasion during pregnancy (idiopathic iliohypogastric syndrome) due to the rapidly expanding abdomen in the third trimester
Ilioinguinal nerve	Lower abdominal incisions
	Pregnancy
	Iliac bone harvesting
	Idiopathically
Genitofemoral nerve	Hernia repair, appendectomy, biopsies, and cesarean delivery.
	Intrapelvic trauma to the posterior abdominal wall, retroperitoneal hematoma, pregnancy, or trauma to the inguinal ligament; fortunately, injury to this nerve is rare
Lateral femoral cutaneous nerve (meralgia paresthetica)	*Intrapelvic causes:* Pregnancy, abdominal tumors, uterine fibroids, diverticulitis, or appendicitis
	Extrapelvic causes: Trauma to the region of the anterior superior iliac spine (ASIS) (e.g., a seatbelt from a motor vehicle accident), tight garments, belts, girdles, or stretch from obesity and ascites
	Mechanical causes: Prolonged sitting or standing and pelvic tilt from leg length discrepancy
	Diabetes: In isolation or in the clinical setting of a polyneuropathy
Sciatic nerve (piriformis syndrome)	Multiple etiologies have been proposed to explain the compression or irritation of the sciatic nerve that occurs with the piriformis syndrome:
	• Hypertrophy of the piriformis muscle.
	• Trauma, direct or indirect, to the sacroiliac or gluteal region can lead to piriformis syndrome and is a result of hematoma formation and subsequent scarring between the sciatic nerve and the short external rotators.
	• A flexion contracture at the hip has been associated with piriformis syndrome. This flexion contracture increases the lumbar lordosis, which increases the tension in the pelvic–femoral muscles as these muscles try to stabilize the pelvis and spine in the new position. This increased tension causes the involved muscles to hypertrophy with no corresponding increase in the size of the bony foramina, resulting in neurological signs of sciatic compression.
	• Females are more commonly affected by piriformis syndrome, with as much as a 6:1 female-to-male incidence.
	• Ischial bursitis.
	• Pseudoaneurysm of the inferior gluteal artery.
	• Excessive exercise to the hamstring muscles.
	• Inflammation and spasm of the piriformis muscle, often in association with trauma, infection, and anatomical variations of the muscle.
	• Local anatomical anomalies may contribute to the likelihood that symptoms will develop.
Femoral nerve	Diabetic amyotrophy
	Trauma such as gunshots, knife wounds, glass shards, or needle puncture in some medical procedures
	Pelvic fractures and acute hyperextension of the thigh may also cause an isolated femoral nerve injury

(continued)

Nerve Involved	Mechanism/Entrapment Site
Saphenous nerve	Inflammation from a sharp angulation of the nerve through the connective tissue at the roof of Hunter canal
	Dynamic forces of the muscles in this region resulting in contraction and relaxation of the fibrous tissue that impinges the nerve
Tibial nerve (entrapment in the popliteal fossa)	Usually caused by an enlarged Baker's cyst (which may also compress the common peroneal and sural nerves)
	Proliferation of the synovial tissue in patients with rheumatoid arthritis
Posterior tibial nerve (entrapment in the tarsal tunnel)	Compression of the nerve behind the medial malleolus

Nerve Injury Classification

Nerve injuries can be classified using the Seddon/Sunderland categories as follows:

- A *first-degree injury* (neuropraxia) involves a temporary conduction block with demyelination of the nerve at the site of injury. Once the nerve has remyelinated at that area, complete recovery occurs. Recovery may take up to 12 weeks. Most carpal or tarsal tunnel injuries are classified as this.
- A *second-degree injury* (axonotmesis) results from a more severe trauma or compression. This causes Wallerian degeneration* distal to the level of injury and proximal axonal degeneration to at least the next node of Ranvier. In more severe traumatic injuries, the proximal degeneration may extend beyond the next node of Ranvier. The endoneurium remains intact, and, therefore, recovery is complete with axons reinnervating their original motor and sensory targets.
- A *third-degree injury* was introduced by Sunderland to describe an injury more severe than second-degree injury. Similar to a second-degree injury, Wallerian degeneration occurs. However, with the increased severity of the injury, the endoneurium is not intact, and regenerating axons therefore may not reinnervate their original motor and sensory targets.
- A *fourth-degree injury* results in a large area of scar at the site of nerve injury and precludes any

axons from advancing distal to the level of nerve injury. No improvement in function is noted, and the patient requires surgery to restore neural continuity, thus permitting axonal regeneration and motor and sensory reinnervation.

- A *fifth-degree injury* is a complete transection (neurotmesis) of the nerve. Similar to a fourth-degree injury, it requires surgery to restore neural continuity.
- A *sixth-degree injury* was introduced by Mackinnon to describe a mixed nerve injury that combines the other degrees of injury. This commonly occurs when some fascicles of the nerve are working normally while other fascicles may be recovering, and other fascicles may require surgical intervention to permit regeneration.

Implications for the PTA

The conservative intervention for mild cases of peripheral nerve injury typically includes protection of the joints including the surrounding ligaments and tendons, activity modification, and passive range of motion. Splints, slings, or both (as appropriate) may be prescribed. For example, a radial nerve injury results in a loss of wrist and finger extension, and wrist drop. A wrist-resting splint may be used to support the hand in a neutral wrist position and place the hand in a more functional position. In patients with brachial plexus nerve injuries, particularly when C5–C6 is affected, or in patients who have suffered a stroke, continued downward stress at the glenohumeral joint may cause the glenohumeral joint to subluxate without the muscle support of the rotator cuff muscles. A sling is helpful to unload this joint, prevent complete shoulder dislocation,

---

*Wallerian degeneration occurs when a nerve fiber is cut or crushed. The part of the axon separated from the neuron's cell nucleus degenerates. This also is known as anterograde degeneration.

and decrease pain. Night splints appear to help to reduce the nocturnal symptoms associated with carpal tunnel syndrome and allow the wrist to rest fully. Splints worn during the day are helpful only if they do not interfere with normal activity. Ergonomic modifications and postural education are important to avoid repetitive motions and sustained positions/postures.

Medical Interventions for Nerve Injury

A number of medical interventions for nerve injury exist, ranging from medication to surgery.

Nerve Repair

With clean sharp injuries to the nerve, a direct repair (neurorrhaphy) is performed. With more crushing or avulsion injuries, the nerve ends are reapproximated so that motor and sensory topography can be realigned. However, if the repair cannot be performed without creating only minimal tension throughout the nerve, nerve grafting is performed. For example, if the median nerve is under tension with a wrist neutral position, a nerve graft is used.

Nerve Graft

In cases in which a gap is present between the proximal and distal end of the nerve, a nerve graft is recommended. Autografts are used in addition to direct adherence of the nerve. The use of a donor nerve results in a sensory loss in the distribution of the donor nerve. This area of sensory loss becomes smaller over 1–3 years with collateral sprouting from the surrounding sensory nerves. In cases in which a large nerve gap is present, the most common autograft for peripheral nerve repair, the sural nerve, is used due to the large length of nerve graft material that can be obtained. For shorter nerve gaps, the anterior branch of the medial antebrachial cutaneous (MABC) nerve is used because the donor site scar is minimal and the resultant sensory loss is on the anterior aspect of the forearm. Other nerves that can be used are the lateral femoral cutaneous nerve of the thigh and the superficial radial sensory nerve.

Nerve Transfer

The concept of a nerve-to-nerve transfer permits a normal neighboring noncritical nerve to be attached to the distal end of the injured nerve. This is particularly useful in cases in which a large nerve gap is present and/or for proximal nerve injuries.

Implications for the PTA

Following surgical repair, the initial goals of therapy are to regain passive range of motion of the joints and soft tissues that have been immobilized. The patient should be instructed in exercises to maintain strength in the unaffected muscles. The patient must adhere to specific protocols. In the later stages of therapy, sensory and motor re-education is recommended to maximize the outcome.

Neurological Testing in Orthopaedics

The PT evaluates the transmission capability of the nervous system to rule out the presence of either an upper motor neuron (UMN) lesion or a lower motor neuron (LMN) lesion. In addition, the neurological examination can often determine the exact site of the lesion.

The examination begins when the PT establishes essential facts about the patient beginning with the chief complaint and continuing through a full, logical sequence of the patient's history of the present illness.[26,27] This is supplemented with a history of past medical disorders, a review of systems, family history, and social history. The neurologic examination is supplemented by a general physical examination to look for medical disorders responsible for all of the contributing factors to the presenting problem.

Deep Tendon Reflex

The PT examines the deep tendon reflex (Figure 3-12) to help determine whether an LMN lesion (hyporeflexive response) or UMN lesion (hyperreflexive response) is present. Deep tendon reflexes may be graded as follows:

0   absent (areflexia)
1+   decreased (hyporeflexia)
2+   normal
3+   hyperactive (brisk)
4+   hyperactive with clonus (hyperreflexive)

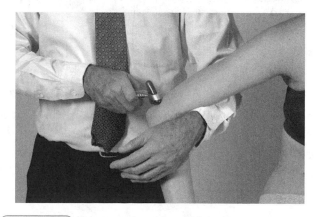

Figure 3-12   Deep tendon reflex testing.

Pathologic Reflexes

Pathologic reflexes involve abnormal or inappropriate motor responses to a controlled stimulus initiated in the sensory organ that is appropriate to the reflex arc. The most important of the pathological reflexes is the Babinski response, which is a superficial reflex that is elicited in the same manner as the plantar response (**Table 3-10**). The Babinski is a primitive withdrawal response that is normal for the first few months of life but is then suppressed by supraspinal activity. Damage to the descending tracts from the brain (either above the foramen magnum or in the spinal cord) promotes a return of this primitive protective reflex, while at the same time abolishing the normal plantar response. The appearance of this reflex therefore suggests the presence of an upper motor neuron lesion.

> ● **Key Point** The Hoffmann sign is the upper limb equivalent of the Babinski. Other pathologic reflexes include the Oppenheimer and clonus—a series of involuntary muscular contractions due to sudden stretching of a muscle.

Sensory Testing

The posterior (dorsal) roots of the spinal nerves are represented by restricted peripheral sensory regions called dermatomes (refer to Figure 3-4). The peripheral sensory nerves are represented by more distinct and circumscribed areas. Sensory testing is performed by the PT throughout the dermatomal areas. For patients with no apparent neurologic symptoms or signs, an abbreviated examination may be substituted by the PT. There are two components to the dermatome tests:

- *Light touch:* Light touch tests for hypoesthesia (decreased sensation) throughout the dermatome. If the light touch test is positive (an area of hypoesthesia is detected), the areas of reduced sensation are mapped out in more detail.[28]
- *Pinprick:* The pinprick test examines for near anesthesia in the autonomous, no-overlap area of a dermatome. When investigating an area of cutaneous sensory loss, it is recommended that the PT begin the pinprick test in the area of anesthesia and work outward until the border of normal sensation is located. The PT stimulates in the aforementioned patterns and asks the patient "Is this sharp or dull?" or, when making comparisons using the sharp stimulus, "Does this feel the same as this?"

A full examination of the sensory system can involve tests for the following:

- *Temperature:* Using two test tubes, filled with hot and cold water, the PT touches the skin and asks the patient to identify "hot" or "cold."
- *Pressure:* Firm pressure is applied to the patient's muscle belly.

TABLE 3-10 Pathological Reflexes

Reflex	Elicitation	Positive Response	Pathology
Babinski	Stroking of lateral aspect of side of foot	Extension of big toe and fanning of four small toes Normal reaction in newborns	Pyramidal tract lesion Organic hemiplegia
Chaddock's	Stroking of lateral side of foot beneath lateral malleolus	Same response as above	Pyramidal tract lesion
Oppenheim's	Stroking of anteromedial tibial surface	Same response as above	Pyramidal tract lesion
Gordon's	Squeezing of calf muscles firmly	Same response as above	Pyramidal tract lesion
Brudzinski's	Passive flexion of one lower limb	Similar movement occurs in opposite limb	Meningitis
Hoffmann's	"Flicking" of terminal phalanx of index, middle, or ring finger	Reflex flexion of distal phalanx of thumb and of distal phalanx of index or middle finger (whichever one was not flicked)	Increased irritability of sensory nerves in tetany Pyramidal tract lesion
Lhermitte's	Neck flexion	An electric shock-like sensation that radiates down the spinal column into the upper or lower limbs	Abnormalities (demyelination) in the posterior part of the cervical spinal cord

- *Vibration:* Using a relatively low-pitched tuning fork, preferably of 128 Hz, the PT taps the fork on the heel of his or her hand and places it firmly over a bony process of the patient, such as the malleoli, patellae, epicondyles, vertebral spinous processes, and iliac crest. The patient is asked what he or she feels and, to be certain, is asked to inform the PT when the vibration stops. The PT then touches the fork to stop the vibration. At this point, the patient should indicate that the vibration has stopped. If vibration sense is absent, the PT should retest, moving proximally along the extremity.

> ● **Key Point**   The posterior (dorsal) medial lemniscus tract conveys impulses concerned with well-localized touch and with the sense of movement and position (kinesthesia). It is important in moment-to-moment (temporal) and point-to-point (spatial) discrimination and makes it possible for a person to put a key in a door lock without light or to visualize the position of any part of his or her body without looking.

- *Proprioception:* The patient is tested for the ability to perceive passive movements of the extremities, especially the distal portions. The PT grasps the involved extremity and moves it into a specific position, and then asks the patient to move the uninvolved extremity into the same position.
- *Movement sense (kinesthesia):* The patient is asked to indicate verbally the direction of movement while the extremity is in motion. The PT must grip the patient's extremity over neutral borders.
- *Stereognosis:* The patient is asked to recognize, through touch alone, a variety of small objects, such as a comb, a coin, a pencil, or a safety pin, that are placed in his or her hand.
- *Graphesthesia:* The patient is asked to recognize letters, numbers, or designs traced on the skin. Using a blunt object, the PT draws an image on the patient's palm, asking the patient to identify the number, letter, or design.
- *Two-point discrimination:* A measure is taken of the smallest distance between two stimuli that can still be perceived by the patient as two distinct stimuli.
- *Equilibrium reactions:* The patient's ability to maintain balance in response to alterations in the body's center of gravity and base of support is tested.
- *Protective reactions:* This tests the patient's ability to stabilize and support the body in response

to a displacing stimulus in which the center of gravity exceeds the base of support (e.g., extension of arms to protect against a fall).

Neuromeningeal Mobility Testing

The neuromeningeal mobility tests examine for the presence of any abnormalities of the dura, both centrally and peripherally. The PT uses these tests if a dural adhesion or nerve irritation is suspected. The tests employ a sequential and progressive stretch to the dura until the patient's symptoms are reproduced (Figure 3-13).[29] Theoretically, if the dura is scarred or inflamed, a lack of extensibility with stretching occurs.

Balance Testing

Good balance requires the dynamic integration of multiple sensory inputs, specifically the visual, somatosensory, and vestibular systems. The PT may decide to perform balance testing if, during the history, the patient described symptoms of dizziness, lightheadedness, a sense of impending faint, or poor balance. Balance can be measured using static or dynamic tests. Static balance analyzes an individual's ability to maintain a stationary position within a base of support. Dynamic balance involves the ability to maintain balance while in motion. The methods for assessing balance range from simple to complex and expensive. Static tests include, but are not limited to:

- *Double-leg stance test (DLST):* The patient stands with feet together, arms by the side, and eyes open. An inability to maintain this

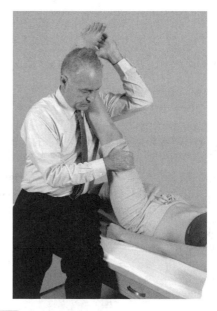

Figure 3-13   Dural stretch of the sciatic nerve using the straight leg raise.

position without swaying or falling is considered a positive test. If this test does not provoke a sway or fall, the patient is asked to repeat the test with their eyes closed.

- *Single-leg stance test (SLST):* This is similar to the DLST except that the patient stands on one leg, first with eyes open and then with eyes closed. This test can be made more challenging by softening the standing surface (using foam padding).
- *Computerized force plate/force platform:* The postural stress test (PST) is designed to measure a patient's ability to maintain balance during a series of progressive and graded destabilizing forces.
- *The reach test:* This test, which can be performed with the patient seated or standing, involves offering the patient a target that is slightly out of reach to test the diagonal component of reaching.[30]

Dynamic balance can be tested using timed agility tests such as the figure-of-eight test,[31,32] carioca or hop test,[33] BESS test for dynamic balance,[34] timed T-band kicks, and timed balance beam walking with eyes open or closed.[35]

Coordination Testing

Coordination is the ability to execute smooth, accurate, controlled motor responses. Efficient motor control includes normal muscle tone and postural response mechanisms, selective movement, and coordination. Abnormalities of coordination are common in motor system disorders. Coordinated movements are characterized by appropriate speed, distance, direction, timing, and muscular tension. Two of the most common tests for coordination are:

- *Finger-nose-finger movements:* The PT holds a finger about 1 meter from the patient's face and asks the patient to use an index finger to touch it repeatedly while alternately touching the nose (Figure 3-14).
- *Heel-knee-shin test:* The patient is positioned in supine, and asked to place the heel of one foot on the knee of the opposite leg and run the heel down the shin across the dorsum of the foot to the great toe.
- *Pronation-supination test:* The patient is positioned in sitting with the arms by the side and the elbows flexed to approximately 90 degrees. The patient is asked to rapidly perform supination and pronation of the forearms.

- *Dorsiflexion-supination test:* The patient is positioned in sitting or in supine. The patient is asked to move the ankles rapidly into dorsiflexion/plantarflexion.

If the patient demonstrates difficulties with these tests, a more in-depth assessment is required.

Upper and Lower Quarter Scanning Examination

The scanning examination is used when there is no history to explain a patient's signs and symptoms, or when the signs and symptoms are unexplainable. The clinician must choose which scanning examination to use, based on the presenting signs and symptoms. The upper quarter scanning examination is appropriate for upper thoracic, upper extremity, and cervical problems, whereas the lower quarter scanning examination is typically used for thoracic, lower extremity, and lumbosacral problems.

Upper Quarter Scanning Examination

The following are the items reviewed during the upper quarter scanning exam:

- *Postural assessment:* The patient's posture is observed from the front, back, and the side for evidence of asymmetry.
- *Range of motion:* The patient performs active range of motion of the cervical spine and upper extremities. The clinician applies passive overpressure at the end of the available active range of motion if the patient does not exhibit signs and symptoms.
- *Resistive testing:* In order to screen the various innervation levels, the following resisted tests are completed: cervical rotation (C1) (Figure 3-15), shoulder elevation (C2–C4) (Figure 3-16), shoulder abduction (C5) (Figure 3-17) or shoulder

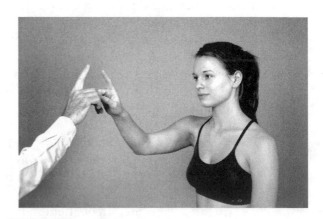

Figure 3-14   Finger to nose test.

external rotation (Figure 3-18), elbow flexion (C5–C6) (Figure 3-19), wrist extension (C6) (Figure 3-20), elbow extension (C7) (Figure 3-21), wrist flexion (C7) (Figure 3-22), thumb extension (C8) (Figure 3-23), and finger adduction (T1) (Figure 3-24).

- *Reflex testing:* Biceps (C5) (Figure 3-25), brachioradialis (C6) (Figure 3-26), and triceps (C7) (refer to Figure 3-12).
- *Dermatomes (Figure 3-4):* Posterior head (C2), posterolateral neck (C3), acromioclavicular joint (C4), lateral arm (C5), lateral forearm and

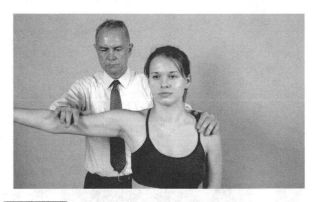

Figure 3-17   Resisted shoulder abduction.

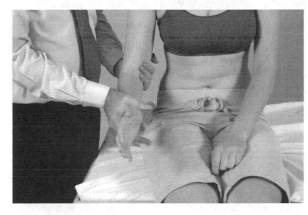

Figure 3-18   Resisted shoulder external rotation.

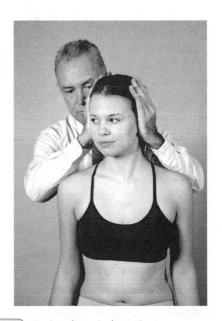

Figure 3-15   Resisted cervical rotation.

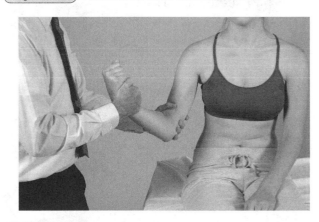

Figure 3-19   Resisted elbow flexion.

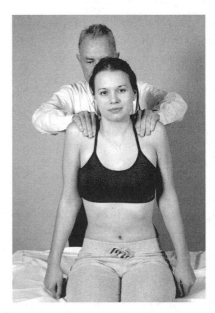

Figure 3-16   Resisted shoulder elevation.

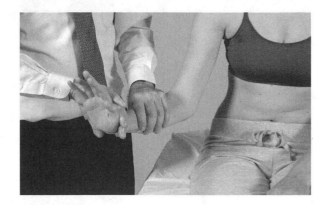

Figure 3-20   Resisted wrist extension.

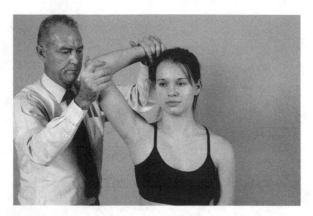

Figure 3-21   Resisted elbow extension.

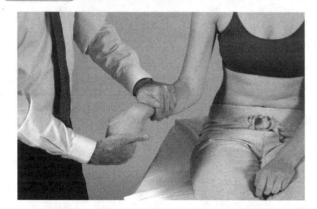

Figure 3-22   Resisted wrist flexion.

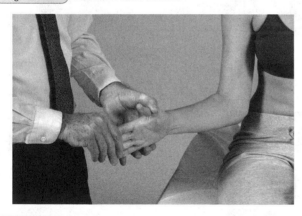

Figure 3-23   Resisted thumb extension.

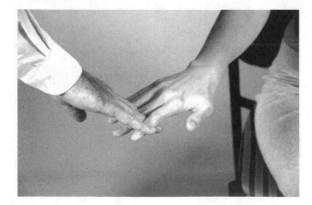

Figure 3-24   Resisted finger adduction.

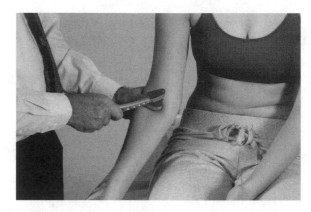

Figure 3-25   Biceps reflex testing.

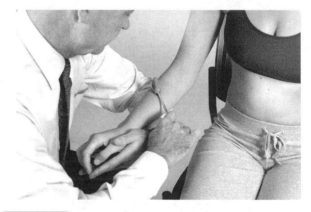

Figure 3-26   Brachioradialis reflex.

thumb (C6), palmar distal phalanx—middle finger (C7), little finger and ulnar border of the hand (C8), and medial forearm (T1).

Lower Quarter Scanning Examination

The following are the items reviewed during the lower quarter scanning exam:

- *Postural assessment:* The patient's posture is observed from the front, back, and the side for evidence of asymmetry.
- *Range of motion:* The patient performs active range of motion of the lumbosacral spine and lower extremities. The clinician applies passive overpressure at the end of the available active range of motion if the patient does not exhibit signs and symptoms.
- *Resistive testing:* In order to screen the various innervation levels, the following resisted tests are completed: heel walking (L4–L5) (Figure 3-27), toe walking (S1) (Figure 3-28), straight leg raise (L4–S1) (refer to Figure 3-13), hip flexion (L1–L2) (Figure 3-29), knee extension (L3–L4) (Figure 3-30), ankle dorsiflexion (L4–L5) (Figure 3-31), and great toe extension (L5) (Figure 3-32).

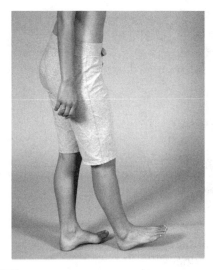

Figure 3-27   Heel walking.

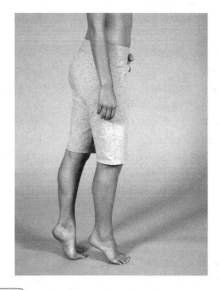

Figure 3-28   Toe walking.

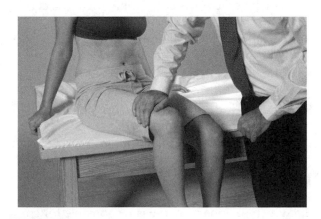

Figure 3-29   Resisted hip flexion.

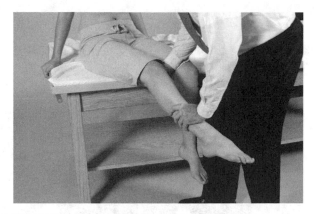

Figure 3-30   Resisted knee extension.

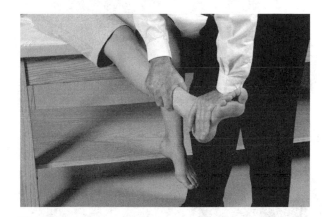

Figure 3-31   Resisted dorsiflexion.

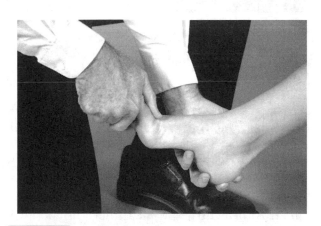

Figure 3-32   Resisted great toe extension.

- *Reflex testing:* Patellar (L4) (Figure 3-33) and Achilles (S1) (Figure 3-34).
- *Dermatomes:* Anterior thigh (L2), middle third of the anterior thigh (L3), patella and medial malleolus (L4), fibular head and dorsum of foot (L5), lateral and plantar aspect of foot (S1), medial aspect of the posterior thigh (S2), and perianal area (S3–S5).

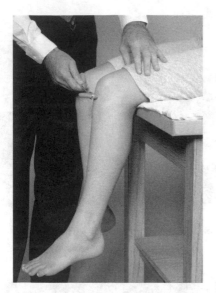

Figure 3-33   Patellar reflex.

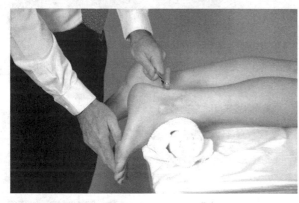

Figure 3-34   Achilles reflex.

Summary

The nervous system of the human body is unique and extremely complex. When operating normally, the nervous system allows for countless skills to be performed, both in the mind and throughout the body. However, given its complexity, the nervous system is prone to failure through either disease or trauma. Although the physical therapist performs the examination and makes note of any irregularity in the physical or nervous system, it is important that the PTA be able to recognize signs and symptoms of neurologic dysfunction that occur after the initial examination. This recognition can only come from a deep understanding of the anatomic structures within the nervous system and their various functions. It is the responsibility of the PTA to alert the PT to any changes that have occurred in the patient that the PTA feels warrants such communication, or communication with the patient's physician.

1. The neuron is composed of which of the following?
   a. Axon
   b. Dendrite
   c. Cell body
   d. All of the above
2. The femoral nerve innervates all but which of the following muscles?
   a. Sartorius
   b. Vastus lateralis
   c. Adductor magnus
   d. Pectineus
3. A patient presents with weak quadriceps muscles with a diagnosis of a lumbar disc herniation. You suspect an L3–L4 problem. What other muscle would you expect to be weak?
   a. Sartorius
   b. Adductor magnus
   c. Biceps femoris
   d. Iliopsoas
4. Which of the following would you expect to find in a patient diagnosed with carpal tunnel syndrome (compression of the median nerve under the transverse carpal ligament of the wrist)?
   a. Tingling in the ulnar side of the hand and reports of pain in the hand with rest
   b. Tingling in the radial side of the hand and pain in the hand at night
   c. A loss of peripheral vision
   d. Pain with elbow extension
5. How many pairs of spinal nerves are there?
   a. 32
   b. 31
   c. 33
   d. 24
6. Which nerve roots commonly form the cervical plexus?
7. Which nerve roots commonly form the brachial plexus?
8. Which two cranial nerves have distributions in other regions than just the head and neck?
9. Which nerve innervates the sternocleidomastoid and the trapezius muscles?
10. Which cord of the brachial plexus supplies the radial nerve?
11. What three arm muscles does the musculocutaneous nerve supply?
12. Which peripheral nerve is responsible for stimulating the muscles that produce dorsiflexion?

13. Which peripheral nerve can be trapped in the arcade of Frohse?
14. Which peripheral nerve can be trapped between the two heads of the pronator teres?
15. Which peripheral nerve can be trapped by the ligament of Struthers?
16. Atrophy of the hypothenar eminence could indicate a lesion to which nerve?
17. Which muscles does the suprascapular nerve innervate?
18. Which nerve innervates the serratus anterior?
19. Which nerve innervates the latissimus dorsi muscle?
20. Which muscles are innervated by the superior gluteal nerve?
21. A herniated disc between the C6 and C7 vertebral levels could impinge upon which nerve root level?
22. Injury to the radial nerve in the spiral groove would result in weakness of which group of muscles?
23. Which of the following muscles is not innervated by the median nerve?
    a. Abductor pollicis brevis
    b. Flexor pollicis longus
    c. Medial heads of flexor digitorum profundus
    d. Superficial head of flexor pollicis brevis
    e. Pronator quadratus
24. Name the nerve that innervates the first lumbrical muscle in the hand.
25. A patient presents with a burning sensation in the anterolateral aspect of the thigh. Dysfunction of which nerve could lead to these symptoms?
    a. Lateral cutaneous (femoral) nerve of the thigh
    b. Femoral
    c. Obturator
    d. Genitofemoral
    e. Ilioinguinal
26. The saphenous nerve supplies cutaneous sensation to the medial aspect of the leg. From which nerve does the saphenous nerve arise?
    a. Obturator.
    b. Deep fibular (peroneal).
    c. Sciatic.
    d. Femoral.
    e. The saphenous nerve arises as a direct branch from the sacral plexus.
27. An injury to the deep branch of the peroneal nerve would result in a sensory deficit to which of the following locations?
    a. Medial side of the foot
    b. Lateral side of the foot

c. Lateral one and one half toes
d. Medial border of the sole of the foot
e. Adjacent dorsal surfaces of the first and second toes

28. Which of the following flexor muscles is not innervated by the median nerve?
    a. Flexor carpi radialis
    b. Flexor carpi ulnaris
    c. Palmaris longus
    d. Flexor digitorum superficialis
    e. Flexor pollicis longus
29. Which two muscles does the anterior interosseous branch of the median nerve innervate?
30. A birth injury that results in injury to the lower portion of the brachial plexus is referred to as:
    a. Bell's palsy
    b. Erb's paralysis
    c. Klumpke's paralysis
    d. Saturday night palsy
    e. Tinel's sign
31. All of the following features may be found in muscle spindles except:
    a. They require a change in length as well as in the rate of change in order to fire.
    b. They demonstrate two kinds of intra-fusal fibers, nuclear bag and nuclear chain fibers.
    c. They are arranged in parallel with the extra-fusal fibers of the muscle itself.
    d. They are innervated by one very large type Ia fiber that serves both fiber types.
32. The perception of the position of the extremities in space is often referred to as:
    a. Depth perception
    b. Spatial discrimination
    c. Paresthesias
    d. Proprioception
33. All of the following are examples of the simple stretch reflex, except:
    a. Knee-jerk reflex
    b. Monosynaptic reflex
    c. Myotatic reflex
    d. Flexor withdrawal reflex
34. A physical therapist assistant working with a patient who has a lower motor neuron injury would expect the patient to present with:
    a. Flaccidity
    b. A positive Babinski reflex
    c. Clonus
    d. Extensor muscle spasms

35. A physical therapist assistant working with a patient who has an upper motor neuron injury would expect the patient to present with:

a. Flaccidity

b. A positive Babinski reflex

c. Clonus

d. B and C

References

1. Waxman SG: Correlative Neuroanatomy (ed 24). New York, McGraw-Hill, 1996

2. Mannheimer JS, Lampe GN: Clinical Transcutaneous Electrical Nerve Stimulation. Philadelphia, FA Davis, 1984, pp 440–445

3. Chusid JG: Correlative Neuroanatomy and Functional Neurology (ed 19). Norwalk, CT, Appleton-Century-Crofts, 1985, pp 144–148

4. Jenkins DB: Hollinshead's Functional Anatomy of the Limbs and Back (ed 7). Philadelphia, WB Saunders, 1998

5. Morgenlander JC: The autonomic nervous system, in Gilman S (ed): Clinical Examination of the Nervous System. New York, McGraw-Hill, 2000, pp 213–225

6. McKnight JT, Adcock BB: Paresthesias: A practical diagnostic approach. Am Fam Phys 56:2253–2260, 1997

7. Wright A, Zusman M: Neurophysiology of pain and pain modulation, in Boyling JD, Jull GA (eds): Grieve's Modern Manual Therapy: The Vertebral Column. Philadelphia, Churchill Livingstone, 2004, pp 155–171

8. Bogduk N: The anatomy and physiology of nociception, in Crosbie J, McConnell J (eds): Key Issues in Physiotherapy. Oxford, Butterworth-Heinemann, 1993, pp 48–87

9. Dray A: Inflammatory mediators of pain. Br J Anaesth 75:125–131, 1995

10. Murphy GJ: Utilization of transcutaneous electrical nerve stimulation in managing craniofacial pain. Clin J Pain 6:64–69, 1990

11. Salar G: Effect of transcutaneous electrotherapy on CSF β-endorphin content in patients without pain problems. Pain 10:169–172, 1981

12. Clement-Jones V: Increased endorphin but not metenkephalin levels in human cerebrospinal fluid after acupuncture for recurrent pain. Lancet 8:946–948, 1980

13. Sterling M, Jull G, Wright A: The effect of musculoskeletal pain on motor activity and control. J Pain 2:135–145, 2001

14. Hides JA, Richardson CA, Jull GA: Multifidus muscle recovery is not automatic after resolution of acute, first-episode low back pain. Spine 21:2763–2769, 1996

15. Hodges P, Richardson C: Inefficient muscular stabilisation of the lumbar spine associated with low back pain: A motor control evaluation of transversus abdominis. Spine 21:2640–2650, 1996

16. Voight M, Weider D: Comparative reflex response times of the vastus medialis and the vastus lateralis in normal subjects and subjects with extensor mechanism dysfunction. Am J Sports Med 10:131–137, 1991

17. Dubner R, Ren K: Endogenous mechanisms of sensory modulation. Pain: 6:S45–S53, 1999 (suppl 6)

18. Voight ML, Cook G, Blackburn TA: Functional lower quarter exercises through reactive neuromuscular training, in Bandy WD (ed): Current Trends for the Rehabilitation of the Athlete—Home Study Course. La Crosse, WI, Sports Physical Therapy Section, American Physical Therapy Association, 1997

19. Borsa PA, Lephart SM, Kocher MS, et al: Functional assessment and rehabilitation of shoulder proprioception for glenohumeral instability. J Sport Rehabil 3:84–104, 1994

20. Lephart SM, Warner JJP, Borsa PA, et al: Proprioception of the shoulder joint in healthy, unstable and surgically repaired shoulders. J Shoulder Elbow Surg 3:371–380, 1994

21. Pierrot-Deseilligny E, Mazieres L: Spinal mechanisms underlying spasticity, in Delwaide PJ, Young RR (eds): Clinical Neurophysiology in Spasticity: Contribution to Assessment and Pathophysiology. Amsterdam, Elsevier BV, 1985, pp 63–76

22. Hoppenfeld S: Orthopedic Neurology—A Diagnostic Guide to Neurological Levels, Philadelphia, JB Lippincott, 1977

23. Ashby P, McCrea D: Neurophysiology of spinal spasticity, in Davidoff RA (ed): Handbook of the Spinal Cord. New York, Marcel Decker, 1987, pp 119–143

24. Brazis PW, Lee AG: Binocular vertical diplopia. Mayo Clinic Proc 73:55–66, 1998

25. Chia L-G, Shen W-C: Wallenberg's lateral medullary syndrome with loss of pain and temperature sensation on the contralateral face: Clinical, MRI and electrophysiological studies. J Neurol 240:462–467, 1993

26. Gilman S: The physical and neurologic examination, in Gilman S (ed): Clinical Examination of the Nervous System. New York, McGraw-Hill, 2000, pp 15–34

27. Gilman S: The mental status examination, in Gilman S (ed): Clinical Examination of the Nervous System. New York, McGraw-Hill, 2000, pp 35–64

28. Meadows J: Orthopedic Differential Diagnosis in Physical Therapy. New York, McGraw-Hill, 1999

29. Butler DS: Mobilization of the Nervous System. New York, Churchill Livingstone, 1992

30. Donahoe B, Turner D, Worrell T: The use of functional reach as a measurement of balance in healthy boys and girls aged 5–15. Phys Ther 73:S71, 1993

31. Fisher A, Wietlisbach S, Wilberger J: Adult performance on three tests of equilibrium. Am J Occup Ther 42:30–35, 1988

32. Newton R: Review of tests of standing balance abilities. Brain Inj 3:335–343, 1992

33. Irrgang JJ, Harner C: Recent advances in ACL rehabilitation: Clinical factors. J Sport Rehabil 6:111–124, 1997

34. Trulock SC: A Comparison of Static, Dynamic and Functional Methods of Objective Balance Assessment. Chapel Hill, NC, The University of North Carolina, 1996

35. Guskiewicz KM: Impaired postural stability: Regaining balance, in Prentice WE, Voight ML (eds): Techniques in Musculoskeletal Rehabilitation. New York, McGraw-Hill, 2001, pp 125–150

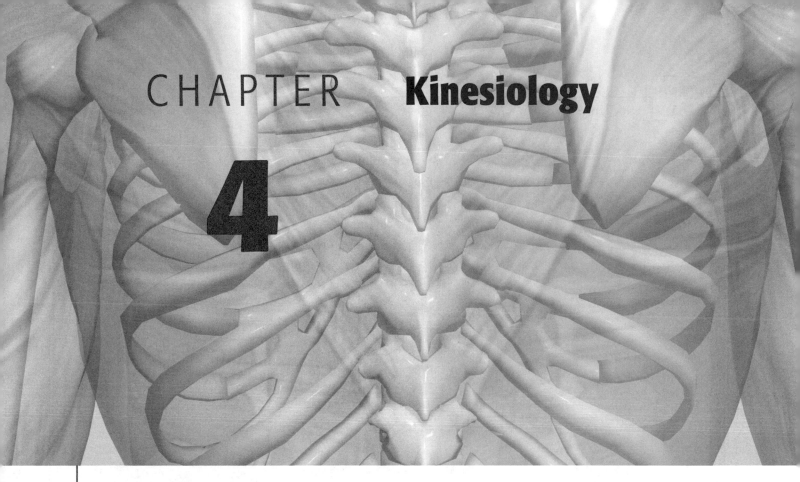

CHAPTER 4   Kinesiology

Chapter Objectives

At the completion of this chapter, the reader will be able to:

1. Give definitions for commonly used biomechanical terms.
2. Describe the various types of loading that can act on the musculoskeletal system.
3. Describe the different planes of the body.
4. Describe the different axes of the body and the motions that occur around them.
5. Describe the different types of levers that exist.
6. Define the terms *osteokinematic motion* and *arthrokinematic motion*.
7. Differentiate between the different types of arthrokinematic motions that can occur at the joint surfaces.
8. Describe the basic biomechanics of joint motion in terms of their concave–convex relationships.
9. Discuss the similarities between range of motion and flexibility and the various factors that determine each.
10. Describe the concept of degrees of freedom.
11. Discuss the differences between open and closed kinematic chain activities and their potential impact on the rehabilitation program.
12. Define the terms *close packed* and *open packed*.

Overview

The word *kinesiology* is derived from the Greek *kinesis*, to move, and *ology*, to study. The science of kinesiology involves the application of mechanical principles in the study of the structure and function of movement. A number of other definitions are worth noting (**Table 4-1**). Most joints in the body are capable of movement, with the synovial joints having the most available range of motion. For the PTA administering rehabilitation programs, a working knowledge of anatomy and kinesiology is essential.

TABLE
4-1
Key Terms Used in Kinesiology

Term	Definition
Biomechanics	The study of the biological and mechanical basis for human motion.
Kinematics	A branch of mechanics that describes the motion of a body in terms of space and time.
Kinetics	The actions or forces applied to the body.
Static	A state of no motion or constant motion.
Dynamic	A state where the motion is changing.
Mass	The quantity of matter composing a body. The mass of an object remains the same wherever it is. Mass influences an object's resistance to a change in linear velocity. The common unit of mass is the kilogram (kg). Weight is measured in units of force such as the Newton.
Force	A push or pull action on an object. Force has both direction and magnitude. Commonly expressed in Newtons (N). *Linear (translatory) motion:* force is applied directly through the center of an object. *Angular (rotational) motion:* force is applied somewhere outside the center of an object. Most forces in the human body cause rotation.
Compression/approximation	A squeezing force.
Tension/traction/distraction	The opposite of a compressive force—a pulling or stretching force.
Pressure	The amount of force acting over a given area.
Weight	The force that a given mass feels because of gravity.
Inertia	The resistance to action or to change. Although inertia has no units of measurement, the amount of inertia a body possesses is directly proportional to its mass.
Center of gravity (COG)	The point around which the weight and mass are equally balanced in all directions. From a kinetic perspective, the location of the COG determines the way in which the body responds to external forces. COG can be referred to as the center of mass (COM), although the COM is technically the mean location of all the mass in a system.
Density	Defined as the mass divided by the volume of an object.
Torque	The measure of a rotary force—when a structure is made to twist about its longitudinal axis, typically when one end of the structure is fixed. The product of force and the perpendicular distance between the line of action for the force and the axis point of rotation (moment arm).
Shear	A force that acts parallel or tangential to a surface.
Displacement	A measure of the change in position of an object. The change in the space of an object from the starting to the ending points.
Translation	When all parts of a body move in the same direction as every other part.
Rotation	The arc of movement of a "body" about an axis of rotation.
Mass moment of inertia	Quantity and distribution of matter in an object. Mass moment of inertia influences an object's resistance to a change in angular velocity.
Distance	Linear or angular displacement.
Velocity	Rate of linear or angular displacement.
Acceleration	Rate of change in linear or angular velocity.
Impulse	The product of the force and the length of time the force was produced.
Momentum	The product of an object's mass and its velocity.
Work	The product of force and the linear displacement of an object.
Power	Rate of linear work.

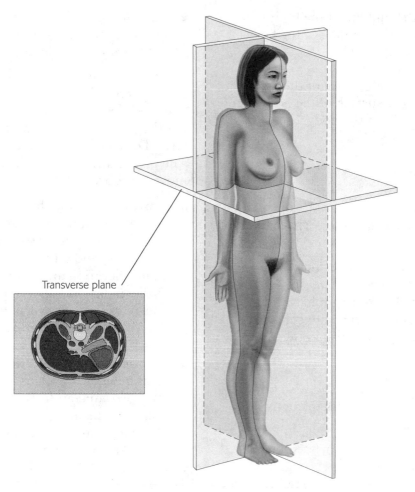

Transverse plane

Figure 4-1 Anatomic position and planes of the body.

To this end, the pertinent anatomy and kinesiology for each of the joints is included in the relevant chapters.

The primary functions of the musculoskeletal system are to transmit forces from one part of the body to another and to protect certain organs (such as the brain) from mechanical forces that could result in damage.[1] The structures involved with human movement include the muscles and tendons, which produce the movement (see Chapter 2); the nervous system, which controls the movement (see Chapter 3); and the joints, around which the movements occur (see Chapter 2).

Anatomic Position

When describing movements, it is necessary to have a starting position. This starting position is referred to as the *anatomic reference position* or *anatomic position*. The anatomic reference position for the

human body is the erect standing position with the feet just slightly separated and the arms hanging by the side, the elbows straight, and the palms of the hands facing forward (Figure 4-1).

Directional Terms

Directional terms are used to describe the relationship of body parts or the location of an external object with respect to the body.[2] The following are commonly used directional terms:

- *Superior or cranial (cephalad):* Closer to the head
- *Inferior or caudal:* Closer to the feet
- *Anterior or ventral:* Toward the front of the body
- *Posterior or dorsal:* Toward the back of the body
- *Midline:* An imaginary line that courses vertically through the center of the body

- *Medial:* Toward the midline of the body
- *Lateral:* Away from the midline of the body
- *Proximal:* Closer to the trunk
- *Distal:* Away from the trunk
- *Superficial:* Toward the surface of the body
- *Deep:* Away from the surface of the body in the direction of the inside of the body

Planes of the Body

There are three cardinal planes of the body corresponding to the three dimensions of space (refer to Figure 4-1):[2]

- *Sagittal:* The sagittal plane, also known as the *anterior–posterior or median plane*, divides the body vertically into left and right halves; the midsagittal plane divides the body into equal halves.
- *Frontal:* The frontal plane, also known as the *lateral* or *coronal plane*, divides the body into front and back halves.
- *Transverse:* The transverse plane, also known as the *horizontal plane*, divides the body into top and bottom halves.

Because each of these planes bisects the body, it follows that each plane must pass through the same point in the body. This point is referred to as the center of gravity (COG).* The COG of the body is located approximately at midline in the frontal plane and slightly anterior to the second sacral vertebra in the sagittal plane.

> **● Key Point** Most movements occur in an infinite number of vertical and horizontal planes parallel to the cardinal planes.

Axes of the Body

Three reference axes are used to describe human motion: frontal, sagittal, and longitudinal. The axis around which the movement takes place is always perpendicular to the plane in which it occurs.

- *Frontal:* The frontal axis, also known as the *transverse axis*, is perpendicular to the sagittal plane.
- *Sagittal:* The sagittal axis is perpendicular to the frontal plane.

---

*The center of gravity is the point at which the three planes of the body intersect. The line of gravity is the vertical line at which the two vertical planes intersect.

- *Longitudinal:* The longitudinal axis, also known as the *vertical axis*, is perpendicular to the transverse plane.

Most movements occur *in* planes and *around* axes that are somewhere in between the traditional planes and axes, with the structure of the joint determining the possible axes of motion that are available (see "Degrees of Freedom" later in this chapter). The planes and axes for the more common planar movements are as follows:

- Flexion, extension, hyperextension, dorsiflexion, and plantarflexion occur in the sagittal plane around a frontal–horizontal axis.
- Abduction and adduction, side bending of the trunk, elevation and depression of the shoulder girdle, radial and ulnar deviation of the wrist, and eversion and inversion of the foot occur in the frontal plane around a sagittal–horizontal axis.
- Rotation of the head, neck, and trunk; internal rotation and external rotation of the arm or leg; horizontal adduction and abduction of the arm or thigh; and pronation and supination of the forearm occur in the transverse plane around a longitudinal axis.
- Arm circling, leg circling, and trunk circling are examples of *circumduction*. Circumduction involves an orderly sequence of circular movements that occur in the sagittal, frontal, and intermediate oblique planes such that the segment as a whole incorporates a combination of flexion, extension, abduction, and adduction. Circumduction movements can occur at the tibiofemoral, radiohumeral, hip, and glenohumeral joints, and in the spine (as a result of the cumulative effects of the various intervertebral joints).

Both the configuration of a joint and the line of pull of the muscle acting at a joint determine the potential motion that can occur at a joint:

- A muscle whose line of pull is lateral to the joint is a potential abductor.
- A muscle whose line of pull is medial to the joint is a potential adductor.
- A muscle whose line of pull is anterior to a joint has the potential to extend or flex the joint. At the knee, an anterior line of pull may cause the knee to extend, whereas at the elbow joint, an anterior line of pull may cause flexion of the elbow.

- A muscle whose line of pull is posterior to the joint has the potential to extend or flex a joint (refer to preceding example).
- A muscle whose line of pull is away from the center of the body has the potential to externally rotate a joint.
- A muscle whose line of pull is toward the center of the body has the potential to internally rotate a joint.

Degrees of Freedom

The number of independent modes of motion at a joint is called the *degrees of freedom (DOF)*. A joint can have up to three DOF, corresponding to the three dimensions of space.[3] If a joint is uniaxial, it is said to have one DOF.[4–7] The proximal interphalangeal joint is an example of a joint with one DOF. If a joint is bi-axial, it is said to have two DOF.[4–7] The temporomandibular joint and metacarpal joint are examples of joints with two DOF. If a joint is tri-axial, then it is said to have three DOF.[4–7] Ball-and-socket joints such as the shoulder and hip have three DOF.

> **● Key Point** Joint motion that occurs only in one plane is designated as one DOF; in two planes, two DOF; and in three planes, three DOF.

Movements of the Body Segments

When a body moves from one position to another, the effect may be described in terms of motion of the COG of the body from a point A to a point B. In general, there are two types of motion: linear motion, or translation, which occurs in either a straight (rectilinear) or curved line (curvilinear), and angular motion, or rotation, which involves a circular motion around a pivot point.

- *Rectilinear motion:* If the center of mass of the body moves along a straight line connecting the points A and B, then the motion of the COG of the body is rectilinear. An example is walking in a straight line.
- *Curvilinear motion:* Motion along a curved path. An example would be performing shoulder abduction.

Movements of the body segments occur in three dimensions along imaginary planes and around various axes of the body.

> **● Key Point** The axis of rotation of a joint may be considered the pivot point about which the joint motion occurs. The axis of rotation is always perpendicular to the plane of motion.

Because of the arrangement of the articulating surfaces—the surrounding ligaments and joint capsules—most motions around a joint do not occur in straight planes or along straight lines. Instead, the bones at any joint move through space in curved paths. This can best be illustrated using *Codman's paradox*:

1. Stand with your arms by your side, palms facing inward, and thumbs extended. Notice that the thumb is pointing forward.
2. Flex one arm to 90 degrees at the shoulder so the thumb is pointing up.
3. From this position, horizontally abduct your arm so the thumb remains pointing up, but your arm is in a position of 90 degrees of glenohumeral abduction.
4. From this position, without rotating your arm, return the arm to your side and note that your thumb is now pointing away from your thigh.

Referring to the start position, and using the thumb as the reference, it can be seen that the arm has undergone an external rotation of 90 degrees. The rotation occurred during the three separate, straight-plane motions or *swings* that etched a triangle in space—an example of a conjunct rotation. Conjunct rotation occurs as a result of joint surface shapes—and the effect of inert tissues rather than contractile tissues. Most habitual movements, or those movements that occur most frequently at a joint, involve a conjunct rotation. However, the conjunct rotations are not always under volitional control. The implications become important when attempting to restore motion at these joints: when choosing mobilizing techniques, the PT must take into consideration both the relative shapes of the articulating surfaces and the conjunct rotation that is associated with a particular motion.

Force

Force is a vector quantity, with magnitude, direction, and point of application to a body. Force, which can be external or internal, may be defined as mechanical disturbance or load.[1] The various units of force are depicted in **Table 4-2**. Kinetics is the branch of mechanics that describes the effect of forces on the

TABLE 4-2	International System of Units (SI) of Force	
Unit	**Definition**	
Dyne	A force magnitude causing an acceleration of 1 cm/s² to a rigid body with 1 g of mass	
Newton (N)	A force magnitude causing an acceleration of 1 cm/s² to a rigid body with 1 kg of mass	
Pound force (lb f)	A force magnitude causing an acceleration of 1 g (32.2 ft/s²) to a mass of 1 lb; 1 kg f = 2.2 lb f	
Kilogram force (kg f)	A force magnitude causing an acceleration of 1 g (9.8 m/s²) to a mass of 1 kg; 1 kg f = 9.8 N	

body. A number of variables determine the degree of force exerted, including:

- *Magnitude:* A measure of the size and strength of a force—the size or length of a vector (Figure 4-2). Vectors are used in kinesiology to represent the magnitude and direction of the force.
- *Direction:* Specifies the direction (positive or negative) in which the resultant force moves along the line of action.
- *Line of action:* Each force has an associated characteristic line that can be described in terms of angle and slope. If the line of action of a force does not pass through the body, then the force attempts to rotate the body. Most forces that act on the body produce rotation.

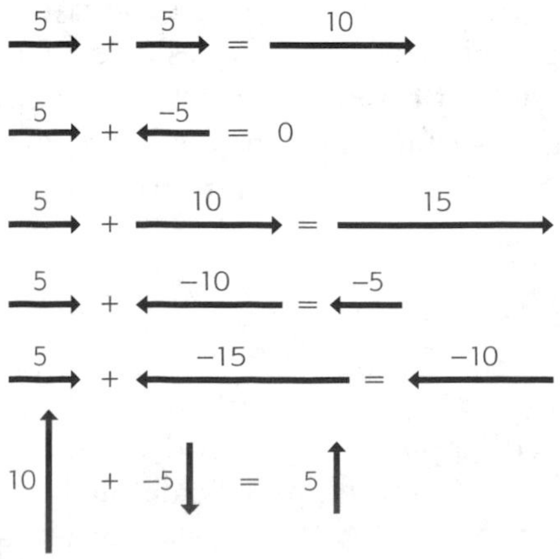

Figure 4-2   Force vectors. Courtesy of Thomas Henderson.

- *Point of application:* The exact location at which a force is applied to a body. This point is usually described by a set of coordinates and is represented graphically by an arrowhead (refer to Figure 4-2). The point of application, which can be more than a single point, is unique to each force.

External forces are produced by forces acting from outside the body, such as gravity or the manual resistance applied by a clinician to a movement. Internal forces are produced from structures located within the body, such as a muscle contraction (active force) or the stretching of connective tissues (passive force). A number of internal forces are recognized. These include compression, tension, shear, and torsion.

- *Compression/approximation:* Can be viewed as a squeezing force. Pressure is defined as the amount of force acting over a given area.

● **Key Point**   Impressive forces cross the joints of the human body. For example, during normal walking, forces of the hip routinely reach three times a person's body weight. Most of this joint force arises from the forces of muscle contraction and are commonly referred to as *joint reaction forces*. In healthy individuals, these forces are absorbed by a thick and moist articular cartilage that dampens the forces while also increasing the surface area of the joint. However, in areas where the cartilage has been worn out, the ability to tolerate even relatively small pressures is reduced, resulting in inflammation (arthritis). In such cases, the PTA teaches the patient joint protection techniques (e.g., good body mechanics, use of an assistive device) to help reduce stress and further wear and tear of the joint.

- *Tension/traction/distraction:* A type of force that is the opposite of a compressive force, and which can be viewed as a pulling or stretching force.
- *Shear:* Shear forces tend to cause one portion of an object to slide or displace with respect to another portion of the object. Whereas compressive and tensile forces act along the longitudinal axis of a structure to which they are applied, shear forces act parallel or tangential to a surface. For example, when bending forward at the waist, shear forces are produced between the lumbar vertebral bodies and their respective intervertebral disks.
- *Torsion:* Torsional forces (torque) occur when a structure is made to twist about its longitudinal axis, typically when one end of the structure is fixed. For example, torsional forces occur through the lower extremity if a directional change is attempted while the sole of the foot is planted firmly on the ground.

● Key Point A system of forces that exerts a resultant moment, but no resultant force, is called a *force couple*. The resultant effect of a force couple is to induce rotation, without any translation. There are a number of important force couples within the human body:

- Hip flexors (iliopsoas, rectus femoris) and the spinal erectors work to produce an anterior tilt of the pelvis.
- Hip extensors and the abdominals work to produce a posterior tilt of the pelvis.
- The upper trapezius, lower trapezius, and serratus anterior work to produce the action of upward rotation of the scapula during arm elevation.

When a force acts on an object, there are two potential effects: acceleration (refer to Table 4-1) and deformation.

● Key Point Friction and gravity are types of forces that commonly act on the body. *Friction* is a force that occurs when two objects are in direct contact and that acts to impede motion of the objects. Once one of the objects begins to move, the frictional force decreases but then remains constant even with additional applied force. *Gravity* is the force that is inversely proportional to the square of the distance between attracting objects and is proportional to the product of their masses. The more mass an object has, the greater the gravitational force.

Load Deformation Curve

The inherent ability of a tissue to tolerate load can be observed experimentally in graphic form. The term *stress* describes the type of force applied to a tissue, whereas *strain* is the deformation that develops within a structure in response to externally applied loads. When any stress is plotted on a graph against the resulting strain for a given material, the shape of the resulting load–deformation curve depends on the kind of material involved. The load–deformation curve, or stress–strain curve, of a structure (Figure 4-3) depicts the relationship between the amount of force applied to a structure and the structure's response in terms of deformation or acceleration. The horizontal axis (deformation or strain) represents the ratio of the tissue's deformed length to its original length. The vertical axis of the graph (load or stress) denotes the internal resistance generated as a tissue resists its deformation, divided by its cross-sectional area. The load–deformation curve can be divided into four regions—toe region, elastic deformation region, plastic deformation region, and failure region—with each region representing a biomechanical property of the tissue.

Toe Region

Collagen fibers have a wavy, or folded, appearance at rest. When a force that lengthens the collagen fibers is initially applied to connective tissue, these folds are affected first. As the fibers unfold, the slack is taken up and tension develops. The length of the toe region depends upon the type of material and the waviness of the collagen pattern.

Elastic Deformation Region

Within the elastic deformation region, the structure imitates a spring—the geometric deformation in the structure increases linearly with increasing load, and after the load is released, the structure returns to its original shape. The ability of a tissue to recover after the stress is removed is extremely important in relation to flexibility. The extensibility of a structure depends on a number of factors. These include the following:

- *Stiffness:* The ratio of stress to strain in an elastic material is a measure of its stiffness. The stiffer the structure, the steeper the slope of its stress–strain curve. All normal tissues within the musculoskeletal system exhibit some degree of stiffness. Stiffness can be defined as the resistance of a structure to deformation, or as the force required to produce a unit of deformation.

● Key Point Connective tissue that is loaded more quickly will behave more stiffly (will deform less) than the same tissue that is loaded at a slower rate.[8] In collagen fibers, the greater the density of the chemical bonds between the fibers or between the fibers and their surrounding matrix, the greater the stiffness. For example, the tendons of the digital flexors and extensors are very stiff, and their length changes very little when muscle forces are applied through them.[9] In contrast, the tendons of some muscles (e.g., the Achilles tendon), particularly those involved in locomotion and ballistic performance, are more elastic.[9]

- *Viscoelasticity:* Viscoelasticity is the time-dependent mechanical property of a material

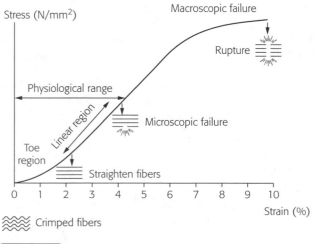

Figure 4-3 Stress–strain curve.

to stretch or shorten over time. The mechanical qualities of a tissue can be separated into categories based on whether the tissue acts primarily like a solid, a fluid, or a mixture of the two. Solids are described according to their elasticity, strength, hardness, and stiffness. Bone, ligaments, tendons, and skeletal muscle are all examples of elastic solids. Biological tissues that demonstrate attributes of both solids and fluids are viscoelastic. The viscoelastic properties of a structure determine its response to loading. A more viscoelastic tissue causes the load–deformation curve to shift further to the right. A number of physical properties of viscoelastic tissues help describe how these tissues elongate with stretching:

- ❑ *Creep:* The ability of a tissue to elongate over time when a constant load is applied to it. For example, when stretching an adaptively shortened biceps that is restricted at 90 degrees of elbow flexion, if a 10 kg load is applied to the elongated muscle, the muscle would gradually lengthen—"creep" a few degrees over a period of time.
- ❑ *Load relaxation:* Describes how less force is required to maintain a tissue at a set length over time. Using the above example, if 10 kg of force is used to achieve 95 degrees of elbow flexion after 15 minutes, less force would be needed to keep the elbow at 95 degrees.
- ❑ *Hysteresis:* Describes the amount of lengthening a tissue will maintain after a cycle of stretching (deformation) and then relaxation. Using the previous example, if an additional 5 degrees of ROM was gained after stretching, that range gain would remain for a period of time after the load is removed.
- *Age:* Age has effects on all aspects of the load–deformation curve. At an early age, a long failure region is observed, which is less evident at a later age.
- *Exercise:* Exercise increases the stiffness and ultimate tensile strength of some structures, such as ligaments, cartilage, bone, and tendons. Conversely, immobility compromises the properties of connective tissue and skeletal muscle.
- *Temperature:* Temperatures in the range of 98.6°F (37°C) to 104°F (40°C) affect the viscoelastic properties of connective tissue.[10] Warmer tissue temperatures result in less microscopic damage when the connective tissue is placed under stress. This is one of the reasons why a structure that is to be stretched is warmed up first, either by using a hot pack or through physical activity.

> **● Key Point** Elastic deformation is similar to the changes that occur with a Thera-Band—after being stretched, the Thera-Band is able to return to its original resting length once the stress is removed.

Plastic Deformation Region

The end of the elastic range and the beginning of the plastic range represent the point where an increasing level of stress on the tissue results in progressive failure, microscopic tearing of the collagen fibers, and permanent deformation. The permanent change results from the breaking of bonds and their subsequent inability to contribute to the recovery of the tissue. Unlike the elastic region, removal of the load in the plastic deformation region will not result in a return of the tissue to its original length.

> **● Key Point** Plastic deformation can be demonstrated using a plastic fork—if a low degree of stress is applied to the fork, it will slowly deform into a new shape. However, if the stress is applied too quickly, the fork breaks.

Failure Region

Deformations exceeding the ultimate failure point (refer to Figure 4-3) produce mechanical failure of the structure, which in the human body may be represented by the fracturing of bone or the rupturing of soft tissues.

> **● Key Point** *Elasticity* is defined as the tendency of a tissue to return to its resting length after passive stretch. *Plasticity* is defined as the tendency of a tissue to assume a new and greater length after passive stretch. *Extensibility* is the ability of a structure to be stretched to its fullest length.[1]

Levers

Biomechanical levers can be defined as rotations of a rigid surface about an axis involving a lever, a load, a fulcrum, and an effort. For simplicity's sake, levers are usually described using a straight bar, which is the lever, and a fulcrum, which is the point on which the bar is resting. The effort force attempts to cause movement of the load. The part of the lever between the fulcrum and the load is the moment arm. There are three types of levers:

- *First class:* Occurs when two forces are applied on either side of an axis and the fulcrum lies between the effort and the load, like a seesaw (Figure 4-4). An example in the human body is the joint between the skull and the atlas vertebrae of the spine: the spine is the fulcrum across which muscles lift the head.

- *Second class:* Occurs when the load is applied between the fulcrum and the point where the effort is exerted (Figure 4-5). This has the advantage of magnifying the effects of the effort so that it takes less force to move the load. Examples of second-class levers in everyday life include a nutcracker and a wheelbarrow—with the wheel acting as the fulcrum. There are a few examples of second-class levers in the human body when only considering

concentric contractions; for example, the Achilles tendon, pushing or pulling across the heel of the foot. When considering both concentric and eccentric contractions, all peripheral joint muscles act as both a third- and a second-class lever—as a third class in concentric contractions and as a second class in eccentric contractions.

- *Third class:* Occurs when the load is located at the end of the lever (Figure 4-6) and the effort lies between the fulcrum and the load (resistance), like a drawbridge or a crane. The effort is exerted between the load and the fulcrum. The effort expended is greater than the load, but the load is moved a greater distance. It is no

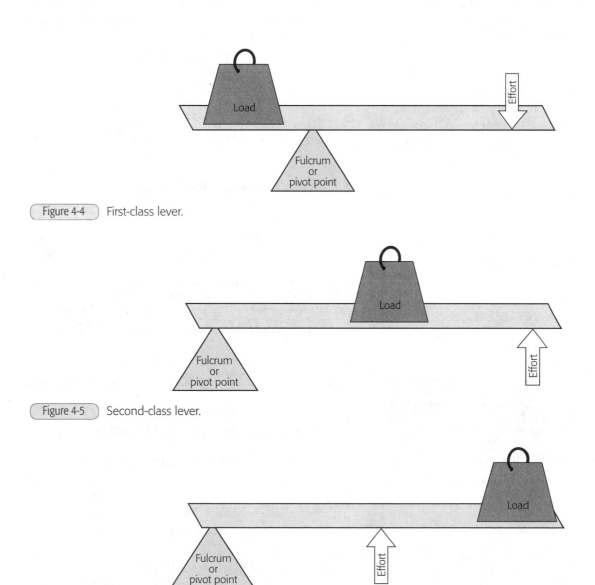

Figure 4-4   First-class lever.

Figure 4-5   Second-class lever.

Figure 4-6   Third-class lever.

accident that the overwhelming majority of bony lever systems in the body are designed as third-class levers because it is usually essential that the distal ends of our limbs move faster than the muscles can physiologically contract (see the following section, "Mechanical Advantage"). For example, great speed and distance of the hand and foot are necessary to impart large power of thrust against objects as well as for rapid advancement of the foot during walking and running.[11] An example of a third-class lever in the body occurs when the hamstrings contract to flex the leg at the knee.

Mechanical Advantage

When a machine puts out more force than is put in, the machine is said to have mechanical advantage (MA). The MA of the musculoskeletal lever is defined as the ratio of the internal moment arm (IMA) to the external moment arm (EMA). For example, muscular forces act about an IMA, whereas gravity could be considered as an EMA. These moment arms convert the forces into rotary torques. Musculoskeletal lever systems that have larger IMAs than EMAs are said to provide good leverage because small muscular (internal) forces are able to move large external loads.[11] In contrast, levers that have smaller IMAs than EMAs favor speed and distance (the distal end of the bone moves at a greater distance and speed than the contracting muscle) but at the expense of requiring increased muscle force.[11] Since MA = IMA / EMA, systems with good mechanical advantage (leverage) will have MA greater than or equal to 1. Depending on the location of the axis of rotation, the first-class lever can have an MA equal to, less than, or greater than 1.[3] Second-class levers always have an MA greater than 1. Third-class levers always have an MA less than 1.

> ● **Key Point** MA relates to the distance of the resistance arm versus the distance of the force arm. Whereas first-class and second-class levers can have a significant mechanical advantage, third-class levers increase distance and speed, but they cannot increase force. Therefore, when a muscle is used as a third-class lever (concentric contraction) it must expend a relatively large force, even for seemingly low-load activities.

Equilibrium

Equilibrium is the condition of a system in which competing forces and torques are balanced. Balance and stability are two aspects related to equilibrium. Balance is the process by which the body's center of mass (COM)[†] is controlled with respect to the base of support, whether that base of support is stationary or moving.[12] Balance testing (see Chapter 3) and balance training (see Chapter 11) are an integral part of physical therapy. According to Berg,[13] balance can be defined as the ability to:

- Maintain a position
- Voluntarily move
- React to a perturbation

The stability of a body is a measure of its ability to return to a position of equilibrium after being disturbed, or the body's resistance to change from a state of equilibrium. From the rehabilitation viewpoint, stability can be defined as the ability to provide a stable base from which to move. Body sway (the slight postural movements made by an individual in order to maintain a balanced position) is an indicator of the presence of postural stability. In patients with poor postural stability, the body sway adaptations (see Chapter 11) are dysfunctional or absent, causing them to fall.

Patients with poor balance and/or stability require a greater base of support (e.g., an assistive device) and a greater level of supervision.

Newton's Laws of Motion

Newton's laws of motion help to explain the relationship between forces and their impact on individual joints, as well as on total body motion (**Table 4-3**).

> ● **Key Point** In accordance with Newton's third law (the law of reaction), the contact between the body and the ground due to gravity is always accompanied by a reaction from it, the so-called ground reaction force (see Chapter 25).[14] The term *center of pressure* is used to describe the location of the vertical projection of the ground reaction force; it is equal and opposite to the weighted average of all the downward forces acting on the air in contact with the ground.[14]

Active Length–Tension Relationship

Muscles are elastic in nature and are therefore constantly being lengthened or shortened. This change in length of a muscle is known as its excursion. Typically, a muscle can only shorten or elongate about half its resting length. In its most basic form, the

---

[†] The center of mass or mass center is the mean location of all the mass in a system or body. The term *center of mass* can be used interchangeably with *center of gravity* because within a uniform gravitational field the two coincide.

TABLE
4-3   Newton's Laws of Motion

	Definition	Description	Real-Life Example
First law	Every object in a state of uniform motion tends to remain in that state of motion unless an external force is applied to it. Also known as the law of inertia.	Describes a body that is in a state of equilibrium—the reluctance of an object to change its movement pattern. The larger the mass or inertia of an object, the more difficult it is to alter its motion.	When a vehicle strikes a large object and is suddenly forced to stop, the driver continues to move forward because of his or her inertia.
Second law	The acceleration of a body is directly proportional to the force causing it. The relationship between an object's mass (m), its acceleration (a), and the applied force (F) is $F = ma$. Acceleration and force are vectors; in this law, the direction of the force vector is the same as the direction of the acceleration vector.	This is the most powerful of Newton's three laws because it allows quantitative calculations of dynamics: how do velocities change when forces are applied?	Because motion is inversely related to mass, gait and weight-bearing exercises are likely to be more challenging for heavier patients.
Third law	For every action there is an equal and opposite reaction.	Describes the forces that occur during all actions.	When stepping off a boat onto the bank of a lake, the boat tends to move in the opposite direction. In rehabilitation, the term ground reaction force is used to describe the reaction of the force patterns that occur when the foot strikes the ground.

length–tension relationship states that isometric tension generated in skeletal muscle is a function of the magnitude of overlap between actin and myosin filaments (see Chapter 2). For each muscle cell, there is an optimum length, or range of lengths, at which the contractile force is strongest. At the optimum length of the muscle, there is near-optimal overlap of actin and myosin, allowing for the generation of maximum tension at this length.

If the muscle is in a shortened position relative to the optimum length, the overlap of actin and myosin reduces the number of sites available for cross-bridge formation. *Active insufficiency* of a muscle occurs when the muscle is incapable of shortening to the extent required to produce full range of motion at all joints crossed simultaneously.[15–18] For example, the finger flexors cannot produce a tight fist when the wrist is fully flexed, as they can when it is in neutral position.

If the muscle is in a lengthened position relative to the optimum length, the actin filaments are pulled away from the myosin heads such that they cannot create as many cross-bridges.[19] *Passive insufficiency* of the muscle occurs when the two-joint muscle cannot stretch to the extent required for full range of motion in the opposite direction at all joints crossed.[15–18] For example, a larger range of hyperextension is possible at the wrist when the fingers are not fully extended.

The length–tension relationship is often represented graphically (Figure 4-7). At short muscle lengths, an increase in length brings an increase in force, giving a positive slope to the length–tension function. At medium lengths, filament overlap allows the largest number of cross-bridges to form, and thus the force is maximum and the slope is zero. At longer lengths, the slope becomes negative in that the force decreases with increasing length because available cross-bridge sites decrease.

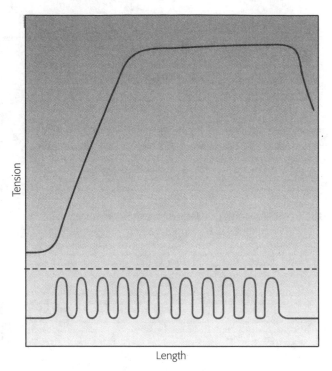

Figure 4-7 Length–tension curve.

Passive Length–Tension Relationship

A muscle generates greater internal elastic force when it is stretched, as demonstrated by a muscle's passive length–tension curve (refer to Figure 4-7). As a muscle is progressively stretched, the tissue is slack until it reaches a critical length where it begins to generate tension. Beyond this critical length, the tension builds exponentially. It is not uncommon for muscles to use active contractions over one joint with passive lengthening over another joint. For example, consider the biceps when pulling an object towards the body, a movement that combines simultaneous and rapid elbow flexion with shoulder extension. As the biceps contracts to perform elbow flexion, it is simultaneously elongated or stretched across the extending shoulder. Such an activity helps maintain a near-constant (and optimal) overall length of the biceps during the activity and allows the biceps to produce a more constant force throughout the range of motion.[20]

Force–Velocity Relationship

The rate of muscle shortening or lengthening substantially affects the force that a muscle can develop during contraction.

Shortening Contractions

As the speed of a muscle shortening increases, the force it is capable of producing decreases.[21,22] The slower rate of shortening is thought to produce greater forces than can be produced by increasing the number of cross-bridges formed. This relationship can be viewed as a continuum, with the optimum velocity for the muscle somewhere between the slowest and fastest rates. At very slow speeds, the force that a muscle can resist or overcome rises rapidly up to 50 percent greater than the maximum isometric contraction.[21,22]

Lengthening Contractions

When a muscle contracts while lengthening (eccentric contraction), the force production differs from that of a shortening (concentric) contraction. Rapid lengthening contractions generate more force than do slower lengthening contractions. During slow lengthening muscle actions, the work produced approximates that of an isometric contraction.[21,22]

Joint Kinematics

A joint is the articulation, or junction, between two or more bones that acts as a pivot point for bony movement (see Chapter 2). In studying joint kinematics, two major types of movements are involved: osteokinematic and arthrokinematic.

Osteokinematic Motion

Osteokinematic motion occurs when any object forms the radius of an imaginary circle about a fixed point. The axis of rotation for osteokinematic motions is oriented perpendicular to the plane in which the rotation occurs.[2] The distance traveled by the motion is measured as an angle, in degrees. All human body segment motions involve osteokinematic motions. Examples of osteokinematic motion include abduction or adduction of the arm, flexion of the hip or knee, and side bending of the trunk.

Center of Rotation

Although muscles produce linear forces, motions at joints are all rotary. For example, some joints can be considered to rotate about a fixed point. A good example of such a joint is the elbow where the humerus and ulna articulate. During flexion or extension at the elbow joint the resulting rotation occurs primarily about a fixed point, referred to as the center of rotation. In the case of the elbow joint, this center of rotation is relatively constant

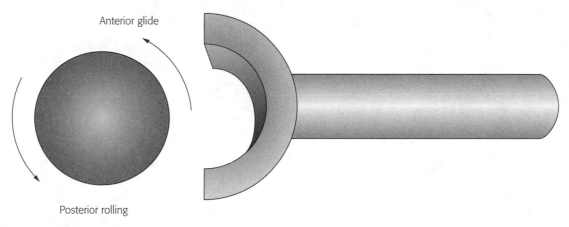

Figure 4-8 Arthrokinematic roll.

throughout the joint range of motion. However, in other joints (for example, the knee) the center of rotation moves in space during movement because the articulating surfaces are not perfect circles.

Arthrokinematic Motion

The involuntary motions that occur at the joint surfaces during activities are termed *arthrokinematic* movements. At each synovial articulation, the articulating surface of one bone end moves relative to the shape of the other articulating surface. For the sake of simplicity, the shapes of these articulating surfaces in synovial joints are described as being *ovoid* or *sellar* in shape (see Chapter 2). Under this concept, an articulating surface can be either concave (female) or convex (male) in shape (ovoid), or a combination of both shapes (sellar).

Osteokinematic and arthrokinematic motions occur simultaneously during movement and are directly proportional to each other, with a small increment of arthrokinematic motion occurring with a larger increment of osteokinematic motion. It therefore follows that if a joint is not functioning correctly, one or both of these motions may be at fault. To improve osteokinematic motion, ROM and flexibility exercises need to be performed, but to improve arthrokinematic motion, a joint mobilization may be required.

Osteokinematic motion is described in terms of planes (e.g., elevation in the sagittal plane) or relative movements (e.g., flexion, adduction). Three fundamental types of arthrokinematic movement exist between joint surfaces:[23]

- *Roll:* A roll occurs when the points of contact on each joint surface are constantly changing (Figure 4-8). This type of movement is

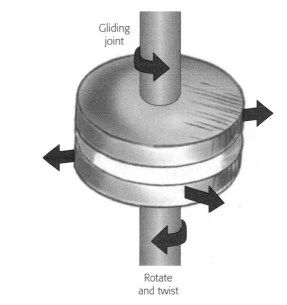

Figure 4-9 Arthrokinematic slide.

analogous to a tire on a car as the car rolls forward. The term *rock* is often used to describe small rolling motions.

- *Slide:* A slide is a pure translation. It occurs if only one point on the moving surface makes contact with varying points on the opposing surface (Figure 4-9). This type of movement is analogous to a car tire skidding when the brakes are applied suddenly on a wet road. This type of motion is also referred to as *translatory* or *accessory* motion. Although the roll of a joint always occurs in the same direction as the swing of a bone, the direction of the slide is determined by the shape of the articulating

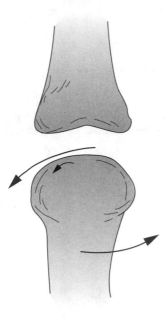

Figure 4-10   Convex on concave.

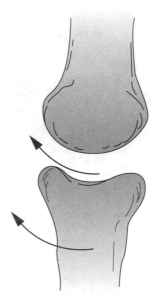

Figure 4-11   Concave on convex.

surface (Figure 4-9). This rule is often referred to as the *concave–convex rule*: If the joint surface that is moving is convex relative to the other stationary surface, the slide occurs in the opposite direction to the osteokinematic motion (Figure 4-10). If, on the other hand, the joint surface of the moving surface is concave, the slide occurs in the same direction as the osteokinematic motion (Figure 4-11). A knowledge of the concave–convex rule is critical when performing joint mobilizations as described in Chapter 6.

● **Key Point** As an example of the concave–convex rule occurring in the clinical setting, consider glenohumeral joint abduction. During this motion the convex humeral head moves on the concave glenoid fossa. The osteokinematic motion occurs as the arm moves superiorly in the frontal plane. However, at the joint surfaces (the arthrokinematic motion), the convex humeral head is sliding inferiorly on the concave glenoid fossa—in the opposite direction to the osteokinematic motion.

■ *Spin*: A spin is defined as any movement in which the bone moves but the mechanical axis remains stationary. A spin involves a rotation of one surface on an opposing surface around a longitudinal axis (Figure 4-12). Spin motions in the body include shoulder flexion/extension

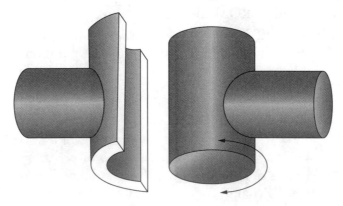

Figure 4-12   Arthrokinematic spin.

and at the radial head during forearm pronation and supination.

> **● Key Point** Most diarthrodial (synovial) joints demonstrate composite motions involving a roll, slide, and spin during activities.

Close-Packed and Open-Packed Positions of the Joint

Joint movements usually are accompanied by a relative compression (approximation) or distraction (separation) of the opposing joint surfaces. These relative compressions or distractions affect the level of *congruity* of the opposing surfaces. The position of maximum congruity of the opposing joint surfaces is termed the *close-packed* position of the joint. The position of least congruity is termed the *open-packed* position. Thus, movements toward the close-packed position of a joint involve an element of compression, whereas movements out of this position involve an element of distraction.

Close-Packed Position

The close-packed position of a joint is the joint position that results in:

- Maximal tautness of the major ligaments
- Maximal surface congruity
- Minimal joint volume
- Maximal stability of the joint

Once the close-packed position is achieved, no further motion in that direction is possible. This is the often-cited reason why most fractures and dislocations occur when an external force is applied to a joint that is in its close-packed position. For example, many of the traumatic injuries of the upper extremities result from falling on a shoulder, elbow, or wrist (FOOSH—a *f*all *o*n an *o*utstretched *h*and) that is in its close-packed position. The close-packed positions for the various joints are presented in **Table 4-4**. From a clinical perspective, the close-packed position is used by the PT for testing the integrity and stability of ligaments and capsular structures.

Open-Packed Position

In essence, any position of the joint, other than the close-packed position, could be considered as an open-packed position. The open-packed position, also referred to as the *loose-packed* or *resting* position of a joint, is the joint position that results in:

- Slackening of the major ligaments of the joint
- Minimal surface congruity
- Minimal joint surface contact
- Maximal joint volume
- Minimal stability of the joint

TABLE 4-4	Close-Packed Position of the Joints
Joint	**Position**
Zygapophysial (spine)	Extension
Temporomandibular	Teeth clenched
Glenohumeral	Abduction and external rotation
Acromioclavicular	Arm abducted to 90 degrees
Sternoclavicular	Maximum shoulder elevation
Ulnohumeral	Extension
Radiohumeral	Elbow flexed 90 degrees; forearm supinated 5 degrees
Proximal radioulnar	5 degrees of supination
Distal radioulnar	5 degrees of supination
Radiocarpal (wrist)	Extension with radial deviation
Metacarpophalangeal	Full flexion
Carpometacarpal	Full opposition
Interphalangeal	Full extension
Hip	Full extension, internal rotation, and abduction
Tibiofemoral	Full extension and external rotation of tibia
Talocrural (ankle)	Maximum dorsiflexion
Subtalar	Supination
Midtarsal	Supination
Tarsometatarsal	Supination
Metatarsophalangeal	Full extension
Interphalangeal	Full extension

The open-packed position permits maximal distraction of the joint surfaces. Because the open-packed position causes the brunt of any external force to be borne by the joint capsule or surrounding ligaments, most capsular or ligamentous sprains occur when a joint is in its open-packed position. For example, at the ankle, which has a close-packed position of dorsiflexion, most ankle sprains occur when the ankle is plantarflexed. The open-packed positions for the various joints are presented in **Table 4-5**.

> **● Key Point** The open-packed position is commonly used during joint mobilization techniques (see Chapter 6).

TABLE 4-5	Open-Packed Position of the Joints
Joint	Position
Zygapophysial (spine)	Midway between flexion and extension
Temporomandibular	Mouth slightly open (freeway space)
Glenohumeral	55 degrees of abduction; 30 degrees of horizontal adduction
Acromioclavicular	Arm resting by side
Sternoclavicular	Arm resting by side
Ulnohumeral	70 degrees of flexion; 10 degrees of supination
Radiohumeral	Full extension; full supination
Proximal radioulnar	70 degrees of flexion; 35 degrees of supination
Distal radioulnar	10 degrees of supination
Radiocarpal (wrist)	Neutral with slight ulnar deviation
Carpometacarpal	Midway between abduction–adduction and flexion–extension
Metacarpophalangeal	Slight flexion
Interphalangeal	Slight flexion
Hip	30 degrees of flexion; 30 degrees of abduction; slight lateral rotation
Tibiofemoral	25 degrees of flexion
Talocrural (ankle)	10 degrees of plantarflexion; midway between maximum inversion and eversion
Subtalar	Midway between extremes of range of movement
Midtarsal	Midway between extremes of range of movement
Tarsometatarsal	Midway between extremes of range of movement
Metatarsophalangeal	Neutral
Interphalangeal	Slight flexion

Range of Motion, Flexibility, and Joint Mobility

Range of motion (ROM) can be defined as the amount of osteokinematic and arthrokinematic movement available to a joint when moving within its anatomic range. *Flexibility* can be defined as the ability of connective tissue (muscles, tendons, ligaments, skin, and joint capsules) to yield to a stretch force. *Joint mobility* can be defined as the amount of arthrokinematic motion available to a joint. Normal range of motion, flexibility, joint mobility, and neuromuscular coordination are required for a joint to function efficiently and effectively.[24] However, a loss of motion at one joint may not prevent the performance of a functional task, although it may result in the task being performed in an abnormal manner. For example, the act of walking can still be accomplished in the presence of a knee joint that has been fused into extension. The amount of available joint motion is based on a number of factors, including:

- Integrity of the joint surfaces and the amount of joint motion
- Mobility and pliability of the soft tissues that surround a joint
- Degree of soft tissue approximation that occurs
- Amount of scarring that is present;[25] interstitial

scarring or fibrosis can occur in and around the joint capsules, within the muscles, and within the ligaments as a result of previous trauma
- Age; joint motion tends to decrease with increasing age
- Gender; in general, females have more joint motion than males

Joint mobility can be assessed using joint mobility testing (see Chapter 2). Range of motion can be measured using standard goniometric instruments. Joint mobility can be improved using joint mobilizations (see Chapter 6). Range of motion and flexibility can be improved using a number of techniques (see Chapter 9).

Hypomobility

If the movement of a joint is less than that considered normal, or when compared with the same joint on the opposite extremity, it may be deemed *hypomobile*. Causes of restricted motion can range from mild muscle shortening to irreversible contractures. Contracture is defined as an adaptive shortening of the soft tissues that cross or surround a joint that results in significant resistance to passive or active stretch and limitation of ROM. Contractures are described by identifying the action of the adaptively shortened muscle. For example, if a patient has adaptively shortened knee flexors and cannot fully extend the knee, he or she is said to have a knee flexion contracture. A number of contractures have been recognized:[26]

- *Arthrogenic and periarticular:* The result of intra-articular pathology, including adhesions, synovial proliferation, joint effusion, irregularities in articular cartilage, or osteophyte formation.
- *Myostatic:* Adaptive shortening of the musculotendinous unit in the presence of no pathology, resulting in significant loss of ROM. These contractures respond well to stretching (see Chapter 9). A pseudomyostatic contracture can result from hypertonicity (i.e., spasticity or rigidity) associated with a central nervous system lesion, or from pain, muscle spasm, or muscle guarding. This type of contracture results in excessive resistance to passive stretch.
- *Fibrotic and irreversible:* Adherence of connective tissue and subsequent development of fibrotic contracture due to fibrous changes. These contractures can be improved through stretching, although it is often difficult to re-establish optimal tissue length.

Hypermobility and Instability

A joint that moves more than is considered normal, when compared with the same joint on the opposite extremity, may be deemed *hypermobile*. Hypermobility may occur as a generalized phenomenon or be localized to just one direction of movement, as follows:

- *Generalized hypermobility:* The more generalized form of hypermobility, as its name suggests, refers to the manifestations of multiple joint hyperlaxity, joint hypermobility, or articular hypermobility. This type of hypermobility can be seen in acrobats, gymnasts, and those individuals who are "double-jointed." In addition, generalized hypermobility occurs with genetic diseases that include joint hypermobility as an associated finding, such as Ehlers-Danlos syndrome, osteogenesis imperfecta, and Marfan's syndrome.
- *Localized hypermobility:* Localized hypermobility is likely to occur as a reaction to neighboring stiffness. For example, a compensatory hypermobility may occur at a joint when a neighboring joint or segment becomes hypomobile secondary to trauma or immobilization.

The term *stability*, specifically related to the joint, has been the subject of much research.[27–42] Joint stability may be viewed as a factor of joint integrity, elastic energy, passive stiffness, and muscle activation.

- *Joint integrity:* Joint integrity is enhanced in those ball-and-socket joints with deeper sockets or steeper sides (e.g., hip), as opposed to those with planar sockets and shallower sides (e.g., shoulder). Joint integrity also depends on the attributes of the supporting structures around the joint and the extent of joint disease. For example, in addition to having a deep acetabulum, the hip joint has a labrum and strong supporting ligaments (see Chapter 19).
- *Elastic energy:* As previously discussed, connective tissues are elastic structures and, as such, are capable of storing elastic energy when stretched. This stored elastic energy may then be used to perform a movement, such as a jump. This is the concept behind an exercise type called *plyometrics*, which uses a combination of eccentric (stretch phase) and then concentric muscle activation (see Chapter 10).
- *Passive stiffness:* Individual joints have passive stiffness that increases toward the joint

end range. An injury to these passive structures causing inherent loss in the passive stiffness results in joint laxity.[43] For example, passive stiffness can exist in the hamstrings prior to stretching and an improvement can be seen with only a few stretches.

■ *Muscle activation:* Muscle activation increases stiffness, both within the muscle and within the joint(s) it crosses.[44] However, the synergist and antagonist muscles that cross the joint must be activated with the correct and appropriate activation in terms of magnitude or timing. A faulty motor control system may lead to inappropriate magnitudes of muscle force and stiffness, allowing a joint to undergo shear translation.[44] For example, following knee surgery, a reflex inhibition of the quadriceps muscle often occurs, requiring the patient to wear a brace to prevent buckling.

Pathologic breakdown of the above factors may result in *instability*. Two types of instability are recognized: articular and ligamentous. In contrast to a hypermobile joint, an unstable joint involves a disruption of the osseous and ligamentous structures of that joint and results in a loss of function.

■ Articular instability can lead to abnormal patterns of coupled and translational movements.[45] For example, in the spine, joint instability can be manifested by permitting sidebending then extension, but not extension followed by sidebending.

■ Ligamentous instability may lead to multiple planes of aberrant joint motion.[46] Consider the amount of aberrant joint motion that occurs at the tibiofemoral joint following a rupture of the anterior cruciate ligament.

Kinematic Chains

The expression *kinematic chain* is used in rehabilitation to describe the function or activity of an extremity or trunk in terms of a series of linked chains. A kinematic chain refers to a series of articulated segmented links, such as the connected pelvis, thigh, leg, and foot of the lower extremity.[3] According to kinematic chain theory, each of the joint segments of the body involved in a particular movement constitutes a link along the kinematic chain. Because each motion of a joint is often a function of other joint motions, the efficiency of an activity can depend on how well these chain links work together.[47] The number of links within a particular kinematic chain

varies, depending on the activity. In general, the longer kinematic chains are involved with more strenuous activities.

Closed Kinematic Chain

A variety of definitions have been proposed for a closed kinematic chain (CKC) activity. Kibler[48] defines a closed-chain activity as a sequential combination of joint motions that have the following characteristics:

■ The distal segment of the kinematic chain meets considerable resistance.

■ The movement of the individual joints, and translation of their instant centers of rotation, occurs in a predictable manner that is secondary to the distribution of forces from each end of the chain.

Examples of closed kinematic chain exercises (CKCEs) involving the lower extremities include the squat (Figure 4-13) and the leg press (**Table 4-6**).[49] The activities of walking, running, jumping, climbing, and rising from the floor all incorporate closed kinematic chain components. Example of CKCEs for the upper extremities are the push-up and using the arms to help rise out of a chair.

● **Key Point**   In most activities of daily living involving the lower extremities, the activation sequence involves a closed chain whereby the activity is initiated from a firm base of support and transferred to a more mobile distal segment.

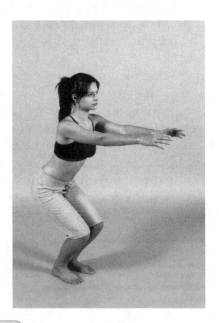

Figure 4-13   Squat.

TABLE 4-6	Differential Features of OKC and CKC Exercises		
Kinematic Chain Mode	Characteristics	Advantages	Disadvantages
Open	Single muscle group	Isolated recruitment	Limited function
	Single axis and plane	Simple movement pattern	Limited eccentrics
	Emphasizes concentric contraction	Minimal joint compression	Less proprioception and joint stability with increased joint shear forces
	Non-weight–bearing		
Closed	Multiple muscle groups	Functional recruitment	Difficult to isolate
	Multiple axes and planes	Functional movement patterns	More complex
	Balance of concentric and eccentric contractions	Functional contractions	Loss of control of target joint
	Weight-bearing exercise	Increased proprioception and joint stability	Compressive forces on articular surfaces

Data from Greenfield BH, Tovin BJ: The application of open and closed kinematic chain exercises in rehabilitation of the lower extremity. *J Back Musculoskel Rehabil* 2:38–51, 1992

Open Kinematic Chain

It is generally accepted that the difference between open kinematic chain (OKC) and CKC activities is determined by the movement of the end segment. The traditional definition for an open-chain activity includes all activities that involve the end segment of an extremity moving freely through space, resulting in isolated movement of a joint.

Examples of an open-chain activity include lifting a drinking glass and waving. Open kinematic chain exercises (OKCEs) involving the lower extremity include the seated knee extension and prone knee flexion. Upper extremity examples of OKCE include the biceps curl (Figure 4-14) and the

military press (refer to Table 4-6).[49] Many activities, such as swimming and cycling, traditionally viewed as OKC activities, include a load on the end segment; yet the end segment is not "fixed" and restricted from movement. This ambiguity of definitions for CKC and OKC activities has allowed some activities to be classified in opposing categories.[50] Thus, there has been a growing need for clarification of OKC and CKC terminology, especially when related to functional activities.

Summary

In kinesiology, the body is often viewed as a machine powered by muscles that produces functional movements by rotating bony levers, some of which are designed to produce large torques, whereas others are designed for speed or endurance. The body, or body segment, moves relative to the three cardinal planes, and the direction of movement is determined by the muscle's line of pull relative to the axis of rotation of the joint around which it is working. In addition, the motion that occurs at a joint follows specific arthrokinematic procedures based on the design and health of the joint. Although it is simpler to describe muscle actions and joint motions as though they occur in isolation, this is extremely uncommon.

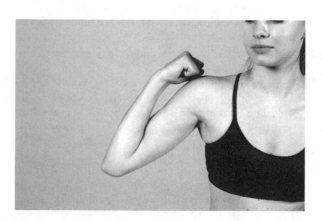

Figure 4-14 Biceps curl.

1. What are the three anatomical planes called?
2. Which of the following motions occurs around the medial-lateral axis of rotation?
   a. Knee flexion
   b. Shoulder extension
   c. Shoulder abduction
   d. A and B
3. Which of the following lever systems is most commonly used by the musculoskeletal system?
   a. First-class
   b. Second-class
   c. Third-class
   d. Fourth-class
4. Which of the following terms describes the proximal attachment of the muscle?
   a. Superior
   b. Inferior
   c. Origin
   d. Insertion
5. What does the term *osteokinematics* describe?
   a. The motion of bones relative to the three cardinal planes
   b. The motion between joint surfaces
   c. The force of a muscle contraction
   d. The direction in which movement takes place
6. Is the shoulder proximal or distal to the elbow?
7. Is a motion such as flexing and extending the elbow with the hand free an example of a closed-chain or an open-chain motion?
8. When a convex joint surface moves about a stationary concave joint surface, does the roll and slide occur in the same direction or in opposite directions?
9. Which of the following motions occurs in the frontal plane?
   a. Hip flexion
   b. Pronation of the forearm
   c. Shoulder adduction
   d. Shoulder flexion

References

1. Goel VK, Khandha A, Vadapalli S: Musculoskeletal Biomechanics, Orthopaedic Knowledge Update 8: Home Study Syllabus. Rosemont, IL, American Academy of Orthopaedic Surgeons, 2005, pp 39–56
2. Hall SJ: Kinematic concepts for analyzing human motion, in Hall SJ (ed): Basic Biomechanics. New York, McGraw-Hill, 1999, pp 28–89
3. Neumann DA: Getting started, in Neumann DA (ed): Kinesiology of the Musculoskeletal System: Foundations for Physical Rehabilitation. St. Louis, MO, Mosby, 2002, pp 3–24
4. Lehmkuhl LD, Smith LK: Brunnstrom's Clinical Kinesiology. Philadelphia, FA Davis, 1983, pp 361–390
5. MacConnail MA, Basmajian JV: Muscles and Movements: A Basis for Human Kinesiology. New York, Robert Krieger, 1977
6. Rasch PJ, Burke RK: Kinesiology and Applied Anatomy. Philadelphia, Lea and Febiger, 1971
7. Steindler A: Kinesiology of the Human Body Under Normal and Pathological Conditions. Springfield, IL, Charles C Thomas, 1955
8. Threlkeld AJ: The effects of manual therapy on connective tissue. Phys Ther 72:893–902, 1992
9. Teitz CC, Garrett WE, Jr., Miniaci A, et al: Tendon problems in athletic individuals. J Bone Joint Surg 79-A:138–152, 1997
10. Tillman LJ, Cummings GS: Biologic mechanisms of connective tissue mutability, in Currier DP, Nelson M (eds): Dynamics of Human Biologic Tissue. Philadelphia, FA Davis, 1992
11. Jackson-Manfield P, Neumann DA: Basic principles of kinesiology, in Jackson-Manfield P, Neumann DA (eds): Essentials of Kinesiology for the Physical Therapist Assistant. St. Louis, MO, Mosby Elsevier, 2009, pp 1–19
12. Voight M, Blackburn T: Proprioception and balance training and testing following injury, in Ellenbecker TS (ed): Knee Ligament Rehabilitation. Philadelphia, Churchill Livingstone, 2000, pp 361–385
13. Federation of State Medical Boards of the United States: Model Guidelines for the Use of Controlled Substances for the Treatment of Pain. Euless, TX, The Federation, 1998
14. Kloos AD, Givens-Heiss D: Exercise for impaired balance, in Kisner C, Colby LA (eds): Therapeutic Exercise. Foundations and Techniques (ed 5). Philadelphia, FA Davis, 2002, pp 251–272
15. Hall SJ: The biomechanics of human skeletal muscle, in Hall SJ (ed): Basic Biomechanics. New York, McGraw-Hill, 1999, pp 146–185
16. Boeckmann RR, Ellenbecker TS: Biomechanics, in Ellenbecker TS (ed): Knee Ligament Rehabilitation. Philadelphia, Churchill Livingstone, 2000, pp 16–23
17. Brownstein B, Noyes FR, Mangine RE, et al: Anatomy and biomechanics, in Mangine RE (ed): Physical Therapy of the Knee. New York, Churchill Livingstone, 1988, pp 1–30
18. Deudsinger RH: Biomechanics in clinical practice. Phys Ther 64:1860–1868, 1984
19. Lakomy HKA: The biomechanics of human movement, in Maughan RJ (ed): Basic and Applied Sciences for Sports Medicine. Woburn, MA, Butterworth-Heinemann, 1999, pp 124–125
20. Jackson-Manfield P, Neumann DA: Structure and function of skeletal muscle, in Jackson-Manfield P, Neumann DA (eds): Essentials of Kinesiology for the Physical Therapist Assistant. St. Louis, MO, Mosby Elsevier, 2009, pp 35–49
21. McArdle W: Exercise Physiology: Energy, Nutrition, and Human Performance. Philadelphia, Lea and Febiger, 1991

22. Astrand PO, Rodahl K: The Muscle and Its Contraction: Textbook of Work Physiology. New York, McGraw-Hill, 1986

23. MacConaill MA: Arthrology, in Warwick R, Williams PL (eds): Gray's Anatomy (ed 35). Philadelphia, WB Saunders, 1975

24. Harris ML: Flexibility. Phys Ther 49:591–601, 1969

25. Gleim GW, McHugh MP: Flexibility and its effects on sports injury and performance. Sports Med 24:289–299, 1997

26. Kisner C, Colby LA: Stretching for impaired mobility, in Kisner C, Colby LA (eds): Therapeutic Exercise. Foundations and Techniques (ed 5). Philadelphia, FA Davis, 2002, pp 65–108

27. Answorth AA, Warner JJP: Shoulder instability in the athlete. Orthop Clin North Am 26:487–504, 1995

28. Bergmark A: Stability of the lumbar spine. Acta Orthop Scand 60:1–54, 1989

29. Boden BP, Pearsall AW, Garrett WE, Jr., et al: Patellofemoral instability: Evaluation and management. J Am Acad Orthop Surg 5:47–57, 1997

30. Callanan M, Tzannes A, Hayes KC, et al: Shoulder instability. Diagnosis and management. Austr Fam Phys 30:655–661, 2001

31. Cass JR, Morrey BF: Ankle instability: Current concepts, diagnosis, and treatment. Mayo Clin Proc 59:165–170, 1984

32. Clanton TO: Instability of the subtalar joint. Orthop Clin N Am 20:583–592, 1989

33. Cox JS, Cooper PS: Patellofemoral instability, in Fu FH, Harner CD, Vince KG (eds): Knee Surgery. Baltimore, Williams & Wilkins, 1994, pp 959–962

34. Freeman MAR, Dean MRE, Hanham IWF: The etiology and prevention of functional instability of the foot. J Bone Joint Surg 47B:678–685, 1965

35. Friberg O: Lumbar instability: A dynamic approach by traction-compression radiography. Spine 12:119–129, 1987

36. Grieve GP: Lumbar instability. Physiotherapy 68:2, 1982

37. Hotchkiss RN, Weiland AJ: Valgus stability of the elbow. J Orthop Res 5:372–377, 1987

38. Kaigle A, Holm S, Hansson T: Experimental instability in the lumbar spine. Spine 20:421–430, 1995

39. Kuhlmann JN, Fahrer M, Kapandji AI, et al: Stability of the normal wrist, in Tubiana R (ed): The Hand. Philadelphia, WB Saunders, 1985, pp 934–944

40. Landeros O, Frost HM, Higgins CC: Post traumatic anterior ankle instability. Clin Orthop 56:169–178, 1968

41. Luttgens K, Hamilton N: The center of gravity and stability, in Luttgens K, Hamilton N (eds): Kinesiology: Scientific Basis of Human Motion (ed 9). Dubuque, IA, McGraw-Hill, 1997, pp 415–442

42. Wilke H, Wolf S, Claes L, et al: Stability of the lumbar spine with different muscle groups: A biomechanical in vitro study. Spine 20:192–198, 1995

43. Panjabi MM: The stabilizing system of the spine. Part 1. Function, dysfunction adaption and enhancement. J Spinal Disord 5:383–389, 1992

44. McGill SM, Cholewicki J: Biomechanical basis for stability: An explanation to enhance clinical utility. J Orthop Sports Phys Ther 31:96–100, 2001

45. Gertzbein SD, Seligman J, Holtby R, et al: Centrode patterns and segmental instability in degenerative disc disease. Spine 10:257–261, 1985

46. Cholewicki J, McGill S: Mechanical stability of the in vivo lumbar spine: Implications for injury and chronic low back pain. Clin Biomech 11:1–15, 1996

47. Marino M: Current concepts of rehabilitation in sports medicine, in Nicholas JA, Herschman EB (eds): The Lower Extremity and Spine in Sports Medicine. St. Louis, MO, Mosby, 1986, pp 117–195

48. Kibler BW: Closed kinetic chain rehabilitation for sports injuries. Phys Med Rehab N Am 11:369–384, 2000

49. Blackard DO, Jensen RL, Ebben WP: Use of EMG analysis in challenging kinetic chain terminology. Med Sci Sports Excr 31:443–448, 1999

50. Dillman CJ, Murray TA, Hintermeister RA: Biomechanical differences of open and closed chain exercises with respect to the shoulder. J Sport Rehabil 3:228–238, 1994

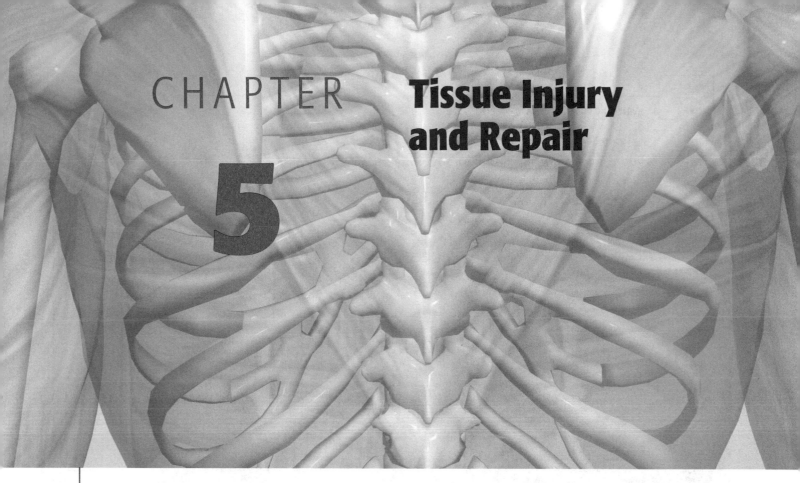

CHAPTER 5

Tissue Injury and Repair

Chapter Objectives

At the completion of this chapter, the reader will be able to:

1. Outline the pathophysiology of the healing process for the various musculoskeletal tissues.
2. Identify techniques that the PTA can use to aid in the healing process.
3. Describe the different major stages of healing for the various musculoskeletal tissues.
4. List the five clinical signs of inflammation that occur in the coagulation and inflammatory phase of healing.
5. Discuss the importance of the application of controlled stresses during the healing process.
6. List the detrimental effects that immobilization can have on tissues of the musculoskeletal system.
7. Describe some of the surgical options available for musculoskeletal tissue injuries.

Overview

The healing process is an intricate phenomenon that occurs following an injury or disease. One of the contributing factors to maintaining musculoskeletal health is the ability of the biological tissues to withstand a wide range of external and internal stresses and strains that are either generated or resisted by the human body during the course of daily activities or recreation. Examples of these forces include gravity, body weight, and friction (see Chapter 4). Maintaining this health is a delicate balance, because insufficient, excessive, or repetitive stresses can prove harmful. Injuries to the musculoskeletal system (**Table 5-1**) can result from a wide variety of causes.[1–4] The purpose of this chapter is to describe the physiology of healing for each of the major components of the musculoskeletal system and how the PTA can help in this process.

TABLE 5-1	Musculoskeletal Injuries: Terms and Definitions
Term	**Definition**
Strain	Overstretching, overexertion, or overuse of the musculotendinous unit; can occur from slight trauma or unaccustomed repeated trauma of a minor degree
Sprain	Severe stress, stretch, or tear of a ligament
Dislocation	Displacement of the bony partners in a joint resulting in loss of the anatomical relationship and leading to soft tissue damage, inflammation, pain, and muscle spasm
Subluxation	An incomplete or partial dislocation of the bony partners in a joint with associated secondary trauma to the surrounding soft tissue
Synovitis	Inflammation of a synovial membrane resulting in an excess of normal synovial fluid in a joint or tendon sheath
Hemarthrosis	Bleeding into a joint, usually due to severe trauma
Ganglion	Ballooning of the wall of the joint capsule or tendon sheath
Contusion	Bruising from a direct blow, resulting in capillary rupture, bleeding, edema, and an inflammatory response
Contracture	Adaptive shortening of skin, fascia, muscle, or joint capsule that prevents normal mobility or flexibility of that structure
Adhesion	Abnormal adherence of collagen fibers to surrounding structures during immobilization, after trauma, or as a complication of surgery

Data from Schrepfer R: Soft tissue injury, repair, and management, in Kisner C, Colby LA (eds): Therapeutic Exercise: Foundations and Techniques (ed 5). Philadelphia, FA Davis, 2002, pp 295–308

Musculotendinous Injuries

Musculotendinous injuries can be categorized according to the cause of injury:

- *Direct:* An injury that is likely to be a result of contact with another player, an object, or the ground (e.g., a contusion)
- *Indirect:* An injury that is likely to be a result of physical impact without contact (e.g., hamstring strain)
- *Overuse:* An injury that is likely to be a result of continual impact on tendon or bone leading to detrimental wear and tear and eventual breakdown (e.g., a tendonitis such as tennis elbow)

Muscle Injuries

Muscle strains can be classified according to their severity as follows:[5,6]

- *Mild (first-degree) strain:* This type involves a tear of a few muscle fibers with minor swelling and local tenderness. Also known as grade I injuries, these are associated with no or minimal loss of strength and restriction of movement. Local tenderness may be present, which is increased when stress is applied to the structure. Patients with a grade I strain usually can continue normal activities as much as possible, but should be monitored for exacerbation of the existing injury.
- *Moderate (second-degree) strain:* This type (also known as grade II) involves greater damage to the muscle and a clear loss of strength. Patients with grade II injuries have pain on activity that often prevents further participation. The pain can be moderate to severe and is often associated with some loss of function and joint stability. Grade II strains typically require 3–28 days of rehabilitation.[7]
- *Severe (third-degree) strain:* This type (grade III) involves a tear extending across the whole muscle belly. Grade III strains are characterized by severe pain or loss of function. Whether pain increases when stress is applied to the structure depends on the integrity of the remaining tissue; for example, there may no pain in cases of a complete tear. Although grade I and II muscle strains are treated conservatively, surgical intervention is often

necessary for grade III injuries.[8] Healing of grade III strains can require up to 3 months of rehabilitation.

Tendon Injuries

Tendon injuries are among the most common overuse injuries. Three major types are recognized:

- *Tendonitis:* By definition, tendonitis is an inflammation of the tendon. Common sites of tendonitis include the rotator cuff of the shoulder (e.g., supraspinatus), the bicipital tendon, the origin of the wrist extensors (e.g., lateral epicondylitis, tennis elbow) and flexors (e.g., medial epicondylitis) at the elbow, the patellar and popliteal tendons and iliotibial band at the knee, the origin of the anterior tibial tendon in the leg (i.e., shin splints), and the Achilles tendon at the heel. Tendonitis most commonly is caused by overuse and can result in pain and loss of function. In specific instances (i.e., calcific tendinitis of the rotator cuff) calcium can be deposited along the course of the tendon. The cause of calcium deposits within the rotator cuff tendon is not entirely understood. Different ideas have been suggested, including blood supply and aging of the tendon, but the evidence to support these conclusions is not conclusive.
- *Tendinosis:* A chronic alteration of the tendon accompanied by tissue degeneration, cell atrophy, and pain, which is often associated with tendon thickening.[9]
- *Paratendonitis:* Encompasses peritendonitis, tenosynovitis, and tenovaginitis and is used to describe an inflammatory disorder of tissues surrounding the tendon, such as the tendon sheath. In most cases, these conditions seem to result from a repetitive friction of the tendon and its sheath.[10]

The goal of rehabilitation is to restore the tendon to its optimal length and cellularity, and to enhance its ability to withstand loads.

Ligament Injury

The most common mechanism of ligament injury is excessive lengthening of the ligament when the associated joint is moved into an excessive range of motion. This results in a ligamentous sprain. Ligament sprains can be classified into three grades:

- *Grade I:* Involves stretching of the ligament, but no fiber damage

TABLE 5-2	Ligament Injuries
Grade	**Signs and Symptoms**
First degree (mild)	Minimal loss of structural integrity
	No abnormal motion
	Little or no swelling
	Localized tenderness
	Minimal bruising
Second degree (moderate)	Significant structural weakening
	Some abnormal motion
	Solid end feel to stress
	More bruising and swelling
	Often associated hemarthrosis and effusion
Third degree (complete)	Loss of structural integrity
	Marked abnormal motion
	Significant bruising
	Hemarthrosis

- *Grade II:* Involves stretching of the ligament and tearing of some fibers
- *Grade III:* Involves almost complete ligament disruption

The signs and symptoms of ligament injuries are outlined in **Table 5-2**.

Musculotendinous Tissue Healing

Tissue repair can be viewed as an adaptive life process in response to both intrinsic and extrinsic stimuli.[11] Research continues to provide an increasing amount of information about the biocellular events that occur as a result of tissue injury, as well as the factors that interfere with the natural progression of these events. The promotion and progression of tissue repair involves a delicate balance between protection and the application of controlled functional stresses to the damaged structure. Physical therapy cannot accelerate the healing process, but with correct education and supervision of the patient, it can ensure that the healing process is not delayed or disrupted, and that it occurs in an optimal environment.[12] The rehabilitation procedures used by the PTA to assist with this repair process differ depending on the type of tissue involved, the extent of the damage, and the stage of healing. Signs and symptoms inform the clinician as to the stage of tissue repair. Aware-ness by the PTA of the various stages of healing is essential for determining the intensity of a particular intervention to avoid doing any harm. Decisions to notify the supervising PT about modifying the plan of care need to be based on the recognition of these signs and symptoms, and on an understanding of the time frames associated with each of the phases.[13,14]

Stages of Soft Tissue Healing

The main stages of soft tissue healing include acute (coagulation and inflammation), which initiates shortly after the initial injury; subacute (migratory and proliferative), which begins within days and includes the major processes of healing; and chronic (maturation and remodeling), which may last for up to a year and is responsible for scar tissue formation and development of new tissue (Figure 5-1).[13–18] Whereas simplification of the complex events of heal-ing into separate categories may facilitate understand-ing of the phenomenon, in reality these events occur as

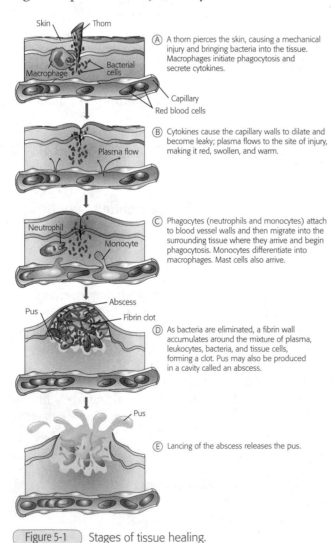

A. A thorn pierces the skin, causing a mechanical injury and bringing bacteria into the tissue. Macrophages initiate phagocytosis and secrete cytokines.

B. Cytokines cause the capillary walls to dilate and become leaky; plasma flows to the site of injury, making it red, swollen, and warm.

C. Phagocytes (neutrophils and monocytes) attach to blood vessel walls and then migrate into the surrounding tissue where they arrive and begin phagocytosis. Monocytes differentiate into macrophages. Mast cells also arrive.

D. As bacteria are eliminated, a fibrin wall accumulates around the mixture of plasma, leukocytes, bacteria, and tissue cells, forming a clot. Pus may also be produced in a cavity called an abscess.

E. Lancing of the abscess releases the pus.

Figure 5-1   Stages of tissue healing.

a continuum, both spatially and temporally.[19] Certain factors appear to determine the prognosis for healing, with the most important regulating factor being suf-ficient blood flow, because it is the blood that supplies oxygen and nutrients to an injured area.[6,14]

Acute (Coagulation and Inflammation) Stage

The reaction that occurs immediately after a soft tissue injury includes a series of defensive events involving the recognition of an invading organism and the mounting of a reaction against it. This reac-tion involves two processes: coagulation and inflam-mation. Following an injury to the tissues, capillary blood flow is disrupted, causing hypoxia to the area. This initial period of vasoconstriction, which lasts 5–10 minutes, limits the blood loss and causes the inflammatory phase to begin, which in turn prompts a period of vasodilation and the extravasation (the movement of white blood cells from the capillaries to the tissues surrounding them) of blood constituents.[14] Extravasated blood contains platelets, which secrete substances that form a clot to prevent further bleed-ing and infection, clean dead tissue, and nourish white cells. These substances include macrophages and fibroblasts.[20] Inflammation is mediated by chemotactic substances, which are bodily cells that direct their movements according to certain chemi-cals in their environment, including anaphylatoxins that attract neutrophils and monocytes.

- *Neutrophils* are white blood cells of the poly-morphonuclear (PMN) leukocyte subgroup that express and release cytokines, which in turn intensify inflammatory reactions by sev-eral other cell types. The function of neutro-phils is to bind to microorganisms, internalize them, and kill them, thereby controlling the spread of infection.
- *Monocytes* are white blood cells of the mono-nuclear leukocyte subgroup that migrate into tissues and develop into macrophages, and provide immunological defenses against many infectious organisms. Macrophages serve to orchestrate a "long-term" response (innate and adaptive immunity) to injured cells subsequent to the acute response.[21]

● **Key Point**   The *innate immune system* comprises the cells and mechanisms that defend the host from infection by other organisms, in a nonspecific manner, but does not confer long-lasting or protective immunity to the host. The *adaptive immune system* is composed of highly specialized, systemic cells and processes that have the ability to recognize and remember specific pathogens (to generate immunity), and to mount stronger attacks each time the pathogen is encountered.

The white blood cells of the inflammatory stage serve to clean the wound debris of foreign substances, increase vascular permeability, and promote fibroblast activity.[21] The extent and severity of the inflammatory response depend on the size and the type of the injury, the tissue involved, and the vascularity of that tissue.[13,22–25] Four systems work together during this phase:

- *Kinin system:* Causes vasodilation and increased permeability and stimulates pain receptors
- *Clotting system:* Leads to fibrin deposition and clot formation
- *Fibrinolytic system:* Leads to the synthesis of plasmin, which functions to degrade/dissolve the fibrin clot and to trigger activation of the complement system
- *Complement system:* Produces a variety of proteins with activities essential to healing

The complete removal of the wound debris marks the end of the inflammatory process, which usually occurs after 4 to 6 days unless the insult is perpetuated.

Clinical findings during the acute (coagulation and inflammatory) stage include swelling, redness and increased warmth of the involved area, and impairment or loss of function. The swelling (edema) is due to an increase in the permeability of the venules, plasma proteins, and leukocytes, which leak into the site of injury.[26,27] During this phase, there is pain at rest or with active motion, or when specific stress is applied to the injured structure. The pain, if severe enough, can result in muscle guarding and loss of function—the body's attempt to immobilize the area. With passive range of motion, pain is reported by the patient before tissue resistance is felt by the clinician (empty end feel). Janda[28] introduced the concept of the direct and indirect effects of neural input on muscle activation, and noted the influence that pain and swelling can have on direct muscle inhibition. According to Janda,[28] muscular development cannot proceed in the presence of pain, because pain has the potential to create a high degree of muscle inhibition that can alter muscle-firing patterns. Therefore, during this stage, the intervention goals are to control pain by reducing the degree of inflammation and swelling.

The short-term goals of the acute phase include:

- Protection of the injury site to allow healing
- Control of pain and inflammation
- Control of and then elimination of edema

- Restoration of pain-free range of motion in the entire kinetic chain
- Improvement of patient comfort by decreasing pain and inflammation
- Retardation of muscle atrophy
- Minimizing detrimental effects of immobilization and activity restriction[29–34]
- Management of scar, if appropriate; the goal of treatment is the formation of a strong, mobile scar at the site of the lesion so there is complete and painless restoration of function[35]
- Maintenance of general fitness with resistive and/or modified aerobic exercises, depending on proximity to associated areas and effect on the primary lesion
- Patient independence with home exercise program

These goals can be achieved by using the principles of PRICEMEM (*p*rotection, *r*est, *i*ce, *c*ompression, *e*levation, *m*anual therapy, *e*arly motion, and *m*edications). The goal of this approach is to decrease early bleeding and facilitate the removal of the inflammatory exudates, which can prevent further damage and inflammation to the area. Limiting the effusion serves to hasten the healing process by minimizing the amount of extracellular fluid and hematoma to be reabsorbed.[36,37] The patient should be reassured that the symptoms are usually of short duration, and instructions are given as to what the patient can do during this stage including any precautions or contraindications.

Protection
Excessive tissue loading must be avoided (**Table 5-3**). For example, in the lower extremity when ambulation is painful, crutches or other assistive devices are advocated until the patient can bear weight painlessly.[38]

Rest
Rest (splint, tape, cast) is defined as absence of abuse, rather than an absence of activity.[39] Complete or continuous immobilization should be avoided whenever possible because it can have detrimental physiologic effects, including loss of muscle, ligament, and bone strength;[40–43] formation of adhesions;[42] and the loss of proprioception[43] (see "Detrimental Effects of Immobilization" later in this chapter).

Ice
The therapeutic application of cold, or cryotherapy, has been used as a healing modality since the days of the ancient Greeks (see Chapter 7).[44] Garrick[38] recommends that ice be used until the swelling

TABLE 5-3	Signs and Symptoms of Excessive Stress with Exercise or Activity

Exercise or activity soreness that does not decrease after 2 to 4 hours and is not resolved after 24 hours

Pain that occurs earlier in the exercise or activity or is increased over the previous session

Progressively increased feelings of stiffness and decreased range of motion over several exercise sessions

Decreased functional usage and progressive weakness of the involved part

Data from Schrepfer R: Soft tissue injury, repair, and management, in Kisner C, Colby LA (eds): Therapeutic Exercise: Foundations and Techniques (ed 5). Philadelphia, FA Davis, 2002, pp 295–308

has ceased. A variety of electrotherapeutic and physical modalities can also be used to help control pain, swelling, and muscle guarding (see Chapter 7).

Compression
The most common method of applying compression is via an elastic bandage.[45] Compression provided by a pneumatic device,[46,47] or by a felt pad incorporated into an elastic wrap or taping,[48] also has been demonstrated to be effective in decreasing effusion.

Elevation
Elevation of an extremity aids in venous return and helps minimize swelling. Elevation and compression should be continued until the swelling has completely dissipated.[38]

Manual Therapy
The controlled application of a variety of manual techniques, described in Chapter 6, can have several therapeutic benefits. These benefits are theoretically achieved through the following:[49,50]

- Stimulation of the large-fiber joint afferents of the joint capsule, soft tissue, and joint cartilage, which aids in pain reduction
- Stimulation of endorphins, which aids in pain reduction
- Decrease of intra-articular pressure, which aids in pain reduction
- Mechanical effect, which increases joint mobility
- Remodeling of local connective tissue
- Increase of the gliding of tendons within their sheaths
- Increase in joint lubrication

The PT, or trained PTA in states where allowable, may perform gentle (grade I) oscillations to the involved joint to improve fluid dynamics, maintain cartilage health, and inhibit the perception of pain. Manual techniques that may be delegated by the supervising PT during this stage include gentle massage to increase blood flow, and passive range of motion. With a muscle lesion, the massage is applied in its shortened position so as not to overstress the damaged fibers.

Early Motion
Tissue-specific movements should be directed to the structure involved to prevent abnormal adherence of the developing fibrils to the surrounding tissue and thus avoid future disruption of the scar.[35] In addition, early motion is advocated to:

- Reduce the muscle atrophy that occurs primarily in type I fibers[29,51,52]
- Maintain joint function
- Reduce the chance of arthrofibrosis or excessive scarring[53–57]
- Enhance cartilage nutrition and vascularization, thereby permitting an early recovery and enhanced comfort[30,52,58]

During the inflammatory stage, it is also important for the patient to function as independently as possible.[11,59,60] Research has demonstrated that joint motion stimulates the healing of torn ligaments around a joint,[61,62] and that early joint motion stimulates collagen bundle orientation in the lines of force, a kind of Wolff's law of ligaments.[61,63] Early ROM exercises are typically performed passively and then actively assisted within the pain-free range. Gentle isometric muscle contractions performed intermittently and at a very low intensity so as to avoid painful joint compression can be used at this time. The pumping action of the contracting muscles assists with the circulation and, therefore, fluid dynamics.[35]

● Key Point
- *Muscle injury:* The exercises are performed with the muscle in the shortened position to help maintain mobility of the actin-myosin filaments without overstressing the damaged tissue.
- *Joint injury:* The usual starting position for the exercises is the resting position of the joint, but the position used should be the one most comfortable for the patient.

Medications
Medications prescribed by the physician can play an important role in the healing process (see the "Musculoskeletal Pharmacology" section in Chapter 1).

Subacute (Migratory and Proliferative) Stage

The criteria to consider advancement from this phase include adequate pain control and tissue healing, near-normal ROM, and tolerance for strengthening.[64] The subacute stage of soft tissue healing, characterized by migration and proliferation, usually occurs from the time of the initial injury and overlaps the inflammation phase. Characteristic changes include capillary growth and granulation tissue formation, fibroblast proliferation with collagen synthesis, and increased macrophage and mast cell activity. This stage is responsible for the development of wound tensile strength. After the wound base is free of necrotic tissue, the body begins to work to close the wound. The connective tissue in healing wounds is composed primarily of collagen, types I and III. Proliferation of collagen results from the actions of the fibroblasts that have been attracted to the area and stimulated to multiply by growth factors. This proliferation produces first fibrinogen and then fibrin, which eventually becomes organized into a honeycomb matrix and walls off the injured site.[65] The wound matrix functions as a glue to hold the wound edges together, giving it some mechanical protection, while also preventing the spread of infection. However, until the provisional extracellular matrix is replaced with a collagenous matrix, the wound matrix has a low tensile strength and is vulnerable to breakdown. The collagenous matrix facilitates angiogenesis by providing time and protection to new and friable vessels. The process of neovascularization during this phase provides a granular appearance to the wound as a result of the formation of loops of capillaries and migration of macrophages, fibroblasts, and endothelial cells into the wound matrix. Once an abundant collagen matrix has been formed in the wound, the fibroblasts stop producing collagen, and the fibroblast-rich granulation tissue is replaced by a relatively acellular scar, marking the end of this stage. This fibrous tissue repair process can last anywhere from 5 to 15 days to several weeks, depending on the type of tissue and the extent of damage.

Clinically, this stage is characterized by a decrease in pain and swelling and an increase in pain-free active and passive ROM. During passive ROM, the subjective report of pain is synchronous with tissue resistance. Although the pain-free ROM may be increased in this phase, it is still not within normal limits, and stress applied to the injured structures still produces pain, although the pain experienced is lessened.[66,67] The decreased ROM is due to the effects of immobilization, pain, muscle inhibition, and weakening of the tissues that occurred during the inflammatory phase. Upon progressing to this stage, the active effusion and local erythema of the inflammation stage are no longer present clinically; however, residual effusion may still be present at this time and resist resorption.[66,67] It seems that the fibroblasts need to be guided during this recovery phase so that the replaced collagen fibers are laid down along the lines of stress. The use of gentle movements to the area provide natural tensions for the healing tissues and help to produce a stronger repair.[26] The goals of this phase are to protect the forming collagen, direct its orientation to be parallel to the lines of force it must withstand, and prevent cross-linking and scar contracture. If these goals are achieved, the scar will be strong and extensible. These goals are achieved by (1) attaining full range of pain-free motion, (2) restoring normal joint kinematics, (3) improving muscle strength to near-normal limits, (4) improving neuromuscular control, and (5) restoring near-normal muscle force couple relationships.

It is important to emphasize to the patient that an overly aggressive approach during this stage can result in a delay or disruption in the repair process through an increase in the stimulation of the inflammatory chemical irritants and exudates. However, the patient should be encouraged to return to normal activities that do not exacerbate symptoms. The exercises, initiated during the acute phase, are progressed to include active motion and stretching based on tissue and patient responses. Criteria for initiating active exercises and stretching during the early subacute stage include decreased swelling, pain that is no longer constant, and pain that is not exacerbated by motion in the available range. The active range of motion (AROM) exercises, performed initially in isolated single-plane motions throughout the pain-free ranges, are used to develop control of the motion. Neuromuscular control exercises during this stage are initially restricted to submaximal isometrics within patient tolerance. The submaximal isometrics are initially performed in the early part of the range and/or in the resting position of the joint, before being performed at multiple angles of the pain-free ROM. The intensity of contraction should be kept below the perception of pain. The isometric exercises not only increase muscle strength and endurance, but also improve the ability of the patient to actively mobilize stiff joints (see Chapter 6).[68] As ROM and joint play improve, resistive exercises are progressed, with the resistance being increased as tolerated. Initially, light resistive, concentric exercises of the involved muscle or muscles are introduced emphasizing control of the motion and proper joint mechanics. Once the single plane motions are tolerated, combined motions or diagonal patterns can be introduced, while ensuring that all of the muscles are effectively participating. As new exercises are introduced, or as the intensity of exercise is progressed, the patient's response must be monitored so that the symptoms determine the intensity of exercise and appropriate modifications can be made. Wherever possible, resistance exercises that strengthen functional muscle groups rather than individual muscles should be selected.[68]

> ● **Key Point** Restoration of normal ROM is essential to allow normal strength and mechanics to be regained.[69] Grade III sustained joint mobilization techniques during this stage include passive traction and/or gliding movements to joint surfaces that maintain or restore the joint play normally allowed by the capsule.

Exercises for muscle endurance are emphasized during the subacute stage because slow twitch muscle fibers are the first to atrophy when there is joint swelling, trauma, or immobilization.[35] Once AROM exercises are tolerated, low intensity, high repetition exercises using light resistance are introduced. The patient should be educated to use correct motor patterns, without substitutions, and to stop the exercise or activity when the involved muscle fatigues or the tissue develops symptoms.[35] For example, if the patient is doing shoulder flexion activities, substitution with scapular elevation or trunk motions must be avoided.

> ● **Key Point** Eccentric exercises are not used in the early subacute stage in the presence of a muscle injury because the tensile quality of the healing tissue is weak. For nonmuscular injuries, eccentric exercises may not reinjure the part, but the resistance should be limited to a low intensity to avoid delayed onset muscle soreness (see Chapter 10).

It is important during this stage to address any muscle length and strength imbalances, including postural stability problems. Other manual therapies that may be utilized during this stage include transverse friction massage (see Chapter 6) and gentle stretching.

Chronic (Maturation and Remodeling) Stage
The criteria for considering advancement to the chronic stage includes no complaints of pain; full, pain-free ROM; good flexibility and balance; and strength of 75 to 80 percent, or greater, compared with the uninvolved side.[64] The chronic phase involves a conversion of the initial healing tissue to scar tissue. This lengthy phase of contraction, tissue remodeling, and increasing tensile strength in the wound can last for up to 1 year. From day 21 to day 60 there is a predominance of fibroblasts that are easily remodeled.[70] Fibroblasts are responsible for the synthesis, deposition, and remodeling of the extracellular matrix. Following the deposition of granulation tissue, some fibroblasts are transformed into myofibroblasts, which congregate at the wound margins and start pulling the edges inward, reducing the size of the wound. Increase in collagen types I and III and other aspects of the remodeling process are responsible for wound contraction and visible scar formation. Epithelial cells migrate from the wound edges and continue to migrate until similar cells from the opposite side are met. This contracted tissue, or scar tissue, is functionally inferior to original tissue and is a barrier to diffused oxygen and nutrients.[71] The remodeling time is influenced by factors that affect the density and activity level of the fibroblasts, including the amount of time to mobilize, the stresses placed on the tissue, the location of the lesion, and the quality of the vascular supply.[35] Imbalances in collagen synthesis and degradation during this phase of healing may result in hypertrophic scarring or keloid formation with superficial wounds.

> ● **Key Point** A *keloid scar* is a result of an overgrowth of granulation tissue at the site of a healed skin injury. The overgrowth extends beyond the boundaries of an injury, damaging healthy tissues. Keloids are firm, rubbery lesions or shiny, fibrous nodules, and they can vary from pink to flesh-colored or red to dark brown in color. A *hypertrophic scar* can occur during the healing process when collagen production greatly exceeds collagen lysis. A hypertrophic scar is raised but remains within the borders of the original injury.

If the healing tissues are kept immobile, the fibrous repair is weak and there are no forces influencing the collagen; if left untreated, the scar formed is less than 20 percent of its original size.[72] Contraction of the scar, due to cross-linking of the collagen fibers and bundles, and the formation of adhesions between the immature collagen and surrounding tissues can cause scar hypomobility. In areas where the skin is loose and mobile, this creates minimal effect. However, in areas such as the dorsum of the hand where there is no extra skin, wound contracture can have a significant effect on function. Despite the presence of an intact epithelium at 3 to 4 weeks after the injury, the tensile strength of the wound has been measured at approximately 25 percent of its normal value. Several months later, only 70–80 percent of the strength may be restored.[73]

This would appear to demonstrate that the remodeling process may last many months or even years, making it extremely important to continue applying controlled stresses in the form of exercise to the tissue long after healing appears to have occurred.[73]

Normally, the remodeling phase is characterized by a progression to pain-free function and activity. The goals during this stage include improving muscle strength to normal levels, returning to normal neuromuscular control, completing a full return to functional activities, and restoring normal muscle force couple relationships.

During this stage, pain is typically felt at the end of range when stress is placed on restricted contractures or adhesions or when there is soreness due to the increased stress of resistive exercise. Musculoskeletal tissues respond to the controlled stresses applied to them by adaptation. This response has been described as a specific adaptation to imposed demand (SAID)[75] (see Chapter 8). Maximum strength of the collagen develops in the direction of the imposed forces. The application of inappropriate stresses during this stage can lead to various forms of tissue dysfunction, such as contracture, laxity, fibrosis, adhesion, diminished function, repeated structural failure, and an alteration in neurophysiologic feedback.[1,76] To avoid chronic or recurring pain, the contractures must be stretched or the adhesions broken up and mobilized. Free joint play within a functional range of motion is necessary to avoid joint trauma. Manual techniques may be required in this stage to emphasize the restoration of joint motion and to increase the extensibility of soft tissues. Techniques to increase soft tissue extensibility include passive and active stretching techniques (see Chapter 6).

In cases of decreased joint mobility, the PT may perform joint mobilizing techniques. Exercises are progressed from isolated, unidirectional, simple movements to complex patterns and multidirectional movements requiring coordination with all muscles functioning for the desired activity.[77] For example, proprioceptive neuromuscular facilitation (PNF) exercises incorporate multiple joints and multiple muscles in functional patterns (see Chapter 10). The progression to advanced functional or sports-specific exercises may also be made, depending on the patient's requirements.

Chronic Recurring Pain

Most episodes of tissue injury resolve normally, provided the condition is not exacerbated through constant reinjury, and that the injured tissue is allowed to progress through the natural stages of healing. If this natural progression does not occur, chronic recurring pain can result. In these cases, the proliferation of fibroblasts with increased collagen production and degradation of mature collagen leads to a predominance of new, immature collagen, which has an overall weakening effect on the tissue. Common causes for chronic recurring pain include:[14,15]

- Overuse, repetitive strain, or trauma
- Reinjury
- Length–strength imbalances
- Tissue weakness or excessive tension at the wound site
- Returning to an activity too soon after injury
- Training errors
- Hypertrophic scarring
- Poor blood supply[78,79]

Implications for the PTA

Conditions involving chronic recurring pain are best treated by initially controlling the inflammation using the principles of PRICEMEM. In addition, the patient should be educated as to the cause of the chronic irritation, and activities and positions to avoid. As with other soft tissue injuries, the patient is progressed through the stages of healing, but special emphasis is placed on addressing any chronic, contracted scar; identifying any faulty muscle and joint mechanics; emphasizing endurance exercises (if the cause is repetitive overuse); and referral to work conditioning and work hardening programs as appropriate.

Articular Cartilage Injury and Disease

Injuries to articular cartilage can be divided into three distinct types:

- Type 1 injuries (superficial) involve microscopic damage to the chondrocytes and extracellular membrane (ECM).
- Type 2 injuries (partial thickness) involve disruption of the articular cartilage surface

(chondral fractures or fissuring).[80] This type of injury has traditionally had an extremely poor prognosis because the injury does not penetrate the subchondral bone and therefore does not provoke an inflammatory response.[80]

- Type 3 injuries (full-thickness) involve disruption of the articular cartilage with penetration into the subchondral bone, which produces a significant inflammatory process.[80]

The intrinsic repair capacity of such defects remains limited to the production of fibrocartilage. When symptomatic, small full-thickness injuries may be successfully treated with minimally invasive techniques designed to permit the efflux of marrow elements into the defect, resulting in fibrocartilage formation (see "Surgical Repair of Cartilage, Bones, and Joints" later in this chapter).[81] However, large defects may respond poorly to such techniques, and may therefore require more sophisticated strategies, including arthroscopic lavage and debridement, microfracture, autologous chondrocyte implantation, or osteochondral grafting (see "Surgical Repair of Cartilage, Bones, and Joints" later in this chapter).[81]

Osteoarthritis

Osteoarthritis (OA), also known as degenerative joint disease, is a clinical condition of synovial joints. OA is characterized by development of fissures, cracks, and general thinning of joint cartilage; bone damage; hypertrophy of the cartilage; and synovial inflammation. The degenerative changes are most pronounced on the articular cartilage in weight-bearing areas of the large joints. Synovitis is minimal in the early stages of the disease but may contribute to joint damage in advanced disease.

● **Key Point**   Diseases such as OA affect the thixotropic properties* of synovial fluid, resulting in reduced lubrication and subsequent wear of the articular cartilage and joint surfaces.[82,83]

The degenerative changes associated with OA may result in pain and stiffness of the affected joints. The two commonly recognized types of OA are primary and secondary.

Primary Osteoarthritis

Primary OA, the most common form, has no known cause, although it appears to be related to aging and

heredity.[84] Most investigators believe that degenerative alterations primarily begin in the articular cartilage as a result of either excessive loading of a healthy joint or relatively normal loading of a previously disturbed joint. External forces accelerate the catabolic effects of the chondrocytes and disrupt the cartilaginous matrix. The diminished elastic return and reduced contact area of the cartilage, coupled with the cyclic nature of joint loading, causes the situation to worsen over time. These changes render the cartilage less resistant to compressive forces in the joint and more susceptible to the effects of stress, eventually leading to mechanical failure. The loss of cartilage results in a decrease of the joint space, and progressive erosion of the damaged cartilage occurs until the underlying bone is exposed. Bone denuded of its protective cartilage continues to articulate with the opposing surface. Eventually, the increasing stresses exceed the biomechanical yield strength of the bone. The subchondral bone responds with vascular invasion and increased cellularity, becoming thickened and dense (eburnation) at areas of pressure. At nonpressure areas along the articular margin of the joint, ossifying cartilaginous protrusions lead to irregular outgrowth of new bone (osteophytes). An osteophyte, which consists of newly formed cartilage and bone, likely forms in response to abnormal stresses on the joint margin, although its formation may also occur as a part of the aging process. There is experimental evidence that osteophyte formation is related to the instability of joints, and its growth has been described as part of the attempt of a synovial joint to adapt to injury, limiting excess movement and helping to re-create a viable joint surface.[85] Fragmentation of these osteophytes or of the articular cartilage itself results in intra-articular loose bodies (joint mice).

Primary OA occurs most commonly in the hands, particularly in the distal interphalangeal (DIP) joints, proximal interphalangeal (PIP) joints, and first carpometacarpal joints. The clinical signs and symptoms of osteoarthritis are described later in this chapter. The pathogenesis of primary OA is multifactorial. Although specific risk factors for OA differ by anatomic joint region, age is the most consistently identified demographic risk factor for all articular sites.[84] Before the age of 50 years, men have a higher prevalence and incidence of this disease than women, but after age 50, women have a higher prevalence and incidence.[86] However, increasing age does not appear to be an absolute risk factor in the development of OA because not

---

*Thixotropy is the property of various gels becoming fluid when disturbed, as by shaking.

every elderly person develops OA. The increase in the incidence and prevalence of OA with age is likely a consequence of several biologic changes that occur with aging, including the following:

- A decreased responsiveness of chondrocytes to growth factors that stimulate repair
- An increase in the laxity of ligaments around the joints, making older joints relatively unstable, and therefore more susceptible to injury
- A failure of major shock absorbers or protectors of the joint with age, including a gradual decrease in strength and a slowing of peripheral neurologic responses,[87] both of which protect the joint[82]

> **● Key Point** *Heberden nodes*, which represent palpable osteophytes in the DIP joints and are characteristic in women but not men, are features of OA, not rheumatoid arthritis. *Bouchard's nodes*, although less common, are similar structures that may be present on the PIP joints. Inflammatory changes are typically absent or at least not pronounced.

Secondary Osteoarthritis

Secondary OA may occur in any joint as a result of articular injury, including fracture, repetitive joint use, obesity, or metabolic disease (osteoporosis, osteomalacia). Secondary OA may occur at any age. OA of the hip and knee represents two of the most significant causes of adult pain and physical disability.[88]

> **● Key Point** OA is not a passive process of joint wear and tear, but a metabolically active process.[89]

Whether OA develops appears to depend on a variety of factors, as follows:[88]

- *Hormone replacement therapy:* Women receiving hormone replacement therapy have a lower prevalence of OA than women who are not receiving this therapy.
- *Obesity:* Studies have repeatedly confirmed the relationship of OA with body mass index. Obesity is more often associated with progressive OA of the knee than of the hip.[89–91]
- *Genetics and family history:* Abundant evidence supports the importance of genetic factors in some subgroups of OA.[91–93]
- *Activity level:* Low activity levels are associated with poorer outcomes, whereas certain forms of exercise are widely believed to increase bone

density (bone mass index) in specific areas of the body. For example, bone mass index can be increased up to 26 percent in some locations by loading the skeleton through physical exercise.[94] Strenuous, high-intensity, and repetitive exercise, both sport and occupational, has been associated with the development of OA, although there appears to be no increased incidence of OA with moderate exercise.

- *Occupation:* Work-related activities that involve repetitive actions have been shown to be correlated with increased rates of OA of the hip, knee, and other joints. Farmers, for example, have high rates of OA of the hip,[95] and epidemiologic studies have shown that firefighters, farmers, construction workers, and miners have a higher prevalence of OA of the knee than does the general population.[96,97] In fact, workers whose jobs require knee bending, as well as lifting or regularly carrying loads of 25 pounds or more, have increased radiologic evidence of OA in the knee compared with those workers who do not.[98] This trend has also been shown to hold true for the upper extremity; for example, jackhammer operators exhibit an increased prevalence of OA of the upper extremity when compared with the general population.[99]
- *Muscle loss:* OA causes atrophy proximal to the involved joints because of progressive weakness and disuse.[89] The loss of supporting muscle may increase the joint load, which can lead to greater cartilage damage, especially in the weight-bearing joints.
- *Trauma:* A prior history of trauma may be an important risk factor in the development of OA in a joint damaged by ligamentous instability or meniscal tear in the knee.

The signs and symptoms common to all types of osteoarthritis generally include the following:

- *Pain and tenderness:* Early in the course of the disease, the pain may be poorly localized, asymmetric, and episodic. Deep, achy joint pain exacerbated by extensive use is the primary symptom in the later stages. The severity and frequency of the pain increase as the disease progresses. More severe reports of pain are usually localized to the joint involved, but the pain may also be referred.[88] For example, with hip OA, pain can be referred to the front of the thigh and knee, and with OA of the knee, pain can be referred into the lower leg. Tenderness to palpation over the joint is common but may be mild or absent.

■ *Crepitus, swelling, inflammation, synovitis, and joint effusion:* All may be present, although swelling and joint effusion are seen in more advanced stages of OA.

■ *Impaired mobility:* This usually includes a characteristic pattern of limitation (capsular pattern), a firm end feel (unless acute; then the end feel may be guarded), decreased and possibly painful joint play, joint malalignment (chronic), and joint swelling (effusion).[100] Early in the disease process, stiffness is experienced in the affected joints following activity resumption after a period of rest. As the disease progresses, pieces of degenerated cartilage may shed into the joint, producing loose bodies that may cause the joint to either lock or give way.[89]

■ *Functional limitations:* The ability to perform activities of daily living may be minimally to significantly restricted. When the knee or hip is involved, gait may be impaired. If the fingers are involved, hand function is likely to be affected.

■ *Impaired balance:* If the weight-bearing joints are involved, patients may develop balance deficits because of altered or decreased sensory input from the joint mechanoreceptors and muscle spindles.[101]

■ *Impaired muscle performance:* The stabilizing muscles are often inhibited when there are swollen or restricted joints, and there may be mechanical imbalances in flexibility and strength of the supporting muscles.[100]

> ● **Key Point** The Western Ontario and McMaster Universities (WOMAC) OA Index is the most widely used disease-specific instrument for the assessment of patients with hip and knee OA (**Table 5-4**).[102,103]

Dramatic spontaneous restoration of the joint space in osteoarthritis is rare, although limited fibrocartilaginous repair is common. Regeneration of the joint space seems to be associated with peripheral osteophyte formation at the joint margin. The physical therapy intervention for hip osteoarthritis is outlined in Chapter 19.

Rheumatoid Arthritis

Rheumatoid arthritis (RA) is an inflammatory disease that affects the entire body and the whole person. It is a life-long disease that, in the majority of people, is modified only somewhat by intervention. The cycle of stretching, healing, and scarring that occurs as a result of the inflammatory process seen in rheumatoid arthritis causes significant damage to the soft tissues and periarticular structures. As a consequence, these events may lead to pain, stiffness, joint damage, instability, and ultimately, deformity. The onset of RA is usually in the small joints of the hands and feet, most commonly in the proximal interphalangeal joints. In the hand, many common deformities can be seen, such as ulnar deviation of the metacarpophalangeal (MCP) joints (ulnar drift), and radial deviation of the carpometacarpal block.

Ulnar Drift

The deformity of the ulnar drift and palmar subluxation of the carpals is a result of a complex interaction of forces and damage to collateral ligaments and extensor mechanism. Clinically, ulnar drift of the MCP articulations often precedes the wrist deformities. The ulnar drift results in an imbalance that has the resultant effect of pulling the fingers into ulnar deviation, pronation, and palmar subluxation.

Radial Deviation of the Carpometacarpal Block

This deformity is the result of the predominant action of the radial tendons (i.e., the flexor carpi radialis and the extensors carpi radialis longus and brevis), which radially deviate the carpometacarpal block. This deviation increases the angle between the radial border of the second metacarpal and the lower border for the distal radius, resulting in an important loss of muscular power in the flexors.

> ● **Key Point** Two finger deformities are associated with RA:
> *Boutonnière deformity:* The PIP joint of the finger is flexed, and the DIP joint is hyperextended (see Chapter 18). *Swan neck deformity:* The DIP is hyperflexed and the PIP is hyperextended (see Chapter 18).

The clinical signs and symptoms of RA include effusion and swelling of the joints, which can cause aching and limited motion. There may be a slight increase in skin temperature over the affected joints. The joint stiffness is prominent in the morning and there is usually pain on motion, with the pain and stiffness worsening after strenuous activity. With progression, the joints may become deformed and may ankylose or subluxate. These alterations can result in muscle atrophy and weakness, asymmetry in muscle strength, and alterations in the line of pull of muscles and tendons further exacerbating the deformity. Because RA can also produce diffuse inflammation in

Name: _____

Primary Care Physician: _____

This survey asks for your views about the amount of pain, stiffness, and disability you are experiencing. Please answer every question by filling in the appropriate response. If you are unsure about how to answer a question, please give the best answer you can. (Please mark your answers with an "X.")

SECTION A: PAIN

The following questions concern the amount of pain you are currently experiencing due to arthritis in your hips and/or knees. For each situation, please enter the amount of pain recently experienced.

Question: How much pain do you have?

	None	Mild	Moderate	Severe	Extreme
1. Walking on a flat surface	☐	☐	☐	☐	☐
2. Going up or down stairs	☐	☐	☐	☐	☐
3. At night while in bed	☐	☐	☐	☐	☐
4. Sitting or lying	☐	☐	☐	☐	☐
5. Standing upright	☐	☐	☐	☐	☐

SECTION B: JOINT STIFFNESS

The following questions concern the amount of joint stiffness (not pain) you are currently experiencing in your hips and/or knees. Stiffness is a sensation of restriction or slowness in the ease with which you move your joints.

	None	Mild	Moderate	Severe	Extreme
1. How severe is your stiffness after first wakening in the morning?	☐	☐	☐	☐	☐
2. How severe is your stiffness after sitting, lying, or resting later in the day?	☐	☐	☐	☐	☐

SECTION C: PHYSICAL FUNCTION

The following questions concern your physical function. By this we mean your ability to move around and to look after yourself. For each of the following activities, please indicate the degree of difficulty you are currently experiencing due to arthritis in your hips and/or knees. (Please mark your answers with an "X.")

Question: What degree of difficulty do you have with:

	None	Mild	Moderate	Severe	Extreme
1. Descending stairs	☐	☐	☐	☐	☐
2. Ascending stairs	☐	☐	☐	☐	☐
3. Rising from sitting	☐	☐	☐	☐	☐
4. Standing	☐	☐	☐	☐	☐
5. Bending to floor	☐	☐	☐	☐	☐
6. Walking on a flat surface	☐	☐	☐	☐	☐
7. Getting in/out of car	☐	☐	☐	☐	☐
8. Going shopping	☐	☐	☐	☐	☐
9. Putting on socks/stockings	☐	☐	☐	☐	☐
10. Rising from bed	☐	☐	☐	☐	☐

(continued)

TABLE 5-4	Western Ontario and McMaster Universities Osteoarthritis Index (WOMAC) (continued)					
		None	Mild	Moderate	Severe	Extreme
11.	Taking off socks/stockings	☐	☐	☐	☐	☐
12.	Lying in bed	☐	☐	☐	☐	☐
13.	Getting in/out of bath	☐	☐	☐	☐	☐
14.	Sitting	☐	☐	☐	☐	☐
15.	Getting on/off toilet	☐	☐	☐	☐	☐
16.	Heavy domestic duties	☐	☐	☐	☐	☐
17.	Light domestic duties	☐	☐	☐	☐	☐

the lungs, pericardium, and pleura, the patient may report nonspecific symptoms such as low-grade fever, loss of appetite and weight, malaise, and fatigue.

Juvenile Rheumatoid Arthritis

Juvenile rheumatoid arthritis (JRA) is described in Chapter 22.

Implications for the PTA

Osteoarthritis
The following guidelines are used in the treatment of osteoarthritis:[100]

- *Patient education:* Includes teaching the patient about the disease process, how to protect the joints while remaining active, and how to manage symptoms.
- *Pain management:* It is important to find a balance between activity and rest and to correct biomechanical stresses in order to prevent, retard, or correct the mechanical limitations. Eventually pain occurs at rest, and at that point cannot be managed with activity modification and analgesics prescribed by the physician, so that surgical intervention becomes an option.
- *Assistive and supportive devices:* The bony remodeling, swelling, and contractures that occur as a result of the progression of the disease alter the transmission of forces to the joint, which further perpetuates the deforming forces and creates joint deformity. Assistive devices such as a walker, cane, or raised toilet seat may be needed to reduce pain and maintain function.
- *Exercise:* The stronger the muscles around the joint the greater the protection. However, resistance exercises must be performed within tolerance of the joint. Aquatic therapy and

group-based exercise in water can decrease pain and improve physical function in patients with lower extremity OA.[104] In addition, the patient should be instructed in low-, moderate-, or high-intensity exercises designed to improve cardiopulmonary function.
- *Joint mobility:* Stretching techniques and joint mobilizations can be used to increase joint mobility.

Rheumatoid Arthritis
The goals of the intervention for RA depend on the stage of the disease process (exacerbation/flare and remission). During the exacerbation stage, the following guidelines should be used:[100]

- *Energy conservation:* The patient should be advised to respect fatigue and, when tired, to rest to minimize undue stress to all body systems.
- *Joint protection:* The patient should be advised to avoid prolonged static positioning, to use stronger and larger muscles and joints during activities whenever possible, to use appropriate adaptive equipment, and to monitor activities and stop the discomfort before fatigue begins to develop. Rest in nondeforming positions is encouraged because inflamed joints are easily damaged. The patient is advised on how to intersperse rest with ROM.
- *Therapeutic modalites:* For control of pain and inflammation using the principles of PRICEMEM.
- *Joint mobility:* Joint mobilizations (grade I and II distraction and oscillation techniques) may be performed during this period to help inhibit pain and minimize fluid status. Stretching techniques are not performed when joints are swollen.

- *Functional training:* Modifications may need to be made to activities of daily living in order to protect joints. If necessary, splints and assistive devices should be used to provide protection.
- *Increase or maintain range of motion:* The patient is encouraged to do active exercises through as much range of motion as possible without stretching. If active exercises are not tolerated, passive range of motion is used.

During the subacute and chronic stages (remission) of RA the intensity of pain, joint swelling, morning stiffness, and systemic effects diminish. These periods may be short in duration, or can last many years. During this time the treatment approach is the same as with any subacute and chronic musculoskeletal disorder, except appropriate precautions must be taken because the pathological changes on the disease process make the structures more susceptible to damage.[100] Emphasis should be placed on improving function, flexibility, muscle performance, and cardiopulmonary endurance using nonimpact or low-impact conditioning exercises such as swimming and bicycling performed within tolerance of the patient.

Fibrocartilage Healing

Fibrocartilage, such as intervertebral discs, the labrum, and the menisci in the knee and temporomandibular joint, differs from hyaline cartilage in that it is composed of type I collagen instead of type II collagen (see Chapter 2), and has a much higher fiber content than other types of cartilage. The nourishment of adult fibrocartilage is largely dependent on diffusion of nutrients through the synovial fluid in synovial joints. In amphiarthrodial joints (e.g., the intervertebral disk [IVD]), nutrients are diffused across the fluid contained in the adjacent trabecular bone, assisted by the "milking" action produced by intermittent weight-bearing. The perichondrium surrounding fibrocartilage is poorly organized and contains small blood vessels located only near the peripheral rim of the tissue. Therefore, injuries to the fibrocartilage lead to abnormal hydration and an irreversible cascade of tissue alteration.[105] Because cartilage is largely aneural, avascular, and devoid of immune system recognition, it has a very low potential of regeneration. However, in adult joints, some repair of damaged fibrocartilage can occur near the vascularized periphery (e.g., the outer one third of the meniscus the knee). Due to these factors, in many cases of fibrocartilage injury, surgical intervention is required. The implications for the PTA when treating IVD lesions are described in Chapters 13 and 15.

Bone Injury and Disease

The skeletal system is prone to injury and disease. Injury can occur by a direct or indirect force applied to the bone or neighboring structure, and disease of bone can occur in many forms.

Osteoporosis

Osteoporosis is a systemic skeletal disorder characterized by decreased bone mass and deterioration of bony microarchitecture. Osteoporosis results from a combination of genetic and environmental factors that affect both peak bone mass and the rate of bone loss. These factors include medications, diet, race, sex, lifestyle, and physical activity. Because osteoclasts require weeks to resorb bone, whereas osteoblasts need months to produce new bone, any process that increases the rate of bone remodeling results in net bone loss over time. This process results in low bone mineral density (BMD) and an associated increased risk of sustaining a fracture.

> ● **Key Point** Calcium, vitamin D, and parathyroid hormone help maintain bone homeostasis. Insufficient dietary calcium or impaired intestinal absorption of calcium can occur due to aging or disease.

BMD peaks by the third decade of life and slowly decreases afterward, so the failure to attain optimal bone strength by this stage in life is one factor that contributes to osteoporosis. Therefore, nutrition and physical activity are important during growth and development. Other factors, such as estrogen levels, also play a part.

> ● **Key Point** Estrogen deficiency can lead to excessive bone resorption accompanied by inadequate bone formation.

Osteoporosis typically involves the hip, distal arm, and spinal vertebrae and is classified as either primary or secondary. Primary osteoporosis is subdivided into types 1 and 2.

- Type 1, or postmenopausal, osteoporosis is thought to result from gonadal (i.e., estrogen, testosterone) deficiency. Estrogen or testosterone deficiency, regardless of age of occurrence, results in accelerated bone loss. After menopause, women experience an accelerated bone loss of 1–5 percent per year for the first 5–7 years. The end result is a decrease in trabecular bone and an increased risk of Colles' and vertebral fractures (see Chapter 14).

- Type 2, or senile, osteoporosis occurs in women and men because of decreased formation of bone and decreased renal production of $1,25(OH)_2 D_3$ occurring late in life. The consequence is a loss of cortical and trabecular bone and increased risk for fractures of the hip, long bones, and vertebrae.

Secondary osteoporosis, also called type 3 osteoporosis, occurs secondary to medications, especially glucocorticoids, or other conditions that cause increased bone loss by various mechanisms.

● **Key Point** Osteoporotic fractures occur when bones fail under excess stress. However, it is important to remember that some osteoporotic fractures may be asymptomatic.

Implications for the PTA

Although the best management of the problems associated with osteoporosis is prevention in susceptible populations, exercise has been found to be a key component in the treatment. In adults, exercise has been shown to maintain or increase bone density; in the elderly, it has been shown to reduce the effects of age-related or disease-related bone loss.[106] In particular, weight-bearing and exercises that apply controlled stresses to the bone have been found to be the most beneficial.[107,108] This is because muscle contraction and mechanical loading deform bone, which in turn stimulates osteoblastic activity and improves bone mineral density.[109–111] However, because osteoporosis changes the shape of the vertebral bodies (they become more wedge-shaped), leading to kyphosis, flexion activities and exercises such as supine curl-ups and sit-ups as well as the use of sitting abdominal machines, which stress the spine into flexion and increase the risk of vertebral compression fracture, should be avoided.[100] Similarly, exercises that combine flexion and rotation of the trunk should also be avoided.

Fractures

A fracture can be defined as a break in the continuity of the bone. Fractures of bone may be due to direct trauma such as a blow, indirect trauma such as a fall on an outstretched hand (FOOSH injury), or a twisting injury.

● **Key Point** Signs and symptoms of acute fracture include:

- Exquisite point tenderness over a bone
- Localized edema not directly associated with joint involvement (e.g., over the midshaft, diaphysis, or body of a long bone, or in the area of the body of a flat bone)
- Reports of grinding or feelings of instability
- Loss of function of the involved area

● **Key Point** Pathological fractures are those that occur from low energy injuries to an area of bone weakness with a preexisting abnormality or disease (osteoporosis, osteomalacia). The typical signs and symptoms of a pathological fracture include:

- Exquisite and localized tenderness upon palpation over the fracture site
- Symptoms aggravated with exertion or prolonged sitting or standing

Fractures are categorized by whether the skin is broken (open) or not (closed), the amount of disruption (displaced if the ends of the bones are not in anatomic alignment with each other, or nondisplaced if the bone on all sides of the fracture remains in anatomic alignment), and the type of fracture (Figure 5-2):

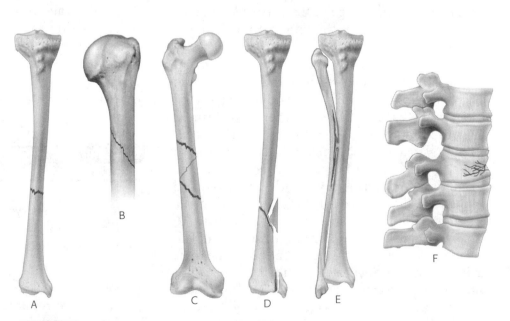

Figure 5-2 Types of fractures. A. Transverse fracture of the tibia. B. Oblique fracture of the humerus. C. Spiral fracture of the femur. D. Comminuted fracture of the tibia. E. Greenstick fracture of the fibula. F. Compression fracture of a vertebral body.

- *Complete fracture:* A fracture in which bone fragments separate completely.
- *Incomplete fracture:* A fracture in which the bone fragments are still partially joined.
- *Linear fracture:* A fracture that is parallel to the bone's long axis.
- *Transverse fracture:* A fracture that is at a right angle to the bone's long axis.
- *Oblique fracture:* A fracture that is diagonal to the bone's long axis.
- *Spiral fracture:* A fracture where at least one part of the bone has been twisted.
- *Compacted fracture:* A fracture caused when bone fragments are driven into each other.
- *Holstein-Lewis fracture:* A fracture of the distal third of the humerus resulting in entrapment of the radial nerve.
- *Comminuted:* A fracture where the bones break into more than two fragments—often the result of significant trauma.
- *Avulsion:* Seen in athletes and children; occurs when a piece of bone attached to a tendon or ligament is torn away.

Pediatric fractures, such as the greenstick fracture, are described in Chapter 22. Fractures commonly occur among seniors for a number of reasons including decreased vision and poor balance, and can have a significant impact on the morbidity, mortality, and functional dependence of this population. Fractures in the elderly have their own set of problems:

- The fractures heal more slowly (taking an average of 6–12 weeks) and are more likely to result in malunion and nonunion.
- There is an increased potential for pneumonia and decubiti if immobilized for long periods.
- There are often changes in mental status.
- The healing of the fracture can be more complicated due to existing comorbidities.

Stress Fractures

Stress fractures are fractures that occur in the absence of a specific acute precipitating traumatic event.[112] Multiple clinical reports have described stress fractures in persons with rheumatoid arthritis, lupus erythematosis, osteoarthritis, pyrophosphate arthropathy, renal disease, osteoporosis, and joint replacements, and in older patients who have no apparent musculoskeletal disease.[112] Stress fractures are also commonly associated with overuse and overtraining.

● **Key Point** In states of increased physical activity where the bone's adaptations do not occur fast enough, bone resorption (bone lysis) occurs faster than it is formed (osteoid synthesis). When bone resorption exceeds bone formation, a reduction in bone mass and strength occurs, resulting in a stress fracture.

Stress fractures can be classified according to cause:[113]

- Fatigue stress fractures are caused by repetitive and abnormally high forces from muscle action and/or weight-bearing torques and are often found in persons with normal bone densities.
- Insufficiency stress fractures are associated with individuals who have compromised bone densities. Because insufficiency stress fractures are associated with decreased bone mineral density (osteoporosis), they tend to be most common in the elderly, especially postmenopausal women. Other predisposing factors for poor bone density include radiation treatments, rheumatoid arthritis due at least in part to the associated disuse secondary to pain and loss of function and either corticosteroid or methotrexate treatment, renal failure, coxa vara (see Chapter 19), metabolic disorders, and Paget's disease.

The clinical presentation of a stress fracture varies according to site:

- *Rib:* There are more reports of stress fractures of the first rib than any other single rib.[114] This injury usually occurs during overhead activities, such as reaching and pulling with the arm held high.[115,116] Pain occurs in the shoulder, anterior cervical triangle, or clavicular region.[116] The pain may radiate to the sternum or pectoral region. The onset is usually insidious, although it may start with acute pain. Pain may occur with deep breathing.[117] Tenderness to palpation may be present medial to the superior angle of the scapula, at the base of the neck, in the supraclavicular triangle, or deep in the axilla.[114] Shoulder movements may be painful or restricted.
- *Femoral neck/head:* Although stress fractures are a relatively uncommon etiology of hip pain, if not diagnosed in a timely fashion, progression to serious complications can occur.[118] It is estimated that up to 5 percent of all stress fractures involve the femoral neck, with another 5 percent involving the femoral head.[119] The fracture typically occurs on the superior side (tension-side fractures) or the

inferior side (compression-side fractures) of the femoral neck.[120] These fractures may develop into a complete and displaced fracture if left untreated. The most frequent symptom is the onset of sudden hip pain, usually associated with a recent change in activity level, training level (particularly an increase in distance or intensity), or training surface. The earliest and most frequent symptom is pain in the deep thigh, inguinal, or anterior groin area.[120] Pain can also occur in the lateral or anteromedial aspect of the thigh. The pain usually occurs with weight bearing or at the extremes of hip motion and can radiate into the knee. Less severe cases may only have pain following a long run. Night pain may occur if the fracture progresses.

- *Tibia:* Tibial stress fractures are a common cause of shin soreness and a very common cause of exertional leg pain. Simple muscle strains are probably the most common cause of acute exercise-induced leg pain, whereas more subacute or chronic pain may be caused by stress fractures or chronic (exertional) compartment syndrome. Recognition of anterior tibial stress fractures is important because these fractures are prone to nonunion and avascular necrosis. They are also at greater risk of becoming displaced than are posterior tibial stress fractures. This increased susceptibility to complication has been attributed to a predominance of tensile forces along the anterior diaphysis rather than compressive forces along the posterior diaphysis.

Bone Healing

The striking feature of bone healing, compared with healing in other tissues, is that repair is by the original tissue, not scar tissue. Regeneration is perhaps a better descriptor than repair. Like other forms of healing, the healing of bone fracture includes the processes of inflammation, repair, and remodeling; however, the type of healing varies, depending on the method of treatment.

The process of bone healing involves a combination of intramembranous and endochondral ossification (Figure 5-3). These two processes participate in the fracture repair sequence by at least four discrete stages of healing:[121]

- *Hematoma formation (inflammatory) phase:* Initially, the tissue volume in which new bone is to be formed is filled with the matrix, generally including a blood clot or hematoma.[80] An effective bone healing response will include an initial inflammatory phase characterized by the release of a variety of products, an increase in regional blood flow, invasion of neutrophils and monocytes, removal of cell debris, and degradation of the local fibrin clot.

- *Soft callus formation (reparative or revascularization) phase:* This phase is characterized by the formation of connective tissues, including cartilage, and formation of new capillaries from preexisting vessels (angiogenesis). During the first 7 to 10 days of fracture healing, the periosteum undergoes an intramembranous bone formation response. By the middle of the second week, abundant cartilage overlies the fracture site, and this chondroid tissue initiates biochemical preparations to undergo calcification.

- *Hard callus formation (modeling) phase:* This phase is characterized by the systematic removal of the initial matrix and tissues that formed in the site, primarily through osteoclastic and chondroclastic resorption, and their replacement with more organized lamellar bone (woven bone) aligned in response to the local loading environment.[80] The calcification of fracture callus cartilage can occur either directly from mesenchymal tissue (intramembranous) or via an intermediate stage of cartilage (endochondral or chondroid routes). Osteoblasts can form woven bone rapidly, but the result is randomly arranged and mechanically weak. Nonetheless, bridging of a fracture by woven bone constitutes so-called *clinical union*. The clinical union is a critical milestone in the healing of a broken long bone because it signals that the woven bone at the fracture site has hardened and become so firmly fixed to the other fragments that they move as a single unit. Usually splinting is reduced at this stage, but the site still requires protection from excessive stresses. Once cartilage is calcified, it becomes a target for the ingrowth of blood vessels.

- *Remodeling phase:* By replacing the cartilage with bone, and converting the cancellous bone into compact bone, the callus is gradually remodeled. During this phase, the woven bone is remodeled into stronger lamellar bone by a

Stage 1: Organization

Procallus (fibrous
connective tissue)

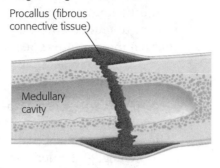

Medullary
cavity

Bleeding and clot formation

Granulation tissue formation
• Fibroblast and blood
  vessel proliferation

Procallus formation

Day 5

Stage 2: Callus formation

Soft callus (fibrous connective tissue
and hyaline cartilage)

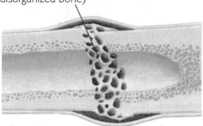

Areas of hyaline cartilage develop
within the procallus, converting it
to a soft callus

Hard callus (weak,
disorganized bone)

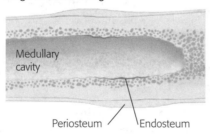

Intramembranous and
endochondrial ossification convert
the soft callus into a hard callus

Day 28

Stage 3: Remodeling

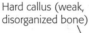

Medullary
cavity

Periosteum   Endosteum

Remodeling has removed the
callus and replaced the fractured
matrix

The only remaining evidence of
former injury may be the slight
thickening of the endosteum and
periosteum

Years later

Figure 5-3 Bone healing.

combination of osteoclast bone resorption and osteoblast bone formation. Radiologically or histologically, fracture gap bridging occurs by three mechanisms:[121]

❏ *Intercortical bridging (primary cortical union):* This mechanism occurs when the fracture gap is reduced by normal cortical remodeling under conditions of rigid fixation. This mode of healing is the principle behind rigid internal fixation.[122]

❏ *External callus bridging by new bone arising from the periosteum and the soft tissues surrounding the fracture:* Small degrees of movement at the fracture stimulate external callus formation.[123] This mode of healing is the aim in functional bracing and intramedullary nailing.

❑ *Intramedullary bridging by endosteal callus:* A remodeling process that substitutes the trabecular bone with compact bone. The trabecular bone is first resorbed by osteoclasts, which creates a small pit. Then osteoblasts deposit compact bone within the pit and the fracture callus begins the remodeling process to return the bone to a close duplication of its original shape and strength.

Implications for the PTA

The correct treatment of fractures requires information about when the fracture occurred and when the immobilization was removed. Continuous immobilization of connective and skeletal muscle tissues can cause some undesirable consequences including cartilage degeneration, decreased mechanical and structural strength of ligaments, decreased bone density, and weakness or atrophy of muscles (see the next section). Normal periods of immobilization following a fracture range from as short as 3 weeks for small bones to about 8 weeks for the long bones of the extremities. During the period of casting, submaximal isometrics are initiated. Once the cast is removed, it is important that controlled stresses continue to be applied to the bone, because the period of bone healing continues for up to 1 year. Successful restoration of osseous morphology and internal architecture is conditional on the remodeling process. According to Wolff's law, bone remodels along lines of stress.[124] Bone is constantly being remodeled as the circumferential lamellar bone is resorbed by osteoclasts and replaced with dense osteonal bone by osteoblasts.[125]

> **● Key Point** Wolff's law is a theory developed by the German anatomist/surgeon Julius Wolff (1836–1902) that states that bone in a healthy person or animal will adapt to the loads applied to it. If loading on the bone increases, the bone remodels over time to become stronger to resist future loading.

Treatment of the edema, pain, and range of motion deficit associated with fractures and bone pathology are important aspects of bone healing. Controlled weight-bearing exercises (based on the weight-bearing status if the lower extremity is involved) during the early stages allows for deposition of cartilage callus and prevents the formation of deep vein thrombosis. Normal joint mobility and mechanics typically need to be restored, and strengthening is initiated and progressed based on patient tolerance and the presence of other factors that demonstrate that healing is continuing.

Possible complications of a fracture that the PTA must be aware of include:

■ *Infection:* Infectious organisms can occur on both implants and the host bone environment, resulting in bone resorption, bone destruction, implant loosening, and reactive periosteal elevation.

■ *Malunion:* Healing results in a nonanatomic position due to ineffective immobilization or a failure to maintain immobilization for an adequate period of time.

■ *Delayed union/nonunion:* The healing process is inhibited or stopped (nonunion) due to an infection or poor blood supply.

■ *Associated injury (e.g., nerve, vessel, soft tissue):* The type and degree of force required to fracture a bone usually injures the surrounding tissues as well.

■ *Deep venous thrombosis/pulmonary embolism:* This can occur in fractures of the pelvis or femur. The risk of pulmonary embolism following acetabular fractures is about 4–7 percent (see Chapter 1).

■ *Acute compartment syndrome:* Compartment syndrome (CS) is a limb-threatening and life-threatening condition observed when perfusion pressure falls below tissue pressure in a closed anatomic space. Long bone fractures are a common cause of compartment syndrome (Volkman's ischemic contracture) (see Chapter 1).

| Detrimental Effects of Immobilization

Continuous immobilization of connective and skeletal muscle tissues in an adaptively shortened state can have some undesirable consequences. These include the following:

■ *Cartilage degeneration:* Immobilization of a joint causes atrophic changes in articular cartilage resulting in cartilage softening.[126] Because the softened articular cartilage is vulnerable to damage during weight bearing, the PTA must be careful during such activities, and the use of an assistive device may be warranted.

■ *Decreased mechanical and structural properties of ligaments:* One study[63] showed that after 8 weeks of immobilization, the stiffness of a ligament decreased to 69 percent of control values; even after 1 year of rehabilitation, the ligament did not return to its prior level of strength. This results in a compromise in the ability of the ligament to provide stabilization, thereby making the joint more susceptible to injury unless protected using splinting, bracing, or an assistive device when weight bearing.

> **● Key Point** Following a period of immobilization, connective tissues are more vulnerable to deformation and breakdown than normal tissues subjected to similar amounts of stress.[127]

- *Decreased bone density:*[32,33,128–130] The interactions among systemic and local factors to maintain normal bone mass are complex. Bone mass is maintained because of a continuous coupling between bone resorption by osteoclasts and bone formation by osteoblasts, and this process is influenced by both systemic and local factors.[131] Mechanical forces acting on bone stimulate osteogenesis (Wolff's law), and the absence of such forces inhibits osteogenesis. Marked osteopenia occurs in otherwise healthy patients in states of complete immobilization or weightlessness.[132,133] In children, bone has a high modeling rate and appears to be more sensitive to the absence of mechanical loading than bone in adults.[134] Decreased bone density results in increased vulnerability of the bone to fracture. Therapeutic exercises, particularly closed-chain exercises, have been shown to be beneficial in strengthening bone.
- *Weakness or atrophy of muscle:* The longer the duration of immobilization, the greater the atrophy of muscle and loss of functional strength. Muscle atrophy is an imbalance between protein synthesis and degradation. After modest trauma, there is a decrease in whole body protein synthesis rather than increased breakdown. With more severe trauma, major surgery, or multiple organ failure, both synthesis and degradation increase, the latter being more enhanced.[135,136] Muscle atrophy can begin within as little as a few days to a week.[137] The composition of muscle affects its response to immobilization, with atrophy occurring more quickly and more extensively in tonic (slow-twitch) postural muscle fibers than in phasic (fast-twitch) fibers.[138]
- *Change in muscle length:* If the muscle is immobilized in a shortened position for several weeks, there is a reduction in the length of the muscle and its fibers and in the number of sarcomeres in series within myofibrils as the result of sarcomere absorption.[139] The absorption rate occurs faster than the muscle's ability to regenerate sarcomeres, resulting in muscle atrophy and weakness and a shift to the left in the length–tension curve (see Chapter 4) of a shortened muscle.[140] This shift decreases the muscle's capacity to produce maximum tension at its normal resting length as it contracts.[141]

The PTA must remember that the restoration of full strength and range of motion may prove difficult if the connective tissues are allowed to heal without early active motion, or in a shortened position, and that the patient may be prone to repeated strains.[142] The cause of muscle damage during exercised recovery from atrophy involves an altered ability of the muscle fibers to bear the mechanical stress of external loads (weight bearing) and movement associated with exercise. Strenuous exercise can result in primary or secondary sarcolemma disruption, swelling or disruption of the sarcotubular system, distortion of the myofibrils' contractile components, cytoskeletal damage, and extracellular myofiber matrix abnormalities.[143] These pathologic changes are similar to those seen in healthy young adults after sprint running or resistance training.[143] It appears that the act of contracting while the muscle is in a stretched or lengthened position, known as an eccentric contraction, is responsible for these injuries.[144] Thus, range-of-motion exercises should be started once swelling and tenderness have subsided to the point that the exercises are not unduly painful, and strengthening exercises introduced as tolerated.[142]

Surgical Interventions

Although surgery is generally elective and used as a treatment of last resort, in cases of fractures, dislocations, and soft tissue ruptures, surgery may be the primary approach.

Surgical Repair of Tendons

Tendon injuries may require operative intervention, depending on the complexity of the injury. The goal of repair is to restore tendon continuity and function. Repair can be accomplished immediately in the emergency department or after a delay of up to 7 days following the injury. The repair involves suturing the two ends of the tendon together using a variety of techniques. The surgical area is then protected using some form of postsurgical splinting or bracing. The postsurgical rehabilitation protocols vary according to site and are not within the scope of this text.

Surgical Repair of Ligaments

Surgical treatment options or indications for ligament injuries are based on the following:[145,146]

- *Degree of injury and the potential for self-repair:* Because of the associated injuries and profound instability with grade III injuries, surgery is often necessary. However, certain ligaments (e.g., the medial collateral ligament [MCL]), because of their anatomic location, have a greater potential for vascular supply and therefore healing, even at the grade III level.
- *Amount of joint instability:* Surgical treatment is usually recommended for young adult athletes because they have more years to develop degenerative joint conditions from chronic instabilities caused by joint ligament deficiencies.
- *Associated injuries:* Oftentimes, due to the level of trauma associated with a ligament injury, some of the surrounding tissues can be injured. For example, a torn anterior cruciate ligament (ACL) can be associated with a meniscal injury, and because the menisci contribute to stability of the knee, the loss of this stabilizing effect appears to predispose these patients to osteoarthrosis.[147–154]
- *Skeletal maturity of patients:* Because of the potential damage to the growth plates that may result in growth arrest following surgery, the decision to perform surgery on children with open growth plates remains questionable.[155,156] The risk of growth disturbance appears to be low if the patient is within 1 year of skeletal maturity at the time of surgery.[157]
- *Expected levels of patients' participation in future sports activities:* The expected future activity levels and participation in sports activities for the younger patient are often more vigorous than those for the middle-aged adult.[158]

Surgical Repair of Cartilage, Bones, and Joints

Current surgical options include those outlined in **Table 5-5**.

TABLE 5-5	Surgical Procedures for Cartilage, Bones, and Joints	
Procedure	**Description**	**Implications for the PTA**
Debridement/abrasion chondroplasty	Debridement procedures are designed to remove loose fragments and other mechanical or chemical irritants. Abrasion chondroplasty is a procedure performed alone or in combination with other procedures for articular cartilage lesions to stimulate a healing response and local fibrocartilage ingrowth.	Rehabilitation varies with the extent and location of the articular cartilage lesion.
Microfracture	Works by creating tiny fractures in the underlying bone, which causes new cartilage to develop from a so-called super-clot.	Rehabilitation varies with the extent and location of the bony lesions.
Osteochondral autograft transplantation (OAT)	Also referred to as mosaicplasty. Designed to restore and preserve articular cartilage by transferring articular cartilage tissue from areas of low loading to areas of high loading.	The general rules about rehabilitating any articular cartilage lesions apply here and are modified based on individual patient factors. PROM is performed as tolerated, whereas AROM varies depending on the size, location, and fixation of the lesion. Patients are typically non-weight-bearing for 3 to 4 weeks, followed by a gradual progression of weight-bearing over the next 3 to 4 weeks.

| TABLE |
| 5-5 |

Surgical Procedures for Cartilage, Bones, and Joints (continued)

Procedure	Description	Implications for the PTA
Autologous chondrocyte implantation	Research is focused on using growth factors to induce the newly attracted or transplanted chondrocytes to mature faster. Bone morphogenic proteins (BMPs) are members of the transforming growth factor superfamily and have a regulatory role in the differentiation of cartilage-forming and bone-forming cells. Used in cases in which the lesion is up to 15 centimeters in diameter. Two to three full-thickness samples of healthy articular cartilage are harvested from the patient, cultivated for 11 to 21 days, and then injected into the site.	Rehabilitation is similar to that following any articular cartilage procedure—full unloaded PROM is initiated early, and the patient is non-weight–bearing for the first 2 to 4 weeks, with progressive weight-bearing over the next 2 to 4 weeks.
Mosaicplasty with either autologous tissue or fresh allograft	Refers to the technique of harvesting small circular (4–8 millimeter) autogenous grafts from regions of a healthy joint and transplanting the grafts in a mosaic pattern until the osteochondral defect is filled.	Rehabilitation is similar to that following any articular cartilage procedure—full unloaded PROM is initiated early, and the patient is non-weight-bearing for the first 2 to 4 weeks, with progressive weight-bearing over the next 2 to 4 weeks.
Open reduction and internal fixation	Commonly performed when closed reduction is impossible or when fracture healing would be protracted if treated without fixation. Fixation may use plates, screws, wires, or other forms of hardware to stabilize the bone and fragments.	Weight-bearing and motion restrictions are specific to the location and severity of the initial fracture. Treatment focuses on associated soft tissue damage and restoration of full function.
Fusion	The operative formation of an ankylosis or arthrodesis. Most commonly performed in the spine or ankle.	The postoperative rehabilitation is focused on the adjacent joints and the procedures necessary to ensure the long-term health of these joints.
Osteotomy	The surgical cutting of the bone to correct bony alignment. Most commonly performed at the knee to correct excessive genu varus or valgus.	The rehabilitation focuses on the preservation or restoration of motion and strength while considering the changing loading patterns on the articular cartilage.
Arthroplasty (joint replacement)	Performed to remedy significant degenerative joint disease. Categorized by component design (constrained, unconstrained, or semiconstrained), fixation (cement or cementless), and materials (titanium alloy, high density polyethylene, or cobalt-chrome alloy).	Rehabilitation protocols are joint- and prosthesis-specific. In general, restoration of motion, strength, and function constitute the rehabilitation framework.

Summary

The three phases of the healing process are the coagulation and inflammation, migratory and proliferative, and maturation and remodeling phases, which occur in sequence but overlap one another in a continuum. The rehabilitation philosophy relative to inflammation and healing after injury is to assist the natural processes of the body while doing no harm. The course of rehabilitation must focus on knowledge of the healing process and its therapeutic modifiers that guide, direct, and stimulate the structural function and integrity of the injured part. This is accomplished by increasing range of motion, muscular strength and endurance, neuromuscular control, and cardiorespiratory endurance while continuing to have a positive influence on the repair process. Finally, focus should be switched to preventing a recurrence of the injury by influencing the structural ability of the injured tissue to resist further overloads by incorporating various therapeutic exercises.

REVIEW Questions

1. What are the three phases of soft tissue healing?
2. How does tendinitis differ from tendinosis?
3. What are the three stages of bone healing?
4. How does Wolff's law apply to bone healing?
5. Name three areas in the body that are prone to tendonopathy.
6. What is the difference between a sprain and a strain?
7. All of the following terms are used to describe fractures, except:
    a. Greenstick
    b. Comminuted
    c. Pathologic
    d. Tangential
8. A disease in which there is deficiency in mineralization of bone matrix is:
    a. Osteogenesis imperfecta
    b. Osteitis deformans
    c. Osteomalacia
    d. Osteoporosis
9. All of the following are considered modifiable risk factors for developing skeletal demineralization, except:
    a. Use of specific medications
    b. Estrogen deficiency
    c. Physical inactivity
    d. Early menopause
10. In differentiating osteoarthritis from rheumatoid arthritis, the latter:
    a. More often involves weight-bearing joints
    b. Involves the distal interphalangeal joints
    c. Is a systemic disease
    d. Is often associated with increasing age

References

1. Barlow Y, Willoughby J: Pathophysiology of soft tissue repair. Br Med Bull 48:698–711, 1992
2. Biundo JJ, Jr., Irwin RW, Umpierre E: Sports and other soft tissue injuries, tendinitis, bursitis, and occupation-related syndromes. Curr Opin Rheumatol 13:146–149, 2001
3. Cailliet R: Soft Tissue Pain and Disability. Philadelphia, FA Davis, 1980
4. Cummings GS: Comparison of muscle to other soft tissue in limiting elbow extension. J Orthop Sports Phys Ther 5:170, 1984
5. Jarvinen TA, Kaariainen M, Jarvinen M, et al: Muscle strain injuries. Curr Opin Rheumatol 12:155–161, 2000
6. Reid DC: Sports Injury Assessment and Rehabilitation. New York, Churchill Livingstone, 1992
7. Watrous BG, Ho G, Jr.: Elbow pain. Prim Care 15:725–735, 1988
8. Glick JM: Muscle strains: Prevention and treatment. Phys Sports Med 8:73–77, 1980
9. Peers KH, Lysens RJ: Patellar tendinopathy in athletes: Current diagnostic and therapeutic recommendations. Sports Med 35:71–87, 2005
10. Backman C, Boquist L, Friden J, et al: Chronic Achilles paratendonitis with tendinosis: An experimental model in the rabbit. J Orthop Res 8:541–547, 1990
11. Dehne E, Tory R: Treatment of joint injuries by immediate mobilization based upon the spiral adaption concept. Clin Orthop 77:218–232, 1971
12. McKenzie R, May S: Introduction, in McKenzie R, May S (eds): The Human Extremities: Mechanical Diagnosis and Therapy. Waikanae, New Zealand, Spinal Publications New Zealand, 2000, pp 1–5
13. Hunt TK: Wound Healing and Wound Infection: Theory and Surgical Practice. New York, Appleton-Century-Crofts, 1980
14. Singer AJ, Clark RAF: Cutaneous wound healing. N Engl J Med 341:738–746, 1999
15. Oakes BW: Acute soft tissue injuries: Nature and management. Austr Fam Phys 10:3–16, 1982
16. Van der Mueulin JHC: Present state of knowledge on processes of healing in collagen structures. Int J Sports Med 3:4–8, 1982
17. Clayton ML, Wier GJ: Experimental investigations of ligamentous healing. Am J Surg 98:373–378, 1959
18. Mason ML, Allen HS: The rate of healing of tendons. An experimental study of tensile strength. Ann Surg 113:424–459, 1941
19. Wong MEK, Hollinger JO, Pinero GJ: Integrated processes responsible for soft tissue healing. Oral Surg Oral Med Oral Pathol Oral Radiol Endod 82:475–492, 1996

20. Heldin C-H, Westermark B: Role of platelet-derived growth factor in vivo, in Clark RAF (ed): The Molecular and Cellular Biology of Wound Repair (ed 2). New York, Plenum Press, 1996, pp 249–273

21. Sen CK, Khanna S, Gordillo G, et al: Oxygen, oxidants, and antioxidants in wound healing: An emerging paradigm. Ann N Y Acad Sci 957:239–249, 2002

22. Kellett J: Acute soft tissue injuries: A review of the literature. Med Sci Sports Exerc 18:5, 1986

23. Amadio PC: Tendon and ligament, in Cohen IK, Diegelman RF, Lindblad WJ (eds): Wound Healing: Biomechanical and Clinical Aspects. Philadelphia, WB Saunders, 1992, pp 384–395

24. Peacock EE: Wound Repair (ed 3). Philadelphia, WB Saunders, 1984

25. Ross R: The fibroblast and wound repair. Biol Rev 43:51–96, 1968

26. Evans RB: Clinical application of controlled stress to the healing extensor tendon: A review of 112 cases. Phys Ther 69:1041–1049, 1989

27. Emwemeka CS: Inflammation, cellularity, and fibrillogenesis in regenerating tendon: Implications for tendon rehabilitation. Phys Ther 69:816–825, 1989

28. Janda V: Muscle strength in relation to muscle length, pain and muscle imbalance, in Harms-Ringdahl K (ed): Muscle Strength. New York, Churchill Livingstone, 1993, pp 83–91

29. Booth FW: Physiologic and biochemical effects of immobilization on muscle. Clin Orthop Relat Res 219:15–21, 1987

30. Eiff MP, Smith AT, Smith GE: Early mobilization versus immobilization in the treatment of lateral ankle sprains. Am J Sports Med 22:83–88, 1994

31. Akeson WH, Amiel D, Mechanic GL: Collagen cross-linking alterations in the joint contractures: Changes in the reducible cross-links in periarticular connective tissue after 9 weeks immobilization. Connect Tissue Res 5:15, 1977

32. Akeson WH, Amiel D, Abel MF, et al: Effects of immobilization on joints. Clin Orthop 219:28–37, 1987

33. Akeson WH, Amiel D, Woo SL-Y: Immobility effects on synovial joints: The pathomechanics of joint contracture. Biorheology 17:95–110, 1980

34. Woo SL-Y, Matthews J, Akeson WH, et al: Connective tissue response to immobility: A correlative study of biochemical and biomechanical measurements of normal and immobilized rabbit knee. Arthritis Rheum 18:257–264, 1975

35. Kisner C, Colby LA: Soft tissue injury, repair, and management, in Kisner C, Colby LA (eds): Therapeutic Exercise. Foundations and Techniques (ed 5). Philadelphia, FA Davis, 2002, pp 295–308

36. Hettinga DL: Inflammatory response of synovial joint structures, in Gould JA, Davies GJ (eds): Orthopaedic and Sports Physical Therapy. St. Louis, MO, CV Mosby, 1985, pp 87–117

37. Thorndike A: Athletic Injuries: Prevention, Diagnosis and Treatment. Philadelphia, Lea and Febiger, 1962

38. Garrick JG: A practical approach to rehabilitation. Am J Sports Med 9:67–68, 1981

39. Nirschl RP: Prevention and treatment of elbow and shoulder injuries in the tennis player. Clin Sports Med 7:289–308, 1988

40. Astrand PO, Rodahl K: Textbook of Work Physiology. New York, McGraw-Hill, 1973

41. Zarins B: Soft tissue injury and repair: Biomechanical aspects. Int J Sports Med 3:9–11, 1982

42. Frank G, Woo SL-Y, Amiel D, et al: Medial collateral ligament healing. A multidisciplinary assessment in rabbits. Am J Sports Med 11:379, 1983

43. Leach RE: The prevention and rehabilitation of soft tissue injuries. Int J Sports Med 3:18–20, 1982 (suppl 1)

44. McMaster WC: Cryotherapy. Phys Sports Med 10:112–119, 1982

45. Maadalo A, Waller JF: Rehabilitation of the foot and ankle linkage system, in Nicholas JA, Hershman EB (eds): The Lower Extremity and Spine in Sports Medicine. St. Louis, MO, CV Mosby, 1986, pp 560–583

46. Quillen WS, Rouillier LH: Initial management of acute ankle sprains with rapid pulsed pneumatic compression and cold. J Orthop Sports Phys Ther 4:39–43, 1981

47. Starkey JA: Treatment of ankle sprains by simultaneous use of intermittent compression and ice packs. Am J Sports Med 4:142–143, 1976

48. Wilkerson GB: Treatment of ankle sprains with external compression and early mobilization. Phys Sports Med 13:83–90, 1985

49. Cole AJ, Farrell JP, Stratton SA: Functional rehabilitation of cervical spine athletic injuries, in Kibler BW, Herring JA, Press JM (eds): Functional Rehabilitation of Sports and Musculoskeletal Injuries. Gaithersburg, MD, Aspen, 1998, pp 127–148

50. Farrell JP: Cervical passive mobilization techniques: The Australian approach. Phys Med Rehab 4:309–334, 1990

51. Booth FW, Kelso JR: The effect of hindlimb immobilization on contractile and histochemical properties of skeletal muscle. Pflugers Arch 342:231–238, 1973

52. Haggmark T, Eriksson E: Cylinder or mobile cast brace after knee ligament surgery. Am J Sports Med 7:48–56, 1979

53. Farmer JA, Pearl AC: Provocative issues, in Leadbetter WB, Buckwalter JA, Gordon SL (eds): Sports-Induced Inflammation: Clinical and Basic Science Concepts. Park Ridge, IL, American Academy of Orthopaedic Surgeons, 1990, pp 781–791

54. Helminen HJ, Jurvelin J, Kuusela T, et al: Effects of immobilization for 6 weeks on rabbit knee articular surfaces as assessed by the semiquantitative stereomicroscopic method. Acta Anat Nippon 115:327–335, 1983

55. Kibler WB: Concepts in exercise rehabilitation of athletic injury, in Leadbetter WB, Buckwalter JA, Gordon SL (eds): Sports-Induced Inflammation: Clinical and Basic Science Concepts. Park Ridge, IL, American Academy of Orthopaedic Surgeons, 1990, pp 759–769

56. Salter RB, Field P: The effects of continuous compression on living articular cartilage. J Bone Joint Surg 42A:31–49, 1960

57. Woo SL-Y, Tkach LV: The cellular and matrix response of ligaments and tendons to mechanical injury, in Leadbetter WB, Buckwalter JA, Gordon SL (eds): Sports-Induced Inflammation: Clinical and Basic Science Concepts. Park Ridge, IL, American Academy of Orthopaedic Surgeons, 1990, pp 189–202

58. Cox JS: Surgical and nonsurgical treatment of acute ankle sprains. Clin Orthop 198:118–126, 1985

59. Bourne MH, Hazel WA, Scott SG, et al: Anterior knee pain. Mayo Clinic Proc 63:482–491, 1988

60. Brody LT, Thein JM: Nonoperative treatment for patellofemoral pain. J Orthop Sports Phys Ther 28:336–344, 1998

61. Akeson WH, Woo SLY, Amiel D, et al: The chemical basis for tissue repair, in Hunter LH, Funk FJ (eds): Rehabilitation of the Injured Knee. St. Louis, MO, CV Mosby, 1984, pp 93–147

62. Tipton CM, James SL, Mergner W, et al: Influence of exercise in strength of medial collateral knee ligaments of dogs. Am J Physiol 218:894–902, 1970

63. Noyes FR, Torvik PJ, Hyde WB, et al: Biomechanics of ligament failure: II. An analysis of immobilization, exercise, and reconditioning effects in primates. J Bone Joint Surg 56A:1406–1418, 1974

64. Herring SA, Kibler BW: A framework for rehabilitation, in Kibler BW, Herring JA, Press JM (eds): Functional Rehabilitation of Sports and Musculoskeletal Injuries. Gaithersburg, MD, Aspen, 1998, pp 1–8

65. Arem A, Madden J: Effects of stress on healing wounds: Intermittent non-cyclical tension. J Surg Res 42:528–543, 1971

66. Safran MR, Zachazewski JE, Benedetti RS, et al: Lateral ankle sprains: A comprehensive review part 2: Treatment and rehabilitation with an emphasis on the athlete. Med Sci Sports Exer 31:S438–S447, 1999

67. Safran MR, Benedetti RS, Bartolozzi AR, III., et al: Lateral ankle sprains: A comprehensive review: Part 1: Etiology, pathoanatomy, histopathogenesis, and diagnosis. Med Sci Sports Exer 31:S429–S437, 1999

68. Stanley BG: Therapeutic exercise: Maintaining and restoring mobility in the hand, in Stanley BG, Tribuzi SM (eds): Concepts in Hand Rehabilitation. Philadelphia, FA Davis, 1992, pp 178–215

69. Pease BJ, Cortese M: Anterior knee pain: Differential diagnosis and physical therapy management, Orthopaedic Physical Therapy Home Study Course 92-1. La Crosse, WU, Orthopaedic Section, American Physical Therapy Association, 1992

70. Tillman LJ, Cummings GS: Biologic mechanisms of connective tissue mutability, in Currier DP, Nelson M (eds): Dynamics of Human Biologic Tissue. Philadelphia, FA Davis, 1992

71. Chvapil M, Koopman CF: Scar formation: Physiology and pathological states. Otolaryngol Clin North Am 17:265–272, 1984

72. Levenson SM, Geever EF, Crowley LV, et al: The healing of rat skin wounds. Ann Surg 161:293–308, 1965

73. Orgill D, Demling RH: Current concepts and approaches to wound healing. Crit Care Med 16:899, 1988

74. Farfan HF: The scientific basis of manipulative procedures. Clin Rheum Dis 6:159–177, 1980

75. Klaffs CE, Arnheim DD: Modern Principles of Athletic Training. St. Louis, MO, CV Mosby, 1989

76. Porterfield JA, DeRosa C: Mechanical Low Back Pain (ed 2). Philadelphia, WB Saunders, 1998

77. Wilk KE, Arrigo CA: An integrated approach to upper extremity exercises. J Orthop Phys Ther Clin North Am 1:337, 1992

78. Garrett WE, Lohnes J: Cellular and matrix response to mechanical injury at the myotendinous junction, in Leadbetter WB, Buckwalter JA, Gordon SL (eds): Sports-Induced Inflammation: Clinical and Basic Science Concepts. Park Ridge, IL, American Academy of Orthopaedic Surgeons, 1990, pp 215–224

79. Di Rosa F, Barnaba V: Persisting viruses and chronic inflammation: Understanding their relation to autoimmunity. Immunol Rev 164:17–27, 1998

80. Vereeke West R, Fu F: Soft tissue physiology and repair, Orthopaedic Knowledge Update 8: Home Study Syllabus. Rosemont, IL, American Academy of Orthopaedic Surgeons, 2005, pp 15–27

81. Lewis PB, McCarty LP, 3rd, Kang RW, et al: Basic science and treatment options for articular cartilage injuries. J Orthop Sports Phys Ther 36:717–727, 2006

82. O'Driscoll SW: The healing and regeneration of articular cartilage. J Bone Joint Surg 80A:1795–1812, 1998

83. Dieppe P: The classification and diagnosis of osteoarthritis, in Kuettner KE, Goldberg WM (eds): Osteoarthritic Disorders. Rosemont, IL, American Academy of Orthopaedic Surgeons, 1995, pp 5–12

84. Lawrence RC, Hochberg MC, Kelsey JL, et al: Estimates of the prevalence of selected arthritic and musculoskeletal diseases in the United States. J Rheumatol 16:427–441, 1989

85. Bullough P, Vigorta V: Atlas of Orthopaedic Pathology. London, Gower, 1984

86. Van Saase JLCM, van Romunde LKJ, Cats A, et al: Epidemiology of osteoarthritis: Zoetermeer survey. Comparison of radiological osteoarthritis in a Dutch population with that in 10 other populations. Ann Rheum Dis 48:271–280, 1989

87. Sharma L, Pai Y-C, Holtkamp K, et al: Is knee joint proprioception worse in the arthritic knee versus the unaffected knee in unilateral knee osteoarthritis? Arthritis Rheum 40:1518–1525, 1997

88. Birchfield PC: Osteoarthritis overview. Geriatr Nurs 22:124-130; quiz 130–131, 2001

89. Townes AS: Osteoarthritis, in Barker LR, Burton JR, Zieve PD (eds): Principles of Ambulatory Medicine (ed 5). Baltimore, Williams & Wilkins, 1999, pp 960–973

90. Birchfield PC: Arthritis: Osteoarthritis and rheumatoid arthritis, in Robinson D, Kidd P, Rogers KM (eds): Primary Care Across the Lifespan. St. Louis, MO, Mosby, 2000, pp 89–95

91. Cardone DA, Tallia AF: Osteoarthritis, in Singleton JK, Sandowski SA, Green-Hernandez C, et al (eds): Primary Care. Philadelphia, Lippincott, 1999, pp 543–548

92. Huang J, Ushiyama KI, Kawasaki T, et al: Vitamin D receptor gene polymorphisms and osteoarthritis of the hand, hip, and knee: A case control study in Japan. Rheumatology 39:79–84, 2000

93. Mustafa Z, Chapman CI, Carr AJ, et al: Linkage analysis of candidate genes as susceptibility loci for arthritis-suggestive linkage of COL9A1 to female hip osteoarthritis. Rheumatology 39:299–306, 2000

94. Sharkey NA, Williams NI, Guerin JB: The role of exercise in the prevention and treatment of osteoporosis and osteoarthritis. Rheumatology 35:209–219, 2000

95. Croft P, Coggon D, Cruddas M, et al: Osteoarthritis of the hip: An occupational disease in farmers. Br Med J 304:1272, 1992

96. Felson DT: The epidemiology of knee osteoarthritis: Results from the Framingham Osteoarthritis Study. Sem Arthritis Rheum 20:42–50, 1990

97. Felson DT, Hannan MT, Naimark A: Occupational physical demands, knee bending and knee osteoarthritis: Results from the Framingham study. J Rheumatol 18:1587–1592, 1991

98. Anderson JJ, Felson DT: Factors associated with osteoarthritis of the knee in the first National Health and Nutrition Examination Survey. Am J Epidemiol 128:179–189, 1988

99. Felson DT: The epidemiology of osteoarthritis: Prevalence and risk factors, in Keuttner KE, Goldberg VM (eds): Osteoarthritic Disorders. Rosemont, IL, American Academy of Orthopaedic Surgeons, 1995, pp 13–24

100. Kisner C, Colby LA: Joint, connective tissue, and bone disorders and management, in Kisner C, Colby LA (eds): Therapeutic Exercise. Foundations and Techniques (ed 5). Philadelphia, FA Davis, 2002, pp 309–327

101. Wegener L, Kisner C, Nichols D: Static and dynamic balance responses in persons with bilateral knee osteoarthritis. J Orthop Sports Phys Ther 25:13–18, 1997

102. Brazier JE, Harper R, Munro J, et al: Generic and condition-specific outcome measures for people with osteoarthritis of the knee. Rheumatology. 38:870–877, 1999

103. Anderson JG, Wixson RL, Tsai D, et al: Functional outcome and patient satisfaction in total knee patients over the age of 75. J Arthroplasty. 11:831–840, 1996

104. Cochrane T, Davey RC, Matthes Edwards SM: Randomised controlled trial of the cost-effectiveness of water-based therapy for lower limb osteoarthritis. Health Technol Assess 9:iii–iv, ix–xi, 2005

105. Alford W, Cole BJ: The indications and technique for meniscal transplant. Orthop Clin North Am 36:469–484, 2005

106. Marcus R: Role of exercise in preventing and treating osteoporosis. Rheum Dis Clin North Am 27:131–141, 2001

107. Ayalon J, Simkin A, Leichter I, et al: Dynamic bone loading exercises for postmenopausal women: Effect on the density of the distal radius. Arch Phys Med Rehabil 68:280–283, 1987

108. Simkin A, Ayalon J, Leichter I: Increased trabecular bone density due to bone-loading exercises in postmenopausal osteoporotic women. Calcif Tissue Int 40:59–63, 1987

109. Sinaki M, Wollan PC, Scott RW, et al: Can strong back extensors prevent vertebral fractures in women with osteoporosis? Mayo Clin Proc 71:951–956, 1996

110. Sinaki M, Itoi E, Rogers JW, et al: Correlation of back extensor strength with thoracic kyphosis and lumbar lordosis in estrogen-deficient women. Am J Phys Med Rehabil 75:370–374, 1996

111. Sinaki M: Effect of physical activity on bone mass. Curr Opin Rheumatol 8:376–383, 1996

112. Buckwalter JA, Brandser EA: Stress and insufficiency fractures. Am Fam Physician 56:175–182, 1997

113. Gurney B, Boissonnault WG, Andrews R: Differential diagnosis of a femoral neck/head stress fracture. J Orthop Sports Phys Ther 36:80–88, 2006

114. Gregory PL, Biswas AC, Batt ME: Musculoskeletal problems of the chest wall in athletes. Sports Med 32:235–250, 2002

115. Jenkins SA: Spontaneous fractures of both first ribs. J Bone Joint Surg 34B:9–13, 1952

116. Lankenner PAJ, Micheli LJ: Stress fractures of the first rib: A case report. J Bone Joint Surg Am 67:159–160, 1985

117. Mintz AC, Albano A, Reisdorff EJ, et al: Stress fracture of the first rib from serratus anterior tension: An unusual mechanism of injury. Ann Emerg Med 19:411–414, 1990

118. Boden BP, Osbahr DC: High-risk stress fractures: Evaluation and treatment. J Am Acad Orthop Surg 8:344–353, 2000

119. Clough TM: Femoral neck stress fracture: The importance of clinical suspicion and early review. Br J Sports Med 36:308–309, 2002

120. Fullerton LR, Jr., Snowdy HA: Femoral neck stress fractures. Am J Sports Med 16:365–367, 1988

121. Marsh DR, Li G: The biology of fracture healing: Optimising outcome. Br Med Bull 55:856–869, 1999

122. Muller ME: Internal fixation for fresh fractures and nonunion. Proc R Soc Med 56:455–460, 1963

123. McKibbin B: The biology of fracture healing in long bones. J Bone Joint Surg 60B:150–161, 1978

124. Monteleone GP: Stress fractures in the athlete. Orthop Clin North Am 26:423, 1995

125. Hockenbury RT: Forefoot problems in athletes. Med Sci Sports Exerc 31:S448–S458, 1999

126. Jurvelin J, Kiviranta I, Tammi M, et al: Softening of canine articular cartilage after immobilization of the knee joint. Clin Orthop 207:246–252, 1986

127. Deyo RA: Measuring functional outcomes in therapeutic trials for chronic disease. Control Clin Trials 5:223, 1984

128. Akeson WH, Woo SL, Amiel D, et al: The connective tissue response to immobility: Biochemical changes in periarticular connective tissue of the immobilized rabbit knee. Clin Orthop 93:356–362, 1973

129. Bailey DA, Faulkner RA, McKay HA: Growth, physical activity, and bone mineral acquisition, in Hollosky JO (ed): Exercise and Sport Sciences Reviews. Baltimore, MD, Williams and Wilkins, 1996, pp 233–266

130. Lane JM, Riley EH, Wirganowicz PZ: Osteoporosis: Diagnosis and treatment. J Bone Joint Surg 78A:618–632, 1996

131. Harris WH, Heaney RP: Skeletal renewal and metabolic bone disease. N Engl J Med 280:193–202, 253–259, 303–311, 1969

132. Donaldson CL, Hulley SB, Vogel JM, et al: Effect of prolonged bed rest on bone mineral. Metabolism 19:1071–1084, 1970

133. Mazess RB, Whedon GD: Immobilization and bone. Calcif Tiss Int 35:265–267, 1983

134. Rosen JF, Wolin DA, Finberg L: Immobilization hypercalcemia after single limb fractures in children and adolescents. Am J Dis Child 132:560–564, 1978

135. Birkhahn RH, Long CL, Fitkin D, et al: Effects of major skeletal trauma on whole body protein turnover in man measured by L-(1,14C)-leucine. Surgery 88:294–300, 1980

136. Arnold J, Campbell IT, Samuels TA, et al: Increased whole body protein breakdown predominates over increased whole body protein synthesis in multiple organ failure. Clin Sci 84:655–661, 1993

137. Kannus P, Jozsa L, Kvist M, et al: The effect of immobilization on myotendinous junction: An ultrastructural, histochemical and immunohistochemical study. Acta Physiol Scand 144:387–394, 1992

138. Lieber RL, Bodine-Fowler SC: Skeletal muscle mechanics: Implications for rehabilitation. Phys Ther 73:844–856, 1993

139. Jokl P, Konstadt S: The effect of limb immobilization on muscle function and protein composition. Clin Orthop Relat Res 174:222–229, 1983

140. Kisner C, Colby LA: Stretching for impaired mobility, in Kisner C, Colby LA (eds): Therapeutic Exercise. Foundations and Techniques (ed 5). Philadelphia, FA Davis, 2002, pp 65–108

141. Gossman MR, Sahrmann SA, Rose SJ: Review of length-associated changes in muscle. Phys Ther 62:1799–1808, 1982

142. Booher JM, Thibodeau GA: The body's response to trauma and environmental stress, in Booher JM, Thibodeau GA (eds): Athletic Injury Assessment (ed 4). New York, McGraw-Hill, 2000, pp 55–76

143. Kasper CE, Talbot LA, Gaines JM: Skeletal muscle damage and recovery. AACN Clin Issues 13:237–247, 2002

144. McNeil PL, Khakee R: Disruptions of muscle fiber plasma membranes: Role in exercise-induced damage. Am J Pathol 140:1097–1109, 1992

145. Williams JS, Bernard RB: Operative and nonoperative rehabilitation of the ACL-injured knee. Sports Med Arth Rev 4:69–82, 1996

146. Keays SL, Bullock-Saxton J, Keays AC: Strength and function before and after anterior cruciate ligament reconstruction. Clin Orthop Rel Res 373:174–183, 2000

147. Frank CB, Jackson DW: The science of reconstruction of the anterior cruciate ligament. J Bone Joint Surg 79:1556–1576, 1997

148. Daniel DM, Stone ML, Dobson BE, et al: Fate of the ACL-injured patient. A prospective outcome study. Am J Sports Med 22:632–644, 1994

149. Ferretti A, Conteduca F, De Carli A, et al: Osteoarthritis of the knee after ACL reconstruction. Int Orthop 15:367–371, 1991

150. Henning CE: Current status of meniscal salvage. Clin Sports Med 9:567–576, 1990

151. Shirakura K, Terauchi M, Kizuki S, et al: The natural history of untreated anterior cruciate tears in recreational ahtletes. Clin Orthop 317:227–236, 1995

152. Sommerlath K, Lysholm J, Gillquist J: The long-term course after treatment of acute anterior cruciate ligament ruptures. A 9 to 16 year followup. Am J Sports Med 19:156–162, 1991

153. Hefzy MS, Grood ES: Ligament restraints in anterior cruciate ligament-deficient knees, in Jackson DW, Arnoczky SP, Woo SL-Y, et al (eds): The Anterior Cruciate Ligament. Current and Future Concepts. New York, Raven Press, 1993, pp 141–151

154. Levy IM, Torzilli PA, Warren RF: The effect of medial meniscectomy on anterior-posterior motion of the knee. Am J Bone Joint Surg 64-A:883–888, 1982

155. Janarv PM, Nystrom A, Werner S, et al: Anterior cruciate ligament injuries in skeletally immature patients. J Ped Orthop 16:673, 1996

156. Parker AW, Drez D, Cooper JL: Anterior cruciate injuries in patients with open physes. Am J Sports Med 22:47, 1994

157. Busch MT: Sports medicine, in Morrissey RT, Weinstein SL (eds): Lovell and Winter's Pediatric Orthopedics (ed 4). Philadelphia, JB Lippincott, 1996, pp 886, 889

158. Micheli LJ, Jenkins M: Knee injuries, in Micheli LJ (ed): The Sports Medicine Bible. Scranton, PA, Harper Row, 1995, pp 42–59

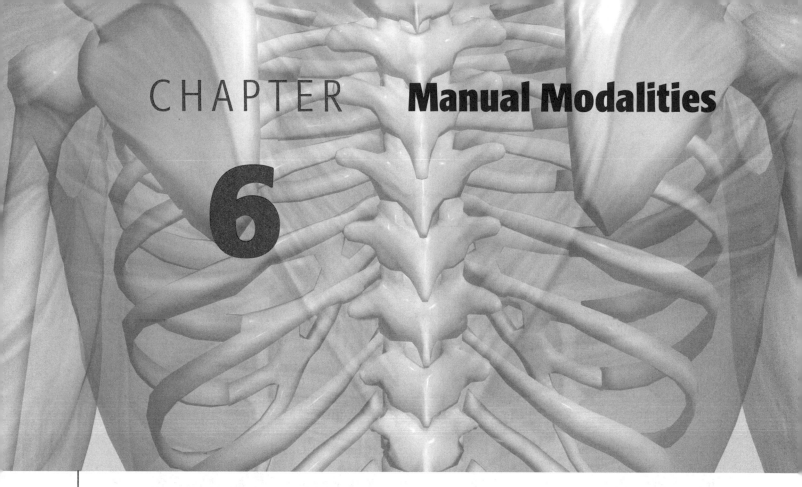

CHAPTER **Manual Modalities**

6

Chapter Objectives

At the completion of this chapter, the reader will be able to:

1. Summarize the various types of manual therapy (MT).
2. Discuss the general and applied concepts of MT.
3. Recognize the role that the various MTs play in the performance of a comprehensive rehabilitation program.
4. Recognize the manifestations of abnormal tissue and develop strategies using MT techniques to treat these abnormalities.
5. Categorize the various effects of MT on the soft tissues.
6. Perform a variety of MT techniques.

Overview

Touch has always been and continues to be a primary healing modality. The techniques of manual therapy (MT) fall under the umbrella of therapeutic touch. MT techniques traditionally have been used to produce a number of therapeutic alterations in pain and soft tissue extensibility through the application of specific external forces.[1–4] MT has become such an important component of the intervention for orthopaedic disorders that it is considered by many as an area of specialization within physical therapy.[5–8]

Within these areas of specialization, a number of major philosophies have dominated. These include the Cyriax,[10] Mennell,[11] and osteopathic techniques,[12,13] which originated from physicians, and the Maitland,[2,14] Kaltenborn,[3] and McKenzie[15] approaches. In addition, a number of MT subsets have emerged, including massage, joint mobilizations, soft tissue techniques, proprioceptive neuromuscular facilitation (PNF), and myofascial trigger point therapy.

At the time of writing, the delegation of many manual techniques is based on the discretion of the supervising physical therapist. There is also the issue of legality, which involves the licensing practice act of the state in which the assistant practices. In the United States, some states still do not have legal rules and regulations covering the service delivery of PTAs in general; other states have laws that limit the performance of specific PTA-related skills. However, whether or not a PTA is permitted to perform manual techniques, it is important that the PTA understands the concepts behind techniques such as joint mobilization so he or she can better understand the rationale of the physical therapist's intervention program.

Correct Application of Manual Techniques

Despite the varied approaches and rationales, there is general agreement concerning criteria that are important for the correct application of a manual technique. These include:[19]

- *Duration, type, and irritability of symptoms:*[2,14] This information can provide the clinician with some general guidelines in determining the intensity of the application of a selected technique (see "Indications for Manual Therapy"

later in this chapter). The more irritable a structure, the gentler the technique needs to be.
- *Patient and clinician position:* Correct positioning of the patient is essential both to help the patient relax and to ensure safe body mechanics from the clinician. When patients feel relaxed, their muscle activity is decreased, reducing the amount of resistance encountered during the technique.
- *Hand placement:* Wherever possible, contact with the patient should be maximized. The hand should conform to the area being treated so the forces are spread over a larger area. A gentle and confident touch inspires confidence from the patient. Accurate hand placement is essential for efficient stabilization and for the accurate transmission of force.
- *Specificity:* Specificity refers to the exactness of the procedure, and is based on its intent. Whenever possible, the forces imparted by a technique should occur at the point where they are needed.
- *Direction of force:* The direction of the force can be either *direct*, which is toward the motion barrier or restriction,[20] or *indirect*, which is away from the motion barrier or restriction.[21,22] Although the rationale for a direct technique is easy to understand, the rationale for using an indirect technique is more confusing. A good analogy is a stuck drawer that cannot be opened. Often the movement that eventually frees the drawer is an inward motion followed by a pull.[19]
- *Reinforcement of any gains made:* It has been demonstrated that movement gained by a specific manual technique performed in isolation will be lost within 48 hours if the motions gained are not reinforced.[23] Thus, motion gained by a manual technique must be reinforced by both the mechanical and the neurophysiologic benefits of active movement.[24] These active movements must be as local and precise as possible to the involved segment or myofascial structure.

If the MT to be used is a joint mobilization, the following criteria are important:

- *Knowledge of the resting (open-packed) position of the joint:* The position of the joint to be treated must be appropriate for the stage of healing and the skill of the clinician. It is recommended that the resting position of the joint be used when the patient has an acute condition or the clinician is inexperienced. The resting position in this case refers to the position that the injured joint adopts, rather than the classic resting (open-packed) position for a normal joint. The resting positions of the joints are outlined in **Table 6-1**. Other positions

TABLE 6-1	Shape, Resting Position, and Treatment Planes of the Joints			
Joint	**Convex Surface**	**Concave Surface**	**Resting Position**	**Treatment Plane**
Sternoclavicular	Clavicle*	Sternum*	Arm resting by side	Parallel to joint
Acromioclavicular	Clavicle	Acromion	Arm resting by side	Parallel to joint
Glenohumeral	Humerus	Glenoid	55 degrees of abduction, 30 degrees of horizontal adduction	In scapular plane
Humeroradial	Humerus	Radius	Elbow extended, forearm supinated	Perpendicular to long axis of radius
Humeroulnar	Humerus	Ulna	70 degrees of elbow flexion, 10 degrees of forearm supination	45 degrees to long axis of ulna
Radioulnar (proximal)	Radius	Ulna	70 degrees of elbow flexion, 35 degrees of forearm supination	Parallel to long axis of ulna
Radioulnar (distal)	Ulna	Radius	Supinated 10 degrees	Parallel to long axis of radius
Radiocarpal	Proximal carpal bones	Radius	Line through radius and third metacarpal	Perpendicular to long axis of radius
Metacarpophalangeal	Metacarpal	Proximal phalanx	Slight flexion	Parallel to joint
Interphalangeal	Proximal phalanx	Distal phalanx	Slight flexion	Parallel to joint
Hip	Femur	Acetabulum	Hip flexed 30 degrees, abducted 30 degrees, slight external rotation	Varies according to goal
Tibiofemoral	Femur	Tibia	Flexed 25 degrees	On surface of tibial plateau
Patellofemoral	Patella	Femur	Knee in full extension	Along femoral groove
Talocrural	Talus	Mortise	Plantarflexed 10 degrees	In the mortise in anterior/posterior direction
Subtalar	Calcaneus	Talus	Subtalar neutral between inversion and eversion	In talus, parallel to foot surface
Intertarsal	Proximal articulating surface	Distal articulating surface	Foot relaxed	Parallel to joint
Metatarsophalangeal	Tarsal bone	Proximal phalanx	Slight extension	Parallel to joint
Interphalangeal	Proximal phalanx	Distal phalanx	Slight flexion	Parallel to joint

*In the sternoclavicular joint, the clavicle surface is convex in a superior/inferior direction and concave in an anterior/posterior direction.
Data from Prentice WE: Joint mobilization and traction, in Prentice WE (ed): Therapeutic Modalities for Allied Health Professionals. New York, McGraw-Hill, 1998, pp 443–478

for starting the mobilization may be used by an experienced and skilled clinician in patients with nonacute conditions.

> **● Key Point** It is worth remembering that the resting position is easily obtainable in a normal joint but is more difficult to obtain in dysfunctional joints due to pain and stiffness. For example, the resting position for the humeroradial joint is elbow extended, forearm supinated, but elbow injuries tend to be held in slight elbow flexion.

- *Knowledge of the relative shapes of the joint surfaces (concave or convex):*[2,3,14,25] If the joint surface is convex relative to the other surface, the joint glide (arthrokinematic) occurs in the direction opposite to the osteokinematic movement (angular motion) (see Chapter 4). If, on the other hand, the joint surface is concave, the joint glide occurs in the same direction as osteokinematic movement. The shape and treatment planes of the joints are outlined in Table 6-1.

Indications for Manual Therapy

MT is generally indicated in the following cases:

- Mild, intermittent musculoskeletal pain that is relieved by rest
- A nonirritable musculoskeletal condition, demonstrated by acute pain that is provoked by motion but that disappears very quickly
- Soft tissue tightness and adhesions
- Contractures
- Edema/effusion
- Pain reported by the patient that is relieved or provoked by particular motions or positions
- Pain that is altered by changes related to sitting or standing posture

Contraindications to Manual Therapy

Contraindications to MT include those that are absolute contraindications and those that are relative.[26,27] Absolute contraindications include the following:

- Bacterial infection
- Malignancy
- Systemic localized infection
- Recent fracture
- Cellulitis
- Febrile state
- Hematoma
- Acute circulatory condition

- An open wound at the treatment site
- Osteomyelitis
- Advanced diabetes
- Hypersensitivity of the skin
- Inappropriate end feel (spasm, empty, and bony)
- Constant, severe pain
- Extensive radiation of pain
- Pain unrelieved by rest
- Severe irritability (pain that is easily provoked and does not go away within a few hours)

Relative contraindications include the following:

- Joint effusion or inflammation
- Rheumatoid arthritis
- Presence of neurologic signs
- Osteoporosis
- Hypermobility
- Pregnancy, if a technique is to be applied to the spine
- Dizziness
- Steroid or anticoagulant therapy

Massage

Massage is a mechanical modality that produces physiologic effects through different types of stroking (Figure 6-1), kneading (Figure 6-2), rubbing, tapotement (Figure 6-3), and vibration (Figure 6-4):

- *Reflexive effects:* An autonomic nervous system phenomenon produced through stimulation of the sensory receptors in the skin and superficial fascia; causes sedation, relieves tension, and increases blood flow
- *Pain reduction:* Most likely regulated by both gate control and the release of endogenous opiates (see Chapter 3)

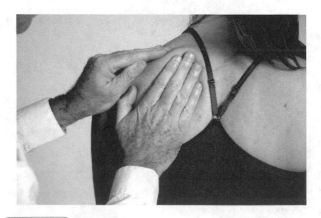

Figure 6-1 Stroking.

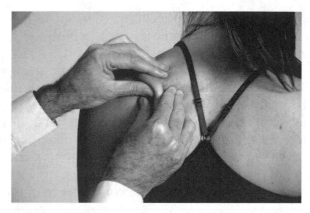

Figure 6-2   Kneading.

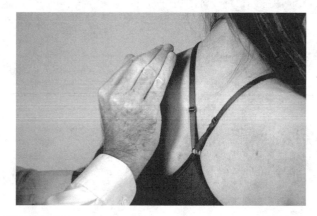

Figure 6-3   Tapotement.

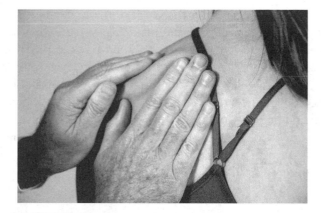

Figure 6-4   Vibration.

- *Circulatory effects:* Increases lymphatic and blood flow
- *Metabolism:* Indirectly affects metabolism due to the increase in lymphatic and blood flow
- *Mechanical effects:* Stretches the intramuscular connective tissue, retards muscle atrophy, and increases range of motion
- *Skin:* Increases skin temperature

Indications for massage include the following:

- To decrease pain
- To decrease neuromuscular excitability
- To stimulate circulation
- To restore skin mobility
- To help remove lactic acid
- To alleviate muscle cramps
- To increase blood flow
- To increase venous return
- To break adhesions
- To alleviate symptoms from myositis, bursitis, fibrositis, or tendonitis

Contraindications for massage include the following:

- Arteriosclerosis
- Thrombosis
- Embolism
- Severe varicose veins
- Acute phlebitis, cellulitis, or synovitis
- Skin infections
- Malignancies
- Acute inflammatory conditions

Specific Massage Techniques

Hoffa, Classic, and Swedish massage are classical massage techniques that use a variety of superficial strokes, including the following:

- *Effleurage:* Produces a reflexive response. Effleurage is typically performed at the beginning and at the end of a massage to allow the patient to relax. It also is used in the management of edema. The massage is begun at the peripheral areas and moves from the extremity toward the heart. At the beginning of the massage, the pressure should be light, using flat hands with fingers slightly bent and thumbs spread apart. In the course of the massage, the pressure can be increased. The direction of the strokes should be towards the heart.
- *Petrissage:* Described as a kneading or working stroke that is directed primarily at the muscle system—the muscle being squeezed and rolled under the clinician's hands. Applied in a distal to proximal sequence, petrissage is used primarily for:
  - Increasing the local blood supply
  - Reducing edema
  - Loosening adhesions
  - Improving lymphatic return
  - Removing metabolic waste

- *Rubbing (friction):* Used primarily in areas of local, deep lying trigger points to produce a strong, hyperemic effect in small surface areas of the muscle. The motion applied is circular to elliptical, or transverse (transverse frictional massage; see details later in this chapter).
- *Tapotement/percussion:* A massage technique that provides stimulation to rapid and alternating movements such as tapping, hacking, cupping, and slapping to enhance circulation and stimulate peripheral nerve endings. This type of massage is used for chest PT techniques and the athletic population.
- *Vibration:* Manual vibration, which is particularly strenuous for the clinician, involves a rapid shaking motion that causes vibration to the treatment area. This type of massage is used primarily for relaxation, but it also can have a stimulating effect.
- *Manual lymphatic drainage (MLD):* According to the Vodder and/or Leduc techniques, this is a gentle technique that stimulates superficial lymphatics and reroutes lymph toward healthy lymphatic vessels. MLD is designed to clear the healthy quadrant (central areas), and then progress systematically down the involved extremity. MLD may be used in cases where there is high-protein edema, as in postsurgical swelling; for wounds that do not heal because of chronic swelling; and to promote a sympathetic and parasympathetic response in those patients who experience chronic pain. Compression garments are essential between treatments. Contraindications specific to this form of therapy include congestive heart failure.

Joint Mobilizations

It is important to note that, at this time, the APTA position statement does not support joint mobilization performed by the PTA. However, it is important to understand the concepts behind joint mobilization and how they relate to the relevant osteokinematics and arthrokinematics (see Chapter 4).

● **Key Point** Some confusion exists regarding the terms *joint mobility* and *joint mobilization*. *Joint mobility* refers to the amount of motion occurring at joint surfaces. The assessment of joint mobility is not within the current scope of PTA practice. *Joint mobilization* is a treatment modality that uses manual passive techniques to enhance arthrokinematic motion (spin, slide, or roll; see Chapter 4). These techniques may or may not be within the scope of the PTA, depending on the state in which he or she practices.

Joint mobilization techniques include a broad spectrum, from the general passive motions performed in the physiologic cardinal planes at any point in the joint range to the semispecific and specific accessory (arthrokinematic) joint glides, or joint distractions, initiated from the resting position of the joint. These techniques form the cornerstone of most rehabilitative programs and involve low- to high-velocity passive movements within or at the limit of joint range of motion, to restore any loss of accessory joint motion as the consequence of joint injury.[5]

● **Key Point** The techniques of joint mobilization are used to improve joint mobility or to decrease joint pain by restoring accessory movements to the joint and thus allowing full, nonrestricted, pain-free range of motion. Additional benefits attributed to joint mobilizations include decreasing muscle guarding, lengthening the tissue around a joint, neuromuscular influences on muscle tone, and increased proprioceptive awareness.[28,29]

● **Key Point** The primary indications for joint mobilizations are:
- Limited passive range of motion
- Limited joint accessory motion, as determined with joint mobility testing
- Tissue texture abnormality in the area of dysfunction
- Pain
- If the symptoms are aggravated by activity but relieved by rest

The PT considers the stage of healing, the direction of force, and the magnitude of force. The joint is positioned in the resting or open-packed position (refer to Table 6-1). Joint mobilizations are applied in a direction that is either parallel or perpendicular to the treatment plane to restore the physiological articular relationship within a joint and to decrease pain.[30] To apply joint mobilizations, a number of components can be utilized, depending on the method employed:

- *Direct method:* An engagement is made against a barrier in several planes.
- *Indirect method:* Maigne[31] postulated the concept of painless and opposite motion, where disengagement from the barrier occurs and a balance of ligamentous tension is sought.
- *Combined method:* Disengagement is followed by direct retracement of the motion.

Joint Mobilization Approaches

Several schools of thought have been put forward to address the concept of increasing joint range of motion.

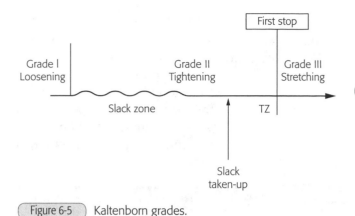

Figure 6-5 Kaltenborn grades.

Kaltenborn

Kaltenborn[3] introduced the Nordic program of manual therapy, which uses Cyriax's[10] method for evaluation and the specific osteopathic techniques of Mennell[11] for intervention. Further influence from Stoddard,[12] an osteopath, cemented the foundations of the Nordic system of manual therapy. Evjenth,[32] who joined Kaltenborn's group, brought a greater emphasis on muscle stretching, strengthening, and coordination training. Kaltenborn's techniques use a combination of traction and mobilization to reduce pain and mobilize hypomobile joints. Three grades of traction are defined (Figure 6-5):

- *Grade I piccolo (loosen):* This involves a distraction force that neutralizes pressure in the joint without producing any actual separation of the joint surfaces. This grade of distraction is used to reduce the compressive forces on the articular surfaces and is used both in the initial intervention session and with all of the mobilization grades. Grade I techniques are used in the inflammatory stage of healing.
- *Grade II (take up the slack):* This grade of distraction separates the articulating surfaces and eliminates the play in the joint capsule.
- *Grade III (stretch):* This grade of distraction actually stretches the joint capsule and the soft tissues surrounding the joint to increase mobility. Grade III traction is used in conjunction with mobilization glides according to the convex-concave

rules to treat joint hypomobility.[3] These techniques are typically used during the remodeling stage of healing.

> **● Key Point** Kaltenborn's piccolo and slack movements are generally used by the PT in the treatment of joint problems in which the predominant feature is pain; stretch is used to improve range of motion in a joint condition whose predominant feature is stiffness.

Australian Techniques

The Australian approach was introduced primarily by Maitland.[14] Under this system, the range of motion is defined as the available range, not the full range, and is usually in one direction only. Each joint has an anatomic limit, which is determined by the configuration of the joint surfaces and the surrounding soft tissues (Figure 6-6). The point of limitation is that point in the range that is short of the anatomic limit and is reduced by either pain or tissue resistance. Maitland advocated five grades of joint mobilization or oscillations, each of which falls within the available range of motion that exists at the joint—a point somewhere between the beginning point and the anatomic limit. Although the relationship that exists between the five grades in terms of their positions within the range of motion is always constant, the point of limitation shifts further to the left as the severity of the motion limitation increases. Grades I through IV are often performed as oscillatory-type movements during treatment. Grade I occurs at the beginning of range, grade II occurs in midrange, grade III is a large-amplitude movement toward the end of range, and grade IV is a small-amplitude movement at the end of range.

> **● Key Point** Many PTs use a combination of Kaltenborn's grade III traction with Maitland's grade IV oscillations to decrease pain and increase joint mobility.

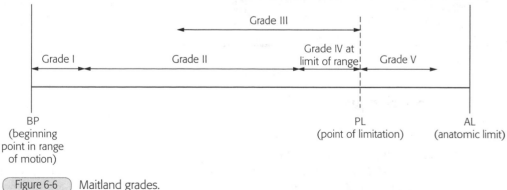

Figure 6-6   Maitland grades.

Source: Dutton M: Orthopaedic Examination, Evaluation and Intervention. New York, McGraw-Hill, 2004.

Maitland's grades I and II are used solely for pain relief and have no direct mechanical effect on the restricting barrier, although they do have a hydrodynamic effect. Mobilization-induced analgesia has been demonstrated in a number of studies in humans[33–35] and is characterized by a rapid onset and a specific influence on mechanical nociception. Grade I and II joint mobilizations theoretically reduce pain by improving joint lubrication and circulation in tissues related to the joint.[36,37] Rhythmic joint oscillations also possibly activate articular and skin mechanoreceptors that play a role in pain reduction.[38,39] Grades III and IV have been further subdivided into III+ (+ +) and IV+ (+ +), indicating that once the end of the range has been reached, a further stretch to impart a mechanical force to the movement restriction is given.[40] Grades III and IV (or at least III+ and IV+) do stretch the barrier and have a mechanical, as well as a neurophysiologic, effect.

Grade III and IV joint distractions and stretching mobilizations may, in addition to the above-stated effects, activate inhibitory joint and muscle spindle receptors, which aid in reducing restriction to movement.[36–39]

Clinical Application

Once the PT has determined the deficient direction of joint motion, the direction of the joint glide mobilization to be used is determined by the concave–convex rule. The clinician then decides which side of the joint is to be stabilized and which side is to be mobilized. For example, if extension of the tibiofemoral joint is restricted, either the femur (convex) can be stabilized and the tibia (concave) glided anteriorly or the tibia can be stabilized and the femur glided posteriorly.

> ● **Key Point** Concave–convex rule:
> • If the joint surface is convex relative to the other surface, the arthrokinematic glide occurs in the opposite direction to the osteokinematic movement.
> • If the joint surface is concave, the arthrokinematic glide occurs in the same direction as the osteokinematic movement.

| Soft Tissue Techniques

Soft tissue techniques are directed towards the muscles and fascia throughout the body to stretch tissues, break adhesions, increase blood flow, and enhance relaxation. The choice of technique is largely based on treatment goals.

Transverse Friction Massage

Transverse friction massage (TFM) is a technique devised by Cyriax, whereby repeated cross-grain massage is applied to muscle, tendons, tendon sheaths, and ligaments. TFM has long been used in physical therapy to increase the mobility and extensibility of individual musculoskeletal tissues, such as muscles, tendons, and ligaments, and to help prevent and treat inflammatory scar tissue.[10,41–46]

> ● **Key Point** TFM is indicated for subacute ligament, tendon, or muscle injuries; chronically inflamed bursae; and adhesions in ligament or muscle, or between tissues. TFM also can be applied before performing a manipulation or a strong stretch to desensitize and soften the tissues.

TFM is contraindicated for acute inflammation, hematomas, debilitated or open skin, and peripheral nerves, and in patients who have diminished sensation in the area.

TFM is purported to have the following therapeutic effects:

- *Traumatic hyperemia:*[10] According to Cyriax, longitudinal friction to an area increases the flow of blood and lymph, which, in turn, removes the chemical irritant by-products of inflammation. In addition, the increased blood flow reduces venous congestion, thereby decreasing edema and hydrostatic pressure on pain-sensitive structures.
- *Pain relief:* The application of TFM stimulates type I and II mechanoreceptors, producing presynaptic anesthesia. This presynaptic anesthesia is based on the gate theory of pain control (see Chapter 3). However, if the frictions are too vigorous, the stimulation of nociceptors will override the effect of the mechanoreceptors, causing the pain to increase. Occasionally, the patient may feel an exacerbation of symptoms following the first two or three sessions of the massage, especially in the case of a chronically inflamed bursa.[47] In these cases, it is important to forewarn the patient to apply ice at home.
- *Decreasing scar tissue:* The transverse nature of the friction assists with the orientation of the collagen in the appropriate lines of stress and also helps produce hypertrophy of the new collagen. Given the stages of healing for soft tissue, light TFM should be applied only in the early stages of a subacute lesion, so as not to damage the granulation tissue. These gentle movements theoretically serve to minimize

cross-linking and so enhance the extensibility of the new tissue. Following a ligament sprain, Cyriax recommends immediate use of TFM to prevent adhesion formation between the tissue and its neighbors, by moving the ligamentous tissue over the underlying bone.[10]

The application of the correct amount of tension to a healing structure is very important. The tissue undergoing TFM should, whenever possible, be positioned in a moderate but not painful stretch. The exception to this rule is when applying TFM to a muscle belly, which is usually positioned in its relaxed position.[10,48] Lubricant is not typically used with the application of TFM; however, ultrasound at the appropriate intensity can be applied to a tissue before TFM.

Beginning with light pressure, and using a reinforced finger (i.e., middle finger over the index finger) or thumb, the clinician moves the skin over the site of the identified lesion back and forth, in a direction perpendicular to the normal orientation of its fibers. It is important that the patient's skin move with the clinician's finger to prevent blistering.

● **Key Point** The application of TFM is condition and patient dependent. The intensity of the application is based on the stage of healing. The pain induced by TFM should be kept within the patient's tolerance. Light pressure should be used in the early stages, before building up the pressure over a few minutes to allow for accommodation.

The amplitude of the massage should be sufficient to cover all of the affected tissue, and the rate should be at two to three cycles per second, applied in a rhythmic manner.

The duration of the friction massage is usually gauged by when desensitization occurs (normally within 3–5 minutes). Tissues that do not desensitize within 3–5 minutes should be treated using some other form of intervention. If the condition is chronic or in the remodeling stage of healing, then the frictions are continued for a further 5 minutes after the desensitization, in an effort to enhance the mechanical effect on the cross-links and adhesions. Following the application of TFM, the involved tissue is either passively stretched or actively exercised, taking care not to cause pain.

Most conditions amenable to TFM should resolve in 6–10 sessions over 2–8 weeks. Tissues that do not show signs of improvement after three treatment sessions should be treated using some other form of intervention.

● **Key Point** Because of their simplicity, TFM techniques are often taught to patients as part of their home exercise program.

Augmented Soft Tissue Mobilization

Augmented soft tissue mobilization (ASTM)[47] is a form of deep massage that uses specially designed handheld devices to assist the clinician in the mobilization of poorly organized scar tissue in and around muscles, tendons, and myofascial planes. ASTM originated from and expanded on the concepts of TFM.[49–51] The instruments used for ASTM are solid, with angled edges, which are guided with the assistance of a lubricant such as cocoa butter. Longitudinal strokes are applied parallel to the fiber alignment, in a stroking motion along the skin, to mobilize the underlying soft tissues. As the instruments move over an area with an underlying fibrotic lesion, a change in texture is palpable. The initial strokes, which are used for screening purposes, are smooth and flowing but become shorter and more concentrated to increase the pressure per unit area once the fibrosis is located. The pressure exerted needs to be firm enough to locate the fibrosis and cause microtrauma, but not so hard that macrotrauma occurs. Patient feedback with regard to pain must guide the treatment. The microvascular trauma and capillary hemorrhage induce a localized inflammatory response and stimulate the body's healing cascade and immune-reparative system.[51]

The stroking motion is sustained for approximately 5–10 minutes. Usually, upon completion of the ASTM, there is immediate erythema and the potential for some transient ecchymosis. Following an application of ASTM, the tissue undergoes a stretching and strengthening program to maintain flexibility and re-establish muscular balance around the area that is being treated, as well as to influence the structural alignment of the remodeling collagen fibers and soft tissue matrix. Subsequently, cryotherapy is applied to the treated area for approximately 5–10 minutes, to limit any posttreatment soreness.

Myofascial Release

Myofasical release (MFR) is a series of techniques designed to release fascial restrictions and is used for the treatment of soft tissue dysfunction. The development of a holistic and comprehensive approach for the evaluation and treatment of the myofascial system of the body is credited to John Barnes, who was strongly influenced by the teachings of Mennell[52] and Upledger.[53]

According to myofascial theory, the collagen provides strength to the fascia, the elastin gives it its elastic properties, and the gel functions to absorb the compressive forces of movement.[35]

MFR is based on the principle that trauma or structural abnormalities may create inappropriate fascial strain, because of an inability of the fascia to absorb or distribute the forces.[54] These strains to the fascia can result in a slow tightening of the fascia, causing the body to lose its physiologic adaptive capacity.[54] Over time, the fascial restrictions begin to pull the body out of its three-dimensional alignment, causing biomechanically inefficient movement and posture.[54] In addition, because of the association of fascia at the cellular level, it is theorized that trauma to or malfunction of the fascia can lead to poor cellular efficiency, disease, and pain throughout the body.[27,54] Three theoretical models for the manifestation of myofascial dysfunction are contraction, contracture, and cohesion–congestion (**Table 6-2**).

Thus, the purpose of MFR techniques is to apply a gentle sustained pressure to the fascia, in order to release fascial restrictions, thereby restoring normal pain-free function.[27] The application of MFR relies entirely on the feedback received from the patient's tissues, with the clinician interpreting and responding to the feedback, so a great deal of practice is required. This rhythm, called the craniosacral rhythm (based on the Upledger concept) is theorized to guide the clinician as to the direction, force, and duration of the technique.

It is not unusual for a patient to experience muscle soreness following MFR techniques. This soreness is thought to result from postural and alignment changes or from the techniques themselves.

Myofascial Stroking

The soft tissue techniques used in MFR are purported to break up cross-restrictions of the collagen of the fascia. Three of the more commonly used techniques involve stroking maneuvers:[27]

- *J stroke:* This technique is used to increase skin mobility. Counterpressure is applied with the heel of the hand, while a stroke in the shape of the letter J is applied using two or three fingers in the direction of the restriction, which creates some torque at the end of the stroke.
- *Vertical stroke:* The purpose of vertical stroking is to open up the length of vertically oriented superficial fascia (Figure 6-7). As in the J stroke, counterpressure is applied with one hand, while the stroking is performed with the other.
- *Transverse stroke.* As its name suggests, the transverse stroke is applied in a transverse direction to the body. Force is applied downward into the muscle with the fingertips of both hands, and the force is applied slowly and perpendicular to the muscle fibers.

The cross-hands technique is used for the release of deep fascial tissues. The clinician places crossed hands over the site of restriction. The elastic component of the fascia is then stretched until the barrier is met. At this point, the clinician maintains consistent gentle pressure at the barrier for approximately 90–120 seconds. Once the release is felt, the clinician reduces the pressure.

TABLE 6-2	Theoretical Models for the Manifestation of Myofascial Disorders	
Model	Manifestation	End Feel
Contraction	Muscle hypertonicity or spasm	Reactive, firm, and painful end feel
Contracture	Inert or noncontractile tissues that have undergone fibrotic alteration	Abrupt, firm, stiff, or hard end feel
Cohesion–congestion	Fluidochemical changes in microcellular transport systems, resulting in impaired lymphatic flow, vascular stasis, or ischemia	Boggy, stiff, or reactive end feel

Data from Ellis JJ, Johnson GS: Myofascial considerations in somatic dysfunction of the thorax, in Flynn TW (ed): The Thoracic Spine and Rib Cage: Musculoskeletal Evaluation and Treatment. Boston, Butterworth-Heinemann, 1996, pp 211–262

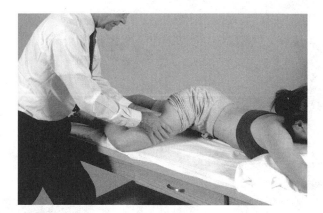

<figure>
Figure 6-7 Myofascial stroking.
</figure>

• Key Point It is important to remember that the claimed benefits and effectiveness of MFR techniques are largely anecdotal, because at the time of writing there is no scientific experimental research to validate these claims.[55]

Proprioceptive Neuromuscular Facilitation

According to the teachings of proprioceptive neuromuscular facilitation (PNF), muscles function as flexors, extensors, rotators, and side benders of joints. Combinations of these components work together to produce diagonals of movement, of which there are two for each major body part: the head, neck, and upper trunk; the lower trunk; the upper extremities (**Table 6-3** and Figure 6-8 through Figure 6-15); and the lower extremities (**Table 6-4** and Figure 6-16 through Figure 6-19). Normal coordinated motions are diagonal with spiral components. The various terms and techniques used in PNF are outlined in Appendix E. PNF techniques can be used to develop muscular strength and endurance; facilitate stability, mobility, neuromuscular control, and coordinated movements; and lay a foundation for the restoration of function.[56] Muscle groups are classified as agonists, antagonists, neutralizers, supporters, and fixators; muscle contractions are classified as dynamic (concentric and eccentric) or static (isometric). In Chapter 9 of this text, the use of PNF stretching techniques—specifically contract-relax and hold-relax techniques or other variations—to increase flexibility are described. In Chapter 10, the PNF techniques that are used to improve muscle performance are described.

• Key Point The intent of PNF is to restore the muscles around a joint to their normal neurophysiologic state, through either stretching or strengthening the agonist and antagonist. PNF techniques used are dependent on the application of sensory cues—specifically proprioceptive, cutaneous, visual, and auditory stimuli—to elicit or augment motor responses.[56]

TABLE 6-3	PNF Patterns for the Upper Extremities			
Joint	D1 Flexion	D1 Extension	D2 Flexion	D2 Extension
Scapulothoracic	Upward rotation, abduction, (protraction) anterior elevation	Downward rotation, adduction, (retraction) posterior depression	Upward rotation, adduction, posterior elevation	Downward rotation, abduction, anterior depression
Glenohumeral	External rotation, adduction, flexion	Internal rotation, abduction, extension	External rotation, abduction, flexion	Internal rotation, adduction, extension
Elbow	Flexion	Extension	Flexion	Extension
Radioulnar	Supination	Pronation	Supination	Pronation
Wrist	Flexion, radial deviation	Extension, ulnar deviation	Extension, radial deviation	Flexion, ulnar deviation
Fingers	Flexion, adduction to the radial side	Extension, abduction to the ulnar side	Extension, abduction to the radial side	Flexion, adduction to the ulnar side
Thumb	Flexion, abduction	Extension, abduction	Extension, adduction	Flexion, abduction

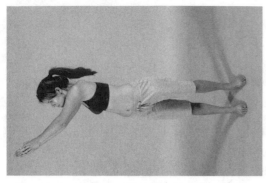

Figure 6-8 | PNF pattern: Flexion with rotation to the right.

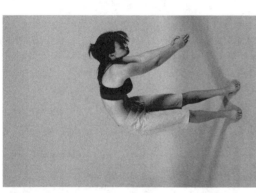

Figure 6-9 | PNF pattern: Extension with rotation to the left.

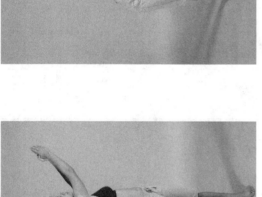

Figure 6-10 | PNF pattern: Flexion with rotation to the left.

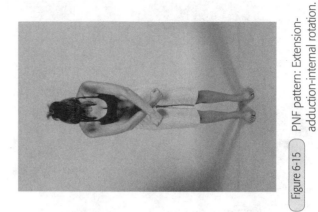

Figure 6-11 | PNF pattern: Extension with rotation to the right.

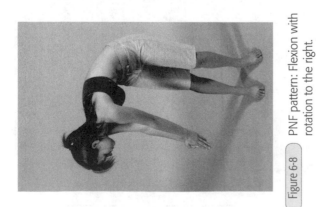

Figure 6-12 | PNF pattern: Flexion-adduction-external rotation (D1 flex).

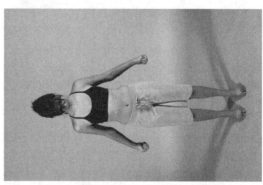

Figure 6-13 | PNF pattern: Extension-abduction-internal rotation (D1 ext).

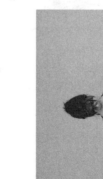

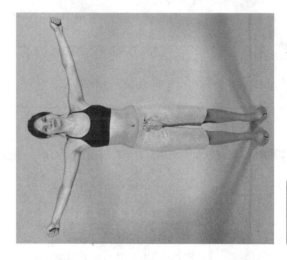

Figure 6-14 | PNF pattern: Flexion-abduction-external rotation.

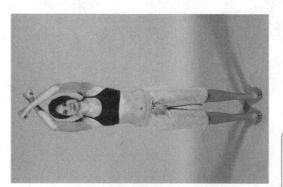

Figure 6-15 | PNF pattern: Extension-adduction-internal rotation.

TABLE 6-4	PNF Patterns for the Lower Extremities			
Joint	D1 Flexion	D1 Extension	D2 Flexion	D2 Extension
Hip	External rotation, adduction, flexion	Internal rotation, abduction, extension	Internal rotation, abduction, flexion	External rotation, adduction, extension
Knee	Flexion or extension	Extension or flexion	Flexion or extension	Extension or flexion
Ankle	Dorsiflexion	Plantarflexion	Dorsiflexion	Plantarflexion
Subtalar	Inversion	Eversion	Eversion	Inversion
Toes	Extension, abduction to the tibial side	Flexion, adduction to the fibular side	Extension, abduction to the fibular side	Flexion, adduction to the tibial side

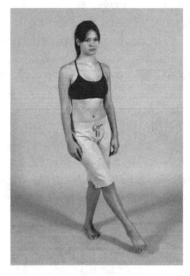

Figure 6-16   PNF pattern: Flexion-adduction-external rotation (D1 flex).

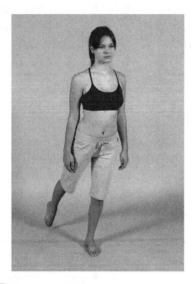

Figure 6-17   PNF pattern: Extension-abduction-internal rotation (D1 ext).

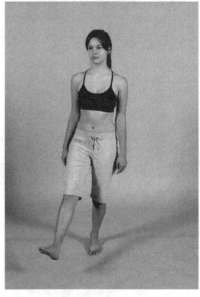

Figure 6-18   PNF pattern: Flexion-abduction-external rotation (D2 flex).

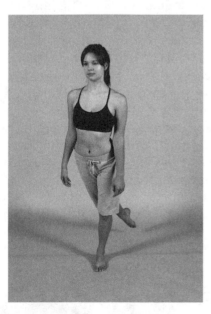

Figure 6-19   PNF pattern: Extension-adduction-internal rotation (D2 ext).

The position of the clinician during the performance of the technique must allow easy access to the structures involved, while maintaining proper body mechanics. The clinician positions the bone or joint so that the muscle group to be used is at its resting length. The patient is then given specific instructions about the direction in which to move, the intensity of the contraction, and the duration of the contraction.[57-60] The amounts of force and counterforce are governed by the length and strength of the muscle group involved, as well as by the patient's symptoms.[57] The clinician's force can match the effort of the patient, thus producing an isometric contraction and allowing no movement to occur, or it may overcome the patient's effort, thus moving the area or joint in the direction opposite to that in which the patient is attempting to move it, thereby using a concentric or isolytic contraction.[58]

Myofascial Trigger Point Therapy

Myofascial pain syndromes are closely associated with tender areas that have come to be known as myofascial trigger points (MTrPs). Dysfunctional joints are also associated with trigger points and tender attachment points.[59]

> **● Key Point**   The term *myofascial trigger point* is a bit of a misnomer, because trigger points can also be cutaneous, ligamentous, periosteal, and fascial.[61]

The major goals of MTrP therapy are to relieve pain and tightness of the involved muscles, improve joint motion, improve circulation, and eliminate perpetuating factors. When treating a patient for a specific muscle syndrome, it is important to explain the function of the involved muscle and to describe or demonstrate a few of the activities or postures that might overstress it, so that the patient can avoid such activities or postures. Ischemic compression is advocated for myofascial trigger points and is achieved by sustaining direct pressure over a trigger point, using the thumb to apply pressure.[62] The procedure is repeated on each trigger point. After all the trigger points have been treated, the clinician returns to the first trigger point. The procedure is repeated three times on each trigger point.[63]

> **● Key Point**   To facilitate self-treatment for inaccessible regions such as the rhomboid muscles, the patient can lie on a tennis ball or use the handle of a cane as substitutes for direct manual compression.[62]

Stretch and Spray or Stretch and Ice

The patient is placed in a position of maximum comfort to enhance muscle relaxation.[61,64] The part of the body affected is then positioned so that a mild stretch is exerted specifically on the taut band. Parallel sweeps of a vapocoolant spray or ice are applied unidirectionally. The spray is held approximately 18 inches away from the skin to allow for sufficient cooling. One or two sweeps of coolant are sprayed over the area of the involved muscle to reduce any pain. Then, while one of the clinician's hands anchors the base of the muscle, the other stretches the muscle to its full length.[65] As the muscle is passively stretched, successive parallel sweeps of the spray are applied over the skin from the MTrP to the area of referred pain, covering as much of the referred pain pattern as possible (Figure 6-20). After each application of the spray-and-stretch technique, the muscle is selectively moved through as full a range of motion as possible to normalize proprioceptive input to the central nervous system.[61] Intense cold stimulates cold receptors in the skin, which tends to inhibit pain. This technique is supposed to help block reflex spasm and pain, allowing for a gradual passive stretch of the muscle, which decreases muscle tension. Several treatments may be needed to eliminate the pain syndrome, and results should be seen after four to six treatments.[61]

It is important to remember that vapor cooling sprays are dangerous if inhaled, are inflammable, and should not be used near the eyes and face or on large areas of damaged skin, puncture wounds, or other wounds. If vaporized coolants are inappropriate or not available, ice may be used in their place, taking care to prevent chilling of the underlying muscles, which is less likely with the use of vaporized coolants.[61]

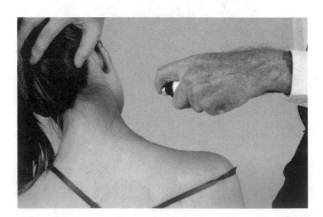

Figure 6-20   Stretch and spray.

Stretching

The following are indications for stretching:

- Loss of soft tissue extensibility due to adhesions, contractures, and scar tissue formation
- Restricted motion in an area that may lead to otherwise preventable structural deformities
- Muscle weakness and adaptive shortening of opposing tissue
- To help minimize postexercise muscle soreness

Contraindications include the following:

- Limited joint motion due to a bony block
- If the adaptive shortened soft tissue is providing necessary joint stability in lieu of normal structural stability or neuromuscular control, or is enabling a patient with paralysis or severe muscle weakness to perform specific functional skills otherwise not possible[66]
- An acute inflammatory or infectious process[66]
- Sharp or acute pain with joint movement or muscle elongation[66]
- A hematoma or other indication of tissue trauma[66]
- Hypermobility[66]

Effects of Manual Stretching

When soft tissue is stretched, a number of changes can occur, depending on the duration of the stretch:

- *Elasticity:* A property of connective tissue that allows the tissue to return to its prestretch resting length directly after a short duration stretch force has been removed.[66,67]
- *Viscoelasticity:* The viscous properties of a tissue allow permanent deformation and are considered time-dependent and rate of change–dependent. The rate of deformation is directly proportional to the force applied. Stress relaxation and creep are examples of viscoelastic properties. Stress relaxation occurs if tissue is stretched to a fixed length tolerable to the patient; the tissue will relax and less force will be necessary for the tissue to remain at the same length (see Chapter 4). If the force is kept constant, the tissue will elongate due to the process known as creep.[66,68]
- *Plasticity:* The tendency of soft tissue to assume a new and greater length after the stretch force has been removed.[66,69] The muscle–tendon unit contains active (contractile) and passive (noncontractile) components. The active components occur as an interaction between the contractile proteins (actin and myosin) within the muscle fibers. The passive components consist of the connective tissue factors within and around the muscle (e.g., perimysium, epimysium, endomysium, sarcolemma), the associated tendon and its insertion, and the connections between the sarcolemma and the tendon. Stretching has its main effect on the passive elements. It is thought that the resistance to stretch is mostly from the extensive connective tissue framework and sheathing within and around the muscle and not from the myofibrillar elements.

Changes in the neurophysiological properties of the muscle–tendon unit also occur with stretching, particularly with the muscle spindle and Golgi tendon organ (see Chapter 3).

Muscle Spindle

When a stretch force is applied, the intrafusal muscle fibers of the muscle spindle sense the length changes and activate the extrafusal muscle fibers, thereby activating the stretch reflex and increasing tension in the muscle being stretched. When the stretch reflex activates the muscle being lengthened, it also may decrease activity in the muscle on the opposite side of the joint. This is referred to as *reciprocal inhibition*.[70–72] To minimize activation of the stretch reflex and the subsequent increase in muscle tension and reflexive resistance to muscle lengthening during stretching procedures, a slowly applied, low intensity, prolonged stretch is considered preferable to a quickly applied, short duration stretch.[66]

Golgi Tendon Organ

When a stretch is produced in a muscle, particularly a prolonged stretch, the Golgi tendon organs (GTOs) in the tendons of that muscle respond to the increase in tension. This response of the GTO has an inhibitory impact (autogenic inhibition) on the level of muscle tension in the muscle tendon unit in which it lies.[73]

Application of a Stretch

The various methods of stretching are described in Chapter 9 and throughout the relevant chapters. When applying a stretch, a number of considerations must be taken into account. Proper alignment or positioning of the patient and the specific muscles and joints to be stretched is necessary for patient comfort and stability during stretching.[66]

For example, to stretch the rectus femoris, the lumbar spine and pelvis should be aligned in a neutral position (to prevent anterior tilting and hyperextension of the spine) as the knee is flexed and the hip is extended. To achieve an effective stretch of the specific muscle or muscle group, the proximal or distal attachment site of the muscle tendon unit being elongated must be stabilized. In addition, the following determinants must be considered:

- *Intensity:* There is general agreement that stretching should be applied at a low intensity by means of a low load to promote patient comfort, minimize voluntary or involuntary muscle guarding, and achieve optimal rates of improvement in ROM.[74]
- *Duration:* The duration (single cycle) refers to the period of time a stretch force is applied and shortened tissues are held in a lengthened position. In general, the shorter the duration of a single stretch cycle, the greater the number of repetitions applied during a stretching session.[66] However, despite numerous studies, there continues to be a lack of agreement on the ideal combination of the duration of a single cycle and the number of repetitions of stretch that should be applied in the daily stretching program to achieve the greatest and most sustained stretch-induced gains in ROM.[66]
- *Speed:* To ensure optimal muscle relaxation and prevent injury to tissues through activity of the stretch reflex, the speed of stretch should be slow and the stretch force should be applied and released gradually.[66]
- *Frequency:* The frequency refers to the number of sessions per day or per week a patient carries out a stretching regimen.[75] To date, it is not possible to draw evidence-based guidelines from the literature as to the ideal frequency.
- *Mode:* The mode refers to the form of stretch or the manner in which stretching exercises are carried out (e.g., manual, mechanical, passive, active, self-stretching).[66]

Summary

A number of manual therapy techniques are at the disposal of the PTA and, when combined with other forms of intervention, such as therapeutic exercise, can be very effective in restoring a patient's function. At present, the number of manual techniques that can be delegated to the PTA remains limited, but as with most things, time brings changes. Until such time, the appropriate application of manual therapy techniques remains at the discretion of the PT.

REVIEW Questions

1. How many grades of physiologic and accessory joint motions has Kaltenborn described?
2. According to Maitland, a large amplitude motion performed by the physical therapist that occurs from the mid-range of motion to the end of the available range is what grade of mobilization?
3. According to Maitland, a small oscillation or small amplitude joint motion performed by the physical therapist that occurs only at the beginning of the available range of motion is what grade of mobilization?
4. What characteristic end-range feel should be felt for knee flexion or elbow flexion?
5. What three benefits are reported to occur with transverse friction massage?
6. What massage technique is typically performed at the beginning and at the end of a massage to allow the patient to relax?
7. Which massage technique provides stimulation through rapid and alternating movements such as tapping, hacking, cupping, and slapping to enhance circulation and stimulate peripheral nerve endings?
8. What specific set of techniques is designed to release fascial restrictions and is used for the treatment of soft tissue dysfunction?

References

1. Threlkeld AJ: The effects of manual therapy on connective tissue. Phys Ther 72:893–902, 1992
2. Maitland G: Vertebral Manipulation. Sydney, Australia, Butterworth, 1986
3. Kaltenborn FM: Manual Mobilization of the Extremity Joints: Basic Examination and Treatment Techniques (ed 4). Oslo, Norway, Olaf Norlis Bokhandel, 1989
4. Jull GA, Janda V: Muscle and motor control in low back pain, in Twomey LT, Taylor JR (eds): Physical Therapy of the Low Back: Clinics in Physical Therapy. New York, Churchill Livingstone, 1987, pp 253–278
5. Di Fabio RP: Efficacy of manual therapy. Phys Ther 72:853–864, 1992
6. Cochrane CG: Joint mobilization principles: Considerations for use in the child with central nervous dysfunction. Phys Ther 67:1105–1109, 1987

7. Brooks SC: Coma, in Payton OD, Di Fabio RP, Paris SV, et al (eds): Manual of Physical Therapy. New York, Churchill Livingstone, 1989, pp 215–238

8. Farrell JP, Jensen GM: Manual therapy: A critical assessment of role in the profession of physical therapy. Phys Ther 72:843–852, 1992

9. Watson T: The role of electrotherapy in contemporary physiotherapy practice. Man Ther 5:132–141, 2000

10. Cyriax J: Textbook of Orthopaedic Medicine, Diagnosis of Soft Tissue Lesions (ed 8). London, Bailliere Tindall, 1982

11. Mennell JM: Back Pain. Diagnosis and Treatment Using Manipulative Techniques. Boston, MA, Little, Brown & Company, 1960

12. Stoddard A: Manual of Osteopathic Practice. New York, Harper & Row, 1969

13. DiGiovanna EL, Schiowitz S: An Osteopathic Approach to Diagnosis and Treatment. Philadelphia, JB Lippincott, 1991

14. Maitland G: Peripheral Manipulation (ed 3). London, Butterworth, 1991

15. McKenzie RA, May S: The lumbar spine: Mechanical diagnosis and therapy (ed 2). Waikanae, New Zealand, Spinal Publication, 2003

16. Nwuga VCB: Relative therapeutic efficacy of vertebral manipulation and conventional treatment in back pain management. Am J Phys Med 61:273–278, 1982

17. Nicholson GG: The effects of passive joint mobilization on pain and hypomobility associated with adhesive capsulitis of the shoulder. J Orthop Sports Phys Ther 6:238–246, 1985

18. Anderson M, Tichenor CJ: A patient with de Quervain's tenosynovitis: A case report using an Australian approach to manual therapy. Phys Ther 74:314–326, 1994

19. Nyberg R: Manipulation: Definition, types, application, in Basmajian JV, Nyberg R (eds): Rational Manual Therapies. Baltimore, MD, Williams & Wilkins, 1993, pp 21–47

20. Kappler RE: Direct action techniques. J Am Osteopath Assn 81:239–243, 1981

21. Mitchell FL, Moran PS, Pruzzo NA: An Evaluation and Treatment Manual of Osteopathic Muscle Energy Procedures. Manchester, MO, Mitchell, Moran and Pruzzo Associates, 1979

22. Greenman PE: Principles of Manual Medicine (ed 2). Baltimore, Williams & Wilkins, 1996

23. Nansel D, Peneff A, Cremata E, et al: Time course considerations for the effects of unilateral cervical adjustments with respect to the amelioration of cervical lateral flexion passive end-range asymmetry. J Manip Physiol Ther 13:297–304, 1990

24. Jull GA: Physiotherapy management of neck pain of mechanical origin, in Giles LGF, Singer KP (eds): Clinical Anatomy and Management of Cervical Spine Pain. The Clinical Anatomy of Back Pain. London, England, Butterworth-Heinemann, 1998, pp 168–191

25. Nitz AJ: Physical therapy management of the shoulder. Phys Ther 66:1912–1919, 1986

26. Kessler RM, Hertling D: Management of Common Musculoskeletal Disorders (ed 2). Philadelphia, Harper and Row, 1983

27. Ramsey SM: Holistic manual therapy techniques. Prim Care 24:759–785, 1997

28. Tanigawa MC: Comparison of hold-relax procedure and passive mobilization on increasing muscle length. Phys Ther 52:725–735, 1972

29. Barak T, Rosen E, Sofer R: Mobility: Passive orthopedic manual therapy, in Gould J, Davies G (eds): Orthopedic and Sports Physical Therapy. St Louis, CV Mosby, 1990

30. Mennel J: Joint Pain and Diagnosis Using Manipulative Techniques. New York, Little, Brown, 1964

31. Maigne R: Orthopedic Medicine. Springfield, IL, Charles C Thomas, 1972

32. Evjenth O, Hamberg J: Muscle Stretching in Manual Therapy, A Clinical Manual. Alfta, Sweden, Alfta Rehab Forlag, 1984

33. Vicenzino B, Collins D, Benson H, et al: An investigation of the interrelationship between manipulative therapy-induced hypoalgesia and sympathoexcitation. J Man Phys Ther 21:448–453, 1998

34. Vicenzino B, Collins D, Wright A: The initial effects of a cervical spine manipulative physiotherapy treatment on the pain and dysfunction of lateral epicondylalgia. Pain 68:69–74, 1996

35. Vicenzino B, Gutschlag F, Collins D, et al: An investigation of the effects of spinal manual therapy on forequarter pressure and thermal pain thresholds and sympathetic nervous system activity in asymptomatic subjects, in Schachlock MO (ed): Moving in on Pain. Adelaide, Australia, Butterworth-Heinemann, 1995

36. Grieve GP: Manual mobilizing techniques in degenerative arthrosis of the hip. Bull Orthop Section APTA 2:7, 1977

37. Yoder E: Physical therapy management of nonsurgical hip problems in adults, in Echternach JL (ed): Physical Therapy of the Hip. New York, Churchill Livingstone, 1990, pp 103–137

38. Wyke BD: The neurology of joints. Ann R Coll Surg Engl 41:25–50, 1967

39. Freeman MAR, Wyke BD: An experimental study of articular neurology. J Bone Joint Surg 49B:185, 1967

40. Meadows JTS: The principles of the Canadian approach to the lumbar dysfunction patient. Management of Lumbar Spine Dysfunction, Independent Home Study Course. La Crosse, WI, American Physical Therapy Association, Orthopaedic Section, 1999

41. Johnson GS: Soft tissue mobilization, in Donatelli RA, Wooden MJ (eds): Orthopaedic Physical Therapy. New York, Churchill Livingstone, 1994

42. Cyriax JH, Cyriax PJ: Illustrated Manual of Orthopaedic Medicine. London, Butterworth, 1983

43. Gersten JW: Effect of ultrasound on tendon extensibility. Am J Phys Med 34:662, 1955

44. Hunter SC, Poole RM: The chronically inflamed tendon. Clin Sports Med 6:371, 1987

45. Palastanga N: The use of transverse frictions for soft tissue lesions, in Grieve GP (ed): Modern Manual Therapy of the Vertebral Column. London, Churchill Livingstone, 1986, pp 819–826

46. Walker JM: Deep transverse friction in ligament healing. J Orthop Sports Phys Ther 6:89–94, 1984

47. Hammer WI: The use of transverse friction massage in the management of chronic bursitis of the hip or shoulder. J Man Physiol Ther 16:107–111, 1993

48. Forrester JC, Zederfeldt BH, Hayes TL, et al: Wolff's law in relation to the healing skin wound. J Trauma 10:770–779, 1970

49. Buckley PD, Grana WA, Pascale MS: The biomechanical and physiologic basis of rehabilitation, in Grana WA, Kalenak A (eds): Clinical Sports Medicine. Philadelphia, WB Saunders, 1991, pp 233–250

50. Harrelson GL: Physiologic factors of rehabilitation, in Andrews JR, Harrelson GL (eds): Physical Rehabilitation of the Injured Athlete. Philadelphia, WB Saunders, 1991, pp 13–39

51. Stauber WT: Repair models and specific tissue responses in muscle injury, in Leadbetter WB, Buckwalter JA, Gordon SL (eds): Sports-Induced Inflammation: Clinical and Basic Science Concepts. Park Ridge, IL, American Academy of Orthopedic Surgeons, 1990, pp 205–213

52. Mennell JB: The Science and Art of Joint Manipulation. London, J & A Churchill, 1949

53. Upledger JE, Vredevoogd JD: Craniosacral Therapy. Chicago, Eastland Press, 1983

54. Barnes J: Myofascial Release: A Comprehensive Evaluatory and Treatment Approach. Paoli, PA, MFR Seminars, 1990

55. Morton T: Panel debates the pros and cons of myofascial release approach. APTA Progress Report, 1988, pp 10–12

56. Kisner C, Colby LA: Resistance exercise for impaired muscle performance, in Kisner C, Colby LA (eds): Therapeutic Exercise. Foundations and Techniques (ed 5). Philadelphia, FA Davis, 2002, pp 140–156

57. Goodridge JP: Muscle energy technique: Definition, explanation, methods of procedure. J Am Osteopath Assoc 81:249–254, 1981

58. Chaitow L: An introduction to muscle energy techniques, in Chaitow L (ed): Muscle Energy Techniques (ed 2). London, Churchill Livingstone, 2001, pp 1–18

59. Liebenson C: Active muscular relaxation techniques (part 2). J Manipulative Physiol Ther 13:2–6, 1990

60. Liebenson C: Active muscular relaxation techniques (part 1). J Manipulative Physiol Ther 12:446–451, 1989

61. Smolders JJ: Myofascial pain and dysfunction syndromes, in Hammer WI (ed): Functional Soft Tissue Examination and Treatment by Manual Methods—The Extremities. Gaithersburg, MD, Aspen, 1991, pp 215–234

62. Dreyer SJ, Boden SD: Nonoperative treatment of neck and arm pain. Spine 23:2746–2754, 1998

63. Cohen JH, Schneider MJ: Receptor-tonus technique. An overview. Chiro Tech 2:13–16, 1990

64. Travell JG, Simons DG: Myofascial Pain and Dysfunction—The Trigger Point Manual. Baltimore, MD, Williams & Wilkins, 1983

65. Simons DG: Muscular pain syndromes, in Fricton JR, Awad E (eds): Advances in Pain Research and Therapy. New York, Raven Press, 1990, pp 1–41

66. Kisner C, Colby LA: Stretching for impaired mobility, in Kisner C, Colby LA (eds): Therapeutic Exercise. Foundations and Techniques (ed 5). Philadelphia, FA Davis, 2002, pp 65–108

67. De Deyne PG: Application of passive stretch and its implications for muscle fibers. Phys Ther 81:819–827, 2001

68. Magnusson SP, Simonsen EB, Aagaard P, et al: A mechanism for altered flexibility in human skeletal muscle. J Physiol 497:291–298, 1996

69. Sapega AA, Quedenfeld T, Moyer R, et al: Biophysical factors in range of motion exercise. Phys Sports Med 9:57–65, 1981

70. Geertsen SS, Lundbye-Jensen J, Nielsen JB: Increased central facilitation of antagonist reciprocal inhibition at the onset of dorsiflexion following explosive strength training. J Appl Physiol 105:915–922, 2008

71. Cutsuridis V: Does abnormal spinal reciprocal inhibition lead to co-contraction of antagonist motor units? A modeling study. Int J Neural Syst 17:319–327, 2007

72. Yang HD, Minn YK, Son IH, et al: Facilitation and reciprocal inhibition by imagining thumb abduction. J Clin Neurosci 13:245–248, 2006

73. Khan SI, Burne JA: Afferents contributing to autogenic inhibition of gastrocnemius following electrical stimulation of its tendon. Brain Res 1282:28–37, 2009

74. Blanton S, Grissom SP, Riolo L: Use of a static adjustable ankle-foot orthosis following tibial nerve block to reduce plantar-flexion contracture in an individual with brain injury. Phys Ther 82:1087–1097, 2002

75. Godges JJ, MacRae H, Longdon C, et al: The effects of two stretching procedures on hip range of motion and gait economy. J Orthop Sports Phys Ther 10:350, 1989

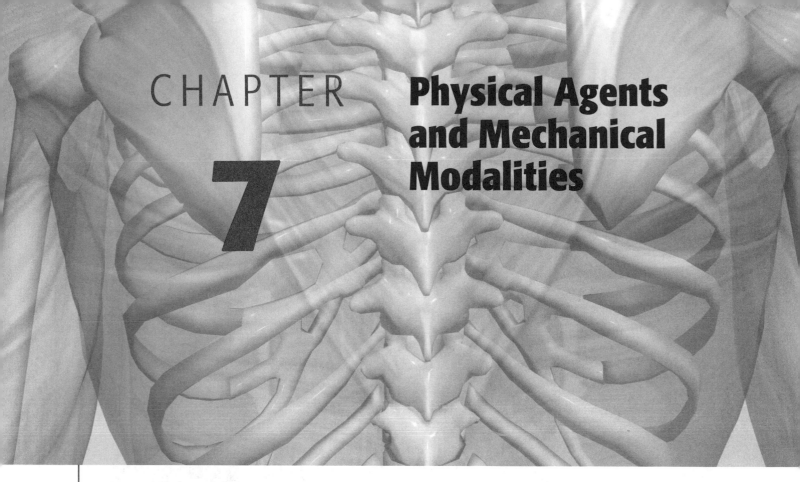

CHAPTER 7

Physical Agents and Mechanical Modalities

Chapter Objectives

At the completion of this chapter, the reader will be able to:

1. List the clinical tools that can be used to control pain, inflammation, and edema and the rationale for each.
2. Discuss the intrinsic and extrinsic stimuli that can be used to promote and progress healing.
3. Describe the physiological effects of a local heat application and of cryotherapy.
4. Describe each of the five types of heat transfer and the modalities that are involved with each.
5. Describe the benefits of each of the physical agents and mechanical modalities.
6. Understand the rationale for use of each of the physical agents and mechanical modalities during each of the three stages of healing.
7. Describe the benefits of each of the electrotherapeutic modalities.
8. Have a working knowledge of the contraindications for each of the physical agents and mechanical modalities.

Overview

A number of modalities are used in physical therapy, the use of which is determined by the goals of the intervention (**Tables 7-1** and **Table 7-2**). Three categories of modalities are recognized:

- Physical agents
- Electrotherapeutic modalities
- Mechanical modalities

If an intervention is delegated to a PTA based on the
physical therapist's plan of care,
the PTA must:

TABLE 7-1	Electrotherapeutic and Thermal Modalities

Modality	Physiologic Responses
Cryotherapy (cold packs, ice)	Decreased blood flow (vasoconstriction)
	Analgesia
	Reduced inflammation
	Reduced muscle guarding/spasm
Thermotherapy (hot packs, whirlpool, paraffin wax)	Increased blood flow (vasodilation)
	Analgesia
	Reduced muscle guarding/spasm
	Increased metabolic activity
Ultrasound	Increased connective tissue extensibility
	Deep heat
	Increased circulation
	Reduced inflammation (pulsed)
	Reduced muscle spasm
Shortwave diathermy and microwave diathermy	Increased deep circulation
	Increased metabolic activity
	Reduced muscle guarding/spasm
	Reduced inflammation
	Facilitated wound healing
	Analgesia
	Increased tissue temperatures over a large area
Electrical stimulating currents: high voltage	Pain modulation
	Muscle re-education
	Muscle pumping contractions (retard atrophy)
	Fracture and wound healing
Electrical stimulating currents: low voltage	Wound healing
	Fracture healing
Electrical stimulating currents: interferential	Pain modulation
	Muscle re-education
	Muscle pumping contractions
	Fracture healing
Electrical stimulating currents: Russian	Muscle strengthening
Electrical stimulating currents: Microelectrical nerve stimulation (MENS)	Fracture healing
	Wound healing

- Adhere to the relevant state practice acts, the practice setting, and any other regulatory agency
- Assess and note the component of the patient's physical therapy plan that is being addressed by the use of a modality to determine whether use of the modality is still warranted
- Ensure that any equipment to be used is correctly functioning and calibrated, and that safety inspections of the device have been performed as per the clinic's policies and procedures
- Adjust or modify an intervention within the established plan of care in response to data collection and patient clinical indications
- Notify the physical therapist of any changing clinical condition that warrants a modification or termination of a particular intervention
- Provide the patient with information about the procedure in addition to describing what the patient may feel during the application of the agent or modality
- Perform the standard pretreatment checks (e.g., skin and sensory integrity, review of contraindications)
- Provide the patient with a call bell if he or she is to be left unattended

> **● Key Point** According to the APTA policy statement, *Direction and Supervision of the Physical Therapist Assistant*, "regardless of the setting in which the service is provided, the determination to utilize physical therapist assistants for selected interventions requires the education, expertise and professional judgment of a physical therapist as described by the Standards of Practice, Guide to Professional Conduct and Code of Ethics."

TABLE 7-2	Clinical Decision Making on the Use of Various Therapeutic Modalities During Various Stages of Healing	
Clinical Presentation	**Possible Modalities Used**	**Examples and Parameters (where applicable)**
Acute: Erythema (rubor), swelling (tumor), elevated tissue temperature (calor), and pain (dolor) Swelling subsides, warm to touch, discoloration, pain to touch, pain on motion	Cryotherapy Electrical stimulation Nonthermal ultrasound	Ice packs, ice massage, cold whirlpool (15–20°C [68°F])
Subacute: Pain to touch, pain on motion, swollen	Cryotherapy/thermotherapy Electrical stimulation Ultrasound	Contrast baths, hot packs, paraffin wax, fluidotherapy, etc. (41–45°C [106–113°F])
Chronic: No more pain to touch, decreasing pain on motion	Thermotherapy (hot packs, ultrasound, paraffin) Electrical stimulation Ultrasound	

Physical Agents

Some physical agents involve the transfer of thermal energy and are referred to as *thermal agents* or *thermal modalities*. Five types of thermal energy transfer are recognized (**Table 7-3**). Thermal agents can either increase tissue temperature (thermotherapy) or lower tissue temperature (cryotherapy).

● Key Point   Temperature conversions:
- Fahrenheit = (Temperature in Celsius × 9/5) + 32 *or* (Temperature in Celsius × 1.8) + 32
- Celsius = (Temperature in Fahrenheit – 32) × 5/9 *or* (Temperature in Fahrenheit – 32) × 0.55

Cryotherapy

Traditionally, cryotherapy has been applied immediately to acute soft tissue injuries and for the first 24–48 hours postinjury. The indications for cryotherapy include the following:

- Acute or subacute pain
- Myofascial pain syndrome
- Muscle spasm
- Bursitis
- Acute or subacute inflammation
- Musculoskeletal trauma (sprains, strains, contusions)
- Tendonitis

TABLE 7-3	Types of Thermal Energy Transfer	
Type	**Description**	**Example**
Evaporation	A liquid changes state to a gas and a resultant cooling takes place.	Vapocoolant sprays
Conduction	Heat is transferred from a warmer object to a cooler object through direct molecular interaction of objects in physical contact.	Cold pack, ice pack, ice massage, cold bath, paraffin bath
Convection	Particles (air or water) move across the body, creating a temperature variation.	Whirlpool
Radiation	The transfer of heat from a warmer source to a cooler source through a conducting medium, such as air.	Infrared lamp
Conversion	The transfer of heat when nonthermal energy (mechanical, electrical) is absorbed into tissue and transformed into heat.	Ultrasound, diathermy

Contraindications include:

- Area of compromised circulation
- Peripheral vascular disease
- Ischemic tissue
- Cold hypersensitivity
- Raynaud's phenomenon
- Cold urticaria
- Hypertension
- Infection
- Cryoglobulinemia

> ● **Key Point** Increased heart rate and blood pressure are associated with cold application to large areas of the body.[1] Conditioned patients should not have a problem with dizziness after cold applications, but care should be taken when transferring any patient from the whirlpool area.

Physiologic Effects

The physiologic effects of a local cryotherapy application include:

- Decreased muscle and intra-articular temperature. This decrease in muscle temperature[2] and intra-articular structures[3–5] occurs because of a decrease in local blood flow,[6–10] and appears to be most marked between the temperatures of 40°C and 25°C (100°F and 77°F).[11] Temperatures below 25°C, which typically occur after 30 minutes of cooling therapy, actually result in an increased blood flow (known as the Hunting effect),[11] with a consequent detrimental increase in hemorrhage and an exaggerated acute inflammatory response.[12]
- Local analgesia.[9,10,13–17] The stages of analgesia achieved by cryotherapy are outlined in **Table 7-4**.[18] It is worth remembering that the timing of the stages depends on the depth of penetration and varying thickness of adipose tissue.[19]

TABLE 7-4	Stages of Analgesia Induced by Cryotherapy	
Stage	**Response**	**Time After Initiation of Cryotherapy (min)**
1	Cold sensation	0–3
2	Burning or aching	2–7
3	Local numbness or analgesia	5–12
4	Deep tissue vasodilation without increase in metabolism	12–15

- Decreased muscle spasm.[13,20–23]
- Decreased swelling.[13,24,25]
- Decreased nerve conduction velocity.[26]

Application

Before the first application, the PTA performs an assessment of skin and sensory integrity, including temperature, and observes for any lesions in the area compared with findings during the initial evaluation. After the first 5 minutes of treatment the PTA visually observes the patient's skin for any adverse effects (e.g., urticaria, facial flush, or anaphylaxis [medical emergency]). The normal response for a cold application, which typically lasts from 10 to 20 minutes, involves the sequence of cold, burning, aching, and numbness (CBAN) (refer to Table 7-4). The patient should be advised about these various stages, especially in light of the fact that the burning or aching phases occur before the therapeutic phases. The patient is given a call bell and instructed to alert the clinician if there are any sensory changes.

Commercial Cold Packs

The commercial cold pack typically contains silica gel and is available in a variety of shapes and sizes. A cold pack requires a temperature of 23°F (–5°C). A towel is dampened with warm water and the excessive water wrung out. The cold pack is taken out of the refrigeration unit, wrapped in the moistened towel, and placed securely on the patient with elastic bandages or towels. One to three dry towels are placed over the cold pack to retard warming. The treatment time is typically 10 to 20 minutes. Cold packs may not maintain uniform contact with the body, so their use requires observation of the skin every 5 minutes. The patient should be kept warm throughout the treatment.

Ice Packs

An ice pack consists of crushed ice folded in a moist towel or placed in a plastic bag covered by a moist towel. The method of application, patient preparation, and treatment time is the same as for the cold packs.

> ● **Key Point** The various methods of applying cryotherapy (ice chips in toweling, cold gel packs, and ice bags) have been examined in different studies. The use of ice chips in toweling has been shown to be more effective in decreasing skin temperature than ice chips in plastic bags or cold gel packs.[5,27]

Ice Massage

Ice massage is recommended for small and contoured areas. It allows for easy observation and is

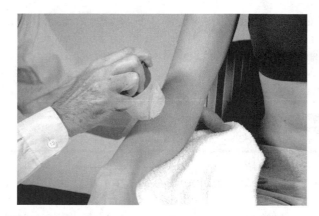

Figure 7-1   Ice massage.

inexpensive to use. Ice massage is typically performed by freezing water in either a commercially available cup (Figure 7-1) or a paper cup that can be torn away to expose the ice block. The ice is then applied directly to the area in small, circular motions for 10 to 15 minutes before and after activity, up to six times a day. Ice massage has been shown to reduce tissue temperature faster than using a cold pack.[28]

Cryokinetics

Cryokinetics is a rehabilitation technique used for the treatment of strains and sprains.[9] The technique involves an initial application of cold for 20 minutes followed by a 3-minute bout of active exercise to the injured area. This is then followed by a 5-minute application of cold. The whole sequence of 3-minute exercise and 5-minute cold applications is repeated for a total of four cycles.

Cryostretching

Cryostretching is a rehabilitation technique that has been advocated to increase flexibility during healing.[9] The technique involves a 20-minute cold application followed by alternating periods of progressive passive stretching with isometric contractions and renumbing using cold for a total of three cycles.

Cold Bath

A cold bath, using a basin or whirlpool, is commonly used for the immersion of the distal extremities. The temperature for a cold whirlpool used for acute conditions is in the range of 55–64°F (13–18°C).[1] Typically the body part is immersed for 5 to 15 minutes, depending on the desired therapeutic effect.

Vapocoolant Spray

Vapocoolant sprays (e.g., Spray and Stretch, which has replaced the non-ozone-layer-friendly Fluori-Methane) are often used in conjunction with passive stretching and in the treatment of muscle spasms, trigger points, and myofascial referred pain (see Chapter 6).[29] The depth of cooling is superficial with this modality. Physiologically the relief is accomplished through the theoretical gate control method of pain control (see Chapter 3).[29]

Thermotherapy

Thermotherapy is the therapeutic application of heat. Thermal modalities generally involve the transfer of thermal energy (refer to Table 7-3). Thermotherapy is used in the later stages of healing, because the deep heating of structures during the acute inflammatory stage may destroy collagen fibers and accelerate the inflammatory process.[30] However, in the later stages of healing, an increase in blood flow to the injured area is beneficial.

Indications for thermotherapy include the following:

- Pain control
- Chronic inflammatory conditions
- Trigger points
- Tissue healing
- Muscle spasm
- Decreased range of motion
- Desensitization

Contraindications include:

- Circulatory impairment
- Area of malignancy; heat can increase the metabolic activity of a tumor and thereby increase the rate of growth[31]
- Acute musculoskeletal trauma
- Bleeding or hemorrhage, including hemophilia
- Sensory impairment; it is important to assess the patient's sensitivity to temperature, pain, and circulation status prior to the use of thermotherapy (see Chapter 3)
- Thrombophlebitis
- Arterial disease
- Pregnancy; the application of heat is contraindicated over the abdominal, pelvic, or low back regions of pregnant women due to the potential risk to the development and growth of the fetus[31]

● **Key Point**   Application of a superficial hot pack over an area with significant subcutaneous fat results in decreased heating of deeper structures.

Physiologic Effects

The physiologic effects of a local heat application include:[7,32–35]

- Dissipation of body heat. This effect occurs through selective vasodilation and shunting of blood via reflexes in the microcirculation, and regional blood flow.[36]
- Decreased muscle spasm.[12,16,36,37] The muscle relaxation probably results from a decrease in neural excitability on the sensory nerves, and hence gamma input.
- Increased capillary permeability, cell metabo-lism, and cellular activity, which have the potential to increase the delivery of oxygen and chemical nutrients to the area while decreasing venous stagnation.[33,38]
- Increased analgesia through hyperstimulation of the cutaneous nerve receptors.
- Increased tissue extensibility.[36] This effect has obvious implications for the application of stretching techniques. The best results are obtained if heat is applied during the stretch, and if the stretch is maintained until cooling occurs after the heat has been removed.

Although the human body functions optimally between 36°C and 38°C (96.8°F and 100.4°F), an applied temperature between 40°C and 45°C (104°F and 113°F) is considered effective for a heat intervention.

Superficial Heating Agents

The area to be treated should be positioned in such a way as to be easily observed and to prevent a depen-dent position of the area, or any areas of the body distal to the treatment site. All clothing and jewelry should be removed from the treatment area. Before the first application, the PTA performs an assessment of skin and sensory integrity, including temperature (see Chapter 3), and observes for any lesions in the area compared with findings during the initial evalu-ation. If any are found, the PT should be notified.

The modality should be positioned correctly and the patient monitored during the application. The patient is given a call bell and instructed to alert the clinician if there are any sensory changes.

Heating Packs

Heating packs are made of a hydrophilic silicate gel encased in a canvas or nylon cover, which is immersed in a thermostatically controlled water unit (hydro-collator) that is typically between 158°F and 167°F (70°C to 75°C). The hot packs are made in vari-ous sizes and shapes designed to fit different body areas. The moist heat pack causes an increase in the local tissue temperature, reaching its highest point about 8 minutes after the application.[41] The depth of penetration for the traditional heating pads (and cold packs) is about 12 centimeters, and it results in changes in the cutaneous blood vessels and the cutaneous nerve receptors.[5] Before applying the hot pack, layers of terrycloth toweling (approximately six to eight depending on the length of treatment and patient comfort) are placed between the skin and the hot pack. Having the patient lie on the pack is not recommended because this position may increase heat transfer beyond therapeutic levels and increase the risk of burn. The skin should be inspected every 5 minutes and the patient should be provided with a call device to notify the clinician of any discomfort.

Treatment times vary from 15 to 20 minutes, depending on the goal established by the evaluating PT. It is important that in every clinic some form of daily monitoring system for the water levels and tem-perature of the hot pack storage units is in place.

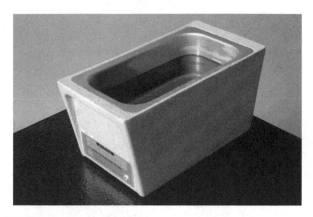

Figure 7-2   Paraffin bath.

Paraffin Bath

Liquid paraffin, heated in a thermostatically controlled paraffin bath unit (Figure 7-2), is used to provide superficial heat to the hands and feet. Paraffin baths are a commonly used modality for stiff or painful joints and for arthritis of the hands and feet, due to the ability of the wax to conform to irregularly contoured areas. It is, however, contraindicated when there is evidence of an allergic rash, open wounds, recent scars or sutures, or a skin infection. In addition, the contraindications for paraffin are essentially the same as for other thermal modalities.

> ● **Key Point**   Paraffin treatments provide six times the amount of heat available in water because the mineral oil in the paraffin lowers the paraffin's melting point.[1] This provides the paraffin with a lower specific heat* than water, allowing for a slower exchange of heat to the skin.

For clinical use, the wax used is a mixture of paraffin wax and mineral oil (approximately 2 pounds of wax mixed with 1 gallon of oil). Paraffin melts rapidly at 118–130°F (48–54°C) and self-sterilizes at 175–200°F (79–93°C).[42,43] The typical paraffin bath unit maintains a temperature of 113–126°F (45–52°C). The patient is asked to remove all jewelry and to wash and dry the area to be treated. (If jewelry cannot be removed it is covered with several layers of gauze.) The clinician inspects the area for infection and open areas. Due to the nature of the paraffin treatment, the treated area cannot be accessed easily for observation, so the PTA must

---

*Specific heat is the amount of heat per unit of mass required to raise the temperature by 1 degree Celsius. The specific heat of water is 1 calorie/gram °C = 4.186 joules/gram °C, which is approximately four times higher than air. Paraffin has a specific heat capacity of 2.14–2.9 joules/gram °C

periodically check the status of the patient and, if the patient is to be left unattended, he or she must be provided with a call bell.

Three different procedures are commonly utilized:

- *Dip-wrap (glove) method:* When dipping into the paraffin, the first layer of wax should be the highest on the body segment, and each successive layer lower than the previous one. This is to prevent subsequent layers from getting between the first layer and the skin and burning the patient.[1] With their fingers/toes apart, the patient is asked to dip the involved part (hand or foot) in the wax bath as far as possible and tolerable, while avoiding touching the sides or bottom of the wax bath to prevent burns. After a few seconds, the patient is asked to remove the hand/foot without moving his or her toes to avoid cracks forming in the wax. The layer of paraffin hardens (becomes opaque). The patient repeats the process five more times. After the paraffin has solidified, the part is then wrapped in a plastic bag, wax paper, or treatment table paper and then in a towel or insulating glove to conserve the heat, thereby slowing down the rate of cooling of the paraffin. The involved extremity is elevated and the paraffin remains on for 15–20 minutes until it cools, after which the clinician peels off the paraffin.
- *Paint:* As its name implies, for this method a brush is used to paint the treatment area with 6–10 layers of paraffin. The area is then covered and the wax remains on for approximately 20 minutes.
- *Dip and immersion:* This method is similar to the dip-wrap method, except the patient's extremity remains comfortably in the bath after the final dip. Extra caution must be taken with this method compared with the other two due to the potential for greater heat exchange to occur.

Fluidotherapy

Fluidotherapy consists of a container (Figure 7-3 and Figure 7-4) that circulates warm air (111–125°F/44–52°C) and small cellulose particles at varying degrees of agitation based on patient comfort. The extremity to be treated is placed into the container and the dry heat is generated through the energy transferred by forced convection for a period of 20 minutes. Unlike a heating pack and paraffin bath, fluidotherapy allows for active movement during treatment and a

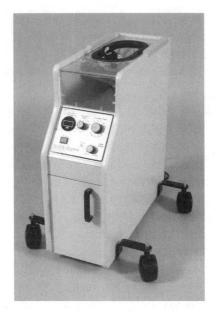

Figure 7-3   Fluidotherapy.

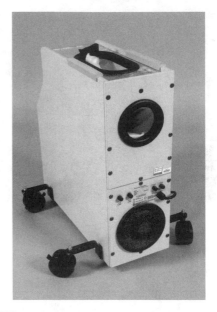

Figure 7-4   Fluidotherapy.

constant treatment temperature. However, the treatment setup may require the extremity to be placed in a dependent position.

Infrared Lamp

The infrared lamp produces superficial heating of tissue through radiant heat with a depth of penetration of less than 1 to 3 millimeters. The patient is positioned approximately 20 inches from the source and a moist towel is placed over the treatment area. The standard parameter for treatment indicates 20 inches in distance should equal 20 minutes of treatment. If the distance decreases, the intensity will increase, and the time of total treatment should decrease. The advantages of infrared are that direct contact with the skin is not required and the area being treated can be easily observed. However, due to the limited depth of penetration, the dehydrating effects on wounds, and the risk of burns during treatment, the use of infrared is declining.

Ultrasound

Indications for ultrasound include the following:

- Soft tissue repair
- Contracture
- Bone fracture healing
- Trigger point
- Dermal ulcer healing
- Scar tissue
- Pain
- Muscle spasm
- Plantar wart

Contraindications include the following:

- Over a pregnant uterus
- Over a cemented prosthetic joint
- Over a cardiac pacemaker
- Over vital areas such as the brain, ear, eyes, heart, cervical ganglia, carotid sinuses, reproductive organs, or spinal cord[44]
- Over epiphyseal areas in children
- Over a malignancy
- Impaired circulation
- Thrombophlebitis
- Impaired pain or temperature sensory deficits
- Infection

Physiologic Effects

Ultrasound (Figure 7-5) can be used to deliver heat to either superficial or deep musculoskeletal tissues

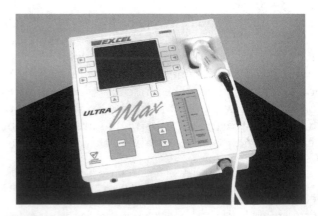

Figure 7-5   Ultrasound.

such as tendon, muscle, and joint structures. The effects of ultrasound are chemical and thermal. The ultrasonic waves are delivered through a transducer, which has a metal faceplate with a piezoelectric crystal cemented between two electrodes. This crystal can vibrate very rapidly, converting electrical energy to acoustical energy. This energy leaves the transducer in a straight line. As the energy travels further from the transducer, the waves begin to diverge. The depth of penetration depends on the absorption and scattering of the beam.

> ● **Key Point** The specific effects and depth of penetration when using ultrasound are affected by the ultrasound wavelength or frequency (1 MHz or 3 MHz), the intensity (W/m^2), the contact quality of the transducer, the treatment surface, and the tissue type (e.g., muscle, skin, fat).[45,46] Scar tissue, tendon, and ligament demonstrate the highest absorption. Tissues that demonstrate poor absorption include bone, tendinous and aponeurotic attachments of skeletal muscle, cartilaginous coverings of joint surfaces, and peripheral nerves lying close to bone.[47]

The portion of the sound head that produces the sound wave is referred to as the *effective radiating area (ERA)*. The ERA, which is always smaller than the transducer, can be found on all transducers, allowing the PTA to determine appropriate treatment time.

Frequency
The depth of penetration of the ultrasound is roughly inversely related to its frequency.[48,49] A frequency of 3 MHz is more superficial, reaching a depth of approximately 2 centimeters, whereas 1 MHz is effective to a depth of 4 or 5 centimeters.[50]

Duty Cycle
A duty cycle refers to the percentage of time (on time ÷ [on time + off time] × 100) that the ultrasound energy is being transmitted with a pulsed waveform to achieve the proposed associated nonthermal effects. Duty cycles less than 100 percent are usually termed *pulsed ultrasound*, whereas a 100 percent duty cycle is referred to as *continuous ultrasound*. Continuous mode ultrasound produces a thermal effect. Pulsed ultrasound with duty cycles of less than 20 percent have no thermal effect, whereas duty cycles of more than 20 percent have a thermal effect.

Acoustic Cavitation
Acoustic cavitation occurs as a result of the acoustic energy generated by ultrasound that develops into microscopic bubbles causing cavities that surround soft tissues. Two types of cavitation can occur:

■ *Stable:* The microscopic bubbles increase and decrease in size but do not burst.

Stabile cavitation produces microstreaming, which is the minute flow of fluid that takes place around the vapor-filled bubbles that oscillate and pulsate.

■ *Transient (unstable):* The microscopic bubbles increase in size over multiple cycles and implode causing brief moments of local temperature and pressure increases in the area surrounding the bubbles. However, this process should not occur during therapeutic ultrasound because the intensities required are much higher than 3 W/cm^2.

The Beam Nonuniformity Ratio
The beam nonuniformity ratio (BNR) of ultrasound is the maximal/average intensity (W/cm^2) found in the ultrasound field. The BNR value should range between 2:1 and 6:1. (Most devices fall in the 5:1 or 6:1 range.) The BNR of a particular unit is required to be listed on the device for consumer education and awareness. Each transducer produces sound waves in response to the vibration of the crystal. This vibration has different intensities at points on the transducer head, having peaks and valleys of intensity. The higher the quality of the transducer, the lower the BNR. The greater ratio difference in the BNR, the more likely the transducer will have *hot spots*. Hot spots are areas of high intensity and increase the likelihood of patient discomfort. High intensities have been shown to cause unstable cavitational effects and to retard tissue repair.[51,52]

Application
A pretreatment and posttreatment assessment of skin and sensory integrity should be completed and any unexpected changes reported to the supervising PT. Ultrasound can be applied directly or indirectly.[44] Direct contact (transducer-skin interface) is used on relatively flat areas.

1. The clinician applies generous amounts of coupling medium (gel/cream) to the treatment area. (If, while performing the ultrasound, a hot spot is encountered, the PTA should apply more coupling agent or decrease the intensity.)
2. The clinician selects an appropriate sound head size. (The ERA should be half the size of the treatment area.)
3. Placing the sound head at a right angle to the skin surface and using relatively light pressure (approximately 1 pound or 450 g), the clinician

maintains the intensity to the desired level while moving the sound head slowly (approximately 1.75 inches/second or 4 cm/s) in overlapping circles or longitudinal strokes and maintaining the sound head/body surface angle. Periosteal pain occurring during treatment may be due to any of the following: high intensity, momentary slowing, or cessation of the moving head.

The area covered should not be greater than two to three times the size of the ERA for 5 minutes of treatment. Areas larger than this will require a separate application of ultrasound or another form of heat.

Intensity for continuous ultrasound is normally set between 0.5 and 2 W/cm² for thermal effects. Pulsed ultrasound for nonthermal effects is normally set between 0.5 and 0.75 W/cm² with a 20 percent duty cycle. The treatment time varies depending on the target tissue (muscle, tendon, and other soft tissues), the size of the area, intensity, condition, and frequency. Indirect contact (water immersion) is used for the application of ultrasound over irregular body parts.

1. The clinician fills a container with water high enough to cover the treatment area. Ideally, a plastic container should be used because it reflects less acoustic energy than a metal one.
2. The body part to be treated is immersed in the water.
3. The sound head is placed in the water, keeping it 1/2 to 1 inch from the skin surface and at right angles to the body part being treated.
4. The clinician moves the sound head slowly, as in the direct contact method, while turning up the intensity to the desired level. If a stationary technique is being applied, the clinician should reduce the intensity or use pulsed ultrasound.

Indirect contact (fluid-filled bag) is an alternative technique to immersion but it is not commonly used. To perform this technique, an ultrasound gel pad, a thin-walled bag such as a balloon, or a surgical glove is needed.

1. The bag is placed around the side of the sound head and the sound head is immersed in water.
2. The clinician applies coupling agent on the skin and then places the bag over the treatment area.
3. While maintaining the sound head within the bag and increasing the intensity to the desired level, the clinician moves the head slowly while keeping a right angle between the sound head and the treatment area. The bag should not slide on the skin.

Phonophoresis

Phonophoresis refers to a specific type of ultrasound application in which pharmacologic agents, such as corticosteroids, local anesthetics, and salicylates, are introduced.[53–60] Phonophoresis has been used clinically since the early 1960s in attempts to drive these drugs transdermally into subcutaneous tissues. Both the thermal and nonthermal (mechanical) properties of ultrasound have been cited as possible mechanisms for the transdermal penetration of the pharmacologic agents. Increases in cell permeability and local vasodilation accompanied by the acoustic pressure wave may result in increased diffusion of the topical agent.[54,55,60]

The indications and contraindications for phonophoresis are the same as for ultrasound, except the clinician needs to be aware of potential allergic reactions to the medications used.

> ● **Key Point** Recent papers have argued that many of the commonly used cream-based preparations do not allow adequate transmission of the acoustic wave.[45,46,61] Gel-based preparations appear to be superior with respect to the transmissivity of ultrasound. Consequently, gel-based corticosteroid compounds might be expected to be superior for phonophoresis applications.

A pretreatment and posttreatment assessment of skin and sensory integrity should be completed and any unexpected changes reported to the supervising PT. It is important that the PTA understands the specific indications and desired effects of the pharmacologic agents being used and that the patient status is monitored to determine the effectiveness of the treatment after every session.

Diathermy

Indications for the use of diathermy include those situations when the aim is to:

- Promote wound care
- Decrease pain and edema
- Increase oxygen to the tissue through vasodilation
- Increase temperature
- Increase metabolic rate
- Decrease nerve conduction latency
- Increase collagen extensibility
- Increase muscle, bone, and nerve tissue repair

via stimulation of protein synthesis at the cell membrane level

- Decrease chronic inflammation

Contraindications include:

- Implanted deep brain stimulators
- Internal or external metal implants
- Cardiac pacemakers
- The presence of malignancy
- Pregnancy
- Use over the eyes, epiphysis of growing bone, or testes
- Acute inflammation

Physiologic Effects

Diathermy, which includes both shortwave (SW) and microwave (MW), is a thermal agent that produces therapeutic effects through conversion. As with ultrasound, diathermy offers both thermal and nonthermal effects through the application of continuous or pulsed modes.

Application

A pretreatment and posttreatment assessment of skin and sensory integrity should be completed and any unexpected changes reported to the supervising PT. The patient needs to be monitored often during treatment because the treated area is not visible. Any conductive material must be removed. This includes jewelry, clothes with zippers, synthetic fabrics, electronic devices, and metal-containing or magnetic equipment.

> ● **Key Point** To avoid any potential exposure to hazardous levels of electromagnetic energy, the operator of the diathermy unit must stand behind the unit console.

Shortwave applicators include inductive coil applicators or capacitive plates. SW delivers a thermal or pulsed electromagnetic field. The most common SW frequency used is 27.12 MHz. In the electrical circuit method, the patient's area to be treated is placed between two conducting electrodes for 15 to 30 minutes. In the inductive field method, the patient's treated area is placed into a magnetic field formed by electrodes, and the current is induced within the patient's body tissues with the tissue resistance to the current producing an increase in temperature of the deep body tissues. Inductive coil applicators utilize a coil that generates alternating electric current, create a magnetic field perpendicular to the coil, and produce eddy currents within the tissues.

As the eddy currents cause an oscillation of ions, tissue temperature is increased.

Microwave is applied using electromagnetic radiation directed through a coaxial cable to an antenna mounted in the treatment applicator. Treatment time is typically 15 to 30 minutes. Caution must be used when energy is reflected at fat/muscle and muscle/bone interfaces because it can increase superficial tissue temperatures (skin or fat).

> ● **Key Point** The choice of heating modality should be made according to the patient's diagnosis, the body part being treated, the onset of the condition, the age of the patient, and the desired goal. For example, if the primary treatment goal is a tissue temperature increase with a corresponding increase in blood flow to the deeper tissues, the clinician should choose a modality, such as diathermy or ultrasound, that produces energy that can penetrate the cutaneous tissues and be directly absorbed by the deep tissues.[1]

Hydrotherapy

Hydrotherapy, formerly called hydropathy, involves the use of warm or cold water for the treatment of musculoskeletal dysfunction. Hydrotherapy, which involves submerging all or part of the body in water, can involve several types of equipment. Various temperatures can be used depending on the desired goal (**Table 7-5**).

Physical Properties of Water

Water has several physical properties:

- *Buoyancy:* The upward force of buoyancy somewhat counteracts the effects of gravity. Archimedes' principle states that any object submerged or floating in water is buoyed upward by a counterforce that helps support the submerged or partially submerged object against the downward pull of gravity, resulting in an apparent loss of weight. The center of buoyancy is the reference point of an immersed object on which the buoyant (vertical) forces of a fluid predictably act. In the vertical position, the human center of buoyancy is located at the sternum. Buoyancy can provide the patient with relative weightlessness and joint unloading, allowing performance of active motion with increased ease.[62] In addition, buoyancy allows the clinician three-dimensional access to the patient.
- *Hydrostatic pressure:* The pressure exerted by fluid on an immersed object is equal on all surfaces of the object (Pascal's law). Therefore, as the density of water and depth of immersion

TABLE 7-5	Clinical Applications of Whirlpool Treatment According to Temperature Ranges	
Temperature	Degrees	Use
Very hot	104–110°F (40–43.5°C)	Used for short exposure of 7–10 minutes to increase superficial temperature
Hot	99–104°F (37–40°C)	Used to increase superficial temperature
Warm	96–99°F (35.5–37°C)	Used to increase superficial temperature where a prolonged exposure is wanted, such as to decrease spasticity of a muscle in conjunction with passive exercise
Neutral	92–96°F (33.5–35.5°C)	Used with patients who have an unstable core body temperature
Tepid	80–92°F (27–33.5°C)	May be used in conjunction with less vigorous exercise
Cool	67–80°F (19–27°C)	May be used in conjunction with vigorous exercise
Cold	55–67°F (13–19°C)	Used for longer exposure of 10–15 minutes to decrease superficial temperature
Very cold	32–55°F (0–13°C)	Used for short exposure of 1–5 minutes to decrease superficial temperature

increase, so does hydrostatic pressure. From a clinical perspective, the proportionality of depth allows patients to perform exercise more easily when closer to the surface. It is important to remember that hydrostatic pressure can result in a number of cardiovascular shifts including decreased peripheral blood flow and vital capacity, increased heart volume, increased stroke volume, increased cardiac output, and a decrease or no change in the heart rate.

- *Viscosity:* Friction that occurs between molecules of liquid resulting in resistance to flow. From a clinical perspective, increasing the velocity of movement increases the resistance. In addition, increasing the surface area moving through the water increases the resistance.
- *Specific gravity:* Any object with a specific gravity less than that of water will float. The buoyant values of different body parts vary according to bone-to-muscle weight and the amount and distribution of fat.
- *Specific heat:* The amount of heat per unit mass required to raise the temperature by 1 degree Celsius. The specific heat of water is higher than any other common substance; as a result,

water plays a very important role in temperature regulation.

- ❏ Water can store four times the heat as compared to air.
- ❏ Water's thermal conductivity is approximately 25 times faster than air at the same temperature.
- *Surface tension:* Formed by the water molecules loosely binding together, whereby the attraction of surface molecules is parallel to the surface. From a clinical perspective, an extremity that moves through the surface performs more work than if kept under the water.
- *Drag force:* A factor of the shape of an object and its speed of movement. Objects that are more streamlined (minimizing the surface area at the front of the object) produce less drag force.

Whirlpool

Whirlpool therapies involve partial or total immersion of a body or body part in an immersion bath in which the water is agitated and mixed with air so that it can be directed against, or around, the involved part. Whirlpool tanks come in various sizes: High-boy (used for upper extremities); low-boy (used for lower extremities); and hubbard tank (used for full body immersion).

A turbine, consisting of a motor secured to the side of the tank, pumps a combination of air and water throughout the tank. The water/air jet can be set in a desired direction and height to increase stimulation, help control pain, or clean an area.[1] If the area is hypersensitive, the pressure can be directed away from it.

> **● Key Point** A ground fault interrupter (GFI) is a safety device that constantly compares the amount of electricity flowing from the wall outlet to the clinical unit with the amount returning to the outlet. If any leakage in the current flow is detected, the GFI unit automatically shuts off current flow to reduce the chances of electrical shock. A GFI should be installed at the circuit breaker at the receptacle of all whirlpools and Hubbard tanks, and the unit should be checked periodically for current leakage.

Application

The tank is filled to the desired level and appropriate temperature (refer to Table 7-5). Whirlpool liners may be used for patients with burns, wounds, or who are infected with bloodborne pathogens. If an antimicrobial is to be used it should be added to the water before the treatment starts. The following are appropriate antimicrobial agents:

- *Sodium hypochlorite (bleach):* Dilution of 200 parts per million (ppm)
- *Povidone-iodine:* Dilution of 4 ppm
- *Chloramine-T:* Dilution of 100–200 ppm

The patient is asked to uncover the treatment area adequately (as appropriate, any wound dressing is removed), and the skin is tested for thermal sensitivity. The checking of vital signs also may be appropriate based on patient history. Patient comfort is ensured by avoiding pressure of the limb on the edge of the whirlpool (which may also compromise circulation). Any pressure points should be padded. Once the patient is comfortable, the turbine direction is adjusted and then turned on. The force, direction, and depth of the jet/agitator are adjusted appropriately. During the treatment, the body part may be exercised. The patient should be accompanied throughout the treatment session and their vital signs monitored as appropriate. Whirlpool treatments can provide a sedative effect, and depending on the temperature of the water, can cause fluctuations in blood pressure.[63]

Once the treatment is completed, the patient is asked to remove the body part from the water, and the area is dried and inspected. If appropriate, a clean dressing is applied. The whirlpool is drained, cleaned, and rinsed. Cleaning procedures vary according to clinical setting. In general, the inside of the tank, outside of the agitator, thermometer, and drains are washed with disinfectant diluted in water. The disinfectant is allowed to stand for at least 1 minute. The agitator is placed in a bucket filled with water and disinfectant, so that all openings are covered with the solution. The agitator is turned on for about 20 to 30 seconds, after which the motor is turned off and the agitator is removed from the bucket. The entire tank and all the equipment is then rinsed until the entire residue is removed. The tank is then drained.

Contrast Bath

Contrast baths are an alternating cycle of warm (38°C to 44°C [100°F to 111°F]) and cold (10°C to 18°C [50°F to 64°F]) whirlpools that create a cycle of alternating vasoconstriction and vasodilation (10 minutes warmth, 1 minute cold, 4 minutes warmth; cycled over a period of 30 minutes). Contrast baths are used most often in the management of extremity injuries to reduce swelling around injuries or to aid recovery from exercise.[64,65] The technique provides good contact over irregularly shaped areas, allows for movement during treatment, and assists with pain management. Disadvantages include potential intolerance to cold and dependent positioning. Contraindications for this modality include both those for thermotherapy and those for cryotherapy.

Aquatic Therapy

In the past decade, widespread interest has developed in aquatic therapy as a tool for rehabilitation. Among the psychological aspects, water motivates movement, because painful joints and muscles can be moved more easily and painlessly in water. The exact proportion and quantity of both land and water activity is determined by the needs and response of the patient.

The indications for aquatic therapy include the following:

- Instances when partial weight-bearing ambulation is necessary
- To increase range of motion
- When standing balance needs to be improved
- When endurance/aerobic capacity needs to be improved
- When the goal is to increase muscle strength via active-assisted, gravity-assisted, active, or resisted exercise[66]

Contraindications to aquatic therapy include:[66]

- Incontinence
- Urinary tract infections
- Unprotected open wounds/menstruation
- Autonomic dysreflexia
- Heat intolerance
- Severe epilepsy/uncontrolled seizures
- Uncontrolled diabetes
- Unstable blood pressure
- Severe cardiac and/or pulmonary dysfunction

Once any contraindications have been ruled out, the patient's water safety skills and swimming ability should be evaluated, as well as their general level of comfort in the water. The following strategies/techniques can be used:[67]

- *Position and direction of movement:* A three-part progression moving from buoyancy-assisted exercises to buoyancy-supported and finally to buoyancy-resisted exercises. As with gravity, patient position and direction of movement can greatly alter the amount of assistance or resistance used.
  - *Buoyancy-assisted exercises:* Involve movements toward the surface of the water and are similar to gravity-assisted exercises on land. For example, in the standing position, shoulder abduction and flexion, as well as the ascent phase of the squat, are considered buoyancy-assisted exercises. In the prone position, hip extension can be buoyancy assisted.
  - *Buoyancy-supported exercises:* Involve movements that are parallel to the bottom of the pool and are similar to gravity-minimized positions on land. In the standing position, horizontal shoulder abduction/adduction is an example of such activity, as are hip and shoulder abduction in the supine position.
  - *Buoyancy-resisted exercises:* Involve movements toward the bottom of the pool. For example, in the supine position, shoulder and hip extension and the descent phase of the squat are considered buoyancy-resisted activities.
- *Depth of water:* Less support is provided by buoyancy in shallow water than in deeper water. In addition, modifications can be made by adding buoyancy equipment or resistance equipment. A study by Harrison and Bulstrode[68] measured static weight bearing in a pool using a population of healthy adults.[69] Results indicated that weight bearing during immersion was reduced to less than land-based weight.

- Immersion to C-7 levels reduced weight to 5.9–10 percent of normal weight.
- Immersion to the xiphosternum reduced weight to 25–37 percent of normal.
- Immersion to the level of the anterior superior iliac spine (ASIS) reduced weight to 40–56 percent of normal.

A follow-up study by Harrison and colleagues[70] compared weight bearing during immersed standing and slow and fast walking.[69] During slow walking, subjects had to be immersed to the ASIS before weight bearing was reduced to 75 percent of normal. Immersion to the clavicle during slow walking reduced weight bearing up to 50 percent of normal values, and immersion above the clavicle resulted in weight bearing of 25 percent of normal or less. During fast walking, mid-trunk immersion produced weight bearing up to 75 percent of actual weight. Subjects had to be immersed deeper than the xiphosternum in order for weight bearing to be less than 50 percent and deeper than C-7 for weight bearing to be less than 25 percent of normal values.

- *Lever arm length:* As with land-based exercises, the lever arm length can be adjusted to change the amount of assistance or resistance. For example, performing buoyancy-assisted shoulder flexion in a standing position is easier with the elbow straight (i.e., long lever) than with the elbow flexed (i.e., short lever). Conversely, buoyancy-resisted shoulder abduction is more difficult with the elbow extended because of the long lever arm.
- *Buoyant equipment:* To further increase the amount of assistance (support for individuals in certain positions) or resistance, buoyant equipment can be added to the lever arm. As the buoyancy of the equipment increases, the resistance also increases. Equipment designed to assist with patient positioning can be applied to the neck, extremities, or trunk.
- *Viscosity:* The viscous quality of water allows it to be used effectively as a resistive medium. When moving through the water, the body experiences a frontal resistance proportional to the presenting surface area. This resistance can be increased by enlarging the surface area or by increasing the velocity of movement.
- *Water temperature:* Variable temperature control for the water should be available and the ambient air temperature should be 3°C (5°F) higher than the water temperature for patient comfort.

The body's ability to regulate temperature during immersion exercise differs from that during land exercise. Water conducts temperature 25 times faster than air, and water retains heat 1000 times more than air. With immersion, less skin is exposed to air, resulting in less opportunity to dissipate heat through normal sweating mechanisms. The following water temperatures are recommended based on activity:

❑ 26°C to 33°C (79°F to 91°F) for aquatic exercises, including flexibility, strengthening, gait training, and relaxation. Therapeutic exercise performed in warm water (33°C [91°F]) may be beneficial for patients with painful musculoskeletal areas.

❑ 26°C to 28°C (79°F to 82°F) should be used for cardiovascular training and aerobic exercise (active swimming).

❑ 22°C to 26°C (71°F to 79°F) should be used for intense and aerobic training.

It is important that the patient enters the water slowly so that all systems have an opportunity to gradually accommodate to the environment.

A variety of aquatic therapy techniques exist (**Table 7-6**). The following is a sample exercise activity for

TABLE 7-6	Aquatic Specialty Techniques
Specialty Technique	**Description**
Ai Chi	Ai Chi is a water-based total body strengthening and relaxation progression that unites the East and West philosophies of T'ai Chi, Shiatsu, and Watsu. Ai Chi is initially performed standing in shoulder-depth water using deep breathing patterns. Progression involves moving from these simple breathing techniques to the incorporation of upper-extremity, trunk, lower-extremity, and finally full torso involvement.
Aquatic proprioceptive neuromuscular facilitation (PNF)	As the name suggests, this technique is based on the principles and movement patterns of PNF while in water. The goal of aquatic PNF is to assist in the restoration of strength and movement through the use of buoyancy, resistance, and heat. The water may be used for use in both active exercise or for passive immersion.
Bad Ragaz ring method (BRRM)	BRRM is an aquatic version of Proprioceptive Neuromuscular Facilitation designed by a German physician that seeks to improve muscle function via patterns of movement and clinician resistance. Exercises are performed while lying horizontal in the water with support provided by rings or floats around the neck, arms, pelvis and knees. By using the extremities as levers, the trunk muscles are activated.
Fluid moves (Aquatic Feldenkrais)	The patient performs Feldenkrais moves, which are based on the early developmental stages of the infant. The movements are performed slowly while the clinician gives verbal (and occasionally tactile) cues. The exercises are usually performed with the patient's back or side against the pool wall to enable feedback from touch receptors. The intent of these exercises is to promote greater flexibility and better body awareness.
Halliwick method	The Halliwick method aims to teach people how to maintain balance control in the water and to teach them to swim by combining the unique qualities of water with rotational control patterns. The Halliwick method uses a ten-point program that is divided into four phases: (1) attempts to address the psychologic aspects of being in water; (2) improves the patient's ability to restore balance from all positions in the water; (3) concentrates on teaching the patient to inhibit undesired movements while maintaining stability in the water; and (4) teaches the patient to move (swim) from a position of stability.
Swim stroke training and modification	Uses swim stroke training to rehabilitate patients.
Task-type training approach (TTTA)	TTTA, which uses a task-oriented approach that emphasizes functional skills performed in functional positions, is designed for patients with neurologic dysfunction.
Watsu	Watsu, or water shiatsu, is a passive technique performed in warm water. The patient is cradled in the clinician's arms (beginning in the fetal position), while stretches and other bodywork are performed.

Adapted from Aquatic Resources Network: How to Define Aquatic Specialty Techniques: Operational Definitions. http://www.aquaticnet.com/Article%20-%20How%20to%20define%20aquatic%20specially%20techniques.htm

a patient with low back pain: In waist-deep water at the side of the pool, the patient is asked to sit in an imaginary chair so that the back is against the pool wall, the thighs are parallel to the bottom of the pool, and the knees are aligned over the ankles. The back remains against the pool wall throughout the exercise. Arms are at the sides with palms facing backward, and shoulders are relaxed. The head faces straight ahead. The patient is asked to begin pumping the arms forward and back about 6 inches while inhaling for five counts and exhaling for five counts.

Design and Special Equipment
Certain characteristics of the pool should be taken into consideration if it is to be used for rehabilitation purposes:

- The pool should not be smaller than 10 feet by 12 feet.
- The pool should have both a shallow (1.25 meter/ 2.5 feet) and a deep (2.5 meter/5+ feet) area to allow for standing exercises and swimming or nonstanding exercises.
- The pool bottom should be flat and the depth gradations clearly marked.

The following equipment will be helpful for aquatic therapy:

- Rescue tubes, inner tubes, and/or wet vests should be purchased to assist in floatation activities, and aqua shoes will help prevent slipping on the bottom of the pool.
- Hand paddles, webbed gloves, and pull-buoys can be used for strengthening the upper extremities.
- Buoyant dumbbells (swim bars), which are available in short and long lengths, can be used for supporting the upper body or trunk in the upright position and the lower extremities in the supine or prone positions.
- Kick boards, boots, and fins are useful for strengthening the lower extremities.

Advantages
The buoyancy of the water allows active exercise while providing a sense of security and causing little discomfort. Early in the rehabilitation process, aquatic therapy is useful in restoring range of motion and flexibility using a combination of the water's buoyancy, resistance, and warmth. Additional advantages include the following:

- The buoyancy provides support.
- The slow-motion effect of moving in water provides extra time to control movement and to react.

- The water provides tactile stimulation and feedback.
- The water allows a gradual transition from non-weight-bearing to full weight-bearing exercises by adjusting the amount the body is submerged.
- The intensity of exercise can be controlled by manipulating the body's position, or through the addition of exercise equipment.

Disadvantages
Disadvantages of aquatic therapy include the following:

- Cost of building and maintenance
- Training and staffing appropriately
- Difficulty treating patients with inherent fear of water
- Cannot treat patients that have open wounds, fever, urinary tract infections, allergies to the pool chemicals, cardiac problems, uncontrolled seizures, contagious skin diseases, or sores
- Difficult to reproduce lower extremity eccentric muscle contractions

Electrotherapeutic Modalities

As their name suggests, electrotherapeutic modalities are those that use electricity to produce a therapeutic effect. There are a variety of electrotherapy devices, each with different current characteristics that result in somewhat different responses. Electrical current that passes through tissue forces nerves to depolarize. Electrotherapeutic devices (Figure 7-6) generate three different types of current:

- *Monophasic or direct (galvanic):* A unidirectional flow of electrons. The energy travels

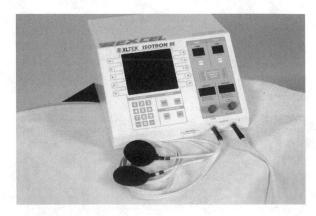

Figure 7-6   Electrical stimulation machine.

only in the positive direction. Direct current produces polar effects. It is important to remember that intact skin cannot tolerate a current density of great than 1 mA/cm^2.[71] Iontophoresis uses direct current.

- *Biphasic or alternating:* The flow of electrons constantly changes direction or, stated differently, reverses its polarity. The energy travels in both a positive and a negative direction. The wave form that occurs will be replicated on both sides of the isoelectric line. Alternating current is used in muscle retraining, spasticity, and stimulation of denervated muscle.
- *Pulsed:* Usually contains three or more pulses grouped together, which are interrupted for short periods of time and repeat themselves at regular intervals. The current can be monophasic or biphasic.

Electrical current tends to choose the path of least resistance in which to flow. Electricity has an effect on each cell and tissue that it passes through. The type and extent of the response depend on the type of tissue and its response characteristics. Typically, tissue that is highest in water content and consequently highest in ion content is the best conductor of electricity.

Good conductors within the body include:

- *Blood:* Composed largely of water and ions, it is consequently the best electrical conductor of all tissues.
- *Muscle:* Composed of about 75 percent water, and therefore a relatively good conductor.
- *Nerves:* The type of nerve and the rate at which the fiber is depolarized will determine the physiologic and, therefore, therapeutic effect achieved.[72,73] Nerves with a larger diameter are depolarized before nerves with smaller diameters.

> **● Key Point** No definitive studies have been done to support the use of electrical muscle stimulation to prevent muscle degeneration. If the nerve does not regenerate in time to reinnervate the muscle, there is no need to stimulate the muscle. With reinnervated muscle, it is theoretically possible to use alternating current stimulation; however, it is necessary to have a large number of reinnervated muscle fibers to stimulate the muscle with alternating current.

Poor conductors include:

- *Skin:* Offers the primary resistance to current flow and is considered an insulator. The greater the impedance (resistance to current) of the skin, the higher the voltage of the electrical current required to stimulate the underlying nerve and muscle.

- *Tendons:* Denser than muscle and contain relatively little water.
- *Fat:* Only about 14 percent water.
- *Bone:* Extremely dense; contains only about 5 percent water—the poorest biological conductor.

The traditional uses of electrical stimulation are listed in **Table 7-7**. Indications for electrotherapeutic modalities include the following:

- Pain relief
- Wound care (The clinician should always use universal precautions when treating a patient with an open wound or lesion, and wear gloves, waterproof gown, goggles, and a mask, particularly when there is a possibility of splashing.)
- Burn care
- Need to facilitate the resorption of effusion (edema control)
- Need to improve range of motion
- Sprain/strain

The following are precautions against electrical stimulation:

- Allergies to tapes and gels
- Areas of absent or diminished sensation
- Electrically sensitive patients
- Need to place electrode over an area of significant adipose tissue, near the stellate ganglion, over the temporal and orbital region, or over damaged skin

Contraindications include the following:

- Decreased temperature sensation
- Impaired cognition
- Recent skin graft
- Incontinence
- Confusion/disorientation
- Deconditioned state
- Bleeding
- Wound maceration
- Cardiac instability
- Profound epilepsy

The key points to remember when using electrical modalities are listed in **Table 7-8**.

Terminology

Before describing the electrical modalities in detail, it is important to provide a basic understanding of the terminology.

- *Electricity:* The force created by an imbalance in the number of electrons at two points: the *negative pole* (an area of high electron

| TABLE 7-7 |

TABLE 7-7 Traditional Uses of Electrical Stimulation

Use	Method	Frequency (Hz)	Pulses per Second	Time (min)
Pain relief	High frequency stimulation (80–120 Hz) and short duration should be used to stimulate the smallest unmyelinated nerve (C and delta) fibers in order to reduce pain (gate control theory).	> 100 (TENS, HVGS, IFC)	70–100	20–60
	Low frequency (longer duration) stimulation, which stimulates the larger myelinated (alpha) fibers, should be used when the goal is to produce muscle contractions.			
	Ultra-low frequencies can increase endorphin production through initiation of the descending inhibition mechanisms (opiate pain control theory).			
Reduce edema	By producing a muscle pump action that increases the lymph and venous flow towards the heart.	100–150 (HVGS, IFC)	120 (negative polarity)	20
	Increasing ion flow by attracting specific ions in a desired direction, because edema is believed to be slightly negatively charged (DC or Hi-volt).			
Wound healing	Through modification of the local inflammatory response (increased polarity produces an increase in inflammation), increasing circulation (negative polarity).	> 100 or 1	Varies but typically 70–100	20
	Pulsed currents (monophasic, biphasic, or polyphasic) with interrupted modulations can increase circulation and thus hasten metabolic waste disposal.			
	Restoration of electrical cell charges through the use of monophasic currents (low-volt continuous modulations and high-volt pulsed currents). May also have a bactericidal effect (cathode) by disrupting DNA or RNA synthesis or the cell transport system of microorganisms.			
	Low-intensity continuous (nonpulsed and low volt) direct current and high-volt pulsed current can be applied for wound healing (by use of ionic effects).			

concentration [cathode]) and the *positive pole* (an area of low electron concentration [anode]).

- *Charge:* An imbalance in energy. The charge of a solution has significance when attempting to "drive" medicinal drugs topically via iontophoresis and in attempting to artificially "fire" a denervated muscle. Cell membranes rest at a *resting potential*, which is an electrical balance of charges. This balance must be disrupted to achieve muscle firing. Muscle depolarization is difficult to achieve with PT modalities, whereas nerve depolarization occurs very easily with PT modalities.

- *Coulomb's law:* Like charges repel; unlike charges attract.
- *Watt:* A measure of electrical power (Watts = volts × amperes).
- *Volt:* The electromotive force that must be applied to produce a movement of electrons—a measure of electrical power. Two modality classifications include high voltage (greater than 100–150 V) and low voltage (less than 100–150 V).
- *Amperes:* A measure of electrical charge/current. Electrons move along a conducting medium as an electrical current. The term *amplitude* refers to the magnitude of current and is associated with the depth

| TABLE 7-7 | Traditional Uses of Electrical Stimulation (continued) |

Use	Method	Frequency (Hz)	Pulses per Second	Time (min)
Muscle re-education	Using electrical stimulation to bring motor nerves and muscle fibers closer to threshold for depolarization. Re-educating muscles to respond appropriately using volitional effort by: • Providing proprioceptive feedback. • Assisting with active exercise to help produce a contraction (active-assisted). • Assisting in the coordination of muscle movement. Current intensity must be adequate for muscle contraction, and pulse duration should be set as close as possible to the duration needed for chronaxie of the tissue to be stimulated. The pulses per second (pps) should be high enough to give a titanic contraction (20–40 pps).	50–60	1–20	Fatigue (1–15)

HVGS, high volt galvanic stimulator; TENS, transcutaneous electrical nerve stimulation; IFC, interferential current.

Data from Riker DK: Assessment: Efficacy of transcutaneous electric nerve stimulation in the treatment of pain in neurologic disorders (an evidence-based review); utility of transcutaneous electrical nerve stimulation in neurologic pain disorders. Neurology 74:1748–1749, author reply 1749, 2010; Cheng JS, Yang YR, Cheng SJ, et al: Effects of combining electric stimulation with active ankle dorsiflexion while standing on a rocker board: A pilot study for subjects with spastic foot after stroke. Arch Phys Med Rehabil 91:505–512, 2010; Dubinsky RM, Miyasaki J: Assessment: Efficacy of transcutaneous electric nerve stimulation in the treatment of pain in neurologic disorders (an evidence-based review): Report of the Therapeutics and Technology Assessment Subcommittee of the American Academy of Neurology. Neurology 74:173–176, 2010; Meade CS, Lukas SE, McDonald LJ, et al: A randomized trial of transcutaneous electric acupoint stimulation as adjunctive treatment for opioid detoxification. J Subst Abuse Treat 38:12–21, 2010; Chan MK, Tong RK, Chung KY: Bilateral upper limb training with functional electric stimulation in patients with chronic stroke. Neurorehabil Neural Repair 23:357–365, 2009; Kumaravel S, Sundaram S: Fracture healing by electric stimulation—biomed 2009. Biomed Sci Instrum 45:191–196, 2009

TABLE 7-8	Key Points to Remember When Using Electrotherapeutic Modalities

The introduction of electricity to a patient affects the whole body.

The physical condition of the patient must be considered before introducing an electrical current.

The electrical current affects the electrically active tissue, such as muscles and nerves.

The response of the tissue is based on the current's density (current amplitude, placement of the electrodes, relative size of the electrodes).

Electrical current affects type II muscle fibers at lower density levels than it does for type I muscle fibers, which results in an abnormal recruitment order.

The current is sensed more by the skin than other tissues, due to the local resistance and ion concentrations in the local areas around the electrodes.

of penetration—the deeper the penetration, the more muscle fiber recruitment possible.

- *Resistance:* The opposition to the flow of current. Factors affecting resistance include material composition (see the "Physiologic Effects" section), length (greater length yields greater resistance), and temperature (increased temperature, increased resistance). Preheating the treatment area may increase patient comfort but also increases resistance and the need for higher output intensities. To minimize resistance, the PTA can:
  - ❏ Reduce the skin–electrode resistance by applying a coupling agent and cleaning the skin with alcohol.
  - ❏ Minimize air–electrode interface by ensuring the electrode has a tight seal.
  - ❏ Keep the electrode and skin clean of oils and the like.

- Use the shortest pathway for energy flow.
- Use the largest electrode that will selectively stimulate the target tissues.

- *Pulse duration (also known as pulse width):* The length of time the electrical flow is "on." It represents the time for one cycle to occur (both phases in a biphasic current). Phase duration is an important factor in determining which tissue is stimulated—if the duration is too short there will be no action potential.
- *Accommodation:* The increased threshold of excitable tissue when a slowly rising stimulus is used. Both nerve and muscle tissues are capable of accommodating to an electrical stimulus, with nerve tissue accommodating more rapidly than muscle tissue. The quicker the rise time, the less the nerve can accommodate to the impulse.
- *Pulse rise time:* The time to peak intensity of the pulse (ramp). Ramping is used to reduce the shock of the current. Rapid rising pulses cause nerve depolarization. Slow rising pulses allow the nerve to accommodate to the stimulus and an action potential is not elicited. This is good for muscle re-education when used with assisted contraction.
- *Pulse Frequency (Hz):* Represents the number of pulses that occur in a unit of time:
  - *Low frequency:* 1 kHz and below (micro-electrical nerve stimulation (MENS) 1 = 1 kHz)
  - *Medium frequency:* 1 to 100 kHz (interferential, Russian stimulation Lo-volt galvanic stimulation [LVGS])
  - *High frequency:* Above 100 kHz (transcutaneous electrical nerve stimulation (TENS), hi-volt galvanic stimulation (HVGS), diathermies)
- *Strength duration curve:* A graphic representation of the relationship between the intensity of an electrical stimulus at the motor point of a muscle and the length of time it must flow to elicit a minimal contraction.
- *Rheobase:* The minimum intensity of an electrical stimulus that will elicit a minimal contraction.
- *Chronaxie:* The minimum time over which an electric current, double the strength of the rheobase, needs to be applied.

- *Duty cycles:* On-off time. May also be called interpulse interval, which is the time between pulses.
  - 1:1 ratio fatigues muscle rapidly.
  - 1:5 ratio causes less fatigue.
  - 1:7 induces no fatigue (passive muscle exercise).
- *Current density:* The amount of charge per unit area. This is usually relative to the size of the electrode. Density will be greater with a small electrode, but the small electrode offers more resistance.

- *Fasciculation:* Involuntary motor unit firing. May see skin move, but no joint motion.
- *Fibrillation:* Involuntary firing of a single muscle fiber; indicative of denervation.
- *Frequency:* Represents the number of cycles or pulses per second (rate of oscillation). Normally described in the unit of Hz.

Physiologic Effects

As electricity moves through the body, changes in physiologic functioning occur at the various levels of the system (**Table 7-9**).

TABLE 7-9	Changes in Physiologic Functioning that Occur Due to Electricity	

Body System Level	Changes
Cellular level	Excitation of nerve cells
	Changes in cell membrane permeability
	Protein synthesis (with DC)
	Stimulation of fibroblasts and osteoblasts (with DC)
	Modification of microcirculation
Tissue level	Skeletal muscle contraction
	Smooth muscle contraction
	Tissue regeneration
Segmental level	Modification of joint mobility
	Muscle pumping action to change circulation and lymphatic activity
	An alteration of the microvascular system not associated with muscle pumping
	An increased movement of charged proteins into the lymphatic channels with subsequent oncotic force bringing increases in fluid to the lymph system
	Transcutaneous electrical stimulation cannot directly stimulate lymph smooth muscle or the autonomic nervous system without also stimulating a motor nerve
Systematic effects	Analgesic effects as endogenous pain suppressors are released and act at different levels to control pain
	Analgesic effects from the stimulation of certain neurotransmitters to control neural activity in the presence of pain stimuli

● **Key Point** The limited studies on postsurgical or acutely injured patients seem to indicate that electrical muscle stimulation is either as effective as, or more effective than, isometric exercises at increasing muscle strength and bulk[74–78] in both atrophied[79] and normal muscles.[80, 81]

According to Taylor and colleagues,[82] the present regimens being used (i.e., one intervention per day or three times per week) may be insufficiently aggressive to provide benefit.

Electrodes and Their Placement

Electrodes are used in the therapeutic application of current. At least two electrodes are required to complete the circuit; the patient's body becomes the conductor. The strongest stimulation is where the current exits the body. Electrodes placed close together will give a superficial stimulation and be of high density, whereas electrodes spaced far apart will penetrate more deeply with less current density (interferential). When stimulating a muscle, electrode orientation should be parallel to the muscle fibers along the line of pull of the muscle group.

Generally, the larger the electrode the less current density. If a large "dispersive" pad is creating muscle contractions there may be some areas of high current concentration and other areas that are relatively inactive, thus functionally reducing the total size of the electrode.

● **Key Point**
- *Large electrodes:* Decreased current density, decreased impedance, and increased current flow
- *Small electrodes:* Increased current density, increased impedance, and decreased current flow

Electrodes may be placed on or around the painful area. The configuration of the electrodes depends on the intent of the intervention:

■ *Monopolar:* Requires one negative electrode and one positive electrode. The stimulating or active electrode is placed over the target area (e.g., motor point). A second dispersive electrode is placed at another site away from the target area. This technique is used with wounds, iontophoresis, and in the treatment of edema.

- *Bipolar:* Two active electrodes of equal size are placed over the target area. This technique is used for muscle weakness, neuromuscular facilitation, spasms, and to increase range of motion.
- *Quadripolar:* Two electrodes from two separate stimulating circuits are positioned so that the individual currents intersect with each other.

Electrical Equipment Care and Maintenance

Electrical safety in the clinical setting should be of maximal concern to the clinician. The typical electrical circuit consists of a source producing electric power, a conductor that carries the power to a resistor or series of given elements, and a conductor that carries the power back to the power source. Safety considerations when using electrical equipment include those listed in **Table 7-10**.

TABLE 7-10	Safety Considerations When Using Electrical Devices

The two-pronged plug has only two leads, both of which carry some voltage. Consequently, the electrical device has no true ground (connected to the earth), and relies instead on the chassis or casing of the power source to act as a ground. This increases the potential for electrical shock.

The third prong of a three-pronged plug is designed to be grounded directly to the earth. However, never assume that all three-pronged wall outlets are automatically grounded. Although three-pronged plugs generally work well in dry environments, they may not provide sufficient protection from electrical shock in a wet or damp area. In such instances, it is mandated that any equipment used in a wet or damp environment should be fitted with a ground fault interrupter (GFI).

Equipment should be visually inspected before each use to check for frayed cords and other safety hazards.

The entire electrical system of the clinic should be designed or routinely evaluated by a qualified electrician.

Equipment should be re-evaluated on an annual basis and should conform to National Electrical Code guidelines. This includes the lead wires.

Any defective equipment should be removed from the clinic immediately.

Do not jerk plugs out of the wall by pulling on the cable.

Extension cords or multiple adapters should never be used.

Transdermal Iontophores

Transdermal iontophoresis is the administration of selected (by the PT or physician) ionic therapeutic agents through the skin by the application of a low-level electrical current. The principle behind iontophoresis is that an electrical potential difference will actively cause ions in solution to migrate according to their electrical charge—negatively charged ions are repelled from a negative electrode and attracted toward the positive electrode. In contrast, the positive ions are repelled from the positive electrode and attracted toward the negative electrode.[83,84] Ionized medications or chemicals do not ordinarily penetrate tissues, and if they do, it is not normally at a rate rapid enough to achieve therapeutic levels.[83] This problem is overcome by using a direct current energy source that provides penetration and transport.[83,84] Iontophoresis has proved to be valuable in the intervention of musculoskeletal disorders because the application of current through the tissue causes an increased penetration of drugs and other compounds into the tissue. Iontophoresis has, therefore, been used for the transdermal delivery of systemic drugs in a controlled fashion.[85] The factors affecting transdermal iontophoretic transport include pH; the intensity of the current, or current density, at the active electrode; ionic strength; concentration of the drug; molecular size; and the duration of the current flow (continuous or pulse current). The proposed mechanisms by which iontophoresis increases drug penetration are as follows:

- The electrical potential gradient induces changes in the arrangement of the lipid, protein, and water molecules.[86]
- Pore formation occurs in the stratum corneum (SC), the outermost layer of the skin.[87] The exact pathway by which ionized drugs are transmitted through the SC has not been elucidated. The impermeability of the SC is the main barrier to cutaneous or transcutaneous drug delivery. If the integrity of the SC is disrupted, the barrier to molecular transit may be greatly reduced.
- Hair follicles, sweat glands, and sweat ducts act as diffusion shunts with reduced resistance for ion transport.[88] Skin and fat are poor conductors of electrical current and offer greater resistance to current flow.

Iontophoresis can be performed using a wide variety of chemicals (**Table 7-11**). For a chemical to be successful in iontophoresis, it must solubilize

TABLE 7-11	Various Ions Used in Iontophoresis			
Ion	Polarity	Solution		Purpose/Condition
Acetate	–	2–5% acetic acid		Calcium deposits
Calcium	+	2% calcium chloride		Myopathy, muscle spasm
Chlorine	–	2% sodium chloride		Scar tissue, adhesions
Dexamethasone	+	4 mg/mL dexamethasone Na-P		Tendonitis, bursitis
Hyaluronidase	+	Wyadase		Edema
Iodine	–	Iodex ointment		Adhesions, scar tissue
Lidocaine	+	4% lidocaine		Trigeminal neuralgia
Potassium iodide	–	10%		Scar tissue
Salicylate	–	2% sodium salicylate		Myalgia, scar tissue
Tap water	+/–	N/A		Hyperhidrosis

+, positive; –, negative.

into ionic components. Following the basic law of physics that *like poles repel*, the positively charged ions are placed under the positive electrode while the negatively charged ions are placed under the negative electrode. If the ionic source is in an aqueous solution, it is recommended that a low concentration be used (2 to 4 percent) to aid in the dissociation.[89] Although electrons flow from negative to positive, regardless of electrode size, having a larger negative pad than a positive one will help shape the direction of flow.

Current intensity is recommended to be at 5 mA or less for all interventions. The duration of the treatment may vary from 15 to 20 minutes. Longer durations have been shown to produce a decrease in the skin impedance, thus increasing the likelihood of burns from an accumulation of ions under the electrodes.[90] The patient is thus monitored during and after the treatment to ensure that the skin is not burned under the electrode. At present, research has been focused on the development of iontophoretic patches for the systemic delivery of drugs. The iontophoretic patch has the option to monitor and control the power supplied during use, thus permitting safer and more reliable operation. The system can also detect the number of times the patch has been used and records the date and time of use, and its microprocessor can detect when the medication is exhausted. Furthermore, the controller can be rendered unusable to avoid abuse once the drug is exhausted.

The indications for the use of transdermal iontophoresis include those situations when the aim is to:

- Decrease inflammation
- Decrease pain
- Decrease calcium deposits
- Facilitate wound healing
- Decrease edema

Contraindications include:

- Cardiac pacemakers or other electrically sensitive implanted devices
- Known sensitivity to the drugs to be administered
- Known adverse reactions to the application of electrical current
- Damaged skin or recent scar tissue
- Use across the temporal regions or for the treatment of the orbital region

Transcutaneous Electrical Nerve Stimulation

Transcutaneous electrical nerve stimulation (TENS) has been used effectively as a safe, noninvasive, drug-free method of treatment for various chronic and acute pain syndromes for many years. Depending on the parameters of electrical stimuli applied, there are several modes of therapy, resulting in different contributions of hyperaemic, muscle-relaxing, and analgesic components of TENS. TENS has been shown to be effective in providing pain relief in the early stages of healing following surgery[75,91–95] and in the remodeling phase of healing.[96–99]

● **Key Point** The percentage of patients who benefit from short-term TENS pain intervention has been reported to range from 50 to 80 percent, and good long-term results with TENS have been observed in 6 to 44 percent of patients.[96,98,100,101] However, most of the TENS studies rely solely on subjects' pain reports to establish efficacy and rarely on other outcome measures such as activity, socialization, or medication use.

TENS units typically deliver symmetric or balanced asymmetric biphasic waves of 100- to 500-millisecond pulse duration, with zero net current to

TABLE 7-12	TENS Parameters and Effects			
Type	Frequency (Hz)	Duration (microseconds)	Amplitude (mA)	Muscle Contraction
Conventional	50–150	20–100	10–30	Yes
Low frequency (acupuncture)	1–4	100–200	30–80	Yes
Burst	70–100/burst	40–75	30–60	Yes
Brief intense (high-intensity)	70–100/burst	15–200	30–60	No

minimize skin irritation,[102] and it may be applied for extended periods (**Table 7-12**). The three modes of action that are theorized for the pain-relieving quality of this modality—gate control mechanism, endogenous opiate control, and central biasing—are described in Chapter 3. There are several guidelines when using electrical stimulation of sensory nerves for pain suppression:

- Electrodes may be placed close to the spinal cord segment that innervates a painful area.
- Placing electrodes over sites where the nerve becomes superficial and can be stimulated easily may stimulate peripheral nerves that innervate a painful area.
- Vascular structures contain neural tissue as well as ionic fluids that would transmit electrical stimulating current and may be most easily stimulated by electrode placement over superficial vascular structures.
- Electrodes can be placed over trigger points and acupuncture locations.
- Electrodes may be placed over specific dermatomes, myotomes, or sclerotomes that correspond to the painful area.

Russian Current or Medium-Frequency Alternating Current

Because medium-frequency stimulation is capable and effective at stimulating deep and superficial tissues, Russian current—a type of neuromuscular electrical stimulation (NMES) or functional electrical stimulation (FES)—is believed to augment muscle strengthening by polarizing both sensory and motor nerve fibers, resulting in tetanic contractions that are painless and stronger than those made voluntarily by the patient. The majority of E-stim units (such

as the one shown in Figure 7-6) provide a variety of treatment modes. The medium frequency used with Russian current makes this type of current more comfortable than some others, especially if the current is delivered in bursts or if an interburst interval is used.

Interferential Current

Interferential current combines two high-frequency alternating waveforms that are biphasic. By using overall shorter pulse widths and higher frequencies of each waveform, interferential current can reach deeper tissues. Interferential current can be used for:[103]

- Muscle contraction (20–50 pps), together with the overall shorter pulse widths (100–200 μs)
- Pain management, using a frequency of 50–120 pps and a pulse width of 50–150 μs AcuStim pain relief, using a frequency of 1 pps

Biofeedback

Biofeedback is a modality that is widely used in musculoskeletal rehabilitation. The clinical conditions for which biofeedback is most commonly used include muscle re-education, which involves regaining neuromuscular control and/or increasing the strength of a muscle; relaxation of muscle spasm or muscle guarding; and pain reduction. The biofeedback units most commonly used in physical therapy measure electromyographic (EMG) activity through skin surface electrodes, indicating the amount of electrical activity during muscle contraction. Specifically, the EMG activity measured is the change in potential difference or voltage associated with depolarization. The biofeedback units provide auditory or visual feedback to give the patient information on timing of recruitment and intensity of muscle contractions. In addition, using biofeedback can help the patient regain function of a muscle that may have been lost or forgotten following injury. It is important to remember that the various EMG biofeedback units do not use a universally accepted standardized measurement scale, so different brands may give different readings for the same degree of muscle contraction. Consequently, EMG readings can be compared only when the same equipment is used for all readings.

EMG skin surface electrodes come in a variety of sizes, and prior to attachment of the surface electrodes, the skin must be appropriately prepared by removing oil and dead skin, along with excessive hair, to reduce skin impedance. The electrodes are placed as near to the muscle being monitored as possible so they are parallel to the direction of the muscle fibers, thereby reducing extraneous electrical activity. Three electrodes are typically used:

- Two active electrodes
- One reference or ground electrode

The electrodes are placed in a bipolar arrangement—the active electrodes are placed in close proximity to one another while the reference electrode is placed between the two active electrodes. As the active electrodes pick up electrical activity, the information is passed into a *differential amplifier*, which basically subtracts the signal from one active electrode from the other active electrode, thereby amplifying the difference between the signals. The ability of the differential amplifier to eliminate the common noise between the active electrodes is called the *common mode rejection ratio*. The external noise can be further reduced by using filters built into the unit. Signal sensitivity or signal gain can be set by the clinician on many units. If a high gain is chosen, the unit will have a high sensitivity for the muscle activity signal. This setting is typically used during relaxation training. Lower sensitivity levels are used more in muscle re-education. Biofeedback units generally provide visual and/or auditory feedback relative to the quantity of electrical activity.

Muscle Re-Education

Biofeedback for muscle re-education is useful in patients who perform poorly on manual muscle tests—those who can elicit only a fair, trace, or zero grade. The sensitivity setting is chosen by having the patient perform a maximum isometric contraction of the target muscle for 6 to 10 seconds. The gain is then adjusted such that the patient will be able to achieve the maximum on about two-thirds of the muscle contraction. The patient should be advised to look at the muscle when trying to contract it. Sometimes it may be necessary to move the active electrodes to the contralateral limb so the patient can practice the muscle contraction. Between each contraction, the patient should be instructed to completely relax the muscle so the feedback mode returns to baseline or zero prior to initiating another contraction. Ideally, a period of 5 to 10 minutes working with a single muscle or muscle group is most desirable to prevent fatigue.

Muscle Relaxation

The purpose of this approach is so that the patient is attempting to reduce the visual auditory feedback to zero. During relaxation training, the patient should be given verbal cues that will enhance relaxation of either individual muscles, muscle groups, or body segments. For example, biofeedback for relaxation is commonly used at the temporomandibular joint where monitoring of the frontal, temporal, and masseter muscles is used. As relaxation progresses, the spacing between the electrodes is increased and the sensitivity setting is adjusted from low to high. Both of these changes require the patient to relax more muscles, thus achieving greater relaxation.

Mechanical Modalities

Mechanical modalities are those that require a physical force to be imparted from either a machine or a clinician and include spinal traction, and intermittent mechanical compression.

Mechanical Spinal Traction

Mechanical spinal traction involves the use of a distraction force applied to the cervical or lumbar spine to separate or attempt to separate the articular surfaces between the zygapophysial joints and the vertebral bodies. A number of methods can be employed to apply a distraction for the spine including positional, gravity-assisted, and inversion techniques, but this discussion will focus on the use of mechanical traction, which can be continuous or intermittent, because this is the most common method. A call bell or cutoff switch is issued to the patient, and the patient should be closely monitored for any adverse reaction. Treatment time varies based on diagnosis and therapeutic goals, and falls between 5 and 20 minutes.

Indications for mechanical spinal traction include:

- Nerve impingement
- Herniated or protruding disk
- Subacute joint inflammation
- Joint hypomobility
- Degenerative joint disease
- Paraspinal muscle spasm

Contraindications include:

- Joint instability or when motion is contraindicated
- Pregnancy (lumbar traction)
- Acute inflammatory response
- Acute sprain
- Osteoporosis
- Fracture
- Impaired cognitive function
- Central spinal stenosis

Cervical Traction

Cervical traction can be applied with the patient in sitting or supine position, although the supine position is generally preferred because it removes the weight of the patient's head and allows the patient to relax more. With intermittent traction, a duty cycle of either 1:1 or 3:1 is used. The treatment time varies according to condition—5 to 10 minutes is recommended for acute conditions and disk protrusion; 15 to 20 minutes is recommended for other conditions.[104–106] Two methods of cervical traction can be used: the halter method or the use of a sliding device (Saunders) (Figure 7-7). The halter device should not be used with patients with TMJ dysfunction or with patients who suffer from claustrophobia.

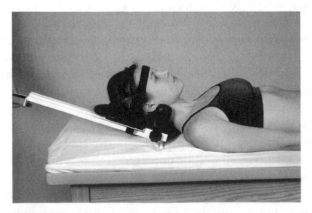

Figure 7-7 Saunders unit for cervical traction.

The traction force used is determined by the treatment goals and by patient tolerance.

Acute Phase
The recommended treatment for disk protrusions, muscle spasm, and elongation of soft tissue is approximately 10–15 pounds of pull initially, with progression up to 7 percent of the patient's body weight, as tolerated.[104–106] Joint distraction requires about 20–30 pounds of force.[104–106]

Halter Method
The head halter is placed under the occiput and the mandible and is then attached to the traction cord directly or to the traction unit through a spreader bar. Generally, a starting position of approximately 20 to 30 degrees of neck flexion is used (a pillow may be used).[104–106] The PT may decide to apply traction more specifically by varying the angle of neck flexion:[104–106]

- To increase the intervertebral space at the C1–C5 levels, approximately 0–5 degrees should be used.
- To increase the intervertebral space at the C5–C7 levels, 25–30 degrees of flexion is recommended.
- 15 degrees of flexion is recommended for zygapophysial joint separation.[107]
- 0 degrees of flexion is recommended for disk dysfunction.

Supine cervical traction has been found to be more efficacious than seated traction in the treatment of cervical spine disorders.[105] The clinician should ensure that the traction force is applied to the occipital region and not to the mandible.

Saunders Device
When using the Saunders device, the clinician places the patient's head on a padded headrest (refer to Figure 7-7) in 20 to 30 degrees of neck flexion. The clinician adjusts the neck yoke so that it fits firmly just below the mastoid processes. A head strap is typically used across the forehead to secure the head in place.

● **Key Point**   The total treatment times to be used in cervical traction are only partially research-based and can range from 5 minutes to 30 minutes.

Lumbar Traction

A split table or other mechanism to eliminate friction between body segments and the table surface is a prerequisite to effective lumbar traction. In addition, a nonslip traction harness is needed to transfer the traction force comfortably to the patient and to stabilize the trunk while the lumbar spine is placed under traction. The patient should be suitably disrobed because clothing between the harness and the skin will promote slipping.

Generally, the harness is applied when the patient is standing next to the traction table, although it can be applied with the patient lying down:

1. The pelvic harness is applied so that the contact pads and upper belt are at or just above the level of the iliac crest.
2. The contact pads are adjusted so that the harness loops provide the required direction of pull, encouraging either lumbar flexion or extension.
3. The rib belt is then applied in a similar manner with the rib pads positioned over the lower rib cage in a comfortable manner. The rib belt is then fitted snugly.

The patient is then asked to lie on the table. For disk protrusions (posterior or posterior lateral), the patient is positioned in the prone position with a normal to slightly flattened lumbar lordosis. For lateral spinal stenosis, the neutral spine position allows for the largest intervertebral foramen opening.

> ● **Key Point** In the supine position, the hip position can affect vertebral separation. As hip flexion increases from 0 to 90 degrees, the traction produces a greater posterior intervertebral and facet joint separation.

Overall, patient positioning should be determined by patient needs and comfort.

As per the PT's instruction, a continuous or intermittent mode is used. The total treatment times to be used in lumbar traction are only partially research-based and can range from 5 minutes to 20 minutes.[108–110] The force of the lumbar traction pull depends on the goals of treatment, and should be set with a force of less than half of the body weight for the initial treatment. Following the treatment session, the patient is re-examined and any changes in their symptoms are noted so the results can be used to determine the parameters for the next session, or whether traction should be discontinued.

Intermittent Mechanical Compression

There are three distinct kinds of tissue swelling that are associated with injury:

- *Joint swelling (effusion):* The presence of blood and joint fluid accumulated within the joint

capsule, which occurs immediately following injury to a joint.
- *Extra-articular edema:* The presence of blood and joint fluid outside of the joint capsule.
- *Lymphedema (also known as lymphatic obstruction):* This type of swelling in the subcutaneous tissues results from an excessive accumulation of lymph and usually occurs over several hours following injury.

Intermittent compression units are designed to keep venous and lymphatic flow from pooling in the interstitial spaces by applying a rhythmic external pressure. This type of external compression is designed to move lymph along and spread the intracellular edema over a larger area, enabling more lymph capillaries to become involved in removing the plasma proteins and water.[111] The most common treatments for lymphedema are a combination of the use of intermittent sequential gradient pumps, lymphatic massage, compression garments, and bandaging. Complex decongestive therapy uses an empiric system of lymphatic massage, skin care, and compressive garments.

Indications for intermittent compression include the following:

- Control of peripheral edema
- Shaping of residual limb following amputation
- Management of scar formation
- Improving lymphatic and venous return
- Prevention of deep vein thrombosis
- Prevention of stasis ulcers

Contraindications include:

- Malignancy of treated area
- Presence of deep vein thrombosis
- Obstructed lymphatic channel
- Unstable or acute fracture
- Heart failure
- Infection of treated area
- Pulmonary edema
- Kidney or cardiac insufficiency
- Patients who are very young, or elderly and frail

Method of Application

The patient is asked to remove all jewelry on the extremity. The clinician checks the patient's blood pressure, measures the extremity, and records the measurement in the patient's chart. The patient is draped appropriately and is placed in a comfortable position with the limb elevated approximately 45 degrees and abducted 20 to 70 degrees. Pretreatment girth measures are taken. A stockinette is placed over the extremity, ensuring that all wrinkles are removed. An appropriate-sized compression appliance is fitted on the extremity. The compression sleeves come as half-leg, full-leg, full-arm, or half-arm. The deflated compression sleeve is connected to the compression unit via a rubber hose and connecting valve.

Once the machine has been turned on, there are three parameters available for adjustment with most intermittent pressure devices:[111]

- *Inflation pressure:* Arterial capillary pressures are 30 mm Hg, so any pressure that exceeds this should encourage reabsorption of the edema and movement of lymph. However, more is not necessarily better. The maximum pressure should correspond to diastolic blood pressure (somewhere around the patient's diastolic blood pressure and based on patient comfort).
- *On-off sequence or inflation/deflation ratio:* This is usually set to approximately 3:1, but can be highly variable, with some protocols calling for a sequence of 30 seconds on, 30 seconds off; 1 minute on, 2 minutes off; and then 4 minutes on, 1 minute off. Patient comfort should be the primary deciding factor. As a general guideline, to reduce edema use 45–90 seconds on/15–30 seconds off.
- *Total treatment time:* This varies. Most of the protocols for primary lymphedema call for 3- to 4-hour treatments. Traumatic edema calls for 2 hours, and residual limb reduction usually receives 1- to 3-hour sessions; however, the average treatment for other conditions can be much shorter, lasting between 20 and 30 minutes.

The patient is issued with a call bell and should be monitored for comfort and blood pressure readings throughout the treatment. At the completion of the treatment, the unit is turned off and the stockinette and appliance removed. The extremity is then measured to see if the desired results have been achieved. If the edema is not reduced, another treatment may be needed after a short recovery time. The part should be wrapped with elastic compression wraps to help maintain the reduction. If not contraindicated, weight bearing should be encouraged to stimulate the venous pump.

CryoCuff and Cryopress

The AirCast CryoCuff combines the therapeutic benefits of controlled compression and cryotherapy to minimize hemarthrosis, edema hematoma, swelling, and pain. The cuff is anatomically designed to completely fit a number of different joints and body parts providing maximum cryotherapy. The cryo-press is a sequential cryocompression unit. Studies have shown that cold therapy and compression combined have a better effect than compression and cryotherapy alone.[6,112]

Summary

Electrotherapeutic modalities, physical agents, and mechanical modalities are best used as adjuncts to other forms of intervention. Decisions on how a particular modality may best be used are established by both theoretical knowledge and practical experience, and, for the PTA, are based on the plan of care. For example, electrical stimulating currents may be used to stimulate sensory nerves to modulate pain, stimulate motor nerves to elicit a muscle contraction, introduce chemical ions into superficial tissues for medicinal purposes, and create an electrical field in the tissues to stimulate or alter the healing process. Modalities used in the initial acute injury phase should be directed at reducing the amount of inflammation and swelling that occurs. During the later stages, the goal is to increase blood flow to the area and increase connective tissue extensibility and strength.

REVIEW Questions

1. In comparing the use of cold pack and hot pack treatments, which of the following statements is false?
   a. Cold packs penetrate more deeply than hot packs.
   b. Cold packs and hot packs can both cause skin burns.
   c. Cold decreases spasm by decreasing sensitivity to muscle spindles, and heat decreases spasm by decreasing nerve conduction velocity.
   d. None of the above.
2. As part of your weekly inspection, you test the temperature of the water in your hydrocollator to make sure it is appropriate to avoid a burn to the patient. What is the ideal temperature range?
3. What is the function of the transducer in an ultrasound machine?
   a. Changes ultrasound waves into heat
   b. Changes electricity into ultrasound waves

c. Changes ultrasound waves into sonic waves

d. Changes light waves into sound waves

4. Which of the following waves are not found on the electromagnetic spectrum, ultraviolet, infrared, or ultrasound?

5. What units are used to measure electrical current?

6. An example of the transmission of heat by conduction is:
   a. Ultrasound
   b. Hot pack
   c. Diathermy
   d. None of the above

7. Which of the following applies to positive ions?
   a. They are attracted to the anode.
   b. They are produced by ionization of acids.
   c. They arc attracted to the cathode.
   d. None of the above.

8. Which of the following tissues provides the best conductivity of electrical current?
   a. Skin
   b. Tendon
   c. Bone
   d. Muscle

9. The unit of power is represented by the:
   a. Ohm
   b. Volt
   c. Watt
   d. Ampere

10. Ultrasound waves cause the greatest rise in temperature in tissues with:
    a. Adipose tissue
    b. Cartilage
    c. Tendon
    d. Protein

11. Ultrasound has what theoretical effect on membrane permeability?
    a. Increases permeability
    b. Decreases permeability
    c. No change
    d. Alternating permeability

12. The minimal amount of current necessary to elicit a threshold contraction of muscle is:
    a. Chronaxie
    b. Rheobase
    c. Rheostat
    d. None of the above

13. In a strength-duration curve, the variable factor is:
    a. Rheobase
    b. Waveform

c. Both A and B

d. Neither A nor B

14. Local effects of a heat application include:
    a. Local analgesia
    b. Decreased blood flow in the area
    c. Decreased tissue metabolism
    d. None of the above

15. Local effects of cold applications include:
    a. Vasoconstriction
    b. Increased local circulation
    c. Increased leukocytic migration
    d. None of the above

16. You are treating a patient who demonstrates mild swelling on the dorsum of the hand and limited flexion of the metacarpophalangeal joints in all digits following an open reduction of a Colles' fracture 6 weeks ago. Which of the following would be the most appropriate heating agent to use?
    a. Hot pack
    b. Ultrasound
    c. Paraffin bath
    d. Massage

17. You are treating a patient with complaints of pain and muscle spasm in the cervical region. Past medical history reveals chronic heart disease and demand-type pacemaker. Which of the following modalities should you avoid in this case?
    a. Hot pack
    b. TENS
    c. Mechanical traction
    d. Ultrasound

18. You are performing an in-service on the use of electrical equipment in the physical therapy department. Which of the following safety precautions would you stress to increase safety to the patient and therapist?
    a. Never use an extension cord.
    b. Check all of the leads for fraying.
    c. When using a device close to water, check that it is fitted with a ground fault interrupter.
    d. All of the above should be stressed.

References

1. Bell GW, Prentice WE: Infrared modalities, in Prentice WE (ed): Therapeutic Modalities for Allied Health Professionals. New York, McGraw-Hill, 1998, pp 201–262
2. Johnson DJ, Moore S, Moore J, et al: Effect of cold submersion on intramuscular temperature of the gastrocnemius muscle. Phys Ther 59:1238–1242, 1979

3. Cobbold AF, Lewis OJ: Blood flow to the knee joint of the dog: Effect of heating, cooling and adrenaline. J Physiol 132:379–383, 1956

4. Wakim KG, Porter AN, Krusen FH: Influence of physical agents and certain drugs on intra-articular temperature. Arch Phys Med Rehab 32:714–721, 1951

5. Oosterveld FGJ, Rasker JJ, Jacobs JWG, et al: The effect of local heat and cold therapy on the intraarticular and skin surface temperature of the knee. Arthritis Rheum 35:146–151, 1992

6. Merrick MA, Knight KL, Ingersoll CD, et al: The effects of ice and compression wraps on intramuscular temperatures at various depths. J Athl Training 28:236–245, 1993

7. Abramson DI, Bell B, Tuck S: Changes in blood flow, oxygen uptake and tissue temperatures produced by therapeutic physical agents: Effect of indirect or reflex vasodilation. Am J Phys Med 40:5–13, 1961

8. Knight KL, Londeree BR: Comparison of blood flow in the ankle of uninjured subjects during therapeutic applications of heat, cold, and exercise. Med Sci Sports Exerc 12:76–80, 1980

9. Knight KL: Cryotherapy in Sports Injury Management. Champaign, IL, Human Kinetics, 1995

10. Knight KL: Cryotherapy: Theory, Technique, and Physiology. Chattanooga, TN, Chattanooga Corp, 1985

11. Pappenheimer SL, Eversole SL, Soto-Rivera A: Vascular responses to temperature in the isolated perfused hind-limb of a cat. Am J Physiol 155:458–451, 1948

12. Kalenak A, Medlar CE, Fleagle SB, et al: Athletic injuries: Heat vs cold. Am Fam Phys 12:131–134, 1975

13. McMaster WC, Liddle S, Waugh TR: Laboratory evaluation of various cold therapy modalities. Am J Sports Med 6:291–294, 1978

14. Daniel DM, Stone ML, Arendt DL: The effect of cold therapy on pain, swelling, and range of motion after anterior cruciate ligament reconstructive surgery. Arthroscopy 10:530–533, 1994

15. Konrath GA, Lock T, Goitz HT, et al: The use of cold therapy after anterior cruciate ligament reconstruction. A prospective randomized study and literature review. Am J Sports Med 24:629–633, 1996

16. Michlovitz SL: The use of heat and cold in the management of rheumatic diseases, in Michlovitz SL (ed): Thermal Agents in Rehabilitation. Philadelphia, FA Davis, 1990, pp 158–174

17. Speer KP, Warren RF, Horowitz L: The efficacy of cryotherapy in the postoperative shoulder. J Shoulder Elbow Surg 5:62–68, 1996

18. Hocutt JE, Jaffee R, Rylander R, et al: Cryotherapy in ankle sprains. Am J Sports Med 10:316–319, 1982

19. Kellett J: Acute soft tissue injuries: A review of the literature. Med Sci Sports Exerc 18:5, 1986

20. McMaster WC: A literary review on ice therapy in injuries. Am J Sports Med 5:124–126, 1977

21. Hartviksen K: Ice therapy in spasticity. Acta Neurol Scand 3:79-84, 1962 (suppl)

22. Basset SW, Lake BM: Use of cold applications in the management of spasticity. Phys Ther Rev 38:333–334, 1958

23. Starkey JA: Treatment of ankle sprains by simultaneous use of intermittent compression and ice packs. Am J Sports Med 4:142–143, 1976

24. Lamboni P, Harris B: The use of ice, air splints, and high voltage galvanic stimulation in effusion reduction. Athl Training 18:23–25, 1983

25. McMaster WC: Cryotherapy. Phys Sports Med 10:112–119, 1982

26. Waylonis GW: The physiological effects of ice massage. Arch Phys Med Rehab 48:42–47, 1967

27. Belitsky RB, Odam SJ, Hubley-Kozey C: Evaluation of the effectiveness of wet ice, dry ice, and cryogen packs in reducing skin temperature. Phys Ther 67:1080–1084, 1987

28. Zemke JE, Andersen JC, Guion WK, et al: Intramuscular temperature responses in the human leg to two forms of cryotherapy: Ice massage and ice bag. J Orthop Sports Phys Ther 27:301–307, 1998

29. Travell JG, Simons DG: Myofascial Pain and Dysfunction—The Trigger Point Manual. Baltimore, Williams & Wilkins, 1983

30. Feibel A, Fast A: Deep heating of joints: A reconsideration. Arch Phys Med Rehab 57, 513–514 1976

31. Cwynar DA, McNerney T: A primer on physical therapy. Lippincott's Prim Care Pract 3:451–459, 1999

32. Clark D, Stelmach G: Muscle fatigue and recovery curve parameters at various temperatures. Res Q 37:468–479, 1966

33. Baker R, Bell G: The effect of therapeutic modalities on blood flow in the human calf. J Orthop Sports Phys Ther 13:23, 1991

34. Knight KL, Aquino J, Johannes SM, et al: A re-examination of Lewis' cold induced vasodilation in the finger and ankle. Athl Training 15:248–250, 1980

35. Zankel H: Effect of physical agents on motor conduction velocity of the ulnar nerve. Arch Phys Med Rehab 47:197–199, 1994

36. Frizzell LA, Dunn F: Biophysics of ultrasound, in Lehman JF (ed): Therapeutic Heat and Cold (ed 3). Baltimore, Williams & Wilkins, 1982, pp 353–385

37. Lehman JF, Masock AJ, Warren CG, et al: Effect of therapeutic temperatures on tendon extensibility. Arch Phys Med Rehabil 51:481–487, 1970

38. Barcroft H, Edholm OS: The effect of temperature on blood flow and deep temperature in the human forearm. J Physiol 102:5–20, 1943

39. Griffin JG: Physiological effects of ultrasonic energy as it is used clinically. J Am Phys Ther Assoc 46:18, 1966

40. Abramson DI, Tuck S, Lee SW, et al: Comparison of wet and dry heat in raising temperature of tissues. Arch Phys Med Rehabil 48:654, 1967

41. Lehmann JF, Silverman DR, Baum BA, et al: Temperature distributions in the human thigh, produced by infrared, hot pack and microwave applications. Arch Phys Med Rehabil 47:291–299, 1966

42. Sandqvist G, Akesson A, Eklund M: Evaluation of paraffin bath treatment in patients with systemic sclerosis. Disabil Rehabil 26:981–987, 2004

43. Stimson CW, Rose GB, Nelson PA: Paraffin bath as thermotherapy: An evaluation. Arch Phys Med Rehabil 39:219–227, 1958

44. Draper DO, Prentice WE: Therapeutic ultrasound, in Prentice WE (ed): Therapeutic Modalities for Allied Health Professionals. New York, McGraw-Hill, 1998, pp 263–309

45. Benson HAE, McElnay JC: Transmission of ultrasound energy through topical pharmaceutical products. Physiotherapy 74:587–589, 1988

46. Cameron MH, Monroe LG: Relative transmission of ultrasound by media customarily used for phonophoresis. Phys Ther 72:142–148, 1992

47. Dyson M: Mechanisms involved in therapeutic ultrasound. Physiotherapy 73:116–120, 1987

48. Lehman JF, deLateur BJ, Stonebridge JB, et al: Therapeutic temperature distribution produced by ultrasound as modified by dosage and volume of tissue exposed. Arch Phys Med Rehabil 48:662–666, 1967

49. Lehman JF, deLateur BJ, Warren CG, et al: Heating of joint structures by ultrasound. Arch Phys Med Rehabil 49:28–30, 1968

50. Goldman DE, Heuter TF: Tabulator data on velocity and absorption of high frequency sound in mammalian tissues. J Acoust Soc Am 28:35, 1956

51. Dyson M, Pond JB: The effect of pulsed ultrasound on tissue regeneration. Physiotherapy 56:136, 1970

52. Dyson M, Suckling J: Stimulation of tissue repair by therapeutic ultrasound: A survey of the mechanisms involved. Physiotherapy 64:105–108, 1978

53. Antich TJ: Phonophoresis: The principles of the ultrasonic driving force and efficacy in treatment of common orthopedic diagnoses. J Orthop Sports Phys Ther 4:99–102, 1982

54. Bommannan D, Menon GK, Okuyama H, et al: Sonophoresis II: Examination of the mechanism(s) of ultrasound-enhanced transdermal drug delivery. Pharm Res 9:1043–1047, 1992

55. Bommannan D, Okuyama H, Stauffer P, et al: Sonophoresis. I: The use of high-frequency ultrasound to enhance transdermal drug delivery. Pharm Res 9:559–564, 1992

56. Byl NN: The use of ultrasound as an enhancer for transcutaneous drug delivery: Phonophoresis. Phys Ther 75:539–553, 1995

57. Byl NN, Mckenzie A, Haliday B, et al: The effects of phonophoresis with corticosteroids: A controlled pilot study. J Orthop Sports Phys Ther 18:590–600, 1993

58. Ciccone CD, Leggin BG, Callamaro JJ: Effects of ultrasound and trolamine salicylate phonophoresis on delayed onset muscle soreness. Phys Ther 71:39–51, 1991

59. Davick JP, Martin RK, Albright JP: Distribution and deposition of tritiated cortisol using phonophoresis. Phys Ther 68:1672–1675, 1988

60. Dinno MA, Crum LA, Wu J: The effect of therapeutic ultrasound on the electrophysiologic parameters of frog skin. Med Biol 25:461–470, 1989

61. Ter Haar GR, Stratford IJ: Evidence for a non-thermal effect of ultrasound. Br J Cancer 45:172–175, 1982

62. Schrepfer R: Aquatic exercise, in Kisner C, Colby LA (eds): Therapeutic Exercise. Foundations and Techniques (ed 5). Philadelphia, FA Davis, 2002, pp 273–293

63. Downey JA: Physiological effects of heat and cold. Phys Ther 44:713–717, 1964

64. Cox JS: The diagnosis and management of ankle ligament injuries in the athlete. Athl Training 18:192–196, 1982

65. Marino M: Principles of therapeutic modalities: Implications for sports medicine, in Nicholas JA, Hershman EB (eds): The Lower Extremity and Spine in Sports Medicine. St. Louis, MO, CV Mosby, 1986, pp 195–244

66. Martin G: Aquatic therapy in rehabilitation, in Prentice WE, Voight ML (eds): Techniques in Musculoskeletal Rehabilitation. New York, McGraw-Hill, 2001, pp 279–287

67. Thein-Brody L: Aquatic physical therapy, in Hall C, Thein-Brody L (eds): Therapeutic Exercise: Moving Toward Function (ed 2). Baltimore, MD, Lippincott Williams & Wilkins, 2005, pp 330–347

68. Harrison RA, Bulstrode S: Percentage weight bearing during partial immersion in the hydrotherapy pool. Physiother Practice 3:60–63, 1987

69. ADA: Americans with Disabilities Act of 1989: 101–336, 1989

70. Harrison RA, Hillma M, Bulstrode S: Loading of the lower limb when walking partially immersed: Implications for clinical practice. Physiotherapy 78:164–166, 1992

71. Pociask FD, Kahn J, Galloway K: Iontophoresis, ultrasound, and phonophoresis, in Placzek JD, Boyce DA (eds): Orthopaedic Physical Therapy Secrets. Philadelphia, Hanley & Belfus, 2001, pp 74–80

72. Scott O: Stimulative effects, in Kitchen S, Bazin S (eds): Clayton's Electrotherapy. London, WB Saunders, 1996, pp 61–80

73. Low J, Reed A: Electrotherapy Explained: Principles and Practice. Oxford, Butterworth-Heinemann, 2000

74. Delitto A, Rose SJ, McKowen JM, et al: Electrical stimulation versus voluntary exercise in strengthening thigh musculature after anterior cruciate ligament surgery. Phys Ther 68:660–663, 1988

75. Gotlin RS, Hershkowitz S, Juris PM, et al: Electrical stimulation effect on extensor lag and length of hospital stay after total knee arthroplasty. Arch Phys Med Rehab 75:957, 1994

76. Laughman RK, Youdas JW, Garrett TR, et al: Strength changes in the normal quadriceps femoris muscle as a result of electrical stimulation. Phys Ther 63:494–499, 1983

77. McMiken DF, Todd-Smith M, Thompson C: Strengthening of human quadriceps muscles by cutaneous electrical stimulation. Scand J Rehabil Med 15:25–28, 1983

78. Snyder-Mackler L, Delitto A, Bailey SL, et al: Strength of the quadriceps femoris muscle and functional recovery after reconstruction of the anterior cruciate ligament. A prospective, randomized clinical trial of electrical stimulation. J Bone Joint Surg 77:1166–1173, 1995

79. Gould N, Donnermeyer BS, Pope M, et al: Transcutaneous muscle stimulation as a method to retard disuse atrophy. Clin Orthop 164:215–220, 1982

80. Selkowitz DM: Improvement in isometric strength of quadriceps femoris muscle after training with electrical stimulation. Phys Ther 65:186–196, 1985

81. Currier DP, Mann R: Muscular strength development by electrical stimulation in healthy individuals. Phys Ther 63:915–921, 1983

82. Taylor K, Fish DR, Mendel FR, et al: Effect of a single 30 minute treatment of high voltage pulsed current on edema formation in frog hind limbs. Phys Ther 72:63–68, 1992

83. Gangarosa LP: Iontophoresis in Dental Practice. Chicago, Quintessence Publishing, 1982

84. Coy RE: Anthology of Craniomandibular Orthopedics. Seattle, International College of Craniomandibular Orthopedics, 1993

85. Burnette RR: Iontophoresis, in Hadgraft J, Guy RH (eds): Transdermal Drug Delivery: Developmental Issues and Research Initiatives. New York, Marcel Dekker, 1989, pp 247–291

86. Chien YW, Siddiqui O, Shi M, et al: Direct current iontophoretic transdermal delivery of peptide and protein drugs. J Pharm Sci 78:376–384, 1989

87. Grimnes S: Pathways of ionic flow through human skin in vivo. Acta Dermatol Venereol 64:93–98, 1984

88. Lee RD, White HS, Scott ER: Visualization of iontophoretic transport paths in cultured and animal skin models. J Pharm Sci 85:1186–1190, 1996

89. O'Malley E, Oester Y: Influence of some physical chemical factors on iontophoresis using radioisotopes. Arch Phys Med Rehabil 36:310–313, 1955

90. Zeltzer L, Regalado M, Nichter LS, et al: Iontophoresis versus subcutaneous injection: A comparison of two methods of local anesthesia delivery in children. Pain 44:73–78, 1991

91. Smith MJ: Electrical stimulation for the relief of musculoskeletal pain. Phys Sports Med 11:47–55, 1983

92. Magora F, Aladjemoff L, Tannenbaum J, et al: Treatment of pain by transcutaneous electrical stimulation. Acta Anaesthesiol Scand 22:589–592, 1978

93. Mannheimer JS, Lampe GN: Clinical Transcutaneous Electrical Nerve Stimulation. Philadelphia, FA Davis, 1984, pp 440–445

94. Woolf CF: Segmental afferent fiber-induced analgesia: Transcutaneous electrical nerve stimulation (TENS) and vibration, in Wall PD, Melzack R (eds): Textbook of Pain. New York, Churchill Livingstone, 1989, pp 884–896

95. Smith MJ, Hutchins RC, Hehenberger D: Transcutaneous neural stimulation use in post-operative knee rehabilitation. Am J Sports Med 11:75–82, 1983

96. Long DM: Fifteen years of transcutaneous electrical stimulation for pain control. Stereotact Funct Neurosurg 56:2–19, 1991

97. Fried T, Johnson R, McCracken W: Transcutaneous electrical nerve stimulation: Its role in the control of chronic pain. Arch Phys Med Rehabil 65:228–31, 1984

98. Eriksson MBE, Sjölund BH, Nielzen S: Long-term results of peripheral conditioning stimulation as an analgesic measure in chronic pain. Pain 6:335–347, 1979

99. Fishbain DA, Chabal C, Abbott A, et al: Transcutaneous electrical nerve stimulation (TENS) treatment outcome in long term users. Clin J Pain 12:201–214, 1996

100. Ishimaru K, Kawakita K, Sakita M: Analgesic effects induced by TENS and electroacupuncture with different types of stimulating electrodes on deep tissues in human subjects. Pain 63:181–187, 1995

101. Eriksson MBE, Sjölund BH, Sundbärg G: Pain relief from peripheral conditioning stimulation in patients with chronic facial pain. J Neurosurg 61:149–155, 1984

102. Murphy GJ: Utilization of transcutaneous electrical nerve stimulation in managing craniofacial pain. Clin J Pain 6:64–69, 1990

103. Hooker DN: Electrical stimulating currents, in Prentice WE (ed): Therapeutic Modalities for Allied Health Professionals. New York, McGraw-Hill, 1998, pp 73–133

104. Colachis SC, Strohm BR: Cervical traction: Relationship of traction time to varied tractive force with constant angle of pull. Arch Phys Med Rehabil 46:815–819, 1965

105. Deets D, Hands KL, Hopp SS: Cervical traction: A comparison of sitting and supine positions. Phys Ther 57:255–261, 1977

106. Harris PR: Cervical traction: Review of literature and treatment guidelines. Phys Ther 57:910–914, 1977

107. Wong AMK, Leong CP, Chen C: The traction angle and cervical intervertebral separation. Spine 17:136–138, 1992

108. Austin R: Lumbar traction a valid option. Aust J Physiother 44:280, 1998

109. Lee RY, Evans JH: Loads in the lumbar spine during traction therapy. Aust J Physiother 47:102–108, 2001

110. Pellecchia GL: Lumbar traction: A review of the literature. J Orthop Sports Phys Ther 20:262–267, 1994

111. Hooker DN: Intermittent compression devices, in Prentice WE (ed): Therapeutic Modalities for Allied Health Professionals. New York, McGraw-Hill, 1998, pp 392–407

112. Aduayom I, Campbell PG, Denizeau F, et al: Different transport mechanisms for cadmium and mercury in Caco-2 cells: Inhibition of Cd uptake by Hg without evidence for reciprocal effects. Toxicol Appl Pharmacol 189:56–67, 2003

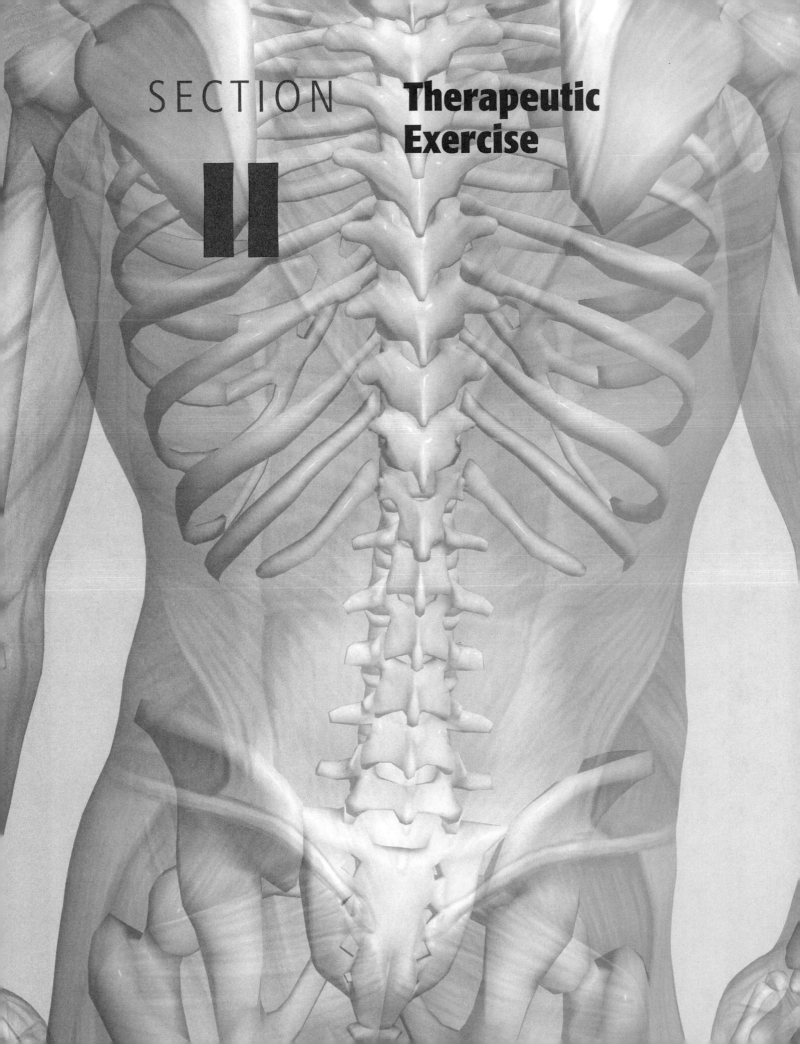

SECTION **II**

Therapeutic Exercise

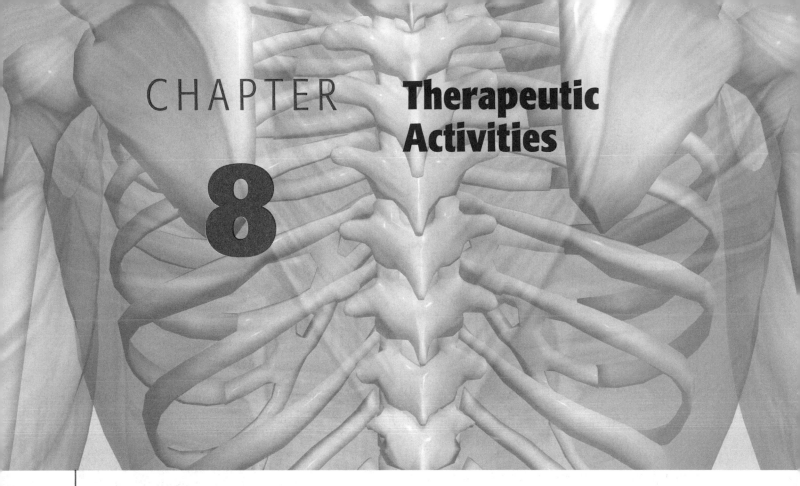

CHAPTER 8 Therapeutic Activities

Chapter Objectives

At the completion of this chapter, the reader will be able to:

1. Describe the most common therapeutic activities used in orthopaedics.
2. Outline how the body creates energy.
3. List some of the methods of measuring energy expenditure.
4. Calculate a person's body mass index (BMI).
5. Describe the concept and importance of specificity of training.

Overview

Therapeutic exercise is the foundation of physical therapy and a fundamental component of the vast majority of interventions. An understanding of how therapeutic exercise can be used to restore, maintain, and improve a patient's functional status by increasing strength, endurance, and flexibility is essential for the PTA. To accomplish this, the PTA must be able to integrate and apply knowledge of anatomy, physiology, kinesiology, pathology, and the behavioral sciences. In addition, the PTA must know and be able to apply principles of motor learning and motor skill acquisition. When prescribed correctly, therapeutic exercise enables the patient/client to:

- Remediate or reduce impairments
- Enhance function
- Optimize overall health
- Enhance fitness and well-being

Exercise Physiology

Exercise physiology is the study of the acute and chronic adaptations of the body in response to a wide-range of physical exercise conditions. Muscles are metabolically active and must generate energy to move. The creation of energy occurs initially from the breakdown of certain nutrients from foodstuffs. The energy required for exercise is stored in a compound called adenosine triphosphate (ATP). ATP is produced in the muscle tissue from blood glucose or glycogen. Fats and proteins can also be metabolized to generate ATP. Glucose not needed immediately is stored as glycogen in the resting muscle and liver. Stored glycogen can later be converted back to glucose and transferred to the blood to meet the body's energy needs. If the duration or intensity of the exercise increases, the body relies more heavily on fat stored in adipose tissue to meet its energy needs. During rest and submaximal exertion, both fat and carbohydrates are used to provide energy in approximately a 60 to 40 percent ratio.

During physical exercise, energy turnover in skeletal muscle can increase by 400 times compared with muscle at rest, and muscle oxygen consumption can increase by more than 100 times.[1] The energy required to power muscular activity is derived from the hydrolysis of ATP to ADP (adenosine diphosphate) and inorganic phosphate (P_i). Despite the large fluctuations in energy demand just mentioned, muscle ATP remains practically constant and demonstrates a remarkable precision of the system in adjusting the rate of the ATP generating processes to the demand.[2] There are three energy systems that contribute to the resynthesis of ATP via ADP rephosphorylation. The relative contribution of these energy systems to ATP resynthesis has been shown to depend upon the intensity and duration of exercise.[3] It is worth noting that at no time during either rest or exercise does any single energy system provide the complete supply of energy. The three energy systems are as follows:

- *Phosphagen system:* The phosphagen system is an anaerobic process; that is, it can proceed without oxygen (O_2). Skeletal muscle cells contain phosphocreatine (PCr), and therefore, at the onset of muscular contraction, PCr represents the most immediate reserve for the rephosphorylation of ATP. The phosphagen system provides ATP primarily for short-term, high-intensity activities (e.g., sprinting) and is active at the start of all exercises regardless of intensity.[4] One disadvantage of the phosphagen system is that because of its significant contribution to the energy yield at the onset of near maximal exercise, the concentration of PCr can be reduced to less than 40 percent of resting levels within 10 seconds of the start of intense exercise.[5]

- *Glycolysis system:* The glycolysis system is an anaerobic process that involves the breakdown of carbohydrates—either glycogen stored in the muscle or glucose delivered in the blood—to produce ATP. Because this system relies upon a series of nine different chemical reactions, it is slower to become fully active than the phosphogen system. However, glycolysis has a greater capacity to provide energy than does PCr, and therefore it supplements PCr during maximal exercise and continues to rephosphorylate ADP during maximal exercise after PCr reserves have become essentially depleted.[4] The process of glycolysis can go one of two ways, termed fast glycolysis and slow glycolysis, depending on the energy demands within the cell. If energy must be supplied at a high rate, fast glycolysis is used primarily. If the energy demand is not as high, slow glycolysis is activated. The main disadvantage of the fast glycolysis system is that during very high-intensity exercise, hydrogen ions dissociate from the glycogenolytic end product of lactic acid.[2] An increase in hydrogen ion concentration is believed to inhibit glycotic reactions and directly interfere with muscle excitation-contraction and coupling, which can potentially impair contractile force during exercise.[4]

- *Oxidative system:* As its name suggests, the oxidative system requires O_2 and is consequently termed the *aerobic system*. The oxidative system is the primary source of ATP at rest and during low-intensity activities. Although unable to produce ATP at an equivalent rate to that produced by PCr breakdown and glycolysis, the oxidative system is capable of sustaining low-intensity exercise for several hours.[4] However, because of an increased complexity, the time between the onset of exercise and when this system is operating at its full potential is around 45 seconds.[6]

Measures of Energy Expenditure

The energy value of the food we eat can be quantified in terms of the calorie. A kilocalorie (kcal) is the amount of heat necessary to raise 1.0 kg of water by 1.0°C. A metabolic equivalent unit, or MET, is defined as the energy expenditure required for sitting quietly, talking on the phone, or reading a book; for the average adult this is approximately 3.5 milliliters of oxygen uptake per kilogram of body weight per minute (3.5 mL O_2/kg/min)—1.2 kcal/min for a 70-kg (154-pound) individual. METs are defined as multiples of resting energy metabolism. For example, a 2-MET activity requires two times the metabolic energy expenditure of sitting quietly. The harder the body works during the activity, the higher the MET (**Table 8-1**). Any activity that burns 3 to 6 METs is considered moderate-intensity physical activity. Any activity that burns more than 6 METs is considered vigorous-intensity physical activity.

Basal Metabolic Rate (BMR)

The basal metabolic rate (BMR), the sum total of cellular activity in all metabolically active tissues while under basal conditions, is the minimum amount of oxygen utilized in order to support life. A person's BMR varies according to overall body size, gender, age, fat-free mass, and endocrine function. In general, the BMR tends to be 5 to 10 percent lower in women than in men. There is a decline in BMR of 2 to 3 percent per decade of life, which is most likely due to the reduction in physical activity associated with aging.

TABLE 8-1	Metabolic Equivalents for Various Activities
Activity	**MET Level**
Mowing the lawn	6–7
Shoveling snow	6–7
Swimming	4–8
Walking (4 mph)	4.5–5.5
Dancing	4–5
Showering	3.5–4
Light gardening	3–4
Light housework	2–4
Cooking	2–3
Bathing	2–3
Walking (2 mph)	2–2.5
Dressing	2
Driving a car	1–2
Eating	1

Body Mass Index (BMI)

Body mass index (BMI) is a measure of body fat based on height and weight. Body fat can be divided into two types:

- *Essential fat:* Necessary for normal physiological function, serving as a source of energy and a storage site for some vitamins
- *Storage fat:* Stored in adipose tissue

Separate calculations are used for boys and girls ages 2–20 and for adult men and women. Further subdivisions can be made according to gender for adults.

The limitations of relying on the BMI include:

- It may overestimate body fat in athletes and others who have a muscular build.
- It may underestimate body fat in older persons and others who have lost muscle mass.

TABLE 8-2 Rating of Perceived Exertion

Traditional Scale	Verbal Rating	Revised 10-Grade Scale	Verbal Rating
6		0	Nothing at all
7	Very, very light	0.5	Very, very weak
8		1.0	Very weak
9	Very light	2.0	Weak (light)
10		3.0	Moderate
11	Fairly light	4.0	Somewhat strong
12		5.0	Strong (heavy)
13	Somewhat hard	6.0	
14		7.0	Very strong
15	Hard	8.0	
16		9.0	
17	Very hard	10.0	Very, very strong (almost maximum)
18			
19	Very, very hard		Maximal

Adapted from Borg GAV: Psychophysical basis of perceived exertion. Med Sci Sports Exerc 14:377–381, 1992

Two methods can be used to calculate BMI:

- BMI (kg/m^2) = weight in kilograms/height in meters^2
- BMI (lbs/inches^2) = (weight in pounds × 703)/ height in inches^2

> **● Key Point** The categories of BMI are as follows:
> - Underweight = < 18.5
> - Normal weight = 18.5–24.9
> - Overweight = 25–29.9
> - Obese = 30 or greater
>
> The standard margin of error when estimating percentage of body fat with the BMI is approximately 5 percent.

Bioelectrical Impedance Analysis

Bioelectrical impedance analysis (BIA) measures body composition by sending a low, safe electrical current through the body fluids contained mainly in the lean and fat tissue. BIA measures the impedance or opposition to the flow of this electric current.

- Impedance is low in lean tissue, where intracellular fluid and electrolytes are primarily contained.
- Impedance is high in fat tissue.

Impedance is thus proportional to total body water volume (TBW). Prediction equations, previously generated by correlating impedance measures against an independent estimate of TBW, may be used subsequently to convert the measured impedance to a corresponding estimate of TBW. Lean body mass is then calculated from this estimate using an assumed hydration fraction for lean tissue. Fat mass is calculated as the difference between body weight and lean body mass.

> **● Key Point** BIA values are affected by numerous variables including body position, hydration status, recent consumption of food and beverages, ambient air and skin temperature, recent physical activity, and conductance of the examining table. Reliable BIA requires standardization and control of these variables.

Motor Learning

Motor learning is a complex set of internal processes that involve the relatively permanent acquisition and retention of a skilled movement or task through practice.[9-11] Motor learning involves the following:

- *Performance:* Acquisition of a skill
- *Learning:* Both acquisition and retention of a skill

- *Motor task:* There are three basic types of motor tasks:[12,13]
  - ❑ *Discrete:* A movement with a recognizable beginning and end; for example, throwing a ball or opening a door
  - ❑ *Serial:* A series of discrete movements that are combined in a particular sequence; for example, getting out of a chair when using crutches
  - ❑ *Continuous:* Repetitive, uninterrupted movements that have no distinct beginning and ending; for example, walking and cycling
- *Action*: The observable outcome resulting from the performer's purposeful interaction with the environment
- *Movement*: The means by which action is realized
- *Neuromotor processes*: The organizational mechanisms within the central nervous system (CNS) that constrain and sequence movement

A number of theories of skill acquisition have been proposed, including open versus closed skills and Gentile's taxonomy.

Open Versus Closed Skills

Open skills are temporal and spatial factors in an unpredictable environment. Closed skills are spatial factors only in a predictable environment. Both involve a single dimensional continuum. Using sports as an example, a closed skill could include shooting a foul shot in basketball. An example of an open skill would be playing a through ball in soccer. Open and closed skills can be viewed as a continuum, where the perceptual and habitual nature of a task determines whether the task is open or closed.

Gentile's Taxonomy of Motor Tasks

Gentile's taxonomy[14] is a two-dimensional classification system for teaching motor skills. Using the concept that motor skills range from simple to complex, Gentile expanded the popular one-dimensional classification system of open and closed skills to combine the environmental context with the function of the action.[13,15] The taxonomy consists of the following:

- *The environmental (closed or open) context in which the task is performed:* Regulatory conditions (other people, objects) in the environment may be either stationary (closed skills) or in motion (open skills).

- *The intertrial variability (absent or present) of the environment that is imposed on the task:* When the environment in which a task is set is unchanging from one performance of a task to the next, intertrial variability is absent—the environmental conditions are predictable. An example is walking on just one type of surface. Intertrial variability is present when the demands change from one attempt or repetition of the task to the next; for example, walking over varying terrain.
- *The need for a person's body to remain stationary (stable) or to move (transport) during the task:* Skills that require body transport are more complex than skills that require no body transport because there are more variables to consider. For example, a body transport task could include walking in a crowded shopping mall.
- *The presence or absence of manipulation of objects during the task:* When a person must manipulate an object, the skill increases in complexity because the person must do two things at once—manipulate the object correctly and adjust the body posture to fit the efficient movement of the object.

Table 8-3 illustrates Gentile's taxonomy of tasks. 1A represents the simplest task, and 4D represents the most complex task.

Stages of Motor Learning

There are three stages of motor learning:[15]

- *Cognitive:* This stage begins when the patient is first introduced to the motor task. The patient must determine the objective of the skill as well as the relational and environmental cues to control and regulate the movement. The patient is more concerned with what to do and how to do it. During this phase, the PTA should provide frequent and explicit positive feedback using a variety of forms of feedback (verbal, tactile, visual), and allow trial and error to occur within safe limits.
- *Associative:* The patient is concerned with performing and refining the skills. The important stimuli have been identified and their meaning is known. Conscious decisions about what to do become more automatic and the patient concentrates more on the task and appears less rushed. During this phase, the PTA should begin to increase the complexity of the task, emphasize problem-solving, avoid manual guidance, and vary the sequence of tasks.

TABLE
8-3

TABLE 8-3 Gentile's Taxonomy

Environmental Context		Body Stability		Body Transport	
		No Object Manipulation	Object Manipulation	No Object Manipulation	Object Manipulation
Stationary regulatory conditions	No intertrial variability	1A	1B	1C	1D
	Intertrial variability	2A	2B	2C	2D
In-motion regulatory conditions	No intertrial variability	3A	3B	3C	3D
	Intertrial variability	4A	4B	4C	4D

■ *Autonomous:* This stage is characterized by a nearly automatic kind of performance; for example, when walking occurs automatically without conscious thought. During this phase, the PTA should set up a series of progressively more difficult activities the patient can do independently, such as increasing the speed, distance, and complexity of the task.

Practice and Feedback

Practice—repeatedly performing a movement or series of movements in a task—is probably the single most important variable in learning a motor skill.[13,15] The various types of practice for motor learning are outlined in **Table 8-4**. Second only to practice, feedback is considered the next most important variable that influences learning. The various types of

TABLE 8-4 Types of Practice for Motor Learning

Type of Practice	Components	Description
Part versus whole	Part	A task is broken down into separate components and the individual components (usually the more difficult) are practiced. After mastery of the individual components, the components are combined in a sequence so the whole task can be practiced.
	Whole	The entire task is performed from beginning to end and is not practiced in separate components.
Blocked, random, and random-blocked	Blocked	The same task or series of tasks is performed repeatedly under the same conditions and in a predictable order; for example, consistently practicing walking in the same environment.
	Random	Slight variations of the same task are carried out in an unpredictable order; for example, a patient could practice on a variety of walking surfaces.
	Random-blocked	Variations of the same task are performed in random order, but each variation of the task is performed more than once; for example, the patient walks on a particular surface and then repeats the same task a second time before moving on to a different surface.
Physical versus mental	Physical	The movements of a task are actually performed.
	Mental (visualization, imagery)	A cognitive rehearsal of how a motor task is to be performed occurs prior to actually doing the task.

Data from Kisner C, Colby LA: Therapeutic exercise: Foundational concepts, in Kisner C, Colby LA (eds): Therapeutic Exercise: Foundations and Techniques (ed 5). Philadelphia, FA Davis, 2002, pp 1–36

TABLE 8-5	Types of Feedback Associated with Motor Learning

Type of Feedback	Description
Intermittent versus continuous	*Intermittent:* Occurs irregularly, randomly. Has been shown to promote learning more effectively than continuous feedback. *Continuous:* Is ongoing. Improves skill acquisition more quickly during the initial stage of learning and intermittent feedback.
Immediate, delayed, and summary	*Immediate:* Is given directly after a task is completed. Used most frequently during the cognitive (initial) stage of learning. *Delayed:* Is given after an interval of time elapses, allowing the learner to reflect on how well or poorly a task was done. Promotes retention and generalizability of the learned skills. *Summary:* Is given about the average performance of several repetitions of the movement or task. Used most frequently during the associative stage of learning.
Knowledge of performance (KP) versus knowledge of results (KR)	*KP:* Can be either intrinsic feedback sense during a task or immediate, post-task, extrinsic feedback (usually verbal) about the nature or quality of the performance of the motor task. *KR:* Immediate, post-task, extrinsic feedback about the outcome of the motor task.
Intrinsic	A sensory cue (proprioceptive, kinesthetic, tactile, visual, or auditory), or set of cues, inherent in the execution of the motor task that arises from within the learner and is derived from performance of the task. May immediately follow completion of a task or may occur even before a task has been completed.
Extrinsic (augmented)	Sensory cues from an external source (mechanical or from another person) that are supplemental to the intrinsic feedback but are not inherent in the execution of the task. Unlike intrinsic feedback, the clinician can control the type, timing, and frequency of extrinsic feedback.

Data from Kisner C, Colby LA: Therapeutic exercise: Foundational concepts, in Kisner C, Colby LA (eds): Therapeutic Exercise: Foundations and Techniques (ed 5). Philadelphia, FA Davis, 2002, pp 1–36

feedback associated with motor learning are outlined in **Table 8-5**.

Therapeutic Exercise

A number of key terms are used when describing therapeutic exercise. They include flexibility, joint mobility, muscle performance, balance, coordination, neuromuscular control, postural control/stability/equilibrium, and joint stability.[13]

Flexibility and Joint Mobility

Joint flexibility is defined as the range of motion (ROM) allowed at a joint. Optimal flexibility is based on physiologic, anatomic, and biomechanical considerations. As outlined in Chapter 4, the range of motion about a joint involves two major types of movements:

1. *Osteokinematic:* Involves the motion of a bone around a fixed point and is measured using a goniometer

2. *Arthrokinematic:* Involves the motion that occurs at the joint surfaces and is measured by the PT using techniques to assess joint mobility

Once the supervising PT determines whether the loss of range of motion is due to an arthrokinematic or an osteokinematic cause, the intervention is designed accordingly.

Static Flexibility

Static flexibility is the passive ROM available to a joint or series of joints.[16,17] Increased static flexibility should not be confused with joint hypermobility (see Chapter 4), or laxity, which is a function of the joint capsule and ligaments. Decreased static flexibility indicates a loss of motion. The end feel encountered may help differentiate between adaptive shortening of the muscle (muscle stretch) versus a tight joint capsule (capsular) or arthritic joint (hard). Static flexibility can be measured by a goniometer or by a number of tests, such as the toe touch and the sit and reach, all of which have been found to be valid and reliable.[18,19]

Dynamic Flexibility

Dynamic flexibility refers to the ease of movement within the obtainable ROM. Dynamic flexibility is measured actively. The important measurement in dynamic flexibility is stiffness, a mechanical term defined as the change in tension per unit change in length (see Chapter 4).[20,21] When passive motion of the joint is assessed, all of the tissues crossing the joint, including ligaments and the joint capsule, contribute to the resistance, which can be referred to as joint stiffness. Therefore, an increase in ROM around a joint does not necessarily equate to a decrease in the passive stiffness of a muscle.[22–24] However, strength training, immobilization, and aging have been shown to increase stiffness.[25–28] The converse of stiffness is pliability. When a soft tissue demonstrates a decrease in pliability, it has usually undergone an adaptive shortening, or an increase in tone, termed *hypertonus*.

Muscle Performance

Muscle performance includes the components of strength, endurance, and power (see Chapter 10).

- *Strength:* The maximum force that a muscle can develop during a single contraction. Muscular strength is derived both from the amount of tension a muscle can generate and from the moment arms of contributing muscles with respect to the joint center. Both sources can be affected by several factors (see Chapter 4).
- *Endurance:* The ability of a muscle to sustain or perform repetitive muscular contractions for an extended period. Cardiopulmonary endurance, sometimes referred to as total body endurance, refers to the ability to perform repetitive activities such as walking, cycling, and swimming, which involve use of the large muscles of the body. The ability to perform these activities is based on the patient's aerobic capacity.
- *Power:* The rate of performing work. Work is the magnitude of force acting on an object multiplied by the distance through which the force acts. Muscular power is the product of muscular force and velocity of muscle shortening.

> **● Key Point** Muscular power is an important contributor to activities requiring both speed and strength. Maximum power occurs at approximately one-third of maximum velocity.[29] Individuals with a predominance of fast twitch fibers (see Chapter 2) generate more power at a given load than those with a high composition of slow twitch fibers.[30] The ratio for mean peak power production by type II B, type II A, and type I fibers in skeletal tissue is 10:5:1.[31]

To what extent each of these three components is altered by exercise depends on how the principles of resistance training are applied and how factors such as the intensity, frequency, and duration of exercise are manipulated.[32] The promotion and progression of tissue repair during healing involves a delicate balance between protection and the application of controlled functional stresses to the damaged structure. The goal of therapeutic exercises is to increase strength, power, and endurance, but the exercises must only be done in ranges that elicit no symptoms, with the long-term goal of enhanced performance through full, pain-free ranges. Patients must be advised to let pain be their guide and that pain-free range of motion activities must be continued to prevent loss of function.

> **● Key Point** The dosage of an exercise refers to:
> - *Intensity:* How much effort is required to perform the exercise.
> - *Duration:* The length of the exercise session or the total number of weeks or months during which a resistance exercise program is carried out.
> - *Rest interval:* To improve muscle performance there must be an appropriate balance of progressive loading and adequate rest intervals. In general, the higher the intensity of exercise, the longer the rest interval.
> - *Frequency:* How often the exercise is performed per day or per week. The optimal frequency has not been determined.
> - *Intensity and duration are inversely proportional:* The higher the intensity, the shorter the duration. Frequency of activity is dependent upon intensity and duration; the lower the intensity, the shorter the duration, the greater the frequency.

All exercise progressions for strength, power, or endurance should include the following:[33]

- *Variation:* Variation to the exercises can be provided by altering:
  - ❑ Plane of motion
  - ❑ Range of motion
  - ❑ Body position
  - ❑ Exercise duration
  - ❑ Exercise frequency
- *A safe progression:* A safe progression is ensured if the exercises are progressed from:
  - ❑ Slow to fast
  - ❑ Simple to complex
  - ❑ Stable to unstable
  - ❑ Low force to high force

Exercise Principles

There are three exercise principles worth mentioning:

- *SAID principle:* The specific adaptation to imposed demand (SAID) principle acknowledges that the human body responds to explicit demands placed upon it with a specific and predictable adaptation. Therefore, the focus of the exercise prescription should be to improve the strength and coordination of functional or sports-specific movements with strengthening and flexibility exercises that approximate the desired activity in terms of its frequency, intensity, and duration.

- *Overload principle:* The principle of overload states that a greater than normal stress or load on the body is required for training adaptation to take place. To increase strength, the muscle must be challenged at a greater level than it is accustomed to. High levels of tension will produce adaptations in the form of hypertrophy and recruitment of more muscle fibers.
- *Reversibility principle:* Any adaptive changes in the body systems, such as increased strength or endurance, in response to a resistance exercise program are temporary unless training-induced improvements are regularly used through functional activities or resistance exercises.[34] These changes can begin within a week or two after the cessation of resistance exercises and will continue until the training effects are lost.[32,35]

Exercise Progression

A number of guidelines can be used to help the clinician in the progression of therapeutic exercise:[36]

- The degree of irritability can be determined by inquiring about the vigor, duration, and intensity of the pain. Greater irritability is associated with very acutely inflamed conditions. The characteristic sign for an acute inflammation is pain at rest that is diffuse in its distribution and often referred from the site of the primary condition, and an empty end feel (see Chapter 5).[37] Chronic conditions usually have low irritability but have an associated loss of active and passive ROM.

> ● **Key Point** If pain is reported by the patient before a resistive activity or before the end feel during passive range of motion, the patient's symptoms are considered irritable. The intervention in the presence of irritability should not be aggressive.[38] If pain occurs after resistance, then the patient's symptoms are not considered irritable and exercise, particularly stretching, can be more aggressive.

- The patient should be taught initially to exercise in cardinal planes before progressing as quickly as allowed to exercising in the functional planes.

- The exercise protocol should initiate with exercises that utilize a short lever arm. These exercises decrease the amount of torque at the joint. Extremity exercises can be adapted to include short levers by flexing the extremity, by exercising with the extremity closer to the body, or if resistance is included, to shorten the lever arm.
- The goal should be to achieve the close packed position at the earliest opportunity. The close packed position of a joint is its position of maximum stability. It also is the position of maximum ligamentous and capsular tautness, so care needs to be taken in achieving this position.
- As the rehabilitation progresses, the prescribed exercises should reproduce the forces and loading rates that will approach the patient's functional demands.

Balance

Balance, or postural stability/equilibrium, involves synchronization among the neurologic system (mechanoreceptor feedback system), the musculoskeletal system, and contextual effects (environment, support surface, lighting, effects of gravity, and task characteristics) in order to maintain a stable weight-bearing and anti-gravity position, or to hold/control a proximal or distal body segment in a stationary position during superimposed movement.[13] In order for balance to be effective, an individual must be able to maintain his or her center of gravity (COG), which is located just above the pelvis, within the body's base of support. Two types of balance are recognized: static and dynamic. Balance and balance training are discussed in Chapter 11.

Coordination

Taber's Cyclopedic Medical Dictionary defines coordination as "the working together of various muscles for the production of a certain movement." Coordination involves an intricate and complex sequence of activities. There are three main stages in coordination refinement:

- *Crude coordination:* Heavy reliance on visual and auditory input systems
- *Fine coordination:* More reliance on proprioceptors and dynamic and static joint receptors
- *Superfine coordination:* The final stage of motor learning that allows the effective execution of the desired movement under a variety of conditions

Coordination demands vary from individual to individual—from the world-class athlete to the patient recovering from a stroke. Thus, the type and focus of the coordination training depends on the presenting condition.

Neuromuscular Control

Neuromuscular control involves the interaction of the sensory and motor systems, which interpret proprioceptive and kinesthetic information to create coordinated movement (see Chapter 3).

Joint Stability

Instability implies that a person has increased joint range of motion but does not have the ability to stabilize and control movement of that joint. Stabilization exercises are dynamic activities that attempt to limit and control any excessive movement (see Chapter 10).

Patient Safety

Many factors can have an impact on patient safety during therapeutic exercise. These include, but are not limited to, the following:[13]

- *The patient's health history and current health status:* Medical clearance is indicated before beginning an exercise program.
- *Medication side effects:* Many medications can adversely affect a patient's cardiopulmonary response to exercise, in addition to having a negative impact on balance and coordination.
- *The environment in which exercises are performed:* Sufficient space, adequate lighting, and safe equipment are minimal requirements.
- *The ability to perform the correct technique at the appropriate intensity, speed, and duration:* Correct technique is important to avoid injury and to focus the exercises on the specific body part. Modifying the intensity, speed, and duration allows the clinician to increase strength, power, or endurance.
- *Ensuring the patient recognizes the instances when they are exercising too aggressively or which signs and symptoms warrant them contacting the PTA or physician (signs and symptoms of infection, severe pain):* The typical signs of overexercising include continued achiness or pain in the muscles and/or joints, fatigue, insomnia, elevated morning pulse rate, headaches, loss of appetite, and increased susceptibility to infections.

Summary

Therapeutic activities are an essential component of the rehabilitation process. When used judiciously, and when designed with specific goals in mind, therapeutic activities can improve overall function by increasing flexibility, joint mobility, and muscle performance. A number of exercise principles and methods of exercise progression must be utilized to ensure patient safety and maximum benefit.

REVIEW **Questions**

1. Name the two energy systems that can be used during anaerobic activity.
2. The energy required for exercise is stored in which compound?
3. What is a metabolic equivalent unit (MET)?
4. What are the two types of fat found in the body?
5. What is considered to be a normal range body mass index score range?
6. Which is the more difficult for a patient to learn—an open skill or a closed skill?
7. What are the two types of flexibility addressed by physical therapy?
8. True or false: Exercises using a long lever arm should be introduced before exercises using a short lever arm.

References

1. Tonkonogi M, Sahlin K: Physical exercise and mitochondrial function in human skeletal muscle. Exerc Sport Sci Rev 30:129–137, 2002
2. Sahlin K, Tonkonogi M, Soderlund K: Energy supply and muscle fatigue in humans. Acta Physiol Scand 162:261–266, 1998
3. Sahlin K, Ren JM: Relationship of contraction capacity to metabolic changes during recovery from a fatiguing contraction. J Appl Physiol 67:648–654, 1989
4. McMahon S, Jenkins D: Factors affecting the rate of phosphocreatine resynthesis following intense exercise. Sports Med 32:761–784, 2002
5. Walter G, Vandenborne K, McCully KK, et al: Noninvasive measurement of phosphocreatine recovery kinetics in single human muscles. Am J Physiol 272:C525–C534, 1997
6. Bangsbo J: Muscle oxygen uptake in humans at onset and during intense exercise. Acta Physiol Scand 168:457–464, 2000
7. Borg GAV: Psychophysical basis of perceived exertion. Med Sci Sports Exerc 14:377–381, 1992
8. Borg GAV: Perceived exertion as an indicator of somatic stress. Scand J Rehabil Med 2:92–98, 1970

9. Winstein CJ, Knecht HG: Movement science and its relevance to physical therapy. Phys Ther 70:759–762, 1990

10. Winstein CJ: Knowledge of results and motor learning—implications for physical therapy. Phys Ther 71:140–149, 1991

11. Winstein CJ: Motor learning considerations in stroke rehabilitation, in Duncan PW, Badke MB (eds): Stroke Rehabilitation: The Recovery of Motor Control. Chicago, Yearbook Medical Publishers, 1987, pp 109–134

12. Schmidt R, Lee T: Motor control and learning (ed 4). Champaign, IL, Human Kinetics, 2005

13. Kisner C, Colby LA: Therapeutic exercise: Foundational concepts, in Kisner C, Colby LA (eds): Therapeutic Exercise. Foundations and Techniques (ed 5). Philadelphia, FA Davis, 2002, pp 1–36

14. Gentile AM: Skill acquisition: Action, movement, and neuromotor processes, in Carr J, Shepherd R (eds): Movement Science: Foundations for Physical Therapy in Rehabilitation. Gaithersburg, MD, Aspen, 2000, pp 111–187

15. Magill RA: Motor learning and control: Concepts and applications (ed 8). New York, McGraw-Hill, 2007

16. American Orthopaedic Society for Sports Medicine: Flexibility. Chicago, American Orthopaedic Society for Sports Medicine, 1988

17. Gleim GW, McHugh MP: Flexibility and its effects on sports injury and performance. Sports Med 24:289–299, 1997

18. Kippers V, Parker AW: Toe-touch test: A measure of validity. Phys Ther 67:1680–1684, 1987

19. Jackson AW, Baker AA: The relationship of the sit and reach test to criterion measures of hamstring and back flexibility in young females. Res Q Exerc Sport 57:183–186, 1986

20. Litsky AS, Spector M: Biomaterials, in Simon SR (ed): Orthopaedic Basic Science. Chicago, American Orthopaedic Society for Sports Medicine, 1994, pp 447–486

21. Johns R, Wright V: Relative importance of various tissues in joint stiffness. J Appl Physiol 17:824–830, 1962

22. Toft E, Espersen GT, Kalund S, et al: Passive tension of the ankle before and after stretching. Am J Sports Med 17:489–494, 1989

23. Halbertsma JPK, Goeken LNH: Stretching exercises: Effect of passive extensibility and stiffness in short hamstrings of healthy subjects. Arch Phys Med Rehab 75:976–981, 1994

24. Magnusson SP, Simonsen EB, Aagaard P, et al: A mechanism for altered flexibility in human skeletal muscle. J Physiol 497:291–298, 1996

25. Klinge K, Magnusson SP, Simonsen EB, et al: The effect of strength and flexibility on skeletal muscle EMG activity, stiffness and viscoelastic stress relaxation response. Am J Sports Med 25:710–716, 1997

26. Lapier TK, Burton HW, Almon RF: Alterations in intramuscular connective tissue after limb casting affect contraction-induced muscle injury. J Appl Physiol 78:1065–1069, 1995

27. McNair PJ, Wood GA, Marshall RN: Stiffness of the hamstring muscles and its relationship to function in ACL deficient individuals. Clin Biomech 7:131–137, 1992

28. McHugh MP, Magnusson SP, Gleim GW, et al: A cross-sectional study of age-related musculoskeletal and physiological changes in soccer players. Med Exerc Nutr Health 2:261–268, 1993

29. Hill AV: The heat and shortening and the dynamic constants of muscle. Proc R Soc Lond B126: 136–195, 1938

30. Tihanyi J, Apor P, Fekete GY: Force-velocity—power characteristics and fiber composition in human knee extensor muscles. Eur J Appl Physiol 48:331–343, 1982

31. Fitts RH, Widrick JJ: Muscle mechanics; adaptations with exercise training. Exerc Sport Sci Rev 24:427–473, 1996

32. Kisner C, Colby LA: Resistance exercise for impaired muscle performance, in Kisner C, Colby LA (eds): Therapeutic Exercise. Foundations and Techniques (ed 5). Philadelphia, FA Davis, 2002, pp 147–229

33. Cook G, Voight ML: Essentials of functional exercise: A four-step clinical model for therapeutic exercise prescription, in Prentice WE, Voight ML (eds): Techniques in Musculoskeletal Rehabilitation. New York, McGraw-Hill, 2001, pp 387–407

34. Connelly DM, Vandervoort AA: Effects of detraining on knee extensor strength and functional mobility in a group of elderly women. J Orthop Sports Phys Ther 26:340–346, 1997

35. Behm DG, Faigenbaum AD, Falk B, et al: Canadian Society for Exercise Physiology position paper: Resistance training in children and adolescents. Appl Physiol Nutr Metab 33:547–561, 2008

36. Litchfield R, Hawkins R, Dillman CJ, et al: Rehabilitation of the overhead athlete. J Orthop Sports Phys Ther 2:433–441, 1993

37. Maitland G: Peripheral Manipulation (ed 3). London, Butterworth, 1991

38. Cyriax J: Textbook of Orthopaedic Medicine, Diagnosis of Soft Tissue Lesions (ed 8). London, Bailliere Tindall, 1982

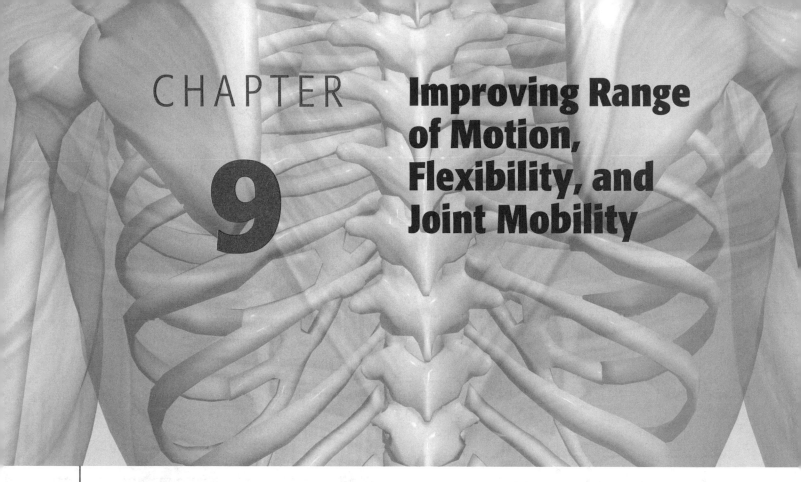

CHAPTER 9

Improving Range of Motion, Flexibility, and Joint Mobility

Chapter Objectives

At the completion of this chapter, the reader will be able to:

1. Define the different types of range of motion (ROM).
2. Describe strategies to increase ROM.
3. Describe the indications and contraindications for the various types of ROM exercises.
4. Outline the indications and contraindications for continuous passive motion.
5. Describe strategies to increase flexibility using different techniques.

Overview

Range of motion (ROM) refers to the distance and direction in which a joint can move. Each specific joint has a normal range of motion that is expressed in degrees. Within the field of physical therapy, goniometry is commonly used to measure the total amount of available motion at a specific joint. Once a determination has been made by the supervising PT that a loss of range of motion is due to an osteokinematic cause, a flexibility program is initiated.

Improving Range of Motion

Movement about the joint, whether passive, active assisted, or active, produces a load in the soft tissues that can maintain the integrity of the connective tissues. Based on these guidelines, in the early stages of the rehabilitation process, range of motion exercises are performed in the following sequence: Passive ROM → Active assisted ROM → Active ROM (**Table 9-1**).

Passive range of motion (PROM) does not prevent muscle atrophy and increase strength or endurance, nor does it assist circulation to the same extent that active, voluntary muscle contraction does. Active range of motion does not maintain or increase strength, or develop skill or coordination except in the movement patterns used.

> ● **Key Point** It is important to remember when making the transition from PROM to AAROM or AROM that gravity has a significant impact, especially on individuals with weak musculature. These individuals may require assistance when the segment moves up against gravity or moves down with gravity.

The mobility activities chosen can be performed in cardinal planes or in multiple planes using functional movement patterns. Once these are tolerated well by the patient, a resistive exercise progression is initiated.

Continuous Passive Motion (CPM)

Continuous passive motion (CPM) refers to passive motion performed by a mechanical device that moves the joint slowly and continuously through a controlled ROM.[1] CPM machines have been designed for use on many body parts, including the hip, knee (most common), ankle, shoulder, elbow, wrist, and hand. The subject of CPM device use following surgery has been debated for years, with some surgeons advocating and others opposing its use.

> ● **Key Point** CPM protocols vary significantly, ranging from 24 hours a day for as long as 1 month to as little as 6 hours a day after surgery. The CPM machine is calibrated in degrees of motion and cycles per minute.

The use of a CPM device has been promoted as a means to facilitate a more rapid recovery by improving ROM, decreasing length of hospital stay, and lowering the amount of narcotic use.[2–12] However, studies have shown that the effect of CPM devices on analgesia consumption, ROM, hospital stay, and complications has been variable:

- Data support the use of CPM to decrease the rate of manipulation for poor ROM after total knee arthroplasty (TKA).
- The use of CPM has not been shown to result in more long-term increases in ROM than other methods of early movement and positioning.
- Although it appears that the use of a CPM device does help regain knee flexion quicker post-TKA, it is not as effective in the enhancement of knee extension.
- Knee impairments or disability are not reduced with the use of a CPM at discharge from hospital.
- Because of standardized inpatient hospital clinical pathways, the length of hospital stay is not decreased by the use of a CPM device but, depending on the hospital involved, the overall cost is not increased.
- Wound complications probably are not increased with the use of CPM, provided good technique is used in wound closure.

> ● **Key Point** It is still not clear whether ROM is achieved faster and whether the prevalence of deep vein thrombosis (DVT) and analgesics use are decreased with CPM.

The desired results for CPM include the following:

- Decrease soft tissue stiffness
- Increase short-term range of motion, which may result in early discharge from the hospital
- Promote healing of the joint surfaces (promotes cartilage growth) and soft tissue
- Prevent adhesions and contractures and thus joint stiffness
- Decrease postoperative pain

Contraindications include:

- Nonstable fracture sites
- Excessive edema
- Patient intolerance

Application and Patient Preparation

First the procedure is explained to the patient. Any wound area must be covered. The clinician adjusts the unit so the patient's anatomical joint is aligned with the mechanical hinge joint of the machine. The patient's limb is secured in the machine using the safety straps. The clinician sets the beginning and end range of motion degrees, and then turns the unit on. Typically a low arc of 20 to 30 degrees is used

Range of Motion Exercise	Description	Examples	Indications	Contraindications
Passive range of motion (PROM)	Movement of a segment within the unrestricted ROM that is produced entirely by an external force; there is little to or no voluntary muscle contraction. PROM and passive stretching are not synonymous.	Pulleys, gravity, another part of the individual's own body, continuous passive motion devices, family members, or various household objects such as the floor, counters, or chairs	Prescribed when mobility must be performed without any muscular activation (acute, inflamed tissue). Exercise is performed within the available ROM to: • Decrease pain and help in the healing process • Prepare a patient for stretching • Maintain joint connective tissue mobility and elasticity • Assist circulation • Prevent joint contracture	Extreme pain at rest Disruption of the healing process
Active assisted range of motion (AAROM)	A type of AROM in which assistance is provided manually or mechanically by an outside force because the prime mover muscle(s) need assistance to complete the motion.	Use of a cane, pulley, or sliding board	Indicated for patients who are unable to complete the ROM actively because of weakness resulting from trauma, neurologic injury, muscular or neuromuscular disease, or pain. Prescribed when mobility must be performed with some muscular activation through the available ROM to: • Increase circulation • Promote healing of connective tissue, including bone • Encourage motor learning, proprioception, and coordination	Extreme pain with movement Disruption of the healing process
Active range of motion (AROM)	Movement of a segment within the unrestricted ROM that is produced by active contraction of the muscles crossing that joint.	Elbow flexion	Prescribed when mobility must be performed with muscular activation through the available ROM to: • Promote healing of connective tissue, including bone • Encourage motor learning, proprioception, and coordination • Prepare connective tissues for functional activities and aerobic conditioning • Initiate strengthening of weak muscles (fair strength [manual muscle grade of 3/5] or less) • Foster independence	Disruption of the healing process

TABLE 9-2	Guidelines for Applying a Low-Load, Prolonged Stretch	
Sequence	**Description**	**Rationale**
I	The involved structure is preheated using either moist heat or ultrasound.	To increase extensibility of connective tissue
II	The involved structure is placed in a gravity-assisted position of slight but not maximum stretch.	To promote relaxation
III	A moist heat application is applied for the entire course of treatment.	To increase extensibility of connective tissue To promote relaxation To increase blood flow
IV	A low-load stress/weight is applied gradually. The patient should be allowed to rest or recover for a few minutes during the course of treatment if the sensation of stretch becomes too uncomfortable.	To enhance a long-lasting change in motion
V	The low-load stress/weight is removed but the moist heat application is continued for a further 5 minutes.	To increase extensibility of connective tissue To promote relaxation To increase blood flow
VI	Isometric contractions and passive stretching are performed.	To enhance strength gains at the new end of range of motion

initially and is progressed 10 to 15 degrees per day as tolerated. The rate of motion is typically one cycle per 45 seconds to 2 minutes. The patient is monitored during the first few minutes to ensure correct fit and patient comfort. Treatment duration varies from 1 hour three times a day to 24 hours a day.

Improving Flexibility

Flexibility training must involve techniques that stretch both the contractile and inert tissues (see Chapter 4). The indications and contraindications for stretching are described in Chapter 6 in addition to the correct dosage and the various effects on the connective tissue.

Methods of Stretching

There are four broad categories of stretching techniques that can be used to increase the extensibility of the soft tissues: static, cyclic, ballistic, and proprioceptive neuromuscular facilitation stretching.

Static Stretching

Static stretching involves the application of a steady force for a sustained period at a point in the range just past tissue resistance. The duration of static stretch is based on the patient's tolerance and response during the stretching procedure. Static stretches can be

applied using a manually applied force, weighted traction, specific low-load braces, or pulley systems that have been modified to provide this type of stretching (**Table 9-2**).[13]

> **Key Point** Small loads applied for long periods produce greater residual lengthening than heavy loads applied for short periods.[14]

The advantages of static stretching include the reduced likelihood of exceeding strain limits of the tissue being stretched and reduced potential for muscle soreness.[15,16] Research has shown that the tension created in muscle during static stretching is approximately half that created during ballistic stretching.[17] Effective stretching, in the early phase, should be performed every hour, but with each session lasting only a few minutes. In healthy young and/or middle-aged adults, stretch durations of 15, 30, 45, or 60 seconds or 2 minutes to lower extremity musculature has been shown to produce significant gains in ROM.[18–22] Longer durations are recommended in older patients due to decreased extensibility in the connective tissues.[18,21] Stretching needs to occur a minimum of two times per week,[23] and approximately 6 weeks of stretching are necessary to demonstrate significant increases in muscular flexibility.[15,16]

> **● Key Point** Heat should be applied to increase intramuscular temperature prior to, and during, stretching.[24,25] This heat can be achieved with either low-intensity warm-up exercises or through the use of thermal modalities.[25]

The question of whether muscle flexibility or stretching before activity results in a decrease in muscle injuries has yet to be answered.[26–31] In addition, there is limited scientific literature to determine the appropriate place for stretching in an exercise program. In one study, static stretching was done before, after, and both before and after each workout. All produced significant increases in range of motion.[32]

Cyclic Stretching

Intermittent cyclic stretching involves a relatively short duration stretch that is repeatedly but gradually applied, released, and then reapplied.[33] The end range stretched force is applied at a slow velocity, with a relatively low intensity, and in a controlled manner. There appears to be no consensus as to the duration of the stretch (5–30 seconds) or the optimal number of repetitions (typically based on patient tolerance) during a treatment session.

Ballistic Stretching

This technique of stretching uses high-velocity, bouncing movements at the end of range to stretch a particular muscle. The bouncing movements at the end of range are slight initially but are progressively increased over several repetitions. Due to the increased potential for injury using this technique, it is not appropriate for all patient populations.

In comparisons of the ballistic and static methods, two studies[34,35] have found that both produce similar improvements in flexibility. However, ballistic stretching appears to cause more residual muscle soreness or muscle strain than those techniques that incorporate relaxation.[36–38]

> **● Key Point** Some areas of the body are difficult to stretch adequately using a lengthening technique. In these instances, techniques of localized, manual release, using varying degrees of manual pressure along the length of the muscle and myofascial tissue, may need to be used.[39]

Proprioceptive Neuromuscular Facilitation Stretching

Proprioceptive neuromuscular facilitation (PNF) stretching is one of the most effective forms of flexibility training for increasing range of motion.[40] PNF techniques (see Chapter 6) can be passive (no associated muscular contraction) or active (performed

with a voluntary muscle contraction). However, PNF stretching techniques are not appropriate in patients with paralysis or spasticity resulting from neuromuscular diseases or injury.

> **● Key Point** The majority of studies have shown the PNF techniques to be the most effective stretching techniques for increasing ROM through muscle lengthening when compared to the static or slow sustained, and the ballistic or bounce techniques.[41–45]

The different techniques of PNF stretching all facilitate muscular inhibition through autogenic inhibition and are therefore more appropriate where muscle spasm limits motion and less appropriate for stretching fibrotic contractures.[40]

> **● Key Point**
> • *Reciprocal inhibition:* The process by which muscles on one side of a joint relax (are inhibited) to accommodate contraction on the other side of the joint.
> • *Autogenic inhibition:* Controlled by the Golgi tendon organ (see Chapter 3), the role of which is to monitor tension within a muscle. The stimulation of the Golgi tendon organ by a muscle contraction causes the inhibition or relaxation of the muscle in which it is located.[46]

Often, in PNF, an isometric contraction is referred to as *hold* and a concentric muscle contraction is referred to as *contract*.

Postisometric Relaxation

A commonly used technique in PNF and other manual techniques is postisometric relaxation (PIR). PIR refers to the effect of the subsequent reduction in tone experienced by a muscle, or group of muscles, after brief periods during which an isometric contraction has been performed.[47] The basis for PIR is related to the theory behind contract–relax in that light, brief isometric contractions of a hypertonic muscle externally stretch the nuclear bag fibers of the muscle spindles. This stretching, in turn, allows a lengthening of muscle during the postisometric phase, without stimulating myostatic reflexes.[48] Phasic muscles that have become adaptively shortened are treated using more forceful isometric contractions.

> **● Key Point** PIR techniques are ideal as an initial method to gain the patient's trust, especially in cases of reflex contraction or trigger point hypertonicity.[49] These techniques can also be used for joint mobilizations when a manipulation is not desirable.[50]

The most common PNF stretching techniques use a combination of contracting, holding, and passive stretching (often referred to as *relaxing*). There appears to be no consensus as to whether to use the relaxation of the agonist or the antagonist to gain motion.[51–55] Each technique, although slightly different, involves starting with a passive stretch held for about 10 seconds. A hamstring stretch can be used to illustrate the different variations. The patient is positioned in supine for each example. The patient places one leg, extended, flat on the floor, and the other extended resting on the clinician's shoulder.

Hold–Relax

The clinician moves the patient's extended leg to a point of mild discomfort. This passive stretch (pre-stretch) is held for 10 seconds. The patient is then asked to isometrically contract the hamstrings by pushing their extended leg against the clinician's shoulder. The clinician applies just enough force so that the leg remains static. This is the hold phase, and it lasts for 6 seconds. The patient is then asked to relax, and the clinician moves the leg into the new range and completes a second passive stretch as the patient's leg is progressively moved further into the range (greater hip flexion) due to the autogenic inhibition of the hamstrings.

● **Key Point** The terms *contract–relax* and *hold–relax* are often used interchangeably, but they are not identical (see Appendix E).

Contract–Relax

The clinician moves the patient's extended leg to a point of mild discomfort. This passive stretch is held for 10 seconds. The patient is then asked to concentrically contract the hamstrings by pushing their extended leg against the clinician's shoulder. The clinician applies just enough force so there is resistance while allowing the patient to push their leg to the floor (i.e., through the full range of motion). This is the contract phase. The patient is then instructed to relax, and the clinician completes a second passive stretch, which is held for 30 seconds. The patient's extended leg should move further into the range (greater hip flexion) due to the autogenic inhibition of the hamstrings.

Hold–Relax with Agonist Contraction

The clinician moves the patient's extended leg to a point of mild discomfort. This passive stretch is held for 10 seconds. The patient is then asked to isometrically contract the hamstrings by pushing their extended leg against the clinician's shoulder. The clinician applies just enough force so the leg remains static. This is the hold phase, and it lasts for

6 seconds. This initiates autogenic inhibition. The clinician completes a second passive stretch held for 30 seconds, and the patient is asked to flex the hip (i.e., move the leg in the same direction as it is being stretched). This initiates the reciprocal inhibition.

Self-Stretching

Self-stretching techniques include any stretching exercise that is carried out independently by the patient after instruction and supervision. Self-stretching techniques are included at the end of each of the joint chapters.

Stretching and warm-up are not synonymous but are often confused by the layman. Warm-up requires activity that raises total body and muscle temperatures to prepare the body for exercise.[56] Research has shown that warm-up prior to stretching results in significant changes in joint range of motion.[57]

● **Key Point** Each exercise session should include a 5- to 15-minute warm-up and a 5- to 15-minute cool-down period. The *warm-up* includes low-intensity cardiorespiratory activities and prepares the heart and circulatory system so they are not suddenly overloaded. The *cool-down* includes low-intensity cardiorespiratory activities and flexibility exercises and helps prevent abrupt physiological alterations that can occur with sudden cessation of strenuous exercise, such as adaptive shortening and lactic acid build-up. The length of the warm-up and cool-down sessions may need to be longer for deconditioned or older individuals.

Anecdotally, it would make sense not to perform stretching at the beginning of the warm-up routine because the tissue temperatures are too low for optimal muscle–tendon function, and are less compliant and less prepared for activity. Some advocate stretching after an exercise session, during the cool-down period, citing that the increased musculotendinous extensibility leads to the potential for improved joint flexibility.[16] Viscoelastic changes are not permanent, whereas plastic changes, which are more difficult to achieve, result in a residual or permanent change in length (see Chapter 4).

It is important for the patient to realize that the initial session of stretching may increase symptoms in the stretched structures[58]; however, this increase in symptoms should only be temporary, lasting for a couple of hours at most.[59,60] The stretch should be performed at the point just shy of pain, although some discomfort may be necessary to achieve results.[61] Connective tissue usually requires a greater stretching force initially, possibly to break up adhesions or cross-linkages, and to allow for viscoelastic and plastic changes to occur in the collagen and elastin fibers (see Chapter 4).[61]

Improving Joint Mobility

Once a determination has been made by the supervising PT that the loss of range of motion is due to an arthrokinematic cause, joint mobilizations are the intervention of choice (see Chapter 6).

Summary

When injury occurs, there is almost always some associated loss of ability to move normally. This loss of motion may be due to pain, swelling, muscle guarding, or spasm; inactivity resulting in shortening of connective tissue and muscle; loss of neuromuscular control; or some combination of these factors. Restoring normal range of motion following injury is one of the primary goals in any rehabilitation program. Flexibility is the ability to move a joint or series of joints smoothly through a full range of motion. Passive range of motion refers to the degree to which a joint may be passively moved to the endpoints in the range of motion, whereas active range of motion refers to movement through the end of a muscle's ability to actively contract.

REVIEW Questions

1. What are the two components of flexibility?
2. What are the two viscoelastic properties of connective tissue related to stretching?
3. List three goals of static stretching.
4. True or false: Tissue temperature does not affect connective tissue extensibility.
5. True or false: Acute exercise has no effect on intramuscular temperature and tissue extensibility.
6. True or false: PNF stretching is superior to other forms of active stretching.
7. In terms of increasing intensity, what is the correct sequence when prescribing range of motion exercises?
8. True or false: Passive range of motion can prevent muscle atrophy.
9. True or false: The use of a continuous passive motion (CPM) machine can increase short-term range of motion, which may result in early discharge from the hospital.
10. What are the four types of stretching techniques described in this chapter?

References

1. Kisner C, Colby LA: Range of motion, in Kisner C, Colby LA (eds): Therapeutic Exercise. Foundations and Techniques (ed 5). Philadelphia, FA Davis, 2002, pp 43–64
2. Johnson DP: The effect of continuous passive motion on wound-healing and joint mobility after knee arthroplasty. J Bone Joint Surg 72A:421–426, 1990
3. Basso M, Knapp L: Comparison of two continuous passive motion protocols for patients with total knee implants. Phys Ther 67:360–363, 1987
4. Colwell, C.W., Morris BA: The influence of continuous passive motion on the results of total knee arthroplasty. Clin Orthop 276:225–228, 1992
5. Coutts RD: Continuous passive motion in the rehabilitation of the total knee patient. Its role and effect. Orthop Rev 15:27, 1986
6. Coutts RD, Toth C, Kaita JH: The role of continuous passive motion in the postoperative rehabilitation of the total knee patient, in Hungerford DS (ed): Total Knee Arthroplasty: A Comprehensive Approach. Baltimore, Williams & Williams, 1984, pp 126–132
7. Jordan LR, Siegel JL, Olivo JL: Early flexion routine, an alternative method of continuous passive motion. Clin Orthop 315:231–233, 1995
8. Maloney WJ, Schurman DJ, Hangen D, et al: The influence of continuous passive motion on outcome in total knee arthroplasty. Clin Orthop 256:162–168, 1990
9. Vince KG, Kelly MA, Beck J, et al: Continuous passive motion after total knee arthroplasty. J Arthroplasty 2:281–284, 1987
10. Wasilewski SA, Woods LC, Torgerson J, et al: Value of continuous passive motion in total knee arthroplasty. Orthopedics 13:291–295, 1990
11. Walker RH, Morris BA, Angulo DL, et al: Postoperative use of continuous passive motion, transcutaneous electrical nerve stimulation, and continuous cooling pad following total knee arthroplasty. J Arthroplasty 6:151–156, 1991
12. McInnes J, Larson MG, Daltroy LH, et al: A controlled evaluation of continuous passive motion in patients undergoing total knee arthroplasty. JAMA 268:1423–1428, 1992
13. Lentell G, Hetherington T, Eagan J, et al: The use of thermal agents to influence the effectiveness of a lowload of prolonged stretch. J Orthop Sports Phys Ther 16:200–207, 1992
14. Yoder E: Physical therapy management of nonsurgical hip problems in adults, in Echternach JL (ed): Physical Therapy of the Hip. New York, Churchill Livingstone, 1990, pp 103–137
15. Zachazewski JE: Flexibility for sports, in Sanders B (ed): Sports Physical Therapy. Norwalk, CT, Appleton and Lange, 1990, pp 201–238

16. Wallman HW: Stretching and flexibility, in Wilmarth MA (ed): Orthopaedic Physical Therapy: Topic—Strength and Conditioning, Independent Study Course 15.3. La Crosse, WI, Orthopaedic Section, American Physical Therapy Association, 2005

17. Walker SM: Delay of twitch relaxation induced by stress and stress relaxation. J Appl Physiol 16:801–806, 1961

18. Bandy WD, Irion JM, Briggler M: The effect of time and frequency of static stretching on flexibility of the hamstring muscles. Phys Ther 77:1090–1096, 1997

19. Cipriani D, Abel B, Pirrwitz D: A comparison of two stretching protocols on hip range of motion: Implications for total daily stretch duration. J Strength Cond Res 17:274–278, 2003

20. de Weijer VC, Gorniak GC, Shamus E: The effect of static stretch and warm-up exercise on hamstring length over the course of 24 hours. J Orthop Sports Phys Ther 33:727–733, 2003

21. Madding SW, Wong JG, Hallum A, et al: Effect of duration of passive stretch on hip abduction range of motion. J Orthop Sports Phys Ther 8:409–416, 1987

22. Willy RW, Kyle BA, Moore SA, et al: Effect of cessation and resumption of static hamstring muscle stretching on joint range of motion. J Orthop Sports Phys Ther 31:138–144, 2001

23. Godges JJ, MacRae H, Longdon C, et al: The effects of two stretching procedures on hip range of motion and gait economy. J Orthop Sports Phys Ther 10:350, 1989

24. Murphy P: Warming up before stretching advised. Phys Sports Med 14:45, 1986

25. Shellock F, Prentice WE: Warm-up and stretching for improved physical performance and prevention of sport-related injury. Sports Med 2:267–278, 1985

26. Worrell TW, Perrin DH, Gansneder B, et al: Comparison of isokinetic strength and flexibility measures between hamstring injured and non-injured athletes. J Orthop Sports Phys Ther 13:118–125, 1991

27. Worrell TW, Perrin DH: Hamstring muscle injury: The influence of strength, flexibility, warm-up, and fatigue. J Orthop Sports Phys Ther 16:12–18, 1992

28. Sutton G: Hamstrung by hamstring strains: A review of the literature. J Orthop Sports Phys Ther 5:184–195, 1984

29. Gleim GW, McHugh MP: Flexibility and its effects on sports injury and performance. Sports Med 24:289–299, 1997

30. Worrell TW: Factors associated with hamstring injuries: An approach to treatment and preventative measures. Sports Med 17:338–345, 1994

31. Jonhagen S, Nemeth G, Eriksson E: Hamstring injuries in sprinters: The role of concentric and eccentric hamstring strength and flexibility. Am J Sports Med 22:262–266, 1994

32. Cornelius WL, Hagemann RW, Jr., Jackson AW: A study on placement of stretching within a workout. J Sports Med Phys Fitness 28:234–236, 1988

33. Kisner C, Colby LA: Stretching for impaired mobility, in Kisner C, Colby LA (eds): Therapeutic Exercise. Foundations and Techniques (ed 5). Philadelphia, FA Davis, 2002, pp 65–108

34. DeVries HA: Evaluation of static stretching procedures for improvement of flexibility. Res Quart 33:222–229, 1962

35. Logan GA, Egstrom GH: Effects of slow and fast stretching on sacrofemoral angle. J Assoc Phys Ment Rehabil 15:85–89, 1961

36. Davies CT, White MJ: Muscle weakness following eccentric work in man. Pflugers Arch 392:168–171, 1981

37. Friden J, Sjostrom M, Ekblom B: A morphological study of delayed muscle soreness. Experientia 37:506–507, 1981

38. Hardy L: Improving active range of hip flexion. Res Q Exerc Sport 56:111–114, 1985

39. Sucher BM: Thoracic outlet syndrome—a myofascial variant: Part 2. Treatment. J Am Osteopath Assoc 90:810–823, 1990

40. Cornelius WL, Hinson MM: The relationship between isometric contractions of hip extensors and subsequent flexibility in males. J Sports Med Phys Fitness 20:75–80, 1980

41. Markos PD: Ipsilateral and contralateral effects of proprioceptive neuromuscular facilitation techniques on hip motion and electromyographic activity. Phys Ther 59:1366, 1979

42. Holt LE, Travis TM, Okita T: Comparative study of three stretching techniques. Percep Motor Skills 31:611–616, 1970

43. Tanigawa MC: Comparison of hold-relax procedure and passive mobilization on increasing muscle length. Phys Ther 52:725–735, 1972

44. Sady SP, Wortman MA, Blanke D: Flexibility training: Ballistic, static or proprioceptive neuromuscular facilitation? Arch Phys Med Rehab 63:261–263, 1982

45. Prentice WE: A comparison of static stretching and PNF stretching for improving hip joint flexibility. Athl Train 18:56–59, 1983

46. Pollard H, Ward G: A study of two stretching techniques for improving hip flexion range of motion. J Man Physiol Ther 20:443–447, 1997

47. Chaitow L: An introduction to muscle energy techniques, in Chaitow L (ed): Muscle Energy Techniques (ed 2). London, Churchill Livingstone, 2001, pp 1–18

48. Mitchell FL, Jr.: Elements of muscle energy techniques, in Basmajian JV, Nyberg R (eds): Rational Manual Therapies. Baltimore, Williams & Wilkins, 1993, pp 285–321

49. Liebenson C: Active muscular relaxation techniques (part 1). J Manipulative Physiol Ther 12:446–451, 1989

50. Lewit K: Manipulative Therapy in Rehabilitation of the Motor System (ed 3). London, Butterworths, 1999

51. Lewit K, Simons DG: Myofascial pain: Relief by postisometric relaxation. Arch Phys Med Rehab 65:452–456, 1984

52. Janda V: Muscles, motor regulation and back problems, in Korr IM (ed): The Neurological Mechanisms in Manipulative Therapy. New York, Plenum, 1978, pp 27–41

53. Janda V: Muscle Function Testing. London, Butterworths, 1983

54. Janda V: Muscle strength in relation to muscle length, pain and muscle imbalance, in Harms-Ringdahl K (ed): Muscle Strength. New York, Churchill Livingstone, 1993, pp 83–91

55. Greenman PE: Principles of Manual Medicine (ed 2). Baltimore, Williams & Wilkins, 1996

56. Anderson B, Burke ER: Scientific, medical, and practical aspects of stretching. Clin Sports Med 10:63–86, 1991

57. Wiktorsson-Moller M, Oberg B, Ekstrand J, et al: Effects of warming up, massage, and stretching on range of motion and muscle strength in the lower extremity. Am J Sports Med 11:249–252, 1983

58. Travell JG, Simons DG: Myofascial Pain and Dysfunction—The Trigger Point Manual. Baltimore, Williams & Wilkins, 1983

59. Swezey RL: Arthrosis, in Basmajian JV, Kirby RL (eds): Medical Rehabilitation. Baltimore, Williams & Wilkins, 1984, pp 216–218

60. Kottke FJ: Therapeutic exercise to maintain mobility, in Kottke FJ, Stillwell GK, Lehman JF (eds): Krusen's Handbook of Physical Medicine and Rehabilitation. Baltimore, WB Saunders, 1982, pp 389–402

61. Joynt RL: Therapeutic exercise, in DeLisa JA (ed): Rehabilitation Medicine: Principles and Practice. Philadelphia, JB Lippincott, 1988, pp 346–371

62. Sapega AA, Quedenfeld T, Moyer R, et al: Biophysical factors in range of motion exercise. Phys Sports Med 9:57–65, 1981

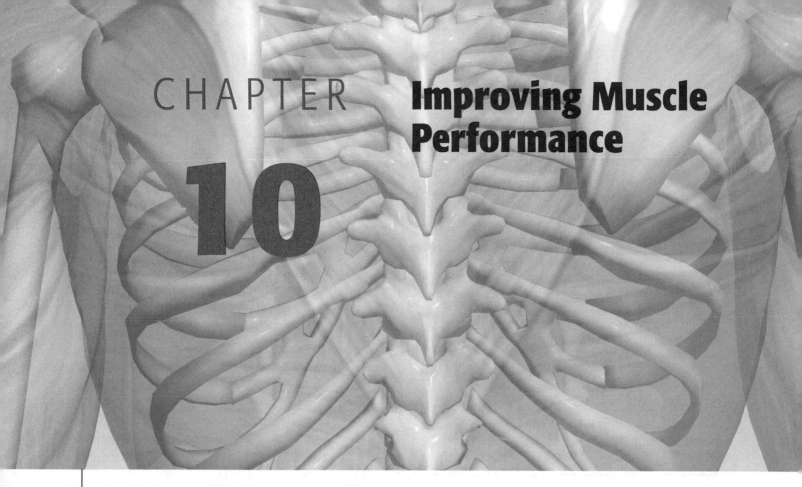

Chapter Objectives

At the completion of this chapter, the reader will be able to:

1. List the different types of muscle contractions and the advantages and disadvantages of each.
2. Differentiate among muscle strength, endurance, and power.
3. Describe strategies to increase muscle strength.
4. List the different types of resistance that can be used to strengthen muscles.
5. Outline the various types of exercise progression and the components of each.
6. Describe strategies to increase muscle endurance.
7. Describe strategies to increase muscle power.
8. Explain the basic principles behind plyometrics.
9. Define delayed onset muscle soreness and explain why it occurs.

Overview

There are three basic types of muscle contraction: isometric, concentric, and eccentric.

- *Isometric contraction:* Provides a static contraction with a variable and accommodating resistance without producing a change in muscle length. Examples of isometric exercise include muscle setting exercises, stabilization exercises, and multiple angle isometrics.
- *Concentric contraction:* Provides a dynamic contraction whereby tension is produced and shortening of the muscle takes place, approximating the origin and insertion of the contracting muscle. An example of a concentric contraction is the raising of a weight during a bicep curl.
- *Eccentric contraction:* Provides a dynamic contraction whereby tension is produced as lengthening of the muscle occurs. The net action is opposite that produced by concentric contraction in that the origin and insertion of the contracting muscle move further apart during the contraction. In reality,

the muscle does not actually lengthen, it merely returns from its shortened position to its normal resting length. An example of an eccentric contraction is the lowering of a weight during a bicep curl.

● Key Point

- *Repetitions:* The number of times a particular movement is repeated against a specific exercise load. The number of repetitions selected depends on the patient's status and whether the goal of the exercise is to improve muscle strength or endurance. No optimal number for strength training or endurance training has been identified.
- *Sets:* A predetermined number of repetitions grouped together. After each set of a specified number of repetitions, there is a brief interval of rest. As with repetitions, there is no optimal number of sets per exercise session, but typically they can vary from one set to as many as six sets.[1]
- *Sequence:* The order in which exercises are performed during an exercise session. It is recommended that large muscle groups should be exercised before small muscle groups and multi-joint muscles before single joint muscles to prevent muscle fatigue and to allow for adaptive training effects.
- *Mode:* The form of exercise, the type of muscle contraction that occurs, and the manner in which the exercise was carried out.[1]
- *Body position:* The body or limb position used for an exercise determines whether the exercise is open chain or closed chain (see Chapter 4) and whether the muscle is working with or against gravity.

Improving Strength

To most effectively increase muscle strength, a muscle must work with increasing effort against progressively increasing resistance.[2,3] If resistance is applied to a muscle as it contracts so that the metabolic capabilities of the muscle are progressively overloaded, adaptive changes occur within the muscle that make it stronger over time.[4,5] These adaptive changes include:[3,6–11]

- An increase in the efficiency of the neuromuscular system. This increased efficiency results in:
  - An increase in the number of motor units recruited
  - An increase in the firing rate of each motor unit
  - An increase in the synchronization of motor unit firing
- An improvement in the endurance of the muscle.
- Stimulation of slow twitch (type I) fibers when performing workloads of low intensity, and stimulation of fast twitch (type IIa) fibers when performing workloads of high intensity and short duration (see Chapter 2).
- The muscle hypertrophies due to an increase in the number and size of the myofilaments (actin and myosin).

- An increase in blood flow to exercising muscles via a contraction and relaxation.
- An improvement in the power of the muscle.
- Improved bone mass (Wolfe's law).
- An increase in metabolism/calorie burning/weight control.
- Increased intramuscular pressure from a muscle contraction of about 60 percent of its force-generating capacity.
- Cardiovascular benefits when using large muscle groups. Strength training of specific muscles has a brief activation period and uses a relatively small muscle mass, thereby producing less cardiovascular metabolic demand than vigorous walking, swimming, and the like.

Conversely, a muscle can become weak or atrophied through:

- Disease
- Neurologic compromise
- Immobilization
- Disuse

Methods of Strengthening Muscles

Physical strength, also known as muscular strength, is the ability of a person to exert force on physical objects using muscles. Increasing muscle strength often is a priority in rehabilitation. A muscle can be strengthened using a variety of methods including exercise and electrical stimulation.

Neuromuscular Electrical Stimulation

Neuromuscular electrical stimulation (NMES), also known as therapeutic (or threshold) electrical stimulation (TES), is a form of electrical stimulation that attempts to strengthen muscles weakened by disuse using a subcontraction stimulus to promote muscle growth. However, in an individual with disuse atrophy, the contracting muscles use the strongest fibers and the weakened fibers deteriorate further. Therefore, NMES is better utilized for muscle re-education, where the patient attempts to actively contract his or her muscle as the electrical stimulation contracts the muscle. NMES often is used for orthopedic rehabilitation in individuals who have disuse weakness, joint restrictions, edema, and spasms.

Isometric Exercises

The amount of tension that can be generated during an isometric muscle contraction depends in part on joint position and the length of the muscle at the time of contraction.[12] A 6- to 10-second hold of 60 to 80 percent of a muscle's force-developing capacity is sufficient to increase strength when performed repetitively.[13] However, typically the rule of tens is used when instructing a patient in isometric exercise. The rule states that the patient must perform 10-second contractions for 10 repetitions with a 10-second rest between each repetition.[14]

> **● Key Point** When instructing a patient on how to perform an isometric exercise, the patient is told to perform the isometric contraction by gradually developing tension for 2 seconds, maintaining a maximal contraction for 6 seconds, and then gradually decreasing tension for 2 seconds.

The advantages of isometric exercises include:

- They can be used in situations where joint movement is restricted, either by pain or by bracing/casting. Their primary role in this regard is to prevent atrophy and prevent a decrease of ligament, bone, and muscle intergrity.
- An overflow of strength occurs approximately 10 degrees above and below the angle at which the exercise is occurring.[13] When using multiple-angle isometrics, they should be performed at 10-degree increments.

The disadvantages of isometric exercises include:

- The strength gains are developed at a specific point in the range of motion and not throughout the range (unless performed at multiple angles).[13]
- Not all of a muscle's fibers are activated—there is predominantly an activation of slow twitch (type I) fibers.
- There are no flexibility or cardiovascular fitness benefits.
- Peak effort can be injurious to the tissues due to vasoconstriction and joint compression forces.
- There is limited functional carryover.[15]
- Considerable internal pressure can be generated, especially if the breath is held during contraction, which can result in further injury to patients with a weakness in the abdominal wall (hernia) and cardiovascular impairment (increased blood pressure through the Valsalva maneuver, even if the exercise is performed correctly). The Valsalva maneuver is performed by forcible exhalation against a closed airway/mouth (a "bearing down" maneuver)

and is particularly relevant in a patient with a cardiac condition because it can result in pressure inside the chest impeding the return of systemic blood to the heart and a reduction in cardiac output and stroke volume.

The typical progression for isometric exercises is:

1. Single-angle submaximal isometrics performed in the neutral position
2. Multiple-angle submaximal isometrics performed at various angles of the range
3. Multiple-angle maximal isometrics

Concentric/Isotonic Exercises

Concentric contractions are commonly used in the rehabilitation process and occur frequently in activities of daily living—the biceps curl and the lifting of a cup to the mouth are examples of each, respectively. (The term *isotonic* is no longer preferred when referring to exercise because it infers that the tension in the muscle remains constant despite changes occurring in muscle length.) A maximum concentric contraction produces less force than a maximum eccentric contraction under the same conditions—that is, greater loads can be lowered than lifted. This is because when the load is lowered, the force exerted by the load is controlled not only by the active, contractile components of the muscle, but also by the connective tissue in and around the muscle. Consequently it requires more effort by a patient to control the same load during concentric exercise than during eccentric exercise.[1] From a clinical perspective, in the presence of substantial muscle weakness, it may be easier for the patient to control lowering a limb against gravity than lifting the limb.

Eccentric Exercises

Eccentric muscle contractions, which are capable of generating greater forces than either isometric or concentric contractions,[3,4,6] are involved in activities that require a deceleration to occur. Such activities include slowing to a stop when running, lowering an object, or sitting down. Because the load exceeds the bond between the actin and myosin filaments during an eccentric contraction, some of the myosin filaments probably are torn from the binding sites on the actin filament while the remainder are completing the contraction cycle.[16] The resulting force is substantially larger for a torn cross-bridge than for one being created during a normal cycle of muscle contraction. Consequently, the combined increase in force per cross-bridge and the number of active cross-bridges results in a maximum lengthening muscle tension that is greater than the tension that could be created during a shortening muscle action.[16,17] A comparison of the three types of muscle actions in terms of maximal force production, according to Elftman's proposal, shows that:[18]

Eccentric maximum tension > Isometric maximum tension > Concentric maximum tension

However, in terms of energy liberated via adenosine triphosphate (ATP) use, eccentric muscle contractions use the least ATP, whereas concentric contractions use the most.[19] Therefore, in terms of energy efficiency, eccentric muscle contractions are more energy-efficient, require less motor unit firing, and produce greater tension per contractile unit than both concentric and isometric contractions, making it the most efficient of all of the contraction types. However, eccentric exercise places greater stress on the cardiovascular system than does concentric exercise.[20]

> **● Key Point** Eccentric muscle contractions stimulate both contractile and noncontractile elements[14] whereas concentric contractions and isometrics focus on the contractile elements.[21]

> **● Key Point** Optimal strength-specific programs include the use of both eccentric and concentric muscle actions and the performance of both single-joint and multi-joint exercises. The hierarchy for the resistive exercise progression is based on patient tolerance and response to ensure that any progress made is done in a safe and controlled fashion. The typical sequence occurs in the following order:[14]
>
> - Small arc submaximal concentric/eccentric
> - Full ROM submaximal concentric/eccentric
> - Full ROM submaximal eccentric
> - Functional/activity-specific plane submaximal concentric
> - Functional ROM submaximal eccentric
> - Full ROM submaximal concentric isokinetic
> - Full ROM submaximal eccentric isokinetic
> - Functional ROM submaximal eccentric isokinetic
>
> Cross-training effects (a slight increase in strength in the same muscle group of the opposite, unexercised extremity) have been shown to occur when a combination of high-intensity concentric and eccentric contractions are used.

Delayed Onset Muscle Soreness

Muscular soreness may result from all forms of exercise and is one of the drawbacks to participating in an exercise program involving activity beyond what one usually experiences. Two types of muscle soreness are commonly reported, acute and delayed onset. Acute soreness is apparent during the later stages of an exercise bout and during the immediate recovery period.[22] This results from an accumulation

of end products that occurs with exercise, H^+ ions, and lactate, but generally disappears between 2 minutes and 1 hour after cessation of exercise.[22] Delayed-onset muscle soreness (DOMS), on the other hand, appears 24–56 hours after the exercise bout.[23] DOMS can present as anything from minor muscle soreness to debilitating pain and swelling, but is most commonly described as causing a reduction in joint range of motion, shock attenuation, and peak torque.[24]

> **● Key Point** Recognized mechanisms that can cause DOMS include lactic acid and potassium accumulation, muscle spasms, mechanical damage to the connective tissues, inflammation, enzyme efflux secondary to muscle cell damage, and edema.[25]

There is certainly a marked increase in the proportion of disrupted muscle fibers after eccentric as compared with concentric exercise, which has been roughly correlated to the degree of DOMS.[26] Eccentric exercise is also linked to morphologic and metabolic signs of muscle alteration: myofibrillar damage along the Z-band,[27,28] mitochondrial swelling,[27,28] increased intramuscular pressure,[27,28] and impaired glycogen resynthesis.

Given the role of eccentric exercise in DOMS, prevention of DOMS involves the careful design of any eccentric program, which should include preparatory techniques, accurate training variables, and appropriate aftercare, including a cool-down period of low-intensity exercise to facilitate the return of oxygen to the muscle.

It is a widely held belief among athletes, coaches, and therapists that massage is an effective therapeutic modality that can enhance muscle recovery and reduce soreness following intense physical activity.[29] However, the actual scientific literature does not tend to support the positive efficacy of manual massage as a postexercise therapeutic modality in the athletic setting.[29–31]

In the presence of DOMS, the intervention should include, as appropriate, rest, local measures to reduce edema (e.g., cryotherapy, elevation of the involved limb[s]), or further exercise (aerobic submaximal exercise with no eccentric component [e.g., swimming, biking, stepper machine], pain-free flexibility exercises, and high-speed [300 degrees per second] concentric-only isokinetic training).[32,33]

Isokinetic Exercise

Isokinetic exercise requires the use of special equipment (Figure 10-1) that produces an accommodating and variable resistance. The main principle behind

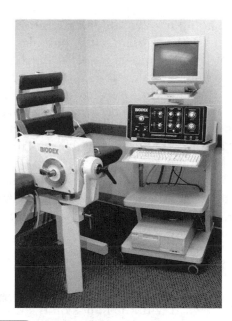

Figure 10-1 Isokinetic machine.

isokinetic exercise is that peak torque (the maximum force generated through the range of motion) is inversely related to angular velocity, the speed that a body segment moves through its range of motion. Thus, an increase in angular velocity decreases peak torque production. Advantages for this type of exercise include the following:

- Both high speed/low resistance and low speed/ high resistance regimens result in excellent strength gains, even though it has been shown the speed of current machines do not come close to matching the actual speed of a joint/ muscle during certain acceleration/deceleration activities.[34-37]
- Both concentric and eccentric resistance exercises can be performed on isokinetic machines.
- The machines provide maximum resistance at all points in the range of motion as a muscle contracts.

The gravity-produced torque created by the machine adds to the force generated by the muscle when it contracts, resulting in a higher torque output than is actually created by the muscle. The disadvantages of this type of exercise include:

- Expense
- The potential for impact loading and incorrect joint axis alignment[38]
- Questionable functional carryover[15]
- Involves open chain exercise only
- Involves a single muscle/motion

Proprioceptive Neuromuscular Facilitation

Proprioceptive neuromuscular facilitation (PNF) techniques utilize manual resistance to strengthen muscles using a variety of muscle contractions:[39]

- *Isometric:* The clinician applies resistance to joint motion that is equal to that provided by the patient, such that no motion occurs. The contraction is held for approximately 30–60 seconds to increase the tone and strength of the muscle or muscle group.
- *Concentric:* The clinician applies resistance to joint motion such that it is less than that provided by the patient, so the patient moves the joint in the desired direction and through the desired range at a speed controlled by the clinician. This is repeated five times and serves to increase the concentric strength of the agonist muscles and relaxation of the antagonists.
- *Eccentric:* The clinician applies resistance to joint motion such that it is greater than that provided by the patient. Thus, the patient is not only unable to move the joint in the desired direction, but also is unable to fully resist the clinician. As a result, even with maximum effort, the joint moves in the opposite direction of the desired movement. This is repeated five times and serves to increase the eccentric strength, and length, of the agonist muscles.

Stabilization Exercises

According to Voight,[40,41] the standard progression for stabilization exercises involves:

- *Static stabilization exercises with closed chain loading and unloading (weight shifting):* This phase initially employs isometric exercises around the involved joint on solid and even surfaces, before progressing to unstable surfaces. The early training involves balance training and joint repositioning exercises, and in the lower extremities is usually initiated (according to weight-bearing restrictions) by having the patient place the involved extremity on a 6- to 8-inch stool, so that the amount of weight bearing can be controlled more easily. The proprioceptive awareness of a joint can also be enhanced by using an elastic bandage, orthotic, or through taping.[42-47] As full weight bearing through the extremity is restored, a number of devices such as a mini-trampoline, balance board, stability ball, and wobble board can be introduced. Exercises on these devices are progressed from double limb support, to single leg support, to support while performing sport-specific skills.

> **● Key Point** One of the advantages of using the stability ball is that it creates an unstable base, which challenges the postural stabilizer muscles more than using a stable base. It is important to choose the appropriate size stability ball, which depends on patient size:
>
> • *45-cm ball:* Shorter than 5'
> • *55-cm ball:* 5' to 5' 8"
> • *65-cm ball:* 5' 9" to 6' 3"
> • *75-cm ball:* Taller than 6' 3"
>
> With the patient sitting on the ball with both feet firmly planted on the ground, the patient's thighs should be parallel to the floor (the knees may be slightly above the hips).
>
> • Pumping up the ball to increase firmness increases the level of difficulty in any given exercise.
> • The further away the ball is from the support points, the greater the demand for core stability.
> • Decreasing the number of support points increases the difficulty of the exercise.

■ *Transitional stabilization exercises:* The exercises during this phase involve conscious control of motion without impact and replace isometric activity with controlled concentric and eccentric exercises throughout a progressively larger range of functional motion. The physiological rationale behind the exercises in this phase is to stimulate dynamic postural responses and to increase muscle stiffness. Muscle stiffness (see Chapter 4) has a significant role in improving dynamic stabilization around the joint by resisting and absorbing joint loads.[48]

■ *Dynamic stabilization exercises:* These exercises involve the unconscious control and loading of the joint, and introduce both ballistic and impact exercises to the patient.

A delicate balance between stability and mobility is achieved by coordination among muscle strength, endurance, flexibility, and neuromuscular control.[49]

The neuromuscular mechanism that contributes to joint stability is mediated by the articular mechanoreceptors. These receptors provide information about joint position sense and kinesthesia.[46,47,50,51] Initially, closed chain exercises are performed within the pain-free ranges or positions. Open chain exercises, including mild plyometric exercises (see "Plyometrics" later in this chapter), can be built upon the base of the closed chain stabilization to allow normal control of joint mobility.

The emphasis during these exercises is to concentrate on functional positioning during exercise rather than isolating open and closed chain activities.[49] The activities should involve sudden alterations in joint positioning that necessitate reflex muscular stabilization coupled with an axial load.[47,49] Such activities include rhythmic stabilization (an isometric contraction of the agonist followed by an isometric contraction of the antagonist) performed in both a closed and open chain position,[52] and in the functional position of the joint.[49] The use of a stable, and then unstable, base during closed chain exercises encourages co-contraction of the agonists and antagonists.[52]

Weight shifting exercises are ideal for this. For example, the following weight shifting exercises may be used for the upper extremity:

■ Standing and leaning against a treatment table or object.
■ In the quadruped position, rocking forward and backward with the hands on the floor or on an unstable object.
■ Kneeling forward in the three-point position (with one hand on the floor). A Body Blade can be added to this exercise to increase the difficulty.
■ Kneeling in the two-point position (high kneeling).
■ Weight shifting on a Fitter while in a kneeling position.
■ Weight shifting on a Swiss ball (see Key Point) with the feet on a chair, and both hands on the Swiss ball in the push-up position.
■ Slide board exercises in the quadruped position moving hands forwards and backwards, in opposite diagonals and in opposite directions.

Periodization

Periodization, a training method used for competitive athletes, consists of an organized and predictable approach to training volume, intensity, and rest periods during a specific period of time. Periodic training systems typically divide time into three cycles:

■ *Microcycle:* Generally up to 7 days. Accumulated microcycles form a mesocycle.
■ *Mesocycle:* May be anywhere from 2 weeks to a few months, but is typically a month. During the preparatory phase, a mesocycle commonly consists of 4–6 microcycles; during the competitive phase it will usually consist of 2–4 microcycles, depending on the competition's calendar.
■ *Macrocycle:* The overall training period, usually representing a year or two.

Using periodization, a competitive athlete is able to achieve peak physical performance at a particular point in time, such as for a major competition.

Although used for competitive athletes, the principles behind periodization can be adapted for the orthopedic population because the same training variables can be manipulated, including:[53]

- The number of sets per exercise
- The repetitions per set
- The types of exercises
- The number of exercises per training session
- The rest periods between sets and exercises
- The resistance used for a set
- The type and tempo of muscle action (e.g., eccentric, concentric, isometric)
- The number of training sessions per day and per week.

Table 10-1 outlines the various types of periodization, and **Table 10-2** outlines the use of periodization depending on the muscle fiber type.

TABLE 10-2	Periodization by Muscle Fiber Type			
	Hypertrophy	Strength and Hypertrophy	Strength	Transition
Sets	1–5	1–5	1–5	1–2
Reps	9–12 (type I, IIa)	6–8 (type IIa)	1–5 (type IIb)	13–20 (type I)
Weeks	2–3	2–3	2–3	1–2

Types of Resistance

Resistance can be applied to a muscle by any external force or mass, including any of the following:

- *Gravity:* Gravity alone can supply sufficient resistance with a weakened muscle. With respect to gravity, muscle actions may occur in:
  - ❏ The same direction of gravity (downward), requiring an eccentric contraction
  - ❏ The opposite direction to gravity (upward), requiring a concentric or isometric contraction
  - ❏ A direction perpendicular to gravity (horizontal), minimizing the effects of gravity and therefore appropriate for weaker muscles
  - ❏ The same or opposite direction as gravity, but at an angle requiring multi-planar concentric/eccentric contractions
- *Body weight:* A wide variety of exercises have been developed that use no equipment and instead rely on the patient's body weight for the resistance (push-up).
- *Small weights:* Cuff weights and dumbbells are economical ways of applying a constant resistance. Small weights are typically used to strengthen the smaller muscles or to increase the endurance of larger muscles by increasing the number of reps. Free weights also provide more versatility than exercise machines, especially for three-dimensional exercises.

● **Key Point** Free weights offer no variable resistance throughout the range of motion, so the weakest point along the length–tension curve of each muscle limits the amount of weight lifted. This factor can be used for those patients in the early stages of rehabilitation who cannot move through the full range of motion using a variable resistance.

- *Surgical tubing/Theraband:* Elastic resistance offers a unique type of resistance because the amount of variable resistance offered by elastic

TABLE 10-1	Periodization Models	
Model	**Description**	
Traditional	Volume and intensity are systematically manipulated. Training cycle begins with a high-volume, low-intensity profile, then progresses to low-volume, high-intensity over time.	
Step wise	Like the traditional model, intensity increases and volume decreases during the training period. Volume is decreased in a stepwise fashion: Repetitions are reduced from eight to five, five to three, and so forth, at specific time intervals.	
Undulating	Training volume and intensity increase and decrease on a regular basis, but do not follow the traditional pattern of increasing intensity and decreasing volume as the mesocycle progresses.	
Overreaching	Volume or intensity is increased for a short period of time (1 to 2 weeks), followed by a return to "normal" training. This method is used primarily with advanced athletes.	

bands or tubing depends on the internal tension produced by the material. This internal tension is a factor of the elastic material's coefficient of elasticity, the surface area of the elastic material, and how much the elastic material is stretched.[54]

● Key Point It is commonly believed that the resistance provided by bands or tubing increases exponentially at the end range of motion. However, the forces produced by elastic resistance are linear until approximately 500 percent elongation, at which point the forces increase exponentially.[54] As a result, Theraband exercises have their limitations, especially in cases when the resistance is greater in those ranges where the muscle tends to be weaker (near end ranges).

■ *Exercise machines:* In situations where the larger muscle groups require strengthening, a multitude of specific indoor exercise machines can be used. These machines are often used in the more advanced stages of a rehabilitation program when more resistance can be tolerated, but they can also be used in the earlier stages depending on the size of the muscle undergoing rehabilitation. Examples of these machines include the multi-hip, the lat pull-down, the leg extension, and the leg curl machines. Exercise machines are often fitted with an oval-shaped cam or wheel that mimics the length of tension curve of the muscle (e.g., Nautilus, Cybex). Although these machines are a more expensive alternative to dumbbell or elastic resistance, they do offer some advantages:
  ❏ Provide more adequate resistance for large muscle groups than can be achieved with free weights/cuff weights or manual resistance
  ❏ Typically safer than free weights, because they provide control throughout the range.
  ❏ Provide the clinician with the ability to quantify and measure the amount of resis. tance the patient can tolerate over time.
  The disadvantages of exercise machines include:
  ❏ The inability to modify the exercise to be more functional or three-dimensional
  ❏ The inability to modify the amount of resistance at particular points of the range
■ *Manual resistance:* A type of active exercise in which another person provides resistance manually. An example of manual resistance is proprioceptive neuromuscular facilitation (PNF). The advantages of manual resistance, when applied by a skilled clinician, are:[55]
  ❏ Control of the extremity position and force applied. This is especially useful in the early

stages of an exercise program when the muscle is weak.
  ❏ More effective re-education of the muscle or extremity through the use of diagonal or functional patterns of movement.
  ❏ Critical sensory input to the patient through tactile stimulation and appropriate facilitation techniques (e.g., quick stretch).
  ❏ Accurate accommodation and alterations in the resistance applied throughout the range; for example, an exercise can be modified to avoid a painful arc in the range.
  ❏ Ability to limit the range. This is particularly important when the amount of range of motion needs to be carefully controlled (postsurgical restrictions or pain).
  The disadvantages of manual resistance include:
  ❏ The amount of resistance applied cannot be measured quantitatively.
  ❏ The amount of resistance is limited by the strength of the clinician/caregiver or family member.
  ❏ No consistency of the applied force throughout the range, and with each repetition.

● Key Point Water can be used as a form of resistance (see Chapter 7). Water provides resistance proportional to the relative speed of movement of the patient and the water and the cross-sectional area of the patient in contact with the water.[56]

Considerations for Strength Training

The greatest amount of tension the muscle can achieve is a 20 percent increase in fiber length measured from the resting length.[57] The clinical implications for this are that the patient can tolerate less resistance in the beginning and at the end of range of a contraction, but can overcome more resistance at a point in the range 20 percent beyond resting contraction.[58]

● Key Point At regular intervals, the clinician should ensure that:
• The patient is adhering to their exercise program at home.
• The patient is aware of the rationale behind the exercise program.
• The patient is performing the exercise program correctly and at the appropriate intensity.
• The patient's exercise program is being updated appropriately based on the functional short- and long-term goals in the plan of care.

A number of precautions must be observed with patients who are performing strength training:

■ *Substitute motions:* Muscles that are weak or fatigued rely on other muscles to produce the movement if the resistance is too high. This results in incorrect stabilization and poor form.

■ *Overworking of the muscles:* This can occur if the exercise parameters (frequency, intensity, duration) are advanced too quickly. Some of the signs of an overloaded muscle include decreased performance and muscle substitutions/compensations. Generally, 24 hours of rest are recommended in between bouts of strength exercise to a particular region to prevent overwork.

■ *Adequate rest:* The patient must rest after each set of vigorous exercise. (Three to four minutes are needed to return the muscle to 90 to 95 percent of pre-exercise capacity, with the most rapid recovery occurring in the first minute.) The rest period between sets can be determined by how long it takes the breathing rate or pulse of the patient to return to the steady state.

Caution must be taken with patients diagnosed with osteoporosis whose bones are unable to withstand normal stresses and are highly susceptible to pathological fracture. Osteoporotic fractures may also occur as a result of prolonged immobilization, bed rest, the inability to bear weight on an extremity, and nutritional or hormonal factors. Other patient populations that require close monitoring include:

■ Patients with an acute illness/fever
■ Patients with an acute injury
■ Postsurgical patients
■ Patients with cardiac/ pulmonary disease (e.g., edema, weight gain, unstable angina)
■ Patients who are obese
■ Patients with diabetes

Strengthening Exercise Programs
Contraindications to Strength Training

Absolute contraindications to strength training include unstable angina, uncontrolled hypertension, uncontrolled dysrhythmias, hypertrophic cardiomyopathy, and certain stages of retinopathy.

Patients with congestive heart failure, myocardial ischemia, poor left ventricular function, or autonomic neuropathies must be carefully evaluated before initiating a strength-training program. A number of programs, however, have been designed for the progression of concentric exercise programs.

Progressive Resistive Exercise

DeLorme[8] introduced a concept called *repetition maximum* (RM) or the greatest amount of weight a muscle can move through the range of motion a specific number of times. One repetition maximum (1 RM) is the maximum amount of weight one person can lift in a single repetition for a given exercise. This is based on the premise that to achieve an increase in the total number of repetitions while maintaining a sufficient effort, the number of sets must also be increased. This increase in sets must occur in conjunction with a reduction in the number of repetitions per set by 10–20 percent,[58] or a reduction in the resistance.

The various programs that utilize the RM concept are summarized in **Table 10-3**.

■ The DeLorme PRE protocol uses three sets of 10 repetitions of resistance after the patient has established a maximum weight that can be lifted for 10 repetitions (10 RM—repetitions maximum). In the first set, the patient uses

TABLE 10-3	The DeLorme, Oxford, and DAPRE (Knight) Exercise Progressions		
	Set(s) of 10	Amount of Weight	Repetitions
DeLorme program (PREs)	1st	50% of 10 RM	10
	2nd	75% of 10 RM	10
	3rd	100% of 10 RM	10
Oxford technique	1st	100% of 10 RM	10
	2nd	75% of 10 RM	10
	3rd	50% of 10 RM	10
DAPRE program	1st	50% of RM	10
	2nd	75% of RM	6
	3rd	100% of RM	Maximum
	4th	Adjusted working weight	Maximum

DAPRE, daily adjustable progressive resistive exercise; RM, repetition maximum.

50 percent of the 10 RM, 75 percent in the second set, and 100 percent of the 10 RM in the third set. In this protocol, the progressive overload occurs by adding resistance.

- The Oxford program begins by establishing the patient's 10 RM. The first set of 10 repetitions is then performed using 100 percent of the 10 RM. The second set is performed at 75 percent of the 10 RM, and the third set is at 50 percent of the established 10 RM. In this protocol, the load is reduced as the session progresses.
- The daily adjustable progressive resistance exercise (DAPRE) protocol uses four sets with variable repetition after establishing the patient's 6 RM. The first set of 10 repetitions is

then performed using 50 percent of the 6 RM. The second set consists of six repetitions at 75 percent of the 6 RM, and the third set consists of as many repetitions as possible at 100 percent of the established 6 RM. The number of repetitions performed in this set is used to determine the weight used in the fourth set, with the patient again performing as many repetitions as possible with this weight. The goal of this protocol is to increase the number of repetitions in the third set, resulting in an increase in weight for the fourth set. The DAPRE adjusted working weight guide is outlined in **Table 10-4**. Two other protocols of note that use the concept of the RM are outlined in **Table 10-5**.

TABLE 10-4   Adjustment Sequence for DAPRE Concentric Program

First Set (at 50% of working weight based on 6 RM)	Second Set (at 75% of working weight)	Third Set (at working weight)	Fourth Set	Next Exercise Session
10 reps	6 reps	As many reps as possible	The adjusted working weight for the fourth set is based on the number of reps in the third set. 0 – 2 = –5 – 10 lb. 3 – 4 = –0 – 5 lb. 5 – 6 = Same weight 7 – 10 = +5 – 10 lb. 11 = +10 – 20 lb.	The next exercise session is based on the number of reps in the fourth set. 0 – 2 = –5 – 10 lb. 3 – 4 = Same weight 5 – 6 = +5 – 10 lb. 7 – 10 = +5 – 15 lb. 11 = +10–20 lb.

TABLE 10-5   The McQueen Technique and the Sander Program

	Sets	Resistance	Repetitions
McQueen technique	3 (beginning/intermediate)	100% of 10 RM	10
	4–5 (advanced)	100% of 2–3 RM	2–3
Sander program	Total of 4 sets (3 times per week)	100% of 5 RM	5
	Day 1: 4 sets	100% of 5 RM	5
	Day 2: 4 sets	100% of 3 RM	5
	Day 3: 1 set	100% of 5 RM	5
	2 sets	100% of 3 RM	5
	2 sets	100% of 2 RM	5

Circuit Training

The term *circuit* refers to a number of carefully selected exercises arranged consecutively. In the original format, 9–12 stations comprised the circuit, but this number may vary according to the circuit's design. Each circuit training participant moves from one station to the next with little (15–30 seconds) or no rest, performing a 15- to 45-second workout of 8–20 repetitions at each station (using a resistance of about 40–60 percent of one repetition maximum [1 RM]). The circuit training workout program may be performed with exercise machines, handheld weights, elastic resistance, calisthenics, or any combination of these. Commonly prescribed exercises for circuit training include bench press, seated row, leg press, seated press, lat pull-down, upright row, leg extension, leg curl, triceps push-down, arm curl, and an abdominal exercise (crunch).

> ● **Key Point** When a 30-second to 3-minute (or longer) aerobics station is added between stations, an aerobic circuit is created. The aim of adding an aerobic circuit is to improve cardiorespiratory endurance as well (although this has not been conclusively supported in experimental research).

Interval Training

Interval training includes an exercise period followed by a prescribed rest interval. It is perceived to be less demanding than continuous training and tends to improve strength and power more than endurance. With appropriate spacing of work and rest intervals, a significant amount of high intensity work can be achieved and is greater than the amount of work accomplished with continuous training. The longer the work interval, the more the anaerobic system is stressed and the duration of the rest interval (a period of low load work rather than actual rest) is not important.

> ● **Key Point** In a short work interval, a work recovery ratio of 1:1 or 1:5 is appropriate to stress the aerobic system.

Tabata Protocol

The Tabata protocol sequence is a high-intensity training regimen involving an interval training cycle of 20 seconds of maximum intensity exercise, followed by 10 seconds of rest, repeated without pause eight times for a total of 4 minutes (14 minutes when including a 5-minute warm-up and a 5-minute cool-down).[59] A study by Tabata showed that moderate-intensity aerobic training that improves the maximal aerobic power does not change anaerobic capacity, and that adequate high-intensity intermittent training may improve both anaerobic and aerobic energy-supplying systems significantly, probably through imposing intensive stimuli on both systems.[59]

Maintaining Strength

In order to maintain the benefits of training, exercise must be maintained. Based on studies of isokinetic and concentric exercise:[60,61]

- The regaining of muscle strength follows a steady and predictable increase over time.[32]
- A lack of training results in decreased muscle recruitment and muscle fiber atrophy (reversibility).
- If an injured patient can maintain some form of strength training, even once per week, their strength can be fairly well maintained over a 3-month period.[62]

> ● **Key Point** When expressed as a weekly percentage, the Albert 5 percent rule states that a 5 percent strength increase in a given week can be maintained for many weeks of resistive training providing that the patient trains three times a week at a minimum resistance load of 70 percent of maximal voluntary muscle contractile force.[32] Although seemingly esoteric, the 5 percent rule can be used in determining the prognosis. For example, a patient with a 40 percent deficit in strength of the biceps can be assumed to take approximately 8 weeks to recover, barring any illness or disease states.[32]

Improving Muscular and Cardiorespiratory Endurance

To increase muscle endurance, exercises are performed against light resistance for many repetitions, so that the amount of energy expended is equal to the amount of energy supplied. This phenomenon, called *steady state*, occurs after some 5 to 6 minutes of exercise at a constant intensity level. Working at a level to which the muscle is accustomed improves the endurance of that muscle, but does not increase its strength. However, exercise programs that increase strength also increase muscular endurance. Muscular endurance programs are typically indicated early in a strengthening program because the high repetition and low load exercises are more comfortable, enhance the vascular supply to muscle, cause less muscle soreness and joint irritation, and reduce the risk of muscle injury.

By definition, cardiorespiratory endurance is the ability to perform whole body activities (e.g., walking, jogging, biking, swimming) for extended periods of time without undue fatigue. A number of adaptations occur within the circulatory system in response to exercise:

■ *Heart rate:* Monitoring heart rate is an indirect method of estimating oxygen consumption because, in general, these two factors have a linear relationship. If a physical therapy intervention requires an increase in systemic oxygen consumption expressed as either an increase in metabolic equivalent unit (MET) levels, kilocalories, or VO_2 max, then heart rate (HR) also should increase.[63]

● **Key Point** The magnitude at which the HR increases with increasing workloads is influenced by many factors including age, fitness level, type of activity being performed, presence of disease, medications, blood volume, and environmental factors such as temperature, humidity, and altitude. Failure of the heart rate to increase with increasing workloads (chronotropic incompetence) should be of concern for the PTA, even if the patient is taking beta-blockers. Beta blockers slow the HR, which can prevent the increase in heart rate that typically occurs with exercise.[63]

■ *Stroke volume:* The volume of blood being pumped out by the left ventricle of the heart with each beat increases with exercise, but only to the point at which there is enough time between beats for the heart to fill up (approximately 110–120 beats per minute). The heart does not pump all the blood out of the ventricle—normally, only about two-thirds. In the normal heart, as workload increases, stroke volume (SV) increases linearly up to 50 percent of aerobic capacity, after which it increases only slightly. Factors that influence the magnitude of change in SV include ventricular function, body position, and exercise intensity.
■ *Cardiac output:* Cardiac output (CO), the product of HR and SV, increases linearly with workload because of the increases in HR and SV in response to increasing exercise intensity. CO is the amount of blood discharged by each ventricle (not both ventricles combined) per minute, usually expressed as liters per

minute. Factors that influence the magnitude of change in CO include age, posture, body size, presence of disease, and level of physical conditioning.

● **Key Point** A long-term beneficial training effect that occurs with regard to cardiac output of the heart is that the stroke volume increases while the exercise heart rate is reduced at a given standard exercise load.

■ *Blood pressure:* Blood pressure, a product of cardiac output and peripheral vascular resistance, is defined as the pressure exerted by the blood on the walls of the blood vessels, specifically *arterial blood pressure* (the pressure in the large arteries). Systolic pressure increases in proportion to oxygen consumption and cardiac output, whereas diastolic pressure shows little or no increase. Long-term aerobic training can result in reduced systolic and diastolic pressure.

● **Key Point** The normal blood pressure response is to observe a progressive increase in systolic blood pressure with no change or even a slight decrease in diastolic blood pressure. A failure of the systolic blood pressure to rise with an increase in intensity (called exertional hypotension) is considered abnormal and may occur in patients with a number of cardiovascular problems. The slight decrease in diastolic blood pressure is due primarily to the vasodilation of the arteries from the exercise bout. Thus, the expansion in artery size may lower blood pressure during the diastolic phase.[63]

■ *Mitochondria:* An increase in size and number of mitochondria.
■ *Hemoglobin concentration:* The concentration of hemoglobin in circulating blood does not change with training; it may actually decrease slightly.
■ *Myoglobin:* Increased myoglobin content.
■ *Fat and carbohydrates:* Improved mobilization and use of fat and carbohydrates.
■ *Lungs:* Lung changes that occur due to exercise include the following:
  ❑ An increase in the volume of air that can be inspired in a single maximal ventilation. Ventilation is the process of air exchange in the lungs.
  ❑ An increase in the diffusing capacity of the lungs.
  ❑ Oxygen consumption rises rapidly during the first minutes of exercise and levels off as the aerobic metabolism supplies the energy required by the working muscles.

Precautions with Aerobic Conditioning

Conditioned individuals have a cardiovascular and pulmonary system that is more capable of delivering oxygen to sustain aerobic energy production at increasingly higher levels of intensity. However, in cases of severe pulmonary disease, the cost of breathing can reach 40 percent of the total exercise oxygen consumption, thereby decreasing the amount of oxygen available for the exercising muscles. A number of precautions need to be taken when exercising patients who have a compromised cardiovascular or pulmonary system. First, an appropriate level of intensity must be chosen. Too high a level can overload the cardiorespiratory and muscular systems and potentially cause injuries. Exercising at this level causes the cardiorespiratory system to work anaerobically, not aerobically. Initially the patient should be exercising so that their heart rate is at 60 percent of his or her maximum (220 – age of patient). If the patient is exercising within their target heart rate, they should be able to carry on a conversation (talk test). A sufficient period of time should be allowed for warm-up and cool-down to permit adequate cardiorespiratory and muscular adaptation.

● **Key Point** Obese individuals should exercise at longer durations and lower intensities.

Techniques for Improving, Maintaining, and Monitoring Cardiorespiratory Endurance

Several different training factors must be considered when attempting to maintain or improve cardiorespiratory endurance. For continuous training, use the FITT (frequency, intensity, type of exercise, and time) principle:

- *Frequency:* To see at least minimal improvement in cardiorespiratory endurance, it is necessary for the average person to engage in no less than three sessions per week. If the intensity is kept constant, there appears to be no additional benefit from exercising more times per week.
- *Intensity:* Recommendations regarding training intensity (overload) vary. Relative intensity for an individual is calculated as a percentage of the maximum function, using VO_2 max or maximum heart rate (HR max). To see minimal improvement in cardiorespiratory endurance, the average person must train with a heart rate elevated to at least 60 percent of his or her maximum HR max. Three common methods of monitoring intensity are employed:
  - ❑ *Monitoring heart rate:* Two formulas are commonly used to monitor heart rate. The Karvonen equation[64] (220 – age) uses the difference between the MHR and the resting heart rate (RHR), referred to as the maximum heart rate reserve. When using this formula, the recommended intensity level range is 50 to 85 percent of VO_2 max. For example, for a 50-year-old with a resting heart rate of 65 bpm who wants to train at an intensity of 70 percent:

    220 – 50 = 170 bpm (maximum heart rate)
    170 – 65 = 105 bpm (maximum heart rate reserve)
    (105 × 0.7) + 65 = 139 bpm

    The age-adjusted maximum heart rate (AAMHR) is calculated using the same formula (220 – age); however, the recommended level of intensity when using this formula is a range between 60 percent and 90 percent of an individual's maximum heart rate. For example, for a 50-year-old the MHR is 220 – 50 = 170. Therefore, the target heart range is between 170 × 0.6 and 170 × 0.9 (102 to 153 bpm).
  - ❑ *Borg rating of perceived exertion (RPE):* A cardiorespiratory training effect can be achieved at a rating of "somewhat hard" or "hard" (13 to 16 on the scale; refer to Table 8-2 in Chapter 8).
  - ❑ *Calculating the VO_2 max or HR directly or indirectly:* This can be done using a 3-minute step test, a 12-minute run, or a 1-mile walk test.
- *Type of exercise:* The type of activity chosen in continuous training must be aerobic, involving large muscle groups activated in a rhythmic manner.
- *Time (duration):* For minimal improvement to occur, the patient must participate in continuous activity with a heart rate elevated to its working level. Three to five minutes per day produces a training effect in poorly conditioned individuals, whereas 20 to 30 minutes, three to five times a week is optimal for conditioned people.

Aerobic Conditioning Programs

Two main types of aerobic conditioning training exist:

- *Continuous training:* Exercise is performed for 20 to 60 minutes with no rest interval at a submaximal energy requirement, and little variation in heart rate. A number of pieces of exercise equipment can be used with continuous training:
  - ❏ *Treadmill walking:* Progressing from slow to fast and short distances to longer distances with or without an incline.
  - ❏ *Ergometers:* These come in a variety of forms for both the upper extremities and the lower extremities. The pace progression is from slow to fast and the goal is to increase the time spent exercising.
  - ❏ *Free weights and elastic resistance:* The use of low resistance and high repetitions can produce an aerobic effect.
- *Discontinuous training:* This type of training, also known as interval training, involves the use of repeated high-intensity exercise bouts that are interspersed with rest intervals. Although endurance levels can be improved with this method, more benefits are seen in the development of strength and power.

Improving Muscle Power

It has been demonstrated that when a concentric contraction is preceded by a phase of active or passive stretching, elastic energy is stored in the muscle. This stored energy is then used in the following contractile phase. During functional activities, the muscles operate with a strong concentric action, which is usually preceded by a *passive* eccentric loading, as part of a stretch shortening cycle.[10] For example, before producing a vertical leap, the Achilles tendon and gastrocnemius muscle undergo a passive eccentric load, before eliciting a strong concentric contraction. The stretch shortening cycle includes the ability of the muscle to absorb or dissipate shock, while also preparing the stretched muscle for response.[65] Plyometric exercises, described next are used to improve the ability of the muscles to perform these actions, by enhancing their power, speed, and agility.

Having a muscle work dynamically against resistance within a specified period increases power. For power development, one to three sets of 30–60 percent of 1 RM for three to six repetitions should be incorporated in the intermediate program. In the context of rehabilitation, plyometric training is the bridge between strength and power exercises.[66]

Plyometrics

The traditional definition of plyometrics was associated with quick rapid movement involving a prestretch of the contracting muscle, which stores elastic energy in the muscle and activates the myotatic reflex.[67–70] The muscle's ability to use the stored elastic energy is affected by time, the magnitude of the stretch, and the velocity of the stretch.[71]

> **● Key Point** The nerve receptors involved in plyometrics are the muscle spindle, the Golgi tendon organ, and the joint capsule/ligamentous receptors (see Chapter 2).

Movement patterns in both athletics and activities of daily living (ADLs) involve repeated stretch shortening cycles, where a downward eccentric movement must be stopped and converted into an upward concentric movement in a desired direction. The degree of enhanced muscle performance is dependent upon the time frame between the eccentric and concentric contractions.[70]

Acceleration and deceleration are the most important components of all task-specific activities.[58] These activities utilize variable speed and resistance throughout the range of contraction, stimulating neurological receptors and increasing their excitability. These neurological receptors play an important role in fiber recruitment and physiologic coordination. A plyometric exercise, such as jumping and landing using one foot (Figure 10-2),

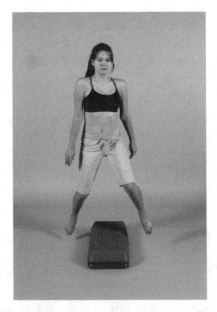

Figure 10-2   Plyometric exercise with one leg.

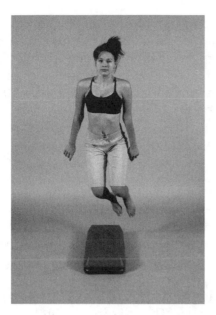

Figure 10-3 Plyometric exercise with both legs.

then both feet (Figure 10-3), serves to improve the reactivity of these receptors by involving muscle stretch-shortening exercises, and consists of three distinct phases:

- A setting or eccentric phase in which the muscle is eccentrically stretched and slowly loaded.[71]
- A rapid amortization (reversal) phase, which is the amount of time between undergo ing the yielding eccentric contraction and the initiation of a concentric force.[71] If the amortization phase is slow, the stretch reflex is not activated.[71]
- A concentric response contraction to develop a large amount of momentum and force.

By reproducing these stretch-shortening cycles at positions of physiologic function, plyometric activities stimulate proprioceptive feedback to fine-tune muscle activity patterns. Stretch-shortening exercise trains the neuromuscular system by exposing it to increased strength loads and improving the stretch reflex.[71]

The goal of plyometric training is to decrease the amount of time required between the yielding eccentric contraction (landing) and the initiation of the overcoming concentric contraction (taking-off). This is particularly useful in activities that require a maximum amount of muscular force in a minimum amount of time. These parameters are difficult to imitate using traditional exercise tools, but are nonetheless a very important component of the rehabilitative process in order for the patient to make a safe return to sport.

Because plyometrics involves ballistic, high velocity movement patterns, before initiating plyometric exercises, the clinician must ensure that the patient has an adequate strength and physical condition base.[71] Minimal performance criteria for safe plyometrics include the ability to perform one repetition of a parallel squat with a load of body weight on the subject's back (for jumps over 12 inches) for the lower extremity, and a bench press with one-third body weight for the upper extremity.[66] In addition, success in the static stability tests[66] and dynamic stability tests (vertical jump for the lower extremities and medicine ball throw for the upper extremities) may be used as a measure of preparation.[32]

Many different activities and devices can be utilized in plyometric exercises. Plyometric exercises can include diagonal and multiplanar motions with tubing or isokinetic machines. These exercises can be used to mimic any of the needed motions and can be performed in the standing, sitting, prone, or supine positions.

Lower Extremity Plyometric Exercises

Lower extremity plyometric exercises involve the manipulation of the role of gravity to vary the intensity of the exercise. Thus, plyometric exercises can be performed horizontally or vertically.

Horizontal plyometrics are performed perpendicular to the line of gravity. These exercises are preferable for most initial clinical rehabilitation plans because the concentric force is reduced, and the eccentric phase is not facilitated.[32] Examples of these types of exercises include pushing a sled against resistance, and a modified leg press that allows the subject to push off and land on the footplate.

Vertical plyometric exercises (against or with gravitational forces) are more advanced. These exercises require a greater level of control.[32] The drop jump is an example—the subject steps off a box, lands, and immediately executes a vertical jump.

The footwear and landing surfaces used in plyometric drills must have shock-absorbing qualities, and the protocol should allow sufficient recovery time between sets to prevent fatigue of the muscle groups being trained.[72]

Upper Extremity Plyometric Exercises

Plyometric exercises for the upper extremities involve relatively rapid movements in planes that approximate normal joint function. For example, at the shoulder this would include 90-degree abduction in shoulder, trunk rotation, and diagonal arm motions, and rapid external/internal rotation exercises.

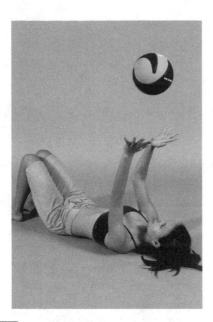

Figure 10-4 Upper extremity plyometric exercise.

Plyometrics should be done for all body segments involved in the activity. Plyometric exercises for the upper extremity include wall push-offs, corner push-ups, box push-offs, the rebounder, and weighted ball throws using medicine (Figure 10-4) and other weighted balls. (The weight of the ball creates a pre-stretch and an eccentric load when it is caught, creating resistance and demanding a powerful agonist contraction to propel it forward again.) The exercises can be performed using one arm or both arms at the same time. The former emphasizes trunk rotation whereas the latter emphasizes trunk extension and flexion, as well as shoulder motion. Although force-dependent motor firing patterns should be re-established, special care must be taken to completely integrate all of the components of the kinetic chain to generate and funnel the proper forces to the appropriate joint.

> **● Key Point**   In general, tonic muscles (e.g., the psoas, erector spinae, upper trapezius) function as endurance (postural) muscles, whereas phasic muscles (e.g., gluteals, triceps, tibialis anterior) function as the power muscles.[73,74]

Summary

Functional strength is the ability of the neuromuscular system to perform the various types of contractions involved with multijoint functional activities in an efficient manner and in a multiplanar environment.[75] Therapeutic exercises must be progressed to include combinations of concentric and eccentric contractions in the performance of activities that relate to a patient's needs and requirements. Effective rehabilitation targets specific muscles with regard to functional muscle activity patterns and overall conditioning, and utilizes a progression of increased activity, while preventing further trauma.[76] Incremental gains in function should be seen as strength increases.

REVIEW Questions

1. What type of contraction occurs when tension is produced in the muscle without any appreciable change in muscle length or joint movement?
2. What type of contraction occurs when a muscle slowly lengthens as it gives in to an external force that is greater than the contractile force it is exerting?
3. Of the three types of muscle actions, isometric, concentric, and eccentric, which one is capable of developing the most force?
4. What are the four biomechanical properties that human skeletal muscle possesses?
5. True or false: Rapid lengthening contractions generate less force than do slower lengthening contractions.
6. Give two disadvantages of isometric exercise.
7. To facilitate muscle control, what is the best way to first exercise the postural (or extensor) musculature when it is extremely weak?
   a. Eccentric exercises
   b. Isometric exercises
   c. Isokinetic exercises
   d. Electrical stimulation
8. What are the four parameters of exercise?
9. What is the best gauge of exercise intensity in a healthy individual?
   a. Blood pressure
   b. Heart rate
   c. Rating of perceived exertion
   d. Rate of perspiration
10. You ask a patient to assess his level of exertion using the Borg rating of perceived exertion (RPE). The patient rates the level of exertion as 9 on the 6–19 scale. A rating of 9 corresponds to which of the following?
    a. Very, very light
    b. Hard
    c. Very light
    d. Somewhat hard

11. The optimal exercise prescription to improve fast movement speeds and enhance endurance (improving fast-twitch fiber function) is:

   a. Low intensity workloads for short durations

   b. High intensity workloads for short durations

   c. Low intensity workloads for long durations

   d. High intensity workloads for long durations

12. A 35-year-old presents with a prescription to improve aerobic conditioning. Which of the following is not a benefit of aerobic exercise?

   a. Improved cardiovascular fitness

   b. Increased high-density lipoprotein (HDL) cholesterol

   c. Improved flexibility

   d. Improved state of mind

13. A high school coach asks you which is the best type of exercise to improve an athlete's vertical jump. Which of the following exercise types would be the best to achieve this goal?

   a. Closed chain

   b. Open chain

   c. Plyometrics

   d. DeLorme's

References

1. Kisner C, Colby LA: Resistance exercise for impaired muscle performance, in Kisner C, Colby LA (eds): Therapeutic Exercise. Foundations and Techniques (ed 5). Philadelphia, FA Davis, 2002, pp 147–229
2. Matsen FA, III, Lippitt SB, Sidles JA, et al: Strength, in Matsen FA, III, Lippitt SB, Sidles JA, et al (eds): Practical Evaluation and Management of the Shoulder. Philadelphia, WB Saunders, 1994, pp 111–150
3. Komi PV: Strength and Power in Sport. London, Blackwell Scientific Publications, 1992
4. McArdle W, Katch, FI, Katch, VL: Exercise Physiology: Energy, Nutrition, and Human Performance. Philadelphia, Lea and Febiger, 1991
5. Kisner C, Colby LA: Therapeutic Exercise. Foundations and Techniques. Philadelphia, FA Davis, 1997
6. Astrand PO, Rodahl K: The Muscle and Its Contraction: Textbook of Work Physiology. New York, McGraw-Hill, 1986
7. Astrand PO, Rodahl K: Physical Training: Textbook of Work Physiology. New York, McGraw-Hill, 1986
8. DeLorme T, Watkins A: Techniques of Progressive Resistance Exercise. New York, Appleton-Century, 1951
9. Soest A, Bobbert M: The role of muscle properties in control of explosive movements. Biol Cybern 69:195–204, 1993
10. Komi PV: The stretch-shortening cycle and human power output, in Jones NL, McCartney N, McComas AJ (eds): Human Muscle Power. Champaign, IL, Human Kinetics, 1986, pp 27–39
11. Bandy W, Lovelace-Chandler V, Bandy B, et al: Adaptation of skeltal muscle to resistance training. J Orthop Sports Phys Ther 12:248–255, 1990
12. Hislop HJ: Quantitative changes in human muscular strength during isometric exercise. J Am Phys Ther Assoc 43:21–38, 1963
13. Knapik JJ, Mawdsley RH, Ramos MU: Angular specificity and test mode specificity of isometric and isokinetic strength training. J Orthop Sports Phys Ther 5:58–65, 1983
14. Davies GJ: Compendium of Isokinetics in Clinical Usage and Rehabilitation Techniques (ed 4). Onalaska, WI, S & S Publishers, 1992
15. Albert MS: Principles of exercise progression, in Greenfield B (ed): Rehabilitation of the Knee: A Problem Solving Approach. Philadelphia, FA Davis, 1993, pp 110–136
16. Lakomy HKA: The biomechanics of human movement, in Maughan RJ (ed): Basic and Applied Sciences for Sports Medicine. Woburn, MA, Butterworth-Heinemann, 1999, pp 124–125
17. Verrall GM, Slavotinek JP, Barnes PG, et al: Clinical risk factors for hamstring muscle strain injury: A prospective study with correlation of injury by magnetic resonance imaging. Br J Sports Med 35:435–439, 2001
18. Elftman H: Biomechanics of muscle. J Bone Joint Surg 48A:363, 1966
19. Albert MS: Eccentric Muscle Training in Sports and Orthopedics (ed 2). New York, Churchill Livingstone, 1995
20. Dean E: Physiology and therapeutic implications of negative work. A review. Phys Ther 68:233–237, 1988
21. Rothstein JM, Lamb RL, Mayhew TP: Clinical uses of isokinetic measurements. Critical issues. Phys Ther 67:1840–1844, 1987
22. Canavan PK: Designing a rehabilitation program related to strength and conditioning, in Wilmarth MA (ed): Orthopaedic Physical Therapy: Strength and Conditioning, Independent Study Course 15.3. La Crosse, WI, Orthopaedic Section, American Physical Therapy Association, 2005
23. Byrnes WC, Clarkson PM, White JS, et al: Delayed onset muscle soreness following repeated bouts of downhill running. J Appl Physiol 59:710, 1985
24. Bennett M, Best TM, Babul S, et al: Hyperbaric oxygen therapy for delayed onset muscle soreness and closed soft tissue injury. Cochrane Database Syst Rev. CD004713, 2005
25. Cheung K, Hume P, Maxwell L: Delayed onset muscle soreness: Treatment strategies and performance factors. Sports Med 33:145–164, 2003
26. Nureberg P, Giddings CJ, Stray-Gundersen J, et al: MR imaging-guided muscle biopsy for correlation of increased signal intensity with ultrastructural change and delayed-onset muscle soreness after exercise. Radiology 184:865–869, 1992
27. Friden J: Delayed onset muscle soreness. Scand J Med Sci Sports 12:327–328, 2002
28. Friden J, Sjostrom M, Ekblom B: Myofibrillar damage following intense eccentric exercise in man. Int J Sports Med 4:170–176, 1983
29. Cafarelli E, Flint F: The role of massage in preparation for and recovery from exercise. Sports Med 14:1–9, 1992
30. Callaghan MJ: The role of massage in the management of the athlete: A review. Br J Sports Med. 27:28–33, 1993

31. Tiidus PM, Shoemaker JK: Effleurage massage, muscle blood flow and long-term post-exercise strength recovery. Int J Sports Med 16:475–483, 1995

32. Albert M: Concepts of muscle training, in Wadsworth C (ed): Orthopaedic Physical Therapy: Strength and Conditioning Applications in Orthopaedics, Home Study Course 98A. La Crosse, WI, Orthopaedic Section, American Physical Therapy Association, 1998

33. Hasson S, Barnes W, Hunter M, et al: Therapeutic effect of high speed voluntary muscle contractions on muscle soreness and muscle performance. J Orthop Sports Phys Ther 10:499, 1989

34. Worrell TW, Perrin DH, Gansneder B, et al: Comparison of isokinetic strength and flexibility measures between hamstring injured and non-injured athletes. J Orthop Sports Phys Ther 13:118–125, 1991

35. Anderson MA, Gieck JH, Perrin D, et al: The relationship among isometric, isotonic, and isokinetic concentric and eccentric quadriceps and hamstrings force and three components of athletic performance. J Orthop Sports Phys Ther 14:114–120, 1991

36. Steadman JR, Forster RS, Silfverskold JP: Rehabilitation of the knee. Clin Sports Med 8:605–627, 1989

37. Montgomery JB, Steadman JR: Rehabilitation of the injured knee. Clin Sports Med 4:333–343, 1985

38. Delsman PA, Losee GM: Isokinetic shear forces and their effect on the quadriceps active drawer. Med Sci Sports Exerc 16:151, 1984

39. Chaitow L: An introduction to muscle energy techniques, in Chaitow L (ed): Muscle Energy Techniques (ed 2). London, Churchill Livingstone, 2001, pp 1–18

40. Voight M, Blackburn T: Proprioception and balance training and testing following injury, in Ellenbecker TS (ed): Knee Ligament Rehabilitation. Philadelphia, Churchill Livingstone, 2000, pp 361–385

41. Voight ML, Cook G: Impaired neuromuscular control: Reactive neuromuscular training, in Prentice WE, Voight ML (eds): Techniques in Musculoskeletal Rehabilitation. New York, McGraw-Hill, 2001, pp 93–124

42. Jerosch J, Prymka M: Propriozeptive Fahigkeiten des gesunden Kniegelenks: Beeinflussung durch eine elastische Bandage. Sportverletz Sportsch 9:72–76, 1995

43. Jerosch J, Hoffstetter I, Bork H, et al: The influence of orthoses on the proprioception of the ankle joint. Knee Surg Sports Traumatol Arthrosc 3:39–46, 1995

44. Perlau R, Frank C, Fick G: The effect of elastic bandages on human knee proprioception in the uninjured population. Am J Sports Med 23:251–255, 1995

45. Robbins S, Waked E, Rappel R: Ankle taping improves proprioception before and after exercise in young men. Br J Sports Med 29:242–247, 1995

46. Barrett DS: Proprioception and function after anterior cruciate ligament reconstruction. J Bone Joint Surg 73B:833–837, 1991

47. Lephart SM, Pincivero DM, Giraldo JL, et al: The role of proprioception in the management and rehabilitation of athletic injuries. Am J Sports Med 25:130–137, 1997

48. McNair PJ, Wood GA, Marshall RN: Stiffness of the hamstring muscles and its relationship to function in ACL deficient individuals. Clin Biomech 7:131–137, 1992

49. Borsa PA, Lephart SM, Kocher MS, et al: Functional assessment and rehabilitation of shoulder proprioception for glenohumeral instability. J Sport Rehabil 3:84–104, 1994

50. Lephart SM, Warner JJP, Borsa PA, et al: Proprioception of the shoulder joint in healthy, unstable and surgically repaired shoulders. J Shoulder Elbow Surg 3:371–380, 1994

51. Fremerey RW, Lobenhoffer P, Zeichen J, et al: Proprioception after rehabilitation and reconstruction in knees with deficiency of the anterior cruciate ligament: A prospective, longitudinal study. J Bone Joint Surg 82:801–806, 2000

52. Irrgang JJ, Whitney SL, Harner C: Nonoperative treatment of rotator cuff injuries in throwing athletes. J Sport Rehabil 1:197–222, 1992

53. Fleck SJ: Periodized strength training: A critical review. J Strength Cond Res 13:82–89, 1999

54. Simoneau GG, Bereda SM, Sobush DC, et al: Biomechanics of elastic resistance in therapeutic exercise programs. J Orthop Sports Phys Ther 31:16–24, 2001

55. Engle RP, Canner GC: Proprioceptive neuromuscular facilitation (PNF) and modified procedures for anterior cruciate ligament (ACL) instability. J Orthop Sports Phys Ther 11:230, 1989

56. Manske RC, Reiman MP: Muscle weakness, in Cameron MH, Monroe LG (eds): Physical Rehabilitation: Evidence-Based Examination, Evaluation, and Intervention. St Louis, MO, Saunders/Elsevier, 2007, pp 64–86

57. Blix M: Length and tension. Scand Arch Physiol 5:93–94, 1892

58. Grimsby O, Power B: Manual therapy approach to knee ligament rehabilitation, in Ellenbecker TS (ed): Knee Ligament Rehabilitation. Philadelphia, Churchill Livingstone, 2000, pp 236–251

59. Tabata I, Nishimura K, Kouzaki M, et al: Effects of moderate-intensity endurance and high-intensity intermittent training on anaerobic capacity and VO$_2$max. Med Sci Sports Exerc 10:1327–1330, 1996

60. Grimby G, Thomee R: Principles of rehabilitation after injuries, in Dirix A, Knuttgen HG, Tittel K (eds): The Olympic Book of Sports Medicine. Oxford, England, Blackwell Scientific Publications, 1984

61. Thomee R, Renstrom P, Grimby G, et al: Slow or fast isokinetic training after surgery. J Orthop Sports Phys Ther 8:476, 1987

62. Graves JE, Pollock SH, Leggett SH, et al: Effect of reduced training frequency on muscular strength. Sports Med 9:316–319, 1988

63. Grimes K: Heart disease, in O'Sullivan SB, Schmitz TJ (eds): Physical Rehabilitation (ed 5). Philadelphia, FA Davis, 2007, pp 589–641

64. Artalejo AR, Garcia-Sancho J: Mobilization of intracellular calcium by extracellular ATP and by calcium ionophores in the Ehrlich ascites-tumour cell. Biochim Biophys Acta 941:48–54, 1988

65. Malone T, Nitz AJ, Kuperstein J, et al: Neuromuscular concepts, in Ellenbecker TS (ed): Knee Ligament Rehabilitation. Philadelphia, Churchill Livingstone, 2000, pp 399–411

66. Voight ML, Draovitch P, Tippett SR: Plyometrics, in Albert MS (ed): Eccentric Muscle Training in Sports and Orthopedics. New York, Churchill Livingstone, 1995, pp 149–163

67. Assmussen E, Bonde-Peterson F: Storage of elastic energy in skeletal muscle in man. Acta Physiol Scand 91:385–392, 1974

68. Bosco C, Komi PV: Potentiation of the mechanical behavior of the human skeletal muscle through prestretching. Acta Physiol Scand 106:467–472, 1979

69. Cavagna GA, Saibene FP, Margaria R: Effect of negative work on the amount of positive work performed by an isolated muscle. J Appl Physiol 20:157, 1965

70. Cavagna GA, Disman B, Margarai R: Positive work done by a previously stretched muscle. J Appl Physiol 24:21–32, 1968

71. Wilk KE, Voight ML, Keirns MA, et al: Stretch-shortening drills for the upper extremities: Theory and clinical application. J Orthop Sports Phys Ther 17:225–239, 1993

72. Wathen D: Literature review: Explosive/plyometric exercises. J Strength Cond Res 15:16–19, 1993

73. Janda V: Muscle Function Testing. London, Butterworths, 1983

74. Jull GA, Janda V: Muscle and motor control in low back pain, in Twomey LT, Taylor JR (eds): Physical Therapy of the Low Back: Clinics in Physical Therapy. New York, Churchill Livingstone, 1987, pp 258–278

75. Clark MA: Integrated Training for the New Millenium. Thousand Oaks, CA, National Academy of Sports Medicine, 2001

76. Lange GW, Hintermeister RA, Schlegel T, et al: Electromyographic and kinematic analysis of graded treadmill walking and the implications for knee rehabilitation. J Orthop Sports Phys Ther 23:294–301, 1996

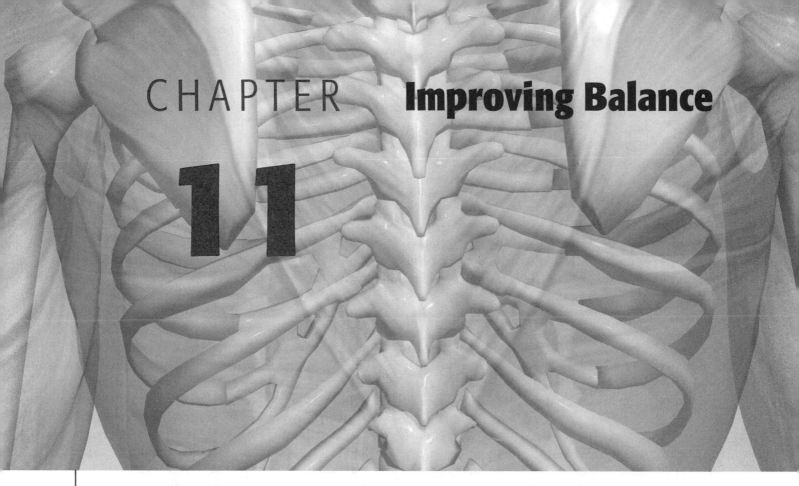

CHAPTER 11   Improving Balance

Chapter Objectives

At the completion of this chapter, the reader will be able to:

1. Define the components of balance.
2. Describe the differences between static and dynamic balance.
3. Describe ways in which balance can be improved through physical therapy.
4. Describe a number of exercises that can be used to improve balance.

Overview

Balance is a complex motor control task involving the detection and integration of sensory information to assess the position and motion of the body in space and the execution of appropriate musculoskeletal responses to control body position within the context of the environment and task.[1]

An individual's balance is greatest when the body's center of gravity (COG) is maintained over its base of support (BOS). Functional tasks require different types of balance control, including:[1]

- *Static balance:* The ability to maintain a stable antigravity position while at rest, such as when standing and sitting
- *Dynamic balance:* The ability to stabilize the body when the support surface is moving or when the body is moving on a stable surface, such as during sit-to-stand transfers or walking
- *Automatic postural reactions:* The ability to maintain balance in response to unexpected external perturbations, such as standing on a bus that suddenly decelerates

To maintain balance, the body must continually adjust its position in space to keep the COG of an individual (see Chapter 4) over the base of support or to bring the COG back to that position after perturbation. A certain amount of anteroposterior and lateral sway normally occurs while maintaining balance; for example, normal anteroposterior sway in adults is 12 degrees from the most posterior to the most anterior position.[2] If the sway exceeds these limits, some strategy must be employed to regain balance.

Impaired Balance

Impaired balance can be caused by injury or disease to any central nervous system structures involved in the stages of information processing (i.e., somatosensory input, visual and vestibular input, sensory motor integration, motor output generation).[1]

Somatosensory System

This system provides information about proprioception (static position) and kinesthesia (positions during movement). The information arises from peripheral sources such as the mechanoreceptors in muscle, the joint capsule, and other soft tissue structures (see Chapter 2). Following soft tissue or joint injury, proprioception and kinesthesia are disrupted and alter neuromuscular control. The alterations in neuromuscular control occur in the normal recruitment pattern and timing of muscular contractions.[3] Any delay in response time to an unexpected load placed on the dynamic restraints (muscles, tendons) can expose the structures that provide static restraint (ligament, joint capsule, bone) to excessive forces, increasing the potential for injury and for falling.[4]

> ● **Key Point** Extremes of joint motion activate the mechanoreceptors of the ligaments, initiating a spinal reflex with contraction of muscles antagonizing the movement through a ligamentomuscular reflex.[5,6] Such contractions are assumed to take place in order to prevent damage to the ligament and cartilage (a joint protective reflex). The reflex pattern most often seen is one of inhibition of knee extension and facilitation of knee flexion following injury or surgery.

> ● **Key Point** Proprioception can play a protective role in an acute injury through reflex muscle splinting via stimulation of the muscle spindles.[7] A common area of the body in which reflex muscle splinting occurs is the spine, particularly the neck and low back.

Visual and Vestibular Input

The visual system provides information about the position of the head relative to the environment and orients the head to maintain level gaze. The system also provides information about the movement of surrounding objects. The vestibular system provides information on the orientation of the head in space and on acceleration.

Sensory Motor Integration

The sensory motor integration involves an analysis of the relative contributions of information from each system. This analysis functions to resolve conflicting input. For example, consider sitting stationary on the plane at an airport when an adjacent plane begins to move backward. The visual input is unable to detect whether one plane is moving backward or forward relative to the other, so the brain must rely on other information, such as information from the somatosensory system.

Motor Output Generation

Following the analysis of the sensory information, a response is selected and then executed. This response programming is influenced by movement and is the stage most often manipulated in treatment.[8] Simple tasks take less time to process and program than complex movements; however, rather than having to determine which of the muscles need to be activated and when, the brain utilizes a number of preprogrammed synergies. Under this system, the brain only needs to decide which synergy to engage, when to engage it, and at what intensity to respond.[9] This is an example of feedforward control or open loop control, in which the responses are preprogrammed and automatic, rather than relying on feedback (feedback control or closed loop control). Healthy individuals use five primary movement strategies to recover balance in response to these sways and sudden perturbations of the supporting surface:

- *Ankle strategy (A-P plane):* Movements of the ankle that are activated during quiet stance and during small perturbations to restore a person's COG to a stable position.
- *Weight-shift strategy (lateral plane):* Involves shifting the body weight laterally from one leg to the other.
- *Suspension strategy:* Occurs during balance tasks when a person quickly lowers his or her body's COG by flexing the knees, causing associated flexion of the ankles and hips.
- *Hip strategy:* Used for rapid and/or large external perturbations or for movement executed with the COG near the limits of stability. For example, hip extension is used with a posterior perturbation (Figure 11-1), and hip flexion is used if the body is perturbed in an anterior direction (Figure 11-2).
- *Stepping strategy:* A forward or backward step that is used when a large force displaces the COG beyond the limits of stability.

In addition, there are a number of reflex mechanisms that produce quick, relatively invariant movements to ensure the response matches the postural challenge.

The PT may choose to use a number of balance tests for an assessment of overall balance, including

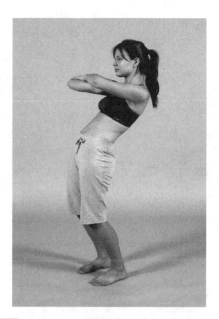

Figure 11-1   Hip strategy following posterior perturbation.

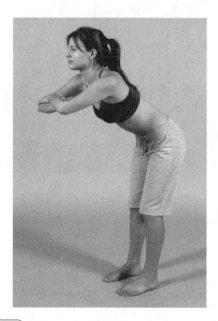

Figure 11-2   Hip strategy following anterior perturbation.

the functional reach test, Tinetti's balance and mobility assessment, timed get up and go, and Berg's balance test.

Improving Balance

Studies have shown that proprioception and kinesthesia do improve following rehabilitation.[3,10] The most important factor in treating balance impairment is determining the cause of the impairment—whether the problem results from musculoskeletal, neuromuscular, sensory, or cognitive (e.g., fear of falling) impairment.[9] In addition, it must be determined whether the patient has adequate strength to maintain balance, particularly core strength. Finally, awareness of posture and the position of the body in space is fundamental to balance training.[9] The patient should receive education about how normal alignment of the spine feels in a variety of positions, and how muscles can be used to control those positions through the provision of verbal, visual, tactile, and proprioceptive cues to enhance learning.

● **Key Point**   Afferent input is altered after joint injury, so the rehabilitation must focus on the restoration of proprioceptive sensibility to retrain these altered afferent pathways and enhance the sensation of joint movement.[11]

Because balance training often involves activities that challenge the patient's limits of stability, it is important that the PTA takes steps to ensure the patient's safety. This includes the use of a gait belt, performing the exercises near a railing, and closely guarding the patient. Balance training to promote static balance control involves changing the base of support of the patient while performing various tasks, first with his or her eyes open and then with the eyes closed. These tasks can be performed with the patient sitting (Figure 11-3), kneeling (Figure 11-4), or standing progressions (Figure 11-5 through Figure 11-11), using one leg or both, depending on the ability of the patient and the goals of the intervention. Dynamic balance activities (Figure 11-12 through Figure 11-15) can then be introduced as appropriate.

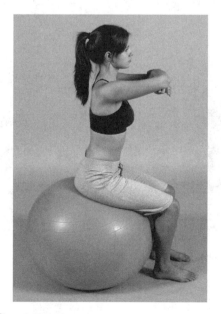

Figure 11-3   Sitting balance.

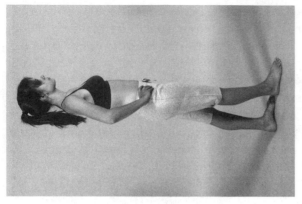

Figure 11-6   Standing balance progression.

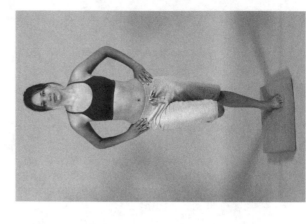

Figure 11-9   Standing balance progression.

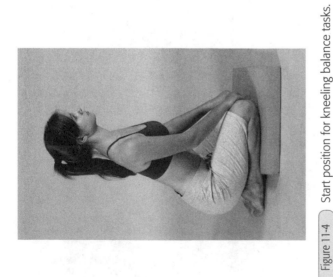

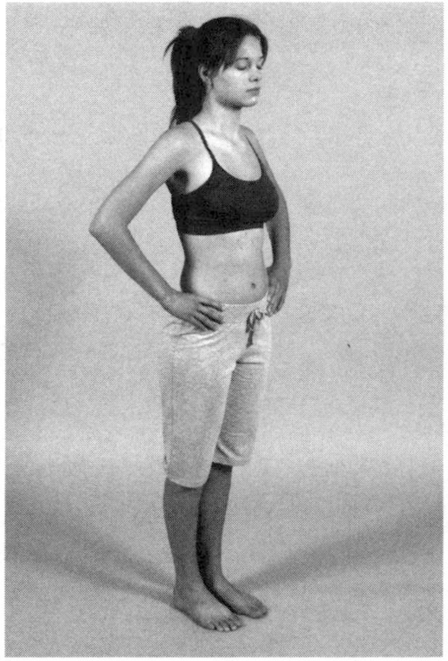

Figure 11-5   Standing balance progression.

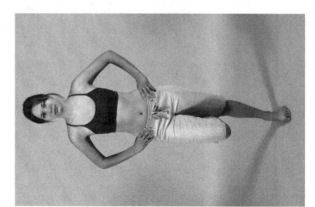

Figure 11-8   Standing balance progression.

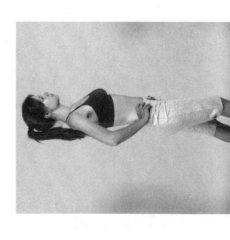

Figure 11-4   Start position for kneeling balance tasks.

Figure 11-7   Standing balance progression.

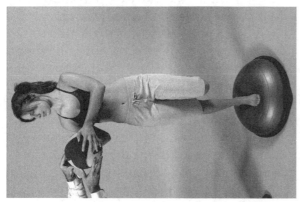

Figure 11-12 Dynamic balance exercise.

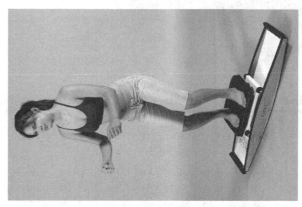

Figure 11-15 Dynamic balance exercise.

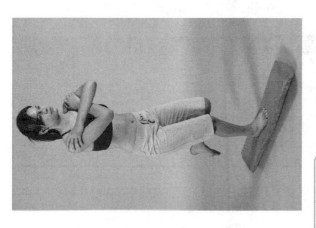

Figure 11-11 Standing balance progression.

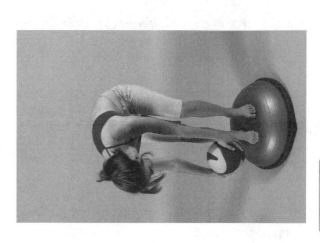

Figure 11-14 Dynamic balance exercise.

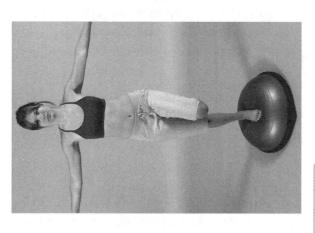

Figure 11-10 Standing balance progression.

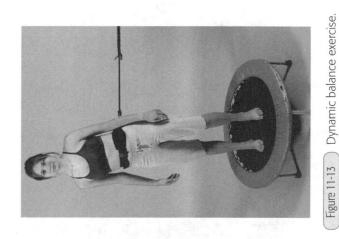

Figure 11-13 Dynamic balance exercise.

The usual progression employed involves a progressive narrowing of the base of support, a rise in the COG, and a change in the weight-bearing surface from hard to soft, or from flat to uneven, while increasing the perturbation (Figure 11-16). Challenges to the patient's position can be added in a variety of ways (**Table 11-1**).

When restoring postural equilibrium, it is important to follow a structured sequence:

1. *Static control of trunk without extremity movement:* A stable base must be provided by proximal segments and trunk onto which functional movements can be superimposed:
   - ❑ Manual perturbation to stable trunk
   - ❑ Weight shifting while maintaining postural equilibrium
2. Dynamic control of trunk without extremity movement:
   - ❑ Fixation of distal segments while proximal segments are moved; for example, maintaining both feet on the ground while bending at the waist
   - ❑ Gradual increase of range of motion from small range to large range

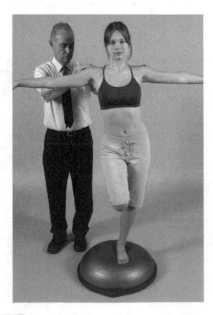

Figure 11-16 Balance activity with perturbation.

3. Static control of trunk with extremity movement:
   - ❑ Maintenance of trunk stability with increasingly ballistic extremity movements; for example, maintain a sitting position while throwing a medicine ball
   - ❑ Exercises to increase strength, endurance, flexibility, and coordination are prescribed in conjunction with equilibrium exercises
   - ❑ Exercises that challenge the endurance capabilities of the core muscles
   - ❑ Progression from extremity exercises with the spine in neutral to extremity exercises with the spine in a variety of functional positions
   - ❑ Emphasis on exercises that involve maintaining functional positions to work the correct muscle groups

At the earliest opportunity functional tasks must be incorporated. A typical functional activity progression includes:

1. *Simple patterns of movements that encourage safe body mechanics:* Once these are mastered, more challenging movements can be introduced.
   - ❑ Closed-chain activities (wall squats, lunges) initially and then open-chain activities superimposed on the closed chain by adding extremity motions to the squats and lunges
   - ❑ Sit-stand-sit activities focusing on moving the body mass forward over the base of support, extending the lower extremities, and raising the body mass over the feet, and then reversing the procedure
   - ❑ Stand-to-sit transitions focusing on balance control while pivoting and changing direction
   - ❑ Floor-to-standing raises using a progression of side-sit to quadruped to kneeling to half-kneeling to standing
2. *Gait activities:* Ambulating forward, backward, and sideways at varying speeds and on varying

TABLE 11-1 Progressive Challenges for Balance Training

Position (in order of increasing difficulty)	Target Muscle Groups	Activities	Progressions and Rationale
Supine/prone	Trunk (all muscles) Neck muscles	Rolling to increase segmentation (using a hook-lying position) Reaching from side lying	Varying speeds can be used to increase the challenge.
Quadruped	Trunk (extensor) Upper extremities Proximal lower extremities	Static holding with applied challenges (e.g., alternating isometrics, rhythmic stabilization) Creeping on all fours	Alternating isometrics applied in a variety of directions—uniplanar (anterior-posterior, medial-lateral) initially and then three-dimensionally.
Sitting	Trunk Lower extremities (hips)	Decreasing upper extremity support Reaching activities Static holding with applied challenges (e.g., alternating isometrics, rhythmic stabilization)	Rhythmic stabilization: produces co-contractions of opposing muscle groups. Reaching activities enhance dynamic control of trunk.
Kneeling (including half-kneeling and tall-kneeling)	Trunk Lower extremities (except the foot and ankle)	Static holding with applied challenges (e.g., alternating isometrics, rhythmic stabilization)	
Standing	Trunk Lower extremities	Static standing Gait: Bilateral support: parallel bars > walker Single hand support: quad cane > straight cane	Varying the base of support widths (wide to narrow).

base of support widths (wide to narrow). These can be progressed to include:

- Cross-step walking and braiding, 360-degree turns, obstacle courses
- Lateral step-ups, stair climbing, walking up and down ramps
- Performing simultaneous activities with the upper extremities (throwing or bouncing a ball, kicking a ball)

3. *Trunk motions:* Uniplanar trunk motions initially, before progressing to three-dimensional trunk motions, such as PNF rotations, in a variety of positions of lumbar flexion and extension.

- The patient uses stability equipment (e.g., stability ball, wobble board).
- The patient performs active weight shifts, upper extremity reaching activities, lower extremity movements such as stepping and marching, and trunk movements with body weight applied through a variety of surfaces.

- Challenges can be added by increasing the range of motion of the movements and by increasing the speed of the movements.

4. Sport-specific progressions as appropriate.

It is important to progress each patient based on the following criteria:

- The required level of strength/endurance is available to perform the activities without fatigue and while maintaining good trunk control.
- The patient has adequate flexibility in those muscles that allow the correct pelvic tilt to occur so that a stable base can be created. (Adaptively shortened hamstrings can hold the pelvis in a posteriorly rotated position; adaptively shortened hip flexors can hold the pelvis in an anteriorly rotated position.)

Summary

Loss of balance and falling are problems that affect individuals with a wide range of diagnoses encountered in physical therapy. The *Guide to Physical Therapist Practice* has designated an entire preferred practice pattern (pattern 5A) to primary prevention/risk reduction for loss of balance and falling. There are many factors to consider when developing an intervention program for balance impairments, and most programs require a multisystem approach. Because balance training often involves activities that challenge the patient's limits of stability, it is important that the PTA takes steps to ensure patient safety.

REVIEW Questions

1. Which two systems provide information concerning joint placement, joint position, pressure and stretch, and pain?
2. List four factors that can contribute to a balance dysfunction.
3. True or false: An individual's balance is greatest when the body's center of gravity is maintained over its base of support.
4. The ability to maintain balance in response to unexpected external perturbations is known as what?
5. Which three components of the central nervous system are critical for good balance?
6. What term is used to describe information in relation to positions during movement?
7. Which three primary movement strategies are used by healthy individuals to recover balance in response to body sways and sudden perturbations of the supporting surface?
8. The functional reach test and timed get up and go are examples of what?
9. Which position is more challenging for a patient with poor balance, quadruped or sitting?
10. True or false: Poor vision, decreased sensation, and medications can all have a negative impact on balance.

References

1. Kloos AD, Givens-Heiss D: Exercise for impaired balance, in Kisner C, Colby LA (eds): Therapeutic Exercise. Foundations and Techniques (ed 5). Philadelphia, FA Davis, 2002, pp 251–272
2. Nashner LM: Sensory, neuromuscular, and biomechanical contributions to human balance. Balance: Proceedings of the American Physical Therapy Association Forum. Nashville, TN, June 13–15, 1989
3. Barrett DS: Proprioception and function after anterior cruciate ligament reconstruction. J Bone Joint Surg 73B:833–837, 1991
4. Voight ML, Cook G: Impaired neuromuscular control: Reactive neuromuscular training, in Prentice WE, Voight ML (eds): Techniques in Musculoskeletal Rehabilitation. New York, McGraw-Hill, 2001, pp 93–124
5. Gardner E: Reflex muscular responses to stimulation of articular nerves in cat. Am J Physiol 161:133–141, 1950
6. Palmer I: On injuries to ligaments of knee joint; clinical study. Acta Chir Scand Supp 53, 520–526, 1938
7. Lephart SM, Henry TJ: Functional rehabilitation for the upper and lower extremity. Orthop Clin North Am 26:579–592, 1995
8. Light KE: Information processing for motor performance in aging adults. Phys Ther 70:820–826, 1990
9. Thein-Brody L, Dewane J: Impaired balance, in Hall C, Thein-Brody L (eds): Therapeutic Exercise: Moving Toward Function (ed 2). Baltimore, MD, Lippincott Williams & Wilkins, 2005, pp 149–166
10. Lephart SM, Pincivero DM, Giraldo JL, et al: The role of proprioception in the management and rehabilitation of athletic injuries. Am J Sports Med 25:130–137, 1997
11. Voight M, Blackburn T: Proprioception and balance training and testing following injury, in Ellenbecker TS (ed): Knee Ligament Rehabilitation. Philadelphia, Churchill Livingstone, 2000, pp 361–385

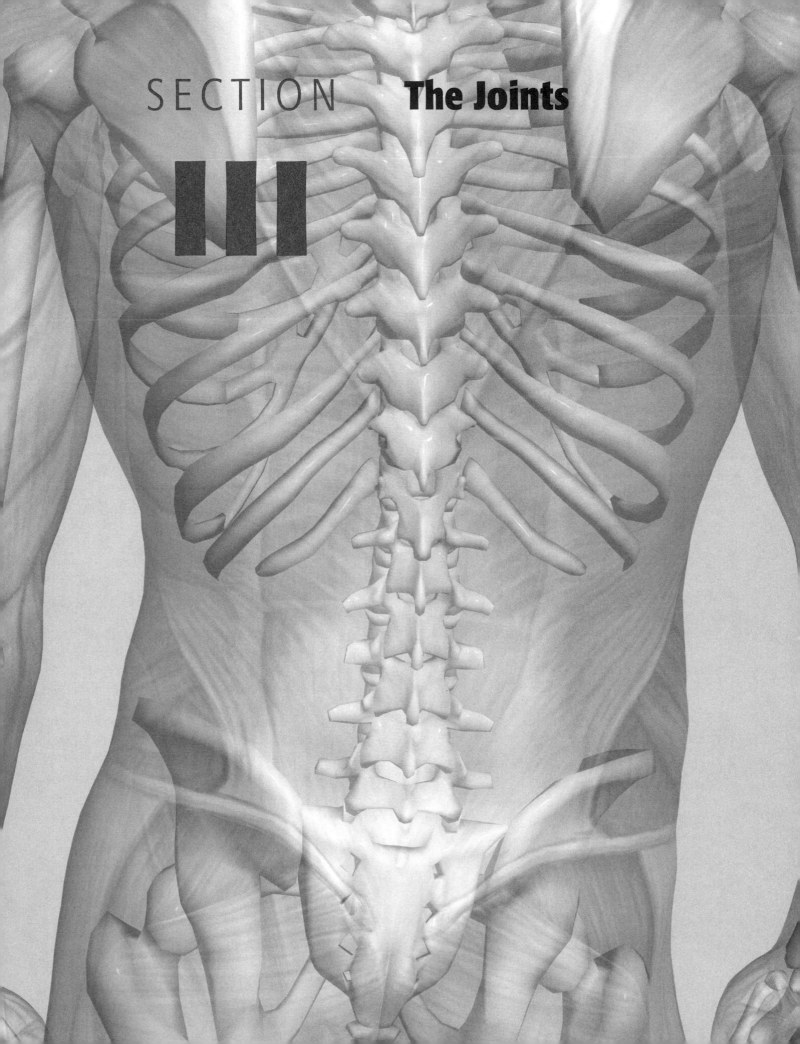

SECTION III

The Joints

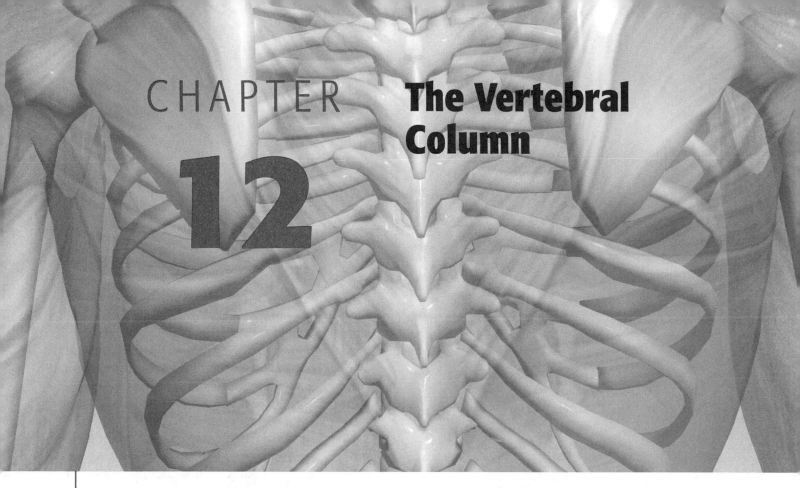

Chapter Objectives

At the completion of this chapter, the reader will be able to:

1. Describe the various components that make up the vertebral column and their various functions.
2. Outline the significance of the zygapophyseal joints and the intervertebral disks and the role they can play in causing a patient's symptoms.
3. Describe the biomechanics of the various regions of the vertebral column, including the coupling motions that occur.
4. Outline how Fryette's Laws can be used to help predict spinal motions.
5. Provide an overview as to the general guidelines for an intervention involving the vertebral column.

Overview

The term *vertebral column* describes the entire set of vertebrae, excluding the ribs, sternum, and pelvis. The vertebral column consists of 33 vertical segments, divided into five regions: cervical, thoracic, lumbar, sacral, and coccygeal. In the normal spine, there are 7 cervical, 12 thoracic, 5 lumbar, 5 sacral, and 4 coccygeal segments (Figure 12-1). The sacrococcygeal segments are fused in the adult, forming individual sacral and coccygeal bones. Individual vertebrae are numbered by region in a cranial to sacral direction; for example, C4 represents the fourth cervical vertebra from the top of the cervical spine, T7 represents the seventh thoracic vertebra (from the top), and L3 describes the third lumbar vertebra from the top.

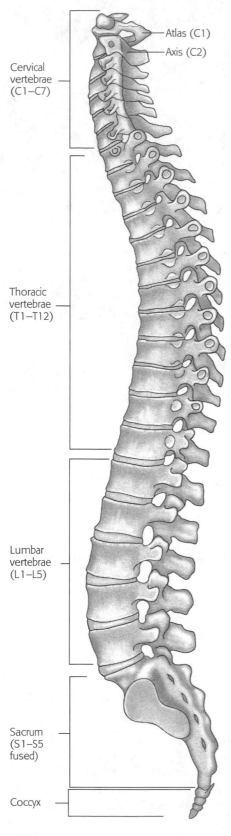

Cervical
vertebrae
(C1–C7)

Atlas (C1)

Axis (C2)

Thoracic
vertebrae
(T1–T12)

Lumbar
vertebrae
(L1–L5)

Sacrum
(S1–S5
fused)

Coccyx

Figure 12-1 The vertebral column (lateral view).

Design

The overall contour of the normal vertebral column in the coronal plane is straight. In contrast, the contour of the sagittal plane changes with development. At birth, a series of primary curves gives a kyphotic posture to the whole spine. With development of the erect posture, secondary curves develop in the cervical and lumbar spines, producing a lordosis in these regions, while the thoracic and sacral regions maintain their kyphosis. The curves in the spinal column are not fixed; they are dynamic and flexible to accommodate a wide variety of different postures and movements and to provide it with shock-absorbing capabilities.[1] Disease, trauma, genetically loose ligaments, or habitual poor posture can lead to an exaggeration (or reduction) of the normal spinal curvatures, placing stress on the local muscles and joints, as well as reducing the volume in the thorax for expansion of the lungs (see Chapter 14).[2]

At the component level, the basic building block of the spine is the vertebra. The vertebra serves as the weight-bearing unit of the vertebral column, and it is well designed for this purpose. Although a solid structure would provide the vertebral body with sufficient strength, especially for static loads, it would prove too heavy and would not have the necessary flexibility for dynamic load bearing.[1] Instead, the vertebral body is constructed with a strong outer layer of cortical bone and a hollow cavity, the latter of which is reinforced by vertical and horizontal struts called *trabeculae*.

Structure

The human vertebral column provides structural stability, affording full mobility as well as protection of the spinal cord and axial neural tissues.[3] While achieving these seemingly disparate objectives for the axial skeleton, the spine also contributes to the functional requirements of gait and to the maintenance of static weight-bearing postures.[3] Functionally, the vertebral column is divided into anterior and posterior pillars (vertebral arch):

- *Anterior pillar:* Consists of the vertebral bodies and intervertebral disks and is the hydraulic, weight-bearing, and shock-absorbing portion of the spinal column.
- *Posterior pillar:* Consists of the articular processes and zygapophyseal (facet) joints, and the two transverse processes and

spinous processes. The function of the posterior pillar is to serve as a gliding mechanism and lever system for muscle attachments.

Motion Segments

A motion segment in the vertebral column is defined as two adjacent vertebrae and the joints in between (typically, two zygapophyseal [facet] joints and one intervertebral disk), forming a three-joint complex. By convention, movement of any spinal region is defined by the direction of the motion of a point on the anterior side of the superior vertebra. For example, rotation of the C4–C5 segment to the left indicates that the anterior side (body) of the C4 vertebra is rotating to the left.

Zygapophyseal Joints

The vertebral column contains 24 pairs of zygapophyseal or facet joints, which are located posteriorly and project from the neural arch of the vertebrae. The regional characteristics of the zygapophyseal joint are described in the relevant chapters. Mechanically, zygapophyseal joints are classified as plane joints because the articular surfaces are essentially flat.[4] The articular surfaces are covered in hyaline cartilage and, like most synovial joints, have small fatty or fibrous synovial meniscoid-like fringes that project between the joint surfaces from the margins.[5] These intra-articular synovial folds act as space fillers during joint displacement and actively assist in the dispersal of synovial fluid within the joint cavity.[3] The articular processes provide mechanical guidance, particularly against excessive torsion and shear, permitting certain movements while blocking others:[4]

- Horizontal articular surfaces favor axial rotation.
- Vertical articular surfaces in the sagittal plane act to block axial rotation.

Most zygapophyseal joint surfaces are oriented somewhere between the horizontal and vertical.

- In the cervical spine, the zygapophyseal joints are relatively horizontal while progressively increasing their surface area, and tend toward 45 degrees to the horizontal at the lower segments. This joint configuration allows fairly free movement in all planes of movement.[6–9]
- In the thoracic region, the joints assume an almost vertical direction while remaining essentially in a coronal (frontal) orientation, which facilitates axial rotation and resists anterior displacement of the vertebral body.[10]

- In the lumbar spine, the zygapophyseal joints are vertical with a curved, J-shaped surface predominantly in the sagittal plane, which helps prevent anterior shear of the vertebral body while restricting rotation.[3]

Understanding the variable structures and functions of the human zygapophyseal joints and their relationship with the other components of the vertebral column is an important requirement in the assessment and intervention of individuals with mechanical spinal pain disorders.[3]

Intervertebral Disks

The intervertebral disks (IVDs) of the vertebral column lie between the adjacent superior and inferior surfaces of the vertebral bodies from C2 to S1 and are similar in shape to the bodies. The intervertebral disks are described by their position between two vertebrae; for example, the L4–L5 disk describes the intervertebral disk located between the fourth and fifth lumbar vertebrae. Each disk is composed of an inner *nucleus pulposus*, an outer *annulus fibrosus*, and limiting cartilage end plates.

- *Annulus fibrosis (AF):* The AF consists of approximately 10–12 (often as many as 15–25) concentric sheets of predominantly type I collagen tissue,[11] bound together by proteoglycan gel.[12] The number of annular layers decreases with age, but there is a gradual thickening of the remaining layers.[13] The fibers of the AF are oriented at about 65 degrees from vertical. The fibers of each successive sheet or lamella maintain the same inclination of 65 degrees, but in the opposite direction to the preceding lamella, resulting in every second sheet having the same orientation. Thus, only 50 percent of the fibers are under stress with rotational forces at any given time. This alteration in the direction of fibers in each lamella is vital in enabling the disk to resist torsional (twisting) forces.[14]
- *Vertebral end plate:* Each vertebral end plate consists of a layer of hyaline and fibrocartilage about 0.6–1 millimeter thick,[15] which covers the top or bottom aspects of the IVD, separating it from the adjacent vertebral body. Peripherally, the end plate is surrounded by the ring apophysis.[2] Nutrition of the IVD comes via a diffusion of nutrients from the anastomosis over the AF and from the arterial plexi underlying the end plate. Although almost the entire AF is permeable to nutrients, only the center

portions of the end plate are permeable. The subchondral bone of the centrum is deficient over approximately 10 percent of the end plate surface. At these points, the bone marrow is in direct contact with the end plate, thereby augmenting the nutrition of the IVD and end plate.[16] It is possible that a mechanical pump action produced by spine motion could aid with the diffusion of the nutrients.

■ *Nucleus pulposus (NP):* The IVDs of a healthy young adult contain an NP that is composed of a semifluid mass of mucoid material. This material is clear, firm, and gelatinous.[2] The overall consistency of the NP changes with increasing age, as the water content of the NP diminishes and it subsequently becomes drier.

The annulus and end plates anchor the disk to the vertebral body. In cervical and lumbar regions, the IVDs are thicker anteriorly, and this contributes to the normal lordosis. In the thoracic region, each of the IVDs is of uniform thickness. The small migrations of the nucleus pulposus with spinal movements are considered normal. However, over time or combined with excessive pressure, the nucleus pulposus may seep through small cracks created within a fragmented annulus fibrosus and may lead to a herniated nucleus pulposus (see Chapter 15).

Intervertebral Foramina

The intervertebral foramina are located between each vertebral segment in the posterior pillar, with the IVD serving as their anterior boundary, the facet joints serving as their posterior boundary, and the pedicles of the superior and inferior vertebrae of the spinal segment serving as their superior and inferior boundaries. A mixed spinal nerve exits the spinal canal by the foramen along with blood vessels and the current meningeal or sinuvertebral nerves.

● **Key Point** The size of the intervertebral foramina is affected by spinal motion, being larger with forward bending and contralateral side bending, and smaller with extension and ipsilateral side bending.

Neutral Zone

From a mechanical point of view, the spinal system is inherently unstable and thus dependent on the contribution of muscles in addition to the passive elements of the spine previously described to maintain stability and control movement.[17,18] Panjabi[19]

divided the full range of motion (ROM) of an intervertebral segment into two zones:

■ *Neutral:* A region of laxity around the neutral resting position of a spinal segment. The neutral zone is the position of the segment in which minimal loading is occurring in the passive structures (IVD, zygapophyseal joints, and ligaments) and the active structures (the muscles and tendons that surround and control spinal motion), and within which spinal motion is produced with minimal internal resistance. The size of the neutral zone, or balance point, is determined by the integrity of the passive restraint and active control systems, which in turn are controlled by the neural system.[17]

■ *Elastic:* Portion of the range of motion from the end of the neutral zone up to the physiologic limits of motion.

● **Key Point** Studies have demonstrated that a larger than normal neutral zone, resulting from an accumulation of microtrauma and muscle weakness, is related to a lack of segmental muscle control and is associated with a higher risk of intersegmental injury and IVD degeneration.

Because the passive system of the spine is known to be unstable at loads far less than that of body weight,[20,21] the muscle and neural systems must fulfill the role of maintaining postural stability while simultaneously controlling and initiating movement. A large number of muscles have a mechanical effect on the spine and pelvis, and all muscles are required to maintain optimal control. The specific muscles that provide stability in the various regions are described in the relevant chapters.

Spinal Motion

The movements of the vertebral column occur in diagonal patterns as a combination of flexion or extension, coupled with motions of side bending and rotation. As stated previously, segmental motion is defined by what is occurring at the anterior portion of the body of the superior vertebra.

■ *Flexion/extension:* The movements of flexion (forward bending) or extension (backward bending) occur in the sagittal plane. With flexion, the anterior portion of the bodies approximate and the spinous processes separate. With extension, the anterior portion of the bodies separate and the spinous processes approximate.

- *Side bending (lateral flexion):* The motion of side bending to the left or right occurs in the frontal plane. With side bending, the lateral edges of the vertebral bodies approximate on the side toward which the spine is bending, and they separate on the opposite side.
- *Rotation:* Rotation of the spine occurs in the transverse plane. Rotation to the right results in relative movements of the body of the superior vertebra to the right and the spinous process to the left, with the opposite occurring with rotation to the left. Even if the motion occurs from the pelvis upward, the motion is still defined by the relative motion of the superior vertebra.
- *Shear:* Shear can occur in a number of directions. When the body of the superior vertebra translates forward on the vertebra below, anterior shearing occurs; if it translates backward, posterior shearing occurs. Lateral shearing occurs when the body of the superior vertebra translates sideways on the vertebra below.
- *Distraction/compression:* Distraction or compression occurs with a longitudinal force, either away from or toward the vertebral bodies.

Movements of the spine, like those elsewhere, are produced by the coordinated action of nerves and muscles. Agonistic and synergistic muscles initiate and perform the movements, whereas the antagonistic muscles control and modify the movements. The *amount* of motion available at each region of the spine is a factor of a number of variables. These include disk–vertebral height ratio; compliance of the fibrocartilage of the IVD; dimensions, orientation, and shape of the adjacent structures; and age, disease, and gender. The *type* of motion available is governed by the shape and orientation of the articulations and the ligaments and muscles of the segment, and the size and location of the vertebral processes.

During spinal motion, the axes of motion for each unit are generally in the nucleus pulposus of the IVD. Although the ROM at each vertebral segment varies, the relative amounts of motion that occur at each region are well documented[22,23] and are described in the relevant chapters.

Coupled Motions

In general, the human zygapophyseal joints of the spine are capable of only two major motions: gliding upward and gliding downward. If these movements occur in the same direction, flexion or extension occurs. If the movements occur in opposite directions, side bending or rotation occurs. Because the orientation of the articular facets of the zygapophyseal joints do not correspond exactly to pure planes of motion, pure motions of the spine occur very infrequently. In fact, most motions of the spine occur three-dimensionally because of the phenomenon of coupling. Coupling involves two or more individual motions occurring simultaneously at the segment, and has been found to occur throughout the lumbar, thoracic, and cervical regions. Descriptions about the types of coupling that occur in these regions are provided in the respective chapters.

Fryette's Laws of Physiologic Spinal Motion

Although listed as laws, Fryette's[24] descriptions of spinal motion are better viewed as concepts, because they have undergone review and modifications over time. However, these concepts serve as useful guidelines in the intervention of spinal dysfunction and are cited throughout many texts describing spinal biomechanics.

Fryette's First Law

"When any part of the lumbar or thoracic spine is in neutral position, side bending of a vertebra will be opposite to the side of the rotation of that vertebra."

The term *neutral*, according to Fryette, is interpreted as any position in which the zygapophyseal joints are not engaged in any surface contact, and the position where the ligaments and capsules of the segment are not under tension. This law describes the coupling for the thoracic and lumbar spines. The cervical spine is not included in this law, because the zygapophyseal joints of this region are always engaged. When a lumbar or thoracic vertebra is side bent from its neutral position, the vertebral body will turn toward the convexity that is being formed, with the maximum rotation occurring near the apex of the curve formed.

Fryette's Second Law

"When any part of the spine is in a position of hyperextension or hyperflexion, the side bending of the vertebra will be to the same side as the rotation of that vertebra."

Put simply, when the segment is under load, the coupling of side bending and rotation occur to the same side. The term *non-neutral*, according to Fryette, is interpreted as any position in which the zygapophyseal joints are engaged in surface contact, the position where the ligaments and capsules of the segment are under tension, or in positions of flexion or extension. This law describes the coupling that occurs in the C2 to T3 areas of the spine.

Fryette's Third Law

"If motion in one plane is introduced to the spine, any motion occurring in another direction is thereby restricted."

For example, there is more rotation available when the spine is in neutral than when the spine is flexed or extended.

General Guidelines for Interventions for Spinal Dysfunction

Based on current evidence, it is not yet possible to give very specific recommendations for the management of patients with spinal dysfunction; however, there is growing evidence to suggest that physical therapy can have a positive impact on spinal dysfunction. For example, a systematic review by the Philadelphia Panel[25] suggested there was "good evidence to include stretching, strengthening, and mobility exercises" in treatment programs directed toward the management of chronic spinal pain.

The most logical approach for intervention is to identify the primary movement or postural dysfunction and focus the intervention on teaching the patient strategies that limit or avoid this motion or posture until safe to do so. This approach should be supplemented with strategies and goals based on the stage of healing (see Chapter 5).

Acute Phase

During the acute phase, the following recommendations for physical therapy intervention should be followed:

- *Decrease pain, inflammation, and muscle spasm.* In cases of severe pain, it may be necessary for the patient to be confined to a bed for a few days (a maximum of 2 days is recommended).[26] For the patient with cervical pain, a cervical collar may be warranted. Pain relief may be accomplished initially by the use of electrotherapeutic modalities, such as electrical stimulation, nonthermal agents, and cryotherapy. Thermal modalities, especially continuous ultrasound, with its ability to penetrate deeply, may be used after 48–72 hours based on the plan of care and patient tolerance.

- *Promote healing of tissues.* Joint protection techniques can reduce and control pain by minimizing repetitive movements into painful ranges of motion. In the lumbar/thoracic spine, a lumbar cushion may be appropriate to support the spine in the position of normal lumbar lordosis/thoracic kyphosis. In the cervical spine, this can be achieved through the use of a cervical collar with appropriate weaning off the collar at the earliest opportunity.

- *Regain soft tissue extensibility and increase pain-free range of segmental motion through therapeutic exercise.* Once the pain and inflammation are under control, the intervention can progress toward the restoration of full strength, ROM, and normal posture. ROM for the lumbar spine is regained initially in the unloaded position of the spine (supine, side lying, or prone). The various exercises recommended for this phase are described in each of the relevant chapters.

- *Aerobic conditioning must be maintained or improved throughout the rehabilitative process as tolerated.* For injuries involving the cervical and thoracic spines, this can be achieved using a stationary cycle, treadmill, or stair-stepper. For low back injuries, an upper body ergometer can be used if the previously mentioned equipment exacerbates the symptoms.

● **Key Point** Tissue loading during walking has been found to be below levels produced by many specific rehabilitation tasks, suggesting that walking is a wise choice as an initial aerobic exercise for general back rehabilitation.

- *Allow progression to the subacute and then chronic (functional) phases of healing.* Patient education is an important component of any rehabilitative process. The patient is taught how to find the neutral position or the position of optimal function of the spine. This position is the least painful and represents the position of minimized biomechanical stresses.[27] The patient also is advised to stay as active as possible and to continue normal daily and work activities whenever possible while maintaining good posture.[26,28]

Subacute and Chronic (Functional) Phases

During the subacute and chronic phases, the following recommendations for physical therapy intervention should be followed:

- *Causative factors associated with the injury must be addressed.* These usually include imbalances in muscle function. Once again, the patient must be taught how to correct these imbalances through correct posture, strengthening exercises, and self-stretches. In individuals suspected to have instability, stretching exercises should be used with caution, particularly ones encouraging end ranges.[29]
- *Progression of strengthening exercises.* The exercises for these phases are described in each of the relevant chapters. Full restoration of spinal function can occur only when the patient is able to progress to dynamic activities involving the trunk and extremities without the provocation of pain or the exacerbation of symptoms.
- *Neuromuscular control must be re-established.* Neuromuscular control of the spine first is taught in static positions and then is advanced to include control during dynamic and functional activities through an appropriate stabilization program.[27,30]
- *Prevention of recurrence.* The patient should be instructed on correct lifting techniques and a maintenance exercise program, and be advised to maintain an appropriate height/weight ratio.

Summary

The vertebral column is involved with many functions. Its semi-rigid structure provides a stable axis for the entire trunk, head, and neck, and also provides the primary source of protection to the delicate spinal cord and exiting spinal nerves. The joints of the vertebral column vary according to location in terms of specialization and available motion. Damage to the vertebral column from fractures, disease, trauma, muscle imbalances, and disk herniation can severely impact the function of the spine. Physical therapy is often the first line of conservative treatment for pain and dysfunction of the vertebral column.

REVIEW Questions

1. What are the five recognized regions of the vertebral column?
2. With development, which two secondary curves of the spine are formed?
3. Which structures are found within the anterior pillar of the spine?
4. How many pairs of zygapophyseal or facet joints are found in the normal spine?
5. What is the name given to the position of the segment in which minimal loading is occurring in the passive structures (IVD, zygapophyseal joints, and ligaments) and the active structures (the muscles and tendons that surround and control spinal motion)?
6. True or False: It is not yet possible to give very specific recommendations for the management of patients with spinal dysfunction; however, there is growing evidence to suggest that physical therapy can have a positive impact on spinal dysfunction.

References

1. Bogduk N, Twomey LT: Anatomy and biomechanics of the lumbar spine, in Bogduk N, Twomey LT (eds): Clinical Anatomy of the Lumbar Spine and Sacrum (ed 3). Edinburgh, Churchill Livingstone, 1997, pp 2–53, 81–152, 171–176
2. Jackson-Manfield P, Neumann DA: Structure and function of the vertebral column, in Jackson-Manfield P, Neumann DA (eds): Essentials of Kinesiology for the Physical Therapist Assistant. St Louis, MO, Mosby Elsevier, 2009, pp 177–225
3. Singer KP, Boyle JJW, Fazey P: Comparative anatomy of the zygapophysial joints, in Boyling JD, Jull GA (eds): Grieve's Modern Manual Therapy: The Vertebral Column. Philadelphia, Churchill Livingstone, 2004, pp 17–29
4. Neumann DA: Axial skeleton: Osteology and arthrology, in Neumann DA (ed): Kinesiology of the Musculoskeletal System: Foundations for Physical Rehabilitation. St Louis, MO, Mosby, 2002, pp 251–310
5. Singer KP, Giles LGF: Manual therapy considerations at the thoracolumbar junction: An anatomical and functional perspective. J Man Physiol Ther 13:83–88, 1990
6. Pal GP, Sherk HH: The vertical stability of the cervical spine. Spine 13:447, 1988
7. Pal GP, Routal RV, Saggu SK: The orientation of the articular facets of the zygapophyseal joints at the cervical and upper thoracic region. J Anat 198:431–441, 2001
8. Pal GP, Routal RV: The role of the vertebral laminae in the stability of the cervical spine. J Anat 188:485–489, 1996
9. Pal GP, Routal RV: A study of weight transmission through the cervical and upper thoracic regions of the vertebral column in man. J Anat 148:245–261, 1986
10. Gregersen GG, Lucas DB: An in vivo study of the axial rotation of the human thoracolumbar spine. J Bone Joint Surg Am 49:247–262, 1967
11. Ghosh P, Bushell GR, Taylor TKF, et al: Collagens, elastin and noncollagenous protein of the intervertebral disc. Clin Orthop 129:124–132, 1977
12. Taylor JR: The development and adult structure of lumbar intervertebral discs. J Man Med 5:43–47, 1990

13. Tsuji H, Hirano N, Ohshima H, et al: Structural variation of the anterior and posterior anulus fibrosus in the development of the human lumbar intervertebral disc: A risk factor for intervertebral disc rupture. Spine 18:204–210, 1993

14. Hickey DS, Hukins DWL: Relation between the structure of the annulus fibrosus and the function and failure of the intervertebral disc. Spine 5:100–116, 1980

15. Eyring EJ: The biochemistry and physiology of the intervertebral disc. Clin Orthop 67:16–28, 1969

16. Nachemson AL: The lumbar spine: An orthopedic challenge. Spine 1:59–71, 1976

17. MM: The stabilizing system of the spine. Part 1. Function, dysfunction adaption and enhancement. J Spinal Disord 5:383–389, 1992

18. Hodges PW: Motor control of the trunk, in Boyling JD, Jull GA (eds): Grieve's Modern Manual Therapy: The Vertebral Column. Philadelphia, Churchill Livingstone, 2004, pp 119–139

19. Panjabi MM: The stabilizing system of the spine. Part II. Neutral zone and instability hypothesis. J Spinal Disord 5:390-396; discussion 397, 1992

20. Nachemson A, Morris JM: In vivo measurements of intradiscal pressure. J Bone Joint Surg 46:1077, 1964

21. Nachemson A: Disc pressure measurements. Spine 6:93–97, 1981

22. White AA, Panjabi MM: Clinical Biomechanics of the Spine (ed 2). Philadelphia, JB Lippincott, 1990

23. American Medical Association: Guides to the Evaluation of Permanent Impairment (ed 5). Chicago, American Medical Association, 2001

24. Fryette HH: Principles of Osteopathic Technique. Colorado, Academy of Osteopathy, 1980

25. Philadelphia Panel evidence-based clinical practice guidelines on selected rehabilitation interventions for low back pain. Phys Ther 81:1641–1674, 2001

26. van Tulder MW, Waddell G: Conservative treatment of acute and subacute low back pain, in Nachemson AL, Jonsson E (eds): Neck and Back Pain: The Scientific Evidence of Causes, Diagnosis, and Treatment. Philadelphia, Lippincott Williams and Wilkins, 2000, pp 241–269

27. Cole AJ, Farrell JP, Stratton SA: Functional rehabilitation of cervical spine athletic injuries, in Kibler BW, Herring JA, Press JM (eds): Functional Rehabilitation of Sports and Musculoskeletal Injuries. Gaithersburg, MD, Aspen, 1998, pp 127–148

28. Waddell G, Feder G, McIntosh A, et al: Low Back Pain Evidence Review. London, Royal College of General Practitioners, 1996

29. Brukner P, Khan K: Core stability, in Brukner P, Khan K (eds): Clinical Sports Medicine (ed 3). Sydney, McGraw-Hill, 2007, pp 158–173

30. Sweeney TB, Prentice C, Saal JA, et al: Cervicothoracic muscular stabilization techniques, in Saal JA (ed): Physical Medicine and Rehabilitation, State of the Art Reviews: Neck and Back Pain. Philadelphia, Hanley & Belfus, 1990, pp 335–359

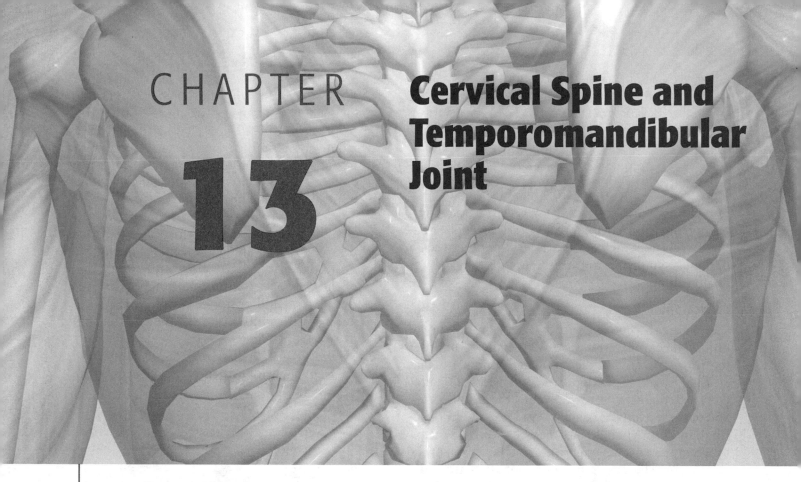

Cervical Spine and Temporomandibular Joint

13

Chapter Objectives

At the completion of this chapter, the reader will be able to:

1. Describe the anatomy of the vertebrae, ligaments, muscles, and blood and nerve supply that comprise the cervical intervertebral segment.

2. Summarize the various causes of temporomandibular dysfunction.

3. Describe the biomechanics of the cervical spine, including coupled movements, normal and abnormal joint barriers, kinesiology, and reactions to various stresses.

4. Describe the close association among the temporomandibular joint, the middle ear, and the cervical spine.

5. Apply a number of manual therapy techniques specific to the cervical spine.

6. Instruct the patient in an effective home program, including spinal care.

7. Help the patient to develop self-reliant intervention strategies through the use of self-stretching.

Overview

The cervical spine consists of 37 joints, which allow for more motion than any other region of the spine. However, with stability being sacrificed for mobility, the cervical spine is rendered more vulnerable to both direct and indirect trauma. As a result, the cervical spine can be the source of many pain syndromes, including neck, upper thoracic, and periscapular syndromes; cervical radiculopathy; and shoulder and elbow syndromes.[1] Indeed, neck and upper extremity pain are common in the general population, with surveys finding the 1-year prevalence rate for neck and shoulder pain to be 16–18 percent.[2,3] This prevalence also is reflected in the incidence of neck pain in the outpatient physical therapy setting, which has been found to be between 15 percent and 34 percent.[2,3] The stomatognathic system comprises the temporomandibular joint (TMJ), the masticatory systems, and the related organs and tissues such as the inner ear and salivary glands.[4] Due to the proximity of this system to the other structures of the head and neck, an intimate relationship exists.

Anatomy and Kinesiology

In order to effectively treat any region of the body, knowledge of anatomy and kinesiology is essential so relationships can be ascertained between a patient's symptoms and the structure that may be responsible.

Cervical Spine

The cervical spine is composed of two functional units. The craniovertebral (CV) complex comprises the bony structures of the foramen magnum, occiput, atlas, axis, and their supporting ligaments. The atlas (C1) articulates with the occiput of the skull above and with the axis (C2) below ((Figure 13-1)). The occipitoatlantal (OA) joint is formed between the occipital condyles and the superior articular facets of the atlas (C1). The paired occipital condyles are ovoid structures with their long axis situated in a posterolateral to anteromedial orientation. The OA joint is inherently stable, reinforced by the joint capsule, which is thickened anteriorly and laterally. The atlantoaxial (AA) joint (C1 and C2) is composed of two lateral facet joints and a median joint (with the dens) complex.

The middle to lower cervical spine consists of the region from the C2–C3 intervertebral segment to the C7–T1 segment. Each mobile segment of the mid-cervical spine consists of several joints, including the paired zygapophyseal (facet) and uncovertebral (UV) joints and the intervertebral disk (IVD).

- *Zygapophyseal (facet) joint:* The joint surfaces are planar, with the orientation gradually changing from approximately 60 degrees from vertical in the upper levels to 30 degrees from vertical in the lower cervical spine (refer to Figure 12-1). Fibroadipose meniscoids are commonly found in the cervical zygapophyseal joints, which can become impinged.
- *Uncovertebral joints:* Consist of nonsynovial clefts between the uncinate processes of adjacent vertebral bodies. They are located at the posterolateral corners of the superior aspect of the C3–C7 vertebrae and function to limit both lateral and posterior translation while guiding the motions of flexion and extension ((Figure 13-2)).
- *Intervertebral disks:* The IVDs lie between the adjacent superior and inferior surfaces of the

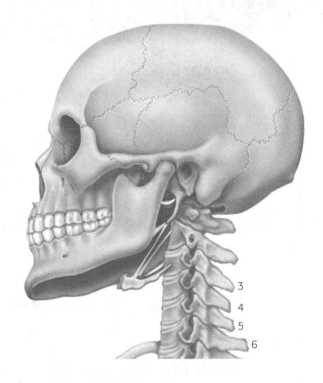

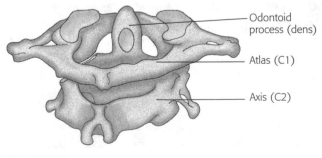

Figure 13-1 The atlas (C1) and axis (C2) (posterosuperior view).

Odontoid process (dens)

Atlas (C1)

Axis (C2)

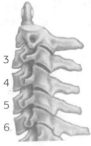

Figure 13-2 The uncovertebral joints.

vertebral bodies and are similar in shape to the bodies. Each disk is composed of an inner *nucleus pulposus*, an outer *annulus fibrosus*, and limiting cartilage end plates (see Chapter 2). The annulus and end plates anchor the disk to the vertebral body. The disks contribute 20–25 percent of the length of the vertebral column. In the cervical region, the IVDs are thicker anteriorly, which contributes to the normal lordosis. One of the functions of the IVDs is to facilitate motion and provide stability. Although IVDs are incapable of independent motion, movement of the IVDs does occur during the clinically defined motions of flexion-extension, side bending, and axial rotation.[5] The major stresses that must be withstood by the IVDs are axial compression, shearing, bending, and twisting, either singly or in combination with each other.

> **● Key Point** In the absence of an IVD at the CV joints, the supporting soft tissues of the joints of C1–C2 must be lax to permit motion, while simultaneously being able to withstand great mechanical stresses.

Eight pairs of cervical spinal nerves exit bilaterally through the intervertebral foramina. Each spinal nerve is named for the vertebra above which it exits; for example, the C6 nerve exits above the C6 vertebra. The nerves are surrounded by several structures including the aforementioned zygapophyseal joints, UV joints, IVD, and bony pedicles. Degenerative changes affecting any of these structures may diminish the foramen size and compromise nerve function.

Osteokinematics of the Cervical Spine

Although it may be clinically useful to describe the motions that occur at the cervical spine as separate motions, these motions correspond to the motion of the head alone, and do not describe what is occurring at the various segmental levels. It should be obvious that the range of head movement bears no relation to the range of neck movement, and that the total range is the sum of both the head and the neck motions.[6]

The upper cervical spine is responsible for approximately 50 percent of the motion that occurs in the entire cervical spine. Motion at the AA joint occurs relatively independently, whereas below C2, normal motion is a combination of motion occurring at other levels. The primary motion that occurs at the OA joint is flexion and extension, although side

bending and rotation also occur. The major motion that occurs at the AA articulations is axial rotation, totaling approximately 40–47 degrees to each side. This large amount of rotation has the potential to cause compression of the vertebral artery if it becomes excessive. Flexion and extension movements of the AA joint amount to a combined range of 10–15 degrees: 10 degrees of flexion and 5 degrees of extension.

At the zygapophyseal (facet) joints of the mid-low cervical spine there is a combined sagittal range of 30 degrees to 60 degrees.[7] Significant flexion occurs at C5–C6, and extension occurs around C6–C7.

> **● Key Point** Panjabi[8] divided the full ROM of an intervertebral segment into two zones: *neutral* (portion of the range of motion that produces little resistance from the articular structures) and *elastic* (portion of the range of motion from the end of the neutral zone up to the physiologic limits of motion). The entire cervical spine, particularly the CV region, has a large neutral zone of motion because of the lack of tension in the capsule or ligamentous system in this middle part of the range.

Arthrokinematics of the Cervical Spine

The only significant arthrokinematics available to the zygapophyseal joint is an inferior, medial glide of the inferior articular process of the superior facet during extension, and a superior, lateral glide during flexion. Segmental side bending is, therefore, extension of the ipsilateral joint and flexion of the contralateral joint. Ipsilateral rotation, coupled with side bending, involves extension of the ipsilateral joint and flexion of the contralateral joint as well.

Muscle Control of the Cervical Spine

The control of head and neck postures and movements is a complicated task, especially in the presence of pain or dysfunction. The muscle groups of the cervical region can be divided into those that produce movement and those that sustain postures or stabilize the segments.[9–11]

There are many muscles in the neck that provide both global and local functions (**Table 13-1**, **Table 13-2**, and **Table 13-3**), with the former having a primary role in torque production and control of the head, and the latter being primarily responsible for the support and control of the spine at a segmental level and as a whole.[11,12] The global muscles of the neck are thought to be the sternocleidomastoid (anteriorly), and the semispinalis capitis and splenius capitis (posteriorly). The local system is thought to comprise the longus capitis and longus colli[13] and semispinalis cervicis and multifidus.[14]

TABLE 13-1 Attachments and Innervation of Cervical Muscles

Muscle	Proximal	Distal	Innervation
Upper trapezius	Superior nuchal line Ligamentum nuchae	Lateral third of clavicle and the acromion process	Spinal accessory
Levator scapulae	Transverse processes of upper four cervical vertebrae	Medial border of scapula at level of scapular superior angle	Dorsal scapular C5 (C3 and C4)
Splenius capitis	Inferior ligamentum nuchae, spinous process of C7 and T1–T4 vertebrae	Mastoid process, occipital bone, and lateral third of superior nuchal line	Cervical spinal nerve and ventral primary rami of cervical spinal nerves
Splenius cervicis	Spinous processes of T3–T6 vertebrae	Posterior tubercles of C1–C3	
Scalenus			
Anterior	Anterior tubercles of C3–C6	Superior crest of first rib	Ventral primary rami of cervical spinal nerves
Middle	Posterior tubercles of C2–C7	Superior crest of first rib	
Posterior	Posterior tubercles of C5–C7	Outer surface of second rib	
Longus colli	Anterior tubercles of C3–C5 Anterior surface of C5–C7, T1–T3	Tubercle of the atlas, anterior tubercles of C5 and C6, anterior surface of C2–C4	Ventral primary rami of cervical spinal nerves
Longus capitis	Anterior tubercles of C3–C6	Inferior occipital bone, basilar portion	Ventral primary rami of cervical spine nerves

TABLE 13-2 Prime Movers of the Cervical Spine: Extensors and Flexors

Prime Extensors	Prime Flexors
Trapezius	Sternocleidomastoid—anterior fibers
Sternocleidomastoid—posterior fibers	Accessory muscles
Iliocostalis cervices	Prevertebral muscles
Longissimus cervices	Longus coli
Splenius cervices	Longus capitis
Splenius capitis	Rectus capitis anterior
Interspinales cervices	Scalene group
Spinalis cervices	Scalenus anterior
Spinalis capitis	Infrahyoid group
Semispinalis cervices	Sternohyoid
Semispinalis capitis	Omohyoid
Levator scapulae	Sternothyroid
Suboccipitals	Thyrohyoid

TABLE 13-3	Prime Movers of the Cervical Spine: Rotation and Side Bending

Ipsilateral Side Bending

Longissimus capitis

Intertransversarii posteriores cervices

Multifidus

Rectus capitis lateralis

Intertransversarii anteriores cervices

Scaleni

Iliocostalis cervicis

Ipsilateral Rotation

Splenius capitis

Splenius cervices

Rotatores breves cervices

Rotatores longi cervices

Rectus capitis posterior major

Obliquus capitis inferior

Contralateral Rotation

Obliquus capitis superior

Ipsilateral Side Bending and Contralateral Rotation

Sternocleidomastoid

Scalenus anterior

Multifidus

Longus colli

Ipsilateral Side Bending and Ipsilateral Rotation

Longus colli

Scalenus posterior

Temporomandibular Joint

The temporomandibular joint (TMJ) is a synovial, compound-modified ovoid bicondylar joint, formed between the articular eminence of the temporal bone, the intra-articular disc, and the head of the mandible. The mandible works like a class-three lever, with its joint as the fulcrum. There is agreement among the experts that postural impairments of the cervical and upper thoracic spine can produce both pain and impairment of the TMJ.[15] Located between the articulating surface of the temporal bone and the mandibular condyle is a fibrocartilaginous disc (sometimes inappropriately referred to as "meniscus"). The TMJ is primarily supplied from three nerves that are part of the mandibular division of the fifth cranial (trigeminal) nerve.

Osteokinematics and Arthrokinematics of the TMJ

The movements that occur at the TMJ are extremely complex.

- Mouth opening (mandibular depression), contralateral deviation, and protrusion all involve an anterior osteokinematic rotation of the mandible and an anterior, inferior, and lateral glide of the mandibular head and disc.
- Mouth closing (mandibular elevation), ipsilateral deviation, and retrusion all involve a posterior osteokinematic rotation of the mandible and a posterior, superior, and medial glide of the mandibular head and disc.

Muscle Control of the TMJ

Working in combinations, the muscles of the TMJ (**Table 13-4**) are involved as follows:

- *Mouth opening (mandibular depression):* Bilateral action of the lateral pterygoid and digastric muscles
- *Mouth closing (mandibular elevation):* Bilateral action of the temporalis, masseter, and medial pterygoid muscles
- *Lateral deviation:* Action of the ipsilateral masseter and temporalis, and contralateral medial and lateral pterygoid muscles
- *Protrusion:* Bilateral action of the lateral pterygoid, medial pterygoid, and anterior fibers of the temporalis muscles
- *Retrusion:* Bilateral action of the posterior fibers of the temporalis muscle, and the digastric, stylohyoid, geniohyoid, and mylohyoid muscles

Examination

The examination of the cervical complex performed by the physical therapist typically follows the outline in **Table 13-5**. The examination of the TMJ complex is outlined in **Table 13-6**. A description of the evidence-based tests of the cervical spine and TMJ are outlined in **Table 13-7**.

Intervention Strategies

Studies have reported that interventions for the cervical spine, which have included manual therapy, postural re-education, neck-specific strengthening and stretching exercises, and ergonomic changes at work, are beneficial in reducing neck pain and

TABLE 13-4 Muscles of the Temporomandibular Joint

Muscle	Proximal	Distal	Innervation
Medial pterygoid	Medial surface of lateral pterygoid plate and tuberosity of maxilla	Medial surface of mandible close to angle	Mandibular division of trigeminal nerve
Lateral pterygoid	Greater wing of sphenoid and lateral pterygoid plate	Neck of mandible and articular cartilage	Mandibular division of trigeminal nerve
Temporalis	Temporal cranial fossa	By way of a tendon into medial surface, apex, and anterior and posterior borders of mandibular ramus	Anterior and posterior deep temporal nerves, which branch from anterior division of mandibular branch of trigeminal nerve
Masseter	Superficial portion: from anterior two-thirds of lower border of zygomatic arch; deep portion from medial surface of zygomatic arch	Lateral surfaces of coronoid process of mandible, upper half of ramus, and angle of mandible	Masseteric nerve from anterior trunk of mandibular division of trigeminal nerve
Mylohyoid	Medial surface of mandible	Body of hyoid bone	Mylohyoid branch of trigeminal nerve, mandibular division
Geniohyoid	Mental spine of mandible	Body of hyoid bone	Ventral ramus of C1 via hypoglossal nerve
Stylohyoid	Styloid process of temporal bone	Body of hyoid bone	Facial nerve
Anterior and posterior digastric	Internal surface of mandible and mastoid process of temporal bone	By intermediate tendon to hyoid bone	Anterior: mandibular division of trigeminal nerve; posterior: facial nerve
Sternohyoid	Manubrium and medial end of clavicle	Body of hyoid bone	Ansa cervicalis
Omohyoid	Superior angle of scapula	Inferior body of hyoid bone	Ansa cervicalis
Sternothyroid	Posterior surface of manubrium	Thyroid cartilage	Ansa cervicalis
Thyrohyoid	Thyroid cartilage	Inferior body and greater horn of hyoid bone	C1 via hypoglossal nerve

improving mobility.[16–18] A study by Hoving and colleagues,[19] who used a pragmatic randomized clinical trial to compare the effectiveness of manual therapy (mainly spinal mobilizations), physical therapy (mainly exercise therapy), and continued care by the general practitioner (analgesics, counseling, and education) for cervical pain over a period of 1 year, found high improvement scores for the manual therapy group for all of the outcomes, followed by physical therapy and general practitioner care.

Acute Phase

The goals during the acute phase for this region:

- *To control pain, inflammation, and muscle spasm:* The usual methods of decreasing inflammation, PRICEMEM (protection, rest, ice, compression, elevation, manual therapy,

early motion, and medications prescribed by the physician), are recommended, although elevation is obviously not applicable. Systematic reviews of physical therapy modalities for neck pain report a lack of high-quality evidence of their efficacy and highlight poor methodological quality in many studies.[20] Although passive modalities have their uses in the acute phase, the clinician should remember that they must only be used as an adjunct to a more active program, and with a specific goal in mind, such as to help in the reduction of pain and inflammation. For example, the patient should be weaned off the use of the following modalities as early as possible.

- *Ultrasound:* Pulsed (at nonthermal levels) ultrasound can be applied to the posterior

TABLE 13-5 — Examination of the Cervical Spine

Observation and Inspection

Upper quarter and peripheral joint scan	Temporomandibular joint, shoulder complex, elbow, forearm, and wrist and hand
	Dermatomes and key muscle tests as appropriate.
Examination of movements; active range of motion with passive overpressure (except extension and rotation)	Flexion, extension, side bending (right and left), rotation (right and left)
	Combined movements as appropriate
	Repetitive movements as appropriate
	Sustained positions as appropriate
	Craniovertebral joint movement testing
Resisted isometric movements	All AROM directions
Palpation	Palpation of bony prominences and superficial structures
Neurological tests as appropriate	Reflexes, key muscle tests, sensory scan, peripheral nerve assessment
	Neurodynamic mobility tests (upper limb tension tests, slump test)
Joint mobility tests	a. Side glides
	b. Anterior and posterior glides
	c. Traction and compression
Special Tests (refer to Table 13-7)	As indicated
Diagnostic Imaging	As appropriate

TABLE 13-6 — Examination of the Temporomandibular Joint

Observation and Inspection

Upper quarter and peripheral joint scan	Cervical spine, shoulder complex, elbow, forearm, and wrist and hand
	Dermatomes and key muscle tests as appropriate.
Examination of movements; active range of motion with passive overpressure (except extension and rotation)	Mouth opening
	Lateral deviation
	Combined movements as appropriate
	Repetitive movements as appropriate
	Sustained positions as appropriate
Resisted isometric movements	All AROM directions
Palpation	
Neurological tests as appropriate	Reflexes, key muscle tests, sensory scan, peripheral nerve assessment
Joint mobility tests	a. Lateral glides
	b. Anterior and posterior glides
	c. Traction and compression
Special Tests (refer to Table 13-7)	As indicated
Diagnostic Imaging	As appropriate

TABLE 13-7 Evidence-Based Special Tests of the Cervical Spine and TMJ

Name of Test	Brief Description	Positive Findings	Sensitivity and Specificity
Temporomandibular joint screen[a]	The patient is asked to open and close the mouth, and to laterally deviate the jaw as the clinician observes the quality and quantity of motion and notes any reproduction of symptoms.	The patient reports tenderness in the masticatory muscles, the preauricular area, or the TMJ area.	Sensitivity: 0.87 Specificity: 0.67
Lateral palpation of TMJ[b]	Clinician palpates the lateral and posterior aspects of the TMJ with the index finger.	Positive for TMJ dysfunction if pain is elicited.	Sensitivity: 0.88 Specificity: 0.36
Auscultation of TMJ using a stethoscope[c]	Clinician auscultates for the presence of sounds during mouth opening/closing.	Presence of a *click* sound is considered positive for TMJ dysfunction.	Sensitivity: 0.69 Specificity: 0.51
Auscultation of TMJ using a stethoscope	Clinician auscultates for the presence of crepitus (grating or grinding) during mouth opening/closing	Presence of *crepitus* is considered positive for TMJ dysfunction.	Sensitivity: 0.70 Specificity: 0.43
Joint mobility testing of TMJ: condylar translation[d]	Clinician palpates condylar movement while patient maximally opens mouth.	Positive for anterior disc displacement if limited motion is detected.	Sensitivity: 0.32 Specificity: 0.83
Spurling (1)[e]	The patient side bends and extends the neck, and the clinician applies compression.	Positive if pain or tingling starts in the shoulder and radiates distally to the elbow.	Sensitivity: 0.30 Specificity: 0.93
Spurling (2)[f]	Patient is seated. Clinician side bends the neck toward the ipsilateral side, and applies 7 kg overpressure.	Positive if symptoms are reproduced.	Sensitivity: 0.50 Specificity: 0.88
Neck compression test[g]	Patient is seated. Clinician side bends and slightly rotates patient's head. A compression force of 7 kg is exerted.	Positive if test aggravates radicular pain, numbness, or paresthesias.	Sensitivity: 0.28 (right), 0.33 (left) Specificity: 0.92 (right), 1.0 (left)
Axial manual traction[h]	With patient supine, clinician provides actual distraction force between 10 and 15 kg.	Positive if symptoms are reduced or disappear.	Sensitivity: 0.26 Specificity: 1.0
Shoulder abduction test[g]	The patient lifts the hand above the head.	Positive if symptoms are reduced or disappear.	Sensitivity: 0.31 (right), 0.42 (left) Specificity: 1.05 (right), 1.0 (left)
Sharp-Purser test[i]	Patient sits with neck in a semi-flexed position. Clinician places palm of one hand on patient's forehead and index finger of the other hand on the spinous process of the axis.	When posterior pressure is applied to the forehead, a sliding motion of the head posteriorly in relation to the axis indicates a positive test for atlantoaxial instability.	Sensitivity: 0.69 Specificity: 0.96

TABLE 13-7

Evidence-Based Special Tests of the Cervical Spine and TMJ (continued)

Name of Test	Brief Description	Positive Findings	Sensitivity and Specificity
Compression of brachial plexus[j]	Clinician applies firm compression and squeezes the brachial plexus with the thumb.	Positive only when the pain radiates to the shoulder or upper extremity.	Sensitivity: 0.69 Specificity: 0.83
Pain provocation using active flexion and extension[k]	The patient performs active flexion and extension to the extremes of the range.	Positive for neck dysfunction if subject reports pain with procedure.	Sensitivity: 0.27 Specificity: 0.90

Data from (a) Cleland J: Temporomandibular joint, Orthopedic Clinical Examination: An Evidence-Based Approach for Physical Therapists. Carlstadt, NJ, Icon Learning Systems, 2005, pp 39–89; (b) Stegenga B, de Bont LG, van der Kuijl B, et al: Classification of temporomandibular joint osteoarthrosis and internal derangement. 1. Diagnostic significance of clinical and radiographic symptoms and signs. Cranio 10:96–106; discussion 116–117, 1992; (c) Manfredini D, Tognini F, Zampa V, et al: Predictive value of clinical findings for temporomandibular joint effusion. Oral Surg Oral Med Oral Pathol Oral Radiol Endod 96:521–526, 2003; (d) Orsini MG, Kuboki T, Terada S, et al: Clinical predictability of temporomandibular joint disc displacement. J Dent Res 78:650–660, 1999; (e) Tong HC, Haig AJ, Yamakawa K: The Spurling test and cervical radiculopathy. Spine 27:156–159, 2002; (f) Wainner RS, Gill H: Diagnosis and nonoperative management of cervical radiculopathy. J Orthop Sports Phys Ther 30:728–744, 2000; (g) Viikari-Juntura E, Porras M, Laasonen EM: Validity of clinical tests in the diagnosis of root compression in cervical disc disease. Spine 14:253–257, 1989; (h) Viikari-Juntura E, Takala E, Riihimaki H, et al: Predictive validity of symptoms and signs in the neck and shoulders. J Clin Epidemiol 53:800–808, 2000; (i) Uitvlugt G, Indenbaum S: Clinical assessment of atlantoaxial instability using the Sharp-Purser test. Arthritis Rheum 31:918–922, 1988; (j) Uchihara T, Furukawa T, Tsukagoshi H: Compression of brachial plexus as a diagnostic test of a cervical cord lesion. Spine 19:2170–2173, 1994; and (k) Sandmark H, Nisell R: Validity of five common manual neck pain provoking tests. Scand J Rehabil Med 27:131–136, 1995

aspects of the zygapophyseal joints or TMJ to control pain and reduce swelling, or applied to a torn muscle.

❑ *Cryotherapy:* Theoretically, ice is the preferred choice in the acute phase; however, ice can often increase pain that arises from trigger points. After several days, the switch can often be made to the use of heat, with its ability to relax musculature and stimulate vasodilation.[21]

The PT may perform grade I and grade II joint mobilization techniques to help provide pain relief.

■ *To promote healing:* Soft cervical collars do not rigidly immobilize the cervical spine, and if used judiciously can provide support for the head and neck in the very acute stages.[22,23] The collar serves a number of functions, among which are the following:

❑ Providing support in maintaining the cervical spine erect

❑ Reminding the patient that the neck is injured, and thereby preventing the patient from engaging in unexpected or excessive movements

❑ Allowing the patient to rest the chin during activities, thereby offsetting the weight of the head

❑ Allowing the patient to perform cervical rotations while the weight of the head is offset

Patients should be weaned off the collar as their recovery progresses (when there is significant improvement in the range of motion and pain levels). In those situations where absolute rest is warranted, the patient is told that rest means just that. Pillows should be adjusted so that the head remains in neutral when sleeping in side-lying or supine position. The patient should be cautioned about prone lying to prevent positions of cervical extension, excessive rotation, and TMJ pressure if these have been found to exacerbate the symptoms.

■ *To increase and maintain the newly attained ranges:* Exercise dosage should be determined on an individual basis, depending on the variables of strength, endurance, and irritability. A better response seems to occur when loads are initially very low (based on tolerance) and progressed slowly. Therefore, most of the initial exercises in the acute stage are performed in a non-weight-bearing position, such as supine, or as gravity assisted, and are performed as gentle repetitions, well within the pain-free range.

> **● Key Point** Although strengthening exercises have been advocated for the intervention of neck pain,[24,25] only a few controlled intervention studies have been conducted to examine their benefit. However, in one randomized study, investigators found that a multimodal intervention of postural, manual, psychological, relaxation, and visual training techniques was superior to traditional approaches involving ultrasound and electrical stimulation.[26] Patients returned to work earlier, and they had better results in pain intensity, emotional response, and postural disturbances.[26]

Cervical exercises that can be prescribed early in the intervention, based on the examination findings and plan of care (POC), include those in the following sections.

Head Nod

The primary exercise to recruit the deep cervical flexors, which are the most common muscles to become weak with neck dysfunction, is the head nod[27] exercise (Figure 13-3). The exercise is performed so that the flexion occurs only at the junction between the head and neck (at the OA joint) and continues segmentally into midcervical flexion. The exercise is initially performed in the upright position (gravity assisted), making sure that no forward movement of the head occurs (thereby changing the exercise into one of eccentric contraction of the cervical extensors), and to reduce the potential of use of the SCM muscle. As the patient slowly nods the chin down, the back of the head should be seen to move up toward the ceiling. The patient can be taught to palpate the SCM and scalene muscles during the exercise for any unwanted contractions. The nod is stopped at the point in the range that can be achieved without superficial muscle activity, held for 10 seconds to encourage the endurance function, and is repeated 10 times. Once the patient is able to tolerate the exercise in this position, they can be asked to perform the exercise in supine on an inclined board, thereby reducing the assistance of gravity as the board is tilted progressively backward toward horizontal. Once in supine, the head is positioned in neutral, resting either on a pillow or on a small folded towel placed under the occiput; support can be provided for the normal cervical lordosis (Figure 13-4). Initially the head nod is performed with no lifting of the head off the surface (the patient can palpate anteriorly to ensure no superficial muscle activity). The exercise is progressed so that the head nod uses the towel roll as a fulcrum and the back of the head may lift just

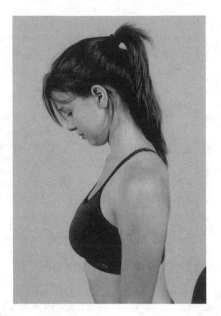

Figure 13-3   The head nod in sitting.

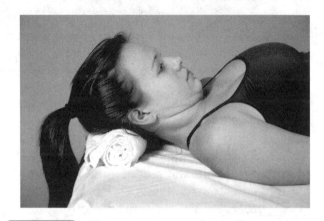

Figure 13-4   The head nod in supine.

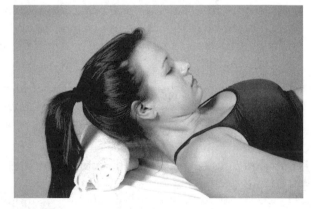

Figure 13-5   The head nod with head lift.

off the bed during the motion. At this time, palpation of the anterior structures is no longer necessary because the superficial muscles must now be active to lift the head off the bed (Figure 13-5). However, the head should not lose contact with the towel, nor should the chin poke forward, because this is a sign of excessive anterior translation caused by a relative dominance of the SCM and scalenes. To emphasize contraction of the flexors more unilaterally in cases of asymmetric weakness, a head nod into a flexion quadrant (e.g., flexion, side bending, rotation to the same side) can be used. The exercise can also be performed in prone over an exercise ball or in the quadruped position (Figure 13-6). In this position, gravity draws the head forward into a position of upper cervical extension, which is opposed by the head nod motion into upper cervical flexion.

Return to Neutral

The return to neutral exercise[27] is designed to recruit the deep cervical segmental extensors. The patient starts in the forward flexed position (Figure 13-7)

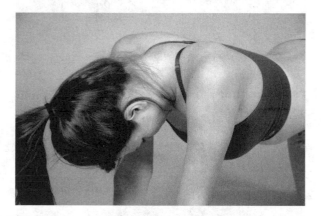

Figure 13-6   The head nod in quadruped.

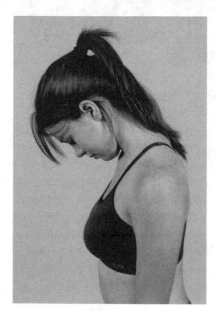

Figure 13-7   Return to neutral.

and initiates extension of the thoracic spine first before the movement reaches the lower cervical spine. If the CV region can be maintained in flexion until the end of the motion, the capitis group of the erector spinae muscles will tend to be inhibited. The exercise is progressed by having the patient perform it on all fours, and then isometrically. In cases of asymmetric weakness, the exercise can be made more specific by working into an extension quadrant (e.g., combined extension, side bending, rotation to the same side).

Coupling Activation

The muscles that are primary side benders and rotators can be recruited by exercising into a quadrant position.[27] For both of the following exercises, the patient is told to perform a preset nod to activate the deep stabilizing muscles prior to performing any motion of the head. A foam wedge (Figure 13-8) with the patient in supine can be used to apply resistance to the combined flexion, side bending, and rotation of the cervical spine. These muscles can be trained more specifically and intensely in the side-lying position, with the head supported on a pillow and a towel roll under the neck (Figure 13-9). As the head

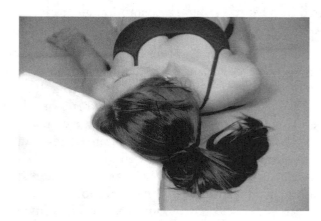

Figure 13-8   Coupling activation.

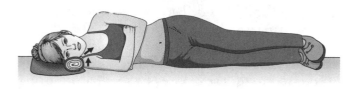

Figure 13-9   Coupling activation in sidelying.

is lifted off the pillow, using the towel roll as a fulcrum, the muscles opposite to the side the patient is lying on contract against gravity. The deeper muscles can be emphasized by ensuring that the neck remains in contact with the towel roll, thereby decreasing the amount of translation.

Active Assisted Range of Motion/Active Range of Motion

Care must be taken in teaching these exercises to ensure that the normal movement pattern is performed and that the pattern is reinforced with repetition.[27] The patient is positioned in supine with the head supported on a pillow. The patient is asked to perform gentle, active, small-range and amplitude rotational movements of the neck, first in one direction, then the other up to a maximum comfortable range. To help relieve muscle tension, the exercises can be done in conjunction with breathing.[28] When the patient reaches the easy end of range (at the point where the neck is about to leave its neutral zone and some tissue resistance is first being felt), the patient takes a moderate breath in and then releases it. At the end of the release, the relaxation of the muscles allows a slight increase in range without stressing any tissues and without causing pain. Once the non-weight-bearing range of motion can be performed without an exacerbation or recurrence of symptoms, active cervical range-of-motion exercises can be initiated in the sitting, and then standing positions.

Global Strengthening

Global strengthening often begins with submaximal isometric contractions throughout all planes using multi-angle isometrics, including flexion (Figure 13-10 and Figure 13-11), extension, side bending, and rotation. These exercises usually are performed initially against manual resistance applied by the clinician and then by the patient. Isolated strengthening of weakened muscle secondary to any radiculopathy is important before advancing to the more complex exercises involving multiple muscles. Although these exercises should not cause sharp pain, they may produce mild delayed-onset muscle soreness. Other movements, such as cervical retraction (Figure 13-12), cervical protrusion (Figure 13-13), extension, flexion, rotation (Figure 13-14), side bending, or a combination of these, can be added to the program, depending on which movements are found to be beneficial during the progression. The weight of the head is gradually introduced to these exercises by gradually moving from the horizontal to vertical position. As with any

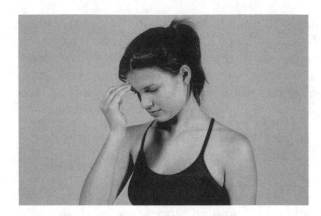

Figure 13-10   Multi-angle isometrics—flexion.

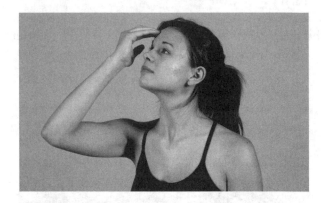

Figure 13-11   Multi-angle isometrics—flexion.

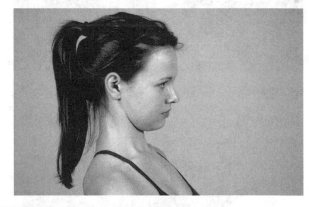

Figure 13-12   Cervical retraction.

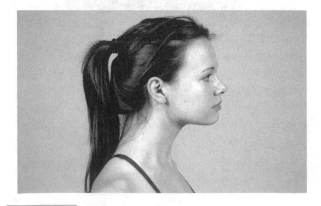

Figure 13-13   Cervical protrusion.

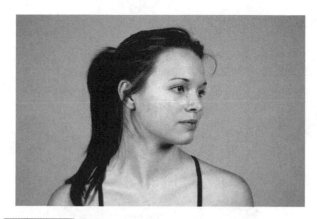

Figure 13-14 Cervical rotation.

exercise progression, as the patient's healing progresses these exercises are replaced with the more challenging exercises of the functional phase.

During this period, patients are encouraged to take up or resume a regular activity such as walking or anything else that will get them back to a normal mindset about their function, without reinjuring the area.

Subacute Through Chronic Phases

The stabilization of this region must include postural stabilization retraining of the entire spine, including the lumbar stabilization progression outlined in Chapter 15. Cervical and cervicothoracic stabilization exercises can help the patient to (1) gain dynamic control of cervical and cervicothoracic spine forces, (2) eliminate repetitive injury to the motion segments, (3) encourage healing of the injured segment, and (4) possibly alter the degenerative process.[29]

Once the patient is able to achieve co-contraction of the anterior and posterior muscles of the cervical spine in resting positions, the next goal is to be able to maintain cervical stabilization during arm motions. Cervical and cervicothoracic stabilization exercises should include those discussed in the following sections.

Upper-Extremity AROM

These exercises consist of initial co-contraction of the cervical musculature (preset nod), which is maintained while the patient performs repetitive motions of the upper extremity (e.g., flexion, abduction, diagonals) in supine and then in various other positions (i.e., quadruped, sitting, standing) while palpating the affected segment for unwanted translation. The pattern of the arm motion, amplitude, and position of the exercises are based on what combination

challenges the patient optimally—only those motions in which the segment can be maintained in neutral are performed. Progression includes adding hand weights or lying on a foam roll, which reduces the stability of the base. The same exercises can be progressed by having the patient perform them in a sitting position with the back to the wall to provide feedback about where the head is in space.

● **Key Point** Bilateral arm motions below 90 degrees often are the least challenging. Unilateral, overhead movements place higher demands on the stabilization system.

Functional Retraining

Many of the movement patterns required for functional activities are multiplanar, so it is beneficial to train muscle groups using these movements.[27] The movement patterns chosen for a particular patient depend on the assessment findings—specific weakness or reproduction of pain—and on the requirements of work and leisure activities. Initially, the patient is taught the correct movement pattern by the clinician, who palpates at the affected level as the patient performs the motion against the resistance of the clinician. The recruitment of the muscles about the segment and any excessive translation can be monitored. Concentric or eccentric muscle contractions can be used. Once the patient can perform these movements correctly (without excessive translation and/or pain), the movements are performed using multi-angle isometrics, then short-arc concentric exercises, progressing to full-arc motions, and then to eccentric contractions. Heavy resistance should be avoided because it tends to encourage faulty movement patterns, as do static maximal isometric contractions.

Strength training can progress to manually resisted cervical stabilization exercises in various planes. Cervical proprioceptive neuromuscular facilitation (PNF) patterns are ideal for this purpose (Figure 13-15 through Figure 13-18). Muscle co-contraction of agonist and antagonist can be used for joint stabilization, by increasing joint stiffness and supporting the independent torque-producing role of the muscles that surround the joint.[30-32] The use of PNF patterns for sport- and work-specific movements introduces a more functional approach. Isokinetic exercises of the neck are not functional and are not recommended as a strengthening tool. Continued efforts must be made to progressively reduce the patient's pain and advance physical function through exercise.[33]

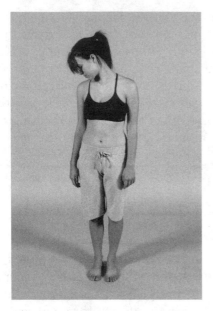

Figure 13-15 Cervical PNF.

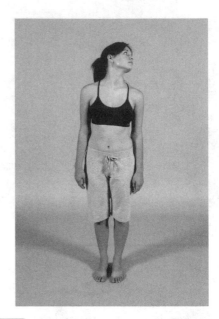

Figure 13-16 Cervical PNF.

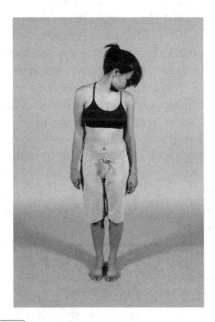

Figure 13-17 Cervical PNF.

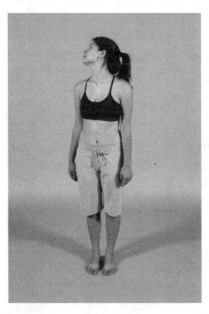

Figure 13-18 Cervical PNF.

Scapular Retractions

Scapular retractions (see Chapter 16) are initially performed supine, with the glenohumeral joint in external rotation. The patient is asked to isometrically retract the shoulders against the bed. Once this exercise can be performed without pain, the patient performs the exercise in prone, sitting, or standing without resistance. Resistance using resistance tubing is added as tolerated.

● **Key Point**   All exercises should be performed without pain, although some degree of postexercise soreness can be expected.

Scapular Stabilizers

The scapular stabilizers (middle and lower fibers of the trapezius, rhomboids, and serratus anterior) should be strengthened (see Chapter 16) using a gradual progression by adding gradual increments of arm load, and by increasing the amount of abduction until segmental control can be maintained in 140 degrees of abduction.[12]

Kinetic Chain Exercises

Strengthening of the entire kinetic chain should always be a consideration and will depend on the physical requirements of the patient. Strengthening exercises for the upper kinetic chain can include lat pull-downs, PREs for the middle trapezius and rhomboid, and upper extremity PNF patterns (see Chapter 16).

Aerobic Exercise

It is important throughout the rehabilitation process for patients to maintain their level of cardiovascular fitness as much as possible. Aerobic exercise, which increases endurance and the general sense of well-being, should be a part of all exercise programs.[34,35] Cardiovascular conditioning should be started as soon as possible to prevent deconditioning. These exercises also serve as a great warm-up prior to a stretching program.

Common Conditions

Some conditions affecting this region are more common than others. While this is not an all-inclusive list, the following information should provide the reader with guidelines for the listed conditions as well as provide help when dealing with similar conditions.

Cervical Strains and Sprains

A cervical strain may be produced by an overload injury to the cervical muscle–tendon unit because of excessive forces. These forces can result in the elongation and tearing of muscles or ligaments, edema, hemorrhage, and inflammation. Many cervical muscles do not terminate in tendons but, instead, attach directly to bone by myofascial tissue that blends into the periosteum.[36] Muscles respond to injury in a variety of ways, including reflex contraction, which further increases the resistance to stretch and serves as a protection to the injured muscle.

A cervical strain may be produced following an injury to the cervical joint capsule[37] and/or ligaments.[38] Pain is the chief complaint. Stiffness, tightness in the upper back or shoulder, and occipital headaches also may occur. Symptoms are typically aggravated by cervical positions that stretch or elongate the involved tissue, or by sustained postural positions, whereas symptoms are typically eased by lying down or supporting the cervical region. Initially, a cervical collar can be prescribed by the physician to reduce muscle guarding. Bed rest, along with analgesics and muscle relaxants, for no more than 2–3 days may also be prescribed by the physician for patients with a severe injury. However, in less severe cases, bed rest has not been shown to improve recovery and, when compared with mobilization or patient education, rest tends to prolong symptoms.[39,40]

Whiplash-Associated Disorders

Despite a great deal of attention, whiplash-associated disorders (WAD), a subset of the cervical sprain/strain diagnosis, remain an enigma. A lack of thorough understanding of WAD is, in part, a result of the nature of the disease itself. The subjective nature and high prevalence of the symptoms have led to controversy over their cause. These subjective complaints are most often characterized by reports of pain and suffering in the absence of focal physical findings and positive imaging studies.[41] In addition, the determination of the diagnosis has been veiled behind issues of appropriate financial compensation.[42–44] The Quebec Task Force on Whiplash-Associated Disorders[45] defines a whiplash as follows:

> Whiplash is an acceleration–deceleration mechanism of energy transfer to the neck. It may result from rear-end or side-impact motor vehicle collisions, but can also occur through diving and other mishaps. The impact may result in bony or soft tissue injuries (whiplash injury), which in turn may lead to a variety of clinical manifestations.

Postmortem studies have found that after whiplash injuries, ligamentous injuries are extremely common in the cervical spine, but that herniation of the nucleus pulposus is a rare event.[46–49]

The symptoms of a WAD usually begin in the neck and interscapular area within a few hours of the injury. These symptoms can develop to include neck swelling, muscle spasms, difficulty moving the neck, cervical radiculopathy, and severe headaches.[50]

A follow-up study, averaging a review time of nearly 11 years,[51] found that 40 percent of patients were still having intrusive or severe symptoms (12 percent severe and 28 percent intrusive). The same study also found that, in general, the symptoms did not alter after 2 years postaccident.

Intervention for Cervical Sprains and Strains

Ice and electrical stimulation are applied to the neck during the first 48–72 hours after injury to help control pain and inflammation. The patient should also receive education about proper resting positions and limitations of activity. Exercises that can be prescribed early in the intervention, based on the examination findings and POC, include those listed in the "Intervention Strategies" section.

At the end of every session, guidelines are provided for safe home exercising by teaching the patient to identify warning signs that could lead to exacerbation or recurrence of symptoms. In the event of an increase of symptoms, the techniques are adjusted by reducing either the amplitude of the movements or the number of movements, or both.

Impaired Posture

Forward head posture is described (in sitting or standing) as the excessive anterior positioning of the head, in relation to a vertical reference line; increased upper cervical spine lordosis and decreased lower cervical spine lordosis; and rounded shoulders with thoracic kyphosis (see Chapter 25). Other postural adaptations associated with the forward head posture include protracted scapulae with tight anterior muscles and stretched posterior muscles, jaw protrusion, and the development of a cervicothoracic kyphosis between C4 and T4.[52–54] These adaptations are further perpetuated by the natural cycle of aging of the spine, which involves degeneration of the disk, vertebral wedging, ligamentous calcification, all of which result in excessive flexion of the lower cervical spine, excessive extension of the upper cervical spine, and adaptively shortened cervical flexors (e.g., SCM and scalenes) and posterior suboccipital muscles. The habitual placement of the head anterior to the center of gravity (COG) of the body places undue stress on the temporomandibular joint, the cervical and upper thoracic facet joints (especially at the cervicothoracic junction), and the supporting muscles.[55,56] For each inch that the head is anterior to the COG, the weight of the head is added to the load borne by the cervical structures.[57] For example, the average head weighs 10 pounds. If the chin is 2 inches anterior to the manubrium, 20 pounds is added to the load. If normal motion is undertaken in this poor postural environment, the result may be abnormal strain placed on the joint capsule, ligaments, IVDs, levator scapulae, upper trapezius, SCM, scalene, and suboccipital muscles. Consequently, patients with a forward head posture can present with head, neck, and TMJ pain, but also mid-back and low-back pain. Few studies have investigated the association between posture and active range of motion. Hanten and colleagues[58] measured resting head posture and total range between full protraction and retraction in the horizontal plane in subjects with and without neck pain and found that the neck pain group had less range than the normal group. Lee and colleagues[59] investigated associations between subclinical neck pain/discomfort and range of motion and physical dimensions of the cervicothoracic spine. Their data suggested there are early range changes associated with the development of neck pain.

Intervention

It is important to retrain the patient to assume a correct upright and neutral spine position and to be able to consciously activate and hold the supporting muscles in a variety of functional positions.[12] The retraining of the cervicothoracic postural muscles usually begins at the lumbopelvic region, ensuring that the patient does not adopt the chest-out, shoulders-back position, which results in an incorrect thoracolumbar or thoracic lordosis, rather than a correct balance among all of the spinal curves.[12] The coordinated activity of the upper thoracic and scapular muscles is important for the maintenance of cervicothoracic posture and for upper limb function. Adaptive shortening of the posterior cervical extensors, scalenes, levator scapulae, upper fibers of the trapezius, and pectoralis major and minor is a common finding,[9,60] as is weakness of the deep, short cervical flexors (upper and mid-cervical), scapular stabilizers (serratus anterior, middle and lower trapezius, and rhomboids), and upper thoracic erector spinae.[12] To correct the forward head posture (FHP), the head must be brought back over the trunk. Patients are initially positioned with front and side mirror views so they are able to see any postural deviations of the spine, and so can see their habitual posture.[33] The clinician first helps the patient to find a neutral and balanced position of the lumbar and cervicothoracic spine, by using verbal and gentle manual cues, and then helps the patient to use this position in a series of basic functional movements.[33] For example, the clinician can direct the patient to "lift the sternum up," thereby decreasing the upper to midthoracic kyphosis. Recommended exercises include the following:

- Head nod exercises in supine lying with the head in contact with the floor with the chin tucked. This is progressed to the nod lift-off exercise, which maintains the neck in a tucked position while raising it off the off the floor and holding it for varying lengths of time.

- A chin drop in sitting (return to neutral exercise), initially with assistance, then without.
- Resisted shoulder retraction exercises in standing using resistance tubing. This is progressed to shoulder retraction in prone using weights.
- Unilateral and bilateral pectoralis stretches.

Maintaining the correct posture while incorporating upper extremity motion is the next progression, with exercises initially done with wall support and then freestanding. Then resistance is added to the upper extremity exercises while continuing to maintain the correct posture. Finally, functional activities are performed while maintaining the correct posture.

Cervical Spondylosis

Cervical spondylosis is a chronic degenerative condition of the cervical spine that affects the joint complexes (IVD, facets, and vertebral bodies) of the neck as well as the contents of the spinal canal (nerve roots and/or spinal cord). The characteristics of degenerative joint disease and degenerative disk disease pertain to bony changes, and the two often occur concurrently.[61] Chronic cervical degeneration is the most common cause of progressive spinal cord and nerve root compression. Abnormalities in the osseous and the fibroelastic boundaries of the bony cervical spinal canal affect the availability of space for spinal cord and nerve roots, resulting in a stenosis. Spondylotic changes can occur in the spinal canal and result in myelopathy, or can occur in the lateral recess and foramina, which can cause radiculopathy.

The clinical presentation of a symptomatic degenerative spine is one of a gradual onset of neck or arm symptoms (radiculopathy), or both, that has increased frequency and severity.[61] The pain is often worse when the patient is in certain positions, and can interfere with sleep. Morning stiffness of the neck, which gradually improves throughout the day, is a common finding.

Intervention

The conservative intervention for cervical spondylosis without radiculopathy or myelopathy involves the use of electrotherapeutic modalities to control pain and inflammation and increase the extensibility of the connective tissue. These modalities usually include moist heat, electrical stimulation, and ultrasound.

Immobilization of the cervical spine may be considered for patients with nerve irritation to limit the motion of the neck and further irritation. In such instances, soft cervical collars are recommended initially. More rigid orthoses (e.g., Philadelphia collar, Minerva body jacket) can significantly immobilize the cervical spine. With the use of any of the braces, the patient's tolerance and compliance are under consideration. The use of the brace should be discontinued as soon as feasible. Molded cervical pillows can better align the spine during sleep and provide symptomatic relief for some patients. Manual techniques may be used to stretch the adaptively shortened tissues. Range-of-motion exercises are performed as tolerated. These exercises initially are performed in the pain-free direction and then in the direction of pain. As the patient regains motion, isometric exercises and cervical stabilization exercises are prescribed (see the "Intervention Strategies" section).

Zygapophyseal Joint Dysfunction

Acute cervical joint lock (facet impingement) is a common condition of the cervical spine. The patient with this condition typically reports an onset of unilateral neck pain, or "neck locking," following sudden backward bending, side bending, or rotation of the neck, or pain that followed a sustained head position. The condition is thought to be the result of entrapment of a small piece of synovial membrane (meniscus) by the facet joint.[38,62,63] Symptoms of facet joint syndrome in the neck include neck pain, headaches, shoulder pain, and difficulty/pain with rotation of the head.

Intervention

The conservative intervention involves the use of electrotherapeutic modalities to control pain and inflammation. Joint mobilization techniques by the PT, involving combinations of flexion or extension and rotation, with traction superimposed, are applied initially in the pain-free direction and then in the direction of pain. As the patient regains motion, range-of-motion and isometric exercises are prescribed until full range of motion is restored, at which time the strengthening exercises are progressed (see the "Intervention Strategies" section).

Thoracic Outlet Syndrome

Thoracic outlet syndrome (TOS) is a clinical syndrome characterized by symptoms attributable to compression of neural or vascular anatomic structures (the brachial plexus and/or the subclavian artery or vein).[64,65] The names used for TOS are based on descriptions of the potential causes for its compression. These names include cervical rib syndrome, scalenus anticus syndrome, hyperabduction syndrome, costoclavicular syndrome, pectoralis minor syndrome, and first thoracic rib syndrome. Symptoms vary from mild to limb threatening and might be ignored by many clinicians, because they mimic common but difficult to treat conditions such as tension headache or fatigue syndromes.

The chief complaint is usually one of diffuse arm and shoulder pain, especially when the arm is elevated beyond 90 degrees. Other potential symptoms include pain localized in the neck, face, head, upper extremity, chest, shoulder, or axilla; and upper extremity paresthesias, numbness, weakness, heaviness, fatigability, swelling, discoloration, ulceration, or Raynaud phenomenon.[65] Neural compression symptoms occur more commonly than vascular symptoms.[66]

Intervention

Common impairments associated with TOS are a muscle length–strength imbalance in the shoulder girdle with tightness in the anterior and medial structures, and weakness in the posterior and lateral structures. The reasons for this imbalance range from faulty postural awareness to poor endurance in the postural muscles to a shallow respiratory pattern characterized by upper thoracic breathing. In addition, there may be poor clavicular and anterior rib mobility. Conservative intervention should be directed toward the cause, and typically focuses on the correction of postural abnormalities of the neck and shoulder girdle, strengthening the weak muscles (i.e., scapular adductors and upward rotators, shoulder external rotators, deep anterior cervical flexor muscles, and thoracic extensors), stretching the adaptively shortened muscles (i.e., scalene, levator scapulae, pectoralis minor, pectoralis major, anterior portion of the intercostals, and short suboccipital muscles), and mobilization by the PT of the hypomobile joints of the shoulder complex, clavicle, and first rib.

Cervical Disk Lesions

The term *disk dysfunction* often is used whenever changes in the IVD alter its biomechanical properties (see Chapter 2) and prevent normal function. Cervical disks may become painful as part of the degenerative cascade, from repetitive microtrauma, or from an excessive single load. Cervical radiculopathy is, by definition, a dysfunction involving compression and irritation of the cervical spinal nerve root. Any pathologic condition that increases the size

of the surrounding zygapophyseal joint, the UV joint, the IVD, and the pedicle can lead to narrowing or stenosis of the foramen, potentially entrapping the nerve root. Foramen size is also reduced by the movements of extension and ipsilateral side bending and rotation. The most common level of cervical nerve root involvement has been reported at the seventh nerve root (60 percent) and sixth nerve root (25 percent).[67,68] The capacity of the disk to self-repair is limited by the fact that only the peripheral aspects of the AF receive blood, and a small amount at that. In the acute stages, there is often painful limitation of active range of motion in all planes, particularly flexion; pain on cough or sneeze; painful cervical muscle contraction resulting from compression loading; and difficulty in maintaining upright postures because of the compression load of the head on the neck.[27]

Intervention

Conservative intervention consists of education about proper resting positions, a cervical collar, and oral corticosteroid "dose packs" and nonsteroidal anti-inflammatory drugs (NSAIDs) prescribed by the physician.[69,70] Electrotherapeutic modalities may be useful to help alleviate the inflammatory response and decrease associated muscle spasm. Manual traction techniques may be performed to help decompress the disk and increase intervertebral foramen size. Joint mobilization may also be used by the PT on hypomobile segments.

A cervical and cervicothoracic stabilization exercise progression, as outlined in the "Intervention Strategies" section, forms the cornerstone of the therapeutic exercise progression. To prevent further disk degeneration, and to reduce the incidence of recurrence, it is important to correct all postural impairments of the cervical spine, thoracic spine, and shoulder girdle.

Cervical Traction

Manual or mechanical traction (see Chapter 7) has long been a preferred intervention throughout the spine with the intent of improving range of motion and treating both zygapophyseal joint impairments and disk herniation.[71-76] The efficacy of traction in reducing radicular pain remains conflicted in the literature;[77,78] however, a clinical prediction rule with the following five variables has recently been developed:[79]

1. Patient-reported peripheralization with lower cervical spine (C4–C7) mobility testing
2. Positive shoulder abduction test

3. Age $\geq$ 55
4. Positive upper limb tension test (a test that places neural structures on stretch)
5. Positive neck distraction test

Having at least three out of five predictors present resulted in increasing the likelihood of success with cervical traction from 44 percent to 79.2 percent. If at least four out of five variables were present, the posttest probability of having improvement with cervical traction increased to 94.8 percent.

The patient position and setup for mechanical traction varies according to the findings (see Chapter 7). Traction is often applied in conjunction with the application of electrotherapeutic modalities, including moist heat and electrical stimulation over the paraspinal muscles, to aid in the relaxation of the muscles and to assist in the pumping of the edema.[80]

Surgical Intervention
In general, the decision to proceed with surgical intervention is made when a patient has significant extremity or myotomal weakness, severe pain, or pain that persists beyond an arbitrary "conservative" intervention period of 2–8 weeks.[81]

Acute Torticollis (Acute Wry Neck)

An acute form of torticollis, known as acute wry neck, typically develops overnight in young and middle-aged adults. The precise etiology is not clear, but because most of these patients appear to experience the symptoms shortly after awakening, it may be the result of an injury to the muscles, joints, or ligaments through simply sleeping with the neck in an unusual position. This unusual position may place the involved joints in a position of extreme motion, stretching the structures and increasing the risk of impingement when the joint position is returned to normal.

Patients with this condition present with painful neck spasms. On examination, cervical muscle spasm is visible and palpable. There is a marked limitation in range of motion of the neck, and the patient may hold the head in a position of comfort toward the side of the involved muscle.

Intervention

The hanging head method is a simple but effective method for treating acute painful wry neck of spontaneous onset.[82] The technique requires a table with a head-down tilt facility. The patient is positioned in supine at the end of the table and a head-down tilt of about 20 degrees is provided. This position, which is maintained for 5–10 minutes, provides a gentle traction force allowing the sternocleidomastoid to

relax. Alternatively, gentle traction can be applied manually by the PT. If this treatment is successful, no further intervention is necessary. In the cases where this technique is unsuccessful, the patient is reassured that they have a self-limiting condition, and that the symptoms will usually resolve significantly within 24–48 hours, with complete resolution within 2 weeks. Treatment during this period is symptomatic and may include:

- Moist heat, massage
- Patient education with regard to maintaining good posture and sleeping with the painful side on a low firm pillow
- Gentle range of motion exercises for the upper limbs and cervical spine
- Cervical collar use, which varies but should be used for only the first 24 hours

The patient's physician may prescribe muscle relaxants and analgesics.

If the symptoms do not resolve significantly after 48 hours, it is important to notify the supervising PT/referring physician to help rule out some of the more serious causes for these signs and symptoms. These include atlantoaxial rotatory displacement, juvenile rheumatoid arthritis, tumor, and bacterial meningitis.

Temporomandibular Joint Dysfunction

There are three cardinal features of temporomandibular joint dysfunction (TMD) that the PT looks for during the examination, which can be local or remote:

- *Restricted jaw function:* A history of limited mouth opening, which may be intermittent or progressive, is a key feature of TMD. Patients may describe a generalized tight feeling, which may indicate a muscular disorder or capsulitis, or have the sensation that the jaw suddenly "catches" or "locks," which usually is related to mechanical interferences in the joint (internal derangement).[83] Associated signs of an internal derangement include pain and deviation of mandibular movements during opening and closing.
- *Joint noises:* The presence of joint noises (crepitus) of the TMJ may or may not be significant, because joint sounds occur in approximately 50 percent of healthy populations.[84] Some joint sounds, such as "soft" crepitus, are not audible to the clinician, so a stethoscope may be required. "Hard" crepitus, often described as gravelly or grating, is a diffuse sustained noise that occurs

during a considerable portion of the opening or closing cycle, or both, and is evidence of a change in osseous contour.[85] Clicking is a brief noise that occurs at some point during opening, closing, or both. Jaw clicking during mouth opening or closing may be suggestive of an internal derangement consisting of an anterior disc displacement with reduction.[86,87]

● **Key Point** TMJ sounds should be described and related to symptoms. Joint noise is, of itself, of little clinical importance in the absence of pain.[88,89]

■ *Orofacial pain*: Approximately half of all cases of TMD are masticatory myalgias.[90] Pain should be evaluated carefully in terms of its onset, nature, intensity, site, duration, aggravating and relieving factors, and, especially, how it relates to the other features such as joint noise and restricted mandibular movements.[83] Orofacial pain associated with mouth opening or closing, and jaw crepitus are suggestive of osteoarthrosis, capsulitis, or internal derangement consisting of an anterior disc displacement with reduction.[86,87,91–94]

Intervention

Conservative intervention for TMD continues to be the most effective way of managing over 80 percent of patients.[95,96] Traditional conservative treatments for TMD have included interocclusal appliances, nocturnal alarms, physical therapy, occlusal calibration (also often termed occlusal equilibration), and cognitive-behavioral skills training (CBST).[97] A number of authors[98,99] have recommended that the intervention for TMD should be directed at the following factors, which are listed in order of importance to the patient:[100]

■ Treatment of symptoms to reduce or eliminate pain or joint noises, or both.
■ Treatment of the underlying cause, and to restore normal mandibular and cervical function. Selected exercises usually are performed by the patient on a regular basis to maintain muscle strength as well as joint arthrokinematic mobility in both the TMJ and cervical spine.[101]
■ Treatment of the predisposing factor. This is best achieved with a comprehensive approach that addresses the contributing factors of poor posture, stress, depression, and oral parafunctional habits.[84,102] Based on a systematic review of 30 studies examining the effectiveness of

exercise, manual therapy, electrotherapy, relaxation training, and biofeedback in the management of TMD, Medlicott and Harris[103] made the following recommendations:

❏ Active exercises and manual mobilizations may be effective.
❏ Postural training may be used in combination with other interventions because the independent effects of postural training are unknown.
❏ Low/mid-laser therapy may be more effective than other electrotherapy modalities.[104]
❏ Programs involving relaxation techniques and biofeedback, electromyography training, and proprioceptive re-education may be more effective than placebo treatment or occlusal splints.
❏ Combinations of active exercises, manual therapy, postural correction, and relaxation techniques may be effective.

It is clear from the studies that the TMD-related pain experience is complex and that there is a clear need for further well-designed randomized controlled trials examining physical therapy interventions for TMD that include valid and reliable outcome measures.

Acute Phase

Acute injuries to the TMJ most frequently have a traumatic origin, such as a direct blow to the masticatory structure[105–107] or a sudden locking of the jaw caused by an internal derangement.[108,109]

The patient with an acute injury typically demonstrates a capsular pattern of restriction (decreased ipsilateral opening and lateral deviation to the involved side), with pain and tenderness on the same side. There may be ligamentous damage, which will be demonstrated on the stress tests, or muscular damage, which will become apparent on isometric testing.

The usual methods of decreasing inflammation—that is, PRICEMEM (protection, rest, ice, compression, elevation, manual therapy, early motion, and medications)—are recommended, although elevation is not applicable with the TMJ. Cold is applied to reduce edema, inflammation, and muscle spasm. The mechanism behind cryotherapy is thought to be a "counter-irritation" and the production of analgesia.[21] The use of ice-filled towels soaked in warm water, applied all around the jaw, may prove beneficial in this phase. The patient should receive instruction on how to obtain the rest position of the TMJ. The rest position can be found by asking the patient to close the mouth so that the lips touch, but the teeth do not, and the tongue is resting gently on the hard palate. Motion of the TMJ should be restricted to pain-free movements. Limitation of mandibular function is encouraged to allow rest or immobilization of the painful muscular and articular structures. Very gentle active exercises, well within the pain-free range, should be performed frequently (every hour or so) to help stimulate the mechanoreceptors and modulate pain, as well as improve vascularization.

Initial exercises during the acute stage include the so-called 6 × 6 exercise protocol of Rocabado.[110] Although the effectiveness of these exercises has not yet been subjected to formal clinical investigation, they are thought to aid in strengthening, coordination, and the reduction of muscle spasm. The goals of these exercises are to:[111]

- Learn a new postural position for the cervical spine, shoulder girdle, and TMJ
- Restore the original muscle length
- Restore normal joint mobility
- Restore normal body balance
- Teach the patient to use these exercises whenever the symptoms of dysfunction return

The patient should be instructed to perform the following exercises six times each at a frequency of six times per day.

- *Tongue rest position and nasal breathing:* The patient places the tip of the tongue on the roof of the mouth, just behind the front teeth. In this position, the patient makes a "clucking" sound and gently holds the tongue against the palate with slight pressure. With the tongue in this position, the patient is asked to breathe through the nose and to use the diaphragm muscle for expiration. The use of accessory breathing muscles (pectoral, scalene, sternocleidomastoid, and intercostals) is discouraged, because they tend to promote and maintain a forward head posture.[111]
- *Controlled opening:* The patient positions the tongue in the rest position and practices opening the mouth to the point where the tongue begins to leave the roof of the mouth. The patient can monitor the joint rotation by placing an index finger over the TMJ region. The patient is encouraged to chew in this nontranslatory manner. In addition, neuromuscular education techniques such as biofeedback can be used to control premature or excessive translation during mouth opening.
- *Rhythmic stabilization:* The patient positions the tongue in the rest position and grasps the chin

with one or both hands. The patient applies a resistance sideways to the right and then to the left. The patient then applies a resistance toward opening and closing. Throughout all of these exercises, the patient must maintain the resting jaw position at all times and should be cautioned against the use of excessive force.

- *Liberation of cervical flexion:* The patient places both hands behind the neck and interlaces the fingers to stabilize the C2–C7 region. The neck is kept upright while the patient nods the head forward without flexing the neck. This motion produces a distraction of the occiput from the atlas and helps to counteract the craniovertebral extension produced by the forward head.
- *Axial neck extension:* In one motion, the patient is asked to glide the neck backward and stretch the head upward. This exercise needs to be monitored closely to prevent a hypermobility of the cervical segments. The goal of this exercise is to improve the functional and mechanical relationship of the head to the cervical spine.
- *Shoulder retraction:* In one motion, the patient is asked to pull the shoulders back and downward while squeezing the shoulder blades together. The goal of this exercise is the restoration of the shoulder girdle to an ideal postural position to establish stability of the entire head–neck–shoulder complex.

Another gentle exercise to increase joint mobility and articulation during this stage is the so-called cork exercise. The size (height) of the cork depends on the available motion. The patient holds the cork between his or her teeth while talking or reading aloud for approximately 2 minutes (Figure 13-19). The reading or talking exercise is then repeated with the cork removed.

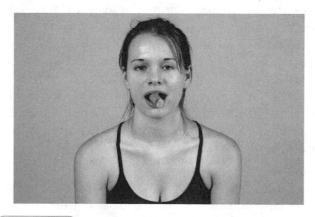

Figure 13-19 Cork exercise.

Patient Education

Perhaps the most important part of the intervention for TMD is to explain to the patient the cause and nature of the disorder, and to reassure him or her of the benign nature of the condition.[102] A successful self-care program may allow healing and prevent further injury, and is often enough to control the problem.[112] A typical self-care program includes the following: limitation of mandibular function (rest), a home exercise program, habit awareness and modification, and stress avoidance.[102] The patient is advised to eat soft foods and avoid those that need a lot of chewing, and is discouraged from wide yawning, singing, chewing gum, and any other activities that would cause excessive jaw movement.[102] The patient's sleeping position must also be addressed. If the intrinsic ligaments are injured, the patient should be advised to sleep on the back, with the mouth open and the neck supported by a cervical pillow.[84] Care must be taken to ensure that the patient does not sleep in the prone position, which stresses the cervical spine by extending and rotating it, and compresses the TMJ. Lastly, patients should be advised to identify source(s) of stress and to try to change their lifestyle accordingly.

Functional Phase

Although the interventions for this phase are discussed separately, for optimal success they are best used in combination and are dependent on the patient's needs.[4,113–115]

Postural Education

Postural education, together with patient education, should form the cornerstone of any physical therapy plan of care for patients with TMD. Because of the association between TMD and poor posture, the prescribed exercises for TMD include strengthening exercises for the cervicothoracic stabilizers and the scapular stabilizers (see Chapter 16). Stretching exercises are prescribed for the scalenes, trapezius, pectoralis minor, and levator scapulae, and the suboccipital extensors. The focus of the postural intervention should be to educate the patient on correct posture of the head, neck, shoulders, and tongue, in order to help minimize symptoms. Oftentimes, the focus of the education is to teach the patient mental reminders to reduce the time spent in habitual positions during work and recreation.[116–118]

Referral for Psychotherapy

Recent studies appear to suggest that TMD may be, on occasion, the somatic expression of an underlying psychological or psychiatric disorder such as depression or a conversion disorder.[102,119–124] Thus, in some cases, the PTA may discuss with the PT the need for a referral to a psychiatrist or clinical psychologist.

Trigger Point Therapy

Masticatory muscle pain is the one symptom for which there is the best overall evidence supporting various physical therapy interventions.[125] The most common intervention for these masticatory muscle disorders is trigger point therapy, which includes deep massage, soft tissue mobilizations, postural exercises, ultrasound, acupuncture, and trigger point injections by the physician.

Exercise

The patient should be encouraged to begin full active range-of-motion exercises as early as tolerated. However, if jaw deviation is occurring, the exercises should be performed in a range in which the patient can control the deviation. Excessive mandibular motion is treated by muscle re-education, with isometrics performed at the desired opening range.

Therapeutic Techniques

A number of techniques exist that can be used to treat the cervical spine based on the goal of treatment. Some of these techniques are performed by the physical therapist assistant while others can be performed by the patient as part of a comprehensive home exercise program.

Techniques to Increase Soft Tissue Extensibility

A variety of soft tissue techniques for the cervical region are available to the clinician. The choice of technique depends on the goals of the treatment and the dysfunction being treated.

Pectoralis Minor

The pectoralis minor can be stretched effectively using a corner and placing the hands on the walls (Figure 13-20). The patient needs to avoid adopting a forward head posture during the stretch. The clinician is cautioned against using this exercise with any patient with shoulder pathology, especially an anterior instability.

Pectoralis Major

The pectoralis major can be specifically stretched if the orientation of its fibers is considered (clavicular and costosternal), by having the patient lie supine and extending the arm off the table in either approximately 140 degrees of shoulder abduction (costosternal fibers) (Figure 13-21) or approximately 90 degrees of abduction (clavicular fibers).

Sternocleidomastoid

The SCM functions to flex and rotate the neck and extend the occipitoatlantal joint. The patient is positioned supine, with the head supported. From this position, the clinician induces side bending of the neck to the contralateral side, and extension of the neck (Figure 13-22). The clinician stabilizes the

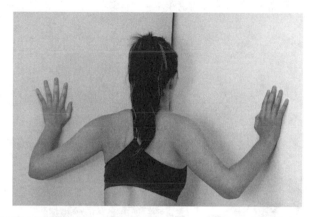

Figure 13-20 Corner stretch.

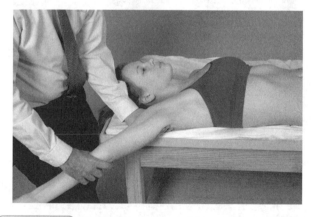

Figure 13-21 Stretch of costosternal fibers of pectoralis major.

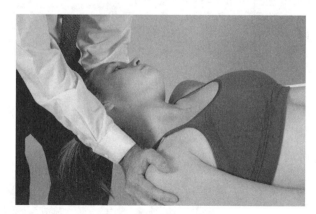

Figure 13-22 Stretch of SCM.

shoulder and rotates the patient's head and neck toward the ipsilateral side. To add a hold-relax stretch, the patient can then be asked to attempt to move the head and neck toward the contralateral side, a motion that is resisted by the clinician. When the patient relaxes, the clinician moves the head and neck further into the range.

Levator Scapulae

The patient is positioned supine, with the head at the edge of the table. The elbow and hand of the side to be treated are placed by the side. The clinician stands at the head of the table and presses his or her hand against the point of the patient's shoulder, fixing it caudally. Using one hand, the clinician then flexes the neck and side flexes the patient's head to the opposite side until resistance is felt (Figure 13-23). To add a hold-relax stretch, the patient can then be asked to look toward the treated side, a motion that is resisted by gravity. When the patient relaxes, the clinician moves the head into further side bending and flexion.

Upper Trapezius

This procedure is similar to that of the levator scapulae except that the amount of neck flexion is reduced. The patient is positioned supine, with the head at the edge of the table. The scapula is stabilized into depression and downward rotation. The clinician stands at the head of the table and presses his or her hand against the point of the patient's shoulder, fixing it caudally. Using both hands, the clinician then flexes the neck and side bends the patient's head to the opposite side. Rotation to the ipsilateral side is then added until resistance is felt (Figure 13-24). To add the PNF technique of hold-relax, the patient is then asked to look toward the treated side, a motion that is

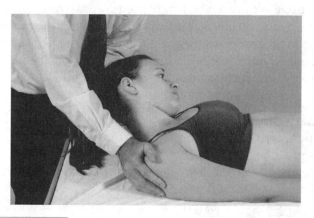

Figure 13-23 Stretch of levator scapulae.

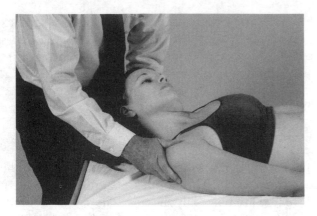

Figure 13-24   Stretch of upper trapezius.

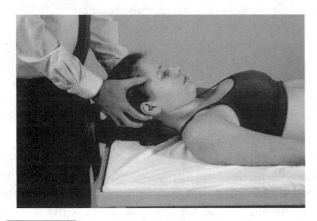

Figure 13-25   Stretch of posterior suboccipitals.

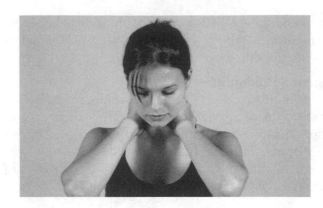

Figure 13-26   Hand-clasp flexion.

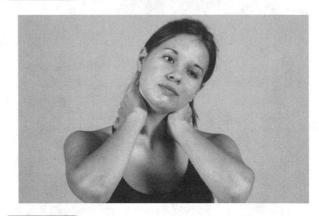

Figure 13-27   Hand-clasp sidebending.

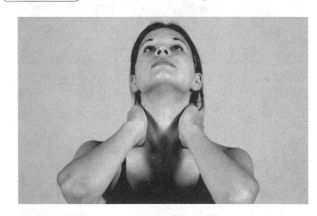

Figure 13-28   Hand-clasp extension.

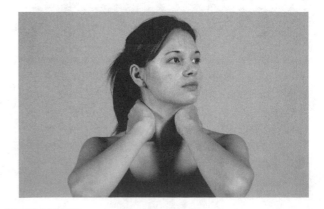

Figure 13-29   Hand-clasp rotation.

resisted by the clinician. When the patient relaxes, the clinician moves the head into further flexion, side bending, and rotation.

Posterior Suboccipital Muscle Group

This group includes the rectus capitis posterior major, the rectus capitis posterior minor, the obliquus capitis inferior, and the obliquus capitis superior. This muscle group can be lengthened by passively flexing the head on the neck (Figure 13-25). The stretch can be localized by supporting the rest of the neck with clasped hands, and further localized by side bending away and rotating toward the tighter side.

Hand-Clasp Exercise

Active range of motion in the cervical spine can be increased through patient participation, using the hand-clasp exercise.[126] The patient clasps his or her hands around the posterior aspect of the neck. The motions of flexion (Figure 13-26), side bending (Figure 13-27), extension (Figure 13-28), and rotation (Figure 13-29) can all be performed.

The patient is cautioned against reproducing sharp pain, while attempting to feel a stretch at the end of the available motion. With a different hand position, cervical extension can be performed in a controlled and safe manner. The fingers are again interlocked and placed behind the neck, but this time with the little fingers placed at the segmental level below the joint restriction. Using the little finger as a fulcrum, the patient extends the cervical spine to the point just shy of pain. This position is held for a few seconds and the neck is returned to the neutral position.

General Soft Tissue Techniques

The theoretical concepts behind soft tissue techniques and the various techniques are described in Chapter 6.

Prone

The patient is positioned prone, with the clinician standing to the side of the patient. The following areas are massaged:

- *Paraspinal gutter:* The clinician uses a thumb to apply a deep massage to the entire length of the paraspinal gutter.
- *Upper trapezius:* The clinician uses the heel of the palm and massages the upper trapezius (Figure 13-30). The clinician can also use the thumb to knead the upper trapezius muscle along the direction of its fibers.

Side Lying

The patient is positioned to be side lying. The following areas are massaged:

- *Scapular distraction:* The patient is in the side-lying position, and the clinician stands

facing the patient. Reaching over the back of the patient, the clinician grasps the scapula by sliding the fingers underneath the medial border and manually distracts the scapula away from the patient's back (Figure 13-31).
- *Scapular rotations:* The patient is in the side-lying position, with the clinician standing to the side of the patient. The clinician takes the patient's arm and rests it on his or her own arm. Reaching over the patient, the clinician grasps the whole shoulder girdle and rotates it in a full circle (Figure 13-32). This is done repeatedly, producing a rhythmic motion.

Self-Stretches

The patient can be instructed on how to self-stretch a number of muscles at home.

- *Upper trapezius:* The patient is seated with good posture. To stretch the right upper trapezius, the patient is asked to use the right

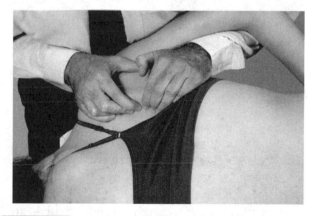

Figure 13-31   Scapular distraction.

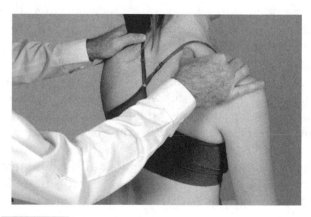

Figure 13-30   Massage to upper trapezius.

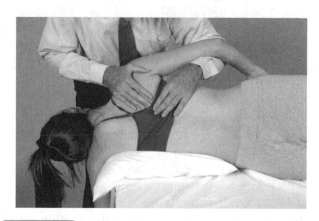

Figure 13-32   Scapular rotations.

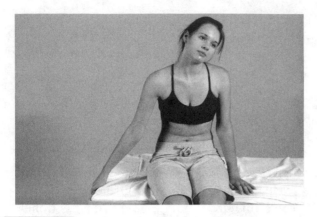

Figure 13-33　Self-stretch to the right upper trapezius.

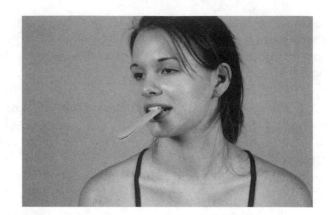

Figure 13-35　Tongue depressor stretch for TMJ.

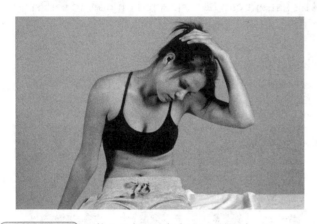

Figure 13-34　Self-stretch to right levator scapulae.

upper extremity to grasp the bottom of the table (Figure 13-33) and learn the head away so that the right shoulder is held in a depressed position. Using the fingers of the left hand, the patient grasps the right aspect of the head. Gentle pressure is applied with the fingers to side bend the head to the right. The side bending continues until a gentle stretch is felt. The stretch is maintained for 30 seconds, and then the patient relaxes. The stretch is repeated 10 times.

- *Levator scapulae:* The patient setup is the same as for the upper trapezius. To stretch the right levator scapula, the patient gently pulls the head and neck forward and to the opposite side, and then rotates the head to the left until the stretch is felt (Figure 13-34). The position of stretch is held for 30 seconds, and the procedure is repeated 10 times.
- *TMJ stretch:* Tongue depressors can be used to progressively increase mouth opening.

The patient is asked to open the mouth as far as is comfortable. A number of tongue depressors are then placed flat in the opening (Figure 13-35) so the stack fits snugly against both the upper and the lower teeth. By adding one depressor at a time to the stack, a gradual and sustained stretch can be applied to the TMJ and the structures restricting the mouth opening. Normal translation begins after 11 millimeters of opening, or about six tongue depressors. With the tongue depressors in position, a patient can mobilize the mandible actively into protrusion and lateral excursion.

Summary

The majority of the anatomy of the cervical spine can be explained in reference to the functions that the head and neck perform on a daily basis. To carry out these various tasks, the head has to be provided with the ability to perform extensive, detailed, and, at times, very quick motions. These motions allow for precise positioning of the eyes and the ability to respond to a host of postural changes that result from stimulation of the vestibular system (see Chapter 3).[127] In addition to providing this amount of mobility, the cervical spine has to afford some protection to several vital structures, including the spinal cord and the vertebral and carotid arteries. Because of the close relationship among the neck, thoracic spine, shoulder girdle, and temporomandibular joint, a complete and successful intervention must also deal with impairments found in these regions.

REVIEW Questions

1. What is the function of the uncinate processes (uncovertebral joint)?
2. Which of the following is not a suboccipital muscle?
    a. Rectus capitis lateralis
    b. Rectus capitis posterior major
    c. Rectus capitis posterior minor
    d. Obliquus capitis inferior
    e. Obliquus capitis superior
3. What is the action of the SCM?
4. What is the name of the second cervical vertebra?
5. In which plane does the craniocervical region allow the most motion?
6. Which of the following motions decreases the diameter of the intervertebral foramen, flexion or extension?
7. In which plane of motion does side bending of the cervical spine occur?
8. True or false: About one-half of the rotation available to the head and neck occurs from motion at the atlantoaxial joint.
9. True or false: The craniocervical region typically allows 90 degrees of axial rotation to each side.
10. True or false: The temporomandibular joint (TMJ) is a synovial, compound-modified ovoid bicondylar joint.
11. Which two muscles are involved with mouth opening?
12. Which muscles are involved with mouth closing?
13. When a patient deviates the jaw laterally to the right, which muscles are being used?
14. Describe the resting position of the TMJ.
15. What is the capsular pattern of the TMJ?

References

1. Maigne J-Y: Cervicothoracic and thoracolumbar spinal pain syndromes, in Giles LGF, Singer KP (eds): Clinical Anatomy and Management of the Thoracic Spine. Oxford, Butterworth-Heinemann, 2000, pp 157–168
2. Kelsey JL: An epidemiological study of the relationship between occupations and acute herniated lumbar intervertebral discs. Int J Epidemiol 4:197–205, 1975
3. Bovim G, Schrader H, Sand T: Neck pain in the general population. Spine 19:1307–1309, 1994
4. McNeill C: Temporomandibular disorders: Guidelines for diagnosis and management. CDA J 19:15–26, 1991
5. Huijbregts PA: Lumbopelvic region: Anatomy and biomechanics, in Wadsworth C (ed): Current Concepts of Orthopaedic Physical Therapy—Home Study Course. La Crosse, WI, Orthopaedic Section, American Physical Therapy Association, 2001
6. Adams CBT, Logue V: Studies in spondylotic myelopathy 2. The movement and contour of the spine in relation to the neural complications of cervical spondylosis. Brain 94:569–586, 1971
7. Penning L: Functional Pathology of the Cervical Spine. Baltimore, Williams & Wilkins, 1968
8. Panjabi MM: The stabilizing system of the spine. Part II. Neutral zone and instability hypothesis. J Spinal Disord 5:390–396; discussion 397, 1992
9. Janda V: Muscles and motor control in cervicogenic disorders: Assessment and management, in Grant R (ed): Physical Therapy of the Cervical and Thoracic Spine. New York, Churchill Livingstone, 1994, pp 195–216
10. Jull GA, Janda V: Muscle and motor control in low back pain, in Twomey LT, Taylor JR (eds): Physical Therapy of the Low Back: Clinics in Physical Therapy. New York, Churchill Livingstone, 1987, pp 258–278
11. Bergmark A: Stability of the lumbar spine. Acta Orthop Scand 60:1–54, 1989
12. Jull GA: Physiotherapy management of neck pain of mechanical origin, in Giles LGF, Singer KP (eds): Clinical Anatomy and Management of Cervical Spine Pain. The Clinical Anatomy of Back Pain. London, Butterworth-Heinemann, 1998, pp 168–191
13. Mayoux-Benhamou MA, Revel M, Valle C, et al: Longus colli has a postural function on cervical curvature. Surg Radiol Anat 16:367–371, 1994
14. Conley MS, Meyer RA, Bloomberg JJ, et al: Noninvasive analysis of human neck muscle function. Spine 20:2505–2512, 1995
15. Bell WE: Orofacial Pains: Classification, Diagnosis, Management (ed 3). Chicago, New Year Medical Publishers, 1985
16. Koes BW, Bouter LM, van Mameren H, et al: The effectiveness of manual therapy, physiotherapy and treatment by the general practitioner for nonspecific back and neck complaints: A randomized clinical trial. Spine 17:28–35, 1992
17. Foley-Nolan D, Moore K, Codd M, et al: Low energy high frequency pulsed electromagnetic therapy for acute whiplash disorders. A double blind randomized controlled study. Scand J Rehabil Med 24:51–59, 1992
18. Giebel GD, Edelmann M, Huser R: Sprain of the cervical spine: Early functional vs. immobilization treatment (in German). Zentralbl Chir 122:512–521, 1997
19. Hoving JL, de Vet HC, Koes BW, et al: Manual therapy, physical therapy, or continued care by the general practitioner for patients with neck pain: Long-term results from a pragmatic randomized clinical trial. Clin J Pain 22:370–377, 2006
20. Gross AR, Aker PD, Goldsmith CH, et al: Physical medicine modalities for mechanical neck disorders. Cochrane Database Syst Rev 2, 2000
21. Michlovitz SL: The use of heat and cold in the management of rheumatic diseases, in Michlovitz SL (ed): Thermal Agents in Rehabilitation. Philadelphia, FA Davis, 1990, pp 158–174

22. Gennis P, Miller L, Gallagher EJ, et al: The effect of soft cervical collars on persistent neck pain in patients with whiplash injury. Acad Emerg Med 3:568–573, 1998
23. Quebec Task Force on Spinal Disorders: Scientific approach to the assessment and management of activity-related spinal disorders: A monograph for clinicians. Report of the Quebec Task Force on Spinal Disorders. Spine 12:1–59, 1987 (Suppl)
24. Berg HE, Berggren G, Tesch PA: Dynamic neck strength training effect on pain and function. Arch Phys Med Rehabil 75:661–665, 1994
25. Dyrssen T, Svedenkrans M, Paasikivi J: Muskelträning vid besvär I nacke och skuldror effektiv behandling för att minska smärtan. Läkartidningen 86:2116–2120, 1989
26. Provinciali L, Baroni M, Illuminati L, et al: Multimodal treatment of whiplash injury. Scand J Rehabil Med 28:105–111, 1996
27. Kennedy CN: The cervical spine, in Hall C, Thein-Brody L (eds): Therapeutic Exercise: Moving Toward Function. Baltimore, MD, Lippincott Williams & Wilkins, 2005, pp 582–609
28. Meadows J: A Rational and Complete Approach to the Sub-Acute Post-MVA Cervical Patient. Calgary, AB, Swodeam Consulting, 1995
29. Cole AJ, Farrell JP, Stratton SA: Functional rehabilitation of cervical spine athletic injuries, in Kibler BW, Herring JA, Press JM (eds): Functional Rehabilitation of Sports and Musculoskeletal Injuries. Gaithersburg, MD, Aspen, 1998, pp 127–148
30. Keshner EA, Campbell D, Katz RT: Neck muscle activiation patterns in humans during isometric head stabilization. Exp Brain Res 75:335–344, 1989
31. Andersson GBJ, Winters JM: Role of muscle in postural tasks: Spinal loading and postural stability, in Winters JM, Woo SL-Y (eds): Multiple Muscle Systems. New York, Springer-Verlag, 1990, pp 375–395
32. O'Connor JJ: Can muscle co-contraction protect knee ligaments after injury or repair? J Bone Joint Surg 75-B:41–48, 1993
33. Sweeney TB, Prentice C, Saal JA, et al: Cervicothoracic muscular stabilization techniques, in Saal JA (ed): Physical Medicine and Rehabilitation, State of the Art Reviews: Neck and Back Pain. Philadelphia, Hanley & Belfus, 1990, pp 335–359
34. Turk DC, Nash JM: Chronic pain: New ways to cope, in Goleman D, Gurin J (eds): Mind Body Medicine. Yonkers, NY, Consumers Union of the United States, 1993, pp 111–131
35. Jette DU, Jette AM: Physical therapy and health outcomes in patients with spinal impairments. Phys Ther 76:930–945, 1996
36. Press JM, Herring SA, Kibler WB: Rehabilitation of Musculoskeletal Disorders. The Textbook of Military Medicine. Washington, DC: Borden Institute, Office of the Surgeon General, 1996
37. McLain RF: Mechanoreceptor endings in human cervical facet joints. Spine 19:495–501, 1994
38. Aprill C, Bogduk N: The prevalence of cervical zygapophysial joint pain: A first approximation. Spine 17:744–747, 1992
39. McKinney LA, Dornan JO, Ryan M: The role of physiotherapy in the management of acute neck sprains following road-traffic accidents. Arch Emerg Med 6:27–33, 1989
40. McKinney LA: Early mobilisation and outcome in acute sprains of the neck. BMJ 299:1006–1008, 1989
41. Spitzer WO, Skovron ML, Salmi LR, et al: Scientific monograph of the Quebec Task Force on Whiplash-Associated Disorders: Redefining "whiplash" and its management. Spine 20, 1-73, 1995 [Erratum, Spine 20:2372, 1995]
42. Reilly PA, Travers R, Littlejohn GO: Epidemiology of soft tissue rheumatism: The influence of the law. J Rheumatol 18:1448–1449, 1991
43. Evans RW: Some observations on whiplash injuries. Neurol Clin 10:975–997, 1992
44. Ferrari R, Russell AS: Epidemiology of whiplash: An international dilemma. Ann Rheum Dis 58:1–5, 1999
45. Scientific monograph of the Quebec Task Force on Whiplash-Associated Disorders. Spine 20:33S, 38S–39S, 1995
46. Jonsson H, Cesarini K, Sahlstedt B, et al: Findings and outcomes in whiplash-type neck distortions. Spine 19:2733–2743, 1994
47. Jonsson H, Bring G, Rauschning W, et al: Hidden cervical spine injuries in traffic accident victims with skull fractures. J Spinal Disord 4:251–263, 1991
48. Rauschning W, McAfee PC, Jonsson H: Pathoanatomical and surgical findings in cervical spinal injuries. J Spinal Disord 2:213–222, 1989
49. Twomey LT, Taylor JR: The whiplash syndrome: Pathology and physical treatment. J Man Manip Ther 1:26–29, 1993
50. Hardin J, Jr.: Pain and the cervical spine. Bull Rheum Dis 50:1–4, 2001
51. Gargan MF, Bannister GC: Long term prognosis of soft tissue injuries of the neck. J Bone Joint Surg 72B:901, 1990
52. Janda V: Muscle Function Testing. London, Butterworths, 1983
53. Refshauge KM, Bolst L, Goodsell M: The relationship between cervicothoracic posture and the presence of pain. J Man Manip Ther 3:21–24, 1995
54. Saunders HD, Ryan RS: Evaluation, Treatment and Prevention of Musculoskeletal Disorders, Vol 1: Spine (ed 4). Chaska, MN, The Saunders Group, 2004
55. Ayub E: Posture and the upper quarter, in Donatelli RA (ed): Physical Therapy of the Shoulder (ed 2). New York, Churchill Livingstone, 1991, pp 81–90
56. Turner M: Posture and pain. Phys Ther 37:294, 1957
57. Cailliet R: Neck and Arm Pain (ed 3). Philadelphia, FA Davis, 1990
58. Hanten WP, Lucio RM, Russell JL, et al: Assessment of total head excursion and resting head posture. Arch Phys Med Rehabil 72:877–880, 1991
59. Lee H, Nicholson LL, Adams RD: Cervical range of motion associations with subclinical neck pain. Spine 29:33–40, 2004
60. White AA, Sahrmann SA: A movement system balance approach to management of musculoskeletal pain, in Grant R (ed): Physical Therapy for the Cervical and Thoracic Spine. Edinburgh, Churchill Livingstone, 1994, pp 339–358
61. Walsh R, Nitz AJ: Cervical spine, in Wadsworth C (ed): Current Concepts of Orthopedic Physical Therapy—Home Study Course. La Crosse, WI, Orthopaedic Section, American Physical Therapy Association, 2001

62. Bogduk N, Lord SM: Cervical zygapophysial joint pain. Neurosurg Q 8:107–117, 1998

63. Dwyer A, Aprill C, Bogduk N: Cervical zygapophyseal joint pain patterns: A study from normal volunteers. Spine 15:453, 1990

64. Nichols AW: The thoracic outlet syndrome in athletes. J Am Board Fam Pract 9:346–355, 1996

65. Thompson JF, Jannsen F: Thoracic outlet syndromes. Br J Surg 83:435–436, 1996

66. Roos DB: The place for scalenectomy and first-rib resection in thoracic outlet syndrome. Surgery 92:1077–1085, 1982

67. Gore DR, Sepic SB, Gardner GM, et al: Roentgenographic findings in the cervical spine of asymptomatic people. Spine 6:521–526, 1987

68. Ward R: Myofascial release concepts, in Nyberg N, Basmajian JV (eds): Rational Manual Therapies. Baltimore, Williams & Wilkins, 1993, pp 223–241

69. Grisoli F, Graziani N, Fabrizi AP, et al: Anterior discectomy without fusion for treatment of cervical lateral soft disc extrusion: A follow-up of 120 cases. Neurosurgery 24:853–859, 1989

70. Gore DR, Sepic SB: Anterior cervical fusion for degenerated or protruded discs. A review of one hundred forty-six patients. Spine 9:667–671, 1984

71. Beurskens AJ, de Vet HC, Koke AJ, et al: Efficacy of traction for nonspecific low back pain: 12-week and 6-month results of a randomized clinical trial. Spine 22:2756–2762, 1997

72. Harris PR: Cervical traction: Review of literature and treatment guidelines. Phys Ther 57:910–914, 1977

73. Licht S: Massage, Manipulation and Traction. Connecticut, E. Licht, 1960, pp 60–92

74. Natchev E: A Manual on Autotraction. Stockholm, Sweden, Folksam Scientific Council, 1984

75. Twomey L: Sustained lumbar traction. An experimental study of long spine segments. Spine 10:146–149, 1985

76. Zylbergold RS, Piper MC: Cervical spine disorders. A comparison of three types of traction. Spine 10:867–871, 1985

77. Young IA, Michener LA, Cleland JA, et al: Manual therapy, exercise, and traction for patients with cervical radiculopathy: A randomized clinical trial. Phys Ther 89:632–642, 2009

78. Dreyer SJ, Boden SD: Nonoperative treatment of neck and arm pain. Spine 23:2746–2754, 1998

79. Raney NH, Petersen EJ, Smith TA, et al: Development of a clinical prediction rule to identify patients with neck pain likely to benefit from cervical traction and exercise. Eur Spine J 18:382–391, 2009

80. Reed BV: Effect of high voltage pulsed electrical stimulation on microvascular permeability to plasma proteins: A possible mechanism of minimizing edema. Phys Ther 68:491–495, 1988

81. Aldrich F: Posterolateral microdiscectomy for cervical monoradiculopathy caused by posterolateral soft cervical disc sequestration. J Neurosurg 72:370–377, 1990

82. Banerjee A: The hanging head method for the treatment of acute wry neck. Arch Emerg Med 7:125, 1990

83. Dimitroulis G: Temporomandibular disorders: A clinical update. BMJ 317:190–194, 1998

84. McNeill C: Temporomandibular Disorders—Guidelines for Classification, Assessment and Management (ed 2). Chicago, Quintessence Books, 1993

85. Kaplan AS: Examination and diagnosis, in Kaplan AS, Assael LA (eds): Temporomandibular Disorders Diagnosis and Treatment. Philadelphia, WB Saunders, 1991, pp 284–311

86. Orsini MG, Kuboki T, Terada S, et al: Clinical predictability of temporomandibular joint disc displacement. J Dent Res 78:650–660, 1999

87. Barclay P, Hollender LG, Maravilla KR, et al: Comparison of clinical and magnetic resonance imaging diagnosis in patients with disk displacement in the temporomandibular joint. Oral Surg Oral Med Oral Pathol Oral Radiol Endod 88:37–43, 1999

88. Green CS, Laskin DM: Long term status of TMJ clicking in patients with myofascial pain dysfunction. J Am Dent Assoc 117:461–465, 1988

89. Dolwick MF: Clinical diagnosis of temporomandibular joint internal derangement and myofascial pain and dysfunction. Oral Maxillofac Surg Clin North Am 1:1–6, 1989

90. Marbach JJ, Lipton JA: Treatment of patients with temporomandibular joint and other facial pain by otolaryngologists. Arch Otolaryngol 108:102–107, 1982

91. Brazeau GA, Gremillion HA, Widmer CG, et al: The role of pharmacy in the management of patients with temporomandibular disorders and orofacial pain. J Am Pharm Assoc (Wash) 38:354-361; quiz 362–363, 1998

92. Cholitgul W, Nishiyama H, Sasai T, et al: Clinical and magnetic resonance imaging findings in temporomandibular joint disc displacement. Dentomaxillofac Radiol 26:183–188, 1997

93. Cholitgul W, Petersson A, Rohlin M, et al: Clinical and radiological findings in temporomandibular joints with disc perforation. Int J Oral Maxillofac Surg 19:220–225, 1990

94. Cholitgul W, Petersson A, Rohlin M, et al: Diagnostic outcome and observer performance in sagittal tomography of the temporomandibular joint. Dentomaxillofac Radiol 19:1–6, 1990

95. Goldstein BH: Temporomandibular disorders: A review of current understanding. Oral Surg Oral Med Oral Pathol Oral Radiol Endod 88:379–385, 1999

96. Carlsson GE: Long-term effects of treatment of craniomandibular disorders. J Craniomand Pract 3:337–342, 1985

97. Gatchel RJ, Stowell AW, Wildenstein L, et al: Efficacy of an early intervention for patients with acute temporomandibular disorder-related pain: A one-year outcome study. J Am Dent Assoc 137:339–347, 2006

98. Ogus HD, Toller PA: Common Disorders of the Temporomandibular Joint. Bristol, John Wright & Son, 1986

99. Guralnik W: The temporomandibular joint: The dentist's dilemma: Parts I and II. Br Dent J 156:315–319; 353–356, 1984

100. Gray RJ, Quayle AA, Hall CA, et al: Physiotherapy in the treatment of temporomandibular joint disorders: A comparative study of four treatment methods. Br Dent J 176:257–261, 1994

101. Dunn J: Physical therapy, in Kaplan AS, Assael LA (eds): Temporomandibular Disorders Diagnosis and Treatment. Philadelphia, WB Saunders, 1991, pp 455–500

102. Dimitroulis G, Gremillion HA, Dolwick MF, et al: Temporomandibular disorders. 2. Non-surgical treatment. Aust Dent J 40:372–376, 1995

103. Medlicott MS, Harris SR: A systematic review of the effectiveness of exercise, manual therapy, electrotherapy, relaxation training, and biofeedback in the management of temporomandibular disorder. Phys Ther 86:955–973, 2006

104. Kulekcioglu S, Sivrioglu K, Ozcan O, et al: Effectiveness of low-level laser therapy in temporomandibular disorder. Scand J Rheumatol 32:114–118, 2003

105. Harkins SJ, Marteney JL: Extrinsic trauma: A significant precipitating factor in temporomandibular dysfunction. J Prosthet Dent 54:271–272, 1985

106. Pullinger AG, Seligman DA: Trauma history in diagnostic groups of temporomandibular disorders. Oral Surg Oral Med Oral Pathol Oral Radiol Endod 71:529–534, 1991

107. Pullinger AG, Monteiro AA: History factors associated with symptoms of temporomandibular disorders. J Oral Rehabil 15:117–124, 1988

108. Weinberg LA, Larger LA: Clinical report on the etiology and diagnosis of TMJ dysfunction-pain syndrome. J Prosthet Dent 44:642–653, 1980

109. Stenger J: Whiplash. Basal facts. J Prosthet Dent 2:5–12, 1977

110. Rocabado M: Physical therapy for the post-surgical TMJ patient. J Craniomand Disord 7:75–82, 1989

111. Rocabado M: Arthrokinematics of the temporomandibular joint, in Gelb H (ed): Clinical Management of Head, Neck and TMJ Pain and Dysfunction. Philadelphia, WB Saunders, 1985

112. Hodges JM: Managing temporomandibular joint syndrome. Laryngoscope 100:60–66, 1990

113. Dimitroulis G, Dolwick MF, Gremillion HA: Temporomandibular disorders. 1. Clinical evaluation. Aust Dent J 40:301–305, 1995

114. Feine JS, Widmer CG, Lund JP: Physical therapy: A critique. Oral Surg Oral Med Oral Pathol Oral Radiol Endod 83:123–127, 1997

115. Feine JS, Lund JP: An assessment of the efficacy of physical therapy and physical modalities for the control of chronic musculoskeletal pain. Pain 71:5–23, 1997

116. Kendall FP, McCreary EK, Provance PG: Muscles: Testing and Function. Baltimore, Williams & Wilkins, 1993

117. Janda V: Muscle strength in relation to muscle length, pain and muscle imbalance, in Harms-Ringdahl K (ed): Muscle Strength. New York, Churchill Livingstone, 1993, pp 83–91

118. Sahrmann SA: Diagnosis and Treatment of Movement Impairment Syndromes. St Louis, Mosby, 2001

119. Moss RA, Adams HE: The class of personality, anxiety and depression in mandibular pain dysfunction subjects. J Oral Rehabil 11:233–237, 1984

120. Rugh JD: Psychological components of pain. Dent Clin North Am 31:579–594, 1987

121. Cohen S, Rodriguez MS: Pathways linking affective disturbances and physical disorders. Health Psychol 14:371–373, 1995

122. Gatchel RJ, Garofalo JP, Ellis E, et al: Major psychological disorders in acute and chronic TMD: An initial examination. J Am Dent Assoc 127:1365–1370, 1372, 1374, 1996

123. Kight M, Gatchel RJ, Wesley L: Temporomandibular disorders: Evidence for significant overlap with psychopathology. Health Psychol 18:177–182, 1999

124. Korszun A, Papadopoulos E, Demitrack M, et al: The relationship between temporomandibular disorders and stress-associated syndromes. Oral Surg Oral Med Oral Pathol Oral Radiol Endod 86:416–420, 1998

125. Clark GT, Adachi NY, Dornan MR: Physical medicine procedures affect temporomandibular disorders: A review. J Am Dent Assoc 121:151–161, 1990

126. Erhard RE: Manual Therapy in the Cervical Spine, Orthopedic Physical Therapy Home Study Course. La Crosse, WI, Orthopaedic Section, American Physical Therapy Association, 1996

127. Pratt N: Anatomy of the Cervical Spine. La Crosse, WI, Orthopaedic Section, American Physical Therapy Association, 1996

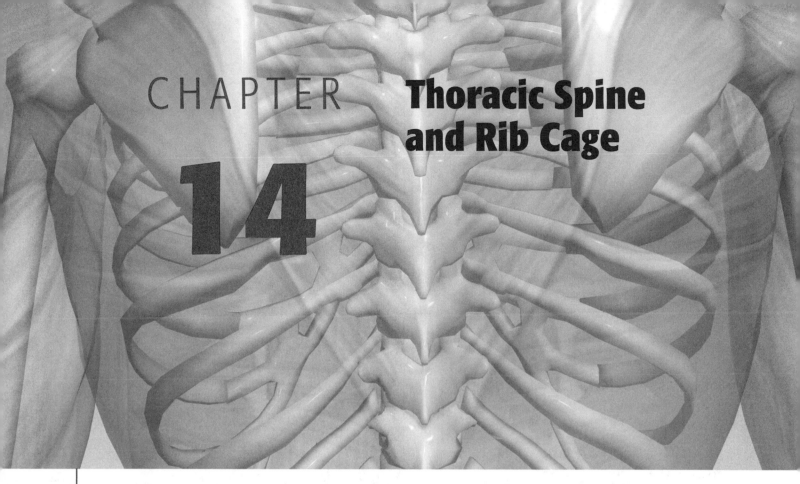

CHAPTER 14

Thoracic Spine and Rib Cage

Chapter Objectives

At the completion of this chapter, the reader will be able to:

1. Describe the vertebrae, ligaments, muscles, and blood and nerve supply that comprise the thoracic intervertebral segment.
2. Outline the coupled movements of the thoracic spine, and the reactions of the various structures to loading.
3. Describe the common pathologies and lesions of this region.
4. Apply a variety of manual techniques to the thoracic spine.
5. Perform an intervention based on patient education, manual therapy, and therapeutic exercise.
6. Evaluate intervention effectiveness in order to progress or modify an intervention.
7. Plan an effective home program, including spinal care and therapeutic exercise, and instruct the patient in this program.

Overview

There are 12 thoracic vertebrae, each of which is involved in at least six articulations. In the thoracic spine, protection and function of the thoracic viscera take precedence over segmental spinal mobility. The posterior thoracic muscles, spinous processes, anterior and posterior longitudinal ligaments, vertebral bodies (Figure 14-1), zygapophyseal and costotransverse joints, inferior articular process, pars interarticularis, intervertebral disk, nerve root, joint meniscus, and dura mater are all capable of producing pain in this region.

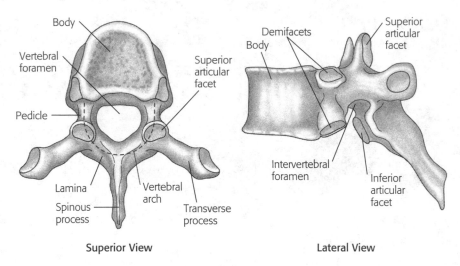

Figure 14-1 Thoracic vertebrae.

Anatomy and Kinesiology

The thoracic spinal segments possess the potential for a unique array of movements. However, there is very little agreement in the literature with regards to the biomechanics of the thoracic spine, and most of the understanding is based largely on the ex vivo studies of White,[1] Panjabi et al.,[2,3] and a variety of clinical models.[4,5]

The rib cage (**Figure 14-2**) and its articulations make the thoracic region less flexible and more stable than the cervical region. This increased stability/reduced mobility of the thoracic segments has been reported to produce three primary effects:[6,7]

- It influences the motions available in other regions of the spine, as well as the shoulder girdle.
- It increases the potential for postural impairments in this region.[8]
- It provides an important weight-bearing mechanism

for the vertebral column.[9] The load-bearing capacity of the spine has been found to be up to three times greater with an intact rib cage.[10,11]

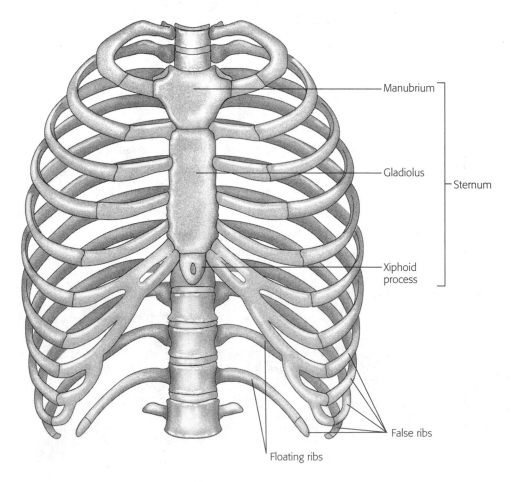

Figure 14-2 The rib cage (anterior view).

Motion in all cardinal planes is possible in the thoracic region, but the magnitude depends on the segmental level:

- Flexion and extension are more limited in the upper thoracic region, where the facets lie closer to the frontal plane. The range of motion of flexion, coupled with anterior translation, in the thoracic spine is 20 to 45 degrees.[12] Flexion is limited by the posterior longitudinal ligament, ligamentum flavum, interspinous ligament, supraspinous ligament, and capsule ligaments. The range of motion of extension, coupled with posterior translation, is 20 to 45 degrees.[12] Extension is limited by the articular and spinous processes.

- Side bending in the frontal plane remains similar throughout, but increases in the lower thoracic region. Side bending of the thoracic spine is approximately 20 to 40 degrees.[12]

- Rotation about the transverse plane is more limited in the lower thoracic region, where the facets lie closer to the sagittal plane. Rotation in the thoracic region is approximately 35 to 50 degrees in each direction.[12]

Respiration

During the rhythmic movements of respiration, the ribs function as levers, with the fulcrum represented by the rib angle, the effort arm represented by the neck, and the load arm represented by the shaft. Because of the relatively small size of the rib neck, a small movement at the rib neck will produce a large degree of movement in the shaft. Although exhalation is typically a passive process, inspiration requires diaphragmatic contraction. In addition, in certain disease states, breathing may require the use of the accessory muscles of respiration (i.e., scalene, sternocleidomastoids, pectoralis minor). The main movement in the upper six ribs during respiration and other movements is one of rotation of the neck of the rib, with only small amounts of superior and inferior motion. In the 7th to 10th ribs, the principal movement is upwards, backwards, and medially during inspiration with the reverse occurring during expiration.[4]

Because the anterior end of the ribs is lower than the posterior, when the ribs elevate they rise upward while the rib neck drops down. In the upper ribs, this

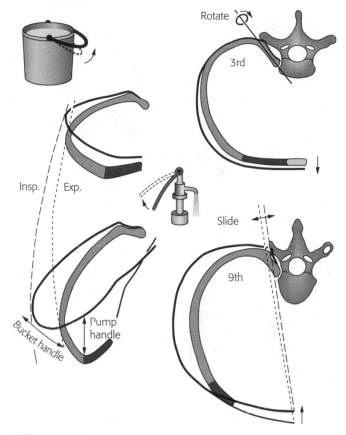

Figure 14-3 Bucket and pump handle rib motions.

results primarily in an anterior elevation (pump handle) and in the middle and lower ribs (excluding the free ribs), primarily a lateral elevation (bucket handle) (**Figure 14-3**), with the former movement increasing the anterior-posterior diameter of the thoracic cavity and the latter increasing the transverse diameter.

Both kinds of rib motion are produced by the action of the diaphragm. The 7th to 10th ribs act to increase the abdominal cavity free space to afford space for the descending diaphragm.

Examination

The examination of the thoracic spine and ribs performed by the physical therapist typically follows the outline in **Table 14-1**.

Intervention Strategies

Because of the complexity of this area, interventions for thoracic and rib dysfunctions require a multifaceted and eclectic approach. It is essential that the impairments, functional limitations, and disability

TABLE 14-1 — Examination of the Thoracic Spine

Observation and Inspection

Upper quarter and peripheral joint scan	Temporomandibular joint, shoulder complex, elbow, forearm, and wrist and hand
	Dermatomes and key muscle tests as appropriate
Examination of movements; active range of motion with passive overpressure	Flexion, extension, side bending (right and left), rotation (right and left)
	Bucket handle and pump handle rib motions
	Combined movements as appropriate
	Repetitive movements as appropriate
	Sustained positions as appropriate
Resisted isometric movements	All AROM directions
	Rectus abdominis, internal and external obliques, quadratus lumborum, back and hip extensors

Palpation

Neurological tests as appropriate	Reflexes, key muscle tests, sensory scan, peripheral nerve assessment
	Neurodynamic mobility tests (straight leg raise, slump test) as appropriate
Joint mobility tests	a. Distraction and compression
	b. Flexion and extension of the zygapophyseal joints
	c. Rib springing
	d. Posteroanterior unilateral vertebral pressure

Special Tests (refer to Special Tests section)

Diagnostic Imaging	As indicated
	As appropriate

found during the examination guide the intervention. The intervention approach for the upper thoracic spine is similar to that of the cervical spine (see Chapter 13), whereas the approach for the lower thoracic spine is similar to that of the lumbar spine (see Chapter 15). The approach to the midthoracic region varies and depends on the cause. The thoracic spine is prone to both postural and biomechanical dysfunctions. Fortunately, there are a number of very effective techniques for the thoracic spine.

Acute Phase

In the acute phase of rehabilitation for the thoracic spine, the intervention goals are to:

- *Decrease pain, inflammation, and muscle spasm:* Pain relief may be accomplished initially by the use of modalities such as cryotherapy and electrical stimulation, gentle exercises, and occasionally the temporary use of a spinal brace. Thermal modalities—especially continuous ultrasound, with its ability to penetrate deeply—may be used after 48–72 hours.

- *Promote healing of tissues:* Ultrasound is the most common clinically used deep-heating modality to promote tissue healing.[13–15] Manual techniques during this phase may include grade I and II joint mobilizations performed by the PT, massage, and gentle stretching.

- *Increase pain-free range of vertebral and costal motion:* Range-of-motion exercises are initiated at the earliest opportunity. These are performed during the early stages in supine and in the pain-free ranges. Diaphragmatic breathing may also need to be included as part of the treatment plan. Diaphragmatic breathing is best learned in supine, followed by practice during sitting, standing, and activity. The patient is asked to place the hands on the stomach and to relax the belly as much as possible. During the first third of inhalation, the belly should be felt to expand slightly (on its own) in an outward direction as the diaphragm pushes down on the contents of the abdomen. Next, the air should move into the middle portion of the lungs, causing the area of the lower and middle ribs to expand (complete inhalation means filling the lungs forward, sideways, and backward). Because the thoracic spine lies between the shoulder girdle and lumbopelvic complex, correction of movement impairment of these regions may be necessary to improve the movement patterns of the thoracic spine.[16]

The exercises in the following sections are recommended to increase vertebral and costal pain-free motion.

Shoulder Sweep

This exercise is used to mobilize the chest wall and to integrate upper extremity function with thoracic spine and rib cage motion.[5] The patient is positioned supine on the floor or on a mat table, with the hips and knees flexed to about 90 degrees (Figure 14-4). A small pillow may be placed under the patient's head for comfort. The patient is asked to place the hand by the side. While maintaining contact with the floor for as long as possible, the patient moves the hand above the head and to the other side of the body, making a large circle around his or her body (refer to Figure 14-4). Manual assistance can be applied to the scapula or rib cage, and deep breathing can be used to move into the restricted ranges.

Thoracic Spine Flexion

The patient is positioned in the quadruped position. The patient arches the thoracic spine as far as is comfortable (Figure 14-5). This position is held for 30 seconds, after which the patient relaxes. The exercise is repeated 8–10 times. The patient can also use deep breathing to increase the stretch, breathing out at the end of available range. In addition, the exercise can be done over a Swiss ball.

Thoracic Spine Extension

It is advised that the clinician monitor this exercise in case the patient loses his or her balance. The patient sits on a Swiss ball, with his or her feet on the ground. Once the patient has good sitting balance, he or she attempts to lie supine on the ball (Figure 14-6). The patient is then instructed to move the top of the head toward the floor, in an attempt to fully extend the thoracic spine. This position is held for 30 seconds, after which the patient relaxes. The exercise is repeated 8–10 times. This exercise can be made more challenging by having the patient hold a small weight and move his or her hands out to the sides and back again while maintaining balance

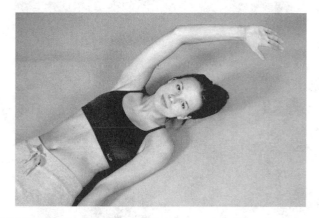

Figure 14-4   Supine shoulder sweep.

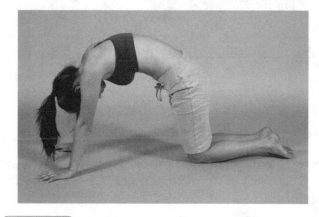

Figure 14-5   Thoracic spine flexion.

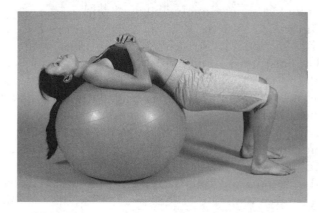

Figure 14-6   Thoracic spine extension.

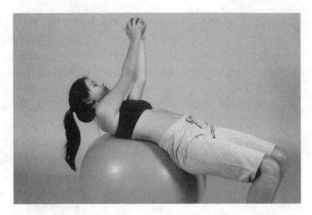

Figure 14-7 — Thoracic spine extension with rotation.

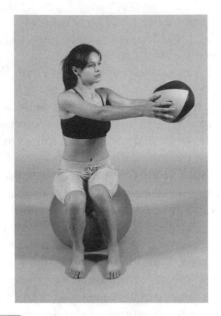

Figure 14-9 — Thoracic spine rotation in sitting.

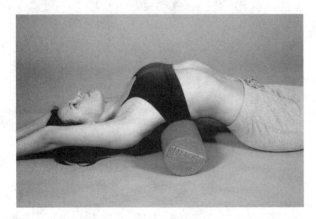

Figure 14-8 — Thoracic spine extension over foam roll.

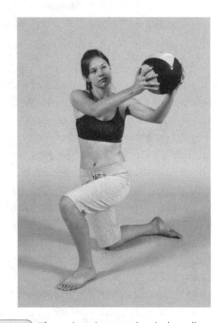

Figure 14-10 — Thoracic spine rotation in kneeling.

(Figure 14-7). If the patient is unable to maintain his or her balance on the Swiss ball, a foam roll may be used (Figure 14-8). The foam roll also allows the clinician to focus the extension exercise on a specific segment.

Thoracic Spine Rotation

Thoracic spine rotation exercises can be performed in a number of positions including sitting (Figure 14-9) and kneeling (Figure 14-10). Thoracic rotation exercises can also be performed in the supine position. The patient lies supine with both knees bent and feet placed on the floor. Keeping the trunk against the floor, the patient lowers the thighs to one side and then the other (Figure 14-11), as far as is comfortable. This position is held for 30 seconds, after which the patient relaxes. The exercise is repeated 8–10 times. To make the exercise more difficult, the arms are abducted to approximately 90 degrees, and one leg is rotated over the other as far as is comfortable (Figure 14-12).

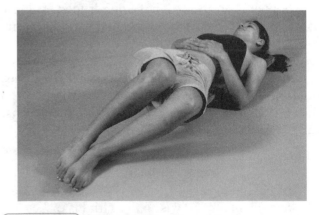

Figure 14-11 — Supine thoracic spine rotation.

Thoracic Spine Side Bending

The patient kneels to the side of a Swiss ball. The patient is asked to lean sideways over the ball and, with the arm closest to the ball, to attempt to touch the floor on the other side of the ball (Figure 14-13) without losing balance. This position is held for 30 seconds, after which the patient relaxes. The exercise is repeated 8–10 times.

Once these exercises can be performed without pain, submaximal isometric exercises are then performed throughout the pain-free ranges. These exercises are progressed as the range of motion and strength increase.

Functional Combinations

In appropriate treatment progressions, component impairments are first addressed, followed by integrated movements with relatively simple activities or techniques, progressed to more challenging activities or techniques, and then progressed to complex, integrated functional movement patterns.[16] For example, normal gait includes simultaneous hip flexion and trunk counterrotation to prepare for the complex movement of the swing phase of gait. These combinations can be taught first in supine to address the hip flexion component (Figure 14-14), and then in side lying combining the hip flexion and trunk rotation (Figure 14-15).

Functional/Chronic Phase

Once the pain and inflammation are controlled, the intervention can progress toward the restoration of full strength, range of motion, and normal posture. The goals of this phase are:

- To achieve significant reduction or the complete resolution of the patient's pain
- Restoration of full and pain-free vertebral and costal range of motion
- Full integration of the entire upper and lower kinetic chains
- Complete restoration of respiratory function
- Restoration of thoracic and upper quadrant strength and neuromuscular control

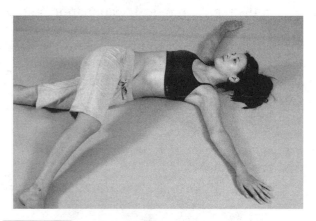

Figure 14-12   Supine thoracic rotation using one leg.

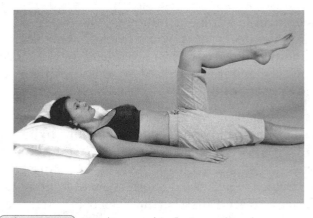

Figure 14-14   Simultaneous hip flexion and trunk counterrotation in supine.

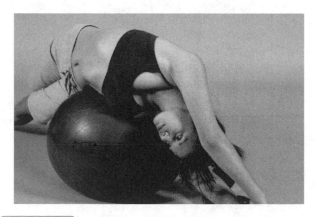

Figure 14-13   Thoracic spine side bending.

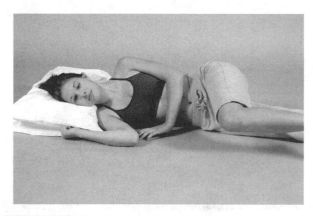

Figure 14-15   Simultaneous hip flexion and trunk counterrotation in side lying.

During this phase, the patient learns to initiate and execute functional activities without pain and while dynamically stabilizing the spine in an automatic manner. The exercises prescribed must challenge and enhance muscle performance, while minimizing loading of the thoracic spine and ribs to reduce the risk of injury exacerbation. The aim is to help the patient to (1) gain dynamic control of spine forces, (2) eliminate repetitive injury to the motion segments, (3) encourage healing of the injured segment, and (4) possibly alter the degenerative process.

Hypermobility

The general plan for excessive motion (hypermobility) is to stabilize with muscle function while addressing biomechanical factors, such as adjacent hypomobile areas. The patient is instructed to hold the spine in ideal alignment during movements of the upper and lower extremities. Exercises can begin in sitting with the back against the wall or in supine and then progress to the quadruped position over a Swiss ball (Figure 14-16) followed by standing. Applying an axial load to the thorax and gauging the response can allow the estimation of ideal optimal alignment in sitting or standing.[16] Home exercises can be performed using a straight back chair for stability and an elastic band or tubing for resistance. The exercises are progressed by adding resistance to the extremities.

Hypomobility

The general plan for reduced motion (hypomobility) is to strengthen the weakened and overstretched muscle group in the shortened range, and to stretch the adaptively shortened muscle groups.[17] Patient-related instruction aimed at correcting posture and movement patterns that perpetuate the length-associated changes is important to prevent recurrence. Treatment of joint restrictions usually requires joint mobilization techniques by the PT, passive stretching, and active range of motion. It is important to teach the patient functional movement patterns that reinforce the mobility gained by the treatment. Cross-body reaching exercises in sitting and then standing (Figure 14-17) can be used to promote independent motion of the shoulder joint from the shoulder blade, torso, and hip.

Postural Dysfunction

A number of authors[18–23] have theorized that postural dysfunctions in this region create an imbalance between agonists and antagonists, producing adaptive shortening and weakness. It is likely that these changes are degenerative in nature, resulting from a change in intervertebral disk height. Postural dysfunctions of the thoracic spine are relatively common. Postural pain is not typically reproducible with the typical physical examination, and the diagnosis is based solely on the history of pain following sustained positions or postures. Occasionally, patients with this type of pain may report that their pain is aggravated by stress, fatigue, or changes in the weather.[24]

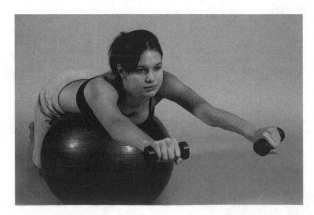

Figure 14-16 Quadruped stabilization exercise.

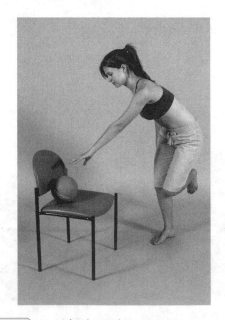

Figure 14-17 Cross-body reaching exercise.

Abnormal Pelvic Tilting

Good mobility of the pelvis in all directions is important for the thoracic spine. Two postural deviations are associated with pelvic tilting:

1. Posterior pelvic tilting in the sitting position produces an increase in the flexion of the lumbar and thoracic spine and a forward head posture. This posture is thought to result in a posterior (dorsal) shifting of the thoracic disk, which places a stress on the posterior longitudinal ligament and the dura mater, producing both local and nonsegmental referrals of pain.

2. Anterior pelvic tilting in the standing position (usually caused by adaptive shortening of the rectus femoris and iliopsoas muscles, and weak abdominals) causes the trunk to lean backward and results in overstretching of the rectus abdominis and a pulling forward of the shoulders, shortening of the posterior neck muscles, and increased extension of the atlanto-occipital joint.[25]

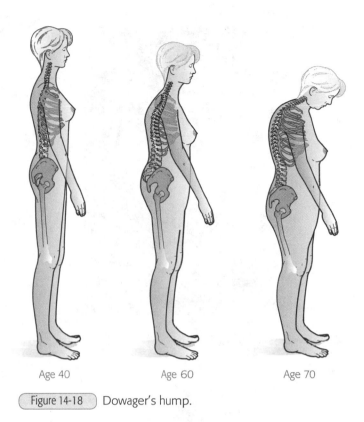

Age 40 Age 60 Age 70

Figure 14-18   Dowager's hump.

Structural Dysfunctions

A number of structural dysfunctions are common to this area, some of which are developmental while others are pathologic or posturally induced.

Kyphosis

The causes of thoracic kyphosis may be either anatomic, resulting from changes in the structure and shape of the spine itself, or postural. Disk height changes commonly are seen in the upper midthoracic segments[26] and may result in an alteration of the kyphotic curve, with subsequent compensatory changes in load bearing and movement. Children may exhibit kyphosis resulting from congenital spinal malformation. In the elderly patient, a kyphotic posture can be acquired from fractures of the anterior aspect of the thoracic vertebral bodies. This is one of the manifestations of osteoporosis. The resultant altered load-bearing patterns may result in a compression of the anterior aspect of the thoracic intervertebral disks and a stretching of the thoracic extensors and the middle and lower trapezius. The posterior ligaments (posterior longitudinal ligament, ligamentum flavum, interspinous ligament, supraspinous ligament, and the capsule ligaments) also are lengthened. In addition, the kyphotic posture is associated with adaptive shortening of the anterior longitudinal ligament, the upper abdominals, and the anterior chest muscles. The common kyphotic deformities include:[27]

- *Dowager's hump:* This deformity (Figure 14-18) is characterized by a severely kyphotic upper dorsal region, which results from multiple anterior wedge compression fractures in several vertebrae of the middle to upper thoracic spine, usually caused by postmenopausal osteoporosis or long-term corticosteroid therapy.[28]
- *Hump back:* This deformity (Figure 14-19) is a localized, sharp, posterior angulation, called *gibbus*, produced by an anterior wedging of one of two thoracic vertebrae as a result of infection (tuberculosis), fracture, or congenital bony anomaly of the spine.[29]
- *Round back:* This deformity (Figure 14-20) is characterized by decreased (20-degree) pelvic inclination (the angle of inclination is measured as the line between the anterior superior iliac spine [ASIS] and the posterior superior iliac spine [PSIS] and its intersection with the horizontal plane, normally 30 degrees) and excessive kyphosis of the thoracic spine.

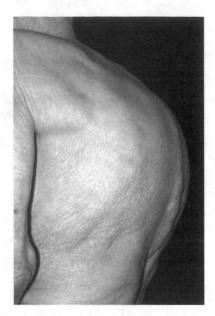

Figure 14-19   Hump back.

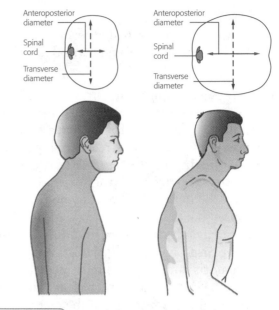

Figure 14-21   Normal chest versus barrel chest.

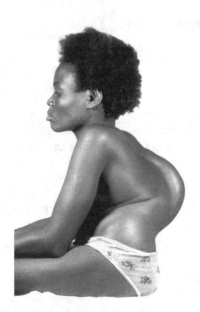

Figure 14-20   Round back.

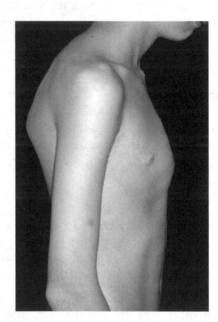

Figure 14-22   Pigeon chest.

Sternal Deformities

Anterior chest deformities include:

- *Barrel chest:* In this deformity, a forward- and upward-projecting sternum increases the anteroposterior diameter (Figure 14-21). The barrel chest results in respiratory difficulty, stretching of the intercostal and anterior chest muscles, and adaptive shortening of the scapular adductor muscles.

- *Pigeon chest:* In this deformity, a forward- and downward-projecting sternum increases the anteroposterior diameter (Figure 14-22). The pigeon chest results in a lengthening of the upper abdominal muscles and an adaptive shortening of the upper intercostal muscles.
- *Funnel chest:* In this deformity, a posterior-projecting sternum occurs secondary to an outgrowth of the ribs (Figure 14-23).[30] The funnel chest results in adaptive shortening of the upper abdominals, shoulder adductors, pectoralis minor, and intercostal muscles, and

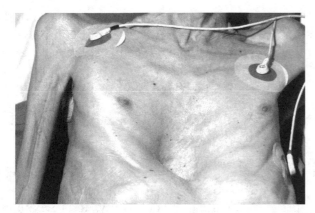

Figure 14-23 Funnel chest.

in lengthening of the thoracic extensors and middle and upper trapezius.

Intervention

Patients with impairments, functional limitations, or disabilities related to muscle imbalance can be treated based on any length-associated strength changes found in the assessment and any positional weakness of one synergist compared with its counterpart or its antagonist muscle group.[16]

> ● **Key Point** Patients with any form of postural dysfunction often benefit from the movement therapies of the Alexander technique, Feldenkrais method, Trager psychophysical integration, Pilates, and tai chi chuan.[31–37]

Muscle Strains

Muscle strains are common in the thoracic region and are characterized by localized pain and tenderness, which is exacerbated with isometric testing or passive stretching of the muscle. Although it is difficult to isolate muscles in this region, the clinician can determine the directions that alleviate the symptoms and those that do not. A gradual strengthening and gentle passive stretching program into the painless directions is initially performed, before progressing as tolerated into the painful directions.

Intercostal Muscles

Injuries to intercostal muscles are mainly caused by trauma after unaccustomed or excessive muscular activity.[38] There may be a specific incident before the onset of pain, such as lifting a heavy object, or symptoms may be of gradual onset with no obvious inciting event.[39] In athletes, a premature return to heavy training after a period of rest or deconditioning may predispose to muscular injuries. Intercostal muscle injuries are more likely in sports in which upper body activity is extreme, such as rowing[39]; however, intercostal pain can occur in the presence of persistent coughing as a result of such conditions as an upper respiratory tract infection.

Diagnosis is based on pain between the ribs that is worse on movement, deep inspiration, or coughing. This pain is associated with tenderness in the same area on palpation. Plain radiographs are normal unless there is underlying lung disease or infection, and diagnosis may be dependent on exclusion of more serious pathology, such as cardiac chest pain, in the absence of a clear history of injury.[39]

Intervention

The intervention for muscle strains is designed to improve muscle performance of underused synergists and address the posture and movement patterns contributing to excessive use.[16] The patient should be instructed to avoid chronic postures of the neck, ipsilateral side bending, and contralateral rotation to avoid overuse of the muscles in the short range.

Rotoscoliosis

Two terms, *scoliosis* and *rotoscoliosis*, are used to describe the lateral curvature of the spine. Scoliosis is the older term and refers to an abnormal side bending of the spine, but gives no reference to the coupled rotation that also occurs. Rotoscoliosis is a more detailed definition, used to describe the curve of the spine by detailing how each vertebra is rotated and side flexed in relation to the vertebra below. For example, with a left lumbar convexity, the L5 vertebra would be found to be side flexed to the right and rotated to the left in relation to the sacrum. The same would be true with regard to the relation between L4 and L5. This rotation, toward the convexity, continues in small increments until the apex at L3. L2, which is above the apex, is right rotated and right side flexed in relation to L3. The small increments of right rotation continue up until the thoracic spine, where the side bending and rotation return to the neutral position.

> ● **Key Point** A slight lateral curve in the coronal plane is thought to result from right-hand dominance, or the presence of the aorta.[40]

Scoliosis is never normal, although most cases are idiopathic (see Chapter 22), manifesting in the pre-adolescent years.[41,42] An abnormal lateral thoracic curve is described as being structural or functional, and can produce a fixed deformity or a changeable adaptation, respectively, with the rib hump occurring on the convex side of the curve.

Intervention

Treatment strategies for idiopathic scoliosis are described in Chapter 22.

Compression Fractures of the Spine

Compression fractures of the vertebral body are common (due to osteoporosis) and range from mild to severe. The signs and symptoms of vertebral fracture include progressive kyphosis of the spine with loss of height, reports of acute back pain (in the midthoracic to lower thoracic or upper lumbar spine, where most vertebral fractures occur), pain after bending, lifting, or coughing. More severe fractures can cause significant pain, leading to inability to perform activities of daily living, and life-threatening decline in the elderly patient who already has decreased reserves. Traditional medical treatment includes bed rest and pain control. Procedures such as vertebroplasty or kyphoplasty can be considered in those patients who do not respond to initial treatment or in those with neurological symptoms or spinal instability. Kyphoplasty and vertebroplasty are two procedures that percutaneously attempt to augment the strength of fractured or weakened vertebrae. Balloon kyphoplasty utilizes orthopedic balloons to create a void in a fractured vertebra, restore vertebral body height, and correct angular deformity. The void allows a viscous cement to be deposited in a controlled manner, stabilizing the fracture. In vertebroplasty, no balloon is used to restore vertebral body height and no cavity is created. Cement is injected into the fractured vertebra, stabilizing it in its current state. However, two trials[43,44] published in 2009 found that vertebroplasty is not effective at relieving pain or deformity and has been associated with more cement leakage than with kyphoplasty.

Intervention

PTs and PTAs can help patients prevent compression fractures by treating predisposing factors, identifying high-risk patients, and educating patients and the public about measures to prevent falls. The intervention should include the following:

- A therapeutic exercise program designed to limit pain and promote mobility. Spinal flexion exercises should be avoided due to the increased risk of spinal wedging or compression fractures.[45] Instead, gentle spinal extension or isometric exercises may be more appropriate to prevent the progression of deformities from osteoporosis.[45]
- Electrotherapeutic and thermal modalities may also be used to help control pain and reduce stiffness.
- Patient education should be provided to address avoidance of forward flexion of the trunk to prevent extending the deformity, and to explain postural awareness.
- The patient should be evaluated for an assistive device to assist with activities of daily living.
- Deep breathing exercises should be performed to maintain or enhance pulmonary function.

Techniques to Increase Soft Tissue Extensibility

A variety of soft tissue techniques for the thoracic region are available to the clinician. The choice of technique depends on the goals of the treatment and the dysfunction being treated.

Manual Stretch into Extension

The patient is positioned supine, and the clinician stands at the head of the bed. The patient elevates both arms over the head and reaches around the back of the clinician's thighs. By having the patient hold a towel in this position, the clinician can place both of his or her hands under the patient's rib cage and pull the rib cage in an anterior and cranial direction, thereby encouraging thoracic extension (Figure 14-24). A belt wrapped around the patient at the correct level can make this technique more specific. The patient can use deep breathing to increase the stretch, breathing out at the end of available range.

Bucket Handle Stretch

The patient is positioned side lying. The clinician fully abducts the patient's uppermost arm, grasping it above the elbow. The arm is taken into hyperabduction, thereby fully expanding the rib cage on the uppermost side (Figure 14-25). The patient can use deep breathing to increase the stretch, breathing out at the end of available range. The patient can also lie over the top of a pillow to enhance the stretch.

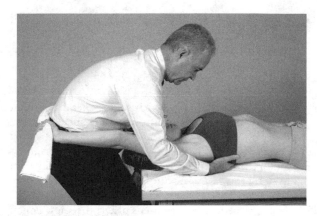

Figure 14-24   Manual stretch into extension.

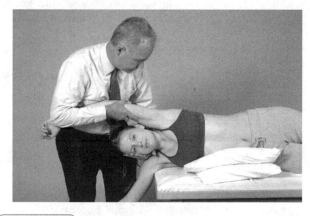

Figure 14-25   Bucket handle stretch.

Summary

The thoracic spine serves as a transitional zone between the lumbosacral region and the cervical spine. Although historically the thoracic spine has not enjoyed the same attention as other regions of the spine, it can be a significant source of local and referred pain. The thoracic spine is the most rigid region of the spine, and in this area, protection of the thoracic viscera takes precedence over segmental spinal mobility. Because each thoracic vertebra is involved in at least six articulations, establishing the specific cause of thoracic dysfunction may not always be immediately possible. This task is made more difficult because of the inaccessibility of most of these joints.[46] Optimal function of the thoracic region requires full and symmetrical cardinal plane

motion as well as combined motions.[16] In addition, full thoracic spine and rib motion during breathing should be the goal.[16]

REVIEW Questions

1. Which motion in the thoracic spine is the least limited: flexion, side bending, or rotation?
2. Which muscle is primarily involved with inspiration?
3. Anterior elevation (pump handle motion) is seen most predominantly in which region of the thoracic spine?
4. Which muscle groups are involved with producing an anterior pelvic tilt?
5. True or false: Normal gait includes simultaneous hip flexion and trunk counterrotation to prepare for the complex movement of the swing phase of gait.
6. True or false: Expiration is normally a passive process.
7. True or false: Rotoscoliosis refers primarily to a frontal plane deviation in the thoracolumbar regions and is named by the convex side of the spinal curve.
8. True or false: The thoracic spine is prone to postural dysfunctions.
9. Which deformity is characterized by decreased (20 percent) pelvic inclination and excessive kyphosis?
10. Describe the characteristics of a pigeon chest deformity.

References

1. White AA: An analysis of the mechanics of the thoracic spine in man. Acta Orthop Scand 127 (Suppl):8–92, 1969
2. Panjabi MM, Hausfeld JN, White AA: A biomechanical study of the ligamentous stability of the thoracic spine in man. Acta Orthop Scand 52:315–326, 1981
3. Panjabi MM, Brand RA, White AA: Mechanical properties of the human thoracic spine. J Bone and Joint Surg 58A:642–652, 1976
4. Lee DG: Biomechanics of the Thorax, in Grant R (ed): Physical Therapy of the Cervical and Thoracic Spine. New York, Churchill Livingstone, 1988, pp 47–76
5. Flynn TW: Thoracic spine and chest wall, in Wadsworth C (ed): Current Concepts of Orthopedic Physical Therapy — Home Study Course. La Crosse, WI, Orthopaedic Section, APTA, 2001

6. Refshauge KM, Bolst L, Goodsell M: The relationship between cervicothoracic posture and the presence of pain. J Man & Manip Ther 3:21–24, 1995

7. Edmondston SJ, Singer KP: Thoracic spine: anatomical and biomechanical considerations for manual therapy. Man Ther 2:132–143, 1997

8. Raine S, Twomey LT: Attributes and qualities of human posture and their relationship to dysfunction or musculoskeletal pain. Crit Rev Phys Rehabil Med 6:409–437, 1994

9. Singer KP, Malmivaara A: Pathoanatomical characteristics of the thoracolumbar junctional region, in Giles LGF, Singer KP (eds): Clinical Anatomy and Management of the Thoracic Spine. Oxford, Butterworth-Heinemann, 2000, pp 100–113

10. Andriacchi T, Schultz A, Belytschko T, et al: A model for studies of mechanical interactions between the human spine and rib cage. J Biomech 7:497–505, 1974

11. Watkins RT, Watkins R, Williams L, et al: Stability provided by the sternum and rib cage in the thoracic spine. Spine (Phila Pa 1976) 30:1283–1286, 2005

12. White AA, Punjabi MM: Clinical Biomechanics of the Spine (ed 2). Philadelphia, PA, J.B. Lippincott Company, 1990

13. Klaffs CE, Arnheim DD: Modern Principles of Athletic Training. St Louis, CV Mosby, 1989

14. Lehmann JF, Silverman DR, Baum BA, et al: Temperature distributions in the human thigh produced by infrared, hot pack and microwave applications. Arch Phys Med Rehabil 47:291, 1966

15. Prentice WE: Using therapeutic modalities in rehabilitation, in Prentice WE, Voight ML (eds): Techniques in Musculoskeletal Rehabilitation. New York, McGraw-Hill, 2001, pp 289–303

16. Landel R, Hall C, Moffat M, et al: The thoracic spine, in Hall C, Thein-Brody L (eds): Therapeutic Exercise: Moving Toward Function. Baltimore, MD, Lippincott Williams & Wilkins, 2005, pp 610–642

17. Cole AJ, Farrell JP, Stratton SA: Functional rehabilitation of cervical spine athletic injuries, in Kibler BW, Herring JA, Press JM (eds): Functional Rehabilitation of Sports and Musculoskeletal Injuries. Gaithersburg, MD, Aspen, 1998, pp 127–148

18. White AA, Sahrmann SA: A movement system balance approach to management of musculoskeletal pain, in Grant R (ed): Physical Therapy for the Cervical and Thoracic Spine. Edinburgh, Churchill Livingstone, 1994, pp 339–358

19. Jull GA, Janda V: Muscle and Motor control in low back pain, in Twomey LT, Taylor JR (eds): Physical Therapy of the Low Back: Clinics in Physical Therapy. New York, Churchill Livingstone, 1987, pp 258–278

20. Jull GA: Physiotherapy management of neck pain of mechanical origin, in Giles LGF, Singer KP (eds): Clinical Anatomy and Management of Cervical Spine Pain. The Clinical Anatomy of Back Pain. London, England, Butterworth-Heinemann, 1998, pp 168–191

21. Crawford HJ, Jull GA: The influence of thoracic posture and movement on range of arm elevation. Physiother Theory Pract 9:143–148, 1993

22. Vasilyeva LF, Lewit K: Diagnosis of muscular dysfunction by inspection, in Liebenson C (ed): Rehabilitation of the Spine: A Practitioner's Manual. Baltimore, Lippincott Williams & Wilkins, 1996, pp 113–142

23. Lewit K: Relation of faulty respiration to posture, with clinical implications. J Amer Osteopath Assoc 79:525–529, 1980

24. Corrigan B, Maitland GD: Practical Orthopaedic Medicine. Boston, Butterworth, 1985

25. Ellis JJ, Johnson GS: Myofascial considerations in somatic dysfunction of the thorax, in Flynn TW (ed): The Thoracic Spine and Rib Cage: Musculoskeletal Evaluation and Treatment. Boston, Butterworth-Heinemann, 1996, pp 211–262

26. Crawford R, Singer KP: Normal and degenerative anatomy of the thoracic intervertebral discs, Proceedings of Manipulative Physiotherapists Association of Australia: 9th Biennial Conference. Gold Coast, 1995, pp 24–29

27. Wiles P, Sweetnam R: Essentials of Orthopedics. London, J.A. Churchill, 1965

28. Deyo RA, Rainville J, Kent DL: What can the history and physical examination tell us about low back pain? JAMA 268:760–765, 1992

29. Bland JH: Diagnosis of thoracic pain syndromes, in Giles LGF, Singer KP (eds): Clinical Anatomy and Management of the Thoracic Spine. Oxford, Butterworth-Heinemann, 2000, pp 145–156

30. Sutherland ID: Funnel chest. J Bone Joint Surg 40B: 244–251, 1958

31. Brennan R: The Alexander Technique: Natural Poise for Health. New York, Barnes & Noble Books, Inc., 1991

32. Buchanan PA, Ulrich BD: The Feldenkrais method: A dynamic approach to changing motor behavior. Res Q for Exercise and Sport 72:315–323, 2001

33. Lake B: Acute back pain: Treatment by the application of Feldenkrais principles. Aust Fam Physician 14:1175–1178, 1985

34. Watrous I: The Trager approach: An effective tool for physical therapy. Physical Therapy Forum 1022–1025, 1992

35. Witt P: Trager psychophysical integration: An additional tool in the treatment of chronic spinal pain and dysfunction. Trager J 2:4–5, 1987

36. Witt P, Parr C: Effectiveness of Trager psychophysical integration in promoting trunk mobility in a child with cerebral palsy, a case report. Phys Occup Ther Pediatr 8:75–94, 1988

37. Blum CL: Chiropractic and pilates therapy for the treatment of adult scoliosis. Journal of Manipulative & Physiological Therapeutics 25:E3, 2002

38. Morgan-Hughes J: Painful disorders of muscle. Br J Hosp Med 360:362–365, 1979

39. Gregory PL, Biswas AC, Batt ME: Musculoskeletal problems of the chest wall in athletes. Sports Medicine 32:235–250, 2002

40. Ombregt L, Bisschop P, ter Veer HJ, et al: A System of Orthopaedic Medicine. London, WB Saunders, 1995

41. Bradford S: Juvenile kyphosis, in Bradford DS, Lonstein JE, Moe JH, et al (eds): Moe's Textbook of Scoliosis and Other Spinal Deformities. Philadelphia, PA, W.B. Saunders, 1987, pp 347–368

42. McKenzie RA: Manual correction of sciatic scoliosis. N Z Med J 76:194–199, 1972

43. Kallmes DF, Comstock BA, Heagerty PJ, et al: A randomized trial of vertebroplasty for osteoporotic spinal fractures. N Engl J Med 361:569–579, 2009

44. Buchbinder R, Osborne RH, Ebeling PR, et al: A randomized trial of vertebroplasty for painful osteoporotic vertebral fractures. N Engl J Med 361:557–568, 2009

45. Sinaki M, Mikkelsen BA: Postmenopausal spinal osteoporosis: flexion versus extension exercises. Arch Phys Med Rehabil 65:593–596, 1984

46. Singer KP, Edmondston SJ: Introduction: the enigma of the thoracic spine, in Giles LGF, Singer KP (eds): Clinical Anatomy and Management of Thoracic Spine Pain. The Clinical Anatomy and Management of Back Pain Series. Oxford, Butterworth-Heinemann, 2000

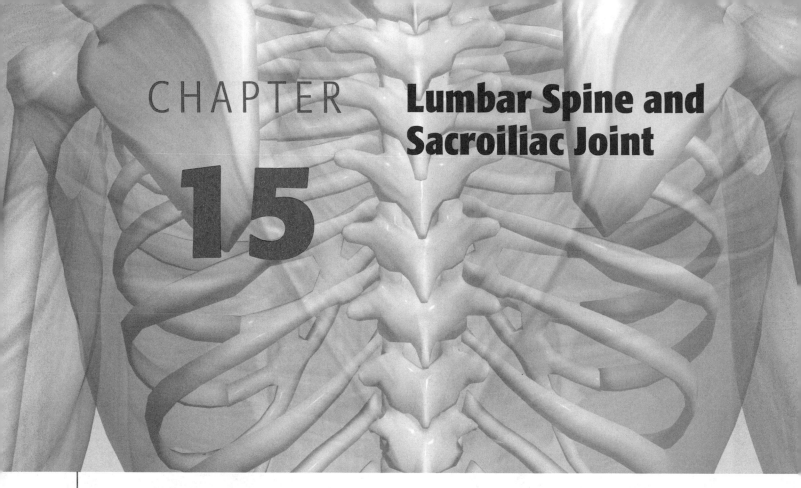

Lumbar Spine and Sacroiliac Joint

15

Chapter Objectives

At the completion of this chapter, the reader will be able to:

1. Describe a number of associated occupational, psychosocial, and environmental factors that can be used to help predict the development of a complicated course of lumbopelvic pain.
2. Describe the structures that comprise the lumbar intervertebral segment.
3. Describe the structures and biomechanics of the sacroiliac joint.
4. Outline the coupled movements of the lumbar spine, the normal and abnormal joint barriers, and the reactions of the various structures to loading.
5. Describe the common pathologies and lesions of this region.
6. Describe intervention strategies based on clinical findings and established goals.
7. Design an intervention based on patient education, manual therapy, and therapeutic exercise.
8. Evaluate intervention effectiveness in order to progress or modify intervention.
9. Perform an effective home program, including spinal care, and instruct the patient in this program.

Overview

Over the past century, lumbopelvic pain has become increasingly problematic, receiving a growing amount of attention and concern due to the burdens placed on health systems and social-care systems.[1,2] A number of associated occupational, psychosocial, and environmental factors can be used to help predict the development of a complicated course of lumbopelvic pain.[3–9] These include the following:

- *Age older than 40 or 50 years:* The relationship between chronic lumbopelvic pain and age over 40 or 50 years, with a decrease of occurrence over 60 years, is considered as an established fact in many reviews.[10,11] The explanation is the presence of a degenerative process and the accumulation of spinal damage associated with increasing age.

- *Physical and psychosocial workload:* A number of studies that examined the relationship between physical and psychosocial load at work and the occurrence of lumbopelvic pain concluded that both work-related physical factors of flexion and rotation of the trunk and lifting at work, and low job satisfaction are risk factors for sickness absence resulting from lumbopelvic pain.[12,13] Physical loading on the back has commonly been implicated as a risk factor for lumbopelvic pain and, in particular, for work-related lumbopelvic pain. Certain occupations and certain work tasks seem to have a higher risk of lumbopelvic pain.[14–17] For example, repeated lifting of heavy loads is considered a risk factor for lumbopelvic pain,[17] especially if combined with side bending and twisting.[18,19] A study of static work postures found that there was an increased risk of lumbopelvic pain if the work involved a predominance of sitting.[20] Kelsey[21] and Kelsey and Hardy[22] found that men who spend more than half their workday driving have a threefold increased risk of disk herniation. Although knowledge is incomplete, a growing body of evidence indicates that exposure to vibration and jolting in workers who operate tractors, excavators, bulldozers, forklift trucks, armored vehicles, lorries, helicopters, and many other vehicles and machines may cause an increased risk of lumbopelvic pain.[21,23–26]

- *Smoking:* In some epidemiologic studies (mostly those of cross-sectional design), smoking has been associated with lumbopelvic pain.[27,28] Several possible pathophysiologic mechanisms have been proposed to explain the association. It has been suggested that smoking accelerates degeneration by impairing the blood supply to the vertebral body and nutrition of the intervertebral disk (IVD).[29] Smoking increases coughing activity, which causes an increase in intradiskal pressure.[30]

- *Obesity:* There are several hypotheses relating to a link between obesity and lumbopelvic pain. Increased mechanical demands resulting from obesity have been suspected of causing lumbopelvic pain through excessive wear and tear,[31–34] and it has been suggested that metabolic factors associated with obesity may be detrimental.[32]

- *Comorbidity:* Comorbidity may slow or interfere with normal recovery from back pain and may affect an individual's general sense of health, leading to a decreased self-perception of capability.[35]

Given the numerous causes and types of lumbopelvic pain, it is imperative that any clinician treating the lower back have a sound understanding and knowledge of the anatomy and biomechanics of this region. Although this knowledge is not the sole determinant of the approach to lumbopelvic pain, it does provide a solid framework on which to build successful management.

● **Key Point** It is worth noting that trunk strength, flexibility, aerobic conditioning, and postural education have all been found to have a significant preventative effect on the occurrence and recurrence of back injuries.[36–43] Thus, physical therapy, with its emphasis on the restoration of functional motion, strength, and flexibility, should be the cornerstone of both the intervention and the preventative processes in lumbopelvic pain.

Anatomy of the Lumbar Spine

The lumbar spine consists of five lumbar vertebral bodies that are distinguished from the thoracic bodies by the absence of rib facets (Figure 15-1). The L1–L3 vertebrae have a similar structure, and the L4–L5 vertebrae have a similar structure.

Ligaments

The primary ligamentous supports for the lumbar spine are the anterior longitudinal ligament, the

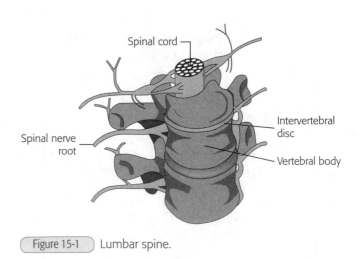

Figure 15-1 Lumbar spine.

TABLE 15-1	Characteristics of the Lumbar Vertebrae	
Structure	**Characteristic**
Pedicles	Project from the upper portion of the vertebral body
Spinous process	Primarily horizontal in orientation; the posterior inferior border projects below the upper level of the spinous process below
Laminae	Thick, and project below the pedicles
Transverse processes	Long and thin with a slant that is both upward and backward

posterior longitudinal ligament, the attachments of the annulus fibrosis, the facet joints, and the interosseous ligaments between the spinous processes.

Vertebrae

The characteristics of the lumbar spine vertebrae are outlined in **Table 15-1**. The zygapophyseal joints (articular facets) of the lumbar spine are heavier than those of the thoracic or cervical spine. The superior facets face medially, whereas the inferior facets face laterally. The angle that each zygapophyseal joint makes with respect to the sagittal plane determines the amount of resistance offered to motion in the sagittal and transverse planes. The more the joint is oriented in the frontal plane, the more it resists sagittal plane (posterior-anterior) motion, but the less it can resist transverse plane (rotation) motion.[44] The zygapophyseal joints adopt a more frontal plane as they move from L1 to L5. At the lumbosacral junction (L5–S1), the point at which the weight of the entire trunk and upper body is transferred to the pelvis, the base of the sacrum is inclined forward about 40 degrees from the horizontal plane. This alignment is referred to as the *sacrohorizontal angle* and serves to prevent the whole lower spine from translating anteriorly relative to the sacrum. Excessive anterior translation of the lumbar spine relative to the base of the sacrum is called *anterior spondylolisthesis* (see "Common Conditions" later in this chapter).

Intervertebral Disk

The lumbar intervertebral disk (IVD), commonly referred to as the interbody joint, is approximately cylindrical, its shape being determined by the

integrity of its outer wall, the annulus fibrosis (AF). The AF consists of approximately 10–12 (often as many as 15–25) concentric sheets (lamellae) of predominantly type I collagen tissue,[45] bound together by proteoglycan gel (see Chapter 2).[46]

● **Key Point** The IVD contains the aggrecans of glycosaminoglycans (GAGs), which imbibe water through the so-called Gibbs-Donnan mechanism on a diurnal basis. More water is imbibed when the spine/IVD is unloaded, such as during sleeping.

Each lamella has an alternating orientation of collagen fibers such that the fibers in adjacent lamellae are at 90 degrees to each other. This orientation effectively resists compression, but horizontal translation and rotation are resisted by only a portion of the fibers.[47] The number of annular layers decreases with age, but there is a gradual thickening of the remaining layers.[48] Contained within the AF is the nucleus pulposus, which is composed of a semifluid mass of mucoid material (see Chapter 2). The IVD is essentially avascular with the exception of the outer AF.[47]

● **Key Point** Although the IVD bears most of the compressive load of the spine in the neutral position and in the very early ranges of flexion and extension, the zygapophyseal joints bear up to 25 percent of the compressive load in the mid-ranges of extension. The contribution of the zygapophyseal joints becomes more significant during prolonged weight bearing, in the presence of IVD space narrowing, or if lumbar extension is combined with rotation.

Kinesiology of the Lumbar Spine

The movement of the lumbar spine is largely confined to flexion and extension with a minor degree of rotation and side bending. Motions at the lumbar spine joints can occur in three cardinal planes: sagittal (flexion and extension), coronal (side bending) and transverse (rotation). The amount of segmental motion at each vertebral level varies. Most of the flexion and extension of the lumbar spine occurs in the lower segmental levels, whereas most of the side bending of the lumbar spine occurs in the mid-lumbar area. Rotation, which occurs with side bending as a coupled motion, is minimal, and occurs most at the lumbosacral junction. The pelvis and hips augment trunk motion by movement of the pelvis over the femoral heads. The amount of range available in the lumbar spine decreases with age.

Flexion

The flexion-extension range of the lumbar spine that occurs between vertebral segments is approximately

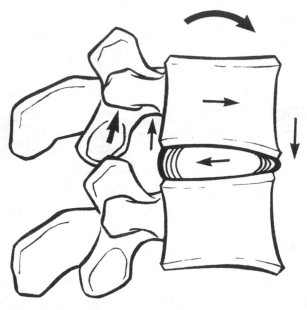

Figure 15-2   Lumbar spine flexion.

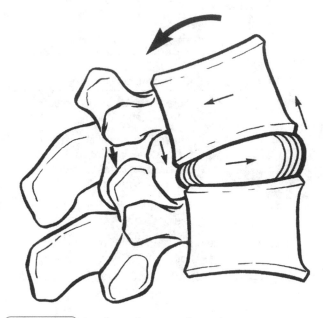

Figure 15-3   Lumbar spine extension.

12 degrees in the upper lumbar spine, increasing by 1–2 degrees per segment to reach a maximum motion of 20–25 degrees between L5 and S1. During lumbar flexion (Figure 15-2), the inferior zygapophyseal joint of the superior vertebra moves upward, producing a stretching of the interspinous ligament between the two spinous processes. A slight amount of anterior sagittal translation also occurs. During lumbar flexion in standing, which is normally initiated by the abdominal muscles, the entire lumbar spine leans forwards, and there is a posterior sway of the pelvis as the hips flex. Bending the trunk forward requires adequate flexibility in the muscles and other soft tissues in both the hip and lower back regions (see "Lumbopelvic Rhythm" in Chapter 19).

● **Key Point**   Flexion of the lumbar spine can also occur with a posterior pelvic tilt. The posterior pelvic tilt, a short-arc posterior rotation of the pelvis about the hip joint, with the trunk held upright and stationary, can be performed voluntarily, or it may occur as a result of weak paraspinal extensor muscles or adaptively shortened hamstring and gluteal muscles, with subsequent lengthening of the hip flexors and back extensors. A patient with lateral spinal stenosis may be instructed in therapeutic exercises that promote a posterior pelvic tilt because such a posture flexes the lumbar spine and thereby widens the intervertebral foramen.

Extension

Extension movements of the lumbar spine produce converse movements of those that occur in flexion (Figure 15-3). Theoretically, true extension of the lumbar spine is pathological, and depends on one's definition—pure extension involves a posterior roll and glide of the vertebrae and a posterior and inferior motion of the zygapophyseal joints, but not necessarily a change in the degree of lordosis.[49] During lumbar extension, the inferior zygapophyseal joint of the superior vertebra moves downward, impacting with the lamina below and producing a buckling of the interspinous ligament between the two spinous processes.

● **Key Point**   An anterior pelvic tilt, a short arc anterior rotation of the pelvis about the hip joints with the trunk held upright and stationary, increases the lumbar lordosis and results in an anterior motion of the vertebrae and their associated structures. An anterior pelvic tilt can be accentuated in patients with adaptively shortened hip flexors/rectus femoris, weak abdominals (particularly the transversus abdominus), weak hip extensors, lengthened hamstrings, and adaptively shortened erector spinae, or in athletic individuals such as gymnasts and dancers. A patient with a posterior disk herniation may be instructed to hold his or her pelvis in a more anteriorly tilted position to help prevent a posterior migration of the nucleus pulposus and to limit or prevent pressure on the nearby neural elements.

Side Bending

Side bending of the spine (Figure 15-4) is a coupled movement involving rotation. How this is achieved, with the exception of L5–S1 where ipsilateral coupling is known to occur, has been the subject of debate for many years, and it is difficult to ascertain how an impaired segment would behave as compared to a healthy one.

Axial Rotation

The axis of rotation passes through the aspect of the IVD and vertebral body. Axial rotation of the lumbar

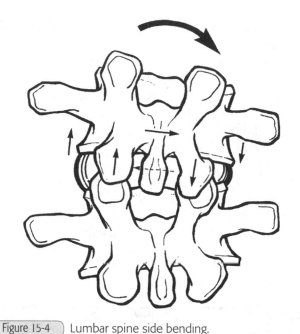

Figure 15-4 Lumbar spine side bending.

spine amounts to approximately 13 degrees to both sides. The greatest amount of segmental rotation, about 5 degrees, occurs at the L5–S1 segment.

The ipsilateral joint does not normally gap during axial rotation. Abnormal gapping has been found to occur in segments with degenerative or traumatic instability.

Axial Loading (Compression)

Even when lifting moderately sized objects, large compression forces can occur in the spine. In intradiskal pressure studies and electromyographic measurements of trunk muscles, in conjunction with mathematical models, investigators have estimated the compressive load on the lumbar spine to reach 1000 Newtons during standing and walking. The compressive load on the lumbar spine is substantially higher in many lifting activities and is estimated to reach several thousand Newtons.[50]

> ● **Key Point** Intradiskal pressure (pressure within the disk) changes according to position or activity:[51,52]
> - *Lying supine:* Disk pressure is equal to 25 percent of body weight.
> - *Lying supine with both knees flexed:* Disk pressure is equal to 35 percent of body weight.
> - *Side lying:* Disk pressure is equal to 75 percent of body weight.
> - *Seated in a flexed position:* Disk pressure is equal to 825 percent of body weight.
> - *Standing:* Disk pressure is equal to 100 percent of body weight.
> - *Standing and bending forward:* Disk pressure is equal to 150 percent of body weight.
> - *Bending forward in a flexed posture and lifting:* Disk pressure is equal to 2750 percent of body weight.

> ● **Key Point** Correct lifting techniques allow the forces on the low back to be shared by muscles of the trunk, legs, and arms. When instructing the patient on correct lifting techniques, the following points should be considered:
> - Whenever possible, use the assistance of a mechanical device or additional people for the lifting task.
> - The load being carried should be held as close to the body as possible.
> - During any lifting, the lumbar spine should be held in as close to a neutral lordotic posture as possible.
> - During the lift, the hip and knee extensor muscles must be fully utilized.
> - Avoid twisting during lifting.
> - Minimize the vertical and horizontal distances that the load must be lifted.

Anatomy of the Sacroiliac Joint

The sacroiliac joint (SIJ) is a true diarthrodial joint that joins the sacrum to the pelvis (innominate) by way of the iliac bones. Each right and left innominate bone is formed by the union of three bones: the ilium, ischium, and pubis. The iliac crest is the palpable ridge of bone that marks the superior border of the ilium. The anterior aspect of the iliac crest ends at the anterior superior iliac spine (ASIS). The posterior aspect of the iliac crest ends at the posterior superior iliac spine (PSIS). The ischium is located on the posteroinferior aspect of the innominate. The ischial tuberosity, the bone on which people sit, serves as the proximal attachment for three of the four hamstring muscles. Including the hamstrings, 35 muscles attach to the sacrum, ilium, or both (**Table 15-2**). The pubis is composed primarily of two rami (arms), the superior and inferior pubic ramus. At the SIJ, hyaline cartilage on the sacral side moves against fibrocartilage on the iliac side. The joint is generally L-shaped with two lever arms that interlock at the second sacral level. The joint contains numerous ridges and depressions, and the sacrum is wedged anteroposteriorly, which allows it to provide resistance to vertical and horizontal translation, indicating its function is for stability more than motion. Stability is also provided by the presence of generously sized ligaments.[53] Stability of the pelvic girdle is important, because it must transmit forces from the weight of the head, trunk, and upper extremities downward and forces from the lower extremities upward.

Posterior Muscle System

The thoracolumbar fascia (TLF) and its muscular attachments (transversus abdominis, internal oblique, gluteus maximus, latissimus dorsi, erector

TABLE 15-2	Muscles that Attach to the Sacrum, Ilium, or Both	
Latissimus dorsi	Gluteus medius
Erector spinae	Gluteus maximus
Semimembranosus	Quadratus femoris
Semitendinosus	Superior gemellus
Biceps femoris	Gracilis
Sartorius	Iliacus
Inferior gemellus	Adductor magnus
Multifidus	Rectus femoris
Obturator internus	Quadratus lumborum
Obturator externus	Pectineus
Piriformis	Psoas minor
Tensor fascia lata	Adductor brevis
External oblique	Adductor longus
Internal oblique	Levator ani
Transversus abdominis	Sphincter urethrae
Rectus abdominis	Superficial transverse perineal ischiocavernosus
Pyramidalis	Coccygeus
Gluteus minimus	

spinae, and biceps femoris) play an important role in stabilization of the lumbopelvic region.[54] These attachments suggests that the hip, pelvic, and leg muscles interact with the arm and spinal muscles through the TLF.[54]

Anterior Muscle System

One of the most important muscle groups contributing to the mobility and stability of the lumbopelvic region is the abdominal wall mechanism. The abdominal wall consists of the following, listed from superficial to deep:

- *Rectus abdominis:* A paired muscle running vertically on each side of the anterior wall of the abdomen, separated by a midline band of connective tissue called the linea alba.
- *Internal and external obliques:* Working synergistically, these muscles provide an anterior oblique sling and, together with the posterior oblique sling (the TLF and associated

structures), assist in stabilization of the lumbar spine and pelvis.

- *Transversus abdominis:* Has attachments to the TLF, the sheath of the rectus abdominis, the diaphragm, the iliac crest, and the lower six costal surfaces. The transversus abdominis activates before the onset of movement in persons without lumbopelvic pain, but this function is lost in those with lumbopelvic pain.[54] Current theory suggests that this muscle is a key background stabilizing muscle for the lumbar spine, and that the emphasis of specific exercises for the abdominal wall should involve specific recruitment of this muscle instead of general strengthening or endurance.[44]

> ● **Key Point** The *lumbar multifidus* is considered to have the greatest potential to provide dynamic control to the motion segment, particularly in its neutral zone. The *transversus abdominis* is primarily active in providing rotational and lateral control to the spine while maintaining adequate levels of intra-abdominal pressure and imparting tension to the thoracolumbar fascia. The *deep erector spinae* have a poor lever arm for spine extension but are in line to provide a dynamic counterforce to the anterior sheer force imparted to the lumbar spine from gravitational force.

Because of the close relationship between the passive anatomical restraints of the lumbar spine and the muscles that control it, it would seem logical to assume that any pain-provoking injury or condition (e.g., muscle strain, ligament sprain, disk herniation) could alter the structural integrity of the lumbopelvic complex. Growing evidence is emerging to support this hypothesis.[56–57] Various studies have demonstrated that coordinated patterns of muscle recruitment are essential between the global and local system muscles of the trunk in order to compensate for the changing demands of daily life and to ensure that the dynamic stability of the spine is preserved.[59–62] A number of studies have highlighted the importance of motor control to coordinate muscle recruitment during functional activities to ensure that mechanical stability is maintained.[59,60,63–66] For example, in standing and walking, the pelvic girdle is stabilized on the femur by the coordinated action of the ipsilateral gluteus medius and minimus and by the contralateral adductor muscles. Indirectly, by maintaining a relationship among the hip, pelvis, and lumbar spine in the frontal plane, the gluteus medius, gluteus minimus, and adductors contribute to lumbar spine stability.

The scientific literature reports varying disruptions in patterns of recruitment and co-contraction within and between different muscles' synergies.[59] Studies also have described subtle changes or shifts in the pattern of abdominal muscle activation, and righting responses in subjects with chronic lumbopelvic pain.[67,68] These changes in the activation patterns result in altered patterns of synergistic control or coordination of the trunk muscles.[69,70] These subtle shifts in the patterns of muscle recruitment can result in some muscles being relatively underused, whereas other muscles relatively dominate, which in turn can increase the size of the neutral zone thereby increasing the potential for injury. In addition to pain, generalized changes to the trunk musculature such as a loss of strength, endurance, and muscle atrophy are also believed to produce changes in the neural control system, affecting the timing of patterns of co-contraction.

Kinesiology of the Sacroiliac Joint

The pelvis is the connecting link between the spine and the lower extremities. The motions at the lumbar spine predominantly occur around the sagittal plane and comprise flexion and extension, whereas the motions occurring at the hip occur in three planes and include the one motion that the lumbar spine does not tolerate well (i.e., rotation). Thus, the pelvic area must function to absorb the majority of the lower extremity rotation, particularly during bipedal gait.[71]

Sacral Motion

There are two primary motions of the sacrum—nutation and counternutation. According to the anatomic-biomechanic model based on the work of Vleeming,[72] Snijders,[73] Lee,[74] Hides, and Richardson and Jull,[75] when the sacrum nutates, or flexes, relative to the innominate, a small linear glide occurs between the two L-shaped articular surfaces of the sacroiliac joint.[76] The shorter of the two lengths, level with S1, lies in a vertical plane, whereas the longer length, spanning S2 to S4, lies in an anteroposterior plane ((Figure 15-5)).

During sacral nutation ((Figure 15-6)), the sacrum glides inferiorly down the short length and posteriorly along the long length. This motion is resisted by a number of factors:

1. The wedge shape of the sacrum
2. The ridges and depressions of the articular surfaces
3. The friction coefficient of the joint surface

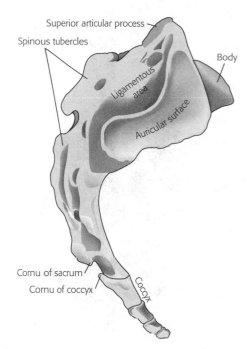

Figure 15-5   The L-shaped articular surface of the sacroiliac joint.

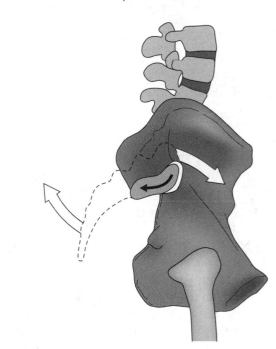

Figure 15-6   Sacral nutation.

Source: Dutton M: Manual Therapy of the Spine an Intergrated Approach. New York, McGraw-Hill Publication Division, 2002.

4. The integrity of the posterior (dorsal), interosseous, and sacrotuberous ligaments, supported by the muscles that insert into the ligaments

During sacral counternutation, or extension ((Figure 15-7)), the sacrum glides anteriorly along the longer length and superiorly up the shorter length.

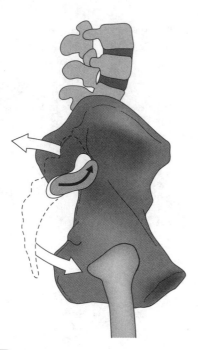

Figure 15-7 Sacral counternutation.

Source: Dutton M: Manual Therapy of the Spine an Intergrated Approach. New York, McGraw-Hill Publication Division, 2002.

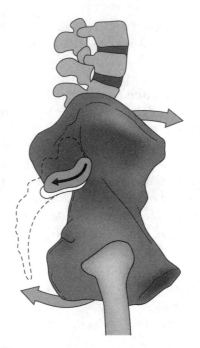

Figure 15-8 Anterior rotation of the innominate.

Source: Dutton M: Manual Therapy of the Spine an Intergrated Approach. New York, McGraw-Hill Publication Division, 2002.

This motion is resisted by the posterior (dorsal) sacroiliac ligament,[76] which is supported by the contraction of the multifidus.

Innominate Motion

Innominate motion is induced by hip and spine motion, as in extension of the lower extremity or during trunk motion when bending forward at the waist. When the innominate rotates anteriorly (Figure 15-8), it theoretically glides in the direction of the short length of the *L* and posteriorly along the longer length of the *L* of the sacroiliac joint, and in exactly the same way as the motion that occurs during counternutation of the sacrum. When the innominate rotates posteriorly (Figure 15-9), it theoretically glides along the longer length of the *L* and superiorly up the short length of the *L* of the sacroiliac joint, exactly the same way as the motion that occurs during nutation of the sacrum. That is, when the inominate anteriorly rotates, the sacrum counternutates; when the inominate posteriorly rotates, the sacrum nutates.

The direction of the innominate rotation depends on the initiating movement.

- During open chain hip flexion, the ipsilateral innominate posteriorly rotates while the sacrum rotates to the same side as the flexed femur. The posterior rotation of the innominate

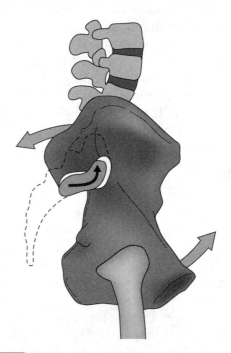

Figure 15-9 Posterior rotation of the innominate.

Source: Dutton M: Manual Therapy of the Spine an Intergrated Approach. New York, McGraw-Hill Publication Division, 2002.

positions the ASIS in an upward position. If the femur is extended, the ipsilateral innominate anteriorly rotates and the sacrum rotates to the contralateral side to the extended femur.

- During an anterior pelvic tilt on a relatively fixed femur (closed chain), an anterior rotation of the innominate occurs. The converse holds true for posterior rotation. Thus, during a posterior pelvic tilt, the innominate posteriorly rotates (refer to Figure 15-9).

> **● Key Point** There is very little agreement, either among disciplines or even within disciplines, about the biomechanics of the pelvic complex. The results from numerous studies on mobility of the sacroiliac joint have led to a variety of different hypotheses and models of pelvic mechanics over the years.

Forward Bending

During closed chain forward bending at the waist, a combination of anterior and outward rotation of both innominates results in the approximation and superior motion of both PSISs, while the sacrum nutates due to the compression effect of the innominates. After about 60 degrees of forward bending, the innominates continue to rotate anteriorly, but the sacrum no longer nutates.[74] If the sacrum remains nutated throughout forward bending, the sacroiliac joint remains compressed and stable. However, if the sacrum is forced to counternutate earlier in the range, as in individuals with tight hamstrings, less compression occurs, thereby increasing the reliance on dynamic stabilization provided by muscles, and thus increasing the potential for sacroiliac joint injury.[74]

Backward Bending

Backward bending at the waist, or extension of the spine, involves a combination of an anterior displacement of the pelvic girdle and an inferior motion of both posterosuperior iliac spines. A slight posterior innominate rotation occurs and the sacrum remains nutated.

Side Bending

During right side bending, the right innominate rotates anteriorly and the sacrum right side bends. Motion of the innominate during side bending likely results from ground reaction forces.[77] As side bending to the right occurs, the right leg takes more weight and so is compressed. This downward body weight force, together with the upward ground reaction force, results in anterior rotation (extension) of the innominate, causing a slight flexion of the hip. This hip flexion, together with the flattening of the foot and hyperextension of the knee, effectively allows the leg to shorten in response to these compressive forces. It is interesting that in non-weight-bearing, anterior innominate rotation results in a leg length increase, whereas in weight bearing, an anterior rotation

produces a leg length decrease. In fact, it is the same mechanism in both cases.[77] In non-weight-bearing, the anterior rotation of the innominate pushes the femur downward. Because there is no resistance under the foot and no force to flex the hip, the leg can lengthen. In weight bearing, ground reaction forces push the innominate superiorly because of the inability of the leg to lengthen during the side bending.

Trunk Rotation

During axial rotation of the trunk to the left, the right innominate rotates anteriorly while the left innominate rotates posteriorly. Simultaneously, counternutation of the sacrum occurs at the right sacroiliac joint, and nutation occurs at the left sacroiliac joint. The motion of the innominates during trunk rotation allows the sacrum to rotate osteokinematically while maintaining a more or less vertical orientation.

Pelvic Tilt

The degree of pelvic tilt, which is measured as the angle between the horizontal plane and a line connecting the ASIS with the PSIS, varies from 5 to 12 degrees in normal individuals.[78] Both a low ASIS in women and a structurally flat back in men can cause structural variations in pelvic alignment, which can be misinterpreted as acquired postural impairments. Actively anteriorly tilting the pelvis is created by force couples involving the hip flexor muscles and erector spinae (low back extensors) in an action that is similar to the push and pull of one's hands when turning a steering wheel—the erector spinae muscles pull upward at the same time the hip flexors pull downward.[79]

Pelvic Stabilization

In upright positions, the sacroiliac joint is subjected to considerable shear force because the mass of the upper body must be transferred to the lower limbs via the ilia.[80,81] The body has two mechanisms to overcome this shear force: one is dependent on the shape and structure of the joint surfaces of the sacroiliac joints (form closure), which is wedge shaped with a high coefficient of friction; the other involves generation of compressive forces across the sacroiliac joint via muscle contraction (force closure).[81]

Form Closure

Form closure refers to a state of stability within the pelvic mechanism, with the degree of stability dependent on its anatomy. No extra forces are needed to maintain the stable state of the system.[73]

The following anatomic structures are proposed to assist with form closure:

- *The congruity of the articular surfaces and the friction coefficient of the articular cartilage:* Both the coarseness of the cartilage and the complementary grooves and ridges increase the friction coefficient, and thus contribute to form closure by resisting against horizontal and vertical translations.[82] In infants, the joint surfaces are very planar, but between the ages of 11 and 15 years, the characteristic ridges and humps that make up the mature sacrum begin to form. By the third decade, the superficial layers of the fibrocartilage are fibrillated and crevice formation and erosion has begun. By the fourth and fifth decades, the articular surfaces increase irregularity and coarseness and the wedging is incomplete.[83]
- The integrity of the ligaments.

Force Closure

Force closure requires intrinsic and extrinsic forces to keep the sacroiliac joint stable.[73] These dynamic forces involve the neurological and myofascial systems and gravity. Together, these components produce a self-locking mechanism for the sacroiliac joint. Critical to the functioning of the self-locking mechanism is the ability of the sacrum to nutate, because nutation of the sacrum winds up most of the SIJ ligaments, particularly the interosseous and posterior (dorsal) ligaments.[73,84,85] These latter ligaments lie posterior to the joint and approximate the posterior iliac bones when placed under tension.[84]

Just as nutation of the sacrum enhances the self-locking mechanism, counternutation of the sacrum, which occurs during activities such as the end range of forward bending, sacral sitting, long sitting, and hip hyperextension, reduces the self-locking mechanism.[84]

In the kinetic analysis of the pelvic girdle, Vleeming et al. identified a number of muscles that resist translational forces and that are specifically important to the force-closure mechanism: the erector spinae, gluteus maximus, latissimus dorsi, and biceps femoris.[55,84] Two other muscle groups, an "inner muscle unit" and an "outer muscle unit," also play an important role.[67,74,75] The inner muscle unit consists of the following:

- The muscles of the pelvic floor (Hemborg et al.[86] have demonstrated that the pelvic floor

muscles coactivate with the transversus abdominis during lifting tasks.)
- Transversus abdominis
- Multifidus
- Diaphragm

The outer muscle unit consists of four systems:[74]

- *The posterior oblique system (latissimus dorsi, gluteus maximus, and thoracolumbar fascia):* The gluteus maximus, which blends with the thoracodorsal fascia, and the contralateral latissimus dorsi contribute to force closure of the sacroiliac joint posteriorly by approximating the posterior aspects of the innominates. This oblique system is a significant contributor to load transference through the pelvic girdle during the rotational activities of gait.
- *The deep longitudinal system (erector spinae, deep lamina of the thoracolumbar fascia, sacrotuberous ligament, and biceps femoris):* This system serves to counteract any anterior shear or sacral nutation forces as well as to facilitate compression through the sacroiliac joints.
- *The anterior oblique system (external and internal obliques, contralateral adductors of the thigh, and the intervening anterior abdominal fascia):* The oblique abdominals, acting as phasic muscles, initiate movements[67] and are involved in all movements of the trunk and upper and lower extremities, except when the legs are crossed.[87]
- *The lateral system (gluteus medius–minimus and contralateral adductors of the thigh):* The lateral system functions to stabilize the pelvic girdle on the femoral head during gait through a coordinated action.

Weakness or insufficient recruitment and/or unbalanced muscle function within the lumbar/pelvic/hip region can reduce the force closure mechanism, which can result in compensatory movement strategies.[88] These compensatory movement strategies and/or patterns of muscle imbalance may produce a sustained counternutation of the sacrum, thereby "unlocking" the mechanism and rendering the SIJ vulnerable to injury. This unlocked position of the pelvis also may increase shear forces at the lumbar spine and cause an abnormal loading of the lumbar disks. Mechanical pain resulting from sacroiliac joint dysfunction may manifest as sacral pain but may also refer pain distally. Sacroiliac joint problems can refer pain to the PSIS, iliac fossa, medial buttock, and superior lateral and posterior thigh.[89] Pain also may be referred to the sacrum from a distant structure, including the contralateral sacrospinalis muscle,[90] the ipsilateral interspinous ligaments of L3 to S2,[91] and the L4 to L5 facet joints.[92] In general, unilateral pain with no referral below the knee may be caused by the sacroiliac joint whereas irritation of a spinal nerve may cause radicular symptoms below the knee.[93] Pubic symphysis dysfunction typically results in localized pain, or groin pain, which is aggravated by activities involving the hip adductor or rectus abdominis muscles.[94]

The following findings are likely to be present with a sacroiliac joint dysfunction:[95–98]

- A history of sharp pain that awakens the patient from sleep upon turning in bed

- Pain with walking, ascending or descending stairs, rising to stand from a sitting position, or hopping or standing on the involved leg
- Pain with a straight leg raise at, or near, the end of range (occasionally early in the range when hyperacute)
- Pain and sometimes limitation on extension and ipsilateral side bending of the trunk

Examination of the Lumbopelvic Complex

The examinations performed by the physical therapist for the lumbar spine and SIJ are summarized in **Table 15-3** and **Table 15-4**. The evidence-based special tests of the lumbar spine and SIJ are outlined in **Table 15-5**. Range of motion of the lumbar spine is best measured using two bubble goniometers (Figure 15-10) through Figure 15-14).

TABLE 15-3	Examination of the Lumbar Spine	
Observation and Inspection		
Lower quarter and peripheral joint scan	Hip, knee, ankle, and foot	
	Dermatomes and key muscle tests as appropriate	
Examination of movements; active range of motion with passive overpressure	Flexion, extension, side bending (right and left), rotation (right and left)	
	Combined movements as appropriate	
	Repetitive movements as appropriate	
	Sustained positions as appropriate	
	Sacroiliac joint movement testing	
Resisted isometric movements	All AROM directions	
	Rectus abdominis, internal and external obliques, quadratus lumborum, back and hip extensors	
Palpation		
Neurological tests as appropriate	Palpation of bony prominences and superficial structures	
Joint mobility tests	Reflexes, key muscle tests, sensory scan, peripheral nerve assessment	
	Neurodynamic mobility tests (straight leg raise, slump test, prone knee flexion)	
	1. Side glides	
	2. Anterior and posterior glides	
	3. Traction and compression	
Special Tests (refer to Table 15-5)	As indicated	
Diagnostic Imaging	As appropriate	

TABLE 15-4   Examination of the Sacroiliac Joint

Observation and Inspection

Lower quarter and peripheral joint scan	Hip, knee, ankle, and foot
	Dermatomes and key muscle tests as appropriate
Examination of movements; active range of motion with passive overpressure	Flexion, extension, side bending (right and left), rotation (right and left) of lumbar spine
	Flexion, extension, adduction and abduction, internal and external rotation of the hip
	Combined movements as appropriate
	Repetitive movements as appropriate
	Sustained positions as appropriate
	Sacroiliac joint movement testing
Resisted isometric movements	Hip flexion, extension, internal and external rotation, abduction and adduction
Palpation	
Neurological tests as appropriate	Palpation of bony prominences and superficial structures
Joint mobility tests	Reflexes, key muscle tests, sensory scan, peripheral nerve assessment
	a. Hip and lumbar spine mobility
	b. Anterior and posterior compression of SIJ
Special Tests (refer to Table 15-5)	As indicated
Diagnostic imaging	As appropriate

TABLE 15-5   Evidence-Based Special Tests of the Lumbar Spine and SIJ

Name of Test	Brief Description	Positive Findings	Evidence-Based
Two-stage treadmill test[a]	Patient ambulates on a level and inclined (15-degree) treadmill for 10 minutes. A 10-minute rest period sitting upright in a chair follows each test.	Positive for lumbar spinal stenosis if symptoms are reproduced based on time to onset of symptoms and prolonged recovery after level walking.	Sensitivity: 0.68–0.82 Specificity: 0.83–0.68
Segmental hypomobility testing[b]	Assessment of AROM, abnormality of segmental motion (AbAROM), passive accessory intervertebral motion (PAIVM), and passive physiologic intervertebral motion (PPIVM).	Presence of hypomobility with any of the tests.	*AROM* Sensitivity: 0.75 Specificity: 0.60 *AbAROM* Sensitivity: 0.43 Specificity: 0.88 *PAIVM* Sensitivity: 0.75 Specificity: 0.35 *PPIVM* Sensitivity: 0.42 Specificity: 0.89

Name of Test	Brief Description	Positive Findings	Evidence-Based
Straight leg raise for detecting disk herniation[c]	Performed with the patient supine, the knee fully extended, and the ankle in neutral dorsiflexion. The clinician then passively flexes the hip while maintaining the knee extension to the point where pain or paresthesia is experienced in the back or lower limb. Various sensitizing maneuvers (dorsiflexion of the ankle and flexion of the cervical spine) are then added.	Positive if the sensitizing maneuvers exacerbate the symptoms.	Sensitivity: 0.91 Specificity: 0.26
Crossed straight leg raise for detecting disk herniation[c]	The clinician performs a straight leg raise on the uninvolved lower extremity.	Reproduction of the patient's symptoms in the involved extremity.	Sensitivity: 0.29 Specificity: 0.88
Patrick test (SIJ pain provocation test)[d]	The patient's hip is flexed, abducted, and externally rotated by placement of the lateral malleolus on the knee of the contralateral leg. The pelvis is stabilized, and overpressure is applied to the medial aspect of the knee.	Positive if buttock and groin pain is reproduced.	Sensitivity: 0.77 Specificity: 1.0
Posterior gapping of the SIJ[e]	Patient side lying. Firm downward pressure is applied by the clinician to the contralateral ilium.	Positive for ankylosing spondylitis if pain over the sacrum or into the buttocks is provoked.	Sensitivity: 0.70 Specificity: 0.90
Anterior gapping of the SIJ[f]	The patient is positioned in supine. The clinician applies cross-over pressure to both anterior superior iliac spines.	Positive if there is a production or increase in familiar symptoms.	Sensitivity: 0.23 Specificity: 0.81
Gaenslen test (SIJ dysfunction)[c]	Patient supine with both legs extended. The leg being tested is passively brought into full knee flexion, while the opposite hip remains in extension. Overpressure is then applied to the flexed extremity.	Positive if pain is reproduced.	Sensitivity: 0.21 Specificity: 0.72
Long sitting test[g]	Patient supine. Clinician palpates inferior border of medial malleoli and makes a determination of symmetry. Patient assumes the long sitting position and the clinician again records symmetry of the malleoli.	Positive for iliosacral dysfunction if asymmetric malleoli lengths reverse from supine to long sit.	Sensitivity: 0.17 Specificity: 0.38
Thigh thrust[h]	The patient is positioned in supine with hip flexed 90 degrees and slightly adducted. The clinician cups the sacrum with one hand and with the other applies a posteriorly directed force to the femur.	Positive for sacroiliac joint dysfunction if familiar symptoms are reproduced or increased.	Sensitivity: 0.88 Specificity: 0.69
Compression test[f]	The patient is positioned in side lying, involved side up, with the hips flexed approximately 45 degrees and the knees flexed approximately 90 degrees. The clinician applies a force vertically downward on the anterior superior iliac crest.	Positive for SIJ dysfunction if there is reproduction or an increase in familiar symptoms.	Sensitivity: 0.22 Specificity: 0.83
Sacral thrust test[h]	The patient is positioned in prone. The clinician applies a force vertically downward to the center of the sacrum.	A positive test for SIJ dysfunction is the production or increase in the familiar symptoms.	Sensitivity: 0.63 Specificity: 0.75

(continued)

TABLE 15-5

Evidence-Based Special Tests of the Lumbar Spine and SIJ (continued)

Name of Test	Brief Description	Positive Findings	Evidence-Based
Mennell's test[f]	The patient is positioned in side lying, involved side down, with the involved side hip and knee flexed toward the abdomen. The clinician puts one hand over the ipsilateral buttock and iliac crest and the other hand grasps the semiflexed ipsilateral knee and lightly forces the leg into extension.	Positive test for SIJ dysfunction is the production or increase of familiar symptoms.	Sensitivity: 0.66 (right), 0.45 (left) Specificity: 0.80 (right), 0.86 (left)
Gillet test[i]	The patient is standing with feet spread 12 inches apart. The clinician palpates the S2 spinous process with one hand and the posterior superior iliac spine (PSIS) with the other. The patient then flexes the hip and knee on the side being tested.	Positive for SIJ dysfunction if the PSIS fails to move in a posteroinferior direction relative to S2.	Sensitivity: 0.08 Specificity: 0.93
Standing flexion test[i]	The patient is standing. The clinician palpates the inferior slope of the PSIS. The patient is asked to forward bend completely.	Positive for sacroiliac hypomobility if one PSIS moves more cranially than the contralateral side.	Sensitivity: 0.17 Specificity: 0.79
Sitting flexion test[i]	The patient is positioned in sitting. The clinician palpates the inferior aspect of each PSIS. The patient is asked to bend forward as far as possible.	Positive for sacroiliac joint dysfunction if inequality of PSIS movement is found.	Sensitivity: 0.09 Specificity: 0.93

Data from (a) Fritz JM, Erhard RE, Delitto A, et al: Preliminary results of the use of a two-stage treadmill test as a clinical diagnostic tool in the differential diagnosis of lumbar spinal stenosis. J Spinal Disord 10:410–416, 1997; (b) Abbot J, Mercer S: Lumbar segmental hypomobility: Criterion-related validity of clinical examination items (a pilot study). N Z J Physiother 31:3–9, 2003; (c) Deville WL, van der Windt DA, Dzaferagic A, et al: The test of Lasegue: Systematic review of the accuracy in diagnosing herniated discs. Spine (Phila Pa 1976) 25:1140–1147, 2000; (d) Broadhurst NA, Bond MJ: Pain provocation tests for the assessment of sacroiliac joint dysfunction. J Spinal Disord 11:341–345, 1998; (e) Russel AS, Maksymowych W, LeClercq S: Clinical examination of the sacroiliac joints: A prospective study. Arthritis Rheum 24:1575–1577, 1981; (f) Ozgocmen S, Bozgeyik Z, Kalcik M, et al: The value of sacroiliac pain provocation tests in early active sacroiliitis. Clin Rheumatol 27:1275–1282, 2008; (g) Bemis T, Daniel M: Validation of the long sitting test on subjects with iliosacral dysfunction. J Orthop Sports Phys Ther 8:336–345, 1987; (h) Laslett M, Aprill CN, McDonald B, et al: Diagnosis of sacroiliac joint pain: Validity of individual provocation tests and composites of tests. Man Ther 10:207–218, 2005; and (i) Levangie PK: Four clinical tests of sacroiliac joint dysfunction: The association of test results with innominate torsion among patients with and without low back pain. Phys Ther 79:1043–1057, 1999

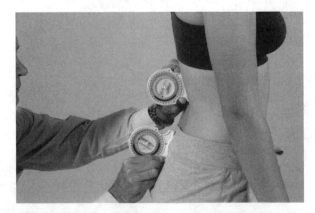

Figure 15-10 Lumbar ROM: start position for flexion/extension.

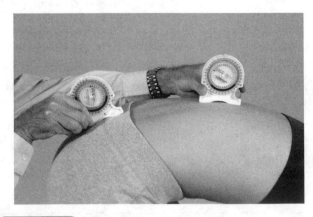

Figure 15-11 Lumbar ROM: flexion.

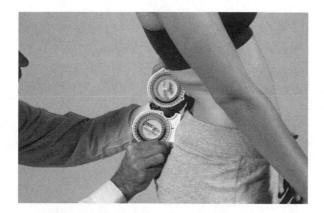

Figure 15-12   Lumbar ROM: extension.

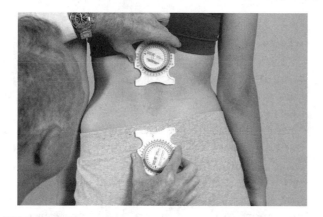

Figure 15-13   Lumbar ROM: start position for side bending.

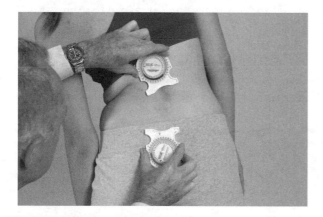

Figure 15-14   Lumbar ROM: end position for side bending.

General Intervention Strategies

The optimal intervention for patients with acute lumbopelvic pain remains largely enigmatic, and a number of clinical studies have failed to find consistent evidence for improved intervention outcomes with many intervention approaches.[99] The decision of whether to treat the low back and SIJ separately or in combination is largely based on training. Because the two joints work in conjunction with each other, this text advocates treating them together. It is essential that the impairments, functional limitations, and disability found during the examination guide the intervention, and that the intervention should be dynamic and should direct the responsibility of the rehabilitative process toward the patient. The recommendations concerning bed rest for common, acute lumbopelvic pain have changed over the years.[100] The most recent guidelines (2000), based on the results of several randomized studies, advise avoiding bed rest to the extent possible.[101] A study by Rozenberg and colleagues[102] found that for patients with acute lumbopelvic pain, normal activity is at least equivalent to bed rest. These authors recommended that prescriptions for bed rest, and thus for sick leaves, should be limited when the physical demands of the job are similar to those for daily life activities.[102]

In the past decade, meta-analysis of the results of randomized clinical trials have provided various degrees of support for the efficacy of specific, nonsurgical physical interventions (that may be delivered by physical therapy) for the management of spine disorders. A number of studies have reported that intensive exercise reduces pain and improves function in patients with chronic lumbopelvic pain.[99,103,104] In addition, exercise programs that combine aerobic conditioning with specific strengthening of the back and legs can reduce the frequency of recurrence of lumbopelvic pain.[105]

Acute Phase

The goals of the acute phase are to:

- Decrease pain, inflammation, and muscle spasm
- Promote healing of tissues
- Increase pain-free range of vertebral and sacral motion
- Regain soft tissue extensibility
- Regain neuromuscular control
- Initiate postural education
- Promote correct body mechanics
- Educate the patient about activities to avoid and positions of comfort
- Allow progression to the functional phase

The exercises described in the following sections can be used for the vast majority of lumbopelvic conditions. In the early phases of rehabilitation, muscle activation is encouraged using one of three exercises, each with its own stabilization activity of the abdominal and multifidus muscles:

Skeletal arrangement in supine

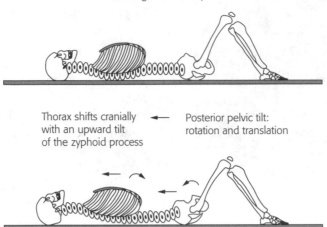

Thorax shifts cranially
with an upward tilt
of the zyphoid process ← Posterior pelvic tilt:
rotation and translation

Figure 15-15   Posterior pelvic tilt.

- *Posterior pelvic tilt:* The posterior pelvic tilt (Figure 15-15) primarily activates the rectus abdominis, which is used mainly for dynamic trunk flexion activity.
- *Abdominal bracing exercise:* This exercise has been shown to activate the oblique abdominal muscles.
- *Drawing-in exercise:* The patient, positioned in hook lying (with knees 70–90 degrees and feet resting on the floor), quadruped, prone, or the semi-reclined position (based on comfort), is asked to take a relaxed breath in and out and then draw the waistline in (towards the spine) without taking a breath (Figure 15-16).[106] The contraction must be performed in a slow and controlled manner. Assessment

of optimal recruitment of the transversus abdominis can be done through palpation just distal to the ASIS and lateral to the rectus abdominis (Figure 15-16), or with the use of biofeedback.[106] When performed correctly, the clinician should feel flat tension of the muscle, rather than a bulge if the internal oblique contracts, and should see no substitute patterns (no movement of the pelvis, no flaring or depression of the lower ribs, no inspiration or lifting of the rib cage, no bulging out of the abdominal wall, and no increased pressure through the feet).[65,75,107]

Once the technique is successfully learned, the patient is encouraged to perform the exercise while in the sitting and standing positions.[65,75,106,107]

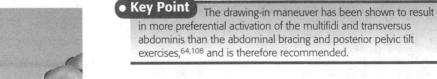

● **Key Point**   The drawing-in maneuver has been shown to result in more preferential activation of the multifidi and transversus abdominis than the abdominal bracing and posterior pelvic tilt exercises,[64,108] and is therefore recommended.

The patient should now be taught how to activate the multifidus. This is performed in prone or side lying. The clinician uses the thumbs or index fingers to palpate immediately lateral to the spinous processes of the lumbar spine, and the patient is asked to bulge the muscle out against the palpating digits (Figure 15-17). Once the multifidus and the drawing-in techniques are mastered, they are performed during lower and upper extremity open-chain activities to improve muscular endurance,[60,109] and the progression to global stabilization occurs.

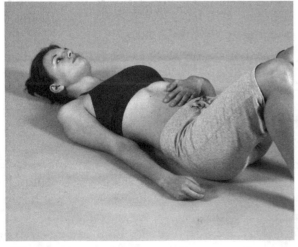

Figure 15-16   Drawing-in exercise.

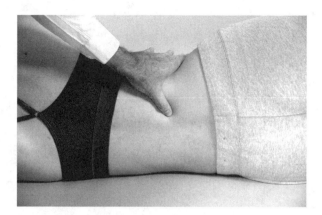

Figure 15-17   Multifidus activation.

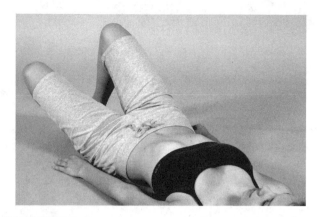

Figure 15-18   Bent-leg fall out.

In general, the global stabilization exercises begin in the recumbent position and progress to sitting. However, the position used should be based on the findings from the clinical examination that minimize symptom reproduction. For example, the quadruped position has a significantly higher center of gravity (COG) and smaller base of support (BOS) than the prone position, making it a more challenging position. All of the following exercises are superimposed on the neutral spine (midrange or functional position) and the drawing-in maneuver, making sure the patient maintains control while applying the extremity motions. If the patient cannot control the position using muscle control, pillows or supports are used.

Emphasis on Abdominals[110]

Bent-Leg Fallout

The patient is positioned in supine hook lying (knees at 90 degrees of flexion) and is asked to separate the knees while preventing pelvic rotation (Figure 15-18).

Progressive Limb Loading

From the supine hook-lying position the patient is asked to:

1. Lift one of the legs to 90 degrees of hip and knee flexion (Figure 15-19).
2. Slide the heel of one leg to extend the knee (Figure 15-20).
3. Lift the straight leg to 45 degrees (Figure 15-21).

The exercise is then repeated using the other leg.

The exercise progression then follows a series of levels of increasing difficulty while performing the same three methods of progressive limb-loading:

■ The opposite leg is held at 90 degrees of hip flexion using both upper extremities (Figure 15-22).

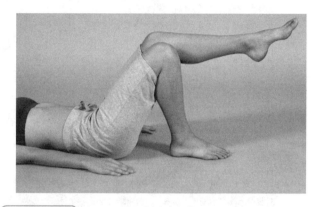

Figure 15-19   Progressive limb loading 1.

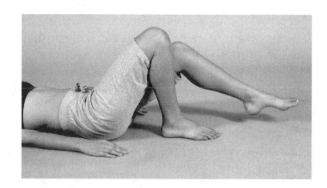

Figure 15-20   Progressive limb loading 2.

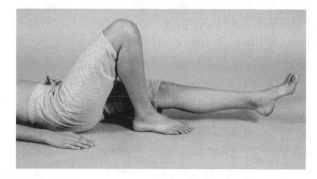

Figure 15-21   Progressive limb loading 3.

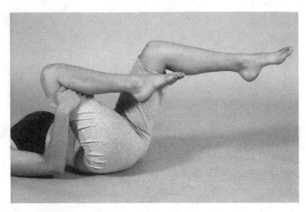

Figure 15-22 Progressive limb loading 4.

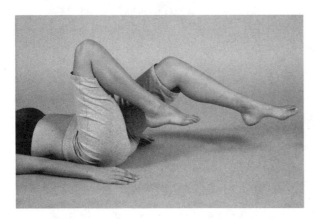

Figure 15-23   Progressive limb loading 5.

- The opposite leg is held at 90 degrees of hip flexion with no upper extremity assistance (Figure 15-23).
- Both legs perform the series of progressive limb loading simultaneously (Figure 15-24).

At this stage, external resistance in the form of weights, elastic resistance, or pulleys can be added for strengthening.

Emphasis on the Trunk Extensors
The following exercises are performed with the patient in prone:[110]

- Extend one lower extremity (Figure 15-25).
- Extend both lower extremities (Figure 15-26).
- Lift the head, arms, and lower extremities (Figure 15-27).

For patients with limited lumbar extension, or those with increased symptoms with lumbar extension, a small pillow can be placed under the hips in prone for starting position, and the patient can lift the upper and lower extremities to the neutral position of the lumbar spine.

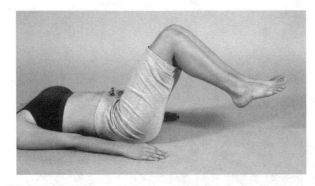

Figure 15-24   Progressive limb loading 6.

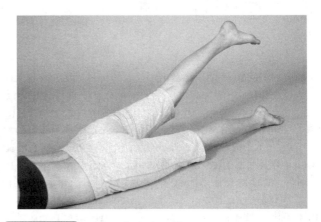

Figure 15-25   Prone single leg raise.

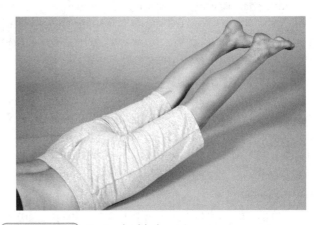

Figure 15-26   Prone double leg raise.

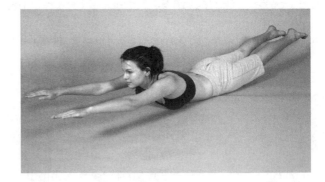

Figure 15-27   Lifting the head, arms, and lower extremities.

At this stage, external resistance in the form of weights, elastic resistance, or pulleys can be added for strengthening. The following exercises are performed in the quadruped position (Figure 15-28) and include the following progression:

- Flex one upper extremity (Figure 15-29).
- Extend one lower extremity by sliding it along the exercise mat and then raising (Figure 15-30).

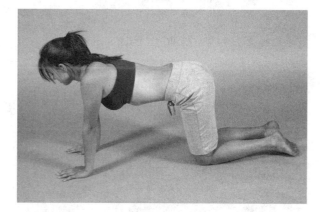

Figure 15-28 Quadruped.

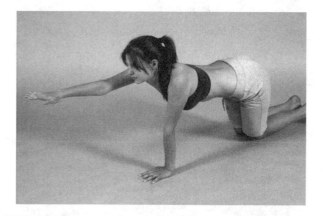

Figure 15-29 Quadruped and upper extremity flexion.

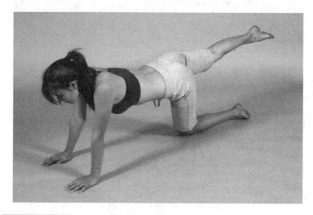

Figure 15-30 Quadruped and lower extremity extension.

- Flex one upper extremity and extend the contralateral lower extremity (Figure 15-31).

Functional/Chronic Phase

The goals of this phase are:

- To achieve significant reduction or to complete resolution of the patient's pain
- Restoration of full and pain-free vertebral range of motion
- Full integration of the entire upper and lower kinetic chains
- Complete restoration of respiratory function
- Restoration of thoracic and upper quadrant strength and neuromuscular control

Emphasis on the Lateral Stabilizers

These exercises are performed in the side-lying position and include the following progression:

- Side plank with hips on bed (Figure 15-32)
- Side plank (Figure 15-33)

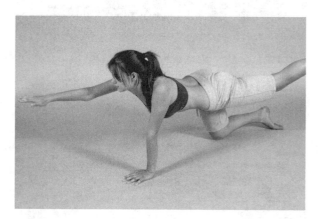

Figure 15-31 Quadruped upper extremity flexion and lower extremity extension.

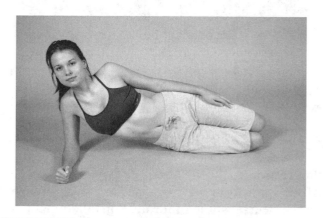

Figure 15-32 Side plank with hips on bed.

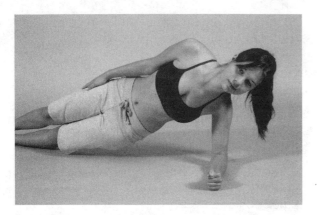

Figure 15-33 Side plank.

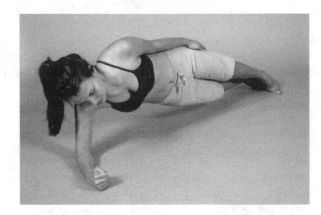

Figure 15-36 Side plank with inward roll: start position.

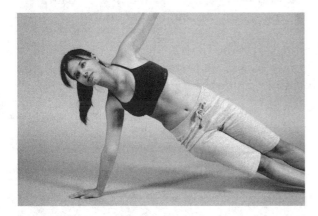

Figure 15-34 Side plank with arm extended.

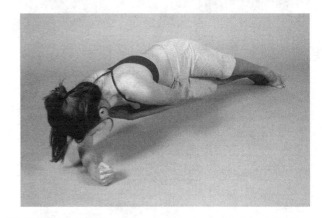

Figure 15-37 Side plank with inward roll: end position.

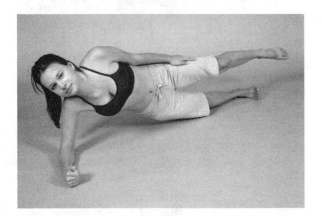

Figure 15-35 Side plank with hip abduction.

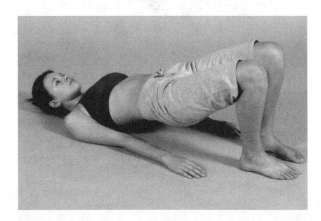

Figure 15-38 Bridging.

- Side plank with arm extended (Figure 15-34)
- Side plank with hip abduction (Figure 15-35)
- Side plank with inward roll (Figure 15-36 and Figure 15-37)

Progression

All of the following exercises are superimposed on the neutral spine (midrange or functional position) and the drawing-in maneuver, making sure the patient maintains control while performing the exercises:

- *Bridging:* The patient is positioned supine, with the arms by the sides. The patient is asked to keep the knees bent and feet flat, and to lift the buttocks from the floor (Figure 15-38). The exercise can be made more challenging by having the patient squeeze a ball with their thighs while performing the bridge

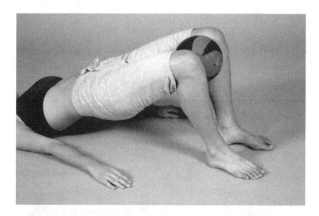

Figure 15-39   Bridging with medicine ball.

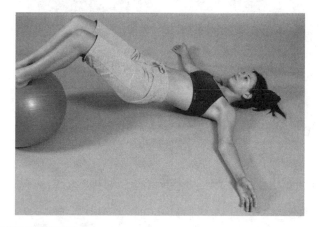

Figure 15-40   Bridging on Swiss ball.

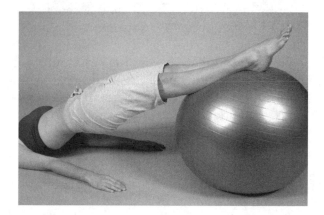

Figure 15-41   Bridging with feet on a Swiss ball, knees straight.

(Figure 15-39). There are variations that use a Swiss ball:

- ❑ Bridging with feet on a Swiss ball, knees bent (Figure 15-40)
- ❑ Bridging with feet on a Swiss ball, knees straight (Figure 15-41)
- ❑ Bridging with shoulders on a Swiss ball (Figure 15-42)

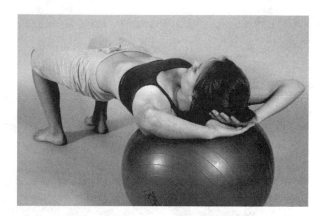

Figure 15-42   Bridging with shoulders on a Swiss ball.

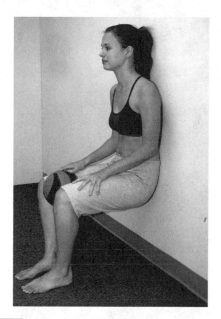

Figure 15-43   Wall slide with medicine ball.

- *Wall slides:* With the back against a wall, the patient is asked to perform a squat and then return to standing while maintaining the neutral zone throughout the exercise. This exercise can be modified by placing a medicine ball between the patient's knees (Figure 15-43).
- *Forward lunge:* While maintaining the neutral zone throughout the exercise, the patient is asked to step forward with one leg and lower the opposite knee toward the ground (Figure 15-44). Hand weights, elastic resistance (Figure 15-45), or dumbbells can be used to make the exercise more challenging.
- *Backward lunge:* While maintaining the neutral zone throughout the exercise, the patient is asked to step backward with one leg and lower the same knee to the ground before returning

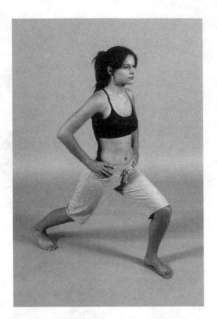

Figure 15-44   Lunge.

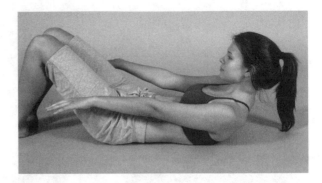

Figure 15-46   Curl-up.

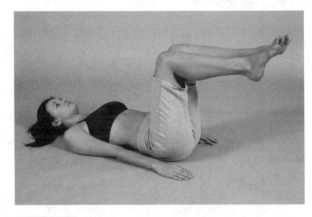

Figure 15-47   Supine with hips and knees at 90 degrees.

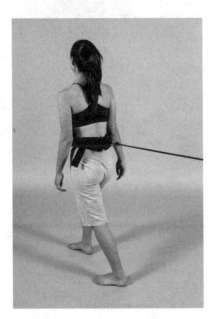

Figure 15-45   Resisted lunge.

to the starting position. Hand weights, elastic resistance, or dumbbells can be used to make the exercise more challenging.

Advanced Techniques

All of the following exercises are superimposed on the neutral spine (midrange or functional position) and the drawing-in maneuver, making sure the patient maintains control while performing the exercises:

- *Curl-up:* The patient is positioned supine, with the legs bent at the knees and the feet flat on the floor. The arms are folded across the chest or

kept by the side (Figure 15-46). Concentrating on curling the upper trunk as much as possible, the patient is asked to perform an abdominal hollowing and then to raise the head and shoulders off the bed by about 30–45 degrees (Figure 15-46). After holding this position for 2–3 seconds, the patient returns to the initial position. The muscles strengthened with this exercise include the rectus abdominis and the internal and external obliques.[111]

- *Hip thrusts:* The patient is positioned supine, with the hips and knees flexed to approximately 90 degrees and the arms by the sides (Figure 15-47). From this position, the patient is asked to perform a posterior pelvic tilt and lift the pelvis off the bed, while maintaining the hip and knee positions. Once the patient is able to do this exercise independently, the exercise can be performed with the hips flexed to 90 percent and the knees extended (Figure 15-48).

- *Rotational partial sit-up:* The patient is asked to lift the chin toward the chest. The patient is then asked to attempt to lift the right shoulder up from the table, while twisting the trunk to the left and touching the outside of the opposite knee (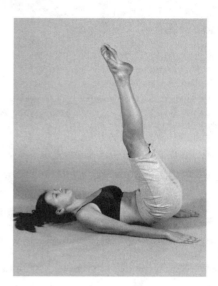Figure 15-49), before slowly lowering the shoulder to the table.

- *Reverse curl-up:* The patient is positioned supine, with the legs bent at the knees and the feet flat on the floor. The arms are by the sides. The patient is asked to raise the feet off the bed until the thighs are vertical (Figure 15-50).

This is the start position. From this position, the patient is asked to raise the pelvis up and toward the shoulders, keeping the knees bent tightly, until the knees are as close to the chest as possible (Figure 15-51). The patient is allowed to push down on the bed with the hands. After holding this position for 2–3 seconds, the patient returns to the start position.

- *Superman:* The patient is positioned prone, with the arms overhead and knees straight. The patient is asked to raise both arms and legs toward the ceiling while also raising the head from the table (Figure 15-52).
- *Prone plank:* This exercise (Figure 15-53) can be made more challenging by asking the patient

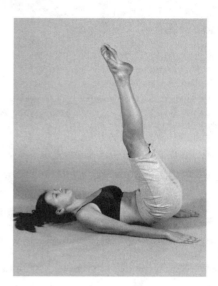

Figure 15-48　Hip thrusts.

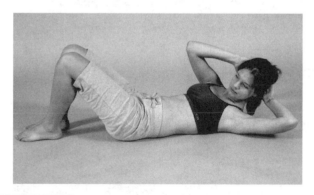

Figure 15-49　Rotational sit-up.

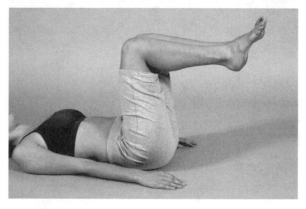

Figure 15-50　Reverse curl-up: start position.

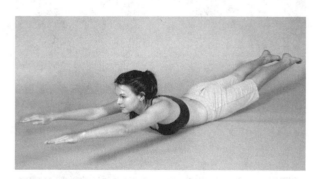

Figure 15-51　Reverse curl-up: end position.

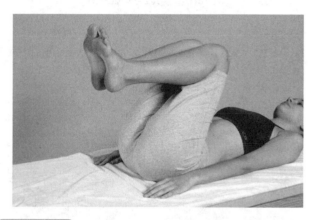

Figure 15-52　Superman.

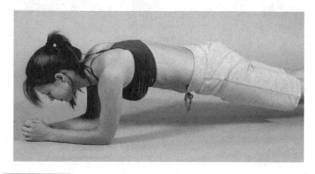

Figure 15-53　Prone plank.

to raise one upper extremity at a time, one lower extremity at a time, or opposite upper extremity and lower extremity simultaneously.

- *Prone lying on a Swiss ball, hands touching floor:* This can be progressed to push-ups with legs on a Swiss ball and to walking in circles around the Swiss ball using only the hands (Figure 15-54).

- *Rhythmic stabilization:* The patient is positioned in quadruped with unilateral hip extension. The clinician applies perturbations to the patient, while the patient attempts to resist using a variety of points of contact (Figure 15-55 and Figure 15-56) and positions (Figure 15-57). This exercise can be progressed by raising both an upper extremity and the contralateral lower extremity.

- *Proprioceptive neuromuscular facilitation (PNF):* A variety of PNF patterns can be applied with manual resistance to help strengthen the lumbar stabilizers. The upper extremity patterns (Figure 15-58 through Figure 15-61), lower extremity patterns (Figure 15-62) through

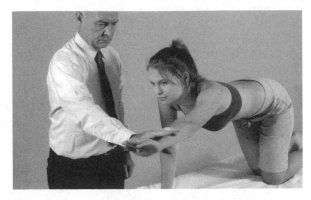

Figure 15-56   Rhythmic stabilization in quadruped with increased challenge to the patient.

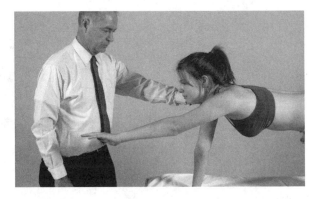

Figure 15-57   Rhythmic stabilization in quadruped while weight bearing through three extremities.

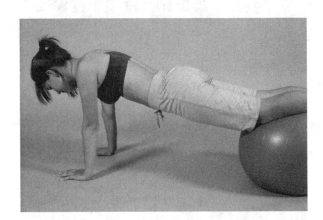

Figure 15-54   Prone lying on a Swiss ball, hands touching floor.

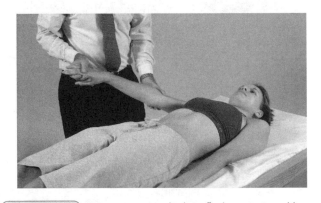

Figure 15-58   D1 upper extemity into flexion: start position.

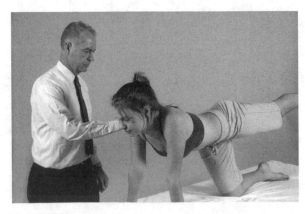

Figure 15-55   Rhythmic stabilization in quadruped.

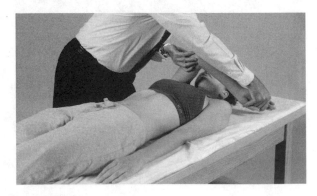

Figure 15-59   D1 upper extemity into flexion: end position.

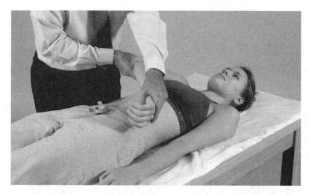

Figure 15-60   D1 upper extemity into extension: start position.

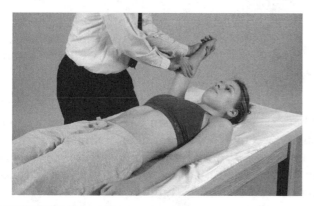

Figure 15-61   D1 upper extemity into extension: end position.

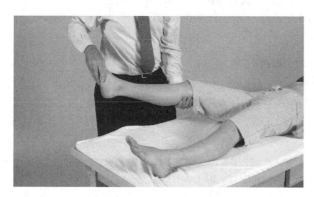

Figure 15-62   D1 lower extemity into flexion: start position.

Figure 15-65), and trunk patterns (Figure 15-66 and Figure 15-67) can all be used.

● **Key Point**   Several important principles must be applied to the exercise progressions. These include multiplanar and dynamic exercises, balance and proprioception drills (progression from a stable surface to a labile surface), power exercises (plyometrics), sport-specific skills as appropriate, and motor programming to integrate the lower and upper kinetic chains.[106]

In addition to addressing core stabilization, muscle imbalances must also be addressed in terms of

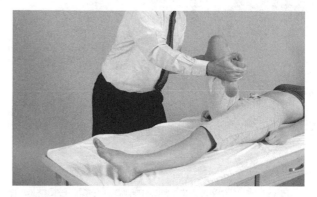

Figure 15-63   D1 lower extemity into flexion: end position.

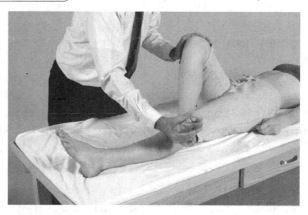

Figure 15-64   D1 lower extemity into extension: start position.

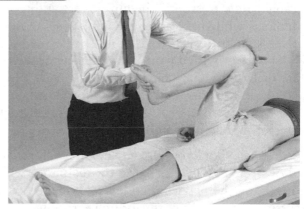

Figure 15-65   D1 lower extemity into extension: mid position.

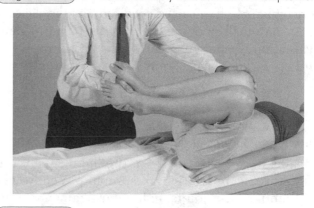

Figure 15-66   Lower trunk pattern moving into extension to the left: start position.

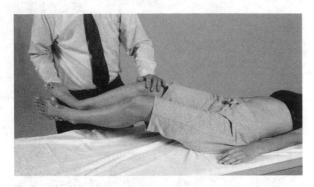

Figure 15-67   Lower trunk pattern moving into extension to the left: end position.

flexibility because poor flexibility may cause excessive stresses to be borne by the lumbar motion segments. For example, adaptively shortened hip flexors and rectus femoris muscles can cause increased anterior shearing of the lumbar spine. Occasionally, stretching both the anterior and the posterior thigh muscles is beneficial. However, most of the time, only one should be stretched, and the decision is based on the diagnosis:

- The patient with spinal stenosis or a painful extension hypomobility, and who responds well to lumbar flexion exercises, should be taught how to stretch the hip flexors and rectus femoris while protecting the lumbar spine from excessive lordosis.
- The patient with a painful flexion hypomobility or IVD herniation, and who responds well to lumbar extension exercises, should be taught how to stretch the hamstrings while protecting the lumbar spine from flexing.

Stretches should be applied and then taught. The goal of stretching is to perform the technique while maintaining the pelvis in its neutral zone, to avoid excessive anterior or posterior pelvic tilting.

The intervention program is only as good as the concomitant home exercise program, and the clinician must continually monitor the home exercise program, evaluating the patient's knowledge of the exercises and upgrading the program when appropriate.

Common Conditions

Strains and Sprains of the Lumbar Spine

Sprains may occur in any of the ligaments of the lumbar spine, but the most common sprain involves the lumbar facet joints. A lumbar ligament sprain typically occurs when bending forward and twisting while lifting and moving some object. The patient will report a sudden acute episode that caused the problem, or they will give a history of a chronic repetitive stress or sustained position that caused the gradual onset of a pain that got progressively worse with continuing activity. The pain is typically local to the structure that has been injured and is often described as a sore pain that gets sharp in response to certain movements or postures. Although similar in their presentation, muscular strains of the lumbar spine have three common characteristics:

- There is tenderness to palpation in the muscular area.
- The muscular pain is provoked with contraction.
- The muscular pain is provoked with stretching of the involved muscle.

Intervention

There is evidence suggesting that therapeutic exercise is effective in the treatment of nonspecific back pain,[112–115] although there is insufficient evidence to conclude with absolute certainty which theoretical mechanism of lumbar stabilization would be most beneficial in the management of patients with segmental lumbar instability.[116] The exercise progressions outlined in the "General Intervention Strategies" section earlier in this chapter can be used with these conditions.

Disk Herniation

Three main types of lumbar disk herniation are recognized.

Herniation

This is a general term used when there is any change in the shape of the annulus that causes it to bulge beyond its normal perimeter.

> ● **Key Point** The patient with a contained injury to the intervertebral disk is likely to report more pain in the morning. The nucleus pulposus (NP) is more swollen because it has imbibed more fluid during the night, and the compressive weight through the spine as the patient gets out of bed increases intradiskal pressure because of this added volume.

Recent attention has been given to the internal disruption of the NP in a herniation.[117] In this condition, the NP becomes inflamed and invaginates itself between the annular layers.

Compression of the disk during sitting and bending increases the pain, because the nociceptive structures within the AF are further irritated.[117]

Protrusion

With a protrusion, the nuclear material bulges outward through the tear to strain, but not escape from, the outer AF or the posterior longitudinal ligament (Figure 15-68). Once a tear to the periphery is opened for the NP, it would seem logical that further stresses can force it to migrate through the tear. However, under normal conditions, the nuclear material is intrinsically cohesive and does not herniate through the AF, even if the AF fibers are weakened by a radial incision.[118] The most common levels of protrusion are the segments between the fourth and fifth lumbar vertebrae and between the fifth lumbar vertebra and the sacrum, although a protrusion may occur at any level.

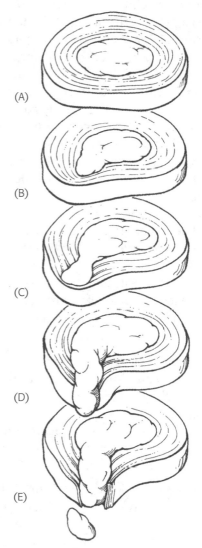

Figure 15-68 Disk herniations. (A) Normal. (B) Herniation. (C) Protrusion. (D) Prolape (extrusion). (E) Prolape (sequestration).

Reprinted from the *Journal of the American Academy of Orthopaedic Surgeons*, Volume 1 (1), pp. 33–40 with permission

> **● Key Point** Centralization of symptoms is the progressive retreat of the most distal extent of referred or radicular pain toward the lumbar spine midline. Peripheralization of symptoms indicates movement in the opposite direction. Centralization of the symptoms normally indicates improvement in the patient's condition.[119]

Prolapse

The migrating nuclear material escapes contact with the disk entirely and becomes a free fragment in the vertebral canal and epidural space (refer to Figure 15-68). Two types of disk prolapse exist:

- *Extrusion:* Extension of nuclear material beyond the confines of the posterior longitudinal ligament or above and below the disk space, as detected on MRI, but still in contact with the disk.[120]
- *Sequestration:* The extruded nucleus has separated from the disk and moved away from the prolapsed area.[120]

The clinical signs and symptoms vary depending on the degree and direction of the protrusion as well as the spinal level of the lesion:

- Posterior or posterolateral protrusions are the most common. With a small posterior or posterolateral lesion, there may be pressure against the posterior longitudinal ligament or against the dura mater or its extensions around the nerve roots. In such cases the patient may describe a severe midline back ache or pain spreading across the back into the buttock and thigh. A large posterior protrusion may cause spinal cord signs (cauda equina syndrome), which results in loss of bowel control, saddle anesthesia, and numbness in the legs. Cauda equina syndrome is considered a medical emergency so the supervising PT or physician must be notified immediately. A large posterolateral protrusion may cause partial cord or nerve root signs.
- An anterior protrusion may cause pressure against the anterior longitudinal ligament, resulting in back pain with no neurologic symptoms.

As part of its unnatural history, the disk may or may not travel through each stage of herniation sequentially. It is also worth remembering that symptoms from a disk lesion may shift if integrity of the annular wall remains because the hydrostatic mechanism is still intact.

The McKenzie examination approach used by the PT attempts to categorize the dysfunction into one of three syndromes: postural, dysfunction, or derangement.

- *Postural syndrome:* The symptoms of the postural syndrome tend to be related to posture and become evident in sustained positions.
- *Dysfunction syndrome:* The symptoms of the dysfunction syndrome tend to be related to movement and become evident in the difficulty or inability of the patient to accomplish end range of movement, most frequently in the extremes of flexion and extension.
- *Derangement syndrome:* McKenzie classifies derangement of the lumbar spine into seven categories on the basis of the location of symptoms and the presentation of fixed antalgias responsive to end-range loading in directions other than that within which complaints are caused.[120,121] Derangements that are considered to be *anterior* require strategies containing a flexion component, whereas those that are considered to be *posterior* involve strategies incorporating an extension component. In most cases, these may be conducted within the sagittal plane, but flexion and extension strategies may, in other cases, be combined with coronal or transverse motions for the best mechanical and symptomatic responses.[122] The theoretical model of the derangement syndrome involves the concept of displacement of the nucleus pulposus/annulus.

Intervention

The natural history of radiculopathy and disk herniation is not quite as favorable as for simple low back pain, but it is still excellent, with approximately 50 percent of patients recovering in the first 2 weeks and 70 percent recovering in 6 weeks.[123] Complete bed rest is not recommended.[124,125]

● **Key Point** Intervention focuses on a return to normal activities as soon as possible, patient education and involvement, and therapeutic exercises.

The McKenzie program can be valuable to the overall intervention strategy and, if centralization of pain occurs, a good response to physical therapy can be anticipated.[119,126] The physical examination component of the McKenzie method involves a comprehensive assessment of the patient, performed in the neutral, flexed, and extended positions of the spine, to gauge the responses, reactions, or effects of spinal loading, and for the presence of the centralization

phenomenon. The same maneuvers are repeated with the trunk in the neutral position, shifted toward the side of pathology, and away from pathology. The end-range exercises theoretically move the NP away from the side of compression loading, with flexion exercises moving the NP posteriorly and extension exercises moving the NP anteriorly.[120,127–132] The midrange exercises are better suited for patients with symptoms of neural compression.[133] The McKenzie approach uses physical signs, symptom behavior, and their relation to end-range lumbar test movements to determine appropriate classification and intervention.

Lateral Pelvic Shift

Patients with disk-related low back pain commonly present with a pelvic shift or list when acute sciatica is present. In these cases, the patient may list away from the side of the sciatica, producing a so-called sciatic scoliosis.[134] The lateral pelvic shift is perhaps the most commonly encountered. Determining the presence of a lateral shift deformity may help speed up the recovery from a derangement by first correcting the lateral shift deformity.[120] The direction of the list, although still controversial, is believed to result from the relative position of the disk herniation to the spinal nerve. Theoretically, when the disk herniation is lateral to the nerve root, the patient may deviate the back away from the side of the irritated nerve, which has the effect of drawing the nerve root away from the disk fragment. When the herniation is medial to the nerve root, the patient may list toward the side of the lesion, in an effort to decompress the nerve root.[135] It is also theorized that this is a protective position resulting from:

- Irritation of a zygapophyseal joint
- Irritation of a spinal nerve or its dural sleeve, caused by disk herniation[136] and the resulting muscle spasm[137]
- Spasm of the quadratus lumborum muscle and, occasionally, the iliacus muscle
- The size of the disk protrusion

To determine the relevance of the shift, a side-glide test sequence is used by the PT with the patient in standing, side lying, or prone. The side-glide test sequence is performed by manually correcting the shift by pushing the pelvis into its correct position (Figure 15-69).[120] If the side-glide produces either a centralization or peripheralization of the patient's symptoms, the test is considered positive for a relevant lateral shift.[138] In addition, for a lateral

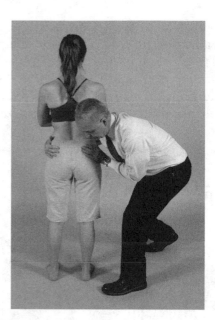

Figure 15-69 Side-glide test.

shift to be significant, the patient must exhibit an inability to self-correct past midline when asked to shift in the direction opposite the shift.[139] It is important to remember that any relevant lateral shift must be corrected, using side-glides, before the patient attempts the McKenzie extension exercises.[140] A lateral shift that is not deemed to be relevant or to be a deformity, per McKenzie's criteria, may be treated with only sagittal plane movements (e.g., extension principles).[120]

Once the centralizing position/motion is identified from examination, the patient is instructed to perform these maneuvers repetitively or sustain certain positions for specific periods throughout the day. Theoretically, the McKenzie program is designed to reduce the disk herniation by altering the position/shape of the nucleus pulposus/annulus using restricted end-range extension loading for a prolonged period of time and then to maintain the reduction and aid recovery of function. In cases of radiculopathy, the goal is to decrease radiating symptoms into the limb and, thus, to centralize the pain using specific maneuvers or positions, such as the lateral shift correction. The McKenzie positions and movements typically involve a series of active and passive movements performed in the beginning, middle, and end ranges of trunk flexion, extension, and combinations of side bending and rotation called *side gliding*.[120] The patient's response to the examination determines a classification and the direction of preference for therapeutic exercise,

with the direction chosen being based on the ability of a position or movement to centralize the patient's symptoms. As mentioned previously, the three major classifications or syndromes are *postural*, *dysfunction*, and *derangement*. Interventions are based on the type of syndrome diagnosed by the PT.

Postural Syndrome

The postural syndrome generally is not affected by mechanical maneuvers performed by the clinician or the patient, so the focus of the intervention is to isolate and subsequently instruct the patient to avoid the offending position(s). The "slouch/overcorrect" maneuver is taught to the patient. The patient should sit on the edge of the chair and allow the lumbar spine to slouch into a fully flexed position and allow the head and chin to protrude. He or she must then smoothly move into a fully erect sitting position, achieving a maximal lumbar lordosis, with the head held directly over the spine and with a retracted chin.[122] This postural motion should be repeatedly performed from the position of "poor" (slouch) posture to the overcorrect position.

Dysfunction Syndrome

The symptoms related to the dysfunction syndrome tend to be related to movement and become evident in the difficulty or inability of the patient to accomplish end range of movement, most frequently in the extremes of flexion and extension. The intervention goal for the dysfunction syndrome is the restoration of function or movement of the adaptively shortened tissue using frequent repetition of restricted end-range exercises. To achieve the lengthening of adaptively shortened soft tissues, the stretches need to be performed daily every 2–3 hours. This usually needs to be continued for a 4- to 6-week period or until the patient can fully stretch without any end-range pain. The following instructions must be given to the patient:[122]

- Stretch in the direction of movement loss and end-range pain.
- Allow elongation without microtrauma.
- Pain produced by stretching must stop shortly after release of stress. (Persisting pain afterward indicates overstretching.)
- Peripheralization of symptoms should never occur.
- Stretching must be strong enough to reproduce discomfort or some pain.
- The stretches must be performed regularly during the day (15 times every 2 hours).

Derangement Syndrome

The intervention goal for the derangement syndrome is to reduce the derangement by altering the position/shape of the nucleus pulposus/annulus using restricted end-range loading for a prolonged period of time and then to maintain the reduction and aid recovery of function.[122] Mechanical treatment is dependent on the mechanical diagnosis for derangements. The sequential extension progression advocated by McKenzie, following correction/self-correction (Figure 15-70) of any lateral deviation, is initiated once the patient is able to tolerate prone lying. The sequence involves prone on elbows (Figure 15-71), prone push-up (Figure 15-72), extension in standing (Figure 15-73), and prone strengthening of the lumbar extensors with arms bent (Figure 15-74) and arms straight (Figure 15-75). The goal of treatment is to prevent and treat any peripheralization of symptoms, with the focus on the centralization of symptoms, and the patient is educated to discontinue any activities/exercises that cause peripheralization.

In addition, the patient is instructed in a lumbar stabilization program, in which neutral zone

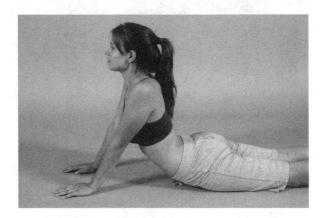

Figure 15-72   Prone push-up.

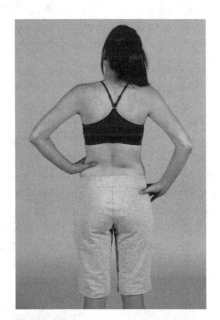

Figure 15-70   Self-correction for lateral shift.

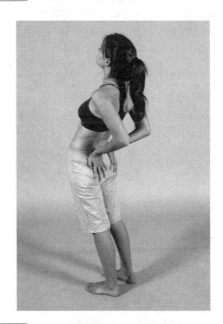

Figure 15-73   Extension in standing.

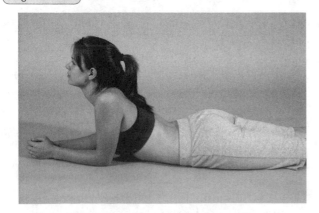

Figure 15-71   Prone on elbows.

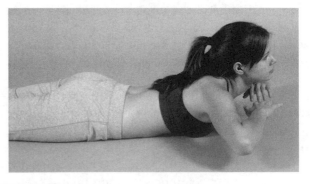

Figure 15-74   Prone strengthening: arms bent.

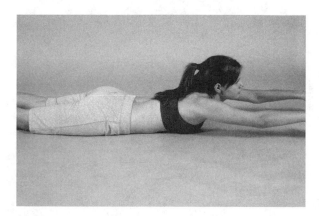

Figure 15-75   Prone strengthening: arms straight.

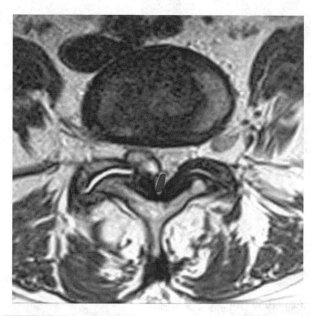

Figure 15-76   Central stenosis.

mechanics are practiced in various positions to decrease stress to the lumbosacral spine. Lumbar stabilizing exercises have been recommended to improve lumbar function in patients with low back injury so that these patients may improve their activities of daily living. It is theorized that these types of exercise may strengthen the stabilizer muscles, which control and limit the free movement of one vertebra on the other, thereby accelerating the recovery process of the herniated disk. The lumbar stabilization exercise progression is described in the "General Intervention Strategies" section earlier in this chapter.

Surgical Intervention

The indications for surgical treatment of symptomatic lumbar disk disease include the following:[141]

- A patient with cauda equina syndrome
- A patient demonstrating progressive neurologic deficit (increased peripheralization of symptoms, increased weakness) during a period of observation
- A patient with persistent sciatic pain, despite conservative management, for a period of 6–12 weeks

There are three common surgical options:

- *Discectomy (also called open discectomy):* The surgical removal of herniated disk material that is impinging a nerve root or the spinal cord. Before the disk material is removed, the lamina from the affected vertebra may be removed (laminotomy or laminectomy)
- *Microdiskectomy:* Requires only a very small incision to remove only that portion of the disk that is impinging on the spinal nerve root. The

recovery time for this particular surgery is usually much less than is required for traditional lumbar surgery. Numerous variations exist.
- *Perculaneous diskectomy:* An instrument is introduced through a needle and placed into the center of the disk where a series of channels are created to remove tissue from the nucleus. Tissue removal from the nucleus acts to decompress the disk and relieve the pressure exerted by the disk on the nearby nerve root.

Degenerative Spinal Stenosis

Degenerative spinal stenosis (DSS) is defined as narrowing of the spinal canal (central stenosis), nerve root canal, or foramen (lateral stenosis).

Central stenosis is characterized by a narrowing of the spinal canal around the thecal sac containing the cauda equina (Figure 15-76). The causes for this type of stenosis include facet joint arthrosis and hypertrophy, thickening and bulging of the ligament enslaving them, bulging of the IVD, and spondylolisthesis.

Lateral stenosis is characterized by encroachment of the spinal nerve in the lateral recess of the spinal canal or in the intervertebral foramen (Figure 15-77). Initially the depth of the canal that constituted narrowing was identified as an anteroposterior measurement,[142] but more recently the lateral width of the spinal canal has been studied.[143] The causes for this type of stenosis include facet joint hypertrophy, loss of IVD height, IVD bulging,

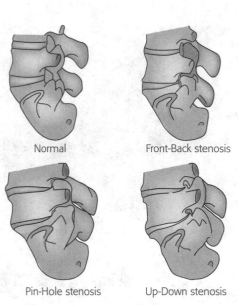

Normal   Front-Back stenosis

Pin-Hole stenosis   Up-Down stenosis

Figure 15-77 Lateral stenosis.

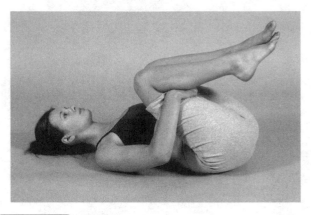

Figure 15-78 Trunk flexion.

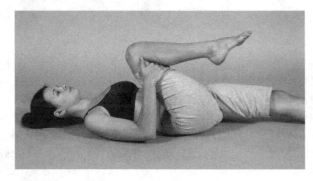

Figure 15-79 Single knee to chest.

and spondylolisthesis. This type is more commonly encountered by the orthopedic PTA.

A compression of the nerve within the canal may result in a limitation of the arterial supply or claudication resulting from the compression of the venous return. Neurogenic claudication, also referred to as pseudoclaudication, may result in nerve root ischemia and symptomatic claudication. Neurogenic claudication is manifested as poorly localized pain, paresthesias, or cramping of one or both lower extremities, which is brought on by walking and relieved by sitting.[144] Compressive loading of the spine can also exacerbate symptoms, such as those that occur with walking. Central stenosis can result in symptoms related to cauda equina compression. Most of the compression occurs when the canal is at its narrowest diameter, with relief occurring when the diameter increases.

> **● Key Point** The compression of the foraminal contents in the canal may occur more often with certain movements or changes in posture:[145]
> • The length of the canal is shorter in lumbar lordosis than kyphosis.
> • Extension and, to a lesser degree, side bending of the lumbar spine toward the involved side produces a narrowing of the canal.
> • Flexion of the lumbar spine reverses the process, returning both the venous capacity and the blood flow to the nerve.

Intervention
Conservative
The therapeutic exercise progression is based on the underlying impairments, and should include:

- Postural education with an emphasis on teaching the patient to maintain a posterior pelvic tilt when standing.

- Hip flexor, rectus femoris, and lumbar paraspinal stretching. There is some controversy as to whether the hamstrings should be stretched because lengthening of these muscles may allow the pelvis to rotate anteriorly, resulting in an increased lordosis and further stenosis.
- Lumbar (core) stabilization exercises targeting the abdominals and gluteals.
- Aerobic conditioning.
- Modified Williams flexion exercises. The goal of some of these exercises is to temporarily widen the intervertebral foramina and gap the zygapophyseal (facet) joints, thereby reducing nerve root compression. There are also strengthening exercises for the abdominal muscles (in order to lift the pelvis from the front) and strengthening exercises for the gluteal muscles (to pull the back of the pelvis down) with the long-term aim of producing a natural posterior tilt/flattening of the lordosis. These exercises are:
  - Trunk flexion or crunch (Figure 15-78)
  - Posterior pelvic tilt (refer to Figure 15-15)
  - Trunk flexion or bilateral/single knee to chest (Figure 15-79)
  - Iliotibial band stretch (see Chapter 19)
  - Stand to squat or stand to sit (Figure 15-80)

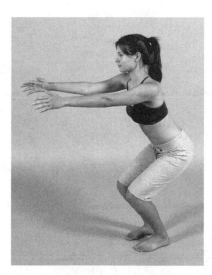

Figure 15-80 Stand to squat.

Medical

Permanent relief in lateral recess stenosis has been reported with an injection of local anesthetic around the nerve root.[146] When injections fail, surgical decompression of the nerve root is often indicated.

Zygapophyseal Joint Dysfunction

Facet joint syndrome (FJS) is a term used to describe a pain-provoking dysfunction of the zygapophyseal joint.[147] This pain is the result of a lesion to the joint and its pain-sensitive structures. The etiology of FJS may be trauma, degenerative, or systemic. The clinical characteristics of FJS include:

- *Pain:* In the acute stage, there is pain and muscle guarding with all motions. In the later stages of healing the pain is related to periods of immobility or excessive activity.
- *Impaired mobility:* This can manifest as either a hypomobility or a hypermobility/instability. Spinal extension is the motion most commonly affected, especially when combined with side bending or rotation.

● Key Point Spondylosis refers to degenerative osteoarthritis of the joints between the center of the spinal vertebrae and/or neural foraminae. If severe, it may cause pressure on nerve roots with subsequent sensory and/or motor disturbances, such as pain, paresthesia, or muscle weakness in the limbs.

Intervention

The conservative intervention for a zygapophyseal dysfunction can include specific joint mobilizations performed by the PT, postural education, and the exercise progression outlined in the "General Intervention Strategies" section.

Spondylolysis

Spondylolysis is a defect of the pars interarticularis of the spine, which lies between the superior and inferior articular facets of the vertebral arch. The actual defect in the pars covers a broad range of etiologies, from stress fracture to a traumatic bony fracture with separation.[148] Patients with bilateral pars defects can progress to spondylolisthesis (see next section). The exact cause of spondylolysis is unclear, but it is likely related to congenital, acquired (repeated microtrauma), or developmental causes. Spondylolysis commonly is asymptomatic, making diagnosis extremely difficult. Those patients with symptoms often have pain with extension and/or rotation of the lumbar spine.

Intervention

Initial therapeutic management of a patient with spondylolysis is conservative. Based on a number of studies,[149–151] the physical therapy intervention should strive to correct any muscle imbalances (adaptively shortened hip flexors), increase trunk muscle strength, and educate the patient to avoid activities involving excessive impact or lumbar hyperextension. Bracing may also be advocated. Surgical intervention is indicated only after patients have failed conservative management.

Spondylolisthesis

Spondylolisthesis, a diagnostic term that identifies anterior slippage and inability to resist shear forces of a vertebral segment in relation to the vertebral segment immediately below it, usually occurs in the lumbar spine, with the most common site being L5–S1.[124] Under normal conditions, any anterior slippage of the vertebra is resisted by the bony block of the posterior facets, by an intact neural arch and pedicle, and, in the case of the L5 vertebra, by the iliolumbar ligament.

● Key Point Frequently, spondylolisthesis leads to spinal instability—the inability of the spine to maintain its normal pattern of displacement when placed under physiological load.[152]

The period of most rapid slipping is between the ages of 10 and 15 years, with no more slipping occurring after the age of 20.[151,153–166] Newman[162] described five groups represented by this deformity, based on etiology:

1. *Congenital spondylolisthesis:* This condition results from dysplasia of the fifth lumbar and sacral arches and zygapophyseal joints (Figure 15-81).

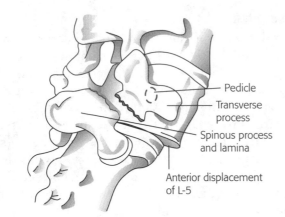

Figure 15-81   Congenital spondylolisthesis.

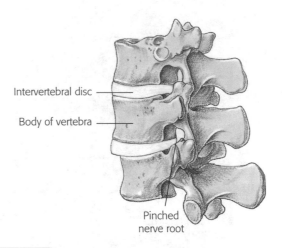

Figure 15-83   Degenerative spondylolisthesis.

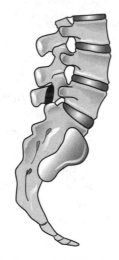

Figure 15-82   Isthmic spondylolisthesis.

2. *Isthmic spondylolisthesis:* This condition is caused by a defect in the pars interarticularis, which can be an acute fracture, a stress fracture, or an elongation of the pars (Figure 15-82). In more advanced slips, there is a palpable soft tissue depression immediately above the L5 spinous process on passing the fingers down the lumbar spine, and a segmental lordosis. If an asymptomatic slip reaches 50 percent, vigorous contact sports and other activities carrying a high risk of back injury should be avoided.

3. *Degenerative spondylolisthesis:* This condition usually affects older people and occurs most commonly at L4–L5 (Figure 15-83). The proposed reasons for this type include dysfunction of the IVD, horizontalization of the lamina and the facets or sacrum morphology,[167] the lumbosacral angle, ligamentous laxity, previous pregnancy, and hormonal factors.[159]

4. *Traumatic spondylolisthesis:* This condition occurs with a fracture or acute dislocation of the zygapophyseal joint. It is fairly rare.

5. *Pathologic spondylolisthesis:* This condition may result from a systemic disease causing a weakening of the pars, pedicle, or zygapophyseal joint, or from a local condition such as a tumor.

Of these categories, degenerative spondylolisthesis is perhaps the most commonly encountered by the PTA. Repetitive motions that cause fatigue may advance to an acute, spontaneous pars interarticularis weakening, stress fracture, or fracture and a predilection for spondylolisthesis.[168]

Clinically, these patients complain of chronic midline pain at the lumbosacral junction, which is mechanical in nature. Mechanical pain is worsened with activity and alleviated with rest. The symptoms can be exacerbated by repetitive extension and torsion activities.[169] Patients may also complain of leg pain, which can have a radicular-type pattern or, more commonly, will manifest as neurogenic claudication.

Intervention

The intervention for spondylolisthesis depends on the severity of the slip and the symptoms, and ranges from conservative to surgical. The symptoms, if they do occur, usually begin in the second decade; however, there is often no correlation with the degree of slip and the level of symptoms.

● **Key Point**   A common clinical manifestation of spondylolisthesis is increased lumbar and hamstring muscular tone, which may be associated with a compensatory response secondary to ineffective stabilization of the painful spinal segment.[169]

Conservative

Conservative intervention is more likely to be successful in the case of a limited slip and sparse clinical findings. Such an approach includes pelvic positioning (usually posteriorly) initially to provide symptomatic relief, followed by an active lumbar stabilization program while avoiding extension past neutral, and stretching of the rectus femoris and iliopsoas muscles to decrease the degree of anterior pelvic tilting.

Surgical

The goals of surgery are to remove pressure on spinal nerves (i.e., decompression) and to provide stability to the lumbar spine. In most cases of spondylolisthesis, the lumbar decompression procedure is performed in conjunction with a spinal fusion. Many patients will require a ready-made or custom-molded brace postoperatively to be worn for 3–6 months.

Rectus Abdominis Strain

Rectus abdominis strains usually occur when the muscle is strongly contracting, as it is being moved into a stretched and lengthened position. These strains are common in such sports as tennis, wrestling, pole vaulting, weight lifting, and soccer, or in activities that involve heavy lifting. Abdominal strains are primarily the result of inadequate abdominal strength and/or incorrect technique.[170] It may be difficult to differentiate this condition from an inflammation of one of the internal abdominal organs, so a physician should be consulted whenever there is any doubt.[171]

Intervention

These are difficult injuries to heal. Although mild strains may take only 2–3 weeks to heal, premature return to play can create large muscle ruptures, leading to hernia formation in the abdominal wall.[170] Conservative intervention involves rest, ice, and compression during the acute phase, progressing to heat and gentle stretching, a graded resistive exercise program, and specific instructions on proper warm-up and cool-down. Training and retraining of the rectus abdominis should include half sit-ups, done slowly with the knees bent, to eliminate compensation by the iliopsoas.[170,171]

Summary

The lumbar region is specialized for two important and interrelated functions. First, the lumbosacral junction and sacroiliac joints must transfer large forces from body weight and activated muscle through the pelvis to the lower extremities.[172] Second, the lumbar spine must interact mechanically with the pelvis and hip joints to maximize the movements of the trunk. A limitation in either region can increase the range of motion demands on the other, which may exceed the physical tolerance of

a structure and result in injury.[172] Pain with limited mobility anywhere within the lumbar region can originate from many sources including torn ligaments, muscle tears, herniated disks, nerve root compression, joint inflammation, or a combination of these.

REVIEW Questions

1. What is the central fluid-filled portion of the intervertebral disk called?
2. The lumbar spine has the most motion in which plane of motion?
3. Which motion of the lumbar spine results in a posterior migration of the nucleus pulposus of an intervertebral disk?
4. True or false: An anterior pelvic tilt decreases the lumbar lordosis.
5. What is the term used to describe anterior slippage, or translation, of one vertebra relative to another?
6. True or false: A posterior pelvic tilt requires activation of the abdominal muscles.
7. True or false: A patient with lateral spinal stenosis is typically prescribed McKenzie extension exercises.
8. Which activity can produce disk pressure that is equal to 2750 percent of body weight?
9. True or false: When lifting a heavy object, the hip and knee extensor muscles must be fully utilized.
10. True or false: The term *sacral nutation* is used to describe sacral flexion.
11. When teaching a group of workers with no history of back injury to lift heavy objects off the floor, the PTA should instruct them to:
    a. Stoop down to the object before trying to lift it.
    b. Keep the lumbar spine flexed during the lift.
    c. Increase the lordotic posture to increase stability when lifting.
    d. Keep objects as far away from the center of gravity as possible.

References

1. Woolf A, Pfleger B: Burden of major musculoskeletal conditions. Bull World Health Organ 81:646–656, 2003
2. Nachemson A: Chronic pain—the end of the welfare state? Qual Life Res Suppl 1:S11–S17, 1994

3. Wipf JE, Deyo RA: Low back pain. Med Clin North Am 79:231–246, 1995
4. Viikari-Juntura E, Jouri J, Silverstein BA, et al: A lifelong prospective study on the role of psychosocial factors in neck, shoulder and low back pain. Spine 16:1056–1061, 1991
5. Bigos SJ, Battié M, Spengler DM, et al: A prospective study of work perceptions and psychosocial factors affecting the report of back injury. Spine 16:1–6, 1991
6. Dehlin O, Berg S: Back symptoms and psychological perception of work. Scand J Rehab Med 9:61–65, 1977
7. Leino PI, Hänninen V: Psychosocial factors in relation to back and limb disorders. Scand J Work Environ Health 21:134–142, 1995
8. Michel A, Kohlmann T, Raspe H: The association between clinical findings on physical examination and self-reported severity in back pain: Results of a population-based study. Spine 22:296–304, 1997
9. Waddell G, Somerville D, Henderson I, et al: Objective clinical evaluation of physical impairment in chronic low back pain. Spine 17:617–628, 1992
10. Burdorf A, Sorock G: Positive and negative evidence of risk factors for back disorders. Scand J Work Environ Health 23:243–256, 1997
11. Riihimaki H: Low-back pain, its origin and risk indicators. Scand J Work Environ Health 17:81–90, 1991
12. Hoogendoorn WE, Poppel MN, Bongers PM, et al: Physical load during work and leisure time as risk factors for back pain. Scand J Work Environ Health 25:387–403, 1999
13. Hemingway H, Shipley MJ, Stansfeld S, et al: Sickness absence from back pain, psychosocial work characteristics and employment grade among office workers. Scand J Work Environ Health 23:121–129, 1997
14. Riihimaki H: Epidemiology and pathogenesis of non-specific low back pain: What does the epidemiology tell us? Bull Hosp Jt Dis 55:197–198, 1996
15. Smedley J, Egger P, Cooper C, et al: Prospective cohort study of predictors of incident low back pain in nurses. BMJ 314:1225–1228, 1997
16. Kraus JF, Gardner LI, Collins J, et al: Design factors in epidemiologic cohort studies of work-related low back injury or pain. Am J Ind Med 32:153–163, 1997
17. Macfarlane GJ, Thomas E, Papageorgiou AC, et al: Employment and physical work activities as predictors of future low back pain. Spine 22:1143–1149, 1997
18. Tichauer ER: The Biomedical Basis of Ergonomics: Anatomy Applied to the Design of the Work Situation. New York, Wiley Inter-Sciences, 1978
19. Magora A: Investigation of the relation between low back pain and occupation: 4. Physical requirements: Bending, rotation, reaching and sudden maximal effort. Scand J Rehabil Med 5:186–190, 1973
20. Magora A: Investigation of the relation between low back pain and occupation: 3. Physical requirements: Sitting, standing and weight lifting. Ind Med Surg 41:5–9, 1972
21. Kelsey JL: An epidemiological study of the relationship between occupations and acute herniated lumbar intervertebral discs. Int J Epidemiol 4:197–205, 1975
22. Kelsey JL, Hardy RJ: Driving of motor vehicles as a risk factor for acute herniated lumbar intervertebral disc. Am J Epidemiol 102:63–73, 1975
23. Backman AL: Health survey of professional drivers. Scand J Work Environ Health 9:30–35, 1983
24. Bongers PM, Boshuizen HC, Hulshof CTJ, et al: Back disorders in crane operators exposed to whole-body vibration. Int Arch Occup Environ Health 60:129–137, 1988
25. Bongers PM, Hulshof CTJ, Dijkstra L, et al: Back pain and exposure to whole body vibration in helicopter pilots. Ergonomics 33:1007–1026, 1990
26. Pietri F, Leclerc A, Boitel L, et al: Low-back pain in commercial drivers. Scand J Work Environ Health 18:52–58, 1992
27. Leboeuf-Yde C, Kyvik KO, Bruun NH: Low back pain and life style: Part I. Smoking information from a population-based sample of 29424 twins. Spine 23:2207–2214, 1998
28. Holmstrom EB, Lindell J, Moritz U: Low back and neck/shoulder pain in construction workers: Occupational workload and psychosocial risk factors. Part 1: Relationship to low back pain. Spine 17:663–671, 1992
29. Miranda H, Viikari-Juntura E, Martikainen R, et al: Individual factors, occupational loading, and physical exercise as predictors of sciatic pain. Spine 27:1102–1109, 2002
30. Kelsey JL: An epidemiological study of acute herniated lumbar intervertebral discs. Rheumatol Rehabil 14:144–159, 1975
31. Heliövaara M: Body height, obesity, and risk of herniated lumbar intervertebral disc. Spine 12:469–472, 1987
32. Aro S, Leino P: Overweight and musculoskeletal morbidity: A ten-year follow-up. Int J Obesity 9:267–275, 1985
33. Böstman OM: Body mass index and height in patients requiring surgery for lumbar intervertebral disc herniation. Spine 18:851–854, 1993
34. Deyo RA, Bass JE: Lifestyle and low-back pain. The influence of smoking and obesity. Spine 14:501–506, 1989
35. Nordin M, Hiebert R, Pietrek M, et al: Association of comorbidity and outcome in episodes of nonspecific low back pain in occupational populations. J Occup Env Med 44:677–684, 2002
36. Bodack MP, Monteiro M: Therapeutic exercise in the treatment of patients with lumbar spinal stenosis. Clin Orthop Relat Res 384:144–152, 2001
37. Caspersen CJ, Powell KE, Christenson GM: Physical activity, exercise and physical fitness. Public Health Rep 100:125–131, 1985
38. Danielsen J, Johnsen R, Kibsgaard S, et al: Early aggressive exercise for postoperative rehabilitation after discectomy. Spine 25:1015–1020, 2000
39. Janeck K, Reuven B, Romano CT: Spinal stabilization exercises for the injured worker. Occup Med 13:199–207, 1998
40. Kendall PH, Jenkins JM: Exercises for back ache: A double blind controlled study. Physiotherapy 54:154–157, 1968
41. O'Sullivan PB: Lumbar segmental 'instability': Clinical presentation and specific stabilizing exercise management. Man Ther 5:2–12, 2000
42. Kahanovitz N, Nordin M, Verderame R, et al: Normal trunk muscle strength and endurance in women and the effect of exercises and electrical stimulation: Part 2. Comparative analysis of electrical stimulation and exercise to increase trunk muscle strength and endurance. Spine 12:112–118, 1987
43. Nachemson A: Work for all. For those with low back pain as well. Clin Orthop 179:77, 1982

44. Hall C: Therapeutic exercise for the lumbopelvic region, in Hall C, Thein-Brody L (eds): Therapeutic Exercise: Moving Toward Function. Baltimore, MD, Lippincott Williams & Wilkins, 2005, pp 349–401

45. Ghosh P, Bushell GR, Taylor TKF, et al: Collagens, elastin and noncollagenous protein of the intervertebral disc. Clin Orthop 129:124–132, 1977

46. Taylor JR: The development and adult structure of lumbar intervertebral discs. J Man Med 5:43–47, 1990

47. Bogduk N, Twomey LT: Anatomy and biomechanics of the lumbar spine, in Bogduk N, Twomey LT (eds): Clinical Anatomy of the Lumbar Spine and Sacrum (ed 3). Edinburgh, Churchill Livingstone, 1997, pp 2–53, 81–152, 171–176

48. Tsuji H, Hirano N, Ohshima H, et al: Structural variation of the anterior and posterior anulus fibrosus in the development of the human lumbar intervertebral disc: A risk factor for intervertebral disc rupture. Spine 18:204–210, 1993

49. White AA, Punjabi MM: Clinical Biomechanics of the Spine (ed 2). Philadelphia, JB Lippincott, 1990

50. Holdsworth F: Fractures, dislocations, and fracture-dislocations of the spine. J Bone Joint Surg 52A:1534–1551, 1970

51. Nachemson A: Lumbar intradiscal pressure, in Jayson MIV (ed): The Lumbar Spine and Back Pain. Edinburgh, Churchill Livingstone, 1987, pp 191–203

52. Sato K, Kikuchi S, Yonezawa T: In vivo intradiscal pressure measurement in healthy individuals and in patients with ongoing back problems. Spine (Phila Pa 1976) 24:2468–2474, 1999

53. Vleeming A, Stoeckart R, Snijders CJ: The sacrotuberous ligament: A conceptual approach to its dynamic role in stabilizing the sacroiliac joint. Clin Biomech 4:201–203, 1989

54. Vleeming A, Pool-Goudzwaard AL, Stoeckart R, et al: The posterior layer of the thoracolumbar fascia: Its function in load transfer from spine to legs. Spine 20:753–758, 1995

55. Hodges PW, Richardson CA: Altered trunk muscle recruitment in people with low back pain: A motor control evaluation of transversus abdominis. Arch Phys Med Rehab 80:1005–1012, 1999

56. O'Sullivan PB, Twomey L, Allison GT: Altered abdominal muscle recruitment in patients with chronic back pain following a specific exercise intervention. J Orthop Sports Phys Ther 27:114–124, 1998

57. O'Sullivan PB, Dankaerts W, Burnett AF, et al: Effect of different upright sitting postures on spinal-pelvic curvature and trunk muscle activation in a pain-free population. Spine 31:E707–E712, 2006

58. O'Sullivan P, Twomey L, Allison G, et al: Altered patterns of abdominal muscle activation in patients with chronic low back pain. Aust J Physiother 43:91–98, 1997

59. O'Sullivan PB: 'Clinical instability' of the lumbar spine: Its pathological basis, diagnosis and conservative management, in Boyling JD, Jull GA (eds): Grieve's Modern Manual Therapy: The Vertebral Column. Philadelphia, Churchill Livingstone, 2004, pp 311–331

60. Stanford ME: Effectiveness of specific lumbar stabilization exercises: A single case study. J Man Manip Ther 10:40–46, 2002

61. Cholewicki J, McGill S: Mechanical stability of the in vivo lumbar spine: Implications for injury and chronic low back pain. Clin Biomech 11:1–15, 1996

62. McGill SM, Cholewicki J: Biomechanical basis for stability: An explanation to enhance clinical utility. J Orthop Sports Phys Ther 31:96–100, 2001

63. Bierdermann HJ, Shanks GL, Forrest WJ, et al: Power spectrum analysis of electromyographic activity. Spine 16:1179–1184, 1991

64. Lindgren K, Sihvonen T, Leino E, et al: Exercise therapy effects on functional radiographic findings and segmental electromyographic activity in lumbar spine stability. Arch Phys Med Rehabil 74:933–939, 1993

65. Hodges P, Richardson C, Jull G: Evaluation of the relationship between laboratory and clinical tests of transversus abdominis function. Physiother Res Int 1:30–40, 1996

66. Hodges P, Richardson C: Inefficient muscular stabilisation of the lumbar spine associated with low back pain: A motor control evaluation of transversus abdominis. Spine 21:2540–2650, 1996

67. Richardson C, Jull G: Muscle control—pain control. What exercises would you prescribe? Man Ther 1:2–10, 1995

68. Hides JA, Richardson CA, Jull GA: Multifidus muscle recovery is not automatic after resolution of acute, first-episode low back pain. Spine 21:2763–2769, 1996

69. O'Sullivan P, Twomey L, Allison G: Altered patterns of abdominal muscle activation in chronic back pain patients. Aust J Physiother 43:91–98, 1997

70. Edgerton V, Wolf S, Levendowski D, et al: Theoretical basis for patterning EMG amplitudes to assess muscle dysfunction. Med Sci Sports Exerc 28:744–751, 1996

71. Basmajian JV, Deluca CJ: Muscles Alive: Their Functions Revealed by Electromyography. Baltimore, Williams & Wilkins, 1985

72. Vleeming A, Mooney V, Dorman T, et al: Movement, Stability and Low Back Pain. Edinburgh, Churchill Livingstone, 1997

73. Snijders CJ, Vleeming A, Stoeckart R, et al: Biomechanics of the interface between spine and pelvis in different postures, in Vleeming A, Mooney V, Dorman T, et al (eds): Movement, Stability and Low Back Pain. Edinburgh, Churchill Livingstone, 1997, pp 103–113

74. Lee DG: The Pelvic Girdle: An Approach to the Examination and Treatment of the Lumbo-Pelvic-Hip Region (ed 2). Edinburgh, Churchill Livingstone, 1999

75. Richardson CA, Jull GA, Hodges P, et al: Therapeutic Exercise for Spinal Segmental Stabilization in Low Back Pain. London, Churchill Livingstone, 1999

76. Vleeming A: The function of the long dorsal sacroiliac ligament: Its implication for understanding low back pain. Spine 21:556, 1996

77. Meadows JTS: Manual Therapy: Biomechanical Assessment and Treatment, Advanced Technique. Calgary, Swodeam Consulting, 1995

78. Deusinger R: Validity of pelvic tilt measurements in anatomical neutral position. J Biomech 25:764, 1992

79. Jackson-Manfield P, Neumann DA: Structure and function of the hip, in Jackson-Manfield P, Neumann DA (eds): Essentials of Kinesiology for the Physical Therapist Assistant. St. Louis, MO, Mosby Elsevier, 2009, pp 227–271

80. Snijders CJ, Vleeming A, Stoeckart R: Transfer of lumbosacral load to iliac bones and legs. Part 1: Biomechanics of self bracing of the sacroiliac joints and its significance for treatment and exercise. Clin Biomech 8:285–294, 1993

81. Snijders CJ, Vleeming A, Stoeckart R, et al: Biomechanical modelling of sacroiliac joint stability in different postures. Spine State Art Rev 9:419–432, 1995

82. Solonen KA: The sacroiliac joint in the light of anatomical roentgenographical and clinical studies. Acta Orthop Scand 26:9, 1957

83. Bowen V, Cassidy JD: Macroscopic and microscopic anatomy of the sacroiliac joint from embryonic life until the eighth decade. Spine 6:620, 1980

84. Vleeming A, Snijders CJ, Stoeckart R, et al: The role of the sacroiliac joints in coupling between spine, pelvis, legs and arms, in Vleeming A, Mooney V, Dorman T, et al (eds): Movement, Stability and Low Back Pain. Edinburgh, Churchill Livingstone, 1997, pp 53–71

85. Franke BA: Formative dynamics: The pelvic girdle. J Man Manip Ther 11:12–40, 2003

86. Hemborg B, Moritz U, Lowing H: Intra-abdominal pressure and trunk muscle activity during lifting. IV. The causal factors of the intra-abdominal pressure rise. Scand J Rehab Med 17:25–38, 1985

87. Snijders CJ, Slagter AHE, van Strik R, et al: Why leg-crossing? The influence of common postures on abdominal muscle activity. Spine 20:1989–1993, 1995

88. Lee DG: Instability of the sacroiliac joint and the consequences for gait, in Vleeming A, Mooney V, Dorman T, et al (eds): Movement, Stability and Low Back Pain. Edinburgh, Churchill Livingstone, 1997, pp 231–233

89. Fortin JD, Dwyer AP, West S, et al: Sacroiliac joint pain referral maps upon applying a new injection/arthrography technique. Part I: Asymptomatic volunteers. Spine 19:1475–1482, 1994

90. Kellgren JH: Observations on referred pain arising from muscle. Clin Sci 3:175–190, 1938

91. Kellgren JH: On the distribution of pain arising from deep somatic structures with charts of segmental pain areas. Clin Sci 4:35–46, 1939

92. McCall IW, Park WM, O'Brien JP: Induced pain referral from posterior lumbar elements in normal subjects. Spine 4:441–446, 1979

93. Hall H: A simple approach to back pain management. Patient Care 15:77–91, 1992

94. LaBan MM, Meerschaert JR, Taylor RS, et al: Symphyseal and sacroiliac joint pain associated with pubic symphysis instability. Arch Phys Med Rehabil 59:470–472, 1978

95. Alderink GJ: The sacroiliac joint: Review of anatomy, mechanics, and function. J Orthop Sports Phys Ther 13:71–84, 1991

96. DonTigny RL: Function and pathomechanics of the sacroiliac joint. A review. Phys Ther 65:35–44, 1985

97. Dreyfuss P, Michaelson M, Pauza K, et al: The value of medical history and physical examination in diagnosing sacroiliac joint pain. Spine 21:2594–2602, 1996

98. Schwarzer AC, Aprill CN, Bogduk N: The sacroiliac joint in chronic low back pain. Spine 20:31–37, 1995

99. van Tulder MW, Koes BW, Bouter LM: Conservative treatment of acute and chronic nonspecific low back pain: A systematic review of randomized controlled trials of the most common interventions. Spine 22:2128–2156, 1997

100. Burton AK, Waddell G: Clinical guidelines in the management of low back pain. Baillere's Clin Rheum 12:17–35, 1998

101. Abenhaim L, Rossignol M, Valat J-P, et al: The role of activity in the therapeutic management of back pain. Report of the International Paris Task Force on back pain. Spine 25:1S–33S, 2000 (Suppl 4S)

102. Rozenberg S, Delval C, Rezvani Y, et al: Bed rest or normal activity for patients with acute low back pain: A randomized controlled trial. Spine 27:1487–1493, 2002

103. Manniche C, Hesselsoe G, Bentzen L, et al: Clinical trial of intensive muscle training for chronic low back pain. Lancet 2:1473–1476, 1988

104. Frost H, Lamb SE, Klaber Moffett JA, et al: A fitness programme for patients with chronic low back pain: 2-year follow-up of a randomised controlled trial. Pain 75:273–279, 1998

105. Lahad A, Malter AD, Berg AO, et al: The effectiveness of four interventions for the prevention of low back pain. JAMA 272:1286–1291, 1994

106. Brukner P, Khan K: Core stability, in Brukner P, Khan K (eds): Clinical Sports Medicine (ed 3). Sydney, McGraw-Hill, 2007, pp 158–173

107. Hodges PW, Richardson CA: Delayed postural contraction of transversus abdominis in low back pain associated with movement of the lower limb. J Spinal Disord 11:46–56, 1998

108. Strohl K, Mead J, Banzett R, et al: Regional differences in abdominal muscle activity during various manoeuvres in humans. J Appl Physiol 51:1471–1476, 1981

109. Hagins M, Adler K, Cash M, et al: Effects of practice on the ability to perform lumbar stabilization exercises. J Orthop Sports Phys Ther 29:546–555, 1999

110. Kisner C, Colby LA: The spine: Exercise interventions, in Kisner C, Colby LA (eds): Therapeutic Exercise. Foundations and Techniques (ed 5). Philadelphia, FA Davis, 2002, pp 439–480

111. Lehman GJ, McGill SM: Quantification of the differences in electromyographic activity magnitude between the upper and lower portions of the rectus abdominis muscle during selected trunk exercises. Phys Ther 81:1096–1101, 2001

112. Hides JA, Jull GA, Richardson CA: Long-term effects of specific stabilizing exercises for first-episode low back pain. Spine 26:E243–E248, 2001

113. van der Velde G, Mierau D: The effect of exercise on percentile rank aerobic capacity, pain, and self-rated disability in patients with chronic low-back pain: A retrospective chart review. Arch Phys Med Rehabil 81:1457–1463, 2000

114. Bentsen H, Lindgarde F, Manthorpe R: The effect of dynamic strength back exercise and/or a home training program in 57-year-old women with chronic low back pain. Results of a prospective randomized study with a 3-year follow-up period. Spine 22:1494–1500, 1997

115. Nelson BW, O'Reilly E, Miller M, et al: The clinical effects of intensive, specific exercise on chronic low back pain: A controlled study of 895 consecutive patients with 1-year follow up. Orthopedics 18:971–981, 1995

116. Cleland J, Schulte C, Durall C: The role of therapeutic exercise in treating instability-related lumbar spine pain: A systematic review. J Back Musculoskel Rehabil 16:105–115, 2002

117. Jonsson B, Stromqvist B: Clinical appearance of contained and non-contained lumbar disc herniation. J Spinal Disord 9:32, 1996

118. Brinckmann P: Injury of the anulus fibrosus and disc protrusions. Spine 11:149–153, 1986

119. Donelson R: The McKenzie approach to evaluating and treating low back pain. Orthop Rev 19:681–686, 1990

120. McKenzie RA, May S: The Lumbar Spine: Mechanical Diagnosis and Therapy (ed 2). Waikanae, NZ, Spinal Publication, 2003

121. Jacob G, McKenzie R: Spinal therapeutics based on responses to loading, in Liebenson C (ed): Rehabilitation of the Spine: A Practitioner's Manual. Baltimore, Lippincott Williams & Wilkins, 1996, pp 225–252

122. Heffner SL, McKenzie R, Jacob G: McKenzie protocols for mechanical treatment of the low back, in Morris C (ed): Low Back Syndromes: Integrated Clinical Management. New York, McGraw-Hill, 2006, pp 611–622

123. Weinstein JN: A 45-year-old man with low back pain and a numb left foot. JAMA 280:730–736, 1998

124. Vroomen PC, de Krom MC, Slofstra PD, et al: Conservative treatment of sciatica: A systematic review. J Spinal Disord 13:463–469, 2000

125. Vroomen PC, de Krom MC, Wilmink JT, et al: Lack of effectiveness of bed rest for sciatica. N Engl J Med 340:418–423, 1999

126. Stankovic R, Johnell O: Conservative management of acute low back pain. A prospective randomized trial: McKenzie method of treatment versus patient education in "mini back school." Spine 15:120–123, 1990

127. Shah JS, Hampson WGJ, Jayson MIV: The distribution of surface strain in the cadaveric lumbar spine. J Bone Joint Surg 60B:246–251, 1978

128. Gill K, Videman T, Shimizu T, et al: The effect of repeated extensions on the discographic dye patterns in cadaveric lumbar motion segments. Clin Biomech 2:205–210, 1987

129. Krag MH, Seroussi RE, Wilder DG, et al: Internal displacement distribution from in vitro loading of human thoracic and lumbar spinal motion segments: Experimental results and theoretical predictions. Spine 12:1001–1007, 1987

130. Schnebel BE, Simmons JW, Chowning J, et al: A digitizing technique for the study of movement of intradiscal dye in response to flexion and extension of the lumbar spine. Spine 13:309–312, 1988

131. Beattie P, Brooks WM, Rothstein J, et al: Effect of lordosis on the position of the nucleus pulposus in supine subjects. Spine 19:2096–2102, 1994

132. Fennell AJ, Jones AP, Hukins DWL: Migration of the nucleus pulposus within the intervertebral disc during flexion and extension of the spine. Spine 21:2753–2757, 1996

133. Schnebel BE, Watkins RG, Dillin W: The role of spinal flexion and extension in changing nerve root compression in disc herniations. Spine 14:835–837, 1989

134. Lorio MP, Bernstein AJ, Simmons EH: Sciatic spinal deformity—lumbosacral list: An "unusual" presentation with review of the literature. J Spinal Disord 8:201–205, 1995

135. DePalma AF, Rothman RH: The Intervertebral Disc. Philadelphia, WB Saunders, 1970

136. Bianco AJ: Low back pain and sciatica. Diagnosis and indications for treatment. J Bone Joint Surg 50A:170, 1968

137. Maigne R: Diagnosis and Treatment of Pain of Vertebral Origin. Baltimore, Williams & Wilkins, 1996

138. Battie MC, Cherkin DC, Dunn R, et al: Managing low back pain: Attitudes and treatment preferences of physical therapists. Phys Ther 74:219–226, 1994

139. Donahue MS, Riddle DL, Sullivan MS: Intertester reliability of a modified version of McKenzie's lateral shift assessment obtained on patients with low back pain. Phys Ther 76:706–726, 1996

140. McKenzie RA: Manual correction of sciatic scoliosis. N Z Med J 76:194-199, 1972

141. Ito T, Takano Y, Yuasa N: Types of lumbar herniated disc and clinical course. Spine 26:648–651, 2001

142. Verbiest H: A radicular syndrome from developmental narrowing of the lumbar vertebral canal. J Bone Joint Surg 26B:230, 1954

143. Huijbregts PA: Lumbopelvic region: Aging, disease, examination, diagnosis, and treatment, in Wadsworth C (ed): Current Concepts of Orthopaedic Physical Therapy—Home Study Course. La Crosse, WI, Orthopaedic Section, American Physical Therapy Association, 2001

144. Katz JN, Dalgas M, Stucki G, et al: Degenerative lumbar spinal stenosis: Diagnostic value of the history and physical examination. Arthritis Rheum 38:1236–1241, 1995

145. Cailliet R: Low Back Pain Syndrome (ed 4). Philadelphia, FA Davis, 1991, pp 263–268

146. Tajima T, Furakawa K, Kuramochi E: Selective lumbosacral radiculography and block. Spine 5:68–77, 1980

147. Mooney V, Robertson J: The facet syndrome. Clin Orthop 115:149–156, 1976

148. Thein-Nissenbaum J, Boissonnault WG: Differential diagnosis of spondylolysis in a patient with chronic low back pain. J Orthop Sports Phys Ther 35:319–326, 2005

149. McNeely ML, Torrance G, Magee DJ: A systematic review of physiotherapy for spondylolysis and spondylolisthesis. Man Ther 8:80–91, 2003

150. Spratt KF, Weinstein JN, Lehmann TR, et al: Efficacy of flexion and extension treatments incorporating braces for low-back pain patients with retrodisplacement, spondylolisthesis, or normal sagittal translation. Spine 18:1839–1849, 1993

151. O'Sullivan P, Twomey L, Allison G: Evaluation of specific stabilizing exercise in the treatment of chronic low back pain with radiologic diagnosis of spondylolysis or spondylolisthesis. Spine 22:2959–2967, 1997

152. Panjabi M, Hult EJ, Crisco J, III, et al: Biomechanical studies in cadaveric spines, in Jayson MIV (ed): The Lumbar Spine and Back Pain. New York, Churchill Livingstone, 1992, pp 133–135

153. Friberg S: Studies on spondylolisthesis. Acta Chir Orthop 60:1, 1939

154. Barash HL: Spondylolisthesis and tight hamstrings. J Bone Joint Surg 52:1319, 1970

155. Bradford DS, Hu SS: Spondylolysis and spondylolisthesis, in Weinstein SL (ed): The Pediatric Spine, Raven, 1994

156. Edelman B: Conservative treatment considered best course for spondylolisthesis. Orthop Today 9:6–8, 1989

157. Grobler LJ, Robertson PA, Novotny JE, et al: Etiology of spondylolisthesis: Assessment of the role played by lumbar facet joint morphology. Spine 18:80–91, 1993

158. Laus M, Tigani D, Alfonso C, et al: Degenerative spondylolisthesis: Lumbar stenosis and instability. Chir Organi Mov 77:39–49, 1992

159. Love TW, Fagan AB, Fraser RD: Degenerative spondylolisthesis: Developmental or acquired? J Bone Joint Surg 81B:670–674, 1999

160. Matsunaga S, Sakou T, Morizonon Y, et al: Natural history of degenerative spondylolisthesis: Pathogenesis and natural course of slippage. Spine 15:1204–1210, 1990

161. Meschan I: Spondylolisthesis: A commentary on etiology and on improved method of roentgenographic mensuration and detection of instability. AJR 55:230, 1945

162. Newman PH: The etiology of spondylolisthesis. J Bone Joint Surg 45B:39–59, 1963

163. Postacchinia F, Perugia D: Degenerative lumbar spondylolisthesis. Part I: Etology, pathogenesis, pathomorphology, and clinical features. Ital J Orthop Traumatol 17:165–173, 1991

164. Rosenberg NJ: Degenerative spondylolisthesis. J Bone Joint Surg 57A:467–474, 1975

165. Seitsalo S, Osterman K, Hyvarinen H, et al: Progression of the spondylolisthesis in children and adolescents. Spine 16:417–421, 1991

166. Spring WE: Spondylolisthesis—a new clinical test. Proceedings of the Australian Orthopedics Association. J Bone Joint Surg 55B:229, 1973

167. Vallois HV, Lozarthes G: Indices lombares et indice lombaire totale. Bull Soc Anthropol 3:117, 1942

168. Clark P, Letts M: Trauma to the thoracic and lumbar spine in the adolescent. Can J Surg 44:337–345, 2001

169. Cook C, Cook A, Fleming R: Rehabilitation for clinical lumbar instability in a female adolescent competitive diver with spondylolisthesis. J Man Manip Ther 12:91–99, 2004

170. Lambert SD: Athletic injuries to the hip, in Echternach J (ed): Physical Therapy of the Hip. New York, Churchill Livingstone, 1990, pp 143–164

171. Peterson L, Renstrom P: Sports Injuries—Their Prevention and Treatment. Chicago, Year Book Medical Publishers, 1986

172. Jackson-Manfield P, Neumann DA: Structure and function of the vertebral column, in Jackson-Manfield P, Neumann DA (eds): Essentials of Kinesiology for the Physical Therapist Assistant. St. Louis, MO, Mosby Elsevier, 2009, pp 177–225

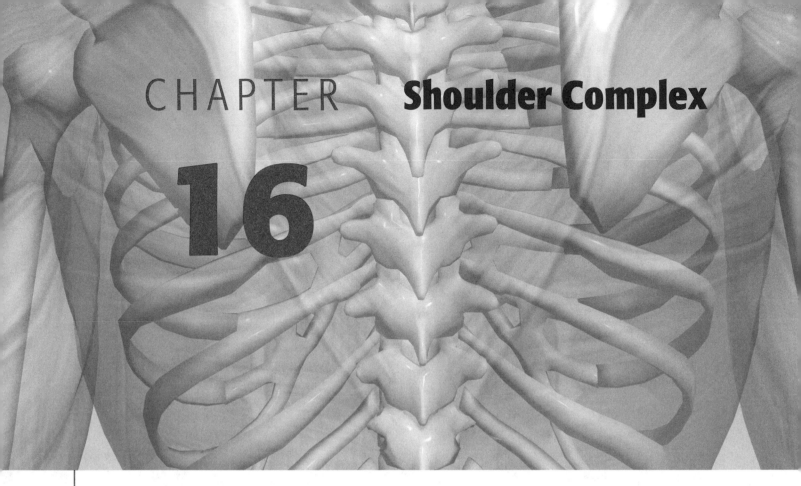

CHAPTER **Shoulder Complex**

16

Chapter Objectives

At the completion of this chapter, the reader will be able to:

1. Describe the anatomy of the joints, ligaments, muscles, blood, and nerve supply that comprise the region.

2. Describe the biomechanics of the shoulder complex, including the open- and close-packed positions, muscle force couples, and static and dynamic stabilizers.

3. Describe the relationship between muscle imbalance and functional performance of the shoulder.

4. Summarize the various factors that can cause shoulder dysfunction.

5. Describe and demonstrate intervention strategies and techniques based on clinical findings and established goals by the physical therapist.

6. Evaluate the intervention effectiveness in order to determine progress and recommend modification as needed.

7. Plan an effective home program, and instruct the patient in its use.

Overview

The shoulder complex is composed of four articulations between the sternum, humerus, scapula, and clavicle (Figure 16-1) and (Figure 16-2) and the surrounding soft tissue structures that connect them. The joints of the shoulder complex are composed of three synovial joints (the glenohumeral joint, the acromioclavicular [AC] joint, and the sternoclavicular [SC] joint) and two functional articulations (suprahumeral/subacromial and scapulothoracic). The shoulder girdle has only one bony attachment to the axial skeleton via the sternoclavicular joint.

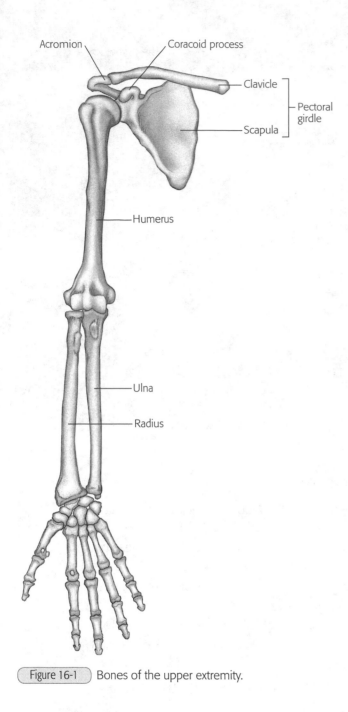

Figure 16-1   Bones of the upper extremity.

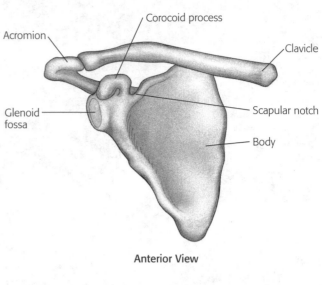

Anterior View

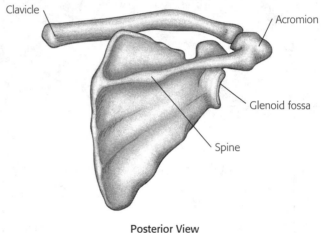

Posterior View

Figure 16-2   The scapula and clavicle.

Anatomy and Kinesiology

The blend of high mobility and low stability of the shoulder complex make this region a challenge for the clinician. Therefore, a sound knowledge of the anatomy and kinesiology is essential.

Sternoclavicular Joint

The SC joint represents the articulation between the medial end of the clavicle, the clavicular notch of the manubrium of the sternum, and the cartilage of the first rib, which forms the floor of the joint. The articulating surfaces of the SC joint are covered with fibrocartilage. Some confusion seems to exist about classification of the SC joint—it has been classified as a ball and socket joint,[1] a plane joint,[2] and a saddle joint.[1] The SC joint is angulated slightly upward approximately 20 degrees in a posterior and lateral direction. The clavicle presents with an irregularly shaped surface to the meniscus, and this lateral part of the joint acts as an ovoid articulation. The SC joint allows motion in all three cardinal planes, and is supported by a network of ligaments (**Table 16-1**), an articular disk, and a joint capsule. Motions at this joint include elevation and depression, protraction and retraction, and axial rotation (**Table 16-2**).

- *Elevation and depression:* Near-frontal plane movements about a near-anterior posterior axis of rotation, allowing approximately 45 degrees of clavicular elevation and 10 degrees of depression.

TABLE 16-1 Ligaments of the Shoulder

Ligament	Description and Function
Clavicular Ligaments	
Coracoclavicular ligament	Composed of the conoid and trapezoid ligaments. Reinforces the connection between the coracoid process and stabilizes the acromioclavicular joint.
Acromioclavicular ligament	Runs between the acromion process and the clavicle. Reinforces the connection between the acromion and the clavicle.
Sternoclavicular Ligaments	
Sternoclavicular ligament	Composed of anterior and posterior ligaments. Reinforces the connection between the sternum and the clavicle.
Interclavicular ligament	Connects the superior-medial sternal ends of each clavicle with the capsular ligaments and the upper sternum. Strengthens the articular capsule and restricts downward forces.
Costoclavicular ligament	The strongest of the sternoclavicular ligaments. Reinforces the connection between the first rib and the clavicle and restricts superior forces.
Glenohumeral Ligaments	Capsular thickenings that limit excessive motion of the humeral head by reinforcing the connection between the glenoid fossa and the humerus.
Inferior glenohumeral ligament	Extends from the under edge of the glenoid cavity to the under part of the anatomical neck of the humerus. Parts include the anterior band, axillary pouch, and posterior band. Provides anterior stabilization, especially during abduction of the arm.
Middle glenohumeral ligament	Strongest of the glenohumeral ligaments. Passes from the medial edge of the glenoid cavity to the lower part of the lesser tubercle of the humerus. Limits external rotation at 45 degrees of abduction.
Superior glenohumeral ligament	Runs from glenoid rim to anatomical neck. Works in conjunction with the coracohumeral ligament to prevent posterior and inferior instability.
Coracohumeral ligament	A broad ligament that reinforces the upper part of the capsule of the shoulder joint. Extends from the lateral end of the coracoid process and inserts on either side of the greater and lesser tuberosities. Provides anterior support by tightening with flexion and provides passive stability when the arm is dependent.
Transverse humeral ligament	Traverses the bicipital groove. Stabilizes the long head of the biceps muscle in the intertubercular groove.
Intrinsic Ligaments of the Scapula	
Superior transverse scapular ligament	Attached by one end to the base of the coracoid process, and by the other to the medial end of the scapular notch. Reinforces the connection between the coracoid process and the medial border of the scapular notch.
Inferior transverse scapular ligament	An inconstant fibrous band that passes from the lateral border of the spine of the scapula to the posterior margin of the glenoid cavity. Reinforces the connection between the lateral aspect of the root of the spine of the scapula and the margin of the glenoid fossa.
Coracoacromial ligament	Runs from the coracoid process to the anterior-inferior aspect of the acromion, with some of its fibers extending to the AC joint. Reinforces the connection between the coracoid process and the acromion, stabilizing the joint.

- *Protraction and retraction:* Occur in the horizontal plane about the vertical axis of rotation, allowing approximately 15 to 30 degrees of clavicular motion in either direction.
- *Axial rotation:* During abduction or flexion of the shoulder, the clavicle rotates posteriorly about its longitudinal axis. As the shoulder is abducted, the coracoclavicular ligament becomes tight and spins the clavicle posteriorly. As the shoulder is extended or adducted back to its rest position, the clavicle rotates anteriorly.

TABLE
16-2   Movements of the Acromioclavicular and Sternoclavicular Complex

Motion	Range of Motion	Motion Limited By	Muscles Involved	Peripheral Nerves Involved
Protraction (sagittal plane: clavicle glides posteriorly, acromion glides anteriorly)	The distal clavicle moves approximately 10 cm.	Anterior SC ligament, costoclavicular ligament (posterior portion), anterior capsule of the SC joint	Serratus anterior, pectoralis minor	Long thoracic, lateral and medial pectoral
Retraction (transverse plane: clavicle glides anteriorly, acromion glides posteriorly)	Distal clavicle moves approximately 3 cm.	Posterior SC ligament, costoclavicular ligament (anterior portion), posterior capsule of the SC joint	Trapezius, rhomboids	Spinal accessory, dorsal scapular
Elevation (frontal plane: clavicle glides superiorly, only slight angular motion occurs at AC joint)	The distal clavicle moves approximately 10 cm.	Costoclavicular ligament, inferior capsule of the SC joint	Upper trapezius, levator scapulae	Spinal accessory, directly via C3–C4 and dorsal scapular
Depression (frontal plane: clavicle glides inferiorly, only slight angular motion occurs at AC joint)	Distal clavicle moves approximately 3 cm.	Interclavicular ligament, SC ligament, articular disk of SC joint, superior capsule of SC joint	Serratus anterior (lower portion), pectoralis minor	Long thoracic, lateral and medial pectoral
Rotation (transverse plane)	30 degrees at AC joint, then 30 degrees at SC joint.	SC: anterior and posterior sternoclavicular ligament, interclavicular ligament, costoclavicular ligament AC: acromioclavicular ligament, coracoclavicular ligament (conoid [limits backward rotation], trapezoid [limits forward rotation])	Upper trapezius, serratus anterior (lower portion)	Spinal accessory, long thoracic

Scapulothoracic Articulation

This articulation is functionally a joint, but it lacks the anatomic characteristics of a true synovial joint. A lack of ligamentous support at this "joint" transfers the function of stability fully to the muscles that attach the scapula to the thorax. An altered position of the scapula and an abnormal motion at this joint have both been linked with shoulder complex dysfunction.[3–5] Motions at this joint are described according to the movement of the scapula relative to the thorax.

- *Elevation, depression, protraction (abduction), and retraction (adduction):* These motions are typically seen with clavicular motions at the SC joint and when the humerus moves, or during shoulder shrugging.
- *Upward and downward rotation:* These motions are seen with clavicular motions at the SC joint and rotation at the AC joint, and with motions of the humerus.

- *Winging and tipping:* These motions are seen with motions of the AC joint and motions of the humerus. Winging normally occurs with horizontal adduction of the humerus, whereas forward tipping of the scapula occurs in conjunction with internal rotation and extension of the humerus, as when reaching behind the back.

● **Key Point**   An important bony landmark of the scapula is the coracoid process, medial to which run the major blood vessels and brachial plexus. The coracoid serves as a muscular attachment for the pectoralis minor, the short head of the biceps, and the coracobrachialis.

Acromioclavicular Joint

The AC joint is a gliding or plane joint, formed by the acromion and the lateral end of the clavicle. When viewed from above, the clavicle is convex anteriorly in the medial two-thirds and convex posteriorly in the lateral one-third. The clavicle serves as the lever by which the upper extremity acts on the torso, and as an attachment site for many soft tissues.[6,7] These include a series of ligaments (refer to Table 16-1), and the pectoralis major, sternocleido-mastoid (SCM), deltoid, and trapezius muscles.[6,8] The AC joint serves as the main articulation that suspends the upper extremity from the trunk, and is the joint about which the scapula moves. The joint has a thin capsule lined with synovium, which is strengthened inferiorly and superiorly by capsular ligaments. Superiorly, the AC ligament gives support to the capsule and serves as the primary restraint to posterior translation and posterior axial rotation at the joint.[7] The motions available at this joint occur in all three planes and include upward and down-ward rotation, rotation in the horizontal plane, and rotation in the sagittal plane (Table 16-2). These relatively slight motions are very important during movements between the scapula and humerus.

Glenohumeral Joint

At the glenohumeral (GH) joint, an incongru-ous, ball-and-socket (spheroidal) joint, the convex humeral head articulates with the concave glenoid of the scapula, allowing for 3 degrees of freedom. The design of this joint (small shallow glenoid fossa, large surplus joint capsule) makes it relatively unstable, so the joint must rely on the static stability provided by a number of structures including a rim of tissue called the labrum, which surrounds the glenoid; the glenohumeral ligaments (superior, middle, inferior); the coracohumeral ligament; the coracoacromial ligament; the coracoclavicular ligaments (Table-16-1); and the joint capsule. It also must rely on the dynamic stability afforded by the muscular dynamic stabilizers, in particular the rotator cuff muscles (supraspinatus, infraspinatus, teres minor, and subscapularis), the biceps tendon, and the muscles of scapular motion (**Table 16-3** and **Table 16-4;** Figure 16-3 through Figure 16-5). Approximate available ranges of motion at the glenohumeral joint are listed in **Table 16-5**.

> ● **Key Point** With the shoulder in roughly 90 degrees of abduction, movement of the humerus toward the midline in the horizontal plane is considered horizontal adduction. Movement away from the midline in the horizontal plane is considered horizontal abduction.

TABLE 16-3 | Muscles of the Shoulder Complex According to Their Actions on the Glenohumeral Joint and Scapula

Action	Muscles
Glenohumeral flexors	Coracobrachialis
	Short and long head of the biceps brachii
	Pectoralis major (clavicular head)
	Anterior deltoid
Glenohumeral extensors	Triceps (long head)
	Posterior deltoid
	Pectoralis major
	Teres major
	Latissimus dorsi
Glenohumeral abductors	Supraspinatus
	Anterior and middle deltoid
Glenohumeral adductors	Pectoralis major
	Latissimus dorsi
	Teres major
	Coracobrachialis
Glenohumeral internal rotators	Pectoralis major
	Subscapularis
	Latissimus dorsi
	Teres major

(continued)

Action	Muscles
Glenohumeral external rotators	Infraspinatus Posterior deltoid Teres minor
Scapular abductors/protractors	Pectoralis minor Serratus anterior (upper fibers)
Scapular adductors/retractors	Levator scapulae Rhomboids Middle trapezius (upper and lower trapezius assist)
Scapular elevators	Upper trapezius Levator scapulae Rhomboids
Scapular depressors	Lower trapezius Latissimus dorsi Pectoralis minor Subclavius
Scapular upward rotators	Serratus anterior Upper trapezius Lower trapezius
Scapular protractors	Serratus anterior Pectoralis minor
Scapular downward rotators	Rhomboids Pectoralis minor Levator scapula
Scapular retractors	Rhomboids Middle trapezius

TABLE 16-4 Shoulder Girdle Muscle Function and Innervation

Muscle	Origin	Insertion	Peripheral Nerve	Nerve Root (Contributing Levels)	Motions
Pectoralis major	Anterior surface of the sternal half of the clavicle; anterior surface of the sternum	Intertubercular groove of humerus	Pectoral	Clavicular head: C5 and C6	Adduction, horizontal adduction, and internal rotation
				Sternocostal head: C7, C8, and T1	Clavicular fibers: Forward flexion Sternocostal fibers: Extension
Pectoralis minor	Ribs 3–5	Medial border and superior surface of coracoid process of scapula	Medial pectoral	C8–T1	Stabilizes scapula by drawing it anteriorly and inferiorly against thoracic wall

TABLE 16-4 Shoulder Girdle Muscle Function and Innervation (continued)

Muscle	Origin	Insertion	Peripheral Nerve	Nerve Root (Contributing Levels)	Motions
Latissimus dorsi	Spinous processes of inferior six thoracic vertebrae, thoracolumbar fascia, iliac crest, and inferior three ribs	Floor of intertubercular groove of humerus	Thoracodorsal	C7 (C6, C8)	Adduction, extension, and internal rotation
Teres major	Dorsal surface of inferior angle of scapula	Medial lip of intertubercular groove of humerus	Subscapular	C5–C8	Adduction, extension, horizontal abduction, and internal rotation
Teres minor	Superior part of lateral border of scapula	Inferior facet on greater tuberosity of humerus	Axillary	C5 (C6)	Horizontal abduction (also a weak external rotator)
Deltoid	Lateral one-third of clavicle, acromion, and spine of scapula	Deltoid tuberosity of humerus	Axillary	C5 (C6)	Anterior: Forward flexion, horizontal adduction Middle: Abduction Posterior: Extension, horizontal abduction
Supraspinatus	Supraspinatus fossa	Superior facet on greater tuberosity of humerus	Suprascapular	C5 (C6)	Abduction
Subscapularis	Subscapularis fossa	Lesser tuberosity of humerus	Upper and lower subscapular	C5–C8	Adduction and internal rotation
Infraspinatus	Infraspinatus fossa	Middle facet on greater tuberosity of humerus	Suprascapular	C5 (C6)	Abduction, horizontal abduction, and external rotation
Serratus anterior	External surfaces of lateral parts of ribs one through eight	Anterior surface of the medial border of scapula	Long thoracic	C5–C7	Protracts and rotates scapula and holds it against thoracic wall
Levator scapula	Posterior tubercles of transverse processes of C1–C4	Superior part of medial border of scapula	Dorsal scapular	C4–C5	Elevates scapula and tilts glenoid cavity inferiorly by rotating scapula
Rhomboids	Ligamentum nuchae and spinous processes of C7–T5	Medial border of scapula from level of spine to inferior angle	Dorsal scapular	C4–C5	Retracts scapula and rotates it to depress glenoid cavity
Coracobrachialis	Tip of coracoid process of scapula	Middle medial border of humerus	Musculocutaneous	C5–C6	Horizontal flexion and adduction of humerus at shoulder
Biceps brachii	Tip of coracoid and supraglenoid tubercle of scapula	Radial tuberosity and lacertus fibrosus	Musculocutaneous	C5–C6	Flexes arm and supinates forearm
Trapezius	Spinous processes of cervical and thoracic vertebrae	Scapula and acromion	Spinal accessory, branches of ansa cervicalis	CN XI	Elevates, retracts, and rotates scapula

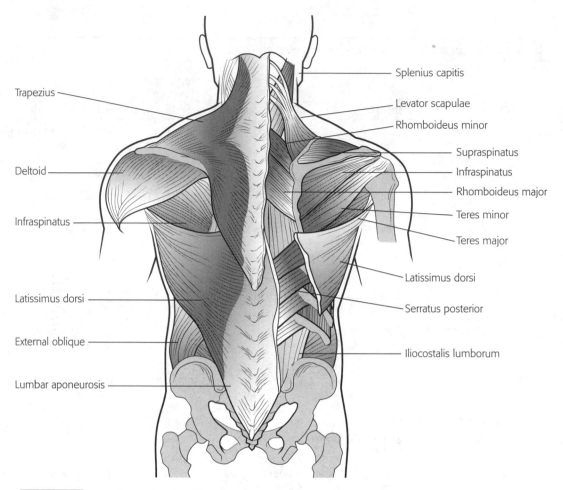

Splenius capitis

Trapezius

Levator scapulae

Rhomboideus minor

Deltoid

Supraspinatus

Infraspinatus

Rhomboideus major

Infraspinatus

Teres minor

Teres major

Latissimus dorsi

Latissimus dorsi

Serratus posterior

External oblique

Lumbar aponeurosis

Iliocostalis lumborum

Figure 16-3 Muscles of the shoulder.

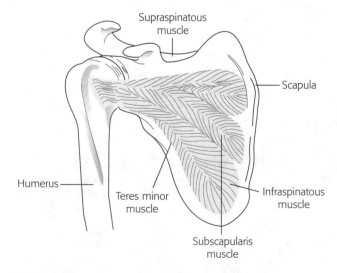

Supraspinatous
muscle

Scapula

Humerus

Teres minor
muscle

Infraspinatous
muscle

Subscapularis
muscle

Figure 16-4 Muscles of the rotator cuff.

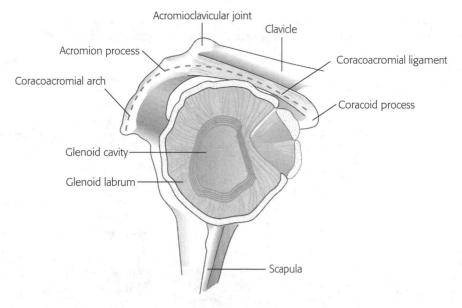

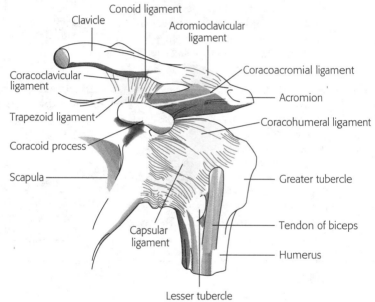

Figure 16-5   Ligaments of the AC and glenohumeral joints.

TABLE
16-5

Movements of the Glenohumeral Joint, Normal Ranges, Kinematics, and Potential Causes of Pain

Motion	Range Norms (Degrees)	Kinematics	Potential Source of Pain
Flexion and extension	Flexion: 0–120 Extension: 0–45	Motions occur in the sagittal plane about a medial-lateral axis of rotation, during which the humeral head spins on the glenoid fossa about a relatively fixed axis. The full 180 degrees of shoulder flexion is obtained by incorporating approximately 60 degrees of scapular upward rotation.	Flexion: • Suprahumeral impingement • Stretching of glenohumeral, acromioclavicular, and sternoclavicular joint capsules • Triceps tendon if elbow flexed Extension: • Stretching of glenohumeral joint capsule • Severe suprahumeral impingement • Biceps tendon if elbow extended
Internal and external rotation	Internal: 0–80 External: 0–90	Motions occur in the horizontal plane about a vertical (longitudinal) axis of rotation. Internal rotation results in the anterior surface of the humerus rotating medially, toward the midline, whereas external rotation results in the anterior surface of the humerus rotating laterally, away from the midline.	Internal: • Anterior glenohumeral instability External: • Suprahumeral impingement • Posterior glenohumeral instability
Abduction	Abduction: 0–120	Motions occur in the frontal plane about an anterior-posterior axis of rotation. Normally, the GH joint allows approximately 120 degrees of abduction; a full 80 degrees of shoulder abduction normally occurs by combining 60 degrees of scapular upward rotation with the abduction of the GH joint. During abduction the complex head of the humerus rolls superiorly while simultaneously sliding inferiorly. The reverse occurs during adduction.	• Suprahumeral impingement • Stretching of glenohumeral, acromioclavicular, and sternoclavicular joint capsule

Coracoacromial Arch

The coracoacromial arch (Figure 16-6) is formed by the anteroinferior aspect of the acromion process, coracoacromial ligament, and inferior surface of the AC joint.[9–11] During overhead motion in the plane of the scapula, the supraspinatus tendon—the region of the cuff most involved in overuse syndromes of the shoulder—can pass directly underneath the coracoacromial arch. If the arm is elevated while internally rotated, the supraspinatus tendon passes under the coracoacromial ligament, whereas if the arm is externally rotated, the tendon passes under the acromion itself.[12]

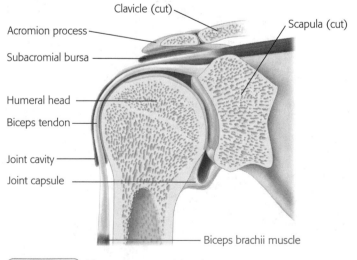

Figure 16-6   The coracoacromial arch.

Suprahumeral/Subacromial Space

As the name suggests, the suprahumeral space is an area located on the superior aspect of the GH joint (Figure 16-7). The boundaries of the space are formed by:

- The greater tuberosity of the humeral head, inferiorly
- The coracoid process, anteromedially
- The coracoacromial arch, superiorly

The structures that are located within the suprahumeral space include (from inferior to superior):

- The head of the humerus
- The long head of the biceps tendon (intra-articular portion)
- The superior aspect of the joint capsule
- The supraspinatus and upper margins of the subscapularis and infraspinatus
- The subdeltoid–subacromial bursae
- The inferior surface of the coracoacromial arch

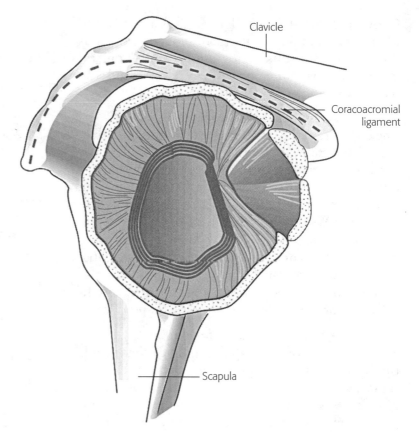

Figure 16-7 The suprahumeral space.

> **● Key Point** Elevating the arm decreases the distance between the acromion and the humerus, with the space at its narrowest between 60 and 120 degrees of scaption (the plane of motion that the scapula moves in).[13] Muscle imbalances or capsular contractures can cause an increase in superior translation of the humeral head, further narrowing the space.

The Scapulohumeral Rhythm

The synchronized motion that occurs between the glenoid cavity and the humerus during arm elevation is referred to as *scapulohumeral rhythm*. Proper rhythm involves a rotation of the scapula during arm elevation, which serves to significantly decrease the shearing effect between the humeral head and the glenoid, thereby increasing stability. By allowing the glenoid to stay centered under the humeral head, the strong tendency for a downward dislocation of the humerus is resisted and the glenoid is maintained within a physiologically allowable range. At full abduction, the glenoid completely supports the humerus. If the scapula cannot be controlled, the glenoid cannot be positioned correctly to allow for the optimal length–tension relationships within the shoulder complex.[14–17]

An early study by Inman[18] determined that a 2:1 ratio existed between the motion occurring at the GH joint and scapula, respectively. This means that for every 2 degrees of GH abduction, the scapula must simultaneously upwardly rotate approximately 1 degree. For example, if the shoulder is abducted to 90 degrees, only about 60 degrees of motion occurs from GH abduction; the additional 30 degrees is achieved through upward rotation of the scapula. At 180 degrees of elevation, the GH joint has contributed approximately 120 degrees, with the other 60 degrees coming from the upward rotation of the scapula. In addition to the GH and scapular motions, full elevation requires a combination of 30 degrees of clavicular elevation at the SC joint with 30 degrees of AC joint upward rotation. Loss of any of these functional components decreases the amount of scapular rotation and thus the ROM of the upper extremity.

> **● Key Point** It is worth noting that the scapulohumeral rhythm has been found to change with external loading of the arm, with increasing ratios of humeral elevation to scapular rotation occurring, depending on which of the five phases is assessed. As high a ratio as 4.3:1 has been noted.[19]

Muscle Function During Shoulder Motions

The muscles of the shoulder complex can be divided into three anatomical groups: thoracoscapular (rhomboids, levator scapulae, serratus anterior, and the trapezius muscles), thoracohumeral (latissimus dorsi and pectoralis major) and scapulohumeral (supraspinatus, infraspinatus, teres minor, and subscapularis [rotator cuff]), and deltoid.

Elevators of the Scapulothoracic Joint

The upper trapezius, levator scapulae, and, to a lesser extent, the rhomboids are responsible for elevating the scapula and supporting proper scapulothoracic posture—a slightly retracted and slightly elevated position with the glenoid fossa facing slightly upward.[20] Weakness or paralysis of the upper trapezius, over time, will likely lead to a depressed and downwardly rotated scapula, increasing the potential for subluxation of the GH joint.[20] Levator scapulae dysfunction often occurs with poor posture, specifically the forward head posture (see Chapter 25).

Depressors of the Scapulothoracic Joint

The depressors of the scapulothoracic joint include the lower trapezius, latissimus dorsi, pectoralis minor, and subclavius. The reverse action of two of these depressors (latissimus dorsi and lower trapezius) can be used to effectively elevate the trunk during such activities as crutch walking, pushing up from sitting to standing, ambulation with a walker, or while transferring to a bed or wheelchair.[20]

Upward Rotators and Protractors of the Scapula

During the first 30 degrees of upward rotation of the scapula, the serratus anterior muscle and the upper and lower divisions of the trapezius muscle are considered the principal upward rotators of the scapula. Together these muscles form two force couples—one formed by the upper trapezius and the upper serratus anterior muscles and the other by the lower trapezius and lower serratus anterior muscles.[18,21,22] A *force couple* is defined as two forces that act in opposite directions to rotate a segment around its axis of motion.[2,23] Weakness or complete paralysis of the serratus anterior or trapezius muscles results in the scapula being rotated downward by the contracting deltoid and supraspinatus as humeral abduction or flexion is attempted. These two muscles then reach active insufficiency, and functional elevation of the arm cannot be reached, even though there may be normal passive ROM and normal strength in the shoulder abductor and flexor muscles.[24]

Scapular protraction occurs primarily as a result of the force generated by the serratus anterior, and it is used in activities such as forward reaching and pushing. A classic sign of serratus anterior weakness is scapular winging, when the medial border of the scapula lifts away from the rib cage during resisted shoulder abduction or during a standard push-up.

> **● Key Point** Although the serratus has been found to be the most effective upward rotator of the scapula during abduction, the trapezius appears to be more critical than the serratus for controlling the scapula during the initial phases of abduction.[18,25] The lower trapezius contributes during the later phase of shoulder abduction by preventing tipping of the scapula and assisting in the stabilization of the scapula through eccentric control of the scapula during scapular upward rotation.[26,27]

Downward Rotators and Retractors of the Scapula

The primary downward rotators of the scapula include the rhomboids and pectoralis minor. In addition, the latissimus dorsi can assist with downward rotation. The primary scapular retractors are the rhomboids and the middle trapezius, although all three parts of the trapezius muscles can assist with protraction.

Muscles of the GH Joint

The main muscles that are used in conjunction with the glenohumeral joint are the group of muscles known as the rotator cuff (supraspinatus, subscapularis, infraspinatus, and teres minor), but other muscles also assist.

Internal Rotation

The primary internal rotators of the GH joint are the teres major, pectoralis major, subscapularis, latissimus dorsi, and anterior deltoid.

External Rotation

The primary external rotators of the GH joint are the teres minor, infraspinatus, and posterior deltoid. The relatively small muscle mass of this group produces the smallest torque of any muscle group of the shoulder.

Abduction

The prime muscles that abduct the GH joint are the anterior and middle deltoid, and the supraspinatus muscles.[28]

- *Deltoid:* Most of the force of the deltoid muscle causes upper translation of the humerus and, if unopposed, can lead to impingement of the soft tissues in the suprahumeral space. The combined effect of the short rotator muscles (infraspinatus, teres minor, and subscapularis) produce a stabilizing compression and then a translation of the humerus in the glenoid.[29]
- *Supraspinatus:* The supraspinatus muscle has a significant superior stabilizing, compressive, and

slight upward translation effect on the humerus. The horizontal line of pull of the supraspinatus allows it to be an important initiator of abduction.[29] During abduction of the GH joint, contraction of the horizontally oriented supraspinatus produces a compression force directly into the glenoid fossa, which stabilizes the humeral head against the fossa during its superior roll. In addition, the three other rotator cuff muscles provide an inferiorly directed force to counteract the tendency of the deltoid to pull the humerus superiorly, which would jam or impinge the humeral head superiorly against the coracoacromial arch.[20] Because of the tangential vector of deltoid contraction, the tendency for superior translation of the humeral head is greatest between 60 and 90 degrees of elevation.[13,30,31] Thus, repetitive overhead activities place a high demand on the rotator cuff to counteract this tendency. In addition, repetitive overhead activities bring the greater tuberosity and supraspinatus insertion into close proximity to the coracoacromial arch.[13,30,31]

Flexion

Elevation of the arm through flexion is performed primarily by the anterior deltoid, pectoralis major, coracobrachialis, and long head of the biceps brachii.[28]

Adduction

The primary adductors of the GH joint are the teres major, latissimus dorsi, and pectoralis major, which work together with the scapula downward rotators to produce adduction of the shoulder.

Extension

The primary extensors of the GH joint are the latissimus dorsi, teres major, pectoralis major, posterior deltoid, and long head of the triceps.

● **Key Point** The muscles that perform shoulder flexion also perform horizontal adduction, and the muscles that perform shoulder extension also perform horizontal abduction. This is because in regard to axes of rotation and lines of pull, the seemingly different actions are actually the same motions, just turned sideways.[20]

Examination

The physical therapist's examination of the shoulder complex typically follows the outline in **Table 16-6**. The evidence-based special tests for the shoulder complex are described in **Tables 16-7** through **16-10**.

TABLE 16-6   Examination of the Shoulder

I. History.
II. Observation and inspection.
III. Upper quarter scan as appropriate.
IV. Examination of movements. Active range of motion with passive overpressure of the following movements:
  a. Elevation (forward flexion, abduction, scaption)
  b. Adduction, extension, horizontal adduction and abduction, circumduction, external rotation, and internal rotation
  c. Scapulohumeral rhythm
V. Resisted isometric movements.
  a. Elevation
  b. Extension
  c. Adduction
  d. Abduction
  e. External rotation
  f. Internal rotation
  g. Elbow flexion
  h. Elbow extension
VI. Palpation.
VII. Neurological tests as appropriate (reflexes, nerve root, and peripheral nerve assessment).
VIII. Joint mobility tests.
  a. Glenohumeral joint
    1. Distraction
    2. Inferior glide of the humeral head
    3. Posterior glide of the humeral head
    4. Anterior glide of the humeral head
  b. Sternoclavicular joint
    1. Superior glide of the clavicle on the sternum
    2. Inferior glide of the clavicle on the sternum
    3. Posterior glide of the clavicle on the sternum
    4. Anterior glide of the clavicle
  c. Acromioclavicular joint
    1. Compression/distraction
    2. Anterior glide of the clavicle on the acromion
    3. Posterior glide of the clavicle
  d. Scapulothoracic joint
    1. Rotation of the scapula
    2. Elevation of the scapula
    3. Depression of the scapula
    4. Retraction of the scapula
    5. Protraction of the scapula
    6. Distraction of the scapula from the thoracic wall
IX. Special tests (refer to Table 16-7).
X. Diagnostic imaging (if any).

TABLE 16-7 Evidence-Based Special Tests for the Shoulder Complex

Name of Test	Brief Description	Positive Finding	Sensitivity	Specificity
Hornblower's sign[a]	Patient is seated. Clinician places patient's arm in 90 degrees of scaption and asks the patient to externally rotate against resistance.	Positive for infraspinatus or teres minor tear if the patient is unable to externally rotate the shoulder.	1.0	0.93
Empty can test for supraspinatus tendon tears[b]	The patient's arm is positioned in the scaption plane—internal rotation and approximately 90 degrees of shoulder flexion. Manual resistance is then applied by the clinician in a direction toward the floor.	Positive for supraspinatus tear if pain, weakness, or both is reproduced.	Pain 0.63 Weakness 0.77 Both 0.89	0.55 0.68 0.50
Full can test for supraspinatus tendon tears[b]	The patient's arm is positioned in the scaption plane—external rotation and approximately 90 degrees of shoulder flexion. Manual resistance then is applied by the clinician in a direction toward the floor.	Positive for supraspinatus tear if pain, weakness, or both is reproduced.	Pain 0.66 Weakness 0.77 Both 0.86	0.64 0.74 0.57
Dropping sign for infraspinatus degeneration[a]	Patient is seated. Clinician places patient's shoulder in 0 degrees of abduction and 45 degrees of external rotation with elbow flexed to 90 degrees. Patient is asked to hold position when clinician releases forearm.	Positive for infraspinatus degeneration if patient is unable to hold position and arm returns to 0 degrees of external rotation.	1.00	1.00
Palm up test (Speed test) for biceps tendon tear[c]	Patient elevates humerus to 60 degrees with elbow extended and forearm supinated. The patient holds this position while the clinician applies resistance against elevation.	Positive if pain is elicited.	0.63	0.35
Combined tests[d]	Clinician tests for supraspinatus and external rotator weakness, and impingement sign.	Positive for subacromial impingement if weakness is found in the supraspinatus and external rotators, and there is a positive impingement sign.	Not applicable	0.00
Trans-deltoid palpation (rent test)[e]	Patient is seated with arm by side. Clinician palpates the anterior margin of the acromion through the deltoid. Clinician then passively extends patient's arm and internally and externally rotates to palpate the rotator cuff tendons.	Positive for rotator cuff tear if clinician palpates eminence or rent.	0.957	0.968
Lift-off test for subscapularis tendon	Patient seated with the arm internally rotated so that the posterior surface of the hand rests on the lower back. The patient is asked to actively lift the hand away from the back.	Positive for subscapularis weakness/subacromial impingement if the patient is unable to lift the hand away from the back.	0.89[6] 0.89[7]	1.00[f] 0.36[g]
Supraspinatus test[g]	Patient is standing, shoulders abducted to 90 degrees in the scapular plane and internal rotation of the humerus. Clinician applies isometric resistance.	Positive if weakness or pain is detected.	1.00	0.53
Combined tests[h]	The clinician performs supraspinatus and infraspinatus manual muscle tests, and palpation.	Positive for rotator cuff involvement if weakness is detected and pain is elicited with palpation.	0.91	0.75

TABLE 16-7

Evidence-Based Special Tests for the Shoulder Complex (continued)

Name of Test	Brief Description	Positive Finding	Sensitivity	Specificity
Neer impingement sign for rotator cuff tear	Patient is seated. Clinician stabilizes the scapula with one hand and forces the patient's arm into maximal elevation with the other hand.	Positive for rotator cuff tear if pain is produced.	0.84[i]	0.51[i]
			0.33[g]	0.61[g]
			0.39[j]	1.0[j]
			0.93[k]	—
			0.00[l]	—
			0.89[m]	—
			0.89[c]	0.31[c]
Neer impingement sign for subacromial bursitis	See above.	Positive for subacromial bursitis if pain is produced.	0.75[i]	0.48[i]
Hawkins impingement sign for rotator cuff tear	Patient's arm is passively flexed to 90 degrees and forcefully moved into internal rotation	Positive for rotator cuff tear if pain is produced.	0.88[i]	0.43[i]
			0.44[g]	0.53[g]
Hawkins-Kennedy test for subacromial impingement	Patient's arm is passively flexed to 90 degrees and forcefully moved into internal rotation.	Positive for subacromial impingement if pain is reproduced.	0.80[j]	0.76[j]
			0.78[l]	1.00[l]
			0.62[g]	0.69[g]
			0.87[m]	—
			0.92[c]	0.25[c]
Horizontal adduction	Clinician flexes shoulder to 90 degrees and then adducts it horizontally across the body.	Positive for an AC lesion if pain is reproduced at the AC joint.	0.82[c]	0.28[c]
Speed test (for subacromial impingement)	Patient elevates humerus to 60 degrees with elbow extended and forearm supinated. The patient holds this position while the clinician applies resistance against elevation.	Positive if pain is elicited.	0.69[c]	0.56[c]
Speed test for biceps or superior labrum anterior and posterior (SLAP)	See above.	Positive if pain is elicited.	0.90[n]	0.14[n]
Yergason test	Patient's elbow is flexed to 90 degrees with forearm in pronation. Patient is then instructed to actively supinate forearm against resistance.	Positive for subacromial impingement if pain is elicited.	0.37[c]	0.86[c]
Painful arc	Patient is instructed to perform straight plane abduction of the arm throughout full range of motion.	Positive if pain occurs between 60 and 100 degrees of abduction.	0.33[c]	0.81[c]

(continued)

TABLE 16-7

Evidence-Based Special Tests for the Shoulder Complex (continued)

Name of Test	Brief Description	Positive Finding	Sensitivity	Specificity
Internal rotation resisted strength test	Patient standing. Clinician positions the patient's arm in 90 degrees of abduction and 80 degrees of external rotation. The clinician applies resistance against external rotation, then internal rotation in the same position.	The test is considered positive for intraarticular disease if the patient exhibits greater weakness in internal rotation when compared with external rotation, and for impingement syndrome if there is greater weakness with external rotation.	0.88[o]	0.96[o]
Anterior apprehension test[p]	The patient is positioned in supine. The clinician passively abducts and externally rotates the humerus.	Positive for shoulder instability if it elicits complaints of pain or instability.	0.62	0.42
Gilcreest test: Palm up test for biceps long head	Patient is asked to elevate arm with elbow extended and forearm supinated against resistance applied by the clinician.	Positive if patient feels pain at anterior aspect of arm along course of biceps brachii.	0.63[m]	0.35[m]
Yocum test	Patient is seated or standing and is asked to place hand of involved shoulder on contralateral shoulder and raise the elbow.	Positive for subacromial impingement if pain is elicited.	0.78[m]	—

Data from (a) Walch G, Boulahia A, Calderone S, et al: The "dropping" and "hornblower's" signs in evaluation of rotator-cuff tears. J Bone Joint Surg Brit 80:624–628, 1998; (b) Itoi E, Tadato K, Sano A, et al: Which is more useful, the "full can test" or the "empty can test" in detecting the torn supraspinatus tendon? Am J Sports Med 27:65–68, 1999; (c) Calis M, Akgun K, Birtane M, et al: Diagnostic values of clinical diagnostic tests in subacromial impingement syndrome. Ann Rheum Dis 59:44–47, 2000; (d) Murrell GA, Walton JR: Diagnosis of rotator cuff tears. Lancet 357:769–770, 2001; (e) Wolf EM, Agrawal V: Transdeltoid palpation (the rent test) in the diagnosis of rotator cuff tears. J Shoulder Elbow Surg 10:470–473, 2001; (f) Gerber C, Krushell RJ: Isolated rupture of the tendon of the subscapularis muscle: Clinical features in 16 cases. J Bone Joint Surg 73B:389–394, 1991; (g) Ure BM, Tiling T, Kirschner R, et al: The value of clinical shoulder examination in comparison with arthroscopy. A prospective study. Unfallchirurg 96:382–386, 1993; (h) Lyons AR, Tomlinson JE: Clinical diagnosis of tears of the rotator cuff. J Bone Joint Surg Br 74:414–415, 1992; (i) MacDonald PB, Clark P, Sutherland K: An analysis of the diagnostic accuracy of the Hawkins and Neer subacromial impingement signs. J Shoulder Elbow Surg 9:299–301, 2000; (j) Bak K, Faunl P: Clinical findings in competitive swimmers with shoulder pain. Am J Sports Med 25:254–260, 1997; (k) Post M, Cohen J: Impingement syndrome: A review of late stage II and early stage III lesions. Clin Orth Rel Res 207:127–132, 1986; (l) Rupp S, Berninger K, Hopf T: Shoulder problems in high level swimmers—impingement, anterior instability, muscular imbalance. Int J Sports Med 16:557–562, 1995; (m) Leroux JL, Thomas E, Bonnel F, et al: Diagnostic value of clinical tests for shoulder impingement. Rev Rheum 62:423–428, 1995; (n) Bennett WF: Specificity of the Speed's test: Arthroscopic technique for evaluating the biceps tendon at the level of the bicipital groove. Arthroscopy 14:789–796, 1998; (o) Zaslav KR: Internal rotation resistance strength test: A new diagnostic test to differentiate intra-articular pathology from outlet (Neer) impingement syndrome in the shoulder. J Shoulder Elbow Surg 10:23–27, 2001; and (p) Oh JH, Kim JY, Kim WS, et al: The evaluation of various physical examinations for the diagnosis of type II superior labrum anterior and posterior lesion. Am J Sports Med 36:353–359, 2008

TABLE 16-8

Diagnostic Test Properties for Labral Injuries

Name of Test	Brief Description	Positive Finding	Sensitivity	Specificity
SLAPrehension test	Patient is standing or seated and is asked to move the humerus into horizontal adduction, internal rotation, and elbow extension. Test is repeated with the patient bringing the humerus into external rotation.	Positive if pain is produced with arm in internal rotation to a greater extent than in external rotation.	0.88[a]	—
Crank test	Patient is supine while the clinician elevates the humerus to 160 degrees in the scapular plane. An axial load is applied to the humerus while the shoulder is internally and externally rotated.	Positive if pain is elicited.	0.91[b]	0.93[b]

TABLE
16-8

Diagnostic Test Properties for Labral Injuries (continued)

Name of Test	Brief Description	Positive Finding	Sensitivity	Specificity
Biceps load test for SLAP lesions in dislocators	Patient is supine. Clinician grasps the wrist and elbow. The arm is abducted to 90 degrees with the elbow flexed to 90 degrees and the forearm supinated. The clinician externally rotates the arm until the patient becomes apprehensive, at which time external rotation is stopped. Patient is asked to flex the elbow against the clinician's resistance.	Positive if patient's apprehension remains or pain is produced.	0.91[c]	0.97[c]
Biceps load test II	Patient is supine with the clinician grasping the wrist and elbow. The arm is elevated 120 degrees and fully externally rotated with the elbow held at 90 degrees of flexion and the forearm supinated. The clinician then resists elbow flexion by the patient.	Positive if resisted elbow flexion causes pain.	0.90[d]	0.97[d]
Anterior slide test	Patient is standing or sitting with hands on hips, thumbs facing posteriorly. The clinician stabilizes the scapula with one hand and, with the other hand on the elbow, applies an anteriorly and superiorly directed force through the humerus. The patient is asked to push back against the force.	Positive if pain or click is elicited in anterior shoulder.	0.78[e]	0.92[e]
Active compression test	Patient is standing. Patient is asked to flex the arm to 90 degrees with the elbow in full extension. The patient then adducts the arm 10 degrees and internally rotates the humerus. The clinician applies a downward force to the arm as the patient resists. The patient then fully supinates the arm and the procedure is repeated.	Positive if pain or painful clicking in the area of the glenohumeral joint is elicited with the first maneuver and reduced with the second maneuver.	1.00[f]	0.985[f]
Pain provocation test for superior labrum	Patient is sitting. Shoulder is abducted 90 degrees to 100 degrees and externally rotated by the clinician. Performed with forearm pronation and supination.	Positive if pain is provoked or is more severe in the pronated position.	1.00[g]	0.90[g]
Speed test for biceps or SLAP lesion	Patient is standing with arm in full elevation and forearm supination, elbow extended. The clinician applies resistance against elevation.	Positive if pain is produced.	0.90[h]	0.14[h]
Bicipital groove tenderness[i]	The clinician gently presses the biceps groove with the shoulder adducted 10 degrees.	Positive for labral tear if pain is reproduced.	0.27	0.66
Biceps palpation[j]	Point tenderness of the biceps tendon in the biceps groove 3–6 cm below anterior acromion.	Positive for labral tear if pain is reproduced.	0.53	0.54
Crank test[k]	Patient is supine. The clinician elevates the humerus 160 degrees in the scapular plane and then applies an axial load to the humerus while the shoulder is internally and externally rotated.	Positive for a labral tear if pain is elicited.	0.61	0.55

(continued)

TABLE 16-8

Diagnostic Test Properties for Labral Injuries (continued)

Name of Test	Brief Description	Positive Finding	Sensitivity	Specificity
O'Brien test[i]	Patient stands and flexes the arm to 90 degrees with the elbow in full extension. The patient then adducts the arm 10 degrees and internally rotates the humerus. The clinician applies a downward force to the arm as the patient resists. The patient then fully supinates the arm and the procedure is repeated.	Positive for labral tear if pain is elicited with the first maneuver and reduced with the second maneuver.	0.63	0.53
Compression rotation test[i]	The patient is in supine with the arm abducted to 90 degrees and the elbow flexed to 90 degrees. The clinician applies an axial force to the humerus. The humerus is circumducted and rotated.	Positive for a labral tear if pain or clicking is elicited.	0.61	0.54

Data from (a) Berg EE, Ciullo JV: A clinical test for superior glenoid labral or "SLAP" lesions. Clin J Sport Med 8:121–123, 1998; (b) Liu SH, Henry MH, Nuccion SL: A prospective evaluation of a new physical examination in predicting glenoid labral tears. Am J Sports Med 24:721–725, 1996; (c) Kim SH, Ha KI, Han KY: Biceps load test: A clinical test for superior labrum anterior and posterior lesions (SLAP) in shoulders with recurrent anterior dislocations. Am J Sports Med 27:300–303, 1999; (d) Kim SH, Ha KI, Ahn JH, et al: Biceps load test II: A clinical test for SLAP lesions of the shoulder. Arthroscopy 17:160–164, 2001; (e) Kibler WB: Specificity and sensitivity of the anterior slide test in throwing athletes with superior glenoid labral tears. Arthroscopy 11:296–300, 1995; (f) O'Brien SJ, Pagnani MJ, Fealy S, et al: The active compression test; a new and effective test for diagnosing labral tears and acromioclavicular abnormality. Am J Sports Med 26:610–613, 1998; (g) Mimori K, Muneta T, Nakagawa T, et al: A new pain provocation test for superior labral tears of the shoulder. Am J Sports Med 27:137–142, 1999; (h) Bennett WF: Specificity of the Speed's test: Arthroscopic technique for evaluating the biceps tendon at the level of the bicipital groove. Arthroscopy 14:789–796, 1998; (i) Oh JH, Kim JY, Kim WS, et al: The evaluation of various physical examinations for the diagnosis of type II superior labrum anterior and posterior lesion. Am J Sports Med 36:353–359, 2008; (j) Gill HS, El Rassi G, Bahk MS, et al: Physical examination for partial tears of the biceps tendon. Am J Sports Med 35:1334–1340, 2007; and (k) Walsworth MK, Doukas WC, Murphy KP, et al: Reliability and diagnostic accuracy of history and physical examination for diagnosing glenoid labral tears. Am J Sports Med 36:162–168, 2008

TABLE 16-9

Diagnostic Test Properties for GH Instability

Name of Test	Brief Description	Positive Finding	Sensitivity	Specificity
Shoulder relocation test (no force on humerus at start position)	Patient is supine with glenohumeral joint at edge of table. Clinician places shoulder in 90 degrees of abduction and 90 degrees of elbow flexion and then externally rotates the shoulder.	The test is considered positive if there is either pain or apprehension.	0.30 for pain[a]	0.58 for pain[a]
Shoulder relocation test (anterior-directed force on humerus at start position)	Patient is supine with glenohumeral joint at edge of table. Clinician places shoulder in 90 degrees of abduction and 90 degrees of elbow flexion and then externally rotates the shoulder and applies an anterior directed force on the humerus.	The test is considered positive if there is either pain or apprehension.	0.57 for apprehension[a] 0.54 for pain[a] 0.68 for apprehension[a]	1.0 for apprehension[a] 0.44 for pain[a] 1.0 for apprehension[a]

TABLE
16-9

Diagnostic Test Properties for GH Instability (continued)

Name of Test	Brief Description	Positive Finding	Sensitivity	Specificity
Anterior release test for anterior instability	Patient is supine with arm in 90 degrees of abduction and external rotation while the clinician applies a posterior force over the humeral head. The clinician quickly releases the posterior force.	The test is considered positive if there is either pain or apprehension.	0.92[b]	0.89[b]
Load and shift[c]	Patient is supine. The clinician grasps the patient's elbow with one hand and the proximal humerus with the other hand. The arm is placed in 90 degrees of abduction in the scapular plane. The clinician attempts to shift the humeral head in anterior, posterior, and inferior directions.	Amount of laxity is graded from 0 to 3, with 0 indicating little or no movement and 3 indicating that the humeral head can be dislocated off the glenoid and remains so when the pressure is released.	Anterior: 0.5 Posterior: 0.14 Inferior: 0.08	Anterior: 1.00 Posterior: 1.00 Inferior: 1.00

Data from (a) Speer KP, Hannafin JA, Altchek DW, et al: An evaluation of the shoulder relocation test. Am J Sports Med 22:177–183, 1994; (b) Gross ML, Distefano MC: Anterior release test: A new test for occult shoulder instability. Clin Orth Rel Res 339:105–108, 1997; and (c) Tzannes A, Murrell GA: Clinical examination of the unstable shoulder. Sports Med 32:447–457, 2002

TABLE
16-10

Diagnostic Utility of Multitest Regimens Consisting of Cross-Body Adduction Stress, Active Compression, and Acromioclavicular Resisted Extension Test for Detecting AC Joint Lesions

	Accuracy	Sensitivity	Specificity
≥ 1 positive test	0.75 (237/315)	0.00 (16/16)	0.74 (221/299)
≥ 2 positive tests	0.89 (279/315)	0.81 (13/16)	0.89 (266/299)
3 positive tests	93 (294/315)	0.25 (4/16)	0.97 (290/299)

Data from Chronopoulos E, Kim TK, Park HB, et al: Diagnostic value of physical tests for isolated chronic acromioclavicular lesions. Am J Sports Med 32:655–661, 2004; and Powell JW, Huijbregts PA: Concurrent criterion-related validity of acromioclavicular joint physical examination tests: A systematic review. J Man Manip Ther 14:E19–E29, 2006

General Intervention Strategies

A number of principles can be used to guide the clinician in the conservative rehabilitation of shoulder injuries:

- Rehabilitate the shoulder according to the stage of healing and degree of irritability. The degree of irritability can be determined by inquiring about the vigor, duration, and intensity of the pain. Greater irritability is associated with very acutely inflamed conditions. The characteristic sign for an acute inflammation of the shoulder is pain at rest, which is described as diffuse and often referred from the site of the primary condition.[32] Pain above the elbow indicates less severity than does pain below the elbow. Chronic conditions usually have low irritability, but have an associated loss of active range of motion (AROM) and passive range of motion (PROM).

- Rehabilitate the shoulder in scapular planes rather than in the straight planes of flexion, extension, and abduction because exercises performed in the scapular plane are more functional.

- Short lever arms (see Chapter 4) should be used with exercises initially, thereby decreasing the torque at the shoulder. This can be achieved by flexing the elbow or by exercising with the arm closer to the body.

- Obtain a stable scapular platform as early as possible. This involves normalizing the relationship between the scapulothoracic upward rotators and the glenohumeral abductors.

- Achieve the close-packed position (full arm elevation) at the earliest opportunity. By definition, the close-packed position of the shoulder is that position which provides the joint with the maximum amount of passive stability.

- Reproduce the forces and loading rates that will approach the patient's functional demands as the rehabilitation progresses. Activities and arm positions that increase or decrease symptoms are helpful in guiding treatment.

Acute Phase

In addition to maintaining or improving general cardiovascular fitness, the goals of the acute phase include the following:

- *Reduce pain and swelling, control inflammation, and protect the injury site.* The reduction of pain and the control of swelling are extremely important. Pain and swelling can both inhibit normal muscle function and control. Pain, swelling, and inflammation are minimized by using the principles of PRICEMEM (protection, rest, ice, compression, elevation, manual therapy, early motion, and medication). Icing for 20–30 minutes, three to four times a day, concurrent with nonsteroidal anti-inflammatory drugs (NSAIDs) or aspirin prescribed by the physician, can aid in reducing pain and swelling.
- *Improve postural awareness.* Due to the close relationships between the cervical spine and scapula, it is important to encourage postural awareness and correction techniques (see Chapter 25).
- *Begin regaining pain-free ROM in the entire kinetic chain.* Early passive and then active assisted exercises are performed in all planes of shoulder movement to nourish the articular cartilage and assist in collagen tissue synthesis and organization.[33–37] These exercises are initiated in pain-free arcs, below 90 degrees of abduction. Recommended ROM exercises for the acute phase include the Codman's or other pendulum exercises (Figure 16-8), passive shoulder flexion (Figure 16-9), abduction, external rotation (Figure 16-10), internal rotation (Figure 16-11), and elbow flexion and extension, progressing to active assisted ROM exercises using a wand or cane (Figure 16-12 and Figure 16-13). Over-the-door pulley exercises are performed later in the acute phase as tolerated. Care must be taken when prescribing pulley exercises in the presence of impingement or adhesive capsulitis because the exercise can reinforce poor scapulohumeral motion.

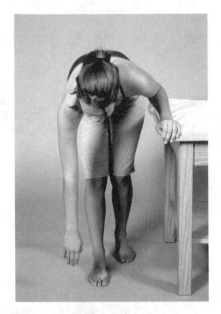

Figure 16-8   Codman's pendulum exercise.

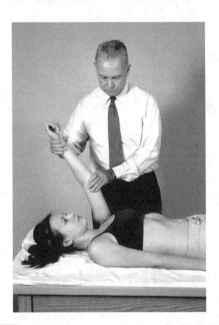

Figure 16-9   Passive shoulder flexion.

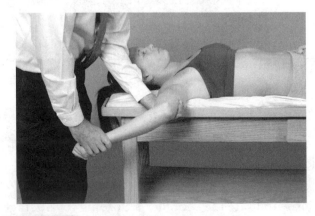

Figure 16-10   Passive shoulder external rotation.

- *Retard muscle atrophy and minimize detrimental effects of immobilization and activity restriction.*[38-43] Jobe and Pink[44] believe that the order of strengthening in the rehabilitation process is important. They advocate strengthening the GH "protectors" (rotator cuff muscles) and scapular "pivoters" (levator scapulae, serratus anterior, middle trapezius, and rhomboids) initially because of the role they play in providing stability, and then the humeral "positioners" (deltoid)

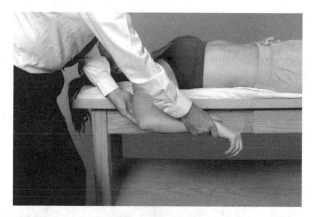

Figure 16-11   Passive shoulder internal rotation.

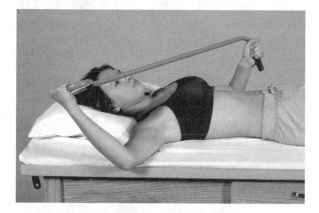

Figure 16-12   Active assisted shoulder external rotation.

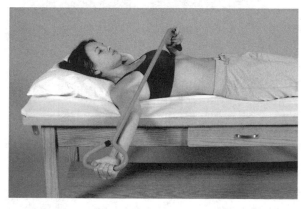

Figure 16-13   Active assisted shoulder abduction.

and the humeral "propellers" (latissimus dorsi and pectoralis major) are introduced. Active exercise can be performed in standing, sitting, or lying. To begin strengthening the shoulder rotators, the face-lying shoulder rotation exercise can be performed, where the patient lies prone close to the edge of the bed so the upper portion (humerus) of the involved arm is supported by a pillow with the shoulder near 90 degrees abduction and the elbow flexed to 90 degrees. The patient then performs active range of motion into external rotation and internal rotation while making sure to keep the upper arm resting on the pillow. Light weights can be added and progressed as tolerated (Figure 16-14). Strengthening exercises at the shoulder in standing or sitting are introduced as tolerated using submaximal isometric exercises, with the arm positioned below 90 degrees of abduction and 90 degrees of flexion. Elbow flexion and extension PREs are introduced as appropriate. Specific scapular rehabilitation exercises are typically initiated with the isometric exercises, such as the scapular retraction (Figure 16-15). Patterns of

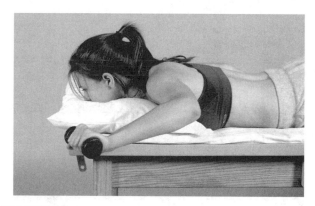

Figure 16-14   PNF pattern: extension-abduction-external rotation.

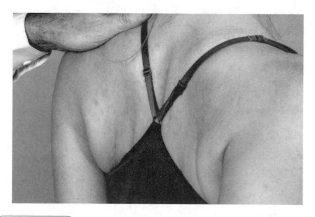

Figure 16-15   PNF pattern: flexion-adduction-internal rotation.

scapular retraction and protraction are started in single planes and then progress to elevation and depression of the entire scapula. It is important to remember that to improve backward reaching, the patient must first learn correct retraction procedures. To begin strengthening the middle and lower trapezius, a series of face-lying arm lifts can be performed:

❏ Prone arm lifts with elbows flexed (Figure 16-16)
❏ Prone arm lifts with elbows extended (Figure 16-17)
❏ Prone arm lifts with arms overhead (Figure 16-18)

Chronic/Functional Phase

The functional phase addresses any tissue overload problems and functional biomechanical deficits. The criteria for progression to the stage include the following:[29]

■ Minimal discomfort when the shoulder is unsupported; arm swing is comfortable during ambulation.

■ Patient demonstrates nearly complete, pain-free, passive range of motion of the shoulder (full mobility of the scapular, at least 150 degrees of shoulder elevation, full rotation).

■ Pain-free active elevation of the arm well above the level of the shoulder in the supine position.

■ Pain-free, active external rotation of the shoulder to about 45 degrees.

■ At least fair (3/5) and preferably good (4/5) muscles testing grade of shoulder musculature.

The goals of the functional phase include the following:

■ *Attain full range of pain-free motion.* Range of motion exercises are progressed as tolerated. In cases where capsular restrictions are limiting the range of motion, the patient can perform external rotation and internal rotation stretches (Figure 16-19).

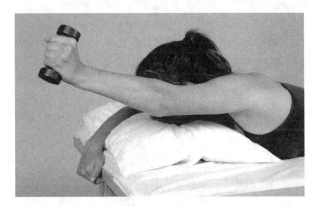

Figure 16-18   Prone arm lifts with arms overhead.

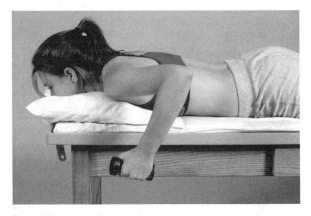

Figure 16-16   Prone arm lifts with elbows flexed.

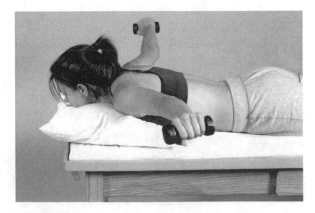

Figure 16-17   Prone arm lifts with elbows extended.

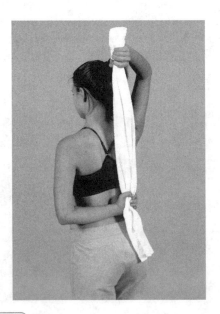

Figure 16-19   Towel stretch.

- *Restore normal joint arthrokinematics.* Normal joint kinematics are restored as joint mobilization techniques are performed.
- *Improve muscle strength and neuromuscular control to within normal limits, and restore normal muscle force couples.* Specific exercises can be given to the rotator cuff muscles in the form of the empty can exercise (Figure 16-20) and the full can exercise (Figure 16-21). In addition to continuing the strengthening of the GH protectors and scapular pivoters, strengthening of the humeral positioners (deltoid) and the humeral propellers (latissimus dorsi and pectoralis major) begins, as well as strengthening of the serratus anterior. The serratus anterior can be strengthened using a progression that starts in the quadruped position and is progressed through prone push-ups while kneeling (Figure 16-22), and finally into the full push-up (Figure 16-23). Other weight-bearing exercises (Figure 16-24 through Figure 16-27), plyometric exercises (Figure 16-28), and sport-specific activities (Figure 16-29 through Figure 16-31) can be introduced if appropriate.

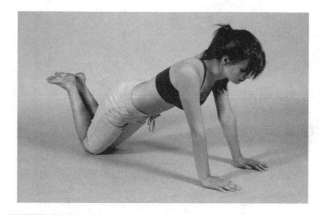

Figure 16-22　Push-up in kneeling.

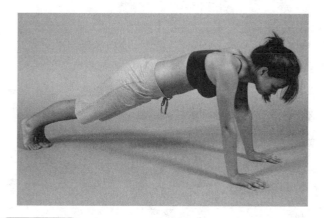

Figure 16-23　Push-up.

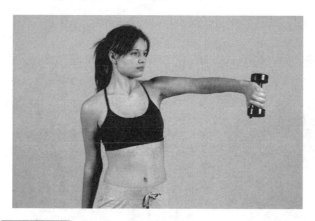

Figure 16-20　Empty can exercise.

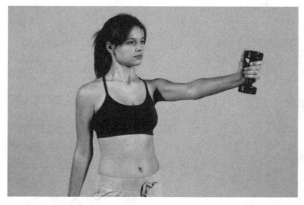

Figure 16-21　Full can exercise.

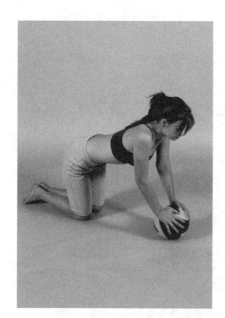

Figure 16-24　Weight bearing through a medicine ball.

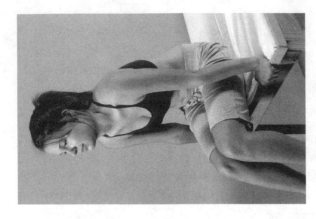

Figure 16-27 Triceps lift.

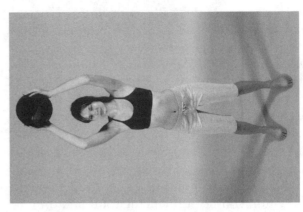

Figure 16-31 Sport-specific exercise.

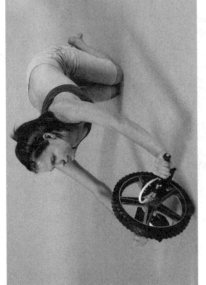

Figure 16-26 Dynamic weight bearing.

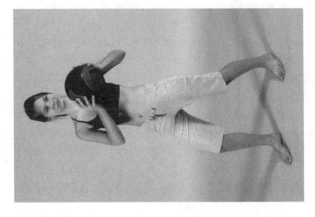

Figure 16-30 Sport-specific exercise.

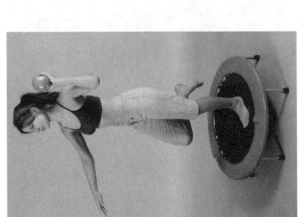

Figure 16-29 Functional drill for athlete.

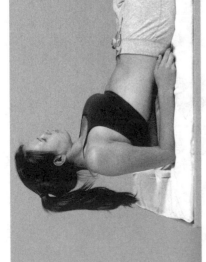

Figure 16-25 Elbow prop.

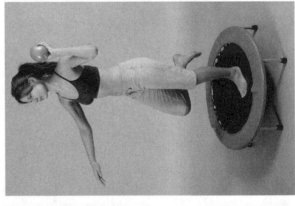

Figure 16-28 Plyometric drill.

Common Conditions

The common conditions that can affect the shoulder include those that relate to poor biomechanics due to weakness, trauma, repetitive overhead activities, or overuse.

Scapular Dyskinesis

Scapular dyskinesis is an alteration in the normal position or motion of the scapula during scapulohumeral movements. Scapular dyskinesis appears to be an unclear response to shoulder dysfunction because no specific pattern of dyskinesis is associated with a specific shoulder diagnosis.[45] It should be suspected in patients with shoulder injury and can be identified and classified by specific physical examination. There are three types of scapular dyskinesis:

- Type I is characterized by a prominence of the inferior medial scapular border.
- Type II has the entire medial border protruding.
- Type III has superior translation of the entire scapula and prominence of the superior medial border.

Once all the factors involved in the dysfunction of the shoulder are identified by the physical therapist, treatment is aimed at restoring normal scapular position and movement.

Intervention

The intervention progression described in the "General Intervention Strategies" section earlier in this chapter can be used for this condition.

Subacromial Impingement Syndrome

The cause of impingement is multifactorial but the mechanism is the same—an increase in superior translation with active elevation that results in encroachment of the coracoacromial arch and produces a compression of the suprahumeral structures against the anteroinferior aspect of the acromion and coracoacromial ligament.[10,30] Repetitive compression of these structures, coupled with other predisposing factors, results in a condition called subacromial impingement syndrome (SIS). SIS is a recurrent and niggling condition that is associated with pathology of one or more of the contents of the subacromial space. Jobe and colleagues[46] and Jobe and Pink[44] proposed two types of impingement, primary and secondary, that relate to chronic disorders of the rotator cuff:

- *Primary impingement* (rotator cuff disease) refers to the intrinsic degenerative process in the structures occupying the subacromial space. It occurs when the superior aspect of the rotator cuff is compressed and abraded by the surrounding bony and soft tissues due to a decreased subacromial space.[47]
- *Secondary impingement* results from GH instability and/or tensile overload of the rotator cuff resulting in poor control of the humeral head during overhead activities.[44,46,48] Secondary impingement is a condition found in both older and younger individuals with varying levels of activity, although patients in this group are usually younger than 35 years, and have a traumatic anterior instability, posterior defect of the humeral head, and damage to the posterior glenoid labrum.[49]

Two other types of impingement are worth mentioning:

- *Internal glenoid impingement:* Also called posterior-superior glenoid impingement (PSGI) or posterior impingement. PGSI is a very common cause of posterior shoulder pain in the throwing or overhead athlete, and is commonly misdiagnosed as rotator cuff tendonitis. PSGI is caused by the impingement of the posterior edge of the supraspinatus and the anterior edge of the infraspinatus against the posterior-superior-glenoid and glenoid labrum. The mechanism of injury is shoulder extension, abduction, and external rotation.
- *Subcoracoid stenosis:* As the name suggests, this condition involves a gradual narrowing of the subcoracoid space. Subcoracoid stenosis may not be pathologic or symptomatic.

The pathophysiology of SIS and rotator cuff disorders may have both intrinsic and extrinsic factors. These intrinsic and extrinsic factors include the following:[9,11,50–52]

- *The shape and form of the acromion:* Acromial morphology is a strong predictor of rotator cuff impingement.[53,54] Bigliani and colleagues[53] studied 140 shoulders in 71 cadavers. The average age was 74.4 years. They identified three acromial shapes: type I (flat) in 17 percent, type II (curved) in 43 percent, and type III (hooked) in 40 percent. Fifty-eight percent of the cadavers had the same type of acromion on each side. Thirty-three percent of the shoulders had full-thickness tears, of which 73 percent were seen in the presence of type III acromia, 24 percent in type II, and 3 percent in type I.

- *The amount of vascularization to the cuff:* The area of the supraspinatus just proximal to its insertion has been found to be markedly under-vascularized in relation to the remainder of the cuff.[52] The work of Rathburn and Macnab[55] noted a consistent zone of poor vascularization near the tuberosity attachment of the supra-spinatus when the arm was adducted; with the arm in abduction, however, there was almost full filling of vessels to the point of insertion. They suggested that some of the previous data suggesting hypovascularity were, in fact, due to this artifact of positioning.[55] Other arm posi-tions, such as raising the arm above 30 degrees, have been shown to increase intramuscular pressure in the supraspinatus muscle to an extent that may impair normal blood perfu-sion.[55,56] Although it is possible that sustained isometric contractions, prolonged adduction of the arm, or increases in subacromial pressure[57] may reduce the microcirculation, it is unlikely that frequent abduction or elevation of the arm would produce selective avascularity of the supraspinatus or biceps tendon.

- *The correct functioning of the dynamic stabiliz-ers:* If the dynamic stabilizers (rotator cuff mus-cles) are weak or injured, increased translation occurs between the humeral head and glenoid labrum.[58]

- *Condition of the AC joint:* Degenerative changes of the AC joint, including narrowing of the joint space and the formation of inferior osteophytes, also can accompany impingement syndrome.[11,59,60]

- *Position of the arm during activities:* The arm position adopted during work activities may contribute significantly to the development of subacromial impingement.[61]

- *Poor endurance of scapular pivoters:* Sustained or repetitive overhead activity requires endur-ance from the scapular pivoters (levator scapu-lae, serratus anterior, middle trapezius, and rhomboids) to maintain appropriate scapular rotation.[9,15,62] Fatigue of the scapular pivoters may lead or contribute to relative subacromial impingement because of poor or asymmetric scapular rotation.[9,15,62] Secondary impingement can occur because of serratus anterior dysfunc-tion, resulting in the forward and downward

movement of the coracoacromial arch. This reduces available freedom for the rotator cuff and greater tuberosity as the shoulder is flexed forward.[15,63] Scapular lag from dysrhythmic scapulothoracic motion can also contribute to subacromial impingement because the acro-mion fails to rotate with the humerus, thereby producing a relative decrease in the acromio-humeral interval.[15,63]

- *Capsular tightness:*[64] Capsular tightness appears to be a common mechanical problem in primary impingement syndrome and has been reported to occur at the posterior,[15] ante-rior,[13] and inferior[65,66] portions of the capsule. Individuals who have poor posture, avoid painful overhead activity, or are predisposed to motion imbalances because of their work or sport can develop capsular tightness.[67] During the period of pain avoidance or unbalanced movement, the capsular connective tissue may lose the ability to lengthen due to decreased critical fiber distance and abnormal collagen fiber cross-linking. This in turn can lead to cap-sular tightness, joint stiffness, painful or limited function, and an earlier onset or greater degree of subacromial compression, particularly in elevated planes of movement.[9,42,68,69] This is particularly true with a posterior capsular contracture, which commonly coexists with SIS and rotator cuff disease. Posterior capsular contracture may add to the abnormal subacro-mial contact by producing an anterosuperior translation during active elevation.[9,70] Tight-ness of the posterior capsule can also cause a decrease in internal rotation of the GH joint, which leads to an increase in the anterior and superior migration of the humeral head. In contrast, tightness of the anteroinferior capsule results in limited external rotation, preventing the greater tuberosity from sufficient external rotation to "clear" the coracoacromial arch.[71] Thus, the restoration of capsular mobility is an important component in the rehabilitation process.

- *Age:* The age of the patient appears to be an important etiologic factor in the development of subacromial impingement in association with repetitive motion.[72–76] In the absence of repetitive motion as a mitigating factor, SIS is more common after the third decade of life and is uncommon in individuals younger than 30 years.[9,10] In addition, there is a normal age-related increase in asymptomatic rotator cuff defects.[72–74,76,77]

Neer[11] divided the age and degenerative changes that occur with the impingement process into three stages, although the condition is a continuum of symptoms with overlap at the margins of each stage.[8] Each impingement stage is managed based on the specific findings and the intrinsic or extrinsic factors contributing to the problem.

- *Stage I:* This stage consists of localized inflammation, slight bleeding, and edema of the rotator cuff. This stage is typically observed in patients under 25 years of age, although it can also be seen in older populations due to overuse. The patient reports pain in the shoulder and a history of acute trauma or repetitive microtrauma. Stage I is a reversible condition.
- *Stage II:* Stage II represents a progressive process in the deterioration of the tissues of the rotator cuff. This stage is generally seen in the 26- to 40-year-old age group. Irritation of the subacromial structures continues as a result of the abnormal contact with the acromion. The subacromial bursa loses its ability to lubricate and protect the underlying rotator cuff, and tendonitis and fibrosis of the bursa and cuff develops. The patient often reports pain as the predominant symptom with specific daily activities aggravating their symptoms, especially an overhead activity. Pain is also reported at night. Stage II is classified as irreversible.
- *Stage III:* Stage III is the end stage, common in the over-40 age group, where destruction of the soft tissue and rupture, or macrotrauma, of the rotator cuff is seen. Localized atrophy can occur with this stage. Osteophytes of the acromion and AC joint develop. The wear of the anterior aspect of the acromion on the greater tuberosity and the supraspinatus tendon eventually results in a full-thickness tear of the rotator cuff.

Intervention

The intervention for SIS follows the progression as outlined in the "General Intervention Strategies" section earlier in this chapter.

Rotator Cuff Repair

The patient with a symptomatic, rotator cuff–deficient glenohumeral joint poses a complex problem for the orthopaedic team, and several surgical options are available, depending on the presentation.[78,79]

There are two broad categories of rotator cuff tears, defined by the depth of the tendon tear: partial thickness and full thickness tears, either of which may require surgical management. The indications for a rotator cuff repair are persistent pain that interferes with activities of daily living (ADLs), work, or sports; patients who are unresponsive to a 4- to 6-month period of conservative care; or active young patients (younger than 50 years of age) with an acute full-thickness tear.[80] Three of the more common repair techniques are the open rotator cuff repair, the mini-open (arthroscopically assisted), and the arthroscopic repair.

- *Traditional open rotator cuff repair:* The open technique involves a vertical incision over the anterior shoulder. The deltoid is divided to allow access to the rotator cuff and subacromial space. An anterior and inferior acromioplasty is performed, and the rotator cuff is inspected because the method of repair is dependent on the extent of the tear. The coracoacromial ligament, an important structure in restraining upward migration of the humerus, is not resected unless major tightness is present or exposure is needed.[81]

> **● Key Point** Subacromial decompression procedures are used to remove the cause of the impingement of the humeral head and the undersurface of the acromion, thereby allowing freer movement. These procedures can include removal of the subacromial bursa (bursectomy), coracoacromial ligament resection, anterior acromioplasty, excision of the outer end of the clavicle, acromionectomy, osteotomies of the glenoid or acromion, and combinations of these procedures. In addition, other procedures may be required including capsular tightening, repair of the biceps brachii (long head), or labral reconstruction.

- *Mini-open:* There are two variations of this type of procedure, both of which involve arthroscopic subacromial decompression and a deltoid splitting approach.
- *Arthroscopic repair:* The role of arthroscopy in the treatment of rotator cuff lesions is evolving. The procedure has advanced remarkably over the past two decades,[82] from its original use as a diagnostic tool to an effective treatment option for patients with stage II impingement and acromioclavicular joint arthritis.[83–85] In the past, arthroscopic techniques were reserved for small or moderately sized partial- or full-thickness tears of the supraspinatus or infraspinatus.[86–88] Recently, repair of full-thickness rotator cuff tears using an arthroscopic

technique has been described.[89–92] The advantages of arthroscopic repair appear to include smaller skin incisions, glenohumeral joint inspection, treatment of intra-articular lesions, avoidance of deltoid detachment, less soft tissue dissection, and less pain.[80,89,92]

Regardless of the technique chosen, open or arthroscopic, the speed of the postsurgical rehabilitation remains unchanged because the limiting factor—tendon-to-bone healing—remains a constant. In addition, the speed of the progression is a factor of the status of the deltoid muscle, the size of the tear, and the ability to move the shoulder without injuring the tissues.[93,94]

Postsurgical Rehabilitation

Following the surgery, there are many factors that influence decisions about the position and duration of immobilization, the selection and application of exercises, and the rate of progression of each patient's postoperative rehabilitation program.[29] Postoperatively, the arm is typically protected in a sling or on a small abduction pillow. The type of immobilization depends on the amount of abduction required to position the affected rotator cuff tendons with little or no tension. A sling may be preferred if the tension on the repair is minimal or none with the arm at the side. Approximate periods of immobilization in a sling, at the discretion of the surgeon, are:

- *Small tears:* 1–3 weeks
- *Medium tears:* 3–6 weeks
- *Large and massive tears:* 6–8 weeks

An abduction orthosis is recommended if the tension through the repair site is minimal or none with the arm in 20–40 degrees of abduction. Approximate periods of immobilization in the orthosis, at the discretion of the surgeon, are:

- *Small tears:* 6 weeks
- *Medium tears:* 6 weeks
- *Large and massive tears:* 8 weeks

Depending on the surgeon, a continuous passive motion machine (CPMM) may be prescribed to prevent the degenerating effects of immobilization, provide nourishment to the articular cartilage, and assist in collagen synthesis and organization.[94–97] However, manual PROM exercises have been found to be more cost-effective and to yield results similar to those of a CPMM.[94] The degree of movement permitted during the first 6 weeks is guided by the

stability of the operative repair and the surgeon's preference.[98] External rotation motion beyond neutral is usually restricted for the first 4 weeks.[81] The rehabilitation progression then closely follows that described in the "General Intervention Strategies" section earlier in this chapter.

● **Key Point** Recommendations for the safest position of the shoulder in which to begin isometric training of the glenohumeral musculature following repair are inconsistent. The PTA should always check with the supervising PT or surgeon.

Glenohumeral Instability

Instability is the abnormal symptomatic motion of the GH joint that affects normal joint kinematics and results in pain, subluxation, or dislocation of the shoulder.[99–102] In the early years of life, the GH joint remains fairly stable due to the active mechanisms stabilizing the joint. However, if the person begins to decondition with time, the dynamic mechanisms become unable to support the joint. The joint becomes involved in a self-perpetuating cycle of more instability, less use, more shoulder dysfunction, and more instability. In addition to shoulder capsular redundancy, underlying causes of GH instability can include genetic, biochemical (collagen), and biomechanical factors.[103] Characteristic of this pattern is the complaint of the shoulder "slipping" or "popping out" during overhead activities.

Instability of the shoulder can be classified by frequency, magnitude, direction, and origin.[8] The frequency of occurrence is classified as acute or chronic. Acute traumatic instability with dislocation of the shoulder is the most striking variety, and often requires immediate manipulative reduction. Shoulder instability is also classified according to the direction of the subluxation. These instabilities can be unidirectional (anterior, posterior, or inferior), bidirectional, or multidirectional. Posterior instability results either from avulsion of the posterior glenoid labrum from the posterior glenoid or from a stretching of the posterior capsuloligamentous structures.

Anterior Instability

Anterior instability of the GH joint is the most common direction of instability. Anterior instability occurs when the abducted shoulder is repetitively placed in the anterior apprehension position of external rotation and horizontal abduction. Such individuals may have pain with overhead movements due to an inability to control their laxity by means of their muscles. They may develop enough instability directed superiorly that they present with impingement-like symptoms (instability–impingement overlap), especially in positions of abduction and external rotation.[104] Unilateral dislocations occurring from acute traumatic events can cause secondary lesions, including the Bankart lesion and the Hill-Sachs lesion (Figure 16-32).

- The Bankart lesion is an avulsion of the anterior inferior labrum from the glenoid rim and requires surgical stabilization (*t*raumatic, *u*nidirectional instability with *B*ankart lesion requiring *s*urgery, or TUBS).
- The Hill-Sachs lesion is a compression fracture on the posterior humeral head at the site where the humeral head impacted the inferior glenoid rim.

Chronic recurrent dislocations of the shoulder can lead to degenerative arthritis. An older person who dislocates a shoulder is likely to have concurrently torn the rotator cuff.[105–107] Lesser traumatic injuries can cause subluxation of the shoulder to such a degree that recurrent subluxation rather than dislocation becomes a source of dysfunction.[102]

The mechanism for a subluxation or recurrent dislocation usually involves a fall on an outstretched hand (FOOSH) injury, whereby the arm is forced into abduction, extension, and external rotation.

Posterior Instability

Posterior instabilities are rare, and comprise approximately 2 percent of all shoulder dislocations.[108] Posterior dislocations are often associated with seizure, electric shock, diving into a shallow pool, or motor vehicle accidents. Patients who have symptoms with the arm in a forward flexed, adducted position, such as when pushing open heavy doors, have a posterior instability pattern. These dislocations are classified as subacromial (posterior and inferior to the acromion process), subglenoid (posterior and inferior to the glenoid rim), and subspinous (medial to the acromion and inferior to the scapular spine), with the former being the more common for posterior dislocations.[8] The classic sign for a posterior dislocation is a loud clunk as the shoulder is moved from a forward flexed position to an abducted and externally rotated

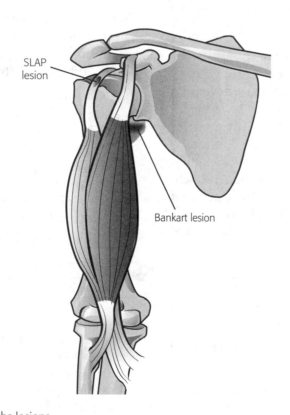

SLAP lesion

Bankart lesion

Figure 16-32   Bankart and Hill-Sachs lesions.

position (due to the relocation of the posteriorly sub-luxed humerus, a positive finding often associated and confused with an anterior dislocation).

Inferior Instability

Inferior dislocations are uncommon. Inferior insta-bility is elicited by carrying heavy objects at one's side (e.g., grocery bag, a suitcase), or by hyperabduc-tion forces that cause a levering of the humeral neck against the acromion.[99,109] Inferior subluxation is common after CNS injury secondary to weakness of the shoulder girdle and the scapular stabilizers.

Multidirectional Instability

Multidirectional instability is symptomatic GH insta-bility in more than one direction (anteriorly, inferiorly, and posteriorly).[99] Multidirectional instability is often described using the abbreviation AMBRII (*a*traumatic onset of *m*ultidirectional instability that is accompa-nied by *b*ilateral laxity or hypermobility. *R*ehabilita-tion is the primary course of intervention to restore GH stability. However, if an operation is necessary, a proce-dure such as a capsulorrhaphy is performed to tighten the *i*nferior capsule and the rotator *i*nterval).[110]

> ● **Key Point** It is commonly believed that females have more joint laxity than males, a fact propagated by the medical literature and medical training.[103] However, with the exception of a few articles, there are inadequate data to confirm this view.

SLAP Lesions

SLAP lesions are defined as *superior *l*abral lesions that are both *a*nterior and *p*osterior. Individuals performing overhead movements may develop a "dead arm" syndrome[111] in which they have a pain-ful shoulder. The main problem is usually a tear of the superior labrum, the so-called SLAP lesion.[112] The lesion can also result from a FOOSH injury, sudden deceleration or traction forces such as catch-ing a falling heavy object, a motor vehicle accident (e.g., drivers who have their hands on the wheel and sustain a rear-end impact), or chronic anterior and posterior instability.[113,114]

> ● **Key Point** The superior aspect of the labrum is more mobile and prone to injury due to its close attachment to the long head of the biceps tendon.[8]

SLAP lesions can be classified into four main types[114] by signs and symptoms:

- *Type I:* This type involves a fraying and degen-eration of the edge of the superior labrum. The patient loses the ability to horizontally abduct

or externally rotate with the forearm pronated without pain.[115]
- *Type II:* This type involves a pathologic detach-ment of the labrum and biceps tendon anchor, resulting in a loss of the stabilizing effect of the labrum and the biceps.[116]
- *Type III:* This type involves a vertical tear of the labrum, similar to the bucket-handle tear of the meniscus, although the remaining portions of the labrum and biceps are intact.[8]
- *Type IV:* This type involves an extension of the bucket-handle tear into the biceps tendon, with portions of the labral flap and biceps tendon displaceable into the GH joint.[8]

Maffet et al.[117] have suggested expanding the clas-sification scale to a total of seven categories, adding descriptions for types V through VII.

- *Type V:* This type is characterized by the pres-ence of a Bankart lesion of the anterior capsule that extends into the anterior superior labrum.
- *Type VI:* This type involves a disruption of the biceps tendon anchor with an anterior or poste-rior superior labral flap tear.
- *Type VII:* This is described as the extension of a SLAP lesion anteriorly to involve the area inferior to the middle GH ligament.

Conservative Approach

The general conservative approach for all forms of GH instability following the period of immobiliza-tion includes the following:

- *Avoidance of provocative positions (those that reproduce the mechanism of dislocation):* While avoiding these positions, the principles of PRICEMEM are followed and active motion exercises are prescribed for the elbow (without compromising the shoulder), wrist, and hand. Submaximal isometrics for the shoulder can be initiated while the arm is maintained in the sling and immobilizer.

> ● **Key Point** Positions to avoid following an anterior shoulder subluxation include shoulder abduction and external rotation.

- *Scapular stability exercises:* These can be started early, and in this early stage the control of the scapula position can be aided by taping the scap-ula in a retracted or elevated position, or by the use of a figure-8 collar, both of which help to normalize the scapular muscle firing pattern.[5]
- *Closed chain exercises:* These exercises,

normally performed with the hand stabilized on a wall or object, simulate normal functional patterns and reorganize and re-establish normal motor firing patterns.[5,118–120] All of the movements of the scapula and shoulder are coupled and are predictable based on arm position.[26,121] Closed chain exercises should involve integration of all the joints in the appropriate kinetic chain with the specific scapular maneuvers of elevation, depression, retraction, and protraction.[5]

- *Early exercises to rehabilitate scapulohumeral rhythm:* These include modified push-ups, and progress to facilitation patterns that include hip extension, trunk extension, and scapular retraction.[122] Clock exercises, in which the scapula is rotated in elevation/depression and retraction/protraction, also develop coordinated patterns for scapular control.[122]

Open chain exercises follow the isometric and gentle closed chain activities because these exercises are more strenuous.[5] The criteria to progress to this phase include full, nonpainful ROM, no palpable tenderness, and uninterrupted progression of shoulder strength. While performing the open chain exercises, care must be taken to avoid the provocative positions of abduction and external rotation. Typical open chain exercises include PNF patterns/diagonals, upright rows, and external rotation and scapular retraction activities as well as machine exercises consisting of lat pull-downs.[5] Weight-bearing exercises through the upper extremities are introduced once the patient has regained sufficient strength in motion, as deemed by the supervising physical therapist.

Surgical Intervention

When the glenohumeral joint subluxes or dislocates, either traumatically or atraumatically, significant capsular stretching can occur. Capsular stretching, in turn, can result in glenohumeral joint laxity or instability, depending on the severity. To regain shoulder stability, these lesions may require surgical repair, with the aim of alleviating pain while permitting the range of motion (ROM) and strength to return to premorbid levels.[48,123–126] Surgical intervention is reserved for patients who remain symptomatic or disabled following the conservative intervention, or those whose instability is so gross that conservative intervention is not deemed appropriate.[127]

A number of surgical procedures exist for instability of the shoulder, including:

- *Bankart:* The Bankart repair involves an open or arthroscopic reattachment of the torn joint capsule to the glenoid. During the repair an anterior capsulolabral reconstruction is performed to reattach the labrum to the surface of the glenoid lip. The proposed advantages of arthroscopic stabilization over the traditional open repairs include smaller skin incisions, more complete inspection of the glenohumeral joint, the ability to treat intra-articular lesions, access to all areas of the glenohumeral joint for repair, less soft tissue dissection, and maximum preservation of external rotation.[128]

- *Capsulorrhaphy:* This technique, which can be performed using either an open or arthroscopic approach, involves tightening the capsule to reduce capsular redundancy and overall capsule volume. The type of procedure used is tailored to the direction of instability, although most procedures are performed because of anterior instability.

- *Electrothermally assisted capsulorrhaphy:*[127] The electrothermally assisted capsulorrhaphy (ETAC) or thermal assisted capsular shift (TACS) is a relatively recent procedure to treat shoulder instability. The thermal capsulorrhaphy technique applies thermal energy, laser, or radiofrequency to the capsular tissues. Ultimately, this shrinks (denatures) the collagen, which tightens the entire anterior and inferior capsule. To resolve posterior instability, the surgeon introduces the thermal capsulorrhaphy probe posteriorly, directly heating the tissue of the posterior capsule. One of the advantages of this procedure is that the patient is often permitted to perform active range of motion (AROM) within 3 days of the surgery.[129,130] Whether this translates into better outcomes has yet to be determined.

> ● **Key Point** The Bristow procedure, no longer in favor, involved the surgical repositioning of the tip of the coracoid process (as well as the attached coracobrachialis and the short head of the biceps) to the anterior glenoid rim to form a bony block.

- *SLAP lesion repair:* An arthroscopic repair that involves debridement of the torn portion of the superior labrum, abrasion of the bony surface of the superior glenoid, and reattachment of the labrum and biceps tendon with tacks and suture anchors. An anterior stabilization procedure may also be performed as appropriate.

Acute Phase Rehabilitation

The goals of the postsurgical rehabilitation process are to restore functional flexibility and to strengthen the rotator cuff muscles and scapular stabilizers while protecting the healing capsule and other tissues involved. The rehabilitation program depends largely on the procedure that was performed and on the surgeon's preferences. There is typically a period of immobilization (ranging from 1 to 3 weeks to as long as 6 to 8 weeks) in a sling or shoulder immobilizer with the position of immobilization determined by the direction of instability prior to the surgery.

- Following the procedure for a recurrent anterior or anteroinferior instability, the shoulder is immobilized in a sling or splint in adduction or varying degrees of abduction and in internal rotation with the arm slightly anterior to the frontal plane of the body.
- Following the procedure for posterior or posteroinferior instability, the upper extremity is supported in an orthosis, and the shoulder is immobilized in neutral rotation to 10 to 20 degrees of external rotation, 20 to 30 degrees of abduction, elbow flexed, and the arm positioned at the side or sometimes with the shoulder in slight extension.

During the period of immobilization, the patient can perform active elbow, wrist, hand, and finger exercises, and pain-free submaximal isometric exercises for the shoulder. With the supervising physical therapist's permission, electrical stimulation can be used for edema reduction, muscle re-education, and pain control.[131–134] A progressive cardiovascular program is initiated, using a walking program or a stationary bike. The time at which the immobilizer may be temporarily removed for exercises varies significantly and depends on a number of factors determined by the surgeon. There are also a number of precautions that must be taken based on the procedure:[29]

- Following an anterior glenohumeral stabilization procedure and/or Bankart repair, care must be taken to limit external rotation, horizontal abduction, and extension during the first 6 weeks. Forward flexion is progressed more cautiously following arthroscopic stabilization as compared to an open stabilization.

  - Following a bony procedure, passive or assisted range of motion is delayed for 6 to 8 weeks to allow time for bone healing.
  - Following a procedure that involved subscapularis detachment and repair, no active or assisted internal rotation is permitted for 4 to 6 weeks.
  - The patient should be advised to avoid functional activities that place stress on the anterior aspect of the capsule for about 4 to 6 weeks. For example, activities that require external rotation, especially if combined with horizontal abduction, should be avoided as should upper extremity weight-bearing, particularly if the shoulder is extended.

- Following a procedure that involved thermally assisted capsular tightening, range of motion exercises should be performed with extreme caution for the first 4 to 6 weeks; additional precautions depend on the direction of instability.
- Following a posterior stabilization procedure and/or reverse Bankart repair, all shoulder exercises are postponed or arm elevation is limited to 90 degrees, internal rotation is limited to neutral or no more than 15 to 20 degrees, and horizontal adduction is restricted to neutral for up to 6 weeks postoperatively.
- Following SLAP lesion repair, progression in cases where the biceps tendon was detached is more cautious than when the biceps remains intact.

  - Passive or assisted elevation of the arm is limited to 60 degrees for the first 2 weeks and to 90 degrees at weeks 3 to 4 postoperatively.
  - Passive assisted humeral rotation is performed in the plane of the scapula for the first 2 weeks (external rotation to only neutral or up to 15 degrees, and internal rotation to 45 degrees); during weeks 3 to 4, external rotation is progressed to 30 degrees and internal rotation to 60 degrees.
  - The patient is educated to avoid positions that create tension in the biceps, such as elbow extension with shoulder extension, and abduction combined with maximum external rotation, during the first 4 to 6 weeks postoperatively.

To help achieve the restoration of shoulder mobility, pendulum exercises (nonweighted) are performed for the first 2 weeks postoperatively. In addition, self-assisted range of motion wand exercises for the glenohumeral joint are performed, initially within protected ranges as early as 2 weeks or as late as 6 weeks postoperatively. Shoulder elevation exercises are begun in the supine position to help stabilize the scapula, and the humeral rotation exercises are performed with the arm supported in the shoulder in a slightly abducted and flexed position.

- *Anterior stabilization:* Gradually progress to near complete range of motion by 6 to 8 weeks, except for external rotation and extension and horizontal abduction past neutral.
- *Posterior stabilization:* Gradually progress to near complete range of motion by 6 to 8 weeks, taking care with forward flexion, horizontal abduction, and internal rotation.

Multiple-angle, low-intensity isometric (muscle setting) exercises are usually initiated as early as the first week or by 3 to 4 weeks postoperatively. The criteria for progression beyond this phase include a well-healed incision, progress in range of motion (active elevation to within 20–30 degrees compared with the uninvolved side, and the rotation to approximately 50–60 percent of the uninvolved side), and minimal pain.

Subacute Phase Rehabilitation

This phase typically begin 6 to 8 weeks postoperatively and continues until approximately 12 to 16 weeks.[127] The following resistive exercises can generally be initiated with an emphasis on internal and external rotation:

- The supraspinatus is exercised actively in isolation using the so-called empty can position (internal rotation of the shoulder, thumb pointing to the floor, and abduction of the shoulder to 90 degrees while maintaining a position of 30 degrees anterior to the midfrontal plane).
- Horizontal abduction is initiated and is typically performed actively in the prone position, whereas horizontal adduction begins 1 week later and is performed in supine.
- Deltoid strengthening and shoulder proprioceptive neuromuscular facilitation (PNF) patterns are introduced based on the patient's tolerance and within the postsurgical range limitations.
- Internal and external rotation strengthening exercises are performed within permitted ranges with the arm at the side. Using an

axillary roll emphasizes the teres minor muscle; omission of the roll emphasizes the infraspinatus muscle.
- Active shoulder extension is performed in the prone position.
- Resisted exercises are added to the elbow and wrist.
- Gentle hands-and-knees rocking is initiated and progressed to gentle three-point rocking. Progressive upper extremity weight bearing is added as tolerated.
- The stretching phase of the program is initiated, taking care to observe the restrictions imposed by the surgery. For anterior instability repairs, external rotation is typically limited to −15 degrees compared with the uninvolved side, and internal rotation is limited similarly for posterior instability repairs. In fact, it is a good idea to allow the patient to achieve the last 15 degrees of each motion at his or her own speed, rather than risk overstretching the capsule too early and possibly compromising the repair.

Eccentric cuff exercises involving internal rotation, abduction, external rotation, adduction, and shoulder flexion are initiated and progressed based on patient tolerance. Functional activities are introduced as tolerated.

Frozen Shoulder/Adhesive Capsulitis

In 1945, Neviaser coined the term *adhesive capsulitis* to describe his findings of a chronic inflammatory process at surgery and autopsy in patients treated for a painful, stiff shoulder.[135] Significant evidence exists[136–139] in support of the hypothesis that the underlying pathologic changes in adhesive capsulitis are synovial inflammation with subsequent reactive capsular fibrosis, making adhesive capsulitis an inflammatory and a fibrosing condition, dependent on the stage of the disease.

> ● **Key Point** Factors associated with adhesive capsulitis include female gender,[140] age older than 40 years,[141] trauma,[141] diabetes,[142–147] prolonged immobilization,[148] thyroid disease,[149–151] stroke or myocardial infarction,[145,152] certain psychiatric conditions,[153,154] and the presence of autoimmune diseases.[136,138]

Nash and Hazelman[155] have described the concept of primary and secondary frozen shoulder.

Primary Adhesive Capsulitis

With primary adhesive capsulitis (PAC), the pathogenesis may be a provoking chronic inflammation in the musculotendinous or synovial tissue such as the rotator cuff, biceps tendon, or joint capsule. PAC, which usually occurs between the ages of 40 and 60 years, is characterized by a progressive and painful loss of active and passive shoulder motion, particularly external rotation, which causes the individual to gradually limit the use of the arm. Difficulty is reported with putting on a jacket or coat, putting objects in back pockets, or hooking garments in the back.[156–159] Inflammation and pain can cause muscle guarding of the shoulder muscles, without true fixed contracture of the joint capsule. Disuse of the arm results in a loss of shoulder mobility, whereas continued use of the arm through pain can result in development of subacromial impingement.[160] Over a period of weeks, compensatory movements of the shoulder girdle develop in order to minimize pain.[160] With time, there is resolution of pain and the individual is left with a stiff shoulder with severe limitation of function.

Secondary or Idiopathic Adhesive Capsulitis

Zuckerman and Cuomo[161] defined idiopathic adhesive capsulitis as a condition characterized by significant restriction of both active and passive shoulder motion that occurs in the absence of a known intrinsic shoulder disorder.

Stages of Progression

Neviaser[135] suggests that adhesive capsulitis passes through three stages based on pathologic changes in the synovium and subsynovium.[8]

- *Freezing:* Patients present with intense pain even at rest. A capsular pattern of motion (loss of external rotation and abduction) is present by 2 to 3 weeks after the onset, as is a more subtle loss of internal rotation and adduction. In this early stage, the majority of motion loss is secondary to the painful synovitis, rather than a true capsular contraction. These acute symptoms may last 10 to 36 weeks.
- *Frozen:* This stage is characterized by pain only with movement. Patients often report a history of an extremely painful phase that has resolved, resulting in a relatively pain-free but stiff shoulder. The motion loss reflects a loss of capsular volume and a response to the painful synovitis. The patient demonstrates a loss of motion in all planes, and pain in all parts of the range. There may be evidence of atrophy of the rotator cuff, biceps, deltoid, and triceps brachii. This stage lasts 4 to 12 months.
- *Thawing:* This stage is characterized by the slow, steady recovery of some of the lost ROM

resulting from capsular remodeling in response to use of the arm and shoulder. Although many people feel less restricted in this phase, objective measurement shows only minor improvement.[162]

Common impairments and functional limitations associated with the various stages of adhesive capsulitis include:

- Pain, which can occur on motion or at rest and disturb sleep during acute flares
- Inability to reach overhead, behind the head, and behind the back, leading to difficulties dressing, reaching, self-grooming, and eating
- Decreased joint play and range of motion
- General muscle weakness and guarded shoulder motions with substitute scapular motions
- Limited ability to sustain repetitive activities

Intervention

Conventional management for adhesive capsulitis includes patient advice, medical intervention (analgesics, NSAIDs, steroid injection), and a wide variety of physical therapy methods.[163] Pajareya and colleagues[163] performed a randomized controlled trial of 122 patients to study the effectiveness of a combination of physical therapy techniques and ibuprofen versus ibuprofen alone. The physical therapy intervention (three times a week for 3 weeks) included short-wave diathermy, joint mobilizations, and passive glenohumeral stretching exercises up to the patient's tolerance. At 3 weeks it was concluded that the treatment group demonstrated more beneficial effects than the group using ibuprofen alone.[163]

The primary goal of conservative intervention is based on the stage of healing:[42,144,160,164–166]

- *Acute/freezing:* Maximum protection through immobilization in a sling and intermittent periods of passive or assisted motion within all pain-free/protected ranges of motion, including the pendulum exercise. The exercises are progressed to include active range of motion using correct joint and muscle mechanics, and gentle (pain-free) muscle setting exercises to all muscle groups of the shoulder and elbow. For example, if the deltoid is overactive, the humeral head may be held superiorly, making it difficult and/ or painful to abduct the shoulder because the greater tuberosity impinges on the coracoacromial arch. Emphasis should be placed on developing control of the weak musculature before progressing to strengthening functional patterns of motion. The trust and confidence of the patient is necessary during this stage, and it is important to ensure that no harm is caused or that the clinician does not indicate any frustration. A sample rehabilitation protocol for adhesive capsulitis is outlined in **Table 16-11**.

- *Subacute/frozen:* The application of controlled tensile stresses to produce elongation of the restricting tissues. The range of motion exercises for the shoulder and scapular motions are progressed to the point of pain. As a general guideline, the patient with capsular restriction and low irritability may require aggressive soft tissue and joint mobilization, whereas patients with high irritability may

TABLE 16-11	Rehabilitation Protocol for Adhesive Capsulitis
Freezing Phase	**Intervention**
Therapeutic exercises	Controlled, pain-free PROM exercises. Focus is on stretching at ROM limits.
	No restrictions on passive range, but PTA and patient have to communicate to avoid injuries.
	Initially focus on forward flexion and external and internal rotation with the arm at the side and the elbow at 90 degrees.
	Active assisted ROM exercises.
	Active ROM exercises.
	A home exercise program should be instituted from the beginning.
	• Patients should perform their ROM exercises three to five times per day.
	• A sustained stretch of 15–30 seconds at the end of the ROM exercises should be part of all ROM routines.
Therapeutic modalities	Ice, nonpulsed ultrasound, electrical stimulation.
Frozen Phase	**Intervention**
Therapeutic exercises	Active ROM exercises.
	Rotator cuff strengthening—three times per week, 8–12 repetitions for three sets.
	Closed-chain isometric strengthening with the elbow flexed to 90 degrees and the arm at the side:
	• External rotation
	• Abduction
	• Forward flexion
	Progress to open-chain strengthening:
	• Internal rotation
	• External rotation
	• Abduction
	• Forward flexion
	Strengthening of scapular stabilizers.
	Closed-chain strengthening exercises:
	• Scapular retraction (rhomboideus, middle trapezius)
	• Scapular protraction (serratus anterior)
	• Scapular depression (latissimus dorsi, trapezius, serratus anterior)
	• Shoulder shrugs (trapezius, levator scapulae)
	Deltoid strengthening.
	Home maintenance exercise program; ROM exercises two times a day.
Thawing Phase	**Intervention**
Therapeutic exercises	Stretching and strengthening exercises are progressed as the joint tissue tolerates. By this time, the patient should be actively involved in self-stretching and strengthening, so emphasis during treatment is on correct mechanics, safe progressions, and exercise strategies for return to function. If the patient is involved in repetitive heavy lifting, exercises are progressed to replicate these demands.

require pain-easing manual therapy techniques.[167] During this stage, the patient can be taught a number of self-stretches, including those in (Figure 16-33) though (Figure 16-35). During the arm elevation exercises, the patient should be taught to avoid hiking the shoulder. The muscle setting exercises introduced during the acute phase are progressed to include protected weight bearing, such as leaning on the hands against the wall or table. These exercises stimulate co-contraction of the rotator cuff and scapular stabilizing muscles. Once tolerated, these exercises can be progressed to include gentle rocking forward/backward and side to side.

- *Chronic/thawing:* Return to function. The goals during this phase are to increase range of motion and progress to strengthening exercises (refer to Table 16-11).

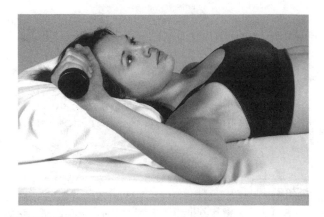

Figure 16-33   Stretch into ER using weight.

● **Key Point**   Complex regional pain syndrome type I is a potential complication after shoulder injury or immobility. Therefore, special attention should be given to the hand, with additional exercises, such as having the patient repetitively squeeze a ball or other soft object.[29]

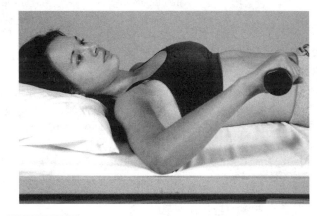

Figure 16-34   Stretch into IR using weight.

Sternoclavicular Joint Sprain

The SC joint is less involved with osteoarthritis or mechanical conditions than is the AC joint.[156] The joint can sustain sprains, dislocations, or physeal injuries, usually secondary to a fall on an outstretched hand (FOOSH) with the arm in either a flexed and adducted position, or an extended and adducted position.[104] The joint also can be injured through motor vehicle accidents and sports.[168] The well-developed interarticular meniscus can be torn and can lead secondarily to degenerative changes. Irritation of this joint may also occur in inflammatory conditions, such as rheumatoid arthritis or repetitive microtrauma.[169] Infection of this joint usually indicates a systemic source, such as bacterial endocarditis.[156] SC sprains are graded according to severity.[170]

- *Type I:* Sprain of SC ligament
- *Type II:* Subluxation, partial tear of capsular ligaments, disk, or costoclavicular ligaments
- *Type IIA:* Anterior subluxation; this is the most common grade
- *Type IIB:* Posterior subluxation; these have the potential to result in circulatory vessel

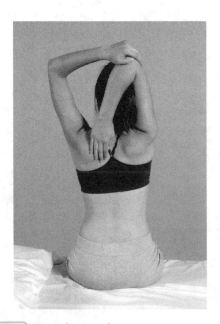

Figure 16-35   Capsular stretch.

compromise, nerve tissue impingement, and difficulty swallowing[169]

- *Type IIIA:* Anterior dislocation
- *Type IIIB:* Posterior dislocation
- *Type IV:* Habitual dislocation (rare)

SC dislocations, although rare, are frequently delayed in their diagnosis. Any trauma to the shoulder girdle may cause an SC dislocation, which is more common and more obvious when it occurs in the anterior direction.[171]

The common impairments associated with these injuries include:[29]

- Pain localized to the involved structure
- Painful arc with shoulder elevation
- Pain with shoulder horizontal adduction or abduction
- Hypomobility (if sustained posture or immobility is involved) or hypermobility (if trauma or overuse is involved)

Intervention

The conservative intervention involves the following:[29]

- Placing the arm in a sling to support the weight of the arm
- Transverse frictional massage to the capsule or ligaments
- Progressive range of motion to the shoulder (PROM, then AAROM, then AROM)

Acromioclavicular Joint Sprain

Disorders of the AC joint are commonly seen in the athletic population. Injuries to this joint can be categorized as either acute traumatic or chronic injuries.[7] The majority of traumatic injuries occur from a fall onto the shoulder with the arm adducted at the side. The chronic disorder may be atraumatic or posttraumatic, with the former being attributed to generalized osteoarthritis, inflammatory arthritis, or mechanical problems of the meniscus of this joint.[156] Injuries to the AC joint were originally classified by Tossy and colleagues[172] and Allman[173] as incomplete (grades I and II) or complete (grade III). This classification has been expanded to include six types of injuries based on the direction and amount of displacement (**Table 16-12**).[174–177]

- Types I–III and V all involve inferior displacement of the acromion with respect to the clavicle. They differ in the severity of injury

to the ligaments and the amount of resultant displacement.[178]

- Types I and II usually result from a fall or a blow to the point on the lateral aspect of the shoulder, or a FOOSH, producing a sprain.
- Types III and IV usually involve a dislocation (commonly called AC separation) and a distal clavicle fracture, both of which commonly disrupt the coracoclavicular ligaments.[7] In addition, damage to the deltoid and trapezius fascia, and rarely the skin, can occur.[7] Type IV injuries are characterized by posterior displacement of the clavicle.
- Type VI injuries have a clavicle inferiorly displaced into either a subacromial or subcoracoid position.[7]

Pain with AC sprains is typically reproduced at the end range of passive elevation, passive external and internal rotation, and passive horizontal adduction, across the chest. This cross-arm test compresses the AC joint and is highly sensitive for AC joint pathology.[6,7,175,179] The ROM available depends on the stage of healing and severity. In the very acute stage, range may be limited by pain, whereas the less acute stage will be painful at the end of range in full elevation or horizontal adduction.

The common impairments associated with these injuries include:[29]

- Pain localized to the involved structure
- Painful arc with shoulder elevation
- Pain with shoulder horizontal adduction or abduction
- Hypomobility (if sustained posture or immobility is involved) or hypermobility (if trauma or overuse is involved)

Intervention

The intervention for these patients depends on the severity of the injury and the physical demands of the patient.

- *Types I and II:* These patients will usually recover full painless function with conservative and medical (NSAIDs and analgesics) intervention.[6] Ice should be used judiciously. Most physicians prescribe a sling for 1–2 weeks. Gentle ROM exercises and functional rehabilitation are started immediately after the period of immobilization, followed by isometric exercises to those muscles with clavicular attachments. The exercises are progressed

Type	Description	Clinical Findings	Recommended Interventions
I	Isolated sprain of acromioclavicular ligaments with intact coracoclavicular ligaments, and deltoid and trapezoid muscles	Include tenderness and mild pain at the AC joint, high (160–180 degrees) painful arc, and pain with resisted horizontal adduction.	TFM, ice, and pain-free AROM
II	The AC ligament is disrupted and there is a sprain of the coracoclavicular ligament.	A wider AC joint gap with possible slight vertical separation when compared to the normal shoulder. In addition, the coracoclavicular interspace may be slightly increased, but the deltoid and trapezoid muscles remain intact. There is moderate to severe local pain and tenderness in the coracoclavicular space. PROM is painful in all end ranges but especially with horizontal adduction. Resisted abduction and adduction are also often painful.	Initiate with ice and pain-free AROM/PROM
III	The AC joint is dislocated and the shoulder complex displaced inferiorly. The AC ligament is disrupted and the coracoclavicular interspace is 25–100 percent greater than the normal shoulder due to coracoclavicular ligament disruption. In addition, the deltoid and trapezoid muscles are usually detached from the distal end of the clavicle.	Clinical findings include the arm is held in an adducted position by the patient and there is an obvious gap visible between the acromion and clavicle. AROM is all painful, but PROM is painless if done carefully.	Initiate with ice and pain-free AROM/PROM
IV	The AC ligament is disrupted and the AC joint is dislocated with the clavicle anatomically displaced posteriorly into or through the trapezius muscle. The deltoid and trapezoid muscles are detached from the distal end of the clavicle. In addition, the coracoclavicular ligaments are completely disrupted. Although the coracoclavicular interspace may be displaced, it may appear normal.	A posteriorly displaced clavicle.	Surgery is indicated
V	The AC and coracoclavicular ligaments are disrupted. The AC joint is dislocated and there is gross disparity between the clavicle and the scapula (300–500 percent greater than normal). In addition, the deltoid and trapezoid muscles are detached from the distal end of the clavicle.	Tenderness over the entire lateral half of the clavicle.	Surgery is indicated
VI	The AC ligaments are disrupted and the coracoclavicular ligaments are completely disrupted. The AC joint is dislocated and the clavicle is anatomically displaced inferior to the clavicle or the coracoid process. In addition, the deltoid and trapezoid muscles are detached from the distal end of the clavicle. Often accompanied by clavicle or upper rib fracture and/or brachial plexus injury.	The coracoclavicular interspace is reversed with the clavicle being inferior to the acromion or the coracoid process. The superior aspect of the shoulder is flatter than the opposite side.	Surgery is indicated

AROM, active range of motion; PROM, passive range of motion.

to progressive resistive exercises (PREs) for the muscles that attach to the clavicle and the scapular pivoters. A graduated return to full activity is very important. Most patients will be back to full sport participation within 12 weeks, although they may have a slight cosmetic deformity.[7]

- *Type III:* The intervention for type III injuries is controversial.[7] The natural history of this injury with conservative intervention suggests that patients have no long-term difficulty with pain or loss of function.[180–184] There is a reported high complication rate with attempts at surgical stabilization.[185,186] Once the sling is removed, pendulum exercises can be initiated. PROM in the extremes of motion are avoided for the first 7 days, but the goal should be for full PROM after 2–3 weeks. A graduated resistance exercise program is initiated once pain is improved and AROM is full. These exercises should emphasize strengthening of the deltoid and upper trapezius muscles and promote dynamic stabilization of the shoulder complex.[187] Full return to sport is expected by 6–12 weeks.[7] If patients are still functionally limited after more than 3 months, a secondary reconstructive procedure may be necessary.[7]
- *Types IV, V, and VI:* These more unusual types of displacement all require surgical intervention.[6] The greater displacement and injury includes damage to the deltoid and trapezius muscle and fascia. Failure to reduce these and repair them may lead to chronic pain and dysfunction.[7] The postsurgical progression involves gaining pain-free ROM prior to advancing to exercises to regain strength, manual techniques to normalize arthrokinematics, and functional training to improve neuromuscular control of the shoulder complex.

Clavicle Fractures

Fractures of the clavicle usually result from a FOOSH, a fall or blow to the point of the shoulder, or less commonly from a direct blow.[173] Patients with a clavicle fracture demonstrate guarded shoulder motions and have difficulty elevating the arm beyond 60 degrees. A clavicular deformity is usually observable. There also is exquisite tenderness to palpation or percussion (bony tap) over the fracture site. Horizontal adduction is painful. The diagnosis is confirmed by radiograph.

Intervention

The intervention for clavicle fractures includes approximation of the fracture ends followed by immobilization with a sling and figure-8 strap for 6–8 weeks. Using pain as a guide, AROM and PROM exercises for the shoulder can be initiated 1 week after the fitting of the figure-8 strap. Joint mobilizations are started immediately after the period of immobilization, and strengthening exercises for the deltoid and upper trapezius muscles are prescribed when appropriate.

Proximal Humeral Fractures

A proximal humeral fracture is the most common fracture of the humerus and typically results from a direct blow to the anterior, lateral, or posterolateral aspect of the humerus, or a FOOSH injury.[188] Like hip fractures, proximal humerus fractures represent a major morbidity in the elderly population. Proximal humeral fractures involve the proximal third of the humerus. These fractures are classified based on severity:

- *Nondisplaced:* The majority of proximal humeral fractures are stable with no significant displacement of the fracture.
- *Displaced:* These types of fractures include:
  - Greater tuberosity fractures
  - Lesser tuberosity fractures
  - Surgical neck fractures
  - Anatomic head fractures
  - Three-part fractures (One tuberosity is displaced and retracted by its attached rotator cuff musculature. The humeral head and the other tuberosity remain attached and are subluxated or dislocated.)
  - Four-part fractures (Detachment of both tuberosities and dislocation of the humeral head from the glenoid.)

Because proximal humeral fractures may result from a fall in the clinic, the PTA needs to be aware of the common findings with this type of fracture:

- *Complaints of pain and loss of function of the involved extremity:* In general, unstable fractures are much more painful and often may require surgical stabilization to allow for adequate pain relief.
- *Swelling and ecchymosis about the shoulder and upper arm:* The presence of extensive ecchymosis may become visible 24–48 hours following injury.

● **Key Point** The axillary nerve is the most common nerve injured in a proximal humerus fracture.

Intervention

Rehabilitation of humerus fractures depends on the severity and complexity of the initial fracture, patient compliance, medical comorbidities, and the means used to secure fixation of the fracture site.

Nondisplaced

This type is typically treated conservatively, with an emphasis on controlling distal edema and stiffness, and early motion at the shoulder to prevent the development of arthrofibrosis (frozen shoulder) secondary to prolonged immobilization.[189] The arm is usually immobilized in a sling until pain and discomfort subsides, often after 2 weeks. AROM exercises for the wrist and hand are initiated immediately. Typically, passive and active assisted exercises for the shoulder can be initiated about 1 week after injury. Clinical unity of the fracture usually occurs after 1–4 weeks.

Once clinical unity has been established, gentle AROM exercises are initiated for the shoulder and elbow. At this point, full PROM exercises to the shoulder and elbow are performed, with progressive resistive exercises typically initiated at 6–8 weeks.

Displaced

If left untreated, displaced fractures have a greater likelihood than nondisplaced fractures of producing limited function. Operative treatment of proximal humerus fractures includes either closed reduction with percutaneous fixation, open reduction and internal fixation (ORIF), or proximal humeral head replacement. The more complex fractures also require prolonged periods of immobilization to allow for bony healing. Once the patient has been managed by an orthopedic surgeon, and the immobilization device has been removed, the physical therapist will perform an examination. One focus of this examination will be to determine whether a concurrent neurovascular injury occurred.

The intervention goals in proximal humerus fractures are to allow bone and soft tissue healing to maximize function of the upper extremity while minimizing risk. The physical therapy intervention includes:

- Gentle range of motion exercises, which may begin after 7–10 days if the fracture is stable. Submaximal isometrics are initiated for the upper arm muscles, rotator cuff, and scapular stabilizers.
- More aggressive passive and active assisted range of motion can begin once bony union has occurred. The fracture is typically healed by the eighth week. As with the rehabilitation of any shoulder condition, the goal should be to achieve a correct scapulohumeral rhythm as compared to the uninvolved side. As healing permits, the rehabilitation program includes functional shoulder activities and resistance exercises.

Total Shoulder Replacement Arthroplasty

A total shoulder replacement (TSR) is a surgical option for elderly patients with cuff-deficient arthritic shoulders.[78] Other patients who may require a TSA include those with bone tumors, rheumatoid arthritis, Paget's disease, avascular necrosis of the humeral head, fracture dislocations, and recurrent dislocations.[190,191] The main indications for surgical intervention are unremitting pain, rather than decreased motion, and a failure of conservative measures. Additional considerations include patient age, loss of function, activity level, job requirements, and general health.[78]

Four types of replacement components traditionally have been used:

1. *Unconstrained:* This is the most widely used component due to its anatomical design. It consists of a shallow glenoid component combined with a stemmed humeral component. Although this type provides the greatest freedom of shoulder motion, it provides little inherent stability.
2. *Semiconstrained:* This type involves the use of a larger glenoid component that is hooded or cup

shaped with a head–neck angle of 60 degrees, which reportedly permits increased ROM while providing some stability.

3. *Reversed ball and socket:* This type, which consists of a small humeral socket that slides on a larger ball-shaped glenoid component, combines some degree of stability with mobility for rotator cuff–deficient shoulders that cannot be repaired.

4. *Constrained:* This type, rarely used because of the high rate of associated complications, was designed for patients who had severe deterioration of the rotator cuff but with a functioning deltoid. The glenoid and humeral components were coupled and fixed to bone.

> **● Key Point** A hemireplacement arthroplasty (hemiarthroplasty) in which one surface, the humeral head, is replaced, is often used when the articular surface and underlying bone of the humeral head have deteriorated but the glenoid fossa is reasonably intact, as seen with necrosis of the head of the humerus.[29,194]

Fixation of the prosthetic components is achieved with a press-fit, bio ingrowth, or cement. The type of fixation depends on the component, the underlying pathology, and the quality of bone stock. Although surgical techniques vary, most involve the dissection of the subscapularis or a rotator cuff repair, or a combination of both. In addition, the procedure may include capsular plication and tightening in cases of chronic glenohumeral subluxation or dislocation, and anterior acromioplasty if there is a history of impingement syndrome. In the operating room, before closing the incision, the surgeon determines the extent of shoulder ROM available, particularly elevation and external rotation that does not place undue stress on periarticular soft tissues or compromise GH joint stability.[29] The patient is usually placed in a sling or an elastic shoulder immobilizer following the operation, which positions the humerus in adduction, internal rotation, and slight forward flexion. An abduction splint may be issued if a rotator cuff repair is performed, and is worn for 6–8 weeks, according to the surgeon's instructions. The shoulder immobilizer is worn between exercise sessions and at night.

> **● Key Point** The amount of external rotation and active internal rotation that the patient can perform in the first 4 to 6 weeks is limited to motion parameters that are achieved at the time of surgery. Typically, the only motions not allowed in the early weeks are active internal rotation and active and passive external rotation beyond 35–40 degrees, but the PTA should always refer to the surgeon's protocol.

The final outcome following shoulder arthroplasty will depend on many factors including the quality of the soft tissue (especially the status of the rotator cuff), the quality of the bone, the type of implant and fixation used, the patient's expectations, and the quality of the rehabilitation program.[193] Only the surgeon knows the extent of soft tissue damage and repair, and the guidelines communicated to the clinician must be strongly adhered to. The goal of the postoperative rehabilitation process is to decrease pain and improve functional status while providing greater joint stability to the patient.

Intervention

Improvements in the surgical approach have allowed the rehabilitation process to occur soon after surgery. However, the rate of progression of the rehabilitation program is influenced by the pre- and postoperative integrity of the rotator cuff mechanism. In cases where there is an intact rotator cuff prior to shoulder arthroplasty, patients can be progressed more rapidly than those patients with a coexisting rotator cuff deficiency. The patient is advised to place a pillow under the humerus, positioning it in slight forward flexion, whenever he or she is lying supine. For a patient with an intact rotator cuff, therapeutic exercise is typically initiated 24–48 hours after the surgery and is usually performed twice daily until the PROM is at 140 degrees of passive forward flexion and scapular plane elevation, and 30–40 degrees of external rotation (humerus positioned in neutral to 30 degrees of abduction). These exercises may be delayed for approximately 3 weeks if subscapularis reattachment or lengthening was performed.[78] Sometimes, a continuous passive motion machine is prescribed by the physician. For a patient with an unconstrained TSR and sufficient postoperative static and dynamic shoulder stability, the goal of the conclusion of rehabilitation is to achieve active ROM equal to intraoperative ROM—ideally 140 to 150 degrees of shoulder elevation and 45 to 50 degrees of external rotation.[29] For a patient with a more constrained TSR, a deficient rotator cuff mechanism, or capsuloligamentous laxity, intraoperative ROM is typically less, and therefore postoperative goals focus more on developing dynamic stability and less on shoulder mobility.[29] The postoperative protocol outlined in **Table 16-13** can be used as a guideline for patients who are rotator cuff deficient, and the protocol outlined in **Table 16-14** can be used as a guideline for a patient without preoperative rotator cuff deficiency; however, the PTA must always use the surgeon's protocol.

TABLE 16-13	Rehabilitation Protocol Following Shoulder Arthroplasty (Rotator Cuff Deficient)

Phase 1	Intervention
Increase range of motion of involved shoulder while maintaining range of motion and strength of elbow, wrist, and hand	Continuous passive motion/passive ROM: • *Forward flexion:* 0–90 degrees • *External rotation at 30 degrees abduction:* 0–20 degrees • *Internal rotation at 30 degrees abduction:* 0–30 degrees Pendulum exercises Active range of motion of elbow and wrist Gripping exercises Pulley exercises (second week)
Initiate strengthening of involved shoulder	Isometric exercises for abductors and external/internal rotators Active assisted motion exercises (as tolerated)
Phase 2 (5–8 weeks)	**Intervention**
Increase range of motion of involved shoulder	AAROM exercises into flexion, external rotation, and internal rotation Pulley exercises Pendulum exercises AROM exercises
Increase strength of involved shoulder	Thera-tubing exercises into internal and external rotation (4–6 weeks) Biceps and triceps PREs using dumbbells
Phase 3 (8–12 weeks)	**Intervention (as appropriate)**
Increase range of motion of involved shoulder	PROM: • *Flexion:* 0–120 degrees • *External rotation at 90 degrees abduction:* 30–40 degrees • *Internal rotation at 90 degrees abduction:* 45–55 degrees
Increase strength of involved shoulder Strength level 4/5: full external and internal rotation abduction	Thera-tubing exercises for external and internal rotation Dumbbell strengthening: abduction, supraspinatus, flexion Stretching exercises using cane: flexion, external rotation, and internal rotation

Data from Cohen BS, Romeo AA, Bach BR: Shoulder injuries, in Brotzman SB, Wilk KE (eds): Clinical Orthopaedic Rehabilitation. Philadelphia, Mosby, 2003, pp 125–250

TABLE 16-14	Rehabilitation Protocol Following Shoulder Arthroplasty (Non–Rotator Cuff Deficient)

Acute Protection Phase

Begins on the first postoperative day and extends for up to 6 weeks. The emphasis is on patient education, pain control, and initiation of ROM exercises within ranges noticed during surgery. In addition, it is important to maintain mobility in the adjacent joints (neck and scapula) and in the involved upper extremity.

Intervention

Continuous passive motion/supine passive ROM:
- *Forward flexion (in the plane of the scapula and with the elbow flexed):* 0–90 degrees. The arm should be resting on a folded towel.
- *External rotation at 30 degrees (no more than 45 degrees) abduction:* 0–20 degrees.
- *Internal rotation at 30 degrees (until the forearm rests on the chest) abduction:* 0–30 degrees.

Later during this phase, the exercises are progressed to self-assisted ROM into elevation and rotation in the supine position, and then the sitting position

Pendulum exercises

Shoulder rolls and postural education

Active range of motion of elbow, wrist, and hand

Gripping exercises

Pulley exercises (second week)

Initiate strengthening of involved shoulder.

Gentle muscle setting exercises for abductors and external/internal rotators

Active assisted motion exercises (as tolerated) using the uninvolved hand, and later using a wand or a cane

Subacute Protection Phase

Criteria to advance to this phase are range of motion of at least 90 degrees of passive elevation, at least 45 degrees of external rotation, and at least 70 degrees of internal rotation in the plane of the scapula with minimal pain. In addition, the patient should be able to perform most waist-level activities of daily living without pain.

Intervention

Progress PROM into AAROM exercises in the following directions: flexion, external rotation, and internal rotation

Gradually transition to AROM exercises and then pain-free, low-intensity resisted isometrics of the shoulder muscles, including the subscapularis or any other repaired muscle tendon units

Pulley exercises

Pendulum exercises

Increase strength of involved shoulder.

Thera-tubing/lightweight exercises into internal and external rotation (4–6 weeks) and from 0 to 90 degrees of shoulder elevation.

Biceps and triceps PREs using dumbbells

Chronic Protection Phase

Usually begins around 12 to 16 weeks postoperatively and typically extends for several more months. The emphasis during this phase is to restore full, active range of motion for functional activities in the presence of adequate stability of the GH joint.

Intervention (as appropriate)

PROM:
- *Flexion:* 0–140 degrees
- *External rotation at least 60 degrees, abduction:* 120 degrees
- *Internal rotation at least 70 degrees, adduction:* 45–55 degrees

Increase strength of involved shoulder to a strength level of 4/5 in the rotator cuff muscles.

Pain-free thera-tubing/lightweight exercises for external and internal rotation

Dumbbell strengthening: abduction, supraspinatus, flexion

End range stretching exercises using cane: flexion, external rotation, and internal rotation

Data from Cohen BS, Romeo AA, Bach BR: Shoulder injuries, in Brotzman SB, Wilk KE (eds): Clinical Orthopaedic Rehabilitation. Philadelphia, Mosby, 2003, pp 125–250

Therapeutic Techniques

A number of therapeutic techniques can be used to assist the patient. These include manual techniques and self-stretches.

Scapular Assist

This technique is designed to apply manual assistance to the scapula during arm elevation. This is a good technique to gain ROM during the period when the scapular controllers are being strengthened but have not reached the point where they are able to work independently. The clinician stands behind the patient. The scapula is stabilized with one hand and, as the patient raises the arm, the scapular motion is assisted by applying a compressive force over the scapula with one hand while stabilizing the AC joint with the other hand (Figure 16-36).

Rhythmic Stabilization

The patient is positioned in supine. The patient raises the involved arm to approximately 90 degrees of flexion and is asked to hold this position (Figure 16-37) while the clinician applies a series of controlled alternating isometric contractions of the agonist and antagonist muscles to stimulate movement of the agonist, and develop stability, while monitoring scapular muscle activity.

Restricted Scapulothoracic Motion

The patient is positioned in side with the lowermost arm over the end of the table. The clinician stands in front of the patient. Using one hand, the clinician grasps the inferior and medial border of the uppermost scapula. The other hand grasps the anterior aspect of the shoulder. The clinician gently brings both hands toward each other, lifting the scapula. This position is held until the muscles are felt to relax (Figure 16-38). Once the muscle relaxation has occurred, the clinician moves the scapula into the PNF patterns for the scapula:

- Elevation with protraction
- Elevation with retraction
- Depression with retraction (Figure 16-39)
- Depression with protraction

At the end range of each of these diagonals, the patient is asked to maintain the position by isometrically holding the scapula. The patient is then asked to resist the clinician as he or she attempts to return the scapula to the start position.

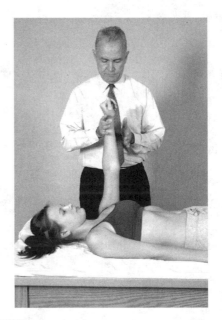

Figure 16-37   Rhythmic stabilization.

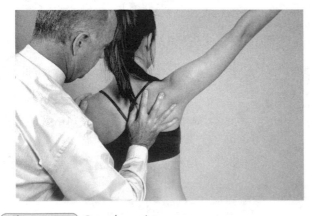

Figure 16-36   Scapular assist.

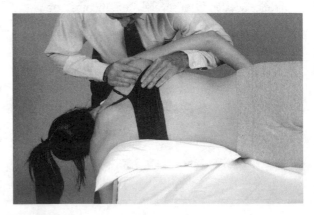

Figure 16-38   Scapular relaxer.

Self-Stretches

The "Saw"

This exercise can be used to stretch the anterior capsule when motion above 90 degrees is restricted. The patient can be positioned in standing or sitting. Maintaining the arm in approximately 90 degrees of elbow flexion, the patient is asked to perform a sawing motion as though cutting through wood (Figure 16-40).

Wall Walking

Wall walking can be used when attempting to regain full range elevation. Clock exercises are a variation of wall walking. The hand is moved to the various positions on an imaginary clock face on the wall, ranging from 8 o'clock, through 12 o'clock, to 4 o'clock. This allows for rotation of the humerus through varying degrees of flexion or abduction to replicate rotator cuff activity. This exercise is first performed against a fixed surface such as a wall or a countertop, and then can be moved to a moveable surface such as a ball or some other moveable implement.

Pulleys

Pulley exercises are commonly used as an active assisted exercise to help regain full overhead motion. However, it is recommended that pulley exercises not be used until the patient has at least 120 degrees of elevation, and then only after ensuring that the patient's scapula is able to upwardly rotate to prevent mechanical impingement.

Wall Corner Stretch

This stretch is used to increase the flexibility of the anterior joint capsule, pectoralis major and minor, anterior deltoid, and coracobrachialis. The patient stands in a corner and places both hands on the wall, level with the shoulders (refer to Figure 13-20 in Chapter 13). The stretch is applied by moving the trunk toward the wall, while keeping it perpendicular to the floor. The exercise can be modified to stretch one shoulder by performing the exercise in a doorway.

Horizontal Abductors

The horizontal abductors (posterior deltoid, infraspinatus, teres minor, rhomboids, and middle trapezius) and the posterior joint capsule are stretched by having the patient pull the arm across the front of the body (Figure 16-41). This exercise should be used with caution for those patients with an impingement syndrome or AC dysfunction.

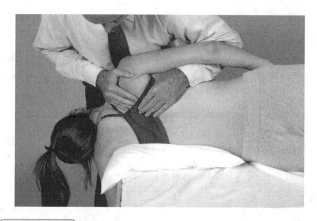

Figure 16-39 Depression with retraction.

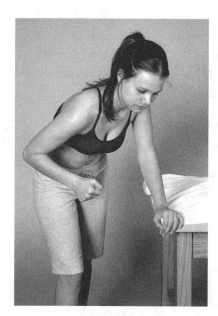

Figure 16-40 The "saw" exercise.

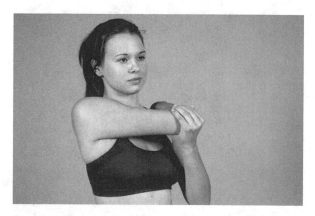

Figure 16-41 Stretch into horizontal adduction.

Inferior Capsule

The inferior capsule stretch is performed by placing the arm in the fully elevated overhead position.

Pectoralis Minor

The pectoralis minor can be stretched by asking the patient to clasp his or her hands behind the head in sitting (Figure 16-42). From this position, the patient attempts to move the elbows in a posterior direction. Initially, the clinician can monitor the exercise to ensure that the stretch is occurring in the correct region.

Transverse Frictional Massage (TFM)

The techniques used in transverse frictional massage are described in Chapter 6.

Biceps

The patient is positioned to expose the biceps tendon. The clinician stands at the patient's side and supports the arm (Figure 16-43). The clinician places his or her thumb on the biceps tendon and alternately applies a medial and lateral glide motion to the tendon to create gentle friction.

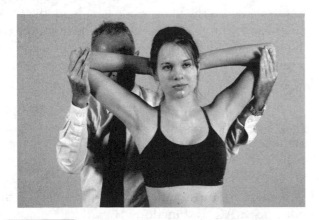

Figure 16-42 Pectoralis minor stretch.

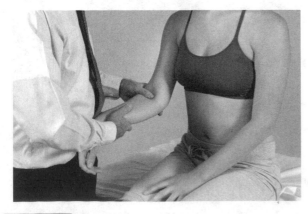

Figure 16-43 TFM of the biceps.

Supraspinatus

The supraspinatus tendon is located just distal to the anterolateral corner of the acromion. The clinician locates the painful location using the thumb (Figure 16-44). The massage is applied perpendicular to the tendon at the point of relative hypovascularity, which is located approximately 1 centimeter proximal to its insertion on the greater tuberosity of the humerus.[195]

Joint Mobilizations

The following techniques can be used with the appropriate grade of mobilization based on the intent of the treatment (see Chapter 6).

- Grade I and II oscillations are used for pain and graded depending on the stage of healing.
- Grade III–V techniques are used to increase range.

Distraction of the GH Joint

The clinician palpates and stabilizes the shoulder girdle and the anterior thorax. With the other hand, the clinician gently grasps the proximal third of the humerus. The clinician distracts the GH joint perpendicular to the plane of the glenoid fossa (30 degrees off the sagittal plane; Figure 16-45).

Inferior Glide of the GH Joint

The clinician stabilizes the GH joint with one hand and gently grasps proximal to the patient's elbow with the other. The humerus is glided inferiorly at the GH joint, parallel to the superoinferior plane of the glenoid fossa.

Anterior Glide of the GH Joint

The patient is positioned in prone or supine (Figure 16-46) and the glenoid fossa is stabilized using the table. One of the clinician's hands supports

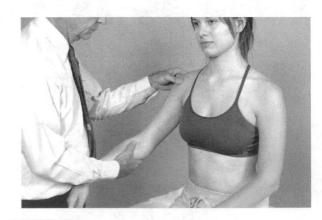

Figure 16-44 TFM of the supraspinatus.

the patient's elbow and the other hand is placed proximal to the humeral head (Figure 16-47). From this position, the clinician glides the humerus anteriorly at the GH joint, parallel to the anteroposterior plane of the glenoid fossa.

Inferior Glide of the Sternoclavicular Joint

With the thumb placed along the superior aspect of the length of the clavicle, the clinician applies an inferior glide to the SC joint (Figure 16-48).

Superior Glide of the Sternoclavicular Joint

Using one hand, the clinician grasps the medial end of the clavicle on the superior and inferior aspect and applies a superior glide to the SC joint (Figure 16-49).

Passive Distraction of the Scapulothoracic Joint

The patient is positioned in side lying (Figure 16-50). The clinician stands in front of the patient. Using both hands, the clinician grasps around the borders

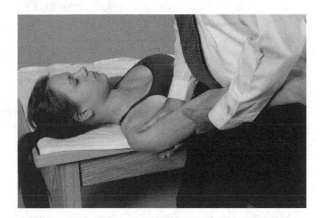
Figure 16-45   Distraction of the GH joint.

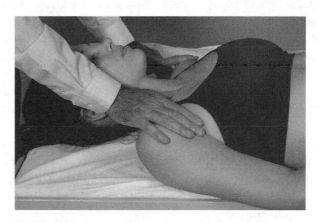
Figure 16-48   Inferior glide of the sternoclavicular joint.

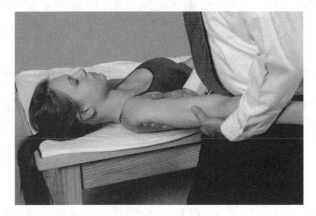
Figure 16-46   Anterior glide of the GH joint.

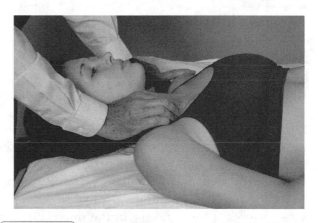
Figure 16-49   Superior glide of the sternoclavicular joint.

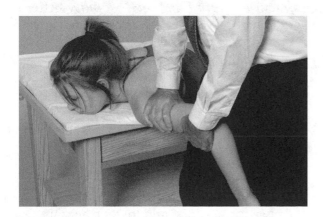
Figure 16-47   Anterior glide of the GH joint.

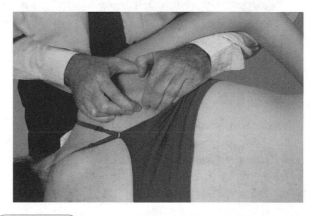
Figure 16-50   Passive distraction of the scapulothoracic joint.

of the scapula. The clinician gently brings both hands together, lifting the scapula off the thoracic wall.

Summary

The shoulder is one of the most complex joints in the body. Complete movement at the shoulder girdle involves a complex interaction among the GH, AC, SC, scapulothoracic, upper thoracic, costal, and sternomanubrial joints, and the lower cervical spine. Within the joints of the shoulder complex, there appear to be no well-defined points within the range where one joint's motion ends and another's begins. Rather, they all blend into a smooth harmonious movement during elevation. Due to this multi-joint arrangement, and the fact that so many muscles must behave in a coordinated fashion during functional movements, dysfunction of the shoulder is relatively common. Therefore, to effectively treat the shoulder, a sound knowledge of its anatomy and kinesiology is essential.

REVIEW Questions

1. Which four joints make up the shoulder complex?
2. Name the two major ligaments of the acromio-clavicular joint.
3. In addition to flexing the shoulder and flexing the elbow, what other function does the biceps perform?
4. Which muscles are capable of producing external rotation at the glenohumeral joint?
5. A brachial plexus injury in the upper portion of the plexus produces winging of the scapula. Weakness of which of the following muscles would produce the winging observed?
   a. Long head of the triceps
   b. Supraspinatus
   c. Deltoid
   d. Serratus anterior
6. Which of the following muscles has the most important function as a downward rotator of the scapula?
   a. Levator scapulae
   b. Upper trapezius
   c. Pectoralis major
   d. Rhomboid major

7. Which of the following muscles does not attach to the humerus?
   a. Teres major
   b. Pectoralis major
   c. Pectoralis minor
   d. Supraspinatus
8. Define the terms *shoulder dislocation* and *shoulder separation*.
9. All of the following are signs and symptoms of a shoulder dislocation, except:
   a. The injured shoulder is held in a flexed position.
   b. The head of the humerus can be palpated.
   c. There is localized pain in the area of injury.
   d. There is a definite sensation of crepitus.
10. Which of the following is frequently injured as a complication of shoulder dislocations?
    a. Axillary artery
    b. Radial artery
    c. Axillary nerve
    d. Radial nerve
11. Which is the only joint that directly attaches the upper extremity to the thorax?
12. The tendons of which muscles attach to the greater tuberosity of the humerus?
13. Which joint is damaged in a shoulder separation?
14. What is a common complication of a proximal humerus fracture?
15. Which of the following muscles is an important stabilizer of the scapula?
    a. Levator scapulae
    b. Latissimus dorsi
    c. Serratus anterior
    d. Deltoid
16. Your first patient of the day has been referred with a prescription stating *Stable humeral neck fracture. Begin functional mobility*. After the examination you decide the best initial intervention for this patient is:
    a. Pendulum exercises
    b. Shoulder isometrics
    c. Manual PNF
    d. Modalities to control pain
17. Which of the following muscles are most important for crutch walking?
    a. Anterior deltoid and biceps
    b. Middle deltoid and triceps
    c. Posterior deltoid and subscapularis
    d. Latissimus dorsi and lower trapezius

18. A 32-year-old patient has a left shoulder injury following a throwing injury. The patient had his upper extremity in an abducted, flexed, and externally rotated position when he felt a sharp pain in their shoulder as he was throwing a baseball. Initial intervention should focus on:

   a. Pendulum exercises
   b. AROM focused on abduction and external rotation
   c. Strengthening of the rhomboids and lower trapezius
   d. Strengthening of the rotator cuff muscles

19. You are treating a patient who has a diagnosis of right shoulder adhesive capsulitis with accessory motion dysfunction and noted loss of proper scapulohumeral rhythm. The intervention most likely to help achieve proper scapulohumeral rhythm of the shoulder complex is to:

   a. Strengthen the parascapular muscles and stretch the glenohumeral structures
   b. Protect joint biomechanics with immobilization
   c. Strengthen the glenohumeral joint at end range
   d. Manually stretch to achieve normal internal and external rotation at the glenohumeral joint

20. A patient presents with limited shoulder abduction secondary to adhesive capsulitis. The supervising physical therapist determines that grade 2 and 3 joint mobilization techniques will assist in promoting the return of normal joint accessory motion and shoulder abduction. Taking into consideration the articular surfaces of the glenohumeral joint, the direction that would be most appropriate for mobilization would be:

   a. Inferior glide of the humerus on the scapula
   b. Superior glide of the humerus on the scapula
   c. Anterior glide of the scapula on the humerus
   d. Posterior glide of the humerus on the scapula

References

1. Moore KL, Dalley AF: Upper limb, in Moore KL, Dalley AF (eds): Clinically Oriented Anatomy. Philadelphia, Williams & Wilkins, 1999, pp 664–830
2. Norkin C, Levangie P: Joint Structure and Function: A Comprehensive Analysis. Philadelphia, FA Davis, 1992
3. Paine RM, Voight M: The role of the scapula. J Orthop Sports Phys Ther 18:386–391, 1993
4. Kibler WB, Chandler TJ, Livingston BP: Correlation of lateral scapular slide measurements with x-ray measurements. Med Sci Sports Exerc 31:S237–243, 1999
5. Kibler BW: The role of the scapula in athletic shoulder function. Am J Sports Med 26:325–337, 1998
6. Gladstone JN, Rosen AL: Disorders of the acromioclavicular joint. Curr Opin Orthop 10:316–321, 1999
7. Turnbull JR: Acromioclavicular joint disorders. Med Sci Sports Exerc 30:S526–532, 1998
8. Brody LT: Shoulder, in Wadsworth C (ed): Current Concepts of Orthopedic Physical Therapy—Home Study Course. La Crosse, WI, Orthopaedic Section, American Physical Therapy Association, 2001
9. Matsen FA, III., Arntz CT: Subacromial impingement, in Rockwood CA, Jr., Matsen FA, III (eds): The Shoulder. Philadelphia, WB Saunders, 1990, pp 623–648
10. Neer CS, II.: Anterior acromioplasty for the chronic impingement syndrome in the shoulder: A preliminary report. J Bone Joint Surg Am 54:41–50, 1972
11. Neer C: Impingement lesions. Clin Orthop 173:71–77, 1983
12. Wickiewicz TL: The impingement syndrome. Postgraduate Advances in Sports Medicine—National Athletic Trainers Association Home Study Course. Omaha, NB, Board of Certification, Inc., 1986
13. Flatow EL, Soslowsky LJ, Ticker JB, et al: Excursion of the rotator cuff under the acromion. Patterns of subacromial contact. Am J Sports Med 22:779–788, 1994
14. Babyar SR: Excessive scapular motion in individuals recovering from painful and stiff shoulders: Causes and treatment strategies. Phys Ther 76:226–247, 1996
15. Warner JJP, Micheli LJ, Arslanian LE, et al: Scapulothoracic motion in normal shoulders and shoulders with glenohumeral instability and impingement syndrome. A study using Moire topographic analysis. Clin Orthop 285:191–199, 1992
16. Warner JJP, Schulte KR, Imhoff AB: Current concepts in shoulder instability, in Stauffer RN, Erlich MG, Kostuik JP, et al (eds): Advances in Operative Orthopedics. St Louis, MO, CV Mosby, 1995, pp 217–248
17. Warner JJ, Navarro RA: Serratus anterior dysfunction. Recognition and treatment. Clin Orthop Relat Res 349:139–148, 1998
18. Inman T, Saunders JR, Abbott LC: Observations on the function of the shoulder joint. J Bone Joint Surg 26:1–18, 1944
19. McQuade KJ, Smidt GL: Dynamic scapulohumeral rhythm: The effects of external resistance during elevation of the arm in the scapular plane. J Orthop Sports Phys Ther 27:125–133, 1998
20. Jackson-Manfield P, Neumann DA: Structure and function of the shoulder complex, in Jackson-Manfield P, Neumann DA (eds): Essentials of Kinesiology for the Physical Therapist Assistant. St Louis, MO, Mosby Elsevier, 2009, pp 51–89
21. Dvir Z, Berme N: The shoulder complex in elevation of the arm: A mechanism approach. J Biomech 11:219–225, 1978
22. Perry J: Normal upper extremity kinesiology. Phys Ther 58:265–278, 1978

23. Schenkman M, De Cartaya VR: Kinesiology of the shoulder complex, in Andrews J, Wilk KE (eds): The Athlete's Shoulder. New York, Churchill Livingstone, 1994, pp 15–35

24. Smith LK, Weiss EL, Lehmkuhl LD: Brunnstrom's clinical kinesiology (ed 5). Philadelphia, FA Davis, 1996

25. Laumann U: Kinesiology of the shoulder: Electromyographic and stereophotogrammetric studies, in Bateman JE, Welsh RP (eds): Surgery of the Shoulder. Philadelphia, BC Decker, 1984, pp 6–11

26. Bagg SD, Forrest WJ: A biomechanical analysis of scapular rotation during arm abduction in the scapular plane. Am J Phys Med 67:238–245, 1988

27. Dunleavy K: Relationship between the shoulder and the cervicothoracic spine. La Crosse, WI, Orthopedic Section, American Physical Therapy Association, 2001

28. Neumann DA: Shoulder complex, in Neumann DA (ed): Kinesiology of the Musculoskeletal System: Foundations for Physical Rehabilitation. St Louis, Mosby, 2002, pp 91–132

29. Kisner C, Colby LA: The shoulder and shoulder girdle, in Kisner C, Colby LA (eds): Therapeutic Exercise. Foundations and Techniques (ed 5). Philadelphia, FA Davis, 2002, pp 481–556

30. Deutsch A, Altchek DW, Schwartz E, et al: Radiologic measurement of superior displacement of the humeral head in the impingement syndrome. J Shoulder Elbow Surg 5:186–193, 1996

31. Flatow E, Soslowsky L, Ticker J, et al: Excursion of the rotator cuff under the acromion: patterns of subacromial contact. Am J Sports Med 22:779–787, 1994

32. Maitland G: Peripheral Manipulation (ed 3). London, Butterworth, 1991

33. Wilk KE, Arrigo C, Andrews JR: Rehabilitation of the elbow in the throwing athlete. J Orthop Sports Phys Ther 17:305–317, 1993

34. Coutts RD: Continuous passive motion in the rehabilitation of the total knee patient. Its role and effect. Orthop Rev 15:27, 1986

35. Dehne E, Tory R: Treatment of joint injuries by immediate mobilization based upon the spiral adaption concept. Clin Orthop 77:218–232, 1971

36. Haggmark T, Eriksson E: Cylinder or mobile cast brace after knee ligament surgery. Am J Sports Med 7:48–56, 1979

37. Noyes FR, Mangine RE, Barber S: Early knee motion after open and arthroscopic anterior cruciate ligament reconstruction. Am J Sports Med 15:149–160, 1987

38. Booth FW: Physiologic and biochemical effects of immobilization on muscle. Clin Orthop Relat Res 219:15–21, 1987

39. Eiff MP, Smith AT, Smith GE: Early mobilization versus immobilization in the treatment of lateral ankle sprains. Am J Sports Med 22:83–88, 1994

40. Akeson WH, Amiel D, Mechanic GL, et al: Collagen cross-linking alterations in the joint contractures: Changes in the reducible cross-links in periarticular connective tissue after 9 weeks immobilization. Connect Tissue Res 5:15–19, 1977

41. Akeson WH, Amiel D, Abel MF, et al: Effects of immobilization on joints. Clin Orthop 219:28–37, 1987

42. Akeson WH, Amiel D, Woo SL-Y: Immobility effects on synovial joints: The pathomechanics of joint contracture. Biorheology 17:95–110, 1980

43. Woo SL-Y, Matthews J, Akeson WH, et al: Connective tissue response to immobility: A correlative study of biochemical and biomechanical measurements of normal and immobilized rabbit knee. Arthritis Rheum 18:257–264, 1975

44. Jobe FW, Pink M: Classification and treatment of shoulder dysfunction in the overhead athlete. J Orthop Sports Phys Ther 18:427–431, 1993

45. Kibler WB, McMullen J: Scapular dyskinesis and its relation to shoulder pain. J Am Acad Orthop Surg 11:142–151, 2003

46. Jobe FW, Kvitne RS, Giangarra CE: Shoulder pain in the overhand and throwing athlete: The relationship of anterior instability and rotator cuff impingement. Orthop Rev 18:963–975, 1989

47. Mohr KJ, Moynes Schwab DR, Tovin BJ: Musculoskeletal pattern F: Impaired joint mobility, motor function, muscle performance, and range of motion associated with localized inflammation, in Tovin BJ, Greenfield B (eds): Evaluation and Treatment of the Shoulder: An Integration of the Guide to Physical Therapist Practice. Philadelphia, FA Davis, 2001, pp 210–230

48. Jobe CM, Pink M, Jobe FW, et al: Anterior shoulder instability, impingement and rotator cuff tear, in Jobe FW (ed): Operative Techniques in Upper Extremity Sports Injuries. St Louis, Mosby-Year Book, 1996, pp 164–176

49. d'Hespeel CG: Current concepts: Rehabilitation of patients with shoulder impingement and tight posterior capsule. Orthop Pract 16:9–13, 2004

50. Moseley HF, Goldie I: The arterial pattern of the rotator cuff of the shoulder. J Bone Joint Surg 45-B:780–789, 1963

51. Neer CS, II, Welsh RP: The shoulder in sports. Orthop Clin North Am 8:583–591, 1977

52. Rothman RH, Parke WW: The vascular anatomy of the rotator cuff. Clin Orthop 41:176–186, 1965

53. Bigliani LU, Morrison D, April EW: The morphology of the acromion and its relationship to rotator cuff tears. Orthop Trans 10:228, 1986

54. Bigliani LU, Ticker JB, Flatow EL, et al: The relationship of acromial architecture to rotator cuff disease. Clin Sports Med 4:823–838, 1991

55. Rathburn JB, Macnab I: The microvascular pattern of the rotator cuff. J Bone Joint Surg Br 52:540–553, 1970

56. Jarvholm U, Styf J, Suurkula M, et al: Intramuscular pressure and muscle blood flow in the supraspinatus. Eur J Appl Physiol 58:219–224, 1988

57. Sigholm G, Styf J, Korner L, et al: Pressure recording in the subacromial bursa. J Orthop Res 6:123–128, 1988

58. Harryman DT, III, Sidles JA, Clark JM: Translation of the humeral head on the glenoid with passive glenohumeral motion. J Bone Joint Surg 72A:1334–1343, 1990

59. Kessel L, Watson M: The painful arc syndrome: Clinical classification as a guide to management. J Bone Joint Surg Br 59:166–172, 1977

60. Neer CS, II., Bigliani LU, Hawkins RJ: Rupture of the long head of the biceps related to subacromial impingement. Orthop Trans 1:111–117, 1977

61. Cohen RB, Williams GR, Jr: Impingement syndrome and rotator cuff disease as repetitive motion disorders. Clin Orthop Relat Res 351:95–101, 1998

62. Sharkey NA, Marder RA, Hanson PB: The role of the rotator cuff in elevation of the arm. Trans Orthop Res Soc 18:137, 1993

63. Perry J: Biomechanics of the shoulder, in Rowe CR (ed): The Shoulder. New York, Churchill Livingstone, 1988, pp 1–15

64. Conroy DE, Hayes KW: The effect of joint mobilization as a component of comprehensive treatment for primary shoulder impingement syndrome. J Orthop Sports Phys Ther 28:3–14, 1998

65. Cofield RH: Current concepts review: Rotator cuff disease of the shoulder. J Bone Joint Surg 67A:974–979, 1985

66. Hjelm R, Draper C, Spencer S: Anterior-superior capsular length insufficiency in the painful shoulder. J Orthop Sports Phys Ther 23:216–222, 1996

67. Donatelli RA: Mobilization of the shoulder, in Donatelli RA (ed): Physical Therapy of the Shoulder. New York, Churchill Livingstone, 1991, pp 271–292

68. Cofield RH, Simonet WT: Symposium on sports medicine: Part 2. The shoulder in sports. Mayo Clin Proc 59:157–164, 1984

69. Morrison DS, Frogameni AD, Woodworth P: Nonoperative treatment of subacromial impingement syndrome. J Bone Joint Surg Am 79:732–737, 1997

70. Harryman DT, III, Sidles JA, Harris SL, et al: The role of the rotator interval capsule in passive motion and stability of the shoulder. J Bone Joint Surg 74A:53–66, 1992

71. Culham E, Peat M: Functional anatomy of the shoulder complex. J Orthop Sports Phys Ther 18:342–350, 1993

72. DePalma AF, Gallery G, Bennett CA: Variational anatomy and degenerative lesions of the shoulder joint, in Blount W (ed): American Academy of Orthopaedic Surgeons Instructional Course Lectures. Ann Arbor, MI, JW Edwards, 1949, pp 255–281

73. De Palma AF, Gallery G, Bennett GA. Variational anatomy and degenerative lesions of the shoulder joint, in Edwards JW (ed): American Academy of Orthopaedic Surgeons Instructional Course Lectures. St Louis, MO, Mosby, 1949, pp 225–281

74. Ozaki J, Fujimoto S, Nakagawa Y, et al: Tears of the rotator cuff on the shoulder associated with pathological changes in the acromion: A study in cadavera. J Bone Joint Surg [Am] 70-A:1224–1230, 1988

75. Petterson G: Rupture of the tendon aponeurosis of the shoulder joint in anterior inferior dislocation. Acta Chir Scand 99:1–184, 1942 (Suppl)

76. Sher J, Uribe J, Posada A, et al: Abnormal findings on magnetic resonance images of symptomatic shoulders. J Bone Joint Surg 77A:10–15, 1995

77. Cotton RE, Rideout DF: Tears of the humeral rotator cuff: A radiological and pathological necropsy survey. J Bone Joint Surg 46B:314–328, 1964

78. Zeman CA, Arcand MA, Cantrell JS, et al: The rotator cuff-deficient arthritic shoulder: Diagnosis and surgical management. J Am Acad Orthop Surgeons 6:337–348, 1998

79. Neer CSI, Watson KC, Stanton FJ: Recent experience in total shoulder replacement. J Bone Joint Surg 64:319–337, 1982

80. Gartsman GM: Arthroscopic rotator cuff repair. Clin Orthop Relat Res 390:95–106, 2001

81. Nirschl RP: Prevention and treatment of elbow and shoulder injuries in the tennis player. Clin Sports Med 7:289–308, 1988

82. Norberg FB, Field LD: Repair of the rotator cuff: Mini-open and arthroscopic repairs. Clin Sports Med 19:77–99, 2000

83. Altchek DW, Warren RF, Wickiewicz TL, et al: Arthroscopic acromioplasty: Technique and results. J Bone Joint Surg 72A:1198–1207, 1990

84. Ellman H: Arthroscopic subacromial decompression: Analysis of one-to three-year results. Arthroscopy 3:173–181, 1987

85. Gartsman GM: Arthroscopic acromioplasty for lesions of the rotator cuff. J Bone Joint Surg 72A:169–180, 1990

86. Ellman H: Diagnosis and treatment of incomplete rotator cuff tears. Clin Orthop 254:64–74, 1990

87. Esch JC: Arthroscopic subacromial decompression: Results according to the degree of rotator cuff tear. Arthroscopy 4:241–249, 1988

88. Gartsman GM, Milne J: Partial articular surface tears of the rotator cuff. J Shoulder Elbow Surg 4:409–416, 1995

89. Gartsman GM, Brinker MR, Khan M: Early effectiveness of arthroscopic repair for full-thickness tears of the rotator cuff: An outcome analysis. J Bone Joint Surg 80A:33–40, 1998

90. Gartsman GM, Hammerman SM: Full-thickness tear: Arthroscopic repair. Orthop Clin North Am 28:83–98, 1997

91. Gleyze P, Thomazeau H, Flurin P, et al: Arthroscopic rotator cuff repair: A multicentric retrospective study of 87 cases with anatomical assessment. Rev Chir Orthop Reparatrice Appar Mot 86:566–574, 2000

92. Gartsman GM, Hammerman SM: Arthroscopic rotator cuff repair: Operative technique. Oper Tech Shoulder Elbow Surg 1:2–8, 2000

93. Marks PH, Warner JJ, Irrgang JJ: Rotator cuff disorders of the shoulder. J Hand Ther 7:90–98, 1994

94. LaStayo PC, Wright T, Jaffe R, et al: Continuous passive motion after repair of the rotator cuff: A prospective outcome study. J Bone Joint Surg 80A:1002–1011, 1998

95. Grieve GP: Manual mobilizing techniques in degenerative arthrosis of the hip. Bull Orthop Section APTA 2:7, 1977

96. Frank C, Akeson WH, Woo SL-Y, et al: Physiology and therapeutic value of passive joint motion. Clin Orthop 185:113, 1984

97. Salter RB, Simmonds DF, Malcolm BW, et al: The biological effect of continuous passive motion on the healing of full-thickness defects in articular cartilage. J Bone Joint Surg 62A:1232–1251, 1980

98. Kibler WB: Shoulder rehabilitation: Principles and practice. Med Sci Sports Exerc 30:40–50, 1998

99. Flatow EL, Warner JJP: Instability of the shoulder: Complex problems and failed repairs: Part I. Relevant biomechanics, multidirectional instability, and severe glenoid loss. Instr Course Lect 47:97–112, 1998

100. Kennedy JC, Alexander IJ, Hayes KC: Nerve supply of the human knee and its functional importance. Am J Sports Med 10:329–335, 1982

101. Rowe CR, Sakellarides HT: Factors related to recurrences of anterior dislocations of the shoulder. Clin Orthop 20:40, 1961

102. Rowe CR, Zarins B: Recurrent transient subluxation of the shoulder. J Bone Joint Surg Am 63:863–872, 1981

103. Brown GA, Tan JL, Kirkley A: The lax shoulder in females. Issues, answers, but many more questions. Clin Orthop Relat Res 372:110–122, 2000

104. Jobe FW, Tibone JE, Jobe CM, et al: The shoulder in sports, in Rockwood CA, Jr., Matsen FA, III (eds): The Shoulder. Philadelphia, WB Saunders, 1990, pp 963–967

105. Berbig R, Weishaupt D, Prim J, et al: Primary anterior shoulder dislocation and rotator cuff tears. J Shoulder Elbow Surg 8:220–225, 1999

106. Sonnabend DH: Treatment of primary anterior shoulder dislocation in patients older than 40 years of age. Clin Orthop 304:74–77, 1994

107. Tijimes J, Loyd HM, Tullos HS: Arthrography in acute shoulder dislocations. South Med J 72:564–567, 1979

108. Matsen FA, Harryman DT, Sidles JA: Mechanics of glenohumeral instability. Clin Sports Med 10:783–788, 1991

109. Cordasco FA, Bigliani LU: Multidirectional shoulder instability: Open surgical treatment, in Warren RF, Craig EV, Altchek DW (eds): The Unstable Shoulder. Philadelphia, Lippincott-Raven, 1999, pp 249–261

110. Lippitt SB, Harryman DT II, Sidles JA, et al: Diagnosis and management of AMBRII syndrome. Tech Orthop 6:61, 1991

111. Burkhart SS, Morgan CD, Kibler WB: Shoulder injuries in overhead athletes: The "dead arm" revisited. Clin Sports Med 19:125–158, 2000

112. Burkhart SS: A 26-year-old woman with shoulder pain. JAMA 284:1559–1567, 2000

113. Snyder SJ, Karzel RP, Del Pizzo W, et al: SLAP lesions of the shoulder. Arthoscopy 6:274, 1990

114. Morgan CD, Burkhart SS, Palmeri M, et al: Type II SLAP lesions: Three subtypes and their relationship to superior instability and rotator cuff tears. Arthroscopy 14:553–565, 1998

115. Berg EE, DeHoll D: Radiography of the medial elbow ligaments. J Shoulder Elbow Surg 6:528–533, 1997

116. Urban WP, Babom DNM: Management of superior labral anterior posterior lesions. Oper Tech Orthop 5:223, 1995

117. Maffet MW, Gartsman GM, Moseley B: Superior labrum-biceps tendon complex lesions of the shoulder. Am J Sports Med 23:93–98, 1995

118. Davies GJ, Dickhoff-Hoffman S: Neuromuscular testing and rehabilitation of the shoulder complex. J Orthop Sports Phys Ther 18:449–458, 1993

119. Kibler WB, Livingston B, Bruce R: Current concepts in shoulder rehabilitation. Adv Op Orthop 3:249–301, 1996

120. Pink MM, Screnar PM, Tollefson KD: Injury prevention and rehabilitation in the upper extremity, in Jobe FW (ed): Operative Techniques in Upper Extremity Sports Injuries. St Louis, Mosby, 1996, pp 3–15

121. Happee R, Van Der Helm FCT: The control of shoulder muscles during goal directed movements. J Biomech 28:1179–1191, 1995

122. Kibler BW: Closed kinetic chain rehabilitation for sports injuries. Phys Med Rehab North Am 11:369–384, 2000

123. Jobe FW, Moynes DR, Brewster CE: Rehabilitation of shoulder joint instabilities. Orthop Clin North Am 18:473–482, 1987

124. Jobe FW, Glousman RE: Anterior capsulolabral reconstruction, in Paulos LE, Tibone JE (eds): Operative Technique in Shoulder Surgery. Gaithersburg, MD, Aspen, 1992, pp 212–234

125. DePalma AF: Surgery of the Shoulder (ed 2). Philadelphia, Lippincott, 1973

126. Jackson D, Einhorn A: Rehabilitation of the shoulder, in Jackson DW (ed): Shoulder Surgery in the Athlete. Rockville, MD, Aspen, 1985, pp 103–118

127. Wirth MA, Groh GI, Rockwood CA, Jr: Capsulorrhaphy through an anterior approach for the treatment of atraumatic posterior glenohumeral instability with multidirectional laxity of the shoulder. J Bone Joint Surg 80A:1570–1578, 1998

128. McIntyre LF, Caspari RB, Savoie FH, III: The arthroscopic treatment of multidirectional shoulder instability: Two-year results of a multiple suture technique. Arthroscopy 13:418–425, 1997

129. Wong KL, Williams GR: Complications of thermal capsulorrhaphy of the shoulder. J Bone Joint Surg 83-A:151–155, 2001 (Suppl 2, Pt 2)

130. Anderson K, Warren RF, Altchek DW, et al: Risk factors for early failure after thermal capsulorrhaphy. Am J Sports Med 30:103–107, 2002

131. Gotlin RS, Hershkowitz S, Juris PM, et al: Electrical stimulation effect on extensor lag and length of hospital stay after total knee arthroplasty. Arch Phys Med Rehab 75:957, 1994

132. Lamboni P, Harris B: The use of ice, air splints, and high voltage galvanic stimulation in effusion reduction. Athl Training 18:23–25, 1983

133. McMiken DF, Todd-Smith M, Thompson C: Strengthening of human quadriceps muscles by cutaneous electrical stimulation. Scand J Rehabil Med 15:25–28, 1983

134. Walker RH, Morris BA, Angulo DL, et al: Postoperative use of continuous passive motion, transcutaneous electrical nerve stimulation, and continuous cooling pad following total knee arthroplasty. J Arthroplasty 6:151–156, 1991

135. Neviaser JS: Adhesive capsulitis of the shoulder. Study of pathological findings in periarthritis of the shoulder. J Bone Joint Surg 27:211–222, 1945

136. Bulgen DY, Binder A, Hazelman BL: Immunological studies in frozen shoulder. J Rheumatol 9:893–898, 1982

137. Grubbs N: Frozen shoulder syndrome: A review of literature. J Orthop Sports Phys Ther 18:479–487, 1993

138. Rizk TE, Pinals RS: Histocompatibility type and racial incidence in frozen shoulder. Arch Phys Med Rehabil 65:33–34, 1984

139. Wiley AM: Arthroscopic appearance of frozen shoulder. Arthroscopy 7:138–143, 1991

140. Binder AI, Bulgen DY, Hazleman BL, et al: Frozen shoulder: A long-term prospective study. Ann Rheum Dis 43:361–364, 1984

141. Lloyd-Roberts GG, French PR: Periarthritis of the shoulder: A study of the disease and its treatment. Br Med J 1:1569–1574, 1959

142. Bridgman JF: Periarthritis of the shoulder and diabetes mellitus. Ann Rheum Dis 31:69–71, 1972

143. Janda DH, Hawkins RJ: Shoulder manipulation in patients with adhesive capsulitis and diabetes mellitus. A clinical note. J Shoulder Elbow Surg 2:36–38, 1993

144. McClure PW, Flowers KR: Treatment of limited shoulder motion: A case study based on biomechanical considerations. Phys Ther 72:929–936, 1992

145. Miller MD, Rockwood CA, Jr.: Thawing the frozen shoulder: The "patient" patient. Orthopedics 19:849–853, 1997

146. Pal B, Anderson JJ, Dick WC: Limitations of joint mobility and shoulder capsulitis in insulin and noninsulin dependent diabetes mellitus. Br J Rheumatol 25:147–151, 1986

147. Fisher L, Kurtz A, Shipley M: Relationship of cheiroarthropathy and frozen shoulder in patients with insulin dependent diabetes mellitus. Br J Rheum 25:141, 1986

148. DePalma AF: Loss of scapulohumeral motion (frozen shoulder). Ann Surg 135:193–197, 1952

149. Bowman CA, Jeffcoate WJ, Patrick M: Bilateral adhesive capsulitis, oligoarthritis and proximal myopathy as presentation of hypothyroidism. Br J Rheumatol 27:62–64, 1988

150. Speer KP, Cavanaugh JT, Warren RF, et al: A role for hydrotherapy in shoulder rehabilitation. Am J Sports Med 21:850–853, 1993

151. Wohlgethan JR: Frozen shoulder in hyperthyroidism. Arthritis Rheum 30:936–939, 1987

152. Mintner WT: The shoulder-hand syndrome in coronary disease. J Med Assoc Ga 56:45–49, 1967

153. Coventry MB: Problem of the painful shoulder. JAMA 151:177, 1953

154. Tyber MA: Treatment of the painful shoulder syndrome with amitriptyline and lithium carbonate. Can Med Assoc J 111:137, 1974

155. Nash P, Hazelman BD: Frozen shoulder. Baillieres Clin Rheumatol 3:551–566, 1989

156. Daigneault J, Cooney LM, Jr.: Shoulder pain in older people. J Am Geriatr Soc 46:1144–1151, 1998

157. Neviaser JS: Adhesive capsulitis and the stiff and painful shoulder. Orthop Clin North Am 11:327–331, 1980

158. Neviaser RJ: Painful conditions affecting the shoulder. Clin Orthop 173:63–69, 1983

159. Reeves B: The natural history of the frozen shoulder syndrome. Scand J Rheumatol 4:193–196, 1975

160. Hannafin JA, Chiaia TA: Adhesive capsulitis. A treatment approach. Clin Orthop Relat Res 372:95–109, 2000

161. Zuckerman JD, Cuomo F: Frozen shoulder, in Matsen FA, III, Fu FH, Hawkins RJ (eds): The Shoulder: A Balance of Mobility and Stability. Rosemont, IL, American Academy of Orthopaedic Surgeons, 1993, pp 253–267

162. Uhthoff HK, Sarkar K: An algorithm for shoulder pain caused by soft tissue disorders. Clin Orthop 254:121, 1990

163. Pajareya K, Chadchavalpanichaya N, Painmanakit S, et al: Effectiveness of physical therapy for patients with adhesive capsulitis: A randomized controlled trial. J Med Assoc Thai 87:473–480, 2004

164. McClure PW, Flowers KR: Treatment of limited shoulder motion using an elevation splint. Phys Ther 72:57, 1992

165. Laska T, Hannig K: Physical therapy for spinal accessory nerve injury complicated by adhesive capsulitis. Phys Ther 81:936–944, 2001

166. Rizk TE, Christopher RP, Pinals RS, et al: Adhesive capsulitis (frozen shoulder): A new approach to its management and treatment. Arch Phys Med Rehabil 64:29–33, 1983

167. Tovin BJ, Greenfield BH: Impairment-based diagnosis for the shoulder girdle, in Tovin BJ, Greenfield BH (eds): Evaluation and Treatment of the Shoulder: An Integration of the Guide to Physical Therapist Practice. Philadelphia, FA Davis, 2001, pp 55–74

168. Omer GE: Osteotomy of the clavicle in surgical reduction of anterior sternoclavicular dislocations. J Trauma 7:584–590, 1967

169. Souza TA: History and examination of the shoulder, in Souza TA (ed): Sports Injuries of the Shoulder—Conservative Management. New York, Churchill Livingstone, 1994, pp 16–219

170. Winkel D, Matthijs O, Phelps V: Pathology of the shoulder, in Winkel D, Matthijs O, Phelps V (eds): Diagnosis and Treatment of the Upper Extremities. Gaithersburg, MD, Aspen, 1997, pp 68–117

171. Clarnette RG, Miniaci A: Clinical exam of the shoulder. Med Sci Sports Exerc 30:1–6, 1998

172. Tossy JD, Mead MC, Simond HM: Acromioclavicular separations: Useful and practical classification for treatment. Clin Orthop 28:111–119, 1963

173. Allman, FL, Jr: Fractures and ligamentous injuries of the clavicle and its articulation. J Bone Joint Surg 49A: 774–784, 1967

174. Rockwood CA, Jr: Injuries to the acromioclavicular joint, in Rockwood CA, Jr, Green DP (eds): Fractures in Adults (ed 2). Philadelphia, JB Lippincott, 1984, pp 860–910

175. Rockwood CA, Jr., Young DC: Disorders of the acromioclavicular joint, in Rockwood CA, Jr, Matsen FA, III (eds): The Shoulder. Philadelphia, WB Saunders, 1990, pp 413–468

176. Williams GR, Nguyen VD, Rockwood CA, Jr.: Classification and radiographic analysis of acromioclavicular dislocations. Appl Radiol 18:29–34, 1989

177. Wirth MA, Rockwood CA, Jr.: Chronic conditions of the acromioclavicular and sternoclavicular joints, in Chapman MW (ed): Operative Orthopaedics (ed 2). Philadelphia, JB Lippincott, 1993, pp 1673–1683

178. Rockwood CA: Rockwood and Green's Fractures in Adults. Philadelphia, Lippincott, 1991, pp 1181–1239

179. Bannister GC, Wallace WA, Stableforth PG, et al: The management of acute acromioclavicular dislocation: A randomized prospective controlled trial. J Bone Joint Surg 71B:848–850, 1989

180. Bjerneld H, Hovelius L, Thorling J: Acromioclavicular separations treated conservatively: A five year follow-up study. Acta Orthop Scand 54:743–745, 1983

181. Dias JJ, Steingold RF, Richardson RA, et al: The conservative treatment of acromioclavicular dislocation: Review after five years. J Bone Joint Surg 69B:719–722, 1987

182. Glick JM, Milburn LJ, Haggerty JF, et al: Dislocated acromioclavicular joint: Follow-up study of thirty-five unreduced acromioclavicular dislocations. Am J Sports Med 5:264–270, 1977

183. Rawes ML, Dias JJ: Long-term results of conservative treatment for acromioclavicular dislocation. J Bone Joint Surg 78B:410–412, 1996

184. Sleeswijk-Viser SV, Haarsma SM, Speeckaert MTC: Conservative treatment of acromioclavicular dislocation: Jones strap versus mitella. Acta Orthop Scand. 55:483, 1984

185. Larsen E, Bjerg-Nielsen A, Christensen P: Conservative or surgical treatment of acromioclavicular dislocation: A prospective, controlled randomized study. J Bone Joint Surg 68A:552–555, 1986

186. Taft TN, Wilson FC, Oglesby JW: Dislocation of the acromioclavicular joint: An end-result study. J Bone Joint Surg 69A:1045–1051, 1987

187. Gladstone J, Wilk KE, Andrews J: Nonoperative treatment of acromioclavicular joint injuries. Op Tech Sports Med 5:78–87, 1998

188. Bigliani LU, Craig EV, Butters KP: Fractures of the shoulder, in Rockwood CA, Green DP, Bucholz RW (eds): Fractures in Adults. Philadelphia, Lippincott, 1991, pp 871–1020

189. Cornell CN, Schneider K: Proximal humerus fractures, in Koval KJ, Zuckerman JD (eds): Fractures in the Elderly. Philadelphia, Lippincott-Raven, 1998, pp 85–92

190. Sisk TD, Wright PE: Arthroplasty of the shoulder and elbow, in Crenshaw AH (ed): Campbell's Operative Orthopaedics (ed 8). St Louis, Mosby, 1992, pp 650–660

191. Bergmann G: Biomechanics and pathomechanics of the shoulder joint with reference to prosthetic joint replacement, in Koelbel R, Helbig B, Blauth W (eds): Shoulder Replacement. Berlin, Spring-Verlag, 1987, pp 33

192. Williams GR, Jr, Rockwood CA, Jr: Massive rotator cuff defects and glenohumeral arthritis, in Friedman RJ (ed): Arthroplasty of the Shoulder. New York, Thieme Medical Publishers, 1994, pp 204–214

193. Brown DD, Friedman RJ: Postoperative rehabilitation following total shoulder arthroplasty. Orthop Clin North Am 29:535–547, 1998

194. Smith KL, Matsen FA: Total shoulder arthroplasty versus hemiarthroplasty: Current trends. Orthop Clin North Am 29:491–506, 1998

195. Codman EA: The Shoulder, Rupture of the Supraspinatus Tendon and Other Lesions in or About the Subacromial Bursa. Boston, MA, Thomas Todd Co, 1934

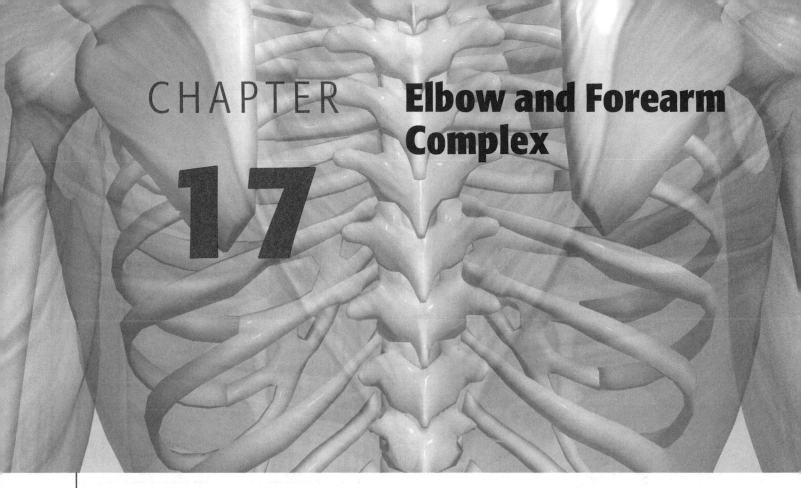

Elbow and Forearm Complex

17

Chapter Objectives

At the completion of this chapter, the reader will be able to:

1. Describe the anatomy of the elbow complex.
2. Describe the biomechanics of the elbow complex, including the open- and close-packed positions, and the static and dynamic stabilizers.
3. Describe the relationship between the joints and functional performance of the elbow.
4. Summarize the various causes of elbow dysfunction.
5. Describe and demonstrate intervention strategies and techniques based on clinical findings and established goals by the physical therapist.
6. Evaluate the intervention effectiveness in order to determine progress and modify an intervention as needed.
7. Plan an effective home program, and instruct the patient in its use.

Overview

The elbow complex is the central link in the kinetic chain of the upper extremity and serves as the intersection for three bones: the humerus, the radius, and the ulna. Functionally, the elbow joint behaves as a constrained hinge, coordinating movements of the upper extremity and facilitating the execution of activities of daily living in areas such as hygiene, dressing, and cooking. The forearm complex permits pronation and supination, motions that rotate the palm upward (supination) or downward (pronation).

Anatomy and Kinesiology

The elbow is composed of three articulations (Figure 17-1):

- *Humeroulnar joint:* The olecranon of the ulna articulates around the trochlea of the humerus. The trochlea is externally rotated 3–8 degrees from a line connecting the medial and lateral epicondyles, resulting in external rotation of the arm when the elbow is flexed 90 degrees. The trochlea normally is tilted in 4 degrees of valgus in males and 8 degrees of valgus in females, thus creating the so-called *carrying angle* of the elbow. A normal carrying angle for men is 10 degrees and is 13 degrees of valgus in women. Any difference in the carrying angle of the elbow is obvious when the elbow is in extension.

> **● Key Point** An increased carrying angle is called cubitus valgus. Cubitus varus, or "gunstock deformity," is the term used to describe a decreased carrying angle. The most common causes of an altered carrying angle are past trauma or epiphyseal growth disturbances. For example, a cubitus valgus can be caused by a lateral epicondylar fracture, whereas a cubitus varus is frequently the result of a supracondylar fracture.

The motions that occur at this joint involve impure flexion and extension. The range of flexion-extension

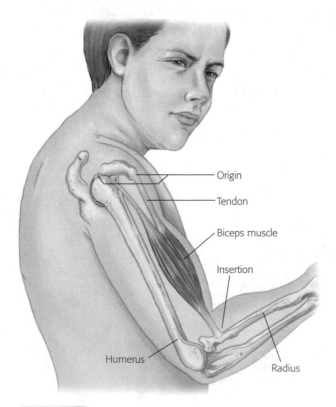

Origin

Tendon

Biceps muscle

Insertion

Humerus

Radius

Figure 17-1 Bony anatomy of the elbow complex.

is from 0–5 degrees beyond extension (hyperextension) to 145–150 degrees of flexion. Full active extension in the normal elbow is some 5–10 degrees short of that obtainable by forced extension, due to passive muscular restraints (biceps, brachialis, and supinator).[1,2] Passive flexion is limited by soft tissue approximation, bony structures (the head of the radius against the radial fossa, and the coronoid process against the coronoid fossa), tension of the posterior capsular ligament, and passive tension in the triceps.[3] Passive extension is limited by the impact of the olecranon process on the olecranon fossa, and tension on the ulnar collateral ligament and anterior capsule.[3] An appreciation and awareness of these end feels can better determine the reason for a joint's lack of motion (or excessive motion). The humeroulnar joint provides most of the structural stability to the elbow as a whole.

> **● Key Point** The resting, or open-packed, position for the humeroulnar joint is 70 degrees of flexion with 10 degrees of forearm supination. The close-packed position is full extension and maximum forearm supination. The capsular pattern is much more limitation in flexion than extension.

- *Humeroradial joint:* The concave head of the radius articulates with the capitulum, which is the convex articular surface of the distal humerus, just lateral to the trochlea. The motions that can occur at this uniaxial hinge joint include flexion and extension of the elbow. Some supination and pronation also occurs at this joint due to a spinning of the radial head (in association with the proximal radioulnar joint [the third articulation of the elbow] and the distal radioulnar joint [see Chapter 18]).

> **● Key Point** The resting, or open-packed, position of the humeroradial joint is extension and forearm supination. The close-packed position is approximately 90 degrees of elbow flexion and 5 degrees of supination. There is no true capsular pattern at this joint.

- *Proximal radioulnar joint:* The proximal or superior radioulnar joint is a uniaxial pivot joint that works in association with the distal or inferior radioulnar joint (see Chapter 18) to form a bicondylar joint. The proximal radioulnar joint is formed between the periphery of the convex radial head and the fibrous osseous ring formed by the concave radial notch of the ulna (which lies distal to the trochlear notch) and the annular ligament (refer to Figure 17-2). An interosseous membrane located between the radius and ulna helps distribute forces (especially compressive forces) throughout the forearm and provide muscle attachment. At the proximal radioulnar joint, one axis of motion exists, permitting pronation and supination. Pronation and supination involve the articulations at the elbow as well as the distal radioulnar joint and the radiocarpal articulation (see Chapter 18). Therefore, a restriction at any of these joints will restrict pronation and supination. There is approximately 0 to 85 degrees of supination and 0 to 75 degrees of pronation available. With the humerus fixed and the forearm free to move, pronation and supination at the proximal radioulnar joint involve the movement of the radius only (the radial head spins in place in the direction of the moving thumb), with the ulna staying essentially stationary. The arthrokinematics of pronation are essentially the same as supination, except that they occur in reverse directions. In full pronation, the shaft of the radius is rotated across the shaft of the ulna, producing a position of relative stability of the forearm.

● **Key Point** Both the humeroulnar and the humeroradial articulations provide approximately 50 percent of the overall stability of the elbow, with the humeroulnar contributing the most.[4–6] Additional support is supplied by ligaments and muscles. The flexor and pronator muscles, which originate at the medial epicondyle, provide additional static and dynamic support to the medial elbow,[7] with the flexor carpi ulnaris (FCU) and flexor digitorum superficialis (FDS) being the most effective in this regard.[8]

● **Key Point** Most activities of daily living require a 100-degree arc of flexion and extension of the elbow, specifically between 30 degrees and 130 degrees, as well as 100 degrees of forearm rotation equally divided between pronation and supination.[9] However, because active internal and external rotation at the shoulder is functionally linked with active pronation and supination of the forearm, a combination of shoulder and forearm rotation can allow the hand to rotate nearly 360 degrees in space, rather than the 170 to 180 degrees by pronation and supination alone.[10] For this reason, the PTA must ensure that no substitute motions are occurring at the shoulder when clinically testing range of motion into pronation and supination.

Ligaments

Support for the elbow complex is provided through strong ligaments (**Table 17-1** and Figure 17-2).

TABLE 17-1 Articular and Ligamentous Contributions to Elbow Stability

Stabilization	Elbow Extended	Elbow Flexed 90 Degrees
Valgus stability	Anterior capsule MCL and bony articular (proximal half of sigmoid notch) *equally divided*	MCL provides 55 percent (primary restraint)
Varus stability	Anterior capsule	Joint articulation (primary restraint)
	Joint articulation (primary restraint)	Anterior capsule
	LCL	LCL
Anterior displacement	Anterior joint capsule	
	Trochlea-olecranon articulation (minimal)	
Posterior displacement	Anterior capsule	
	Radial head against capitellum	
	Coracoid against trochlea	
Distraction	Anterior capsule (primary restraint)	LCL 10 percent
	LCL	MCL (primary restraint)
	MCL	Capsule
	Triceps, biceps, brachial, brachioradial, forearm muscles	

MCL, medial collateral ligament; LCL, lateral collateral ligament.

Data from Sobel J, Nirschl RP: Elbow injuries, in Zachazewski JE, Magee DJ, Quillen WS (eds): Athletic Injuries and Rehabilitation. Philadelphia, WB Saunders, 1996, pp 543–583

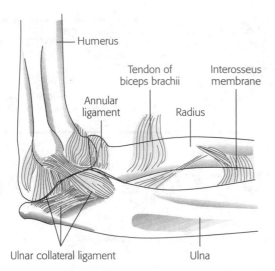

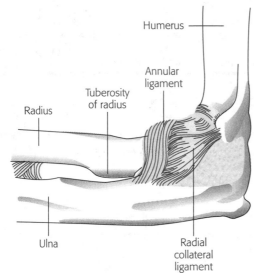

Figure 17-2 Elbow structures.

Medial (Ulnar) Collateral Ligament

The fan-shaped medial collateral ligament (MCL) is functionally the most important ligament in the elbow for providing stability against valgus stress, particularly in the range of 20–130 degrees of flexion and extension,[11] with the humeroradial joint functioning as a secondary stabilizer to valgus loads. In full elbow extension, valgus stability of the elbow is provided equally by the MCL, the joint capsule, and the joint relationships.[7] Anatomically, there are three distinct components of the MCL: anterior bundle, transverse bundle, and posterior bundle. The various bundles of the ligaments are taut in different ranges of motion, providing medial support to the elbow against valgus stresses and limiting end-range elbow extension while keeping the joint surfaces in approximation.

Lateral (Radial) Collateral Ligament

The lateral, or radial, collateral ligament (LCL) consists of the annular ligament, a fan-like ligament that originates from the lateral humerus at the center of the trochlea and capitellum, and the accessory collateral ligament. The LCL provides stability to the lateral aspect of the elbow against varus forces and prevents posterior translation of the radial head. Secondary restraints of the lateral elbow consist of the bony articulations, the joint capsule, and the extensor muscles with their fascial bands and intermuscular septa.

Annular Ligament

The annular ligament functions to maintain the relationship between the head of the radius and the humerus and ulna.

Muscles

The movements of the elbow complex, produced by muscle action, include flexion and extension of the elbow and pronation and supination of the forearm.

Elbow Flexors

The prime movers of elbow flexion are the biceps, brachialis, and brachioradialis (**Table 17-2** and Figure 17-3).[12] The pronator teres, flexor carpi radialis (FCR), flexor carpi ulnaris (FCU), and extensor carpi radialis longus (ECRL) muscles are considered to be weak flexors of the elbow.[13] Most elbow flexors, and essentially all the major supinator and pronator muscles, have their distal attachments on the radius.[14] Whether the brachioradialis is considered a pronator or a supinator depends entirely on the position of the forearm at the start of the muscle contraction. Contraction of these muscles, therefore, pulls the radius proximally against the humeroradial joint.[15,16] The combined efforts of all the elbow flexors can create large amounts of elbow flexion torque. The interosseous membrane transfers a component of this muscle force to the radius and the ulna, thereby dissipating some of the force.[14] The reverse action of the elbow flexors can be used in a closed chain perspective by bringing the upper arm closer to the forearm, such as when performing a pull-up.[10]

> **● Key Point** The brachialis is often referred to as the "workhorse" of elbow flexion because its distal attachment to the ulna (and not the radius like the biceps) prevents any influence on the muscle's length or force-producing capability, whether the forearm is pronated or supinated.

TABLE 17-2	Muscles of the Elbow and Forearm		
Action	**Muscles Acting**	**Peripheral Nerve Supply**	**Nerve Root Deviation**
Elbow flexion	Brachialis	Musculocutaneous	C5–C6, (C7)
	Biceps brachii	Musculocutaneous	C5–C6
	Brachioradialis	Radial	C5–C6, (C7)
	Pronator teres	Median	C6–C7
	Flexor carpi ulnaris	Ulnar	C7–C8
Elbow extension	Triceps	Radial	C7–C8
	Anconeus	Radial	C7–C8, (T1)
Forearm supination	Supinator	Posterior interosseous (radial)	C5–C6
	Biceps brachii	Musculocutaneous	C5–C6
Forearm pronation	Pronator quadratus	Anterior interosseous (median)	C8, T1
	Pronator teres	Median	C6–C7
	Flexor carpi radialis	Median	C6–C7

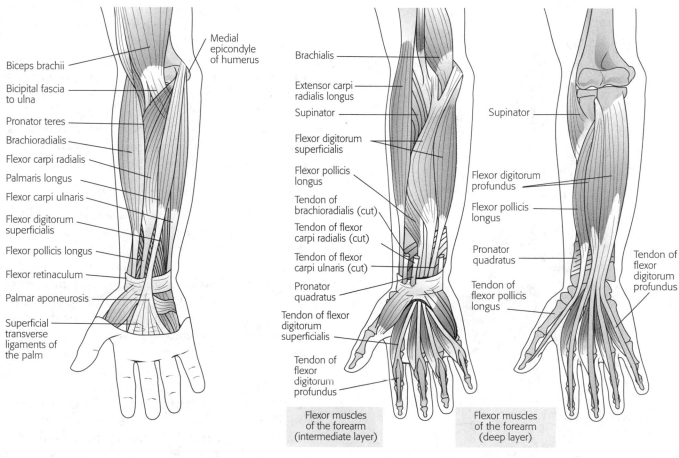

Figure 17-3   Flexor muscles of the forearm.

Elbow Extensors

There are two muscles that extend the elbow: the triceps and the anconeus (Figure 17-4).

- *Triceps brachii:* The triceps brachii has three heads of origin. Like the biceps, it is a two-joint muscle. All three heads of the triceps can extend the elbow, and the long head, which crosses the shoulder, can also perform shoulder extension. The triceps has its maximal force in movements that combine both elbow extension and shoulder extension. The medial head of the triceps is the workhorse of elbow extension, with the lateral and long head recruited during heavier loads.[17] During strong contractions of the triceps—for example a push-up, which involves a combination of elbow extension and shoulder flexion—as the triceps strongly contracts to extend the elbow, the shoulder simultaneously flexes by action of the anterior deltoid, which overpowers the shoulder extension torque of the long head of the triceps.[10]

- *Anconeus:* It has been suggested that in addition to assisting with elbow extension, the anconeus functions to stabilize the ulna in all directions (except valgus) and to pull the subanconeus bursa and the joint capsule out of the way during extension, thus avoiding impingement.[7,18] The anconeus has also been found to help stabilize the elbow during forearm pronation and supination.[19]

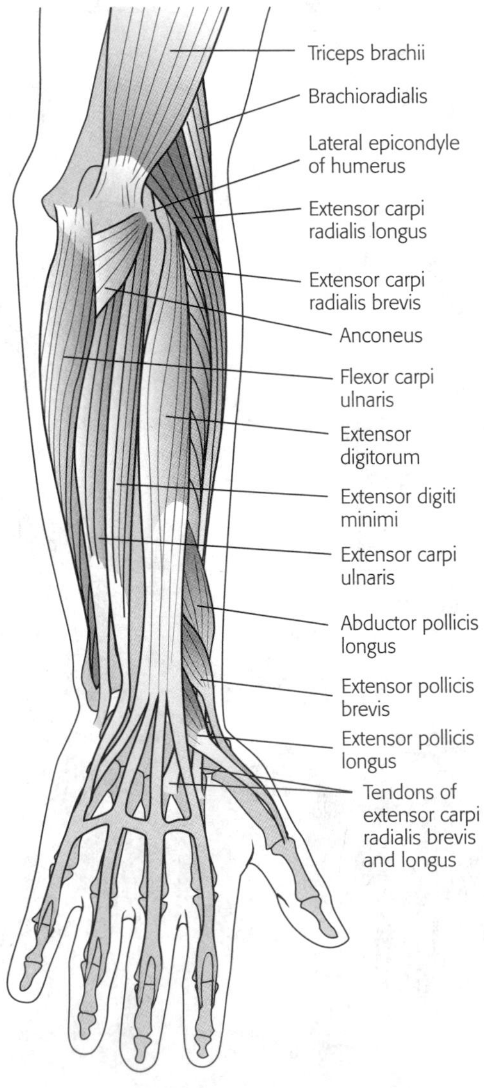

Forearm Pronators

There are two primary pronators:

- *Pronator teres:* The pronator teres has two heads of origin: a humeral head and an ulnar head. The humeral head arises from the medial epicondylar ridge of the humerus and common flexor tendon, whereas the ulnar head arises from the medial aspect of the coronoid process of the ulna. The pronator teres inserts on the anterolateral surface of the midpoint of the radius. The muscle functions predominantly to pronate the forearm, but can also assist with elbow flexion.[7,20,21]

- *Pronator quadratus:* The pronator quadratus is the main pronator of the forearm, in addition to assisting with elbow flexion.

The secondary pronators include the following:

- *Flexor carpi radialis:* The flexor carpi radialis, a forearm muscle, acts to flex and radially deviate the hand.

- *Palmaris longus:* This is a small tendon between the flexor carpi radialis and the flexor carpi ulnaris, although it is not always present. It arises from the medial epicondyle of the humerus by the common flexor tendon, from the intermuscular septa between it and the adjacent muscles, and from the antebrachial fascia. The palmaris longus muscle is the most popular for use in tendon grafts for the wrist due to the length and diameter of the palmaris longus tendon and the fact that it can be used without producing any functional deficits.

Triceps brachii
Brachioradialis
Lateral epicondyle of humerus
Extensor carpi radialis longus
Extensor carpi radialis brevis
Anconeus
Flexor carpi ulnaris
Extensor digitorum
Extensor digiti minimi
Extensor carpi ulnaris
Abductor pollicis longus
Extensor pollicis brevis
Extensor pollicis longus
Tendons of extensor carpi radialis brevis and longus

Figure 17-4   Extensor muscles of the forearm.

Forearm Supinators

There are two forearm supinators:

- *Biceps:* In addition to being an elbow flexor, the biceps assists with supination. The combined action of elbow flexion and forearm supination provided by the biceps is important in bringing the palm of the hand toward the face, such as when eating. The effectiveness of the biceps as a supinator is greatest when the elbow is flexed to 90 degrees, placing the biceps tendon at a 90-degree angle to the radius. In contrast, with the elbow flexed only 30 degrees, much of the rotational efficiency of the biceps is lost.[10]

- *Supinator:* The supinator muscle is a relentless forearm supinator, similar to the brachialis with elbow flexion. The supinator functions to supinate the forearm in any elbow position, while the previously mentioned ECRL and brevis work as supinators during fast movements and against resistance.

Nerve Supply

The elbow has complex innervation (refer to Table 17-2). In general, the musculocutaneous nerve innervates most of the elbow flexors (except the brachioradialis and pronator teres), the radial nerve innervates all the muscles that extend the elbow, and the median nerve supplies all the pronators of the forearm.

The Cubital Tunnel

The cubital tunnel is a fibro-osseous canal, through which the ulnar nerve passes and in which the nerve can be compressed. The volume of the cubital tunnel is greatest with the elbow held in extension and the least in full elbow flexion. A number of factors have been associated with a decrease in the size of the cubital tunnel: space-occupying lesions, bulging of the medial collateral ligament (MCL), osteoarthritis, rheumatoid arthritis, heterotopic bone formation, or trauma to the nerve. Patients with systemic conditions such as diabetes mellitus, hypothyroidism, alcoholism, and renal failure also may have a decreased tunnel diameter.

The Cubital Fossa

The cubital fossa (Figure 17-5) represents the triangular space, or depression, located over the anterior surface of the elbow joint, and which serves as an "entrance" to the forearm, or antebrachium. The boundaries of the fossa are:

- *Lateral:* Brachioradialis and extensor carpi radialis longus muscles
- *Medial:* Pronator teres muscle
- *Proximal:* An imaginary line that passes through the humeral condyles
- *Floor:* Brachialis muscle

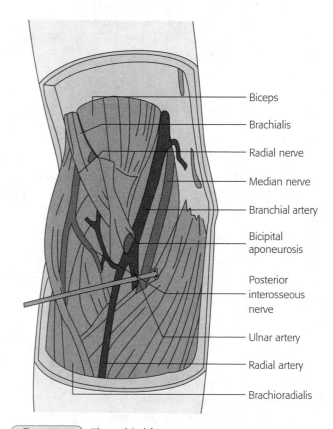

Figure 17-5 The cubital fossa.

The contents of the fossa include:

- The tendon of the biceps brachii, which lies as the central structure in the fossa.
- The median nerve, which runs along the lateral edge of the pronator teres muscle, running between the two heads of the muscle. Entrapment of the median nerve may occur between the heads of the pronator teres muscle, mimicking carpal tunnel syndrome (see Chapter 18).
- The brachial artery, which enters the fossa just lateral to the median nerve and just medial to the biceps brachii tendon.
- The radial nerve, which runs along the medial edge of the brachioradialis and extensor carpi radialis longus (ECRL) muscles, is vulnerable to injury here.
- The median cubital or intermediate cubital cutaneous vein crosses the surface of the fossa.

Bursae

There are numerous bursae in the elbow region:

- *Olecranon bursa:* The main bursa of the elbow complex, which lies posteriorly between the skin and the olecranon process.
- *Deep intratendinous bursa and deep subtendinous bursa:* These are present between the triceps tendon and olecranon.
- *Bicipitoradial bursa:* This separates the biceps tendon from the radial tuberosity.

Examination of the Elbow Complex

The physical therapist's examination of the elbow complex typically follows the outline in **Table 17-3**. The evidence-based special tests for the elbow are outlined in **Table 17-4**.

Intervention Strategies

Due to the unique orientation of the elbow complex, the clinician is faced with multiple clinical challenges to successfully rehabilitate the injured elbow.[22] It is important that the elbow is able to move freely and painlessly throughout its available motion. Throughout all phases of rehabilitation and exercise, training should be within physiologic limits for cellular response and homeostasis.[23] Therefore, relative rest is sometimes advised during painful periods.

TABLE 17-3	Examination of the Elbow

I. History.

II. Observation and inspection.

III. Upper quarter scan as appropriate.

IV. Examination of movements. Active range of motion with passive overpressure of the following movements:
   a. Flexion and extension of the elbow
   b. Pronation and supination of the forearm
   c. Wrist flexion and extension

V. Resisted isometric movements:
   a. Elbow flexion and extension
   b. Pronation and supination of the forearm
   c. Wrist flexion and extension
   d. Radial and ulnar deviation of the wrist

VI. Palpation.

VII. Neurological tests as appropriate (reflexes, sensory scan, peripheral nerve assessment).

VIII. Joint mobility tests:
   a. Distraction/compression of the ulnohumeral joint
   b. Medial and lateral glide of the ulnohumeral joint
   c. Distraction of the radiohumeral joint
   d. Anterior and posterior glide of the radial head
   e. Anterior and posterior glide of the proximal radioulnar joint
   f. Anterior and posterior glide of the distal radioulnar joint

IX. Special tests, including functional testing (refer to Table 17-4).

X. Diagnostic imaging.

Acute Phase

In addition to maintaining general fitness and getting the patient to be independent with a home exercise program, the goals of the acute phase of elbow rehabilitation include the following:

- *Decrease pain and inflammation.* The principles of PRICEMEM (protection, rest, ice, compression, elevation, manual therapy, early motion, and medication) are applied as appropriate. The elbow may need to be immobilized using a splint.
- *Protect the injury site and promote healing.* Early passive and then active assisted exercises are performed in all planes of shoulder, elbow, and wrist motions, to nourish the articular cartilage and assist in collagen tissue synthesis and organization.[22,24–27] Provoking activities, such as strong or repetitive gripping, are avoided. The formation of an elbow flexion contracture must also be avoided.[28] One of the

TABLE 17-4	Evidence-Based Special Tests for the Elbow Complex		
Name of Test	**Brief Description**	**Positive Findings**	**Evidence-Based**
Elbow extension test[a]	With the patient seated with the arms supinated, the patient flexes his or her shoulders to 90 degrees and then extends both elbows.	Positive for bony or joint injury if the involved elbow has less extension than the contralateral side.	Sensitivity: 0.96 Specificity: 0.48
Pressure provocative test[b]	The patient's elbow is positioned in 20 degrees of flexion and forearm supination. The clinician applies pressure to the ulnar nerve just proximal to the cubital tunnel for 60 seconds.	Positive for cubital tunnel syndrome if the patient reports symptoms in the distribution of the ulnar nerve.	Sensitivity: 0.89 Specificity: 0.98
Moving valgus stress test[c]	The patient's shoulder is abducted to 90 degrees with maximal external rotation. The clinician maximally flexes the elbow and applies a valgus stress and then quickly extends the elbow to 30 degrees.	If the patient experiences maximal medial elbow pain between 120 degrees and 70 degrees of elbow flexion, the test is considered positive.	Sensitivity: 1.0 Specificity: 0.75

Data from (a) Appelboam A, Reuben AD, Benger JR, et al: Elbow extension test to rule out elbow fracture: Multicentre, prospective validation and observational study of diagnostic accuracy in adults and children. BMJ 337:a2428, 2008; (b) Novak CB, Lee GW, Mackinnon SE, et al: Provocative testing for cubital tunnel syndrome. J Hand Surg [Am] 19:817–820, 1994; and (c) O'Driscoll SW, Lawton RL, Smith AM: The "moving valgus stress test" for medial collateral ligament tears of the elbow. Am J Sports Med 33:231–239, 2005

most common causes of joint contracture at the elbow is scar formation at the anterior capsule and at the insertion site of the brachialis.[22] This scarring can be minimized with joint mobilizations to the humeroulnar and humeroradial joints. The anterior capsule can also be stretched using long-duration, low-intensity stretching to produce a plastic response of the collagen tissue.[22,29,30] This can be accomplished by positioning the patient in supine, with a towel roll placed posterior and slightly proximal to the elbow joint, and the forearm hanging over the edge of the bed (Figure 17-6). A light weight (2–4 pounds) is placed in the hand or around the wrist, and the elbow is extended as far as is comfortable. This procedure becomes an important component of the patient's home exercise program.

- *Restore pain-free range of motion in the entire kinetic chain.* As the available range at the elbow occurs at the humeroulnar, humeroradial, and proximal and distal radioulnar joints, restrictions or laxities at any of these joints can affect the eventual outcome of the rehabilitative process. Range of motion exercises begin with passive range of motion, progressing to active assisted range of motion, and then active range of motion based on patient tolerance.

Hold-relax and passive stretching techniques can be used to elongate the adaptively shortened muscle to the end of range. In addition, the patient can be taught a number of self-stretches (see the "Therapeutic Techniques" section later in this chapter).

- *Retard muscle atrophy and minimize detrimental effects of immobilization and activity restriction.*[31–36] Patients are initially instructed to perform submaximal isometric exercises at multiple angles for the elbow flexors and extensors, the forearm supinators and pronators, and the wrist flexors and extensors as appropriate.

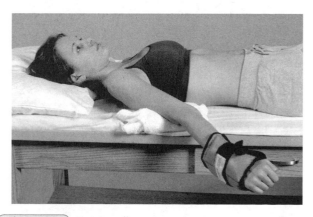

Figure 17-6   Passive elbow extension.

Chronic/Functional Phase

The functional phase addresses any tissue overload problems and functional biomechanical deficits. The goals of the functional phase include:

- *Improve neuromuscular control.* Once full range of pain-free motion has been achieved, the patient's strengthening program is progressed to using dumbbells or surgical tubing through pain-free ranges. Initially low intensity resistance with multiple repetitions are used for muscular endurance, with progression to more intense resistance to strengthen the muscles in preparation for functional demands.[37] Any unused or underused part of the extremity or trunk should be incorporated into the training program, and exercises simulating the desired activity are progressed from slow, controlled motions to high speed with low resistance to improve timing.[37] Co-contraction of the muscles around the elbow can be produced with closed chain exercises such as with the push-up, and quadruped exercises (see Chapter 16).

- *Improve muscle strength to within normal limits (WNL).* Exercises to increase strength should include:
  - ❑ Concentric exercises for the wrist flexors and extensors (see Chapter 18), elbow flexors (Figure 17-7) and extensors (Figure 17-8) through (Figure 17-10), and radial and ulnar deviators (see Chapter 18), performed at varying speeds.
  - ❑ Mechanical resistance using a small bar or hammer with asymmetrically placed weight for strengthening the pronators (Figure 17-11) and supinators (Figure 17-12).
  - ❑ The broom-handle exercise, a recommended exercise for the wrist flexors and extensors. A weight is tied to a rope or piece of string

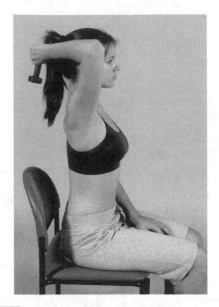

Figure 17-8 Strengthening exercise for elbow extensors: triceps press start position.

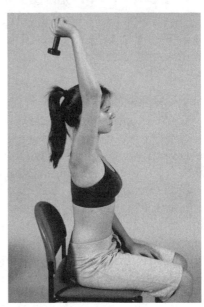

Figure 17-9 Strengthening exercise for elbow extensors: triceps press end position.

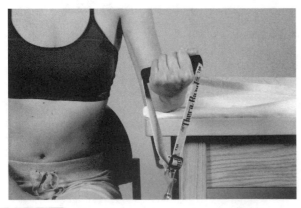

Figure 17-7 Elbow flexor strengthening.

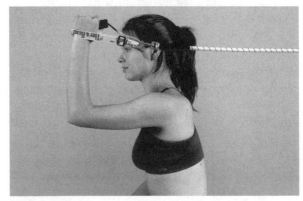

Figure 17-10 Strengthening exercise for elbow extensors using elastic resistance.

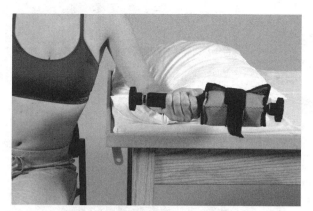

Figure 17-11   Strengthening exercise for forearm pronators.

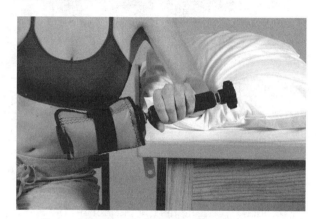

Figure 17-12   Strengthening exercise for forearm supinators.

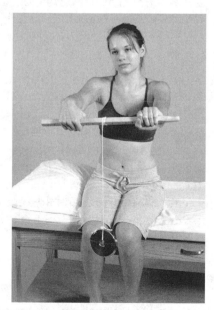

Figure 17-13   Wrist extensor strengthening.

approximately 3 feet in length, which is then tied to a broom handle or dowel. The broom handle is held out in front of the patient with the palms down (for wrist extensors; Figure 17-13) or palms up (for

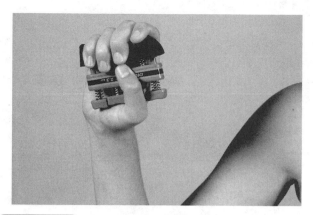

Figure 17-14   Grip stengthening.

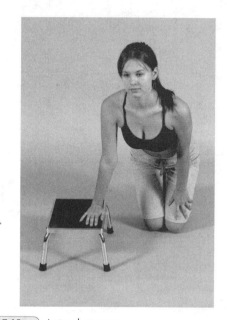

Figure 17-15   Lateral step up.

wrist flexors). The patient then rolls the string onto the handle/dowel to raise and then lower the weight.

❑ Tennis ball squeezes or Gripmaster Digiflex (Figure 17-14) to improve grip strength (once symptoms have subsided).

❑ Exercises to increase the strength in opposing muscles, such as the flexors of the wrist and digits (see Chapter 18), in order to balance the force couple.

❑ Incorporation of the entire upper kinetic chain. Examples of such exercises include the lateral step up using the hand (Figure 17-15), where the patient moves the hand from the floor to the step while applying as much weight as tolerated through the arm, and weight shifting

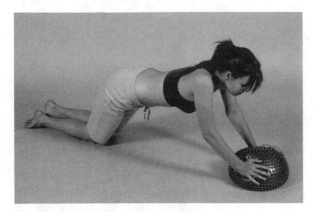

Figure 17-16   Weight shifting and joint loading.

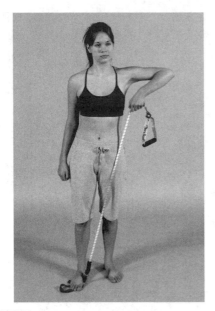

Figure 17-17   PNF exercise for the upper kinetic chain.

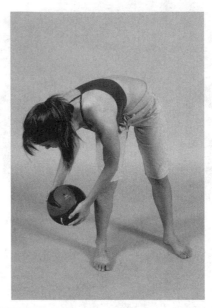

Figure 17-18   Exercise incorporating the trunk and upper kinetic chain.

and joint loading (Figure 17-16) (see also upper kinetic chain exercises in Chapter 16). Caution should be used with shoulder external rotation exercises because of the potential for valgus stress to the elbow.[22,38–40] Stability at the shoulder and the elbow is extremely important for those patients returning to overhead sports, and it can be addressed using proprioceptive neuromuscular facilitation (PNF) patterns with increasing resistance (Figure 17-17). In addition, PNF exercises can be prescribed that incorporate the trunk and upper kinetic chain (Figure 17-18).

❑ Once the functional tests are pain free, an eccentric strengthening program based on the principles of healing can be initiated. These exercises are an essential component of the rehabilitation program with conditions such as medial or lateral epicondylitis. Cryotherapy should be used immediately following these exercises.

■ *Increase muscular endurance:* Endurance is developed over time, as the patient becomes able to tolerate more repetitions and sustained activities. If endurance is not developed and the muscle–tendon unit becomes fatigued, the muscular portion can no longer absorb the stresses and greater stresses are absorbed by the tendon.[41]

There should be a gradual transition back to strenuous activities requiring elbow and forearm power. In such cases, plyometrics that closely simulate the anticipated demands should be added to the program. In order to return to strenuous activities, the minimum requirements are that the elbow has full, pain-free range of motion; no pain or tenderness on physical examination; and adequate muscle strength, power, and endurance that is 70 percent of the uninvolved side.[22]

Common Conditions

The common conditions that can affect the elbow include those that relate to poor biomechanics due to weakness, trauma, repetitive activities involving the wrist and hand, or overuse.

Tendon Ruptures

Tendon ruptures around the elbow require significant forces.

Biceps Tendon Rupture

The biceps brachii may be injured either at the musculotendinous junction or at the radial tuberosity, being avulsed partially or completely. These distal injuries account for 3–10 percent of all biceps tendon ruptures, with the remainder occurring at the shoulder.[42] Avulsions of the biceps tendon at the elbow occur almost exclusively in males.[43] Most typically it affects the dominant elbow of a muscular male in his fifth decade of life.[44] Clinical findings vary depending on whether the rupture is partial or complete. The history may include a report of either a sharp, tearing-type pain coincident with an acute injury or swelling and activity-related pains in the antecubital fossa from chronic injury.[44] The physical examination may reveal ecchymosis in the antecubital fossa (and sometimes also in the distal ulnar part of the arm), a palpable defect of the distal biceps, loss of strength of elbow flexion and grip, but especially a loss of forearm supination strength.[45] In active individuals, primary repair of the acute tendon avulsion is the treatment of choice. If not repaired, a 30 percent loss of elbow flexion and a 40 percent loss of supination strength can be expected.[45]

Triceps Tendon Rupture

Triceps tendon ruptures usually occur with a deceleration force during extension or an uncoordinated contraction of the triceps muscle against the flexing elbow.[46] As with rupture of the biceps tendon, the physical findings depend on whether the avulsion is partial or complete. Loss of elbow extension strength, inability to extend overhead against gravity, and a tendon defect are findings if the tear is complete.[44]

Intervention for Tendon Ruptures

Surgical repair is the treatment of choice in acute complete ruptures. Partial injury may be treated conservatively with immobilization for about 3 weeks, followed by a gradual progression of range of motion and strengthening.

Overuse Injuries

Chronic overuse injuries are the result of multiple microtraumatic events that cause disruption of the internal structure of the tendon and produce tendonitis or tendonosis.

Bicipital Tendonosis

Bicipital tendonosis is an overuse injury resulting from repetitive hyperextension of the elbow with pronation, or repetitive flexion combined with stressful pronation-supination.[47] The condition is common in weightlifters, bowlers, gymnasts, and those involved in heavy lifting. Typically there are complaints of pain located at the anterior aspect of the distal part of the arm. There is tenderness to palpation of the distal biceps belly, the musculotendinous portion of the biceps, or the bicipital insertion of the radial tuberosity.[3,47] Other findings include pain on resisted elbow flexion and supination, and pain with passive shoulder and elbow extension.

The rehabilitation focuses on strength, endurance, and flexibility of the flexor/supinator mechanism (see the "Intervention Strategies" section earlier in this chapter) and on strengthening the shoulder stabilizers (see Chapter 16). In addition, electrotherapeutic and thermal modalities, transverse friction massage, trigger point treatment, and specific elbow joint mobilizations can also be used.

Triceps Tendonosis

Triceps tendon overload injury results from repetitive extension. The patient reports tenderness localized to the triceps insertion at the olecranon, which is aggravated with resisted elbow extension. The initial stages of the intervention emphasize the principles of PRICEMEM. Therapeutic exercises emphasize strength of the elbow extensor mechanism. Closed chain exercises are particularly effective.[48] Additional emphasis is placed on shoulder strength and scapular stabilization exercises (see Chapter 16).

Brachialis Strain

A strain to the brachialis is relatively rare but can occur from overuse in activities such as heavy lifting. The brachialis is also prone to myositis ossificans, a pathologic bone formation, due to the fact that it is likely to hemorrhage when injured. If myositis ossificans is suspected due to signs and symptoms including a painless, enlarging mass, the PT should be notified and therapy placed on hold.

As in the lesion of the biceps, the pain is felt on the anterior aspect of the distal part of the arm. There is palpable tenderness in the muscle belly of the brachialis, at the level of the musculotendinous junction of the biceps. Resisted supination is not painful, although resisted elbow flexion with the forearm pronated is.

Epicondylitis

Defined literally, epicondylitis suggests an inflammation at one of the epicondyles of the elbow. Two types of epicondylitis are commonly described: tennis elbow (lateral epicondylitis) and golfer's elbow (medial epicondylitis; see the following sections). Both types of epicondylitis are common in persons who frequently overuse the upper arm, particularly with activities that involve rotation of the arm with flexion and extension. However, lateral epicondylitis has been found to be four to seven times more common than medial epicondylitis.[49]

Lateral Epicondylitis (Tennis Elbow)

Lateral epicondylitis, more commonly known as tennis elbow, represents a pathologic condition of the common extensor muscles at their origin on the lateral humeral epicondyle. Although the terms *epicondylitis* and *tendonitis* are commonly used to describe tennis elbow, histopathologic studies have demonstrated that tennis elbow is often not an inflammatory condition; rather, it is a degenerative condition, a tendonosis.[49,50] Specifically, the condition involves the tendons of the muscles that control wrist extension and radial deviation resulting in pain on the lateral side of the elbow with contraction of these muscles.[51]

Tennis elbow affects between 1 percent and 3 percent of the population, and occurs most commonly between 35 and 50 years of age with a mean age of 45.[52] More than 25 conditions have been suggested as causes of tennis elbow,[53] including periostitis,[53–56] infection,[57,58] bursitis,[53,56,59–63] fibrillation of the radial head,[64] radioulnar joint disease,[65] annular ligament lesion,[66–68] nipped synovial fringe,[69–74] calcific tendonitis,[75] neurogenic causes,[76,77] osteochondritis dissecans, and radial nerve entrapment.[76,78–82]

Whatever the source of the symptoms, tennis elbow is usually the result of overuse but can be traumatic in origin. Whereas macrotramatic injuries can be clearly explained by excessive forces overwhelming tissue tensile strength, overuse injuries are somewhat more controversial in their pathogenesis. The tendons involved in locomotion and ballistic performance, which transmit loads under elastic and eccentric conditions, are susceptible to injury. Some tendons, such as those that wrap around a convex surface or the apex of a concavity, those that cross two joints, those with areas of scant vascular supply, and those that are subjected to repetitive tension, are particularly vulnerable to overuse injuries.[83–88] Occupations or sports that involve repetitive grasping, with the wrist positioned in extension, place the elbow particularly at risk because it is the wrist extensors that must contract during grasping activities to stabilize the wrist.[44]

Diffuse achiness and morning stiffness are common complaints.[51] Occasionally the pain is experienced at night and the patient may report frequent dropping of objects, especially if they are carried with the palm facing down.

The exact location of the pain is revealed by palpation, and tenderness is usually found over the extensor carpi radialis brevis (ECRB) and extensor carpi radialis longus (ECRL), especially at the lateral epicondyle. The resisted tests typically reproduce symptoms with resisted wrist extension and radial deviation with the elbow extended. Pain on resisted finger extension has also been reported.

Intervention for Lateral Epicondylitis

The lack of agreement in the literature regarding the pathogenesis of tennis elbow has led to a proliferation of interventions, both medical and surgical.[89] Recent literature has demonstrated a trend toward treatment of the cervical and thoracic spine with this disorder. A retrospective study by Cleland and colleagues[90] demonstrated that patients receiving manual therapy techniques directed at the cervical spine achieved similar success rates as a group who received treatment solely directed at the elbow; however, they achieved this success in significantly fewer visits ($p = 0.01$). A more recent pilot clinical trial by Cleland et al.[91] that compared the outcomes of 10 patients with lateral epicondylalgia who were randomly assigned to receive localized treatment or localized treatment plus manual therapy to the cervicothoracic spine found that the latter group demonstrated greater improvement in all outcome measures as compared to the localized treatment group. Although promising, replication of these results is needed in a large-scale randomized clinical trial with a control group and a longer-term follow-up before any meaningful conclusions can be drawn.

The patient may be prescribed an orthotic device as a treatment strategy; many different types of braces and other orthotic devices are available. The main type is a band or strap around the muscle belly of the wrist extensors. Theoretically, binding the muscle with a clasp, band, or brace should limit expansion and thereby decrease the contribution to force production by muscle fibers proximal to the band.[92] Counterforce bracing[93] has been shown to:

- Have a beneficial effect on the force couple imbalances and altered movements associated with tennis elbow[38,94,95]
- Decrease elbow angular acceleration[96]
- Decrease electromyographic activity[96]

However, contrary to popular belief, tennis-elbow braces have been shown to have little effect in vibrational dampening.[97] As an alternative to elbow bracing, Gellman[98] recommends a protective 20-degree wrist extension splint for tennis elbow to help offload the ECRB.[51] The results from a study by Struijs and colleagues[92] would tend to indicate that brace treatment might be useful as an initial therapy.

Cyriax recommends the Mill's manipulation to treat true tennis elbow, a thrust technique by the physical therapist that is intended to maximally stretch the ECRB tendon, in order to try to pull apart the two surfaces of the painful scar.[53] Manipulation of this kind has also been advocated in other studies.[99–101]

Johnson[102] recommends an exercise regimen consisting of progressive resistance exercise to the wrist extensors, with the elbow flexed to 90 degrees and also with the elbow straight. This should be performed as a 10-repetition maximum, morning and night. Gradually, the weight must be increased so that the 10-repetition maximum is always maintained. Pain will be increased for the first 1 to 3 weeks, but by the fifth or sixth weeks, the elbow pain will be better. An ice pack or heating pad can be a mitigating modality during the painful period.[102]

Wilk and Andrews[103] recommend the guidelines outlined in **Table 17-5**.

If the symptoms are not controlled with the above measures, a local injection of corticosteroid by the physician may be helpful.[104–106]

Surgical Intervention for Lateral Epicondylitis

Surgery is indicated if the symptoms do not resolve despite properly performed nonoperative treatments lasting 6 months.[44] The goals of operative treatment

---

TABLE 17-5 Conservative Rehabilitation for Lateral Epicondylitis

Phase 1	Intervention
Increase flexibility	Stretches into: • Wrist extension–flexion • Elbow extension–flexion • Forearm supination–pronation
Decrease inflammation/pain	Cryotherapy Phonophoresis Iontophoresis (with an anti-inflammatory such as dexamethasone)
Promote tissue healing	Avoid painful movements (such as gripping) Friction massage

Phase 2	Intervention
Improve flexibility	Continue flexibility exercises
Increase muscular strength and endurance	Emphasize concentric–eccentric strengthening Initiate shoulder strengthening (if deficiencies are noted)
Increase functional activities and return to function	Use counterforce brace Continue use of cryotherapy after exercise or function Initiate gradual return to stressful activities Gradually reinitiate previously painful movements

Phase 3	Intervention
Improve muscular strength and endurance	Continue strengthening exercises (emphasize eccentric–concentric) Continue to emphasize deficiencies in shoulder and elbow strength
Gradually return to high-level sport activities	Gradually diminish use of counterforce brace Use cryotherapy as needed Equipment modifications (grip size, string tension, and playing surface)

Data from Wilk KE, Andrews JR: Elbow injuries, in Brotzman SB, Wilk KE (eds): Clinical Orthopaedic Rehabilitation. Philadelphia, Mosby, 2003, pp 85–123

of tendonosis of the elbow are to resect pathologic material, to stimulate neovascularization by producing focused local bleeding, and to create a healthy scar while doing the least possible structural damage to surrounding tissues. Postoperatively, a carefully guided resistance-based rehabilitation program is recommended (**Table 17-6**).

Medial Epicondylitis (Golfer's Elbow)

Medial epicondylitis primarily involves a tendinopathy of the common flexor origin, specifically the FCR and the origin of the pronator teres.[8,52,107] To a lesser extent, the palmaris longus, FCU, and flexor digitorum superficialis may also be involved.[108]

The mechanism for medial epicondylitis is not usually related to direct trauma, but rather to overuse. This commonly occurs for three reasons:

- The flexor–pronator tissues fatigue in response to repeated stress, particularly with activities involving repetitive flexing of the fingers and thumb, and flexing and pronating of the wrist.
- There is a sudden change in the level of stress that predisposes the elbow to medial ligamentous injury, such as repetitive throwing/pitching.[109]
- The ulnar collateral ligament fails to stabilize the valgus forces sufficiently.[110]

Similar to lateral epicondylitis, medial epicondylitis usually begins as a microtear. The microtear in medial epicondylitis frequently occurs at the interface between the pronator teres and FCR origins with subsequent development of fibrotic and inflammatory granulation tissue.[111] Chronic symptoms result from a loss of extensibility of the tissues, leaving the tendon unable to attenuate tensile loads. The symptoms are typically reported to be exacerbated with either resisted wrist flexion and pronation or passive wrist extension and supination.[107,111]

Intervention

Conservative intervention for medial epicondylitis, which is similar to that of lateral epicondylitis, has been shown to have success rates as high as 90 percent.[107] The intervention for this condition initially involves rest, activity modification, and local modalities. Complete immobilization is not

TABLE 17-6	Rehabilitation Protocol Following Lateral Epicondylitis Surgery
Phase 1	**Intervention**
Protect surgical site	Extremity positioned in a sling (sling removed at 2–4 weeks)
Control inflammation and edema	Cryotherapy
Maintain range of motion	Gentle (pain-free) passive/active assisted hand, wrist, elbow, and active shoulder ROM exercises
Phase 2 (weeks 2–4)	**Intervention**
Increase range of motion	Continue progression of ROM exercises
Initiate strengthening	Active motion
	Submaximal isometrics
	Shoulder and scapular strengthening: manual D1 and D2 PNF with patient supine
Phase 3 (weeks 5+)	**Intervention**
Strengthening	PREs with weights or Theraband
	Return to sport at weeks 8–12
Functional training	Modified activities (task-specific functional training at weeks 8–12)
Scar formation	Gentle massage along and against fiber orientation

ROM, range of motion; PRE, progressive resistive exercise; PNF, proprioceptive neuromuscular facilitation.

Data from Wilk KE, Andrews JR: Elbow injuries, in Brotzman SB, Wilk KE (eds): Clinical Orthopaedic Rehabilitation. Philadelphia, Mosby, 2003, pp 85–123

recommended, even in the acute phase, because it eliminates the stresses necessary for maturation of new collagen tissue, resulting in healed tissue that is not strong enough to withstand the stresses associated with a return to activity. However, the patient may need to stop activities that produce tension overload. Once the acute phase has passed, the focus is to restore the range of motion and correct imbalances of flexibility and strength. The strengthening program is progressed to include concentric and eccentric exercises of the flexor–pronator muscles. Splinting or the use of a counterforce brace may be a useful adjunct.[111]

Medial (Ulnar) Collateral Ligament Sprain (Medial Valgus Stress Overload)

The most common mechanisms of MCL insufficiency are a chronic attenuation of valgus and external rotation forces,[112–116] as seen in the tennis serve or in the baseball throwing pitch,[117,118] and posttraumatic, usually after a fall on an outstretched hand (FOOSH injury).[11] Associated injuries after trauma may include fractures of the radial head, olecranon, or medial humeral epicondyle.[115,116] MCL injury can also occur during surgery for cubital tunnel syndrome.[119,120] Irritation of the ulnar nerve, with symptoms of ulnar neuritis, may be present secondary to inflammation of the ligamentous complex.[112,121,122]

The most common complaint from the patient is medial elbow pain at the ligament's origin,[51] or at the insertion site if there is an acute avulsion.[11] The primary restraint to valgus stress is the anterior bundle of the MCL,[4,5,116,123–126] so the physical examination by the physical therapist focuses on palpation of the course of the MCL.[11] Valgus stress testing of the elbow is also performed (refer to Table 17-4).

Conservative Approach

The intervention for early symptoms of MCL injury includes rest and activity modification or restriction for about 2–4 weeks, range of motion exercises, physical therapy modalities, and NSAIDs prescribed by the physician.[111]

Strengthening and stretching of the FCU, pronator teres, and flexor digitorum superficialis are initiated once the acute inflammatory stage has subsided; they are performed in the pain-free mid-range of motion.[8,117,127,128] Emphasis is placed on isometric exercises of the forearm flexors, ulnar deviators, and pronators, in order to enhance their role as secondary stabilizers of the medial joint. In addition, strengthening of the shoulder and elbow muscles may help prevent or minimize injury and may facilitate rehabilitation.[8,51] For those returning to sports, a well-supervised throwing and conditioning program is initiated, as appropriate, at approximately 3 months, once the athlete has regained full range of motion and strength.[111]

Surgical Intervention

The anterior oblique band of the ulnar collateral ligament is particularly vulnerable to microtearing, attenuation, weakening, and eventual rupture in those involved in heavy manual labor. Reconstruction of this ligament centers on the restoration of the anterior oblique band of the ulnar collateral ligament with the use of an autologous free tendon graft. Additional considerations include patient age, activity level, job requirements, general health, and general integrity of the uninvolved elbow.[112,129,130]

The surgical repair or reconstruction can be performed with or without ulnar nerve transposition.[131] The palmaris longus tendon is the most frequently used graft for elbow reconstruction,[132] although the plantaris and toe extensor tendons can also be used.[113] The surgical procedure in which a ligament in the medial elbow is replaced with a tendon from elsewhere in the body is also known as the Tommy John surgery. The postsurgical rehabilitation begins immediately with the patient's involved upper extremity immobilized in a brace to protect against valgus stress. Active range of motion of the shoulder (taking care with external rotation because this motion produces valgus stress on the elbow), hand, and wrist begins immediately. Following the period of immobilization, forearm and elbow range of motion exercises are begun, and by the third week postoperatively, range of motion of the elbow should approach 20 to 110 degrees. At this time, concentric and eccentric exercises are used for the wrist, and submaximal isometrics are used for elbow flexion and extension. By 4 to 6 weeks, elbow range of motion should be 0 to 130 degrees. At this time, concentric and eccentric exercises are introduced for elbow flexion and extension and are progressed as tolerated. In addition, forearm pronation and supination resistance exercises are introduced. Functional training begins around 2 to 4 months postsurgery, although a return to heavy manual labor or sport takes approximately 12 months.

Olecranon Bursitis

Because of its location, the olecranon bursa is easily bruised through direct trauma or is irritated through repetitive grazing and weight bearing, causing bursitis.[133]

Acute bursitis presents as a swelling over the olecranon process that can vary in size from a slight distension to a mass as large as 6 centimeters in diameter.[134] An inflamed bursa can occasionally become infected, requiring differentiation between septic and nonseptic bursitis.[135]

Pain and swelling can be gradual as in the chronic cases, or sudden as in acute injury or an infection.[134] Redness and heat suggest infection, whereas exquisite tenderness indicates trauma or infection as the underlying cause. Patients often note a decreased range of motion or an inability to don a long-sleeved shirt.[136]

Intervention

Although the simple posttraumatic bursitis can be treated with the principles of PRICEMEM, the infected bursa needs prompt medical attention.[136] If the patient is experiencing significant pain or discomfort with movement of the elbow, a sling helps to reduce these symptoms and calm the joint.[134]

Supracondylar Fractures

Supracondylar fractures are caused by direct trauma to the arm or shoulder or by axial loading transmitted through the elbow. The fracture pattern produced is related to the degree of elbow flexion and the direction and magnitude of the force applied. Indications for surgery are to prevent further injury, restore anatomy, and provide an optimal environment for healing.

Intervention

The choice of operative exposure depends on the fracture pattern and surgeon preference. The chevron olecranon osteotomy allows for stable fixation and early range of motion. Following the procedure, a posterior long-arm splint is applied with the elbow at 60–90 degrees of flexion, depending on the amount of swelling. At 10–14 days postoperatively the sutures are removed; if the wound is stable, the patient is placed in a hinged elbow orthosis and protected active range of motion is allowed. Passive, then active assisted range of motion is allowed to the point of discomfort, not pain. The orthosis is worn until both clinical and radiographic evidence of fracture union is present, at approximately 6–12 weeks postoperatively; after this, orthosis use is discontinued.

> ### ● Key Point
> One of the serious complications arising from supracondylar fractures is *Volkmann's ischemic contracture,* which occurs as the result of increased tissue fluid pressure within a fascial muscle compartment that reduces capillary blood perfusion below a level necessary for tissue viability.[137] Clinical findings include:[138]
>
> - A swollen and tense tender compartment
> - Severe pain, exacerbated by passive stretch of the forearm muscles
> - Sensibility deficits
> - Motor weakness or paralysis
>
> However, there is no absence of radial and ulnar pulses at the wrist.

Intercondylar Fractures

The intercondylar fracture of the distal end of the humerus is one of the most difficult of all fractures to manage. Recommendations for treatment have ranged widely, from essentially no treatment to operative reduction and extensive internal fixation. Typically occurring following high-energy injury, intercondylar fractures can lead to significant functional impairment. Much of the difficulty encountered with these fractures lies in the complex anatomy of the elbow joint and the high potential for articular comminution. Operative intervention for distal humerus fractures is based on many factors, including fracture type, intra-articular involvement, fragment displacement, bone quality, joint stability, and soft tissue quality and coverage. In addition, individual factors, such as patient age, overall health condition, functional extremity demands, and patient compliance, are all considered.

Conservative Approach

Nonoperative treatment depends on the fracture type. Casting and immobilization can be used for nondisplaced fractures, particularly with medial, lateral, and supracondylar process fractures (extra-articular and extracapsular).

- Medial epicondylar fractures are typically immobilized for 7 days, with the elbow flexed at 90 degrees, the forearm pronated, and the wrist flexed at 30 degrees to relax the common flexor–pronator muscle group.
- Lateral epicondylar fractures are typically immobilized with the elbow in 90 degrees of flexion, the forearm in supination, and the wrist extended slightly to relax the extensor muscles.

Surgical Intervention

The rehabilitation for an intercondylar fracture is similar to that for a supracondylar fracture:

- A period of immobilization to avoid all stress to the involved arm

- A general conditioning program during the period of immobilization and active exercises prescribed for the wrist, hand, and shoulder
- Active range of motion exercises for elbow flexion and extension, and forearm pronation/supination once prescribed by the physician and supervising physical therapist
- Initiation of strength training once stable union of the fracture has been established

Radial Head Fractures and Dislocations

Radial head fractures and dislocations are traumatic injuries that require adequate treatment to prevent disability from stiffness, deformity, post-traumatic arthritis, nerve damage, or other serious complications.[139] Radial head fractures and dislocations may be isolated just to the radial head (and neck) and the lateral elbow (and proximal forearm), or they may be part of a combined complex fracture injury pattern, involving the other structures of the elbow, distal humerus, or forearm and wrist. Radial head fractures and dislocations are typically as a result of trauma, usually from a FOOSH with the force of impact transmitted up the hand through the wrist and forearm to the radial head, which is forced into the capitellum. The wrist, especially the distal radioulnar joint, may be damaged simultaneously.

Monteggia Fracture

Monteggia fracture–dislocations are a special type of radial head injury, involving a combination of a fracture of the ulna and a dislocation of the proximal end of the radius. Instead of the radial head dislocation, the radial head or neck may be fractured as an equivalent injury. These lesions typically result from a direct blow to the forearm or a FOOSH injury with the arm positioned in either hyperextension or hyperpronation. Although relatively rare, these fractures can present with serious problems and poor functional outcomes if mismanaged.[140,141] The complications include damage to the posterior branch of the radial nerve, anterior interosseous nerve (AIN), and ulnar nerve as well as nonunion and poor AROM.[140]

Essex–Lopresti Fracture

This type of fracture is defined as a fracture of the radial head with proximal radius migration and disruption of the distal radioulnar joint and interosseous membrane,[142] which typically results from a FOOSH injury.[143]

Intervention

Radial head fractures present several challenges during the rehabilitative process, because the radial head is a secondary stabilizer for valgus forces at the elbow and resists longitudinal forces along the forearm.[144] Compromise of the medial (ulnar) collateral ligament makes the radial head a more important stabilizer of the elbow.[7,144,145] A successful outcome for this condition correlates directly with accuracy of anatomic reduction, restoration of mechanical stability that allows early motion, and attention to the soft tissues. Treatment options for radial head fractures or dislocations include closed reduction with casting or early motion or open reduction with internal fixation (ORIF), replacement, or resection. Closed reduction and casting often have associated high rates of stiffness, and closed reduction and early motion may still have high rates of nonunion and malunion in comminuted or unstable fractures, resulting in generally poor functional results. Open treatment (including internal fixation, replacement, or excision depending on the fracture) is associated with better long-term function.

> ● **Key Point** For Monteggia fracture–dislocations, the optimum treatment includes ORIF of the ulna diaphyseal fracture. Following the surgery, the elbow is immobilized for about 4 weeks in 90–120 degrees of elbow flexion, after which AROM exercises for elbow flexion and forearm supination are initiated. AROM into extension beyond 90 degrees begins 4–6 weeks postoperatively.

Using the Mason classification, the fracture is type I if it is undisplaced, type II if a single fragment is displaced, and type III if it is comminuted. Type I (nondisplaced) is generally treated nonoperatively. Type II may be treated nonoperatively if the displacement is minimal. Type III fractures usually require operative intervention but may occasionally be treated closed with early motion if the radial head is not reconstructible. If a mechanical block to motion is present, then nonsurgical treatment cannot be used.

Use of a splint or a sling for 3 days is indicated in type I fractures, with active elbow flexion exercises being initiated immediately. As much early mobilization as the patient can tolerate is the key to a favorable outcome. Strengthening, initially involving isometric exercises, begins at 3 weeks and progresses to concentric exercises at 5–6 weeks. Heavy resistance is not performed until after 8 weeks, or when adequate healing is demonstrated on radiographs.

Fractures with radial head surface involvement of more than 30 percent, fracture fragment displacement, and type III characteristics require management by an orthopaedic surgeon.[134]

Rehabilitation following elbow fractures that undergo internal fixation usually lasts for 12 weeks. Immediately following the immobilization of elbow fractures, active and passive motion exercises are initiated. The goal is to achieve 15–105 degrees of motion by the end of week 2. Isometric exercises for elbow flexion and extension and forearm pronation/supination are started within the first week. Active assisted pronation/supination exercises do not begin until week 6. Concentric exercises are given for the shoulder and the wrist and hand. Joint mobilizations, which, if needed, begin in the second week, are used to help regain elbow extension.

By the third week, the patient should be performing lightweight concentric exercises for elbow flexion and extension, and beginning at week 7, eccentric and plyometric exercises are prescribed. At about the same time, neuromuscular re-education exercises and functional training exercises are added.

> ● **Key Point** For Essex–Lopresti fractures, conservative intervention involves rest from throwing or impact-loading stress, with a short period of splint immobilization in a Muenster cast sometimes being necessary. Gentle AROM for forearm rotation is initiated about 6 weeks after surgery and immobilization. The exercise progression is based on clinical findings and patient tolerance.

Olecranon Fracture

An olecranon process fracture is not uncommon due to its subcutaneous position, and may be caused by either a high- or a low-energy injury.[146,147] The high-energy mechanism is usually a fall backward onto the elbow or a FOOSH injury, which produces passive elbow flexion with the forearm in a supinated position. Recognition of an avulsion fracture involving the triceps is through loss of active extension; a palpable gap, pain, and swelling at the fracture site; and a large hematoma developing into diffuse ecchymosis.[148]

Intervention

The goals of olecranon fracture treatment must be customized based on the needs of the patient. In young active individuals, restoration of the articular surface, preservation of strength and power, restoration of stability, and prevention of joint stiffness are important. In older patients, minimization of morbidity is the most important goal.

Nondisplaced fractures with intact extensor mechanisms may be treated nonoperatively. Three weeks of casting usually is sufficient. The elbow can be placed at any degree of flexion. The focus of the intervention for minimally displaced fractures is to allow restoration of the articular surfaces and maintenance of triceps function, while allowing early range of motion. The elbow is immobilized in a posterior splint or elbow immobilizer, with the elbow flexed at 90 degrees for 6 to 8 weeks (sometimes for as little as 3 weeks). Pronation and supination are started at 2–3 days, and easy flexion and extension motions begin at 2 weeks. Early range of motion exercise is performed in mid-ranges, specifically avoiding full flexion for up to 2 months. Protected immobilization should continue until there is evidence of union (approximately 6 weeks). Muscle strengthening is not emphasized until bone healing is visualized radiographically in order to ensure healing of the olecranon. Patients may return to work involving vigorous use of the extremity at 3–4 months postoperatively. Resistance exercises are avoided for up to 3 months.

All other fractures require ORIF or excision of the bone fragments with repair of the extensor mechanism.[140,146,147,149] Rehabilitation following surgery is dependent on the extent of the surgery and the length of the immobilization, although the emphasis on regaining early motion remains the same. Range of motion exercises start at around 10 days.

Elbow Dislocation

Posterior elbow displacement is much more common than anterior displacement. With posterior displacements, the ulna is displaced posteriorly in relation to the distal humerus. Posterior displacements can be further subdivided into three types: posterior-lateral (most common), lateral, and posterior-medial (least common).[150,151] Elbow subluxations and dislocations can be associated with fractures and neurovascular injuries (median, ulnar, and radial nerves; brachial artery) about the elbow. Three other conditions have been associated with elbow dislocations:

- Compartment syndrome may develop in the forearm fascia or biceps tendon due to substantial swelling. Symptoms include the presence of persistent pain, particularly with passive finger and wrist extension of the dislocated arm.
- Ectopic calcification, such as myositis ossificans.
- Ulnar collateral ligament (anterior oblique band) involvement.

Intervention

Isolated posterior elbow dislocations are managed using closed reduction and immobilization. Early ROM exercises in stable, reduced elbow dislocations have been shown to be associated with an improved outcome.[152] However, immobilization of the affected elbow for longer than 3 weeks in patients following an elbow dislocation has been associated with loss of ROM compared with patients who start early ROM exercises.[152]

● **Key Point** The most common sequela after elbow dislocation is a loss (5–15 degrees) of extension.

A sample protocol for the conservative intervention following an elbow dislocation is outlined in **Table 17-7**.

Surgical intervention is reserved for patients with signs of neurovascular compromise, associated fractures, or nonreducible dislocations.

TABLE 17-7	**Conservative Intervention Following an Elbow Dislocation**
Phase 1 (1–4 days)	**Intervention**
Protection of injury site	Immobilization of elbow at 90 degrees of flexion in a well-padded posterior splint for 3–4 days
	Avoid valgus stresses to the elbow
Initiation of range of motion	Avoid any passive ROM (patient to perform active ROM when the posterior splint is removed and replaced with a hinged elbow brace or sling)
Strengthening of uninvolved areas	Begin light gripping exercises (putty or tennis ball)
Control of inflammation and edema	Use cryotherapy and high-voltage galvanic stimulation
Phase 2 (days 5–14)	**Intervention**
Protection of injury site	Replace the posterior splint with a hinged elbow brace initially set at 15–90 degrees
Range of motion	Wrist and finger active ROM in all planes.
	Active elbow ROM (*avoid valgus stress*)—flexion-extension-supination-pronation
Strengthening	Multiangle flexion isometrics
	Multiangle extension isometrics (avoid valgus stress)
	Wrist curls/reverse wrist curls
	Light biceps curls
	Shoulder exercises (avoid external rotation of shoulder, because this places valgus stress at the elbow); the elbow is stabilized during shoulder exercises
Phase 3 (weeks 2–8)	**Intervention**
Protection of injury site	Hinged brace settings 0 degrees to full flexion
Strengthening	PRE progression of elbow and wrist exercises
	Initiation of gentle low-load, long-duration stretching around 5–6 weeks for the patient's loss of extension
	Gradual progression of weight with curls, elbow extensions, and so on
	Sport-specific exercises and drills initiated as appropriate
	External rotation and internal rotation exercises of the shoulder may be incorporated at 6–8 weeks
	Interval throwing program initiated at around 8 weeks (in the asymptomatic patient)
	No return to play until strength is 85 to 90 percent of the uninvolved limb

Data from Wilk KE, Andrews JR: Elbow injuries, in Brotzman SB, Wilk KE (eds): Clinical Orthopaedic Rehabilitation. Philadelphia, Mosby, 2003, pp 85–123

Therapeutic Techniques

A number of therapeutic techniques can be used to assist the patient. These include manual techniques and self-stretches.

Techniques to Increase Soft Tissue Extensibility

An increase in flexibility is achieved through a routine stretching program that may be instituted early in the course of treatment, with emphasis on stretching not only the elbow, but also the entire hand, forearm, and shoulder complex. Stretching should follow the application of local heat, such as that afforded by ultrasound or transverse friction massage. Patients should be taught how to perform these techniques on themselves at the earliest opportunity.

In each of the following techniques, the left arm is being treated and the stretch is maintained for approximately 30 seconds:

- *Biceps:* The patient stands by a table and places the back of the hand on the tabletop with the forearm pronated. The elbow is gradually extended and the forearm is moved into further pronation (Figure 17-19).
- *Elbow and wrist flexors:* The patient is positioned in standing. A stretching strap is secured to the patient's foot and grasped by the hand of the involved side. Maintaining the forearm in a supinated position and the elbow extended as far as possible, the patient raises their arm out to the side (Figure 17-20) until a stretch it felt.
- *Wrist and finger extensors:* Stretching of the ECRB is always combined with stretching of the ECRL and extensor digitorum and is indicated in all types of tennis and golfer's elbow. The patient is positioned in sitting with the elbow flexed 90 degrees, the forearm pronated, and the wrist flexed. The patient uses the right hand to grasp his or her left hand and position the wrist in maximal flexion and maximal forearm pronation (Figure 17-21). The elbow is then brought very slowly into extension.
- *Stretch for golfer's elbow:* The function of the long wrist flexors is flexion of the elbow, pronation of the forearm, and flexion of the wrist. The patient sits on a chair, with the elbow slightly flexed, the forearm supinated, and the wrist extended (Figure 17-22). The patient uses the right hand to bring the wrist and fingers into as much extension as possible. While holding the wrist in maximal

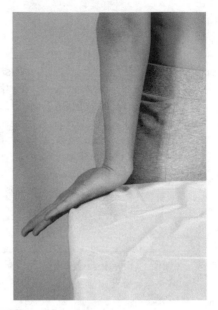

Figure 17-19   Biceps stretch.

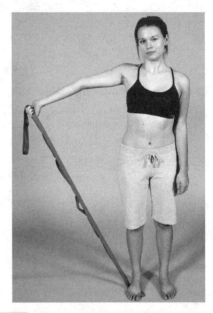

Figure 17-20   Elbow and wrist flexor stretch with strap.

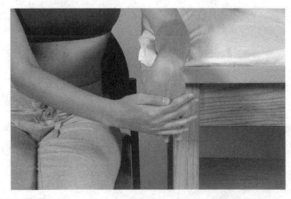

Figure 17-21   Wrist and finger extensor stretch.

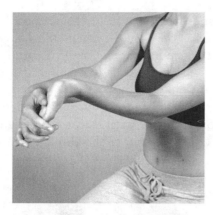

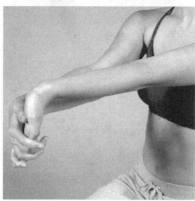

Figure 17-22 Golfer's elbow stretch (start and end positions).

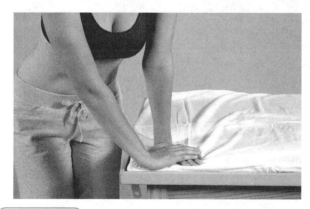

Figure 17-23 Weight-bearing wrist flexor stretch.

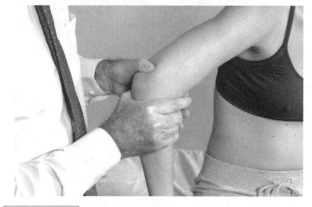

Figure 17-24 TFM of the triceps.

extension, the patient very slowly extends the elbow. As soon as pain or muscle guarding occurs, the motion is stopped and the elbow is brought slightly back into more flexion. If the pain disappears after a few seconds, the elbow can be brought further into extension.

■ *Weight-bearing wrist flexor stretch:* This stretch is performed by asking the patient to position the hand palm side down on a table and to position the elbow in slight flexion, the wrist in neutral radial-ulnar deviation (Figure 17-23). Being careful to avoid pain and muscle splinting, the patient slowly straightens the elbow. The stretch should be held for approximately 40 seconds. At this point, the patient can gently pull the fingers up from the table to stretch the flexor muscles of the palm. Against very slight resistance, performed by the other hand, the arm is then brought back to the original position. This stretching procedure is repeated 6–10 times. The exercise can be modified by placing the wrist in maximal ulnar deviation or radial deviation, and/or the forearm in maximal pronation or supination.

Transverse Frictional Massage

The techniques used in transverse frictional massage are described in Chapter 6.

The Biceps

The patient is positioned to expose the biceps tendon. The clinician stands at the patient's side and supports the arm. The clinician places his or her thumb on the biceps tendon and alternately applies a medial and lateral glide motion to the tendon to create gentle friction (refer to Figure 16-43).

Insertion Tendinopathy of the Triceps

Transverse friction massage is indicated for lesions in the musculotendinous junction (rare), the tendon, or the teno-osseous insertion of the triceps. Insertion tendinopathy of the triceps can occur as a result of chronic abuse or macrotrauma. Objective findings for this condition typically include pain with resisted elbow extension.

The patient is positioned with the upper arm supported. The clinician is positioned at the patient's involved side. The exact site of the lesion is confirmed by palpation. With one hand, the clinician holds the patient's elbow in slightly more than 90 degrees of flexion. The thumb of the other hand is placed at the site of the lesion (Figure 17-24). Static stretching of the triceps is combined with the transverse friction, while taking care at the teno-osseous insertion to avoid friction over the ulnar or radial nerve or bursa.

Medial Humeral Epicondyle (Golfer's Elbow)

To determine the most painful site of the lesion, the clinician palpates the anterior plateau of the medial humeral epicondyle. The patient sits with the elbow extended and the forearm supinated. Using one hand, the clinician grasps the patient's forearm just distal to the elbow and holds the elbow in extension. The tip of the thumb is positioned in slight flexion over the treatment site (Figure 17-25). The massage is applied perpendicular to the tendon.

Lateral Epicondyle (Tennis Elbow)

The patient is positioned with the upper arm adducted, with the elbow in approximately 80 degrees of flexion, and the forearm in pronation. The tendon of the extensor carpi radialis brevis is located and TFM is performed by moving the thumb in a medial-to-lateral direction over the tendon (Figure 17-26).

Selective Joint Mobilizations

The theoretical concepts behind joint mobilizations are described in Chapter 6.

- *Proximal radioulnar glide:* The patient is positioned in sitting with the elbow and forearm resting comfortably on the table. Using the index fingers and thumbs of both hands, the clinician grasps the radial head and applies a glide in the anterior direction, and then the posterior direction (Figure 17-27). Anterior glides increase flexion, while posterior glides increases extension.
- *Inferior humeroulnar glide:* The patient is positioned supine with the arm resting on the

table and the elbow flexed to about 90 degrees. Using one hand, the clinician stabilizes the distal end of the humerus. Using the other hand, the clinician grasps the forearm and applies an inferior glide (Figure 17-28).
- *Inferior humeroradial glide:* The patient is positioned supine with the arm resting on the table. Using one hand, the clinician stabilizes

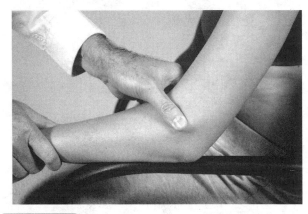

Figure 17-26   TFM of lateral epicondyle.

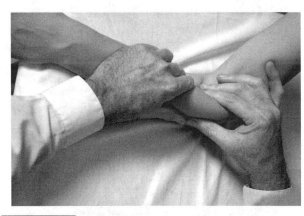

Figure 17-27   Proximal radioulnar glide.

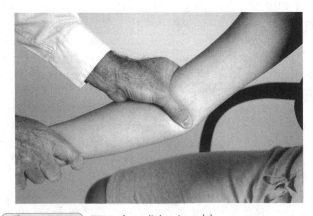

Figure 17-25   TFM of medial epicondyle.

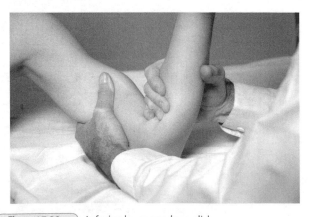

Figure 17-28   Inferior humeroulnar glide.

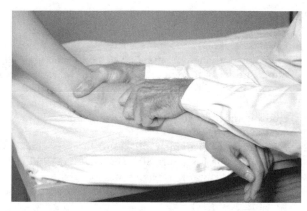

Figure 17-29 Inferior humeroradial glide.

the distal end of the humerus. Using the other hand, the clinician grasps the radius and applies a longitudinal traction force in an inferior direction (Figure 17-29).

Summary

The elbow complex, located between the shoulder and the hand, contributes highly to the overall function of the upper extremity. Forces that are transmitted between the hand and shoulder must be stabilized at the elbow through muscular action and static restraints, while simultaneously allowing ample mobility to adjust the functional length of the arm and place the hand in a position of function. Although the structure of the four joints at the elbow and forearm complex allow for both mobility and stability, the elbow joint is a common place for overuse and traumatic injuries. A working knowledge of anatomy and kinesiology of the elbow joint is a minimal requirement to provide effective treatment.

REVIEW Questions

1. What is the close-packed position of the humeroulnar joint?
2. What is the resting position of the humeroulnar joint?
3. What is the resting position of the proximal radioulnar joint?
4. Injury to the radial nerve will likely result in significant weakness of which elbow action?
5. How many degrees of freedom are there at the humeroulnar joint?
6. What is the normal cubitus valgus angle at the elbow?

7. Which two elbow flexors have their distal attachment on the radius?
8. On which bone is the trochlea found?
9. Using the anatomic position as a reference, is the radius medial or lateral to the ulna?
10. True or false: The biceps brachii and the brachialis are both innervated by the musculocutaneous nerve?
11. A patient presents with lateral elbow pain that has persisted for several months as a result of repetitive use of power tools. The patient complains of aching in the forearm and sharp pain when gripping an object tightly. The supervising PT completed the examination and recommended a treatment program addressing chronic lateral epicondylitis (tennis elbow). The most appropriate treatment protocols for this patient would be:
    a. Heat therapy prior to activities, practice using power tools with review of proper ergonomic positioning and body mechanics, and cryotherapy postactivities
    b. Cryotherapy, cross-friction massage followed by electrical stimulation, then flexibility exercises.
    c. Cryotherapy prior to activities, practice using power tools with review of proper ergonomic positioning and body mechanics, and heat therapy postactivities
    d. Heat therapy, then ultrasound followed by strengthening activities
12. A patient has muscle weakness in elbow flexion; however, pronation and supination strength of the forearm is normal. The muscle that requires strengthening in this case is the:
    a. Brachialis
    b. Biceps brachii
    c. Brachioradialis
    d. Coracobrachialis
13. A patient has rheumatoid arthritis in her elbows and is having difficulty tolerating the long hours required at her desk job. Initial physical therapy treatment would include:
    a. Use of heat or cold modalities and joint protection
    b. Use of cold and avoidance of active elbow flexion
    c. Application of topical analgesics and light resistance strengthening
    d. Splinting in 90 degrees of flexion and isometric exercise at 80 percent effort

References

1. Cummings GS: Comparison of muscle to other soft tissue in limiting elbow extension. J Orthop Sports Phys Ther 5:170, 1984
2. Kapandji IA: The Physiology of the Joints, Upper Limb. New York, Churchill Livingstone, 1991
3. Hammer WI: Functional Soft Tissue Examination and Treatment By Manual Methods. Gaithersburg, MD, Aspen, 1991
4. Morrey BF, Tanaka S, An KN: Valgus stability of the elbow: A definition of primary and secondary constraints. Clin Orthop 265:187–195, 1991
5. Sojbjerg JO, Ovesen J, Nielsen S: Experimental elbow instability after transection of the medial collateral ligament. Clin Orthop Relat Res 218:186–190, 1987
6. Jobe FW, Kvitne RS: Elbow instability in the athlete. Inst Course Lect 40:17–23, 1991
7. An KN, Morrey BF: Biomechanics of the elbow, in Morrey BF (ed): The Elbow and Its Disorders (ed 2). Philadelphia, WB Saunders, 1993, pp 53–73
8. Davidson PA, Pink M, Perry J, et al: Functional anatomy of the flexor pronator muscle group in relation to the medial collateral ligament of the elbow. Am J Sports Med 23:245–250, 1995
9. Morrey BF, Askew LJ, Chao EYS: A biomechanical study of normal functional elbow motion. J Bone Joint Surg 63A:872–877, 1981
10. Jackson-Manfield P, Neumann DA: Structure and function of the elbow and forearm complex, in Jackson-Manfield P, Neumann DA (eds): Essentials of Kinesiology for the Physical Therapist Assistant. St Louis, MO, Mosby Elsevier, 2009, pp 91–122
11. Cohen MS, Bruno RJ: The collateral ligaments of the elbow: Anatomy and clinical correlation. Clin Orthop Relat Res 1:123–130, 2001
12. Jobe FW, Nuber G: Throwing injuries of the elbow. Clin Sports Med 5:621, 1986
13. Ryan J: Elbow, in Wadsworth C (ed): Current Concepts of Orthopedic Physical Therapy—Home Study Course. La Crosse, WI, Orthopaedic Section, American Physical Therapy Association, 2001
14. Neumann DA: Elbow and forearm complex, in Neumann DA (ed): Kinesiology of the Musculoskeletal System: Foundations for Physical Rehabilitation. St Louis, MO, Mosby, 2002, pp 133–171
15. Schuind F, Garcia-Elias M, Cooney WP, et al: Flexor tendon forces: In vivo measurements. J Hand Surg 17A:291–298, 1992
16. Schuind FA, Goldschmidt D, Bastin C, et al: A biomechanical study of the ulnar nerve at the elbow. J Hand Surg [Br] 20:623–627, 1995
17. Basmajian JV, Deluca CJ: Muscles Alive: Their Functions Revealed by Electromyography. Baltimore, Williams & Wilkins, 1985
18. Reid DC: Functional Anatomy and Joint Mobilization (ed 2). Edmonton, University of Alberta Press, 1975
19. Funk DA, An KA, Morrey BF, et al: Electromyographic analysis of muscles across the elbow joint. J Orthop Res 5:529–538, 1987
20. Basmajian JV, Deluca CJ: Muscles Alive: Their Functions Revealed by Electromyography (ed 5). Baltimore, Williams & Wilkins, 1985, pp 268–269
21. Thepaut-Mathieu C, Maton B: The flexor function of the muscle pronator teres in man: A quantitative electromyographic study. Eur J Appl Physiol 54:116–121, 1985
22. Wilk KE, Arrigo C, Andrews JR: Rehabilitation of the elbow in the throwing athlete. J Orthop Sports Phys Ther 17:305–317, 1993
23. Novacheck TF: Running injuries: A biomechanical approach. J Bone Joint Surg 80-A:1220–1233, 1998
24. Coutts RD: Continuous passive motion in the rehabilitation of the total knee patient. Its role and effect. Orthop Rev 15:27, 1986
25. Dehne E, Tory R: Treatment of joint injuries by immediate mobilization based upon the spiral adaption concept. Clin Orthop 77:218–232, 1971
26. Haggmark T, Eriksson E: Cylinder or mobile cast brace after knee ligament surgery. Am J Sports Med 7:48–56, 1979
27. Noyes FR, Mangine RE, Barber S: Early knee motion after open and arthroscopic anterior cruciate ligament reconstruction. Am J Sports Med 15:149–160, 1987
28. Andrews JR, Frank W: Valgus extension overload in the pitching elbow, in Andrews JR, Zarins B, Carson WG (eds): Injuries to the Throwing Arm. Philadelphia, WB Saunders, 1985, pp 250–257
29. Kottke FJ: Therapeutic exercise to maintain mobility, in Kottke FJ, Stillwell GK, Lehman JF (eds): Krusen's Handbook of Physical Medicine and Rehabilitation. Baltimore, WB Saunders, 1982, pp 389–402
30. Warren CG, Lehmann JF, Koblanski JN: Elongation of rat tail: Effect of load and temperature. Arch Phys Med Rehabil 52:465–474, 1971
31. Booth FW: Physiologic and biochemical effects of immobilization on muscle. Clin Orthop Relat Res 219:15–21, 1987
32. Eiff MP, Smith AT, Smith GE: Early mobilization versus immobilization in the treatment of lateral ankle sprains. Am J Sports Med 22:83–88, 1994
33. Akeson WH, Amiel D, Mechanic GL, et al: Collagen cross-linking alterations in the joint contractures: Changes in the reducible cross-links in periarticular connective tissue after 9 weeks immobilization. Connect Tissue Res 5:15, 1977
34. Akeson WH, Amiel D, Abel MF, et al: Effects of immobilization on joints. Clin Orthop 219:28–37, 1987
35. Akeson WH, Amiel D, Woo SL-Y: Immobility effects on synovial joints: The pathomechanics of joint contracture. Biorheology 17:95–110, 1980
36. Woo SL-Y, Matthews J, Akeson WH, et al: Connective tissue response to immobility: A correlative study of biochemical and biomechanical measurements of normal and immobilized rabbit knee. Arthritis Rheum 18:257–264, 1975
37. Kisner C, Colby LA: The elbow and forearm complex, in Kisner C, Colby LA (eds): Therapeutic Exercise. Foundations and Techniques (ed 5). Philadelphia, FA Davis, 2002, pp 557–587
38. Kibler WB: Concepts in exercise rehabilitation of athletic injury, in Leadbetter WB, Buckwalter JA, Gordon SL (eds): Sports-Induced Inflammation: Clinical and Basic Science Concepts. Park Ridge, IL, American Academy of Orthopaedic Surgeons, 1990, pp 759–769

39. Kibler WB, Chandler TJ, Pace BK: Principles of rehabilitation after chronic tendon injuries. Clin Sports Med 11:661–671, 1992

40. Nirschl RP, Sobel J: Arm Care. A Complete Guide to Prevention and Treatment of Tennis Elbow. Arlington, VA, Medical Sports, 1996

41. Woo SL-Y, Tkach LV: The cellular and matrix response of ligaments and tendons to mechanical injury, in Leadbetter WB, Buckwalter JA, Gordon SL (eds): Sports-Induced Inflammation: Clinical and Basic Science Concepts. Park Ridge, IL, American Academy of Orthopaedic Surgeons, 1990, pp 189–202

42. Hempel K, Schwencke K: About avulsions of the distal insertion of the biceps brachii tendon. Arch Orthop Unfallchir 79:313–319, 1974

43. McReynolds IS: Avulsion of the insertion of the biceps brachii tendon and its surgical treatment. J Bone Joint Surg 45A:1780–1781, 1963

44. Kandemir U, Fu FH, McMahon PJ: Elbow injuries. Curr Opin Rheumatol 14:160–167, 2002

45. Morrey BF, Askew LJ, An KN, et al: Rupture of the distal tendon of the biceps brachii: A biomechanical study. J Bone Joint Surg 67A:418–421, 1985

46. Farrrar EL, Lippert FG: Avulsion of triceps tendon. Clin Orthop 161:242–246, 1981

47. Morrey BF, An KN, Chao EYS: Functional evaluation of the elbow, in Morrey BF (ed): The Elbow and Its Disorders (ed 2). Philadelphia, WB Saunders, 1993, pp 86–97

48. O'Connor FG, Wilder RP, Sobel JR: Overuse injuries of the elbow. J Back Musculoskel Rehabil 4:17–30, 1994

49. Nirschl RP: Elbow tendinosis: Tennis elbow. Clin Sports Med 11:851–870, 1992

50. Nirschl RP: Tennis elbow tendinosis: Pathoanatomy, nonsurgical and surgical management, in Gordon SL, Blair SJ, Fine LJ (eds): Repetitive Motion Disorders of the Upper Extremity. Rosemont, IL, American Academy of Orthopaedic Surgeons, 1995, pp 467–479

51. Field LD, Savoie FH: Common elbow injuries in sport. Sports Med 26:193–205, 1998

52. Nirschl RP: Muscle and tendon trauma: Tennis elbow, in Morrey BF (ed): The Elbow and Its Disorders (ed 2). Philadelphia, WB Saunders, 1993, pp 681–703

53. Cyriax JH: The pathology and treatment of tennis elbow. J Bone Joint Surg 18:921–940, 1936

54. Runge F: Zur genese und behandlug des schreibekrampfs. Berliner klinische Wochenschrift 10:245–246, 1873

55. Vulliet H: Die Epicondylitis humeri. Zentralbl Chir 40:1311–1312, 1910

56. Fischer AW: Üeber die Epicondylus: Und Styloidesneuralgie, ihre Pathogenese und zweckmäßige therapie. Archiv Klin Chir 125:749–775, 1923

57. Franke F: Ueber Epicondylitis humeri. Dtsch Med Wochenschr 36:13, 1910

58. Elmslie RC: Tennis elbow. Proc Royal Soc Med 23 (Part 1): 328, 1929

59. Osgood RB: Radiohumeral bursitis, epicondylitis, epicondylalgia (tennis elbow): A personal experience. Arch Surg 4: 420–433, 1922

60. Gruber W: Monographie der Bursae Mucosae Cubitales. St Petersburg, Mém. de l'Acad. Imp. d. Science de St Petersburg, 1866

61. Schmitt J: Bursitis calcarea am Epicondylus externus humeri: Ein beitrag zur Pathogenese der epicondylitis. Archiv für Orthopädie und Unfall-Chirurgie 19:215–221, 1921

62. Crawford HD: Discussion to epicondylitis humeri (Hansson). NY State J Med 43:32–33, 1943

63. Swensen L: Tennis elbow. J Mich State Med Soc 48:997, 1949

64. Neuman JH, Goodfellow JW: Fibrillation of head of radius as one cause of tennis elbow. BMJ 2:328–330, 1975

65. Preiser G: Ueber 'Epicondylitis humeri.' Dtsch Med Wochenschr 36:712, 1910

66. Major HP: Lawn-tennis elbow. BMJ 15:557, 1883

67. Mills PG: The treatment of "tennis elbow." BMJ 1:12–13, 1928

68. Bosworth DM: The role of the orbicular ligament in tennis elbow. J Bone Joint Surg Am 37A:527–533, 1955

69. Trethowan WH: Tennis elbow. BMJ 2:1218, 1929

70. Trethowan WH: Minor injuries of the elbow joint. BMJ 2:1109, 1929

71. Ogilvie WH: Tennis elbow. Proc Royal Soc Med 23:306–322, 1929

72. Bell Allen JC: Epicondylitis: Traumatic radio-humeral synovitis. Med J Aust 1:273–274, 1944

73. Moore M: Radiohumeral synovitis, a cause of persistent elbow pain. Surg Clin North Am 33:1363–1371, 1953

74. Murley AHG: Tennis elbow: Treated with hydrocortisone acetate. Lancet 2:223–225, 1954

75. Paul NW: Radio-humeral bursitis—Is it traumatic? Analysis and report of 314 cases. Ind Med Surg 26:383–390, 1957

76. Winkworth CE: Lawn-tennis elbow. BMJ 6:708, 1883

77. Kaplan EB: Treatment of tennis elbow (epicondylitis) by denervation. J Bone Joint Surg Am 41A:147–151, 1959

78. O'Sullivan S: Tennis-elbow. BMJ 8:1168, 1883

79. Roles NC, Maudsley RH: Radial tunnel syndrome: Resistant tennis elbow as a nerve entrapment. J Bone Joint Surg Br 54B:499–508, 1972

80. Moss SH, Switzer HE: Radial tunnel syndrome: A spectrum of clinical speculations. J Hand Surg 8:414–418, 1983

81. Lister GD, Belsoe RB, Kleinert HE: The radial tunnel syndrome. J Hand Surg Am 4:52–59, 1979

82. Morrison DL: Tennis elbow and radial tunnel syndrome: Differential diagnosis and treatment. J Am Osteopath Assoc 80:823–826, 1981

83. Curwin S, Stanish WD: Tendinitis, Its Etiology and Treatment. Lexington, MA, Collamore Press, 1984

84. Leadbetter WB: Cell-matrix response in tendon injury. Clin Sports Med 11:533–578, 1992

85. Nirschl RP: Patterns of failed tendon healing in tendon injury, in Leadbetter WB, Buckwalter JA, Gordon SL (eds): Sports-Induced Inflammation: Clinical and Basic Science Concepts. Park Ridge, IL, American Academy of Orthopaedic Surgeons, 1990, pp 609–618

86. Teitz CC, Garrett WE, Jr., Miniaci A, et al: Tendon problems in athletic individuals. J Bone Joint Surg 79A:138–152, 1997

87. Woo SL-Y, Gomez MA, Woo YK, et al: Mechanical properties of tendons and ligaments. II. The relationships of immobilization and exercise on tissue remodeling. Biorheology 19:397–408, 1982

88. Woo SL-Y, An K-N, Arnoczky SP, et al: Anatomy, biology, and biomechanics of tendon, ligament, and meniscus, in Simon SR (ed): Orthopaedic Basic Science. Rosemont, IL, American Academy of Orthopaedic Surgeons, 1994, pp 45–87

89. Friedlander HL, Reid RL, Cape RF: Tennis elbow. Clin Orthop 51:109–116, 1967

90. Cleland J, Whitman JM, Fritz J: Effectiveness of manual physical therapy to the cervical spine in the management of lateral epicondylalgia: A retrospective analysis. J Orthop Sports Phys Ther 34:713–724, 2004

91. Cleland JA, Flynn TW, Palmer JA: Incorporation of manual therapy directed at the cervicothoracic spine in patients with lateral epicondylalgia: A pilot clinical trial. J Man Manip Ther 13:143–151, 2005

92. Struijs PA, Kerkhoffs GM, Assendelft WJ, et al: Conservative treatment of lateral epicondylitis: Brace versus physical therapy or a combination of both—a randomized clinical trial. Am J Sports Med 32:462–469, 2004

93. Nirschl RP, Pettrone FA: Tennis elbow. J Bone Joint Surg [Am] 61A:832–839, 1979

94. Froimson A: Treatment of tennis elbow with forearm support. J Bone Joint Surg 43:100–103, 1961

95. Ilfeld FW, Field SM: Treatment of tennis elbow: Use of special brace. JAMA 195:67–71, 1966

96. Groppel J, Nirschl RP: A biomechanical and electromyographical analysis of the effects of counter force braces on the tennis player. Am J Sports Med 14:195–200, 1986

97. Chiumento AB, Bauer JA, Fiolkowski P: A comparison of the dampening properties of tennis elbow braces. Med Sci Sports Exerc 29:123, 1997

98. Gellman H: Tennis elbow (lateral epicondylitis). Orthop Clin North Am 23:75–79, 1992

99. Marlin T: Treatment of "tennis elbow": With some observations on joint manipulation. Lancet 1:509–511, 1930

100. Bryce A: A case of "tennis elbow" treated by luminous heat. Br J Actinother Physiother 5:55, 1930

101. Kininmonth DA: (Discussion on manipulation.) Tennis elbow. Ann Phys Med 1:144, 1953

102. Johnson EW: Tennis elbow. Misconceptions and widespread mythology. Am J Phys Med Rehabil 79:113, 2000

103. Wilk KE, Andrews JR: Elbow injuries, in Brotzman SB, Wilk KE (eds): Clinical Orthopaedic Rehabilitation. Philadelphia, Mosby, 2003, pp 85–123

104. Clarke AK, Woodland J: Comparison of two steroid preparations to treat tennis elbow using the hypospray. Rheumatol Rehabil 14:47–49, 1975

105. Day BH, Govindasamy N, Patnaik R: Corticosteroid injections in the treatment of tennis elbow. Practitioner 220:459–462, 1978

106. Hughes GR, Currey HL: Hypospray treatment of tennis elbow. Ann Rheum Dis 28:58–62, 1969

107. Jobe FW, Ciccotti MG: Lateral and medial epicondylitis of the elbow. J Am Acad Orthop Surgeons 2:1–8, 1994

108. Nirschl RP: Prevention and treatment of elbow and shoulder injuries in the tennis player. Clin Sports Med 7:289–308, 1988

109. Krischek O, Hopf C, Nafe B, et al: Shock-wave therapy for tennis and golfer's elbow—1 year follow-up. Arch Orthop Trauma Surg 119:62–66, 1999

110. Glousman RE, Barron J, Jobe FW, et al: An electromyographic analysis of the elbow in normal and injured pitchers with medial collateral ligament insufficiency. Am J Sports Med 20:311–317, 1992

111. Chen FS, Rokito AS, Jobe FW: Medial elbow problems in the overhead-throwing athlete. J Am Acad Orthop Surgeons 9:99–113, 2001

112. Conway JE, Jobe FW, Glousman RE, et al: Medial instability of the elbow in throwing athletes: Treatment by repair or reconstruction of the ulnar collateral ligament. J Bone Joint Surg 74A:67–83, 1992

113. Azar FM, Andrews JR, Wilk KE, et al: Operative treatment of ulnar collateral ligament injuries of the elbow in athletes. Am J Sports Med 28:16–23, 2000

114. Jobe FW, Stark H, Lombardo SJ: Reconstruction of the ulnar collateral ligament in athletes. J Bone Joint Surg 68A:1158–1163, 1986

115. Kuroda S, Sakamaki K: Ulnar collateral ligament tears of the elbow joint. Clin Orthop 208:266–271, 1986

116. Schwab GH, Bennett JB, Woods GW, et al: Biomechanics of elbow instability: The role of the medial collateral ligament. Clin Orthop 146:42–52, 1980

117. Jobe FW, Tibone JE, Moynes DR, et al: An EMG analysis of the shoulder in pitching and throwing: A preliminary report. Am J Sports Med 11:3–5, 1983

118. Jobe FW, Radovich M, Tibone JE, et al: An EMG analysis of pitching—a second report. Am J Sports Med 12:218–220, 1984

119. Froimson AI, Anouchi YS, Seitz WH, et al: Ulnar nerve decompression with medial epicondylectomy for neuropathy at the elbow. Clin Orthop 265:200–206, 1991

120. Heithoff SJ, Millender LH, Nalebuff EA, et al: Medial epicondylectomy for the treatment of ulnar nerve compression at the elbow. J Hand Surg Am 15A:22–29, 1990

121. Glousman RE: Ulnar nerve problems in the athlete's elbow. Clin Sports Med 9:365–370, 1990

122. Ciccotti MG, Jobe FW: Medial collateral ligament instability and ulnar neuritis in the athlete's elbow. Instr Course Lect 48:383–391, 1999

123. Hotchkiss RN, Weiland AJ: Valgus stability of the elbow. J Orthop Res 5:372–377, 1987

124. Morrey BF, An KN: Functional anatomy of the ligaments of the elbow. Clin Orthop 201:84–90, 1985

125. Morrey BF: Applied anatomy and biomechanics of the elbow joint. Inst Course Lect 35:59–68, 1986

126. Regan WD, Korinek SL, Morrey BF, et al: Biomechanical study of ligaments around the elbow joint. Clin Orthop 271:170–179, 1991

127. Glousman R, Jobe FW, Tibone JE: Dynamic EMG analysis of the throwing shoulder with glenohumeral instability. J Bone Joint Surg 70:220–226, 1988

128. Sisto DJ, Jobe FW, Moynes DR, et al: An electromyographic analysis of the elbow in pitching. Am J Sports Med 15:260–263, 1987

129. Zeman CA, Arcand MA, Cantrell JS, et al: The rotator cuff-deficient arthritic shoulder: Diagnosis and surgical management. J Am Acad Orthop Surgeons 6:337–348, 1998

130. Thompson WH, Jobe FW, Yocum LA, et al: Ulnar collateral ligament reconstruction in athletes: Muscle-splitting approach without transposition of the ulnar nerve. J Shoulder Elbow Surg 10:152–157, 2001

131. Smith GR, Altchek DW, Pagnani MJ, et al: A muscle split-ting approach to the ulnar collateral ligament of the elbow: Neuroanatomy and operative technique. Am J Sports Med 24:667–673, 1996

132. Wright PE: Flexor and extensor tendon injuries, in Cren-shaw AH (ed): Campbell's Operative Orthopaedics (ed 8). St Louis, Mosby-Year Book, 1992, pp 3003–3054

133. Reilly J, Nicholas JA: The chronically inflamed bursa. Clin Sports Med 6:345–370, 1987

134. Onieal M-E: Common wrist and elbow injuries in primary care. Lippincott's Primary Care Practice. Musculoskeletal Conditions 3:441–450, 1999

135. Shell D, Perkins R, Cosgarea A: Septic olecranon bursi-tis: Recognition and treatment. J Am Board Fam Pract 8:217–220, 1995

136. Reid DC, Kushner S: The elbow region, in Donatelli RA, Wooden MJ (eds): Orthopaedic Physical Therapy (cd 2). New York, Churchill Livingstone, 1994, pp 203–232

137. Benjamin A: The relief of traumatic arterial spasm in threatened Volkmann's ischemic contracture. J Bone Joint Surg 39:711–713, 1957

138. Botte MJ, Gelberman RH: Acute compartment syndrome of the forearm. Hand Clin 14:391–403, 1998

139. Rabin SI: Radial head fractures, 2005. http://www.emedicine.com/orthoped/topic276.htm

140. Crenshaw AH: Shoulder and elbow injuries, in Crenshaw AH (ed): Campbell's Operative Orthopaedics (ed 8). St Louis, MO, Mosby-Year Book, 1992, pp 2515–2519

141. Bado JL: The Monteggia lesion. Clin Orthop 50:71, 1967

142. Bowers WH: The distal radioulnar joint, in Green DP, Hotchkiss RN (eds): Operative Hand Surgery (ed 3). New York, Churchill Livingstone, 1993, pp 973–1019

143. Morgan WJ, Breen TF: Complex fractures of the forearm. Hand Clin 10:375, 1994

144. Hotchkiss RN: Displaced fractures of the radial head: Internal fixation or excision. J Am Acad Orthop Surgeons 5:1–10, 1997

145. King GJW, Morrey BF, An K-N: Stabilizers of the elbow. J Shoulder Elbow Surg 2:165–170, 1993

146. Rettig AC, Waugh TR, Evanski PM: Fracture of the ole-cranon: A problem of management. J Trauma 19:23–28, 1979

147. Horne JG, Tanzer TL: Olecranon fractures: A review of 100 cases. J Trauma 21:469–472, 1981

148. Bach BR, Warren RF, Wickiewicz TL: Triceps rupture: A case report and literature review. Am J Sports Med 15:285–289, 1987

149. O'Driscoll SW: Technique for unstable olecranon fracture-subluxations. Oper Tech Orthop 4:49–53, 1994

150. O'Driscoll SW: Elbow instability. Hand Clin 10:405–415, 1994

151. Nestor BJ, O'Driscoll SW, Morrey BF: Ligamentous re-construction for posterolateral rotatory instability of the elbow. J Bone Joint Surg 74A:1235–1241, 1992

152. Geertsen SS, Lundbye-Jensen J, Nielsen JB: Increased cen-tral facilitation of antagonist reciprocal inhibition at the onset of dorsiflexion following explosive strength training. J Appl Physiol 105:915–922, 2008

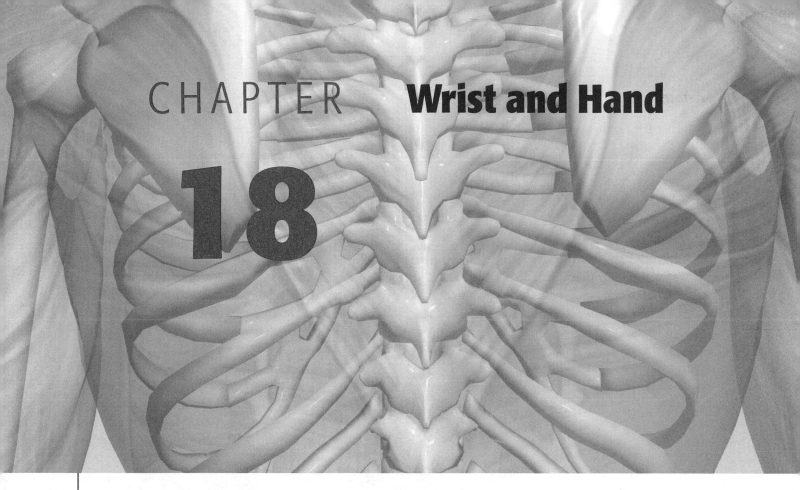

CHAPTER 18   **Wrist and Hand**

Chapter Objectives

At the completion of this chapter, the reader will be able to:

1. Describe the anatomy of the joints, ligaments, muscles, blood, and nerve supply that comprise the region.
2. Describe the biomechanics of the wrist and hand complex, including the open- and close-packed positions, muscle force couples, and the static and dynamic stabilizers.
3. Summarize the various causes of wrist and hand dysfunction.
4. Describe and demonstrate intervention strategies and techniques.

Overview

The human wrist joint is a complex arrangement of eight small bones and numerous ligaments that form a mobile yet stable link from the powerful forearm to the hand. In order to effectively treat hand problems, the clinician must have a sound understanding of both the anatomy and kinesiology.

Anatomy

The distal forearm and hand have three major articulations:

- The distal radioulnar joint
- The radiocarpal joint
- The midcarpal joint

Distal Radioulnar Joint

The distal radioulnar joint (DRUJ) is a double pivot joint that unites the distal radius and ulna and an articular disc (Figure 18-1), and functions to transmit the loads from the hand to the forearm. An articular disc, known as the triangular fibrocartilaginous complex (TFCC), assists in binding the distal radius and is the main stabilizer of the distal radioulnar joint. It improves joint congruency and cushions against compressive forces.

Radiocarpal (Wrist) Joint

The radiocarpal (wrist) joint is composed of the distal concave surface of the radius and ulna, which articulate with the adjacent articular disk (TFCC), which in turn articulates with the convex articular surfaces of the scaphoid and the lunate (Figure 18-2).

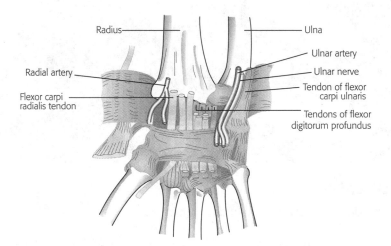

Figure 18-1   The distal radioulnar joint.

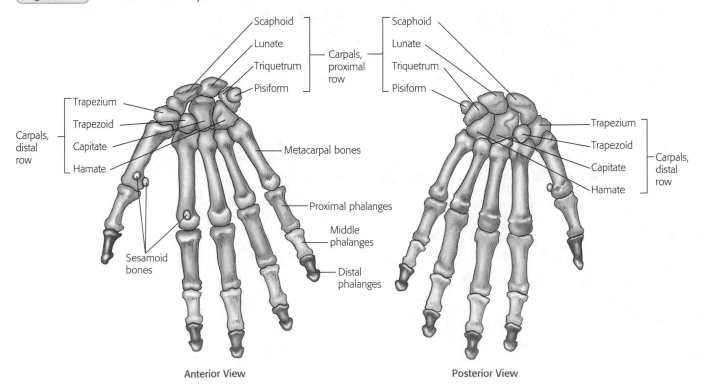

Figure 18-2   Bones of the hand.

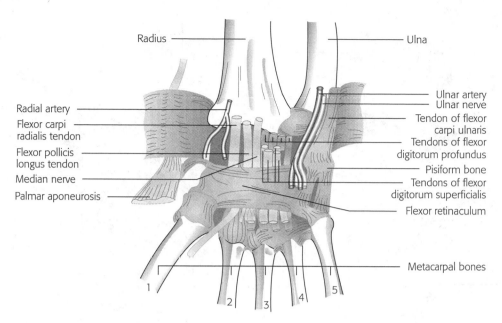

Radius

Ulna

Radial artery

Flexor carpi
radialis tendon

Flexor pollicis
longus tendon

Median nerve

Palmar aponeurosis

Ulnar artery
Ulnar nerve

Tendon of flexor
carpi ulnaris

Tendons of flexor
digitorum profundus

Pisiform bone

Tendons of flexor
digitorum superficialis

Flexor retinaculum

Metacarpal bones

Figure 18-3 Ligaments of the anterior aspect of the wrist.

The distal end of the ulna expands slightly laterally into a rounded head, and medially into the ulnar styloid process. The ulnar styloid process is approximately one-half inch shorter than the radial styloid process, resulting in more available ulnar deviation than radial deviation.[1] There are eight carpal bones, which lie in two transverse rows. The proximal row contains (lateral to medial) the scaphoid (navicular), lunate, triquetrum, and pisiform (a sesamoid bone that develops within the tendon of the flexor carpi ulnaris). The distal carpal row, which articulates with the bases of five metacarpals, holds the trapezium, trapezoid, capitate, and hamate.

● Key Point

• The precarious blood supply to the scaphoid bone predisposes a person to aseptic necrosis after fracture to the proximal aspect of this bone.[2]
• The lunate is the most commonly dislocated carpal bone.
• With its central location, the capitate serves as the keystone of the proximal transverse arch. This arch is important to prehensile activity of the hand.

The major ligaments of the wrist (Figure 18-3 and Figure 18-4) include the following:

■ *Dorsal radiocarpal ligament:* Resists extremes of wrist flexion
■ *Radial collateral ligament:* Resists extremes of ulnar deviation

■ *Palmar radiocarpal ligament:* Resists extremes of wrist extension
■ *Ulnar collateral ligament:* Resists extremes of radial deviation

● Key Point When relaxed, the palmar surface of the hand adopts a natural arched curvature. This concavity is supported by three arch systems: two transverse and one longitudinal.

Midcarpal Joint

The midcarpal joint lies between the proximal and distal rows of carpal bones. It is referred to as a *compound* articulation because each row has both a concave and a convex segment.

Antebrachial Fascia

The antebrachial fascia is a dense connective tissue "bracelet" that encases the forearm and maintains the relationships of the tendons that cross the wrist.

Extensor Retinaculum

Where the tendons cross the wrist, a ligamentous structure called a retinaculum prevents the tendons from "bow-stringing" when the tendons turn a corner at the wrist.[3] The tunnel-like structures formed by the retinaculum and the underlying bones are called *fibro-osseous compartments.* There are six fibro-osseous compartments, or

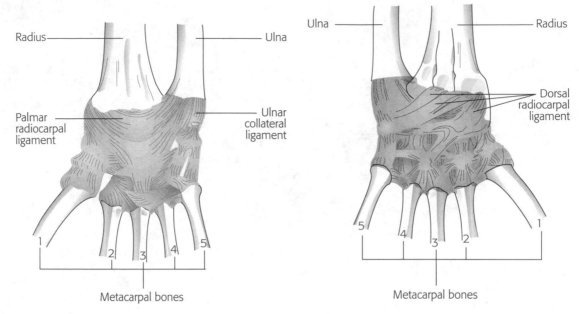

Figure 18-4   Ligaments of the posterior aspect of the wrist.

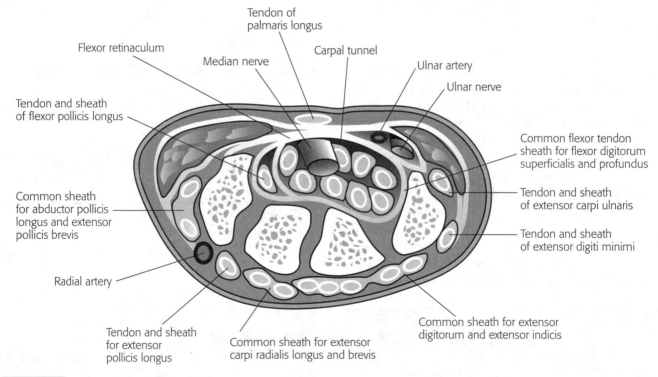

Figure 18-5   The six fibro-osseous compartments of the dorsal wrist.

tunnels, on the dorsum of the wrist (Figure 18-5). The compartments, from lateral to medial, contain the following tendons:

- Abductor pollicis longus (APL) and extensor pollicis brevis (EPB)
- Extensor carpi radialis longus (ECRL) and extensor carpi radialis brevis (ECRB)

- Extensor pollicis longus (EPL)
- Extensor digitorum and extensor indicis
- Extensor digiti minimi (EDM)
- Extensor carpi ulnaris

● Key Point   The mnemonic 2 2 1 2 1 1 can be used to remember the number of tendons in each compartment.

Flexor Retinaculum

The flexor retinaculum spans the area between the pisiform, hamate, scaphoid, and trapezium. It transforms the carpal arch into a tunnel, through which pass the median nerve and some of the tendons of the hand. Proximally, the retinaculum attaches to the tubercle of the scaphoid and the pisiform. Distally it attaches to the hook of the hamate and the tubercle of the trapezium. The tendons that pass *deep* to the flexor retinaculum include the following (Figure 18-6):

- Flexor digitorum superficialis (FDS)
- Flexor digitorum profundus (FDP)
- Flexor pollicis longus (FPL)
- Flexor carpi radialis (FCR)

Structures that pass *superficial* to the flexor retinaculum include the following:

- Ulnar nerve and artery
- Tendon of the palmaris longus
- Sensory branch (palmar branch) of the median nerve

Carpal Tunnel

The carpal tunnel serves as a conduit for the median nerve and nine flexor tendons. The palmar radiocarpal ligament and the palmar ligament complex form the floor of the canal. The roof of the tunnel is formed by the flexor retinaculum (transverse carpal ligament). The ulnar and radial borders are formed by carpal bones (trapezium and hook of hamate, respectively). Within the tunnel, the median nerve divides into a motor branch and distal sensory branches.

Tunnel of Guyon

The tunnel of Guyon is a depression superficial to the flexor retinaculum, located between the hook of the hamate and the pisiform bones. The tunnel serves as a passageway for the ulnar nerve and artery into the hand.

Metacarpophalangeal Joints of the Second to Fifth Digits

The metacarpophalangeal (MCP) joints of digits 2–5 allow flexion/extension and abduction/adduction associated with a slight degree of axial rotation.

- Approximately 90 degrees of flexion is available at the second MCP. The amount of available flexion progressively increases towards the fifth MCP.
- Active extension at these joints is 25–30 degrees; up to 90 degrees is obtainable passively.
- Approximately 20 degrees of abduction/adduction can occur in either direction, with more being available in extension than in flexion.[4]

The joint capsule of these joints is relatively lax and redundant, endowed with collateral ligaments, which pass posterior to the joint axis for flexion/extension of the MCP joints. Although lax in extension, these collateral ligaments become taut in approximately 70–90 degrees of flexion of the MCP joint.

Carpometacarpal Joints of the Second to Fifth Digits

The carpometacarpal (CMC) joints progress in mobility from the second to the fifth digit.

First Carpometacarpal Joint

The thumb is the most important digit of the hand in terms of function, and the sellar (saddle-shaped) CMC joint is the most important joint of the thumb. Motions that can occur at this joint include flexion/extension, adduction/abduction, and opposition (all of which include varying amounts of flexion, internal rotation, and palmar adduction).

Metacarpophalangeal Joint of the Thumb

Unlike the MCP joints of the fingers, the MCP joint of the thumb is a hinge joint. Approximately

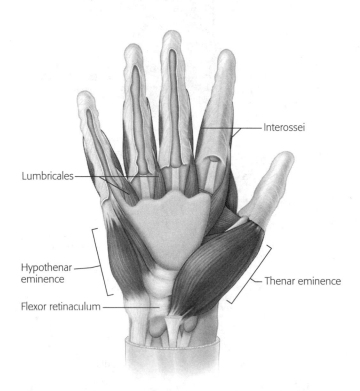

Lumbricales

Interossei

Hypothenar eminence

Thenar eminence

Flexor retinaculum

Figure 18-6   The flexor retinaculum and muscles of the palm.

75–80 degrees of flexion is available at this joint. The extension movement as well as the abduction and adduction motions are negligible.

Interphalangeal Joints

Adjacent phalanges articulate in hinge joints that allow motion in only the sagittal plane, producing flexion and extension. The congruency of the interphalangeal (IP) joint surfaces contributes greatly to finger joint stability.

- *Proximal interphalangeal (PIP) joints:* Approximately 110 degrees of flexion and 0 degrees of extension
- *Thumb interphalangeal joint:* Approximately 90 degrees of flexion and 25 degrees of extension
- *Distal interphalangeal (DIP) joints:* Approximately 90 degrees of flexion and 25 degrees of extension

Palmar Aponeurosis

The palmar aponeurosis is located just deep to the subcutaneous tissue. It is a dense fibrous structure continuous with the palmaris longus tendon and fascia covering the thenar and hypothenar muscles.

● **Key Point** *Dupuytren's contracture* is a fibrotic condition of the palmar aponeurosis that results in nodule formation or scarring of the aponeurosis, and which may ultimately cause finger flexion contractures (see "Common Conditions" later in this chapter).

Anatomic Snuff Box

The anatomic snuffbox (Figure 18-7) is represented by a depression on the dorsal surface of the hand at the base of the thumb, just distal to the radius. The tendons of the APL and EPB form the radial border of the snuffbox, while the tendon of the EPL forms the ulnar border. Along the floor of the snuffbox are the deep branch of the radial artery and the tendinous insertion of the ECRL. Underneath these structures are the scaphoid and trapezium bones.

● **Key Point** Tenderness with palpation in the anatomic snuffbox suggests a scaphoid fracture, but also can present in minor wrist injuries or other conditions.

Muscles of the Wrist and Forearm

The muscles of the forearm (Figure 18-8 and Figure 18-9), wrist, and hand (Figure 18-10 and **Table 18-1**) can be subdivided into the 19 intrinsic muscles that arise and insert within the hand and the 24 extrinsic muscles that originate in the forearm and insert within the hand. The three peripheral nerves that supply the skin and muscles of the wrist and hand are the median, ulnar, and radial nerves.

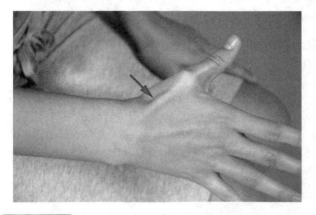

Figure 18-7 Anatomic snuffbox.

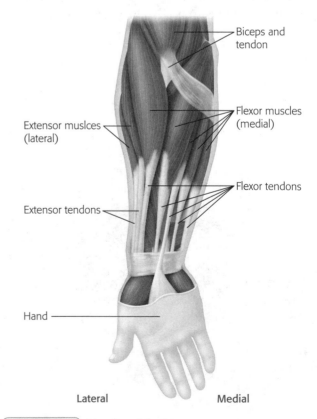

Biceps and tendon

Flexor muscles (medial)

Extensor muslces (lateral)

Flexor tendons

Extensor tendons

Hand

Lateral   Medial

Figure 18-8 Muscles of the forearm.

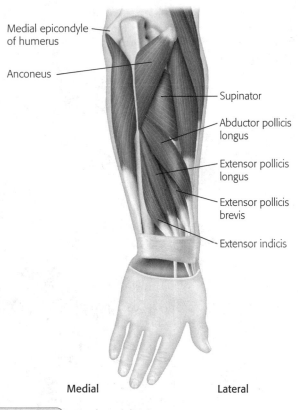

Figure 18-9 Muscles of the forearm.

Labels for Figure 18-9:
- Medial epicondyle of humerus
- Anconeus
- Supinator
- Abductor pollicis longus
- Extensor pollicis longus
- Extensor pollicis brevis
- Extensor indicis
- Medial
- Lateral

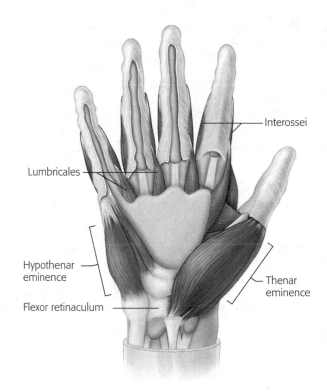

Figure 18-10 Muscles of the hand.

Labels for Figure 18-10:
- Interossei
- Lumbricales
- Hypothenar eminence
- Flexor retinaculum
- Thenar eminence

TABLE 18-1	**Muscles of the Wrist and Hand: Their Actions and Nerve Supply**	
Action	**Muscles**	**Nerve Supply**
Wrist extension	Extensor carpi radialis longus	Radial
	Extensor carpi radialis brevis	Posterior interosseous
	Extensor carpi ulnaris	Posterior interosseous
Wrist flexion	Flexor carpi radialis	Median
	Flexor carpi ulnaris	Ulnar
Ulnar deviation of wrist	Flexor carpi ulnaris	Ulnar
	Extensor carpi ulnaris	Posterior interosseous
Radial deviation of wrist	Flexor carpi radialis	Median
	Extensor carpi radialis longus	Radial
	Abductor pollicis longus	Posterior interosseous
	Extensor pollicis brevis	Posterior interosseous
Finger extension	Extensor digitorum communis	Posterior interosseous
	Extensor indicis	Posterior interosseous
	Extensor digiti minimi	Posterior interosseous
Finger flexion	Flexor digitorum profundus	Anterior interosseous, lateral two digits
		Ulnar, medial two digits

(continued)

Action	Muscles	Nerve Supply
	Flexor digitorum superficialis	Median
	Lumbricals	First and second: median
		Third and fourth: ulnar
	Interossei	Ulnar
	Flexor digiti minimi	Ulnar
Abduction of fingers	Dorsal interossei	Ulnar
	Abductor digiti minimi	Ulnar
Adduction of fingers	Palmar interossei	Ulnar
Thumb extension	Extensor pollicis longus	Posterior interosseous
	Extensor pollicis brevis	Posterior interosseous
	Abductor pollicis longus	Posterior interosseous
Thumb flexion	Flexor pollicis brevis	Superficial head: median
		Deep head: ulnar
	Flexor pollicis longus	Anterior interosseous
	Opponens pollicis	Median
Abduction of thumb	Abductor pollicis longus	Posterior interosseous
	Abductor pollicis brevis	Median
Adduction of thumb	Adductor pollicis	Ulnar
Opposition of thumb	Opponens pollicis	Median
Thumb flexion	Flexor pollicis brevis	Superficial head: median
Opposition of little finger	Opponens digiti minimi	Ulnar

Kinesiology

The movements of the forearm, wrist, and hand are a function of a close relationship between the proximal and distal radioulnar joints and the joints of the wrist.

Pronation and Supination

Approximately 75 degrees of forearm pronation are available, and approximately 85 degrees of forearm supination are available. Congruency of the distal radioulnar joint (DRUJ) surfaces is maximal at mid-range of motion, although the joint is not considered to be truly locked in this position. The open-packed position is 10 degrees supination. The proximal and distal radioulnar joints are intimately related biomechanically, with the function and stability of both joints dependent on the configuration of, and distance between, the two bones.

Movement of the Hand on the Forearm

There are two major factors that influence the motion that occurs between the hand and the forearm:

- *Morphology:* Due to the morphology of the wrist, movement at this joint complex involves a coordinated interaction among a number of articulations including the radiocarpal joint, the proximal row of carpals, and the distal row of the carpals. Because the concave trapezium and trapezoid slide in a posterior direction on the scaphoid, and the complex capitate and hamate slide in an anterior direction on the lunate and triquetrum during wrist extension and radial deviation, the resulting motion is a supination twist of the distal row on the proximal row.[5] Conversely, a pronation twist occurs during flexion and ulnar deviation as the trapezium and trapezoid slide anteriorly and the capitate and hamate slide posteriorly.[5]

- *Length-tension:*[6] The position of the wrist controls the length of the extrinsic muscles of the digits, so as the fingers or thumb flex, the wrist must be stabilized by the wrist extensor muscles to prevent the flexor digitorum profundus and flexor digitorum superficialis, or the flexor pollicis longus, from simultaneously flexing the wrist. As the grip becomes stronger, synchronous wrist extension lengthens the extrinsic flexor tendons across the wrist and maintains a more favorable overall length of the musculotendinous unit for a stronger contraction. During strong finger or thumb extension, the wrist flexor muscles stabilize or flex the wrist so the extensor digitorum communis, extensor indices, extensor digiti minimi, or extensor pollicis longus muscles can function more efficiently.

Functional Use of the Hand

The hand serves many important functions that allow us to interact with others and the environment. In addition to providing a wealth of sensory information, the hand grasps objects. A loss of grip is a measurable factor used in the determination of permanent disability by compensation boards in some states.[7] The grip is typically divided into the following stages:[8,9]

- Opening of the hand.
- Positioning and closing of the fingers to grasp an object and adapt to the object's shape.
- Controlled approach and purposeful closing of the fingers and/or palm. The amount of force exerted is determined by the weight, surface characteristics, and fragility of the object.[10]
- Maintenance and stabilization of the grip. This phase is not used in precision tasks.[11,12]
- The release of the object.[11,12]

Hand functions have been further categorized by adding the terms *grasp* and *prehension*, which are used to describe functions of power or precision.[13,14]

Power Grasp

The power grasp involves the use of force to stabilize an object in the hand. Power grasps include the fist, cylindrical, ball, hook (see the "General Intervention Strategies" section later in this chapter), pincer, and pliers grasps. The strength and power of a grasp comes from a combination of:

- Thumb adduction
- Isometric flexion
- An approximation of the thenar and hypothenar eminences
- Intact function of the ulnar side of the hand

Participation of the intrinsic muscles follows specific patterns in the various power grasps.

Precision Grasp

In the precision grasp, the muscles primarily function to provide exact control of finger and thumb position, so the position of the handled object can be changed either in space or about its own axis.[8,11] Due to the higher levels of sensory input required during these tasks, the areas with the most sensory receptors are used. A number of precision grasps are recognized:[4,15]

- *Pulp-to-pulp pinch:* The pad of the thumb is opposed to the pad of one or more fingers.
- *Lateral prehension:* The palmar aspect of the thumb presses against the radial aspect of the first phalanx of the index finger.
- *Tip prehension:* The extreme tip of the thumb pad is opposed to the tip of the index or middle finger.
- *Three-fingered pinch:* Involves the thumb, index finger, and middle finger, as in sprinkling herbs.
- *Five-fingered pinch:* Uses all five fingers, as in picking up a face towel.

The radial side of the hand and the MCP joints are involved more in the precision or prehensile types of grasps.[4,15]

Flexion and Extension Movements of the Wrist

Wrist movements occur around a combination of three functional axes: frontal, sagittal, and longitudinal (or vertical). In a neutral wrist position, the scaphoid contacts the radius, and the lunate contacts the radius and disc.

The movements of flexion and extension of the wrist are shared between the radiocarpal articulation and the intercarpal articulation, in varying proportions.

- During wrist flexion, most of the motion occurs in the midcarpal joint (60 percent or 40 degrees versus 40 percent or 30 degrees at the radio-carpal joint) and is associated with slight ulnar deviation and pronation of the forearm.[16]

■ During wrist extension, most of the motion occurs at the radiocarpal joint (66.5 percent or 40 degrees versus 33.5 percent or 20 degrees at the midcarpal joint) and is associated with slight radial deviation and supination of the forearm.[16]

Frontal Lateral Movements of the Wrist

There is a physiological ulnar deviation at rest, easily demonstrated clinically and radiographically. The amount of deviation available is approximately 40 degrees of ulnar deviation and 15 degrees of radial deviation.[16]

Radial Deviation

Radial deviation occurs primarily between the proximal and distal rows of the carpal bones. The motion of radial deviation is limited by the impact of the scaphoid onto the radial styloid and ulnar collateral ligament. The abductor pollicus longus and extensor pollicis brevis are best suited to produce radial deviation of the wrist.

Ulnar Deviation

Ulnar deviation occurs primarily at the radiocarpal joint and is limited by the radial collateral ligament.[15] Although ulnar deviation brings the triquetrum into contact with the disc on the ulnar side, the lack of direct ulnar-triquetral articulation permits a greater range of ulnar deviation. The muscle with the best biomechanical advantage to produce ulnar deviation of the wrist in pronation is the extensor carpi ulnaris.

● **Key Point** The position of the wrist in flexion or extension influences the tension of the long or "extrinsic" muscles of the digits. Neither the flexors nor the extensors of the fingers are long enough to allow maximal range of motion at the wrist and the fingers simultaneously.

The open-packed and close-packed positions of the wrist and hand articulations, in addition to the capsular patterns of each joint, are described in **Table 18-2**.

Thumb Movements

Thumb flexion and extension occur around an anterior-posterior axis in the frontal plane that is perpendicular to the sagittal plane of finger flexion and extension. In this plane, the metacarpal surface is concave and the trapezium surface is convex. Flexion occurs with a conjunct internal rotation of the metacarpal. Extension occurs with a conjunct external rotation of the metacarpal. A total range of 50–70 degrees is available at the CMC joint.

Thumb abduction and adduction occur in the sagittal plane, which is perpendicular to the frontal plane of finger abduction and adduction, around a medial-lateral (frontal) axis. During thumb abduction

TABLE 18-2	The Open-Packed and Close-Packed Positions and Capsular Patterns for the Articulations of the Wrist and Hand		
Joint	Open-Packed	Close-Packed	Capsular Pattern
Distal radioulnar	10 degrees of supination	5 degrees of supination	Minimal to no limitation with pain at the end ranges of pronation and supination
Radiocarpal (wrist)	Neutral with slight ulnar deviation	Extension	Equal limitation of flexion and extension
Intercarpal	Neutral or slight flexion	Extension	None
Midcarpal	Neutral or slight flexion with ulnar deviation	Extension with ulnar deviation	Equal limitation of flexion and extension
Carpometacarpal	*Thumb:* Midway between abduction and adduction and midway between flexion and extension	*Thumb:* Full opposition	*Thumb:* Abduction then extension
	Fingers: Midway between flexion and extension	*Fingers:* Full flexion	*Fingers:* Equal limitation in all directions
Metacarpophalangeal	Slight flexion	*Thumb:* Full opposition	Flexion then extension
		Fingers: Full flexion	
Interphalangeal	Slight flexion	Full extension	Flexion, extension

and adduction, the convex metacarpal surface moves on the concave trapezium. Abduction occurs with a conjunct internal rotation. Adduction occurs with a conjunct external rotation. A total range of 40–60 degrees is available.

Opposition of the thumb involves a wide arc motion composed of sequential palmar abduction and flexion from the anatomic position, accompanied by internal rotation of the thumb. Retroposition of the thumb returns the thumb to the anatomic position, a motion that incorporates elements of adduction with extension and external rotation of the metacarpal.

Examination

The physical therapist's examination of the wrist and hand typically follows the outline in **Table 18-3**. A number of evidence-based special tests also can be used at the wrist and hand (**Table 18-4**).

TABLE 18-3	**Examination of the Forearm, Wrist, and Hand**

I. History.
II. Observation and inspection.
III. Upper quarter scan as appropriate.
IV. Examination of movements. Active range of motion with passive overpressure of the following movements:
    a. Forearm pronation and supination
    b. Wrist flexion and extension
    c. Wrist radial deviation and ulnar deviation
    d. Finger flexion and extension (MCP, PIP, and DIP joints)
    e. Finger abduction and adduction
    f. Thumb flexion, extension, abduction, and adduction
    g. Opposition of the thumb and little finger
V. Resisted isometric movements:
    a. Forearm pronation and supination
    b. Wrist flexion and extension
    c. Wrist radial deviation and ulnar deviation
    d. Finger flexion and extension (MCP, PIP, and DIP joints)
    e. Finger abduction and adduction
    f. Thumb flexion, extension, abduction, and adduction
    g. Opposition of the thumb and little finger
VI. Palpation.
VII. Neurological tests as appropriate (reflexes, sensory scan, peripheral nerve assessment).
VIII. Joint mobility tests:
    a. Distraction of the radiohumeral joint
    b. Anterior and posterior glide of the radial head
    c. Anterior and posterior glide of the proximal radioulnar joint
    d. Anterior and posterior glide of the distal radioulnar join
    e. Long-axis extension at the wrist and fingers (MCP, PIP, and DIP joints)
    f. Anteroposterior glide at the wrist and fingers (MCP, PIP, and DIP joints)
    g. Side glide at the wrist and fingers (MCP, PIP, and DIP joints)
    h. Anteroposterior glides of the intermetacarpal joints
    i. Rotation of the MCP, PIP, and DIP joints
    j. Individual carpal bone mobility
IX. Special tests, including functional testing (refer to Table 18-4).
X. Diagnostic imaging.

TABLE 18-4

Evidence-Based Tests for the Wrist and Hand

Name of Test	Brief Description	Positive Findings	Evidence-Based
Scaphoid fracture test[a]	Clinician exerts passive overpressure into ulnar deviation of wrist while forearm is pronated.	Positive if patient reports pain in the anatomical snuffbox.	Sensitivity: 1.0 Specificity: 0.34
Longitudinal compression of thumb[b]	Clinician holds the patient's thumb and applies a long axis compression through the metacarpal bone into the scaphoid.	Positive for a scaphoid fracture if patient reports pain in the anatomical snuffbox.	Sensitivity: 0.98 Specificity: 0.98
Tinel sign[c]	The clinician taps the median nerve at the wrist 4–6 times.	Positive for carpal tunnel syndrome if patient reports pain or paresthesias in the distribution of the median nerve.	Sensitivity: 0.68 Specificity: 0.90
Phalen's test[c]	The patient is asked to hold the wrist in complete flexion with the elbow extended and the forearm pronated for 60 seconds.	Positive if symptoms are reproduced.	Sensitivity: 0.68 Specificity: 0.91
Carpal compression test[d]	The patient is seated with the elbow flexed to 30 degrees, the forearm supinated, and the wrist in neutral. The clinician places both thumbs over the transverse carpal ligament and applies 6 pounds of pressure for a maximum of 30 seconds.	Positive for carpal tunnel syndrome if the patient experiences exacerbation of symptoms in the median nerve distribution.	Sensitivity: 0.64 Specificity: 0.30
Scaphoid shift (Watson) test[e]	Patient elbow is stabilized on the table with forearm in slight pronation. With one hand, the clinician grasps the radial side of the patient's wrist with the thumb on the palmar prominence of the scaphoid. With the other hand, the clinician grasps the patient's hand at the metacarpal level to stabilize the wrist. The clinician maintains pressure on the scaphoid tubercle and moves the patient's wrist into ulnar deviation with slight extension, then radial deviation with slight flexion. The clinician releases pressure on the scaphoid while the wrist is in radial deviation and flexion.	Positive for instability of the scaphoid if the scaphoid shifts or the patient's symptoms are reproduced when the scaphoid is released.	Sensitivity: 0.69 Specificity: 0.66
Ballottement (Reagan's) test[e]	The clinician stabilizes the patient's lunate bond between the thumb and index finger of one hand, while the other hand moves the pisotriquetral complex in a palmar and dorsal direction.	The test is positive for instability of the lunotriquetral joint if the patient's symptoms are reproduced or excessive laxity of the joint is revealed.	Sensitivity: 0.64 Specificity: 0.44

Data from (a) Powell JM, Lloyd GJ, Rintoul RF: New clinical test for fracture of the scaphoid. Can J Surg 31:237–238, 1988; (b) Waeckerle JF: A prospective study identifying the sensitivity of radiographic findings and the efficacy of clinical findings in carpal navicular fractures. Ann Emerg Med 16:733–737, 1987; (c) Ahn DS: Hand elevation: A new test for carpal tunnel syndrome. Ann Plast Surg 46:120–124, 2001; (d) Wainner RS, Fritz JM, Irrgang JJ, et al: Development of a clinical prediction rule for the diagnosis of carpal tunnel syndrome. Arch Phys Med Rehabil 86:609–618, 2005; and (e) LaStayo P, Howell J: Clinical provocative tests used in evaluating wrist pain: a descriptive study. J Hand Surg 8:10–17, 1995

General Intervention Strategies

Due to the integrated nature of the wrist and hand in functional activities, the rehabilitation is organized around a common framework for most wrist and hand pathologies.

Acute Phase

The goals of the acute phase include:

- *Maintain or improve general fitness.* The overall cardiovascular fitness of each patient is important, especially in cases where function and overall activity level may be impacted by an injury in the extremity.
- *Provide independence with a home exercise program.* At the earliest opportunity, the patient must become independent with the home exercise program.
- *Maintain pain-free range of motion and strength in the rest of the kinetic chain.* Due to the fact that the wrist and hand requires the normal function of the rest of the upper kinetic chain, exercises must be designed to incorporate elbow, shoulder, and trunk exercises at the earliest opportunity.
- *Improve patient comfort by decreasing pain and inflammation.* This can be accomplished using the principles of PRICEMEM (protection, rest, ice, compression, elevation, manual therapy, early motion, and medication prescribed by the physician).
- *Protect the injury site to allow healing.* Movement is the activity necessary to maintain joint mobility and gliding tendon function. Range-of-motion exercises are introduced as early as tolerated. These may be passive, active assisted, or active, as appropriate and based on patient tolerance. If protected motion is necessary, it can be provided with taping, bracing, splinting, or, in extreme cases, casting. Protected range-of-motion exercises are performed to selectively mobilize joints and tendons, while minimizing stress on repairing structures. As their name suggests, protected range-of-motion exercises are accomplished by placing the repaired structure in a protected position, while adjacent tissues are carefully mobilized. An example of a protective exercise can be seen following a radial nerve injury, where the protective active motion exercises include MCP joint flexion, and then PIP and DIP joint flexion with the MCP joint maintained in extension.[17]

- *Control and then eliminate edema.* One of the most significant problems the PTA faces with a hand-injured patient is the control and elimination of edema. Edema can increase the risk of infection, decrease motion, and inhibit arterial, venous, and lymphatic flow.[18] Methods to control edema include cryotherapy, elevation of the extremity and hand above the level of the heart, active exercise, retrograde massage, intermittent compression, continuous compression wrapping, and contrast baths.
- *Provide scar management, if appropriate.* Scar tissue management focuses on the control of stresses placed on healing tissues. Early active and passive motion provides controlled stress, encouraging optimal remodeling of scar tissue.[18] Methods to control scarring include the use of thermal agents, transverse friction massage (see Chapter 6), mechanical vibration, compressive techniques, and splinting. Although it is not within the scope of this text to provide comprehensive detail with regard to splinting (entire texts are devoted to the subject),[19–22] the PTA needs to be aware of the purposes of splinting as well as some of the options available. The general purposes of a splint are to:[23,24]
  - *Immobilize/stabilize:* Splinting is especially useful for stabilizing mobile joints so the corrective exercise force can be directed to the stiff joint or adherent tendon.[17]
  - *Protect:* Static splints have no moveable parts and maintain joints in one position to promote healing and minimize friction.
  - *Correct deformity or dysfunction:* Splints can maintain or re-establish normal tissue length, balance, and excursion.
  - *Control/modify scar formation.*
  - *Substitute for dysfunctional tissue:* This thereby enhances function.
- *Provide exercise: Dropout splints* block joint motion in one direction but allow motion in another. *Articulated splints* contain at least two static components and are connected in such a way as to allow motion in one plane at a joint. *Dynamic splints* are used to provide active resistance in the direction opposite to their line of pull to increase muscle strength, as well as to apply a corrective passive stretch to tendon adhesions and joint contractures.[17] *Static-progressive* splints involve the use of inelastic components, such as hook-and-loop tapes, Dacron line, turnbuckles, and screws, to allow

progressive changes in joint position as PROM changes without changing the structure of the splint. *Serial static splints* differ from static progressive splints in that they require the clinician to remold the splint to accommodate increases in mobility.

- *Retard muscle atrophy and minimize the detrimental effects of immobilization and activity restriction:*[25-30] Therapeutic exercises are performed with the goal of adequate soft tissue rebalancing of the wrist to restore the alignment of the extensor and flexor tendons as near to normal as possible, and to prevent scarring or soft tissue contractures by influencing the physiologic process of collagen formation. Passive range-of-motion exercises are performed through the available range of motion to maintain joint and soft tissue mobility, or a passive stretch can be applied at the end range of motion to lengthen pathologically shortened soft tissue structures, thereby increasing motion. Depending

on the focus of the intervention, the passive/active range-of-motion exercises may include:

- ❏ MP flexion and extension (Figure 18-11)
- ❏ PIP flexion and extension (Figure 18-12)
- ❏ DIP flexion and extension (Figure 18-13)

Active range-of-motion exercises are performed throughout the available range. Active exercises should include specific and composite exercises. Composite exercises, which reproduce normal functional activities, include fisting and thumb opposition to each digit in addition to exercises involving the wrist, elbow, and shoulder. Passive overpressure should be applied as appropriate. When active exercises are used to restore mobility in the presence of increasing tissue resistance, fast ballistic movements are discouraged.[17] Examples of active range-of-motion exercises include:

- Wrist and finger flexion and extension; thumb opposition, flexion, extension, abduction, and adduction (Figure 18-14); wrist ulnar

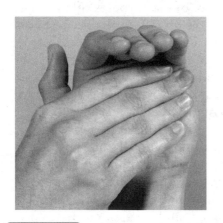 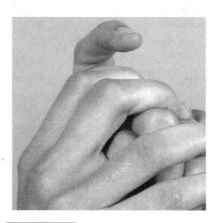 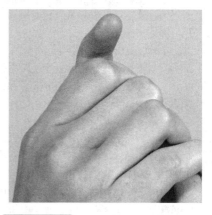

Figure 18-11 MP flexion and extension.   Figure 18-12 PIP flexion and extension.   Figure 18-13 DIP flexion and extension.

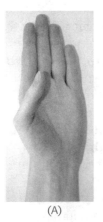 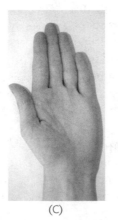 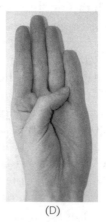 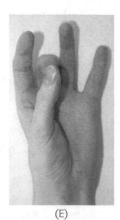

(A)   (B)   (C)   (D)   (E)

Figure 18-14 Active thumb motions. (A) Abduction. (B) Extension. (C) Flexion. (D) Hyperflexion. (E) Opposition.

(Figure 18-15) and radial deviation (Figure 18-16); and finger adduction and abduction. The wrist and hand muscles are usually exercised as a group if their strength is similar. If one muscle is weaker, the clinician should exercise that muscle in isolation, in a similar fashion as that used when isolating the muscle for manual muscle testing.

- Active exercises of forearm pronation and supination (Figure 18-17 and Figure 18-18), and elbow flexion and extension.

Active range-of-motion exercises are progressed to submaximal isometrics and muscle co-contractions. Isometric exercise allows for strengthening early in the rehabilitative process, without the stress to joints and soft tissue produced by other forms of exercise. These early strengthening exercises are performed initially in the available pain-free ranges and are gradually progressed so that they are performed throughout the entire range.

Functional/Chronic Phase

The functional phase of rehabilitation usually commences when normal wrist positions and co-contractions of the wrist flexors and extensors can be performed. The goals of the functional phase include:

- *Attain full range of pain-free motion.* The AROM exercises, initiated during the acute phase, are progressed until the patient demonstrates that they have achieved the maximum range anticipated.
- *Restore normal joint kinematics.* Normal joint arthrokinematics are restored by performing joint mobilization techniques.
- *Improve muscle strength to within normal limits and restore normal muscle force couple relationships.* Specific exercises for the wrist and hand include:
  - ❏ Resisted exercises into pronation and supination (see Chapter 17).
  - ❏ Resisted exercises into radial (Figure 18-19 and Figure 18-20) and ulnar (Figure 18-21 and Figure 18-22) deviation.
  - ❏ Resisted exercises into wrist extension (Figure 18-23) and flexion (same position except palm up).
  - ❏ Hand and finger dexterity exercises (Figure 18-24 and Figure 18-25).
  - ❏ Power and prehension grasp activities (Figure 18-26 through Figure 18-29).

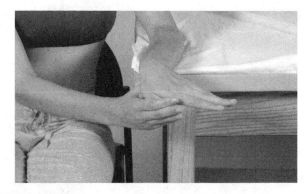

Figure 18-15 Active ulnar deviation with passive overpressure.

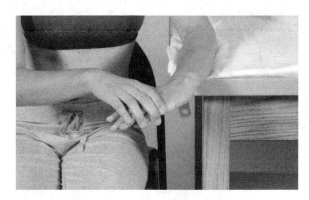

Figure 18-16 Active radial deviation with passive overpressure.

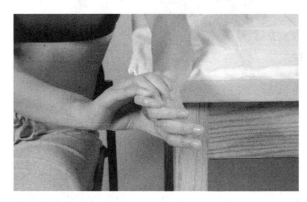

Figure 18-17 Active forearm pronation with passive overpressure.

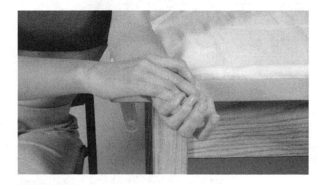

Figure 18-18 Active forearm supination with passive overpressure.

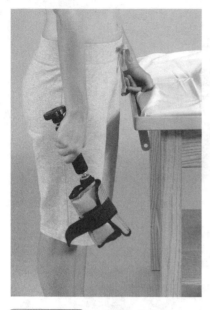

Figure 18-19   Radial deviation PRE: start position.

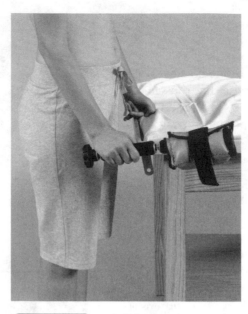

Figure 18-20   Radial deviation PRE: end position.

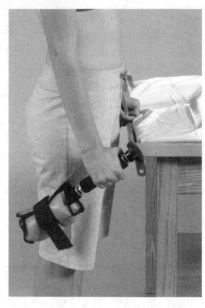

Figure 18-21   Ulnar deviation PRE: start position.

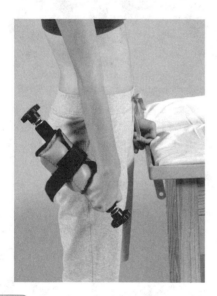

Figure 18-22   Ulnar deviation PRE: end position.

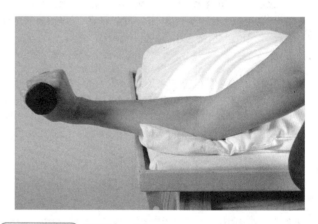

Figure 18-23   PRE for wrist extensors.

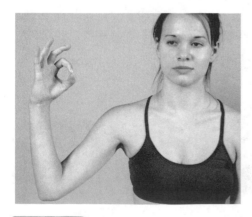

Figure 18-24   Finger dexterity exercise.

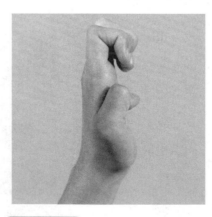

Figure 18-25   Finger dexterity exercise.

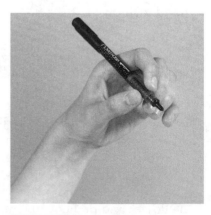

Figure 18-26   Tip-to-tip grasp.

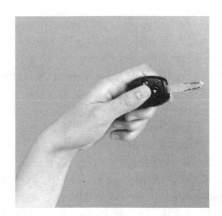

Figure 18-27   Thumb tip to lateral index finger grasp.

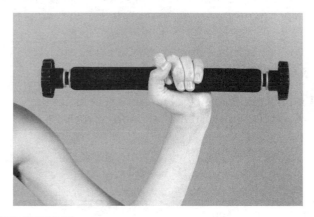

Figure 18-28   Hook grasp.

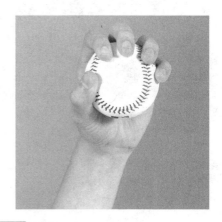

Figure 18-29   Ball grasp.

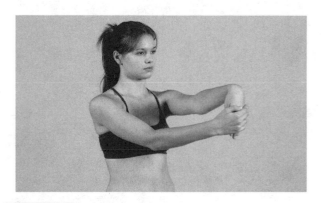

Figure 18-30   Wrist extensor stretch.

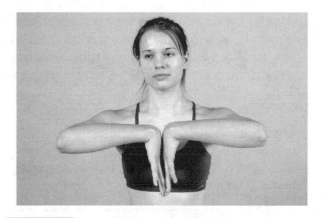

Figure 18-31   Bilateral wrist extensor stretch.

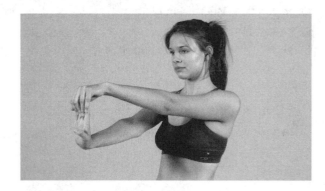

Figure 18-32   Wrist flexor stretch.

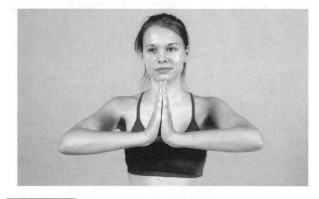

Figure 18-33   Bilateral wrist flexor stretch.

❑ Passive stretching of the wrist into flexion (Figure 18-30) and (Figure 18-31)), extension (Figure 18-32) and (Figure 18-33)), radial deviation (refer to Figure 18-16), and ulnar deviation (refer to Figure 18-15).

Resisted exercises can be performed using gripping with light resistive putty, a washcloth or sponge, or a hand exerciser (see Chapter 17). Care must be

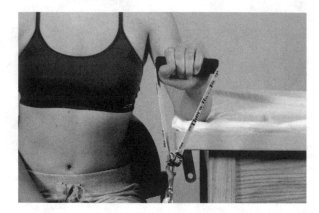

Figure 18-34 PRE using elastic tubing.

taken with gripping or squeezing exercises, because they typically restrict the use of the full range of motion. Resisted exercises also can be performed using elastic resistance (Figure 18-34), a soup can, or dumbbells.

Wrist extension can be performed in pronation to work against gravity or in neutral forearm rotation to eliminate gravity. This exercise encourages the involvement of the ECRL, ECRB, and ECU. MCP flexion can be employed to eliminate any contribution from the ECU, thereby isolating the wrist musculature. Wrist flexion can be performed in supination to work against gravity or in neutral forearm rotation to eliminate gravity. Wrist flexion works the FCU and FCR. Proprioceptive neuromuscular facilitation (PNF) patterns of the upper extremity are performed actively and then with resistance (see Chapter 16 and 17). These patterns incorporate the conjunct rotations involved with finger, hand, and wrist motions. Modified push-ups encourage full wrist extension, and full push-ups require full, or close to full, wrist extension.

Common Conditions

A number of common conditions that affect the wrist and hand are described here and in **Table 18-5**.

TABLE 18-5	Common Causes of Wrist and Hand Pain		
Condition	**Mechanism of Injury**	**Symptoms Aggravated By**	**AROM**
Carpal tunnel syndrome	Gradual overuse Wide variety of factors	Repetitive activities of wrist	Full and pain free
Wrist extensor tendonitis	Repetitive or prolonged activities, forceful exertion, awkward and static postures, vibration, and localized mechanical stress	Sustained positioning of wrist in flexion	Pain with wrist and finger flexion
Wrist flexor tendonitis	Forceful gripping, rapid wrist movements, and moving the wrist and fingers to the extremes of range	Activities involving wrist extension	Pain with wrist and finger extension
OA of the first CMC joint	Repetitive trauma Degeneration	Repetitive use of thumb Strong gripping	Mid-limitation of all thumb movements
Trigger finger	Disproportion between the flexor tendon and its tendon sheath	Finger flexion/extension	Decreased finger extension Clicking or jerking with movements
De Quervain's tenosynovitis	Repetitive finger–thumb gripping combined with radial deviation	Overuse, repetitive tasks that involve overexertion of the thumb	Decreased ulnar deviation Decreased thumb flexion
Dupuytren's contracture	Multifactorial (alcohol, diabetes, epilepsy, smoking, and trauma)	Pain initially with ring and little finger extension.	Decreased finger extension
Thumb ulnar collateral ligament injury	Forced hyperabduction and/or hyperextension stress of the thumb MCP joint	Extension of the thumb	Usually unremarkable
Wrist sprain	Trauma (FOOSH injury)	Taking weight through the hand	Pain with extremes of all ranges

OA, osteoarthritis; CMC, carpometacarpal; FOOSH, fall on an outstretched hand; MCP, metacarpophalangeal; AROM, active range of motion.

Peripheral Nerve Entrapment

Peripheral nerve entrapments are common in the forearm and wrist. Neurogenic syndromes are usually incomplete, indicating the absence of severe motor or sensory deficits, but in the typical case they are accompanied by a history of pain or vague sensory disturbances.[31] As a result, nerve injuries are frequently overlooked as a source of acute, or more commonly chronic, symptomatology.[32] Loss of vibration sensibility has been suggested as an early indicator of peripheral compression neuropathy.[33] The intervention for nerve compression can be surgical or conservative, depending on the severity. Conservative intervention for mild compression involves the application of a protective splint and patient education to avoid positions and postures that could compromise the injured nerve.

Median Nerve

Median nerve compression, as it passes through the carpal tunnel, is a cause of chronic wrist pain and functional impairment of the hand. CTS is the most common compression neuropathy, with a prevalence of 9.2 percent in women and 0.6 percent in men.[34,35] Although it occurs in all age groups, CTS more commonly occurs between the fourth and sixth decades. Compression of the nerve in the carpal tunnel is compounded by an increase in synovial fluid pressure and tendon tension, which decreases the available volume. CTS may result from a wide variety of factors, several of which can easily be remembered using the mnemonic PRAGMATIC:

- Pregnancy secondary to fluid retention.[36]
- Renal dysfunction.
- Acromegaly.
- Gout and pseudogout.[37]
- Myxedema or mass.
- Amyotrophy. Neuralgic amyotrophy is the most likely diagnosis in patients who suddenly develop arm pain, followed within a few days by arm paralysis in the distribution of single or multiple nerves or extending over multiple myotomes.[38]
- Trauma (repetitive or direct). About half of the cases of CTS are related to repetitive and cumulative trauma in the workplace, making it the occupational epidemic syndrome of our time.[39,40] Frequent repetitive wrist flexion and extension or motions that cause repeated palmar trauma may be a factor in the development of CTS. Forceful and repetitive contraction of the finger flexors can also provoke CTS, as demand

for tendon lubrication overwhelms the ability of the sheath to respond, producing an inflammatory reaction.[41] Acute wrist trauma has also been associated with CTS. A FOOSH injury or other trauma can cause a palmar subluxation of the lunate[42] or a distal radius fracture.[43,44]

- Infection.[45,46]
- Collagen disorders. The incidence of CTS in patients with polyarthritis is high; 60–70 percent of patients at some time have a significant CTS.[47,48] This usually is seen in association with a flexor tenosynovitis.[49]

Other causes include RA,[50] diabetes, hypothyroidism, and hemodialysis.[51] Less common causes include incursion of the lumbrical muscles within the tunnel during finger movements[52,53] and hypertrophy of the lumbricales.[54]

The diagnosis of CTS is most reliably made by an experienced PT after a review of the patient's history and a physical examination.[55] The clinical features of this syndrome include intermittent pain and paresthesias in the median nerve distribution of the hand, which can become persistent as the condition progresses.[47,56–58] Muscle weakness and paralysis can occasionally occur. The symptoms are typically worse at night, exacerbated by strenuous wrist movements, and can be associated with morning stiffness. The pain may radiate proximally into the forearm and arm. The physical assessment by the PT focuses on an examination of the motor and sensory functions of the hand as compared to the uninvolved hand.[56,59,60]

Conservative Approach

The conservative intervention for mild cases of CTS typically includes the use of splints, activity modification, exercise, diuretics, and nonsteroidal anti-inflammatory drugs (NSAIDs) prescribed by the physician.[61]

- Splints: The rationale for splints was originally based on observations that CTS symptoms improve with rest and worsen with activity.[62] Splints during the day are helpful only if they do not interfere with normal activity. Rigid splints have been found to be superior to flexible ones in controlling carpal tunnel pressure,[63] although the softer flexible ones enhance compliance in rheumatoid arthritis patients.[64] However, prescription parameters for the type of splint are not standardized,[65] with some advocating neutral positioning[66] and some recommending 10 to 20 degrees of wrist extension. The length of time for wearing the splint is also uncertain, with some recommending day and night use,[67] whereas others instruct patients to wear the brace only at night and during activities stressful to the wrist.[68] Still others recommend only night use.[66] Night splints appear to help reduce the nocturnal symptoms by preventing excessive wrist flexion, although one study found that night splints did not significantly reduce intracarpal pressure when compared to controls who did not wear them.[69]

- *Joint mobilization:* If there is restricted joint mobility, the carpals can be mobilized for increased carpal tunnel space.

- *Activity modification:* Ergonomic modifications can help reduce the incidence of CTS and alleviate symptoms in the already symptomatic patient. Patient education is also important to avoid sustained pinching or gripping, repetitive wrist motions, and sustained positions of full wrist flexion. Patients should also be instructed to observe areas with decreased sensitivity to avoid tissue injury.

- *Exercise:* Isolated tendon excursion exercises for the finger flexor tendons and nerve gliding of the median nerve exercises are performed. These include isolated tendon gliding of the FDS and FDP of each digit (Figure 18-35) through (Figure 18-38). The exercises may have a positive effect by facilitating venous return or edema dispersion in the median nerve.[66] After a period of approximately 4–5 weeks, AROM of the wrist, hand, and fingers and gentle resistance exercise can be introduced.

● **Key Point** Contrast baths can be used in 10-minute sessions to assist in the reduction of inflammation and edema.

Surgical Intervention

Patients with CTS who do not improve with conservative measures are often referred for surgical decompression of the carpal tunnel.[51] Various surgical techniques are available for the carpal tunnel release; however, there has been considerable discussion about which method is most effective. The technique can be endoscopic or open, with the

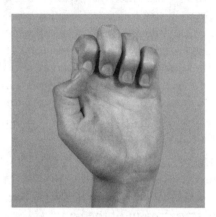

Figure 18-36 Isolated tendon excursion exercise for the finger flexor tendons.

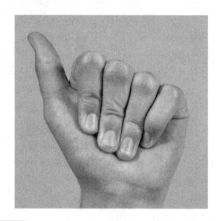

Figure 18-37 Isolated tendon excursion exercise for the finger flexor tendons.

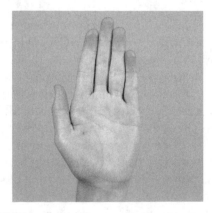

Figure 18-35 Isolated tendon excursion exercise for the finger flexor tendons.

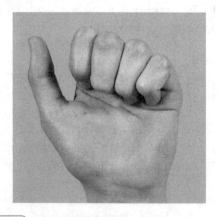

Figure 18-38 Isolated tendon excursion exercise for the finger flexor tendons.

former being used more commonly recently. The advantages of the endoscopic technique are that it offers decreased scar formation and the ability to avoid an incision directly over the carpal tunnel between the thenar and hypothenar muscles, which is a sensitive region of the hand.[70]

Whichever technique is used, a carpal tunnel release generally involves a division of the transverse carpal ligament, thereby increasing the tunnel volume[71] and reducing the compression of the median nerve.[72] In the presence of thenar muscle atrophy, constant loss of sensibility along the median nerve distribution, and severe pain, an internal neurolysis may be performed in addition to the carpal tunnel release.

Following carpal tunnel release procedures, a bulky dressing is applied immediately after surgery, which is changed to a smaller dressing after several days.[70] The patient may be fitted with a splint to keep the wrist in slight extension but leaving the MCP and IP joints free. If used, the splint remains in place for approximately 10 days. It has been proposed that the positioning of the splint may be associated with differential outcomes,[57] although studies have demonstrated no significant difference in outcome between patients treated with and without immobilization after surgery.[73]

Once the sutures are removed after 10–14 days, the patient can progress to AROM exercises of the wrist including extension, radial deviation, and ulnar deviation. Wrist flexion is usually avoided until at least 3 weeks after the surgery to prevent bowstringing of the flexor tendons through the healing carpal ligament. Strengthening of the forearm, elbow, and shoulder girdle is initiated on the twenty-eighth day after surgery.

By the third to sixth week, the patient should be performing gentle strengthening with a foam ball or therapeutic putty, and isometrics in the neutral wrist position, for wrist extension and flexion.[74]

The patient performs sensory retraining through scar desensitization once the surgical incision is closed. This can include manual self-massage of the scar or the use of a mini-vibrator, gripping of different textured materials, and rubbing the scar with different textured materials.[75] Fluidotherapy and rice gripping also can be used.

The following soft tissue techniques are advocated:

- Soft tissue mobilization of the thenar eminence
- Gentle friction massage to reduce scar adhesion to tendons, skin, and nerves following suture removal, usually after 2 weeks

- Manual lymphatic drainage using a light retrograde massage

Ulnar Nerve

Entrapment of the ulnar nerve at the wrist can occur at Guyon's canal. The clinical features of an ulnar nerve entrapment at the wrist include:[76]

- Claw hand resulting from unopposed action of the extensor digitorum (ED) communis in the fourth and fifth digits.
- An inability to extend the second and distal phalanges of any of the fingers.
- An inability to adduct or abduct the fingers, or to oppose all the fingertips, as in making a cone with the fingers and thumb.
- An inability to adduct the thumb.
- A loss of sensation on the ulnar side of the hand, the ring finger, and most markedly over the entire little finger. The posterior (dorsal) ulnar aspect of the hand should be normal because that is innervated by the posterior (dorsal) cutaneous branch.

Atrophy of the interosseous spaces (especially the first) and of the hypothenar eminence can occur in long-standing cases.

Conservative Intervention

The same guidelines as outlined for carpal tunnel syndrome should be used with an emphasis on modifying the provoking activity, avoiding pressure to the base of the palm of the hand, and the provision of rest with a cock-up splint.

Tendonitis/Tenosynovitis

Tendonitis is a term that clearly indicates an inflammation of the tendon or tendon–muscle attachment, whereas *tenosynovitis* involves an inflammation of the tendon sheath. Because the majority of muscles entering the wrist and hand have long tendons, surrounded by tendon sheaths, tenosynovitis is quite common in this region. Most commonly, the tendons of the APL and EPB are involved (De Quervain's disease—see details later in this section). There are, however, some uncommon locations and types of tendonitis. There has been a marked increase in reports of the so-called repetitive strain injury of the upper extremity.[32] Tenosynovitis is frequently seen in inflammatory rheumatic diseases, diabetes mellitus, or hypothyroid conditions.

Extensor Pollicis Longus Tendonitis

This condition is rare except in rheumatoid arthritis (RA), but occurs when the EPL muscle extends into a tight third compartment.[77] Overuse (drummer boy palsy), direct trauma, forced wrist extension, and distal radius fractures may cause EPL tendonitis, which presents with the clinical signs and symptoms of decreased thumb flexion, pain, swelling, and crepitus at Lister's tubercle.[78]

Extensor Indicis Proprius Syndrome

An increase in muscle size of the extensor indices, caused by swelling or hypertrophy from repetitive exercise, may cause stenosis of the fourth posterior (dorsal) compartment, and resultant tenosynovitis.[78] A simple test of a resistance applied to active index finger extension while holding the wrist in a flexed position is a reliable provocative test to reproduce the pain.[79]

Extensor Carpi Ulnaris Tendonitis

ECU tendonitis, a tenosynovitis of the sixth posterior (dorsal) compartment, usually presents as chronic dorsoulnar wrist pain, which is aggravated with forearm supination and ulnar deviation, which causes the tendon to sublux palmarly.[78,80]

Flexor Carpi Ulnaris Tendonitis

The FCU is the most common wrist flexor tendon to become inflamed and is often associated with repetitive trauma and racquet sports.[81] The clinical signs and symptoms include pain and swelling localized just proximal to the pisiform, which is aggravated with wrist flexion and ulnar deviation.[78]

Flexor Carpi Radialis Tendonitis

FCR tendonitis usually develops due to stenosis and tenosynovitis in the FCR fibro-osseous tunnel within the transverse metacarpal ligament. FCR tendonitis usually produces localized pain and swelling, and painful deviation of the wrist.[78] It frequently coexists with other conditions, including fracture or arthritis around the CMC joint of the thumb.[78]

De Quervain's Disease

De Quervain's disease[82] is a progressive stenosing tenosynovitis or tenovaginitis that affects the tendon sheaths of the first posterior (dorsal) compartment of the wrist, resulting in a thickening of the extensor retinaculum, a narrowing of the fibro-osseus canal, and an eventual entrapment and compression of the tendons, especially during radial deviation.[83] Although originally thought of as an active inflammatory condition, recent histological studies have found that the disorder is characterized by degeneration and thickening of the tendon sheath.[84] In most circumstances, the first posterior (dorsal) compartment is a single compartment, which contains the tendons and

synovial sheaths of the APL and the EPB tendons. These tendons allow the thumb to abduct, extend, and grip objects. Overuse, repetitive tasks that involve overexertion of the thumb or radial and ulnar deviation of the wrist, and arthritis are the most common predisposing factors, because they cause the greatest stresses on the structures of the first posterior (dorsal) compartment.[85,86] Such activities include painting, scraping wallpaper, hammering, golfing, fly fishing, typing, sewing, knitting, and cutting.[85,87–90]

Frequently, patients report a gradual and insidious onset[85,86,91] of a dull ache over the radial aspect of the wrist, made worse by turning doorknobs or keys.[92] Patients may also note a "creaking" in the wrist as the tendon moves. Observation of the wrist may reveal a localized swelling and tenderness in the region of the radial styloid process.[86,91] The Finkelstein test is often used to help confirm the diagnosis. The patient is asked to tuck the thumb into a closed fist (Figure 18-39) and then to ulnarly deviate the hand (Figure 18-40). The test is considered positive if this maneuver reproduces the patient's pain.

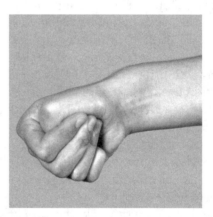

Figure 18-39   Finkelstein test: start position.

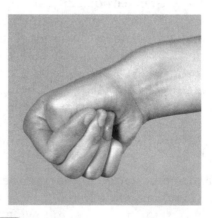

Figure 18-40   Finkelstein test: end position.

Intervention

The typical intervention for tendon injuries can be broken down into two phases:

- *Protection phase:* Usually involves splinting related joints to rest the involved tendon, applying transverse friction massage while the tendon is in an elongated position (if the tendon is in a sheath), use of multi-angle muscle setting techniques in the pain-free positions followed by pain-free range of motion, and instruction in tendon gliding exercises to prevent adhesions.
- *Controlled motion and return to function phase:* Involves a progression of the intensity of massage, exercises, and stretching techniques; an assessment of the functional activity provoking the symptoms; and integration of the entire upper kinetic chain.

Surgical intervention commonly involves a tendon sheath release.[92] The postsurgical rehabilitation plan of care closely parallels the care provided following a carpal tunnel release.

Intersection Syndrome

Intersection syndrome is a tenosynovitis of the radial wrist extensors (ECRL and ECRB) where they cross under the more obliquely oriented APL and EPB.[78] It can also be located over the mid-dorsum of the distal forearm, approximately a hand's breadth proximal to the wrist joint. At this site, there is no actual tenosynovium; rather, the tendons are aligned by peritenon. The cause of intersection syndrome is typically repetitive wrist flexion and extension,[93] and the condition is common in rowers, weightlifters, and canoeists.[94] Although similar to de Quervain's, differentiation is made by the PT using the pain distribution. With the intersection syndrome, the pain is located over the distal forearm, 4–8 centimeters proximal to Lister's tubercle (a small, mast-like protuberance in the center of the distal radius that is identified by palpating the distal radius while the patient flexes the wrist).[78] Symptoms are exacerbated by wrist flexion and extension and by resisted wrist extension. Intervention, in addition to NSAIDs prescribed by the physician, involves the following:[78,95]

- Splint immobilization of the wrist and thumb, with the wrist in 15–20 degrees of extension
- Iontophoresis/phonophoresis
- Deep transverse friction massage followed by exercises for stretching and strengthening

- Patient education to emphasize the importance of avoiding repetitive wrist flexion and extension in combination with a power grip

Digital Flexor Tendonitis and Trigger Digits

Painful snapping or triggering of the fingers and thumb is due to a disproportion between the flexor tendon and its tendon sheath.[78,96–98] The condition is more common in the fibrous flexor sheath of the thumb or ring or middle finger.[99,100] The etiology for this condition is unknown, although it shows a predilection for patients with diabetes, young children, and menopausal women.[99,100] Trigger finger also commonly coexists with rheumatic changes of the hand and may be the earliest sign of RA.[101] In the absence of connective tissue disease, most cases are idiopathic. The first sign is usually the trigger phenomenon—pain on digital motion, with or without associated triggering or locking. (The joint "locks" or "snaps" into flexion when the patient actively flexes that joint; the patient frequently has to physically move the joint back into extension manually or it will remain flexed.) The base of the affected finger is often tender. Over time, the condition becomes very painful, and digital motion may be limited or absent, especially in the PIP joint.[102] Conservative intervention involves the fitting of a hand-based MP flexion block splint for the involved digit only, with only the MP joint being immobilized in full extension, for up to 6 weeks.[103] This immobilization theoretically alters the mechanical forces and encourages maximal differential tendon gliding. The patient should be advised to eliminate such provocative movements as repetitive grasping or the use of tools that apply pressure over the area.

Medical intervention usually involves one or a series of steroid injections,[104] with surgical release of the trigger finger being reserved for the recalcitrant cases.[78]

Dupuytren Contracture (Palmar Fasciitis)

Dupuytren disease, an active cellular process in the fascia of the hand, is characterized by the development of nodules in the palmar and digital fascia. These nodules occur in specific locations along longitudinal tension lines.[105,106] The appearance of the nodules is followed by the formation of tendon-like cords, which are due to the pathologic change in normal fascia.[107–109] The thickening and shortening of the fascia causes contracture (Figure 18-41), which behaves similarly to the contracture and maturation of wound healing.[106] The contractures form at the MCP joint,

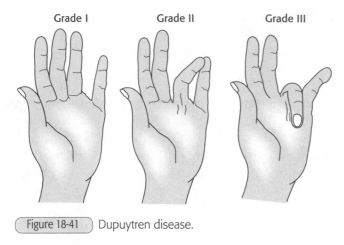

Grade I   Grade II   Grade III

Figure 18-41 Dupuytren disease.

Source: Image reprinted with permission from Medscape.com, 2011.
Available at: http://emedicine.medscape.com/article/1285422-overview

the PIP joint, and occasionally the DIP joint.[110] The etiology of Dupuytren's disease is thought to be multifactorial. There is a higher incidence in the alcoholic population, the diabetic population, and the epileptic population.[106,111,112] Dupuytren's disease can be classified into three biologic stages:[108]

- *First stage:* The first stage is the proliferative stage, characterized by an intense proliferation of myofibroblasts (the cells believed to generate the contractile forces responsible for tissue contraction) and the formation of nodules.
- *Second stage:* The second, involutional, stage is represented by the alignment of the myofibroblasts along lines of tension.
- *Third stage:* During the third, residual, stage the tissue becomes mostly acellular and devoid of myofibroblasts, and only thick bands of collagen remain.[113]

The disease is usually bilateral, with one hand being more severely involved. However, there appears to be no association with hand dominance. The patient may have one, two, or three rays involved in the more severely affected hand. The most commonly involved digit is the little finger, which is involved in approximately 70 percent of patients.

Intervention

Conservative interventions have not yet proven to be clinically useful or of any long-term value in the treatment of established Dupuytren contractures.[114] The goal of surgical care is to excise or incise the diseased fascia. This treatment does not cure the disease but is meant to prevent progression to severe debilitating joint contractures.[106,115] Postoperatively, the hand is maintained in the original dressing and

splint and strictly elevated for 2 days. Scar management and splinting are an important part of the postoperative management. The initial static dorsal forearm splint is positioned to provide slight MCP joint flexion of 10–20 degrees with PIP joint extension to allow maximal elongation of the wound.[106] Active, active-assisted, and passive exercises are usually initiated at the first treatment session. Rehabilitation is a gradual process of increasing activity and decreasing splinting to achieve optimal restoration of movement: restoration of preoperative flexion and maintenance of the extension gained at the time of surgery. The splint may be removed several times daily beginning on postoperative day 2 to allow active and passive range of motion of the digits. Activity may be increased as tolerated, and heat applied prior or during (whirlpool) therapy may improve tissue elasticity and patient comfort.

● **Key Point** Silastic pads, stretching, and scar massage are useful adjuncts to promote scar softening and maturation.

The PTA should regularly record objective measurements of function to monitor progress, facilitate communication with the hand surgeon, and encourage patient compliance. The patient should be instructed to perform the following simple exercises at regular intervals every day:

- Opening and closing the hand
- Thumb–fingers opposition
- Full flexion of the PIP joints
- Flexion of each finger at the distal palmar crease
- Finger adduction/abduction
- Elbow, wrist, and hand motions

After about 6 weeks, patients should wear the splint nightly for an additional 3–6 months, at the discretion of the supervising PT and hand surgeon, to maintain extension and prevent scar contracture. The patient can expect to return to normal activities within 2–3 months.

Tendon Ruptures

Tendon ruptures can occur anywhere along the route of the tendon, including at the wrist, in the palm of the hand, or along the finger.

Flexor Tendon

One of the main purposes of the hand is to grasp; therefore, the loss of flexor tendons imposes a catastrophic functional loss.[116] Most flexor tendon ruptures occur silently after prolonged inflammatory tenosynovitis, although the causes can also be traumatic. When all nine flexor tendons to the digits have ruptured, little can be done. Single tendon ruptures are more common, and the flexor pollicis longus tendon is the most vulnerable to attrition rupture where it crosses the scaphotrapezial joint, and where local synovitis can create a sharp spike of bone that abrades against this spur and ruptures during use. The flexor digitorum profundus (FDP) tendon to the index finger is also at risk from this bony spur.[117] The indications for surgical repair are normally based on the level of functional loss.

Mallet Finger Deformity

Mallet finger deformity (Figure 18-42) is a traumatic disruption of the terminal tendon of the extensor hood, resulting in a loss of active extension of the DIP joint. This is one of the most common hand injuries sustained by the athletic population and is especially common in the baseball catcher and football receiver. The deformity usually results from the delivery of a longitudinal force to the tip of the finger.[118] The sudden acute flexion force that is produced results in a rupture of the extensor tendon just proximal to its insertion into the third phalanx, or a fracture at the base of the distal phalanx. The primary goal of treatment is to promote healing of the tendon so as to maximize function and range of motion of the involved DIP joint. Conservative intervention involves 6 weeks of immobilization of the DIP joint, during which time the patient is instructed on exercises for all of the noninvolved joints of the upper extremity. During the sixth to eighth weeks, active exercises are initiated for the involved DIP joint with the patient performing gentle active DIP flexion to 20 degrees to avoid excessive stretching of the healing tendon. In subsequent weeks, active flexion is progressed in 5- to 10-degree increments.

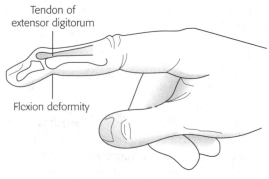

Tendon of
extensor digitorum

Flexion deformity

Figure 18-42 Mallet finger.

Mallet deformities with an associated large fracture fragment are typically treated with 6 weeks of immobilization following open reduction and internal fixation (ORIF), usually with K-wires.[118] Closed reduction is used for other types, followed by 6 weeks of continuous posterior (dorsal) splinting of the DIP in 0 degrees of extension to 15 degrees of hyperextension.[118] The PIP joint should be free to move. If splinted, the splint is removed once a day, while simultaneously holding the DIP joint in extension to allow air to reach the palmar aspect of the middle and distal phalanx. Following the period of immobilization, the splint or fixators are removed and the terminal tendon is evaluated. If the tendon is unable to maintain extension of the DIP joint, a splint is reapplied and the tendon is retested periodically. Once the tendon has healed sufficiently to perform active extension of the DIP, AROM exercises to 20–35 degrees are initiated to the DIP joint. Gentle progressive resistive exercises (PREs) using putty or a hand exerciser are initiated at week 8. Usually, the splint is discontinued at 9 weeks if the DIP extension remains at 0–5 degrees and there is no extensor lag. Unrestricted use usually occurs after 12 weeks.

Rupture of the Terminal Phalangeal Flexor (Jersey Finger)

The rupture of the FDP tendon from its insertion on the distal phalanx (Jersey finger) is often misdiagnosed as a sprained or "jammed" finger because there is no characteristic deformity associated with it.[118]

The injury is typically caused by forceful passive extension while the FDP muscle is contracting. A common example is in football, when the flexed finger is caught in a jersey while the athlete is attempting to make a tackle, hence the term *jersey finger*. Although this condition can occur in any finger, the most commonly injured is the ring finger.[119] The injury usually occurs with forced passive extension of a flexed finger. The intervention can involve doing nothing, if function is not seriously affected, or surgical reattachment of the tendon, which requires a 12-week course of rehabilitation.

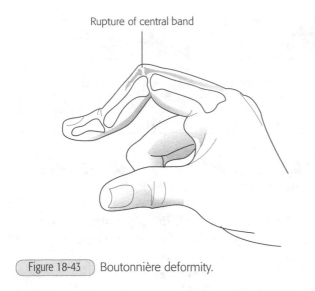

Rupture of central band

Figure 18-43 Boutonnière deformity.

Boutonnière Deformity

Boutonnière deformity, which results from deformity or disruption of the central extensor tendon at the proximal interphalangeal (PIP) joint (Figure 18-43), can manifest acutely following trauma, but most cases are found weeks following the injury or as the result of progressive arthritis. The PIP of the finger is flexed, and the DIP joint is hyperextended. The basis of conservative management for tendon rupture with no associated avulsion fracture is splinting. A variety of techniques have been described, all requiring a minimum of 4 weeks (preferably 6 weeks) of immobilization of the PIP in extension to be effective. The DIP is not immobilized so the patient is able to perform both passive and active DIP flexion during this time.

Wrist Sprains

Wrist sprains are more common than wrist fractures, with the most common wrist sprain resulting from a downward force to the wrist exceeding its normal range of motion. In ligament injuries, the injury usually is to the middle of the ligament.[120]

In the common presentation of a wrist injury, forced movement of the joint is followed immediately by intense pain that subsides and then returns.[92] Swelling occurs within 1–2 hours of the injury. The degree of joint swelling indicates the degree of injury. Ecchymosis develops in severe injuries in 6–12 hours.

Conservative Approach

Conservative intervention includes immobilization of the wrist, depending on the degree of the sprain, to avoid exacerbating the injury. Custom splints made from casting material allow for proper hand and wrist contouring and should cover the palm, allowing the fingers to move freely, and extend to about midforearm.[92] Cocking the wrist up about 10 degrees places the wrist in a position of rest.

Slight sprains should remain splinted for 3–5 days. Icing for 20–30 minutes, three to four times a day, concurrent with NSAIDs prescribed by the physician, can aid in reducing pain and swelling. More severe sprains take longer to recover but should still be removed from the splint in 3–5 days to avoid stiffness.[92] During the period of immobilization, the shoulder, elbow, and fingers of the upper extremity are exercised with active motion and resistance exercises, taking care to apply no stress to the healing ligaments.

After splint removal, a rehabilitation program of wrist curls without weights should be started. Until the pain and swelling subside, wrist curls can be done in water to reduce muscle effort.[120]

Surgical Intervention

The integrity of the carpal relationship depends on the stability provided by both the interosseous ligaments and the midcarpal ligaments.[121] This relationship ensures that the carpal bones move as a unit. Conversely, disruption of this relationship allows abnormal independent motion of one or two carpal bones. The surgical intervention for carpal instability is complex and usually specific to the type of instability. Options include closed reduction with percutaneous pinning and open reduction and internal fixation (ORIF). During the period of immobilization the shoulder, elbow, wrist, and fingers of the involved side should be exercised with active pain-free motion progressing to resistance exercises (**Table 18-6**).

Distal Radius Fractures

Fracture of the distal radius is the most common wrist injury for all age groups. The older patient usually sustains an extra-articular metaphyseal fracture, whereas the younger patient experiences the more complicated intra-articular fracture.[122]

Colles' Fracture

Colles' fracture[92] is defined as a complete fracture of the distal radius with posterior (dorsal) displacement of the distal fragment (Figure 18-44). The typical mechanism of injury is a FOOSH injury. Management of this fracture requires an accurate reduction of the fracture and maintenance of the normal length of the radius. The method of reduction, as well as the position of immobilization, is quite variable. In

TABLE 18-6	Rehabilitation Protocol Following Surgery for Ligament Injury
Phase 1	**Intervention**
Protection of surgical site	Immobilization, protection, rest
Control of pain, inflammation, and swelling	Nonsteroidal anti-inflammatory drugs
	Ice packs
Maintenance of uninvolved areas	Shoulder, elbow, and hand active range of motion and resistance exercise
	General conditioning
Phase 2	**Intervention**
Protection of surgical site	Gradual reduction in immobilization
Initiation of range of motion	Active assisted range of motion
Strengthening exercises	Resistance exercises for the hand and fingers
	Submaximal isometric wrist exercises
	Continuation of shoulder, elbow, and hand exercises together with general conditioning
Phase 3	**Intervention**
Protection of surgical site	Functional splint for protection
Strengthening exercises	Active motion
	Concentric, eccentric resistance
	Hand and finger resistance exercise

most cases, closed reduction and a cast are effective. In other cases, open reduction and external fixation are necessary.[123] Loss of full rotation of the forearm is a common sequelae of this fracture. Occasionally,

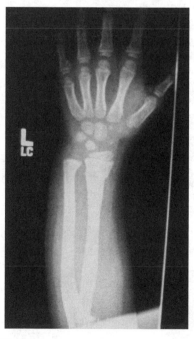

Figure 18-44   Colles' fracture.

patients with distal radius fractures will be prescribed physical therapy during the period of immobilization so that exercises for the shoulder, elbow, and fingers can be performed throughout the involved upper extremity. Upon the removal of the immobilization device (after between 4 and 6 weeks), active range of motion exercises are initiated. Joint mobilization of the wrist and carpal bones may be performed if the PT found joint mobility tests to be positive for joint limitation. Functional exercises for the wrist and hand are begun early in the rehabilitation program and include gripping and squeezing exercises. Usually by the sixth to eighth week more aggressive stretching and strengthening can begin.

Smith's Fracture

A Smith's fracture, sometimes called a reverse Colles' fracture, is a complete fracture of the distal radius with palmar displacement of the distal fragment (refer to Figure 18-44).[124] The usual mechanism for this type of fracture is a fall on the back of a flexed hand. Smith's fractures are classified into three types:[125]

- *Type I:* This is a transverse fracture through the distal radial shaft.

- *Type II:* This is an oblique fracture through the distal shaft starting at the posterior (dorsal) articulating lip.
- *Type III:* This type (also referred to as a reverse Barton's fracture, see next section) is an oblique fracture beginning further down on the articular surface of the radius.

Customary management for a Smith's fracture is with closed reduction and long arm casting in supination for 3 weeks, followed by 2–3 weeks in a short-arm cast.[124] Types II and III are frequently unstable, however, and thus require an ORIF.

Barton's Fracture

A Barton's fracture involves a posterior (dorsal) or volar articular fracture of the distal radius, resulting in a subluxation of the wrist.[124] The mechanism of injury for this type of fracture usually includes some form of direct and violent injury to the wrist, or a sudden pronation of the distal forearm on a fixed wrist. Seventy percent of these fractures occur in young men. Once the fracture has been reduced, an above-elbow cast is applied for 4 weeks, followed by a forearm cast for a further 3 weeks, with the wrist in ulnar deviation. Other techniques include performing an ORIF, with 16 weeks being the average healing time.

Buckle Fracture

A buckle fracture is an incomplete, undisplaced fracture of the distal radius commonly seen in children. The fracture is treated with a cast, ORIF, or external fixation. The fracture site is immobilized for 6 weeks if cast, 8 weeks with an external fixator, or 2 weeks if an ORIF with plate and screws is performed. If the fracture is nondisplaced, rehabilitation may last 2–6 weeks, whereas displaced fractures typically require 8–12 weeks.

Intervention

Successful treatment of a fracture of the distal radius must take into account maintaining the integrity of the soft tissues by not relying on tight casts or restricting the gliding structures that control the hand, while restoring anatomic alignment of the bones (**Table 18-7**). The wrist should not be distracted or placed in a flexed position, because these abnormal positions diminish the mechanical advantage of the extrinsic tendons, increase pressure in the carpal canal, exacerbate carpal ligament injury, and contribute to stiffness. With all of the distal

---

TABLE 18-7 Intervention-Based Classification of Distal Radius Fractures

Type and Description	Management
I: Undisplaced, extra-articular	Splinting or casting with the wrist in a neutral position for 4–6 weeks (based on physician preference and patient condition/compliance)
II: Displaced, extra-articular	Fracture reduced under anesthesia
IIA: Stable	Splinted, then casted
IIB: Unstable, reducible	Remanipulation; may need percutaneous pinning for improved stability
IIC: Unreducible	Open reduction and internal fixation (ORIF)
III: Intra-articular, undisplaced	Immobilization and possible percutaneous pinning for stability
IV: Intra-articular, displaced	Adjunctive fixation with percutaneous pinning/external fixation
IVA: Stable, reducible	
IVB: Unstable, reducible	Percutaneous pinning/external fixation to improve rigidity and immobilization
IVC: Unreducible	Open reduction and internal fixation/external fixation
IVD: Complex	Open reduction with internal fixation/external fixation

Data from Brotzman SB, Calandruccio JH, Jupiter JB: Hand and wrist injuries, in Brotzman SB, Wilk KE (eds): Clinical Orthopaedic Rehabilitation. Philadelphia, Mosby, 2003, pp 1–83; and Cooney WP: Fractures of the distal radius. A modern treatment-based classification. Orthop Clin North Am 24:211–216, 1993

radius fractures, rehabilitation can begin while the fracture is immobilized and involves AROM of the shoulder in all planes, elbow flexion and extension, and finger flexion and extension. The finger exercises must include isolated MCP flexion, composite flexion (full fist), and intrinsic minus fisting (MCP extension with IP flexion). If a fixator or pins are present, pin site care should be performed according to the physician's preference. Following the period of immobilization, an immobilization capsular pattern will initially be present. Extension and supination are commonly limited and need to be mobilized. AROM exercises of wrist flexion and extension and ulnar and radial deviation are initiated. Wrist extension exercises are performed with the fingers flexed, especially at the MCP joints. PROM is performed according to the physician's preference, either immediately or after 1–2 weeks. The AROM exercises of the wrist and forearm are progressed to strengthening exercises, using light weights and tubing. Putty can be used to increase grip strength if necessary.

Plyometrics and neuromuscular re-education exercises are next, followed by return to function or sports activities.

Fractured Scaphoid

Of all the wrist injuries encountered in the emergency department, fracture of the scaphoid is one of the most commonly missed.[126,127] This is unfortunate, given that the scaphoid is the most commonly fractured carpal bone due to its location and is the only bone fractured in approximately 70 percent of all carpal-fracture cases.[36,120,128,129]

> **Key Point** Accurate early diagnosis of scaphoid fracture is critical, because the morbidity associated with a missed or delayed diagnosis is significant, and can result in long-term pain, loss of mobility, and decreased function.[2]

The degree of morbidity associated with scaphoid fractures is related to its scant blood supply, which results in a high incidence of delayed healing or nonunion, and the fact that scaphoid fractures are inherently unstable.

> **Key Point** Although a fracture can occur in any part of the scaphoid, the common areas are at the waist and at the proximal pole.

Classically, the injury results from a FOOSH, with the wrist pronated. Patients typically complain of posterior (dorsal) wrist pain and have tenderness over the anatomic snuffbox. Even with appropriate radiographs, fractures of the scaphoid can be subtle and difficult to visualize.[127]

Intervention

Conservative management of a scaphoid fracture is controversial. There is no agreement on the optimum position for immobilization. Current management is immobilization in a long-arm or short-arm thumb spica cast, with the wrist position and length of immobilization being dependent on the location of the fracture:

- *Proximal pole:* Immobilization is for 16–20 weeks in a long- or short-arm thumb spica, with the wrist in slight extension and radial deviation.
- *Central third:* Immobilization is for 6 weeks in a long-arm thumb spica, followed by a further 6 weeks in a short-arm thumb spica. Some physicians advocate splinting the wrist in radial deviation and mild flexion for 6 weeks.[36,128,130] After 6 weeks, if healing is evident on radiographs, a short-arm thumb spica cast is applied for 2–4 weeks. If after 6 weeks the fracture line seems greater or the fracture appears displaced, evaluation for possible surgery is in order.[128,131]
- *Distal third:* Immobilization is for 6–8 weeks in a short-arm thumb spica.
- *Tuberosity:* Immobilization is for 5–6 weeks in a long- or short-arm thumb spica.

A suggested protocol to use for scaphoid fracture treated with ORIF is outlined in **Table 18-8**.

Chronic pain, loss of motion, and decreased strength from prolonged immobilization or early arthritis are common following a scaphoid fracture. Following the removal of the splint, a capsular pattern of the wrist (an equal limitation of flexion and extension) will dominate. In addition, there will be a painful weakness of the thumb and/or wrist extension/radial deviation, and compression of the first metacarpal on the scaphoid will be painful. AROM exercises for wrist flexion and extension and radial and ulnar deviation are initiated as early as possible after the splint removal, with PROM to the same motions beginning after 2 weeks. A wrist and thumb immobilization splint can be fabricated to wear between exercises and at night for comfort and protection.

At about the same time as the PROM exercises, gentle strengthening exercises are begun with 1- to 2-pound weights or putty. Over a period of

TABLE 18-8	Conservative Intervention for Scaphoid Fracture Treated with ORIF
Time Frame	**Recommended Intervention**
0–10 days	Elevate sugar-tong thumb spica splint, ice
	Shoulder ROM
	MCP/PIP/DIP joint active ROM exercises
10 days to 4 weeks	Suture removal
	Sugar-tong thumb spica cast (immobilizing elbow)
	Continue hand/shoulder ROM
4–8 weeks	Short-arm thumb spica cast
	Elbow active/assisted extension, flexion/supination/pronation; continue fingers two through five active ROM and shoulder active ROM

ORIF, open reduction and internal fixation; MCP, metacarpophalangeal; PIP, proximal interphalangeal; DIP, distal interphalangeal; ROM, range of motion.

Data from Brotzman SB, Calandruccio JH, Jupiter JB: Hand and wrist injuries, in Brotzman SB, Wilk KE (eds): Clinical Orthopaedic Rehabilitation. Philadelphia, Mosby, 2003, pp 1–83

several weeks, the exercise program is progressed to include weight-bearing activities, plyometrics, open and closed chain exercises, and neuromuscular re-education, before finally progressing to functional and sport-specific exercises and activities.

The most common complication of scaphoid fracture is nonunion. Missed and therefore untreated scaphoid fractures often progress to nonunions. Because of the precarious nature of the blood supply and potential for movement at the fracture line, nonunion can occur in 8–10 percent of cases.[126,132] The rate of nonunion varies with the actual fracture site. Nonunion complicates up to 20–30 percent of proximal third fractures, and 10–20 percent of middle third fractures.[127] Nonunion of distal third fractures is relatively rare.[126,132]

Ulnar Collateral Ligament Sprain of the Thumb

A UCL injury, also known as *gamekeeper's thumb*, *skier's thumb*,[133] and *breakdancer's thumb*, involves injury to the ulnar collateral ligament of the MCP joint of the thumb and is the most common ligament injury of the hand.[134]

Key Point The MCP joint of the thumb is primarily stabilized by the UCL. The origin of this ligament is on the ulnar aspect of the metacarpal head, whereas the insertion of the UCL is located distally on the proximal phalanx.

The most common cause of UCL injury is an acute abducting (radially directed) force upon the thumb, but the injury may also result from a combination of torsion, abduction, and hyperextension at the first MCP joint. The patient typically complains of pain or tenderness on the ulnar aspect of the MCP joint.

Key Point The PT can test the stability of the joint by applying an abduction stress with the thumb in full extension, and then in full flexion, which stresses the accessory collateral ligament and the UCL, respectively. An angulation of greater than 35 degrees or 15 degrees greater than the uninvolved side indicates instability and the need for surgical intervention.

Intervention

For the purposes of intervention, these injuries can be divided into two categories:

- *Grade I and II sprains:* The majority of the ligament remains intact. The intervention for grade I and II tears is immobilization in a thumb spica cast for 3 weeks, with additional protective splinting for 2 weeks. Thumb spica splints, which are forearm-based splints fabricated from a palmar or radial approach, are designed to immobilize the wrist, CMC, and MCP joints of the thumb, thereby permitting the radial wrist extensors and the proximal thumb to rest. The splint is worn at all times except for removal for hygiene and exercise. AROM of flexion and extension begins at 3 weeks and progresses to strengthening exercises by 8 weeks, taking care not to apply any abduction stress to the MCP joint during the first 2–6 weeks.

- *Grade III tears and displaced bony avulsions:* These injuries are treated with surgery and immobilization.[135] Postsurgical rehabilitation involves wearing a thumb spica cast or splint for 3 weeks, with an additional 2 weeks of splinting, except during the exercises of active flexion and extension. Otherwise the exercise progression is the same as for the grade I and II sprains.

Radial collateral sprains are classified and treated in a similar manner.

Metacarpal Fractures

Injury to the metacarpals is the result of either direct or indirect trauma. The nature and direction of the applied force determines the exact type of fracture or dislocation, with the specific injury patterns as follows:

- *Carpometacarpal (CMC) injuries:* Metacarpal base fractures and dislocations of the CMC joint commonly result from an axial load or other stress on the hand with the wrist flexed.
- *Metacarpal shaft and neck injuries:* Typically, metacarpal shaft fractures are produced by torsion, axial loading, or direct trauma. Metacarpal neck fractures, the most common metacarpal fractures, usually result from striking a solid object with a clenched fist. A Bennett's fracture is a fracture dislocation of the proximal first metacarpal.
- *Metacarpal head injuries:* Metacarpal head (boxer's) fractures are intra-articular injuries and result from axial loading or direct trauma.
- *Metacarpophalangeal (MCP) dislocations:* These result from forced hyperextension of the digits. Dorsal MCP dislocations are the most frequent dislocations.

Intervention

Treatment of metacarpal fractures and dislocations is primarily nonoperative. The goals of nonoperative management are to obtain alignment and stability and to begin motion of the fingers and wrist as soon as possible. Following a closed reduction of the fracture or dislocation, a forearm-based splint/cast is then applied. Generally, the wrist is placed in 20–30 degrees of extension; the MCP joints are immobilized in 70–90 degrees of flexion, with the dorsal aspect of the splint extending to the IP joints and the volar aspect ending at the distal palmar crease. Throughout the immobilization period, the patient is instructed on AROM exercises for the shoulder, elbow, and fingers of the involved upper extremity. After approximately 3–5 weeks, the splint/cast is removed and AROM exercises of the hand are initiated as per the physician's instructions. Hand PREs are initiated based on healing and patient tolerance.

Although closed management of these injuries is typical, certain fractures and dislocations require operative intervention (ORIF) to ensure satisfactory restoration of function and cosmesis. Once the cast is removed, AROM exercises of the hand are initiated as per the physician's instructions. Hand PREs are initiated based on healing and patient tolerance.

Finger Fractures

Phalangeal fractures represent approximately 46 percent of fractures of the hand and wrist and are more common than metacarpal or carpal fractures.[136] These fractures can be divided into base, shaft, and neck and head fractures. Unstable displaced articular fractures require surgical intervention.

Intervention

Conservative intervention of the more stable fractures involves closed reduction in as near normal a position as possible with an appropriate cast or splint:[137]

- *Distal phalanx fractures:* A protective splint is worn for 2–4 weeks until the fracture site is nontender. AROM begins at 2–4 weeks, or earlier if the fracture is stable enough. PROM begins at 5–6 weeks. PREs normally begin at 7–8 weeks.
- *Middle phalanx fractures:* If nondisplaced, these fractures are splinted in the intrinsic plus position for approximately 3 weeks. In the intrinsic plus position, the MCP joints are flexed at 60–70 degrees and the IP joints are fully extended. The wrist is held in extension at 10 degrees less than maximal. Buddy splinting, the taping of a neighboring finger to the involved finger, may also be an option. AROM is initiated when pain and edema subside. PROM begins at 4–6 weeks, with PREs normally beginning at 6–8 weeks.
- *Proximal phalanx fractures:* Nondisplaced extra-articular fractures are splinted with buddy tape. AROM is initiated immediately, with PROM being initiated at 6–8 weeks. Nondisplaced intra-articular fractures are splinted in the intrinsic plus position for 2–3 weeks.

AROM begins at 2–3 weeks, with PROM being initiated at 4–8 weeks. PREs normally begin at clinical union (8–12 weeks).

Complex Regional Pain Syndrome

The term *complex regional pain syndrome (CRPS)*, formerly known as reflex sympathetic dystrophy (RSD), refers to a classification of disorders that can occur even after minor injury to a limb. It is a major cause of disability.[138] CRPS can occur in any of the extremities.

> **Key Point** CRPS, originally termed *causalgia*, has since been referred to by a number of names, including posttraumatic osteoporosis, Sudeck's atrophy, transient osteoporosis, algoneurodystrophy, shoulder–hand syndrome, gardenalic rheumatism, neurotrophic rheumatism, reflex neurovascular dystrophy, and reflex sympathetic dystrophy (RSD).[139]

There are three variants of CRPS, previously thought of as stages, and patients are likely to have one of the following three types of disease progression:

- *Type one:* Characterized by severe, burning pain at the site of the injury. Signs and symptoms include muscle spasm, joint stiffness, restricted mobility, and rapid hair and nail growth. Vasospasm (constriction of the blood vessels) that affects the color and temperature of the skin can also occur.
- *Type two:* Characterized by more intense pain, an increase in the spread of the swelling, diminishing hair growth, and the nails becoming cracked, brittle, grooved, and spotty. Associated osteoporosis becomes severe and diffuse, the joints thicken, and the muscles atrophy.
- *Type three:* Characterized by irreversible changes in the skin and bones, while the pain becomes unyielding and may involve the entire limb. There is marked muscle atrophy, severely limited mobility of the affected area, and flexor tendon contractions (contractions of the muscles and tendons that flex the joints). Occasionally the limb is displaced from its normal position, and marked bone softening and thinning is more dispersed.

Intervention

The most effective intervention for CRPS is disputed; however, most agree that the intervention requires a team approach, in which physical therapy plays a pivotal role, and that the earlier the intervention is instituted, the better the prognosis. Immobilization and overprotecting the affected limb may produce or exacerbate demineralization, vasomotor changes, edema, and trophic changes.[140] Topical capsaicin is helpful, as are NSAIDs prescribed by the physician. Physical therapy is the first line of intervention, whether it be the sole intervention or performed immediately following a sympathetic nerve block to reduce hypersensitivity and pain.[141,142]

> **Key Point** The most important rule is to minimize pain while employing physical therapy. When excessive pain is created, sympathetically mediated pain may worsen.[142] It is vital to not reinjure the region or aggravate the problem with aggressive physical rehabilitation.[143]

The patient's involved limb must be elevated as often as possible and actively mobilized several times per day.[142] Recovery from muscle dysfunction, swelling, and joint stiffness requires appropriate physical activity and exercise, and pressure and motion are necessary to maintain joint movement and prevent stiffening.[142] The progression should occur slowly and gently with strengthening, active assisted range-of-motion exercises, and active range-of-motion exercises.

Active stress loading exercises, such as scrubbing and carrying, should also be incorporated:

- *Scrubbing:* Scrubbing is performed with the patient in quadruped for upper extremity involvement and in elevated sitting or standing for lower extremity involvement. For upper extremity involvement, the patient holds a scrub brush with the affected hand.[144] For lower extremity involvement, a long Velcro strap can assist in fastening the brush to the bottom of the affected foot.[144] Modifications can be made to enhance performance or compliance. For example, upper extremity scrubbing may be done standing at a table or counter.[144] Persons with limited wrist extension may benefit from using a handled brush.
- *Carrying:* Small objects are carried in the hand on the affected side, progressing to a handled bag loaded with increasingly heavier weight. The lower extremity can be loaded in a variety of ways. Walking is an important loading technique if care is taken to ensure weight bearing through the affected leg during gait. Increased weight bearing can be accomplished by having the patient carry a weighted object or bag on the affected side. Loading can also be facilitated

by engaging the patient in activities that promote weight shifting and balance (e.g., ball toss) or by placing the nonaffected foot onto a small footstool during static standing tasks.[145]

Sensory threshold techniques including fluidotherapy (see Chapter 7), vibration desensitization, transcutaneous electrical nerve stimulation (TENS), contrast baths, and desensitization, using light and heavy pressure of various textures over the sensitive area, should be used.

Affected joints should be rested and elevated to counteract the vascular stasis, but the joint also should be mobilized gently several times per day.[146] Physical therapy is advised as long as the patient works within his or her pain threshold.[142] Complete rest to the affected region, particularly immobilization in a cast, is harmful.[143,146]

Therapeutic Techniques

A number of therapeutic techniques can be used to assist the patient. These include exercises and manual techniques.

To Improve Hand Dexterity

The patient is asked to practice touching the thumb to each of the fingers (Figure 18-45), first in one direction and then another.

To Improve Hand Strength

The patient is asked to perform hand squeezing exercises using Theraputty (Figure 18-46).

Joint Mobilizations

The techniques for the wrist and hand have much in common—using a pinch grip of the index finger and thumb of one hand, the clinician palpates and stabilizes the proximal bone of the joint to be mobilized. With a pinch grip of the index finger and thumb of the other hand, the clinician palpates and then mobilizes the distal bone.

- *Distal radioulnar joint (anterior/posterior glides):* Using one hand, the clinician stabilizes the ulna and with the other hand glides the radius in a posterior and an anterior direction (Figure 18-47). Alternatively, the clinician can stabilize the radius and mobilize the ulna.
- *Radiocarpal joint anterior glide:* The patient sits at the end of the table, with his or her wrist at the edge of the table, palm facing downward. The clinician uses one hand to stabilize the radius and ulna. Using the other hand, the clinician performs an anterior glide in a downward

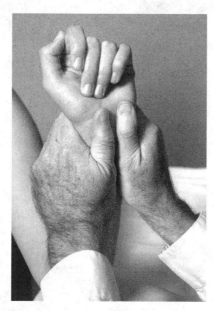
Figure 18-46 Hand strengthening with Theraputty.

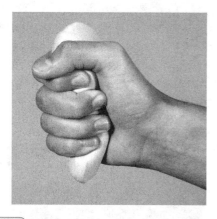

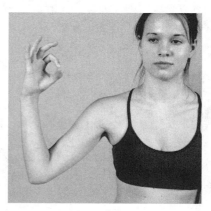
Figure 18-45 Hand dexterity exercise.

Figure 18-47 Distal radioulnar joint (anterior/posterior glides).

direction (Figure 18-48). This joint mobilization is designed to increase wrist extension.

- *Radiocarpal joint posterior glide:* The patient sits at the end of the table, with his or her wrist at the edge of the table, palm facing upward. The clinician uses one hand to stabilize the radius and ulna. Using the other hand, the clinician performs a posterior glide in a downward direction (Figure 18-49). This joint mobilization is designed to increase wrist flexion.

- *Radiocarpal joint ulnar glide:* The patient sits at the end of the table, with his or her wrist at the edge of the table, thumb side uppermost. The clinician uses one hand to stabilize the radius and ulna. Using the other hand, the clinician performs a posterior glide in a downward direction (Figure 18-50). This joint mobilization is designed to increase radial deviation.

- *Radiocarpal joint radial glide:* The patient sits at the end of the table, with his or her wrist at the edge of the table, little finger uppermost. The clinician uses one hand to stabilize the radius and ulna. Using the other hand, the clinician performs a posterior glide in a downward

direction (Figure 18-51). This joint mobilization is designed to increase ulnar deviation.

- *Carpometacarpal joint anterior/posterior glide:* Using both hands, the clinician cradles the patient's hand. Using the index fingers of both hands to stabilize the proximal segment (distal row of the carpals) on the palmar side of the patient's hand, the clinician superimposes one thumb on top of the other and supplies the mobilizing force at the proximal end of the specific metacarpal in a downward direction (Figure 18-52).

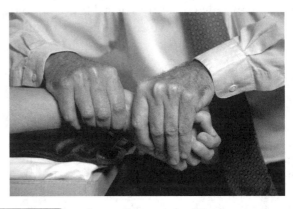

Figure 18-50   Radiocarpal joint ulnar glide.

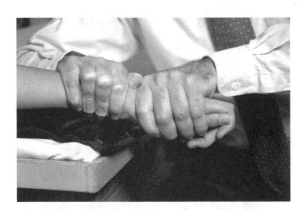

Figure 18-48   Radiocarpal joint anterior glide.

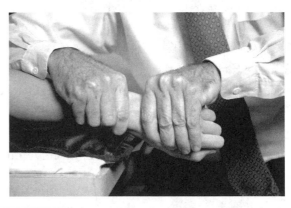

Figure 18-51   Radiocarpal joint radial glide.

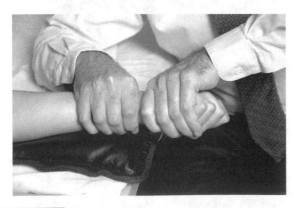

Figure 18-49   Radiocarpal joint posterior glide.

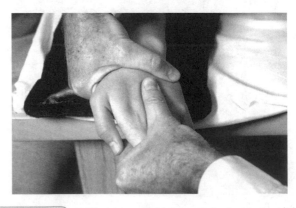

Figure 18-52   Carpometacarpal joint anterior/posterior glide.

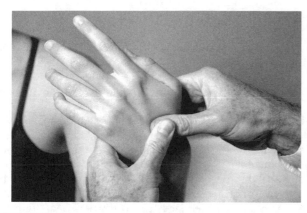

Figure 18-53 Intercarpal joint glides.

- *Intercarpal glides:* Using the same technique as the previous, the clinician stabilizes the proximal row of carpals with the index fingers and mobilizes the specific carpal in a downward direction using both thumbs (Figure 18-53).

Summary

The wrist joint is actually composed of two separate joints: the radiocarpal joint and the midcarpal joint. Working with an extensive array of ligaments, the primary muscles of the wrist effectively stabilize and mobilize the wrist for a variety of different functions.

When functioning normally, the 19 bones and 19 joints of the hands produce remarkably diverse functions. However, an injured hand can dramatically reduce the overall function of the entire upper limb. Injuries to the hand are common because the hand is used to explore and interact with the environment, placing it at potential risk.

REVIEW Questions

1. What is the triangular fibrocartilage complex?
2. What is a Colles' fracture?
3. Which carpal bone is the most commonly fractured?
4. A fracture to the scaphoid can cause what complication?
5. What motions do the lumbricals perform?
6. The flexor digitorum profundus muscle is primarily a flexor of which joints?

7. While palpating a patient's wrist and hand you elicit tenderness on a line between the radial tubercle and the base of the third metacarpal. Which bones are probably affected?
   a. Scaphoid and capitate
   b. Capitate and hamate
   c. Trapezium and scaphoid
   d. Trapezium and trapezoid
8. Atrophy of the muscles of the thenar eminence would indicate injury to which nerve?
   a. Musculocutaneous
   b. Median
   c. Radial
   d. Ulnar
9. You are treating a patient who demonstrates an inability to fully flex the index finger and middle finger, thumb opposition is lost, and the sensory deficit includes the lateral one-half of the ring finger, the middle and index finger, and the thumb. Which nerve do you suspect is involved?
   a. Ulnar nerve
   b. Radial nerve
   c. Median nerve
   d. None of the above
10. An injury to which part of the brachial plexus would cause weakness of the biceps, coracobrachialis, and finger flexors?
11. Which of the following muscles is not supplied by the median nerve?
   a. Flexor carpi radialis
   b. Flexor digitorum superficialis
   c. Flexor pollicus longus
   d. Abductor pollicus longus
12. All of the following muscles have an action at the wrist except the:
   a. Flexor carpi radialis
   b. Extensor carpi ulnaris
   c. Flexor carpi ulnaris
   d. Extensor digitorum communis
13. You are reading a plan of care for a 74-year-old patient with the diagnosis of rheumatoid arthritis. The clinical presentation of this patient will most closely follow:
   a. Complaints of morning stiffness; nodules over bony prominences; joints of the cervical spine, hand, and elbow involved
   b. Complaints of morning stiffness; Herberden's nodules; joints of the hand, knee, and hip involved
   c. Complaints of pain with weight bearing; ulnar drift and subluxation of the wrist joint;

joints of the wrist and hand, elbow, and cervical spine involved

    d. Complaints of stiffness following periods of rest; deformities of interphalangeal joints; joints of the lumbar spine, hips, and knees involved

14. A patient who has rheumatoid arthritis would more likely benefit from which of the following?

    a. Cock-up splint

    b. Airplane splint

    c. Dynamic wrist extension splint

    d. Milwaukee brace

15. Following removal of a cast for a fracture of the distal third of the radius, a patient now has limited wrist extension. To increase wrist extension, gentle stretching can be initiated by:

    a. Pronating the forearm and extending the wrist while allowing the fingers to flex

    b. Supinating the forearm and extending the wrist and fingers

    c. Supinating the forearm and extending the wrist while allowing the fingers to flex

    d. Pronating the forearm and extending the wrist and fingers

References

1. Wadsworth CT: Anatomy of the hand and wrist, in Wadsworth CT (ed): Manual Examination and Treatment of the Spine and Extremities. Baltimore, MD, Williams & Wilkins, 1988, pp 128–138

2. Wackerle JF: A prospective study identifying the sensitivity of radiographic findings and the efficacy of clinical findings in carpal navicular fractures. Ann Emerg Med 16:733–737, 1987

3. Moore JS: De Quervain's tenosynovitis: Stenosing tenosynovits of the first dorsal compartment. J Occup Environ Med 39:990–1002, 1997

4. Tubiana R, Thomine J-M, Mackin E: Examination of the Hand and WriSt London, Mosby, 1996

5. Austin NM: The wrist and hand complex, in Levangie P, Norkin C (eds): Joint Structure and Function: A Comprehensive Analysis. Philadelphia, FA Davis, 2005, pp 305–336

6. Kisner C, Colby LA: The wrist and hand, in Kisner C, Colby LA (eds): Therapeutic Exercise. Foundations and Techniques (ed 5). Philadelphia, FA Davis, 2002, pp 589–642

7. Stokes HM: The seriously uninjured hand—weakness of grip. J Occup Med 25:683–684, 1983

8. Landsmeer JMF: The anatomy of the dorsal aponeurosis of the human finger and its functional significance. Anat Rec 104:31–45, 1949

9. Bendz P: Systematization of the grip of the hand in relation to finger motion systems. Scand J Rehabil Med 6:158–165, 1974

10. Magee DJ: Orthopedic Physical Assessment (ed 2). Philadelphia, WB Saunders, 1992

11. Long C, Conrad DW, Hall EA: Intrinsic–extrinsic muscle control of the hand in power grip and precision handling. J Bone Joint Surg 52A:853–867, 1970

12. Griffiths HE: Treatment of the injured worker. Lancet 1:729–731, 1943

13. Tylor C, Schwartz R: The anatomy and mechanics of the human hand. Artifical Limbs 2:49–62, 1955

14. Napler JR: The prehensile movements of the human hand. J Bone Joint Surg 38B:902–913, 1956

15. Kapandji IA: The Physiology of the Joints, Upper Limb. New York, Churchill Livingstone, 1991

16. Sarrafian SK, Melamed JL, Goshgarian GM: Study of wrist motion in flexion and extension. Clin Orth Rel Res 126:153–159, 1977

17. Stanley BG: Therapeutic exercise: Maintaining and restoring mobility in the hand, in Stanley BG, Tribuzi SM (eds): Concepts in Hand Rehabilitation. Philadelphia, FA Davis, 1992, pp 178–215

18. Walsh M, Muntzer E: Wound management, in Stanley BG, Tribuzi SM (eds): Concepts in Hand Rehabilitation. Philadelphia, FA Davis, 1992, pp 153–177

19. Fess EE, Phillips CA: Hand Splinting: Principles and Methods (ed 2). St Louis, CV Mosby, 1987

20. Malick MH: Manual on Static Hand Splinting. Pittsburgh, Harmarville Rehabilitation Center, 1972

21. Lohman H, Schultz-Johnson K, Coppard BM: Introduction to Splinting: A Clinical–Reasoning and Problem-Solving Approach. St Louis, Mosby, 2001

22. Cannon NM: Manual of Hand Splinting. New York, Churchill Livingstone, 1985

23. Gribben MG: Splinting principles for hand injuries, in Moran CA (ed): Hand Rehabilitation: Clinics in Physical Therapy. New York, Churchill Livingstone, 1986, pp 166–179

24. Schultz-Johnson K: Splinting—A problem-solving approach, in Stanley BG, Tribuzi SM (eds): Concepts in Hand Rehabilitation. Philadelphia, FA Davis, 1992, pp 238–271

25. Booth FW: Physiologic and biochemical effects of immobilization on muscle. Clin Orthop Relat Res 219:15–21, 1987

26. Eiff MP, Smith AT, Smith GE: Early mobilization versus immobilization in the treatment of lateral ankle sprains. Am J Sports Med 22:83–88, 1994

27. Akeson WH, Amiel D, Abel MF, et al: Collagen crosslinking alterations in the joint contractures: Changes in the reducible cross–links in periarticular connective tissue after 9 weeks immobilization. Connect Tissue Res 5:15, 1977

28. Akeson WH, Amiel D, Abel MF, et al: Effects of immobilization on joints. Clin Orthop 219:28–37, 1987

29. Akeson WH, Amiel D, Woo SL-Y: Immobility effects on synovial joints: The pathomechanics of joint contracture. Biorheology 17:95–110, 1980

30. Woo SL-Y, Matthews J, Akeson WH, et al: Connective tissue response to immobility: A correlative study of biochemical and biomechanical measurements of normal and immobilized rabbit knee. Arthritis Rheum 18:257–264, 1975

31. Weinstein SM: Nerve problems and compartment syndromes in the hand. Clin Sports Med 11:161–188, 1992

32. van Vugt RM, Bijlsma JWJ, van Vugt AC: Chronic wrist pain: Diagnosis and management. Development and use of a new algorithm. Ann Rheum Dis 58:665–674, 1999

33. Brain WR, Wright AD, Wilkinson M: Spontaneous compression of both median nerves in the carpal tunnel: Six cases treated surgically. Lancet 1:277–282, 1947

34. DeKrom MC, Knipschild PG, Kester AD, et al: Carpal tunnel syndrome: Prevalence in the general population. J Clin Epidemiol 45:373–376, 1992

35. Stevens JC, Sun S, Beard CM, et al: Carpal tunnel syndrome in Rochester, Minnesota, 1961–1980. Neurology 38:134–138, 1988

36. Gates SJ, Mooar PA: Orthopaedics and Sports Medicine for Nurses: Common Problems in Management. Baltimore, Williams & Wilkins, 1999

37. Ogilvie C, Kay NRM: Fulminating carpal tunnel syndrome due to gout. J Hand Surg 13:42–43, 1988

38. Rosenbaum R: Disputed radial tunnel syndrome. Muscle Nerve 22:960–967, 1999

39. Centers for Disease Control and Prevention: Occupational diseases surveillance: Carpal tunnel syndrome. JAMA 77:889, 1989

40. Rempel DM, Harrison RJ, Barnhart S: Work-related cumulative trauma disorders of the upper extremity. JAMA 267:838–842, 1992

41. Rowe L: The diagnosis of tendon and tendon sheath injuries. Semin Occup Med 1:1–6, 1987

42. Robbins H: Anatomical study of the median nerve in the carpal canal and etiologies of the carpal tunnel syndrome. J Bone Joint Surg 45:953–956, 1963

43. Bauman TD, Gelberman RH, Mubarak SJ, et al: The acute carpal tunnel syndrome. Clin Orthop 156:151–156, 1981

44. Paley D, McMurtry RY: Median nerve compression by volarly displaced fragments of the distal radius. Clin Orthop 215:139–147, 1987

45. Flynn JM, Bischoff R, Gelberman RH: Median nerve compression at the wrist due to intracarpal canal sepsis. J Hand Surg 20A:864–867, 1995

46. Gerardi JA, Mack GR, Lutz RB: Acute carpal tunnel syndrome secondary to septic arthritis of the wrist. JAOA 89:933–934, 1989

47. Barnes CG, Curry HLE: Carpal tunnel syndrome in rheumatoid arthritis: A clinical and electrodiagnostic survey. Ann Rheum Dis 26:226–33, 1970

48. Stanley JK: Conservative surgery in the management of rheumatoid disease of the hand and wrist. J Hand Surg Am 17B:339–342, 1992

49. Vainio K: Carpal canal syndrome caused by tenosynovitis. Acta Rheumatoid Scand 4:22–27, 1957

50. Gelberman RH: Carpal tunnel syndrome, in Gelberman RH (ed): Operative Nerve Repair. Philadelphia, JB Lippincott, 1991, pp 939–948

51. Von Schroeder HP, Botte MJ: Carpal tunnel syndrome. Hand Clin 12:643–655, 1996

52. Cobb TK, An K, Cooney WP, et al: Lumbrical muscle incursion into the carpal tunnel during finger flexion. J Hand Surg 19B:434–438, 1994

53. Yii NW, Elliot D: A study of the dynamic relationship of the lumbrical muscles and the carpal tunnel. J Hand Surg 19B:439–443, 1994

54. Robinson D, Aghasi M, Halperin N: The treatment of carpal tunnel syndrome caused by hypertrophied lumbrical muscles. Scand J Plast Reconstr Surg 23:149–151, 1989

55. Katz JN, Larson MG, Sabra A, et al: The carpal tunnel syndrome: Diagnostic utility of the history and physical examination findings. Ann Intern Med 112:321–327, 1990

56. D'Arcy CA, McGee S: Does this patient have carpal tunnel syndrome? JAMA 283:3110–3117, 2000

57. Feuerstein M, Burrell LM, Miller VI, et al: Clinical management of carpal tunnel syndrome: A 12 year review of outcomes. Am J Ind Med 35:232–245, 1999

58. Szabo RM: Carpal tunnel syndrome-general, in Gelberman RH (ed): Operative Nerve Repair and Reconstruction. Philadelphia, JB Lippincott, 1991, pp 882–883

59. Heller L, Ring H, Costeff H, et al: Evaluation of Tinel's and Phalen's signs in diagnosis of the carpal tunnel syndrome. Eur Neurol 25:40–42, 1986

60. Kenneally M, Rubenach H, Elvey R: The upper limb tension test: The SLR of the arm, in Grant R (ed): Physical Therapy of the Cervical and Thoracic Spine. New York, Churchill Livingstone, 1988

61. Chang MH, Chiang HT, Lee SSJ, et al: Oral drug of choice in carpal tunnel syndrome. Neurology 51:390–393, 1998

62. Roaf R: Compression of median nerve in carpal tunnel [letter to the editor]. Lancet 1:387, 1947

63. Rempel D, Manojlovik R, Levinsohn DG, et al: The effect of wearing a flexible wrist splint on carpal tunnel pressure during repetitive hand activity. J Hand Surg 19:106–110, 1994

64. Callinan NJ, Mathiowetz V: Soft versus hard resting hand splints in rheumatoid arthritis: Pain relief, preference and compliance. Am J Occup Ther 50:347–353, 1995

65. Sailer SM: The role of splinting and rehabilitation in the treatment of of carpal and cubital tunnel syndromes. Hand Clin 12:223–241, 1996

66. Burke DT, Burke MM, Stewart GW, et al: Splinting for carpal tunnel syndrome: In search of the optimal angle. Arch Phys Med Rehab 75:1241–1244, 1994

67. Kruger VL, Kraft GH, Deitz JC, et al: Carpal tunnel syndrome: Objective measures and splint use. Arch Phys Med Rehab 72:517–520, 1991

68. Dolhanty D: Effectiveness of splinting for carpal tunnel syndrome. Can J Occup Ther 53:275–280, 1986

69. Luchetti R, Schoenhuber R, Alfarano M, et al: Serial overnight recordings of intracarpal canal pressure in carpal tunnel syndrome patients with and without wrist splinting. J Hand Surg 19:35–37, 1994

70. Trumble TE, Gilbert M, McCallister WV: Endoscopic versus open surgical treatment of carpal tunnel syndrome. Neurosurgery Clin North Am 12:255–266, 2001

71. Richman JA, Gelberman RH, Rydevik BL, et al: Carpal tunnel syndrome: Morphologic changes after release of the transverse carpal ligament. J Hand Surg 14A:852–857, 1989

72. Okutsu I, Ninomiya S, Hamanaka I, et al: Measurement of pressure in the carpal canal before and after endoscopic management of carpal tunnel syndrome. J Bone Joint Surg 71A:679–683, 1989

73. Bury TF, Akelman E, Weiss AP: Prospective, randomized trial of splinting after carpal tunnel release. Ann Plast Surg 35:19–22, 1995

74. Kasch M: Therapist's evaluation and treatment of upper extremity cumulative trauma disorders, in Hunter

JM, Mackin EJ, Callahan AD (eds): Rehabilitation of the Hand: Surgery and Therapy (ed 4). St Louis, Mosby, 1995, pp 1745–1763

75. Waylett–Rendall J: Use of therapeutic modalities in upper extremity rehabilitation, in Hunter JM, Mackin EJ, Callahan AD (eds): Rehabilitation of the Hand: Surgery and Therapy (ed 4). St Louis, Mosby, 1995, pp 1764–1799

76. Chusid JG: Correlative Neuroanatomy and Functional Neurology (ed 19). Norwalk, CT, Appleton-Century-Crofts, 1985, pp 144–148

77. Mogensen BA, Mattson HS: Stenosing tenovaginitis of the third compartment of the hand. Scand J Plast Reconstr Surg 14:127, 1980

78. Thorson E, Szabo RM: Common tendinitis problems in the hand and forearm. Orthop Clin North Am 23:65–74, 1992

79. Spinner M, Olshansky K: The extensor indicis proprius syndrome. Plast Reconstr Surg 51:134, 1973

80. Hajj AA, Wood MB: Stenosing tenosynovitis of the extensor carpi ulnaris. J Hand Surg 11A:519, 1986

81. Helal B: Racquet player's pisiform. Hand 10:87, 1978

82. de Quervain F: Uber eine Form von chronischer Tendovaginitis. Cor-Bl f schweiz Aertze 25:389–394, 1895

83. Lapidus PW, Fenton R: Stenosing tenovaginitis at the wrist and fingers: Report of 423 cases in 269 patients. Arch Surg 64:475–487, 1952

84. Clarke MT, Lyall HA, Grant JW, et al: The histopathology of de Quervain's disease. J Hand Surg [Br] 23:732–734, 1998

85. Muckart RD: Stenosing tendovaginitis of abductor pollicis brevis at the radial styloid (de Quervain's disease). Clin Orthop 33:201–208, 1964

86. Finkelstein H: Stenosing tenovaginitis at the radial styloid process. J Bone Joint Surg 12A:509, 1930

87. Patterson DC: DeQuervain's disease: Stenosing tendovaginitis at the radial styloid. N Engl J Med 214:101–102, 1936

88. Cotton FJ, Morrison GM, Bradford CH: DeQuervain's disease: Radial styloid tendovaginitis. N Engl J Med 219:120–123, 1938

89. Diack AW, Trommald JP: DeQuervain's disease: A frequently missed diagnosis. West J Surg 47:629–633, 1939

90. Wood CF: Stenosing tendovaginitis at the radial styloid. South Surgeon 10:105–110, 1941

91. Lamphier TA, Crooker C, Crooker JL: DeQuervain's disease. Ind Med. Surg 34:847–856, 1965

92. Onieal M-E: Common wrist and elbow injuries in primary care. Lippincotts Prim Care Pract 3:441–450, 1999

93. Grundberg AB, Reagan DS: Pathologic anatomy of the forearm: Intersection syndrome. J Hand Surg 10A:299, 1985

94. Williams JG: Surgical management of traumatic noninfective tenosynovitis of the wrist extensors. J Bone Joint Surg 59B:408, 1977

95. Hunter SC, Poole RM: The chronically inflamed tendon. Clin Sports Med 6:371, 1987

96. Hueston JT, Wilson WF: The aetiology of trigger finger. Hand 4:257, 1972

97. Kolin–Sorensen V: Treatment of trigger fingers. Acta Orthop Scand 41:428, 1970

98. Lipscomb PR: Tenosynovitis of the hand and wrist: Carpal tunnel syndrome, de Quervain's disease, trigger digit. Ann Surg 134:110, 1951

99. Nasca RJ: "Trigger finger:" A common hand problem. J Ark Med Soc 76:388–390, 1980

100. Medl WT: Tendonitis, tenosynovitis, "trigger finger," and Quervain's disease. Orthop Clin North Am 1:375–382, 1970

101. Pulvertaft RG: Clinical Surgery of the Hand. London, Butterworths, 1966

102. Kolind-Sorensen V: Treatment of trigger fingers. Acta Orthop Scand 41:428–432, 1970

103. Evans BE, Hunter JM, Burkhalter WE: Conservative management of the trigger finger: A new approach. J Hand Ther 1:59–68, 1988

104. Newport ML, Lane LB, Stuchin SA: Treatment of the trigger finger by steroid injection. J Hand Surg 15A:748, 1990

105. McFarlane RM, Albion U: Dupuytren's disease, in Hunter JM, Schneider LH, Mackin EJ, et al (eds): Rehabilitation of the Hand (ed 3). St Louis, CV Mosby, 1990, pp 867–872

106. Saar JD, Grothaus PC: Dupuytren's disease: An overview. Plast Reconstr Surg 106:125–136, 2000

107. Hill NA, Hurst LC: Dupuytren's contracture, in Doyle JR (ed): Landmark Advances in Hand Surgery. Hand Clinics. Philadelphia, WB Saunders, 1989, pp 349–362

108. Luck JV: Dupuytren's contracture: A new concept of the pathogenesis correlated with surgical management. J Bone Joint Surg Am 41:635, 1959

109. Rayan GM: Clinical presentation and types of Dupuytren's disease. Hand Clin 15:87, 1999

110. Strickland JW, Leibovic SJ: Anatomy and pathogenesis of the digital cords and nodules. Hand Clin 7:645, 1991

111. Noble J, Arafa M, Royle SG, et al: The association between alcohol, hepatic pathology and Dupuytren's disease. J Hand Surg Br 17:71, 1992

112. Yi IS, Johnson G, Moneim MS: Etiology of Dupuytren's disease. Hand Clin 15:43–51, 1999

113. Tomasek JJ, Vaughan MB, Haaksma CJ: Cellular structure and biology of Dupuytren's disease. Hand Clin 15:21, 1999

114. Hurst LC, Badalamente MA: Nonoperative treatment of Dupuytren's disease. Hand Clin 15:97, 1999

115. Gosset J: Dupuytren's disease and the anatomy of the palmodigital aponeuroses, in Hueston JT, Tubiana R (eds): Dupuytren's Disease. Edinburgh, Churchill Livingstone, 1985, pp 75–81

116. Ertel AN, Millender LH, Nalebuff E: Flexor tendon ruptures in patients with rheumatoid arthritis. J Hand Surg Am 13A:860–866, 1988

117. Mannerfelt L, Norman O: Attrition rupture of flexor tendons in rheumatoid arthritis caused by bony spurs in the carpal tunnel: A clinical and radiological study. J Bone Joint Surg 51B:270–277, 1969

118. Burton RI, Eaton RG: Common hand injuries in the athlete. Orthop Clin North Am 4:809–838, 1973

119. Lubahn JD, Hood JM: Fractures of the distal interphalangeal joint. Clin Orthop Rel Res 327:12–20, 1996

120. Onieal M-E: Common wrist and ankle injuries. Adv Nurse Pract 4:31–36, 1996

121. Waggy C: Disorders of the wrist, in Wadsworth C (ed): Orthopaedic Physical Therapy Home Study Course—The Elbow, Forearm, and Wrist. La Crosse, WI, Orthopaedic Section, American Physical Therapy Association, 1997

122. Chin HW, Visotsky J: Wrist fractures in the hand in emergency medicine. Emerg Med Clin North Am 11:703–735, 1993

123. McLatchie GR: Essentials of Sports Medicine (ed 2). Edinburgh, Churchill Livingstone, 1993

124. Wilson RL, Carter MS: Management of hand fractures, in Hunter J, Schneider LH, Mackin EJ, et al (eds): Rehabilitation of the Hand. St Louis, CV Mosby, 1990, pp 284–294

125. Sorenson MK: Fractures of the wrist and hand, in Moran CA (ed): Hand Rehabilitation: Clinics in Physical Therapy. New York, Churchill Livingstone, 1986, pp 191–225

126. Ring D, Jupiter JB, Herndon JH: Acute fractures of the scaphoid. J Am Acad Orthop Surg 8:225–231, 2000

127. Perron AD, Brady WJ, Keats TE, et al: Orthopedic pitfalls in the ED: Scaphoid fracture. Am J Emerg Med 19:310–316, 2001

128. Onieal M-E: Essentials of musculoskeletal care (ed 1). Rosemont, IL, American Academy of Orthopaedic Surgeons, 1997

129. Onieal M-E: The hand: Examination and diagnosis, American Society for Surgery of the Hand (ed 3). New York, Churchill Livingstone, 1990

130. Weber ER, Chao EY: An experimental approach to the mechanism of scaphoid waist fractures. J Hand Surg 3:142–153, 1978

131. Onieal M-E: Athletic Training and Sports Medicine (ed 2). Park Ridge, IL, American Academy of Orthopaedic Surgeons, 1991

132. Ritchie JV, Munter DW: Emergency department evaluation and treatment of wrist injuries. Emerg Med Clin North Am 17:823–842, 1999

133. Husband JB, McPherson SA: Bony skier's thumb injuries. Clin Orthop Rel Res 327:79–84, 1996

134. Rettig AC: Current concepts in management of football injuries of the hand and wrist. J Hand Ther 4:42–50, 1991

135. Stener B: Displacement of the ruptured ulnar collateral ligament of the metacarpophalangeal joint of the thumb. J Bone Joint Surg 44B:869–879, 1962

136. Hove LM: Fractures of the hand. Distribution and relative incidence. Scand J Plast Reconstr Surg Hand Surg 27:317–319, 1993

137. Hritcko G: Finger fracture rehabilitation, in Clark GL, Aiello B, Eckhaus D, et al (eds): Hand Rehabilitation: A Practical Guide (ed 2). Philadelphia, Churchill Livingstone, 1998, pp 319–327

138. Subarrao J, Stillwell GK: Reflex sympathetic dystrophy syndrome of the upper extremity: Analysis of total outcome of management of 125 cases. Arch Phys Med Rehab 62:549–554, 1981

139. Veldman PHJM, Reynen HM, Arntz IE, et al: Signs and symptoms of reflex sympathetic dystrophy: Prospective study of 829 patients. Lancet 342:1012–1016, 1993

140. Walker SM, Cousins MJ: Complex regional pain syndromes: Including "reflex sympathetic dystrophy" and "causalgia." Anaesth Intens Care 25:113–125, 1997

141. Kingery WS: A critical review of controlled clinical trials for peripheral neuropathic pain and complex regional pain syndromes. Pain 73:123–139, 1997

142. Dunn D: Chronic regional pain syndrome, type 1: Part I. AORN J 72:421–424,426,428–432,435,437–442,444–449,452–458, 2000

143. Wilson PR: Post-traumatic upper extremity reflex sympathetic dystrophy: Clinical course, staging, and classification of clinical forms. Hand Clinics 13:367–372, 1997

144. Phillips ME: OT treatment for complex regional pain syndrome. OT Pract August 20, 2001

145. Watson HK, Carlson L: Treatment of reflex sympathetic dystrophy of the hand with an active "stress loading" program. J Hand Surg Am 12:779–785, 1987

146. Gordon N: Review article: Reflex sympathetic dystrophy. Brain Dev 18:257–262, 1996

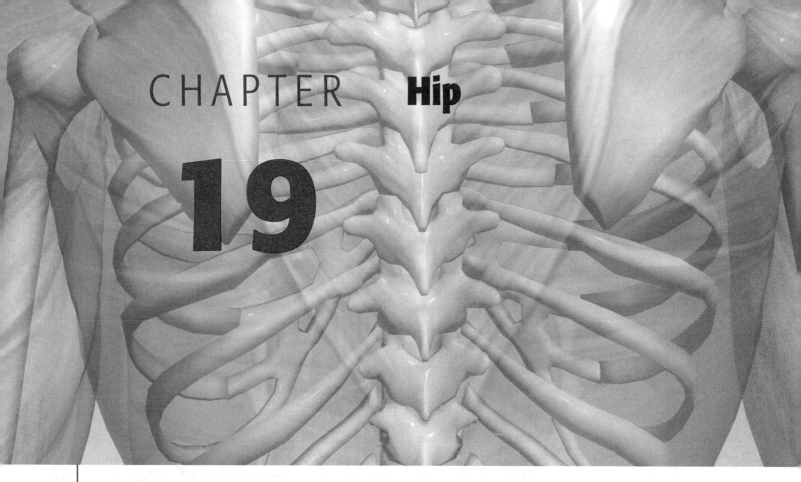

CHAPTER 19 **Hip**

Chapter Objectives

At the completion of this chapter, the reader will be able to:

1. Describe the anatomy of the joints, ligaments, muscles, blood, and nerve supply that comprise the region.
2. Describe the biomechanics of the hip complex, including the open- and close-packed positions, muscle force couples, and the static and dynamic stabilizers.
3. Describe the relationship between muscle imbalance and functional performance of the hip.
4. Summarize the various causes of hip dysfunction.
5. Describe and demonstrate intervention strategies and techniques based on clinical findings and established goals by the physical therapist.
6. Evaluate the intervention effectiveness in order to determine progress and modify an intervention as needed.
7. Teach an effective home program, and instruct the patient in its use.

Overview

The hip joint is the articulation between the rounded head of the femur and the acetabulum of the pelvis. Due to its location, design, and function, the hip joint transmits truly impressive loads, both tensile and compressive. Loads of up to eight times body weight have been demonstrated in the hip joint during jogging, with potentially greater loads present during vigorous athletic competition.[1] Fortunately, the structures about the hip are uniquely adapted to transfer such forces.

Anatomy

The anatomy of the hip provides this complex with a fine balance between mobility and stability. Any imbalance between these two variables can leave the hip joint and surrounding tissues prone to soft tissue injuries, impingement syndromes, and joint dysfunctions.

Bones

Three bones—the ilium, ischium, and pubis—fuse to form each of the two innominate bones. The two innominate bones form an anatomic ring with the pelvis.

Acetabulum

The acetabulum of the innominate is formed at the point where the ilium, ischium, and pubis converge. The acetabulum encloses the head of the femur at the hip joint. The superior surface of the acetabulum, the lunate surface, is heavily lined with articulate cartilage, and is the only part of the acetabulum that normally contacts the femoral head. The acetabular labrum, a ring of fibrocartilage that surrounds the outer rim of the acetabulum, deepens the acetabulum and increases articular congruence by creating a partial vacuum.

Proximal Femur

The femur is the longest bone in the body. The proximal aspect of the femur is composed of a head, neck, and shaft. The proximal shaft of the femur and the femoral neck have a plentiful blood supply from the medial circumflex femoral artery and its branches. The vascular supply to the femoral head is tenuous and provided largely by two sources:

- Branches of the medial and lateral circumflex femoral arteries
- The artery of the ligament of the head of the femur (foveal artery), a branch of the obturator artery, which is typically present within the ligament of the head of the femur

A loss of blood supply to the femoral head can lead to avascular necrosis (AVN). AVN may occur after hip fracture in about 65 to 85 percent of patients.[2]

Muscles

The hip joint is surrounded by a large number of muscles (Figure 19-1), which enable the joint to move through a wide range of motion (ROM), but which are prone to strains. The hip actions and muscles are outlined in **Table 19-1**.

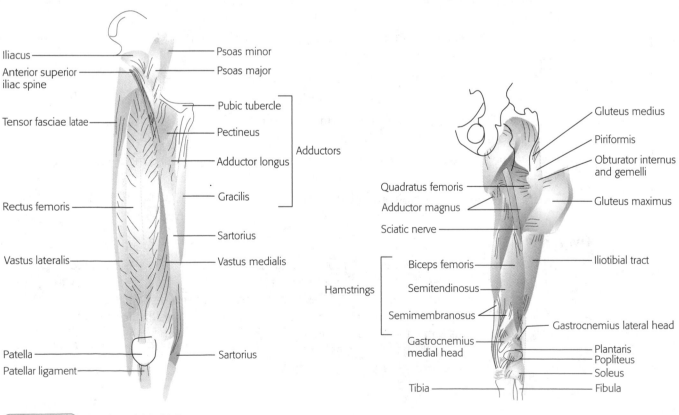

Figure 19-1 Muscles of the thigh.

**TABLE
19-1**   Muscles Acting Across the Hip Joint

Muscle	Origin	Insertion	Innervation
Adductor brevis	External aspect of the body and inferior ramus of the pubis	By an aponeurosis to the line from the greater trochanter of the linea aspera of the femur	Obturator nerve, L3
Adductor longus	Pubic crest and symphysis	By an aponeurosis to the middle third of the linea aspera of the femur	Obturator nerve, L3
Adductor magnus	Inferior ramus of the pubis, ramus of the ischium, and inferolateral aspect of the ischial tuberosity	By an aponeurosis to the linea aspera and adductor tubercle of the femur	Obturator nerve and tibial portion of the sciatic nerve, L2–L4
Biceps femoris (long head)	Arises from the sacrotuberous ligament and posterior aspect of the ischial tuberosity	By way of a tendon, on the lateral aspect of the head of the fibula, the lateral condyle of the tibial tuberosity, the lateral collateral ligament, and the deep fascia of the leg	Tibial portion of the sciatic nerve, S1
Gemelli (superior and inferior)	Superior-dorsal surface of the spine of the ischium, inferior-upper part of the tuberosity of the ischium	Superior and inferior-medial surface of the greater trochanter	Sacral plexus, L5–S1
Gluteus maximus	Posterior gluteal line of the ilium, iliac crest, aponeurosis of the erector spinae, dorsal surface of the lower part of the sacrum, side of the coccyx, sacrotuberous ligament, and intermuscular fascia	Iliotibial tract of the fascia lata, gluteal tuberosity of the femur	Inferior gluteal nerve, S1–S2
Gluteus medius	Outer surface of the ilium between the iliac crest and the posterior gluteal line, anterior gluteal line, and fascia	Lateral surface of the greater trochanter	Superior gluteal nerve, L5
Gluteus minimus	Outer surface of the ilium between the anterior and inferior gluteal lines, and the margin of the greater sciatic notch	A ridge laterally situated on the anterior surface of the greater trochanter	Superior gluteal nerve, L5
Gracilis	The body and inferior ramus of the pubis	The anterior-medial aspect of the shaft of the proximal tibia, just proximal to the tendon of the semitendinosus	Obturator nerve, L2
Iliacus	Superior two-thirds of the iliac fossa, upper surface of the lateral part of the sacrum	Fibers converge with tendon of the psoas major to lesser trochanter	Femoral nerve, L2
Obturator externus	Rami of the pubis, ramus of the ischium, medial two-thirds of the outer surface of the obturator membrane	Trochanteric fossa of the femur	Obturator nerve, L4
Obturator internus	Internal surface of the anterolateral wall of the pelvis, and obturator membrane	Medial surface of the greater trochanter	Sacral plexus, S1
Pectineus	Pecten pubis	Along a line leading from the lesser trochanter to the linea aspera	Femoral or obturator or accessory obturator nerves, L2
Piriformis	Anterior sacrum, gluteal surface of the ilium, capsule of the sacroiliac joint, and sacrotuberous ligament	Upper border of the greater trochanter of the femur	Sacral plexus, S1

(continued)

TABLE
19-1

Muscles Acting Across the Hip Joint (continued)

Muscle	Origin	Insertion	Innervation
Psoas major	Transverse processes of all the lumbar vertebrae, bodies, and intervertebral discs of the lumbar vertebrae	Lesser trochanter of the femur	Lumbar plexus, L2–L3
Quadratus femoris	Ischial body next to the ischial tuberosity	Quadrate tubercle on femur	Nerve to quadratus femoris
Rectus femoris	By two heads, from the anterior inferior iliac spine, and a reflected head from the groove above the acetabulum	Base of the patella	Femoral nerve, L3–L4
Sartorius	Anterior superior iliac spine and notch below it	Upper part of the medial surface of the tibia in front of the gracilis	Femoral nerve, L2–L3
Semimembranosus	Ischial tuberosity	Posterior-medial aspect of the medial condyle of the tibia	Tibial nerve, L5–S1
Semitendinosus	Ischial tuberosity	Upper part of the medial surface of the tibia behind the attachment of the sartorus and below that of the gracilis	Tibial nerve, L5–S1
Tensor fasciae latae	Outer lip of the iliac crest and lateral surface of the anterior superior iliac spine	Iliotibial tract	Superior gluteal nerve, L4–L5

Hip Flexors

The hip flexors are used for a variety of everyday functional activities such as advancing the lower extremity during running and lifting the leg to go upstairs.[3] Efficient execution of these hip flexion activities is highly dependent on the stabilizing forces provided by the abdominal muscles.[3]

Iliopsoas

The iliopsoas muscle, formed by the iliacus and psoas major muscles, is the most powerful of the hip flexors. This muscle also functions as a weak adductor and external rotator of the hip. The iliopsoas attaches to the hip joint capsule, thereby affording it some support. It is worth remembering that any muscle with the potential to flex the hip has the same potential to anteriorly tilt the pelvis because, from a closed-chain perspective, an anterior pelvic tilt is hip flexion.[3]

Rectus Femoris

The reflected head of the rectus femoris attaches to the hip capsule; therefore, an injury to it can cause a capsular adhesion of the hip. The rectus femoris combines movements of flexion at the hip and extension at the knee. It functions more effectively as a hip flexor when the knee is flexed, as when a person kicks a ball.[4]

Tensor Fascia Latae

The tensor fascia latae (TFL) arises from the outer lip of the iliac crest and the lateral surface of the anterior superior iliac spine (ASIS). Over the flattened lateral surface of the thigh, the fascia latae thickens to form a strong band, the iliotibial tract (see Chapter 20).[5] When the hip is flexed, the TFL is anterior to the greater trochanter and helps maintain the hip in flexion by counteracting the backward pull of the gluteus maximus. As the hip extends, the TFL moves posteriorly over the greater trochanter to assist in hip extension. The TFL also assists in abducting and internally rotating the hip.

Sartorius

The sartorius muscle is the longest muscle in the body. The sartorius is responsible for flexion, abduction, external rotation of the hip, and some degree of knee flexion.[6]

Hip Extensors

The powerful hip extensors are used for functional activities involving upward and forward propulsion of the body such as for jumping, running, stair climbing, and transitioning from sitting to standing. With the femur well stabilized, activation of a force couple between the hip extensors and abdominal muscles can also posteriorly tilt the pelvis.[3]

Gluteus Maximus

The gluteus maximus is the largest and most important hip extensor and external rotator of the hip. The muscle consists of a superficial and deep portion. The larger, superficial portion of this muscle inserts at the proximal part of the iliotibial band (ITB), while the deep portion inserts into the gluteal tuberosity of the femur. The inferior gluteal nerve, which innervates the muscle, is located on the deep portion. The gluteus maximus is usually active only when the hip is in flexion, as during stair climbing or cycling, or when extension of the hip is resisted.[4] In addition to extending the hip, the gluteus maximus can also perform the last 20 or 30 degrees of knee extension, provided the foot is in firm contact with the ground, by thrusting the hips forward to move the line of gravity and hence the femur forward, producing an extension movement at the knee. The use of such proximal musculature to help extend the knee is a valuable substitution technique for those with knee extensor paralysis or a prosthetic leg who lack true knee extensors.[3]

Hamstrings

The hamstrings muscle group consists of the biceps femoris, the semimembranosus, and the semitendinosus (see also Chapter 20). All three muscles of the hamstring complex (except for the short head of the biceps) work with the posterior adductor magnus and the gluteus maximus to extend the hip. The hamstrings also flex the knee and weakly adduct the hip. The long head of the biceps femoris aids in external rotation of the thigh and leg; the more medial semimembranosus and semitendinosus muscles assist with internal rotation of the thigh and leg. When the hamstrings contract, their forces are exerted at both the hip and knee joints simultaneously, although they can move only one of these joints at any one time. Both the extensibility and maximal force generated by the hamstrings are highly dependent on the position of the hip.

- *Extensibility:* Adaptive shortening of the hamstrings is a common occurrence, and in extreme cases can produce either a knee flexion contracture or an extreme posterior pelvic tilt and flattened lumbar spine, which increases the likelihood of a posterior herniated intervertebral disk. Due to these potential stresses, it is important that the PTA stabilize the pelvis while stretching the hamstrings to avoid posteriorly tilting the pelvis and overstretching the connective tissue in the lumbar region.

- *Maximal force generated:* Most functional activities of the lower extremity combine the motions of either hip flexion and knee flexion, or hip extension and knee extension. For example, when climbing a hill, the combination of hip flexion and knee flexion is used, followed by hip extension and knee extension. A similar combination is used during running.

Adductor Magnus: Extensor Head

The extensor head portion of the adductor magnus is sometimes considered functionally as a hamstring due to its anatomic alignment.

Hip Abductors

The most frequent demands placed on the hip abductors occur while walking (see Chapter 25). In addition, the hip abductors can hike the hip when working concentrically and can lower the pelvis when working eccentrically.

Gluteus Medius

The gluteus medius is the main abductor of the hip and a primary stabilizer of the hip and pelvis. Due to its shape and function, the gluteus medius is known as the deltoid of the hip. On the deep surface of this muscle is located the superior gluteal nerve and the superior and inferior gluteal vessels. The muscle can be divided into two functional parts: an anterior portion and a posterior portion. The anterior portion works to flex, abduct, and internally rotate the hip. The posterior portion extends and externally rotates the hip. The muscle also provides pelvic support during one-legged stance[7] and functions as a decelerator of hip adduction.

Gluteus Minimus

The gluteus minimus is a rather thin muscle situated between the gluteus medius muscle and the external surface of the ilium. In addition to abducting the hip, it is a major internal rotator of the femur. During internal rotation, it receives assistance from the TFL, semitendinosus, semimembranosus, and gluteus medius.[4]

> **● Key Point** The attachments of the gluteus medius and gluteus minimus to the greater trochanter of the femur significantly increase the internal moment arm of these muscles for abduction. This makes such activities as single limb support during gait based more on the moment arm length and less on muscle force.[3]

The tensor fascia latae is also considered a hip abductor.

Hip External Rotators

The external rotators express their primary function when the lower limb is in contact with the ground. For example, during cutting motions while running, the necessary rotation of the pelvis is performed by this muscle group. In addition to the gluteus maximus, the hip external rotators include the following muscles.

Piriformis

The piriformis is the most superior of the external rotators of the hip. The piriformis is an external rotator of the hip at less than 60 degrees of hip flexion. At 90 degrees of hip flexion, the piriformis reverses its muscle action, becoming an internal rotator and abductor of the hip.[8] The piriformis, with its close association with the sciatic nerve, can be a common source of buttock and leg pain.[9–12]

Obturator Internus

The obturator internus is normally an external rotator of the hip and an internal rotator of the ilium, but becomes an abductor of the hip at 90 degrees of hip flexion.[13]

Obturator Externus

The obturator externus, named for its location external to the pelvis, is an adductor and external rotator of the hip.[14]

Gemelli

The superior and inferior gemelli muscles are considered accessories to the obturator internus tendon. The superior gemellus is the smaller of the two. Both the gemelli function as minor external rotators of the hip.[14]

Quadratus Femoris

The quadratus femoris muscle is a flat, quadrilateral muscle, located between the inferior gemellus and the superior aspect of the adductor magnus. The quadratus femoris is an external rotator of the hip.

Hip Adductors

The adductors of the hip are found on the medial aspect of the joint. The primary function of this muscle group is to create an adduction torque, bringing the lower extremity toward the midline.[3] This adduction torque can also bring the pubis symphysis region of the pelvis closer to the femur.[3] From the anatomic position, the adductors are also considered hip flexor muscles.

Adductor Magnus

The adductor magnus is the most powerful adductor, and it is active to varying amounts in all hip motions except abduction. In addition, regardless of the position of the hip, the extensor head of the adductor magnus is a powerful hip extensor. Due to its size, the adductor magnus is less likely to be injured than the other hip adductors.[15]

Adductor Longus

During resisted adduction, the adductor longus is the most prominent muscle of the adductors and forms the medial border of the femoral triangle. The adductor longus can function as either a hip flexor or a hip extensor, depending on the position of the hip, which affects the line of pull of the muscle, placing it either posterior to the medial lateral axis of the hip (extensor) or anterior to the medial lateral axis of the hip (flexor).[3] The adductor longus also assists with external rotation, extension, and internal rotation in other positions. The adductor longus is commonly strained.[16]

Adductor Brevis

The adductor brevis, which is the smallest and shortest of the three short adductor muscles, occupies the middle layer of the adductors, just deep to the adductor longus. The adductor brevis assists with hip adduction and hip flexion.

Gracilis

The gracilis is the most superficial and medial of the hip adductor muscles. It is also the longest. The gracilis functions to adduct and flex the thigh, and flex and internally rotate the leg.

Pectineus

The pectineus is an adductor, flexor, and internal rotator of the hip. Like the iliopsoas, the pectineus attaches to and supports the joint capsule of the hip.

Ligaments

The femur is held in the acetabulum by five separate ligaments.

- The iliofemoral ligament attaches to the anterior inferior iliac spine of the pelvis and the intertrochanteric line of the femur. By limiting the range of hip extension, this ligament, with the assistance of the pubofemoral ligament, allows maintenance of the upright posture and reduces the need for contraction of the hip extensors in balanced stance. The ligament is also thought to limit external rotation, and the superior portion tightens with hip adduction.
- The pubofemoral ligament originates at the superior ramus of the pubis, also attaching to

the intertrochanteric line of the femur. Its fibers tighten in extension and abduction, and reinforce the joint capsule along the medial surface.

- The ischiofemoral ligament connects the ischium to the greater trochanter of the femur. This ligament, which tightens with internal rotation of the hip, is more commonly injured than the other hip ligaments. When the hip is flexed, the ligament serves to limit hip adduction.
- The transverse acetabular ligament consists of the labrum covering the acetabular notch.
- The femoral head ligament joins the femoral head with the transverse ligament and acetabular notch.

Most people can stand for long periods of time using only minimal amounts of muscular energy about the hip. This is because of the relationship between the ligaments of the hip and the line of gravity, the latter of which, when standing in the full upright posture, normally travels just posterior to the medial lateral axis of rotation of the hips. Due to this arrangement, gravity provides a passive extension torque at the hip, which if not opposed by the hip ligaments that tighten in hip extension, would cause a backward bending of the pelvis over the femurs.[3] This balancing act between the tension in the stretched ligaments and the action of gravity is so effective that it can enable an individual with paralysis of the lower extremities to stand with the aid of crutches and braces at the knees and ankles.[3]

Kinesiology

The hip joint is classified as an unmodified ovoid (ball and socket) joint. This arrangement permits motion in three planes: sagittal (flexion and extension around a transverse axis), frontal (abduction and adduction around an anterior-posterior axis), and transverse (internal and external rotation around a vertical axis), with all three of the axes passing through the center of the femoral head. During these motions, the convex femoral head slides in the direction of the osteokinematic motion. In addition to providing mobility, the hip joint permits a great deal of stability. Most activities involving the hip incur a combination of mobility and stability stresses, but, providing there are no biomechanical imbalances, the hip joint and surrounding tissues deal with these stresses efficiently and effectively.

> **● Key Point** Motions about the hip can occur in one of two ways:
> - By rotating the femur relative to a stationary or otherwise fixed pelvis (e.g., straight leg raise)
> - By rotating the pelvis relative to a fixed or stationary femur (e.g. bending forward at the waist)

Motions about the hip joint can occur independently; however, the extremes of motion require motion at the pelvis.[17] End range hip flexion is associated with a posterior rotation of the ilium bone. The end range of hip extension is associated with an anterior rotation of the ilium. Hip abduction and adduction are associated with a lateral tilt of the pelvis.

In the anatomic position, the orientation of the femoral head causes the contact force between the femur and acetabulum to be high in the anterior-superior region of the joint.[18] Because the anterior aspect of the femoral head is somewhat exposed in this position, the joint has more flexibility in flexion than in extension.[19] The hip joints allow six basic motions. Hip flexion averages 110–120 degrees, extension 10–15 degrees, abduction 30–50 degrees, and adduction 25–30 degrees. Hip external rotation averages 40–60 degrees and internal rotation averages 30–40 degrees (**Table 19-2**).

> **● Key Point** A hip flexion contracture is a limitation of passive hip extension caused by a lack of extensibility of the muscles or ligaments of the hip. Hip flexion contractures are more common in sedentary individuals or those confined to a wheelchair. The hip flexed posture prevents the hip from dissipating the compression forces that act through it, creating abnormal wear and tear on the joint.

The most stable position of the hip is the normal standing position: hip extension, slight abduction, and slight internal rotation.[14,20,21] The commonly

TABLE 19-2	Normal End Feels at the Hip
Motion	**End Feel**
Flexion	Tissue approximation or tissue stretch
Extension	Tissue stretch
Abduction	Tissue stretch
Adduction	Tissue approximation or tissue stretch
External rotation	Capsular stretch
Internal rotation	Capsular stretch

cited open-packed (resting) positions of the hip are between 10 and 30 degrees of flexion, 10 and 30 degrees of abduction, and 0 and 5 degrees of external rotation. According to Cyriax,[22,23] the capsular pattern of the hip is a marked limitation of flexion, abduction, and internal rotation. Kaltenborn[20] considers the capsular pattern at the hip to be extension more limited than flexion, internal rotation more limited than external rotation, and abduction more limited than adduction. Most studies indicate a total hip joint reaction force of three times body weight when standing on one leg. This total force is created by the body weight itself and the contraction force of the hip abductor muscles (which generates a force two times body weight). These large forces are tolerated well in the healthy hip, but in a person with painful osteoarthritis in the hip, these forces can aggravate the joint and lead to further inflammation and degeneration. To offset these joint reaction forces, the patient can be given a cane to hold in the hand opposite the painful hip. The cane serves to reduce the demands on the hip abductor muscles of the involved hip, and thereby reduces the compression forces through the involved hip.

Lumbopelvic Rhythm

Bending forward at the waist requires a coordinated movement among the lumbar spine, pelvis, and hips. As the head and upper trunk initiate flexion, the pelvis shifts posteriorly to maintain the center of gravity over the base of support. The trunk continues to forward bend, being controlled by the extensor muscles of the spine, until approximately 45 degrees, at which point the posterior ligaments become taut and the facets of the zygapophyseal joints approximate. Once all of the vertebral segments are at the end of the range and stabilized by the posterior ligaments and facets, the pelvis begins to rotate forward (anterior pelvic tilt), being controlled eccentrically by the gluteus maximus and hamstring muscles. The pelvis continues to anteriorly rotate until the full length of the muscles is reached. The return to the upright position begins with the hip extensor muscles rotating the pelvis posteriorly through reverse muscle action, then the back extensor muscles extending the spine from the lumbar region upward. An assessment of the lumbopelvic rhythm can alert the clinician to the primary area of a particular limitation. During normal forward bending, the patient should be able to touch his or her toes without bending the knees and with a flattening of the lordosis. However, if the hamstrings are adaptively shortened, toe touching cannot be accomplished even with a flattening of the lordosis. If the tightness is located in the low back, as the patient bends forward, no flattening of the lordosis occurs, and the patient is unable to touch the toes even with good hamstring flexibility.

Collum/Inclination Angle

The frontal plane angle between the femoral shaft and the neck is called the collum/inclination angle. This angle is approximately 125 degrees (Figure 19-2),[8] but can vary with body types. The collum angle has an important influence on the hips. In a tall person the collum angle is larger; the opposite is true with a shorter individual. An increase in the collum angle causes the femoral head to be directed more superiorly in the acetabulum, and is known as coxa valga. Coxa valga has the following effects at the hip joint:

- It changes the orientation of the joint reaction force from the normal vertical direction to one that is almost parallel to the femoral shaft.[24,25] This lateral displacement of the joint reaction force reduces the weight-bearing surface, resulting in an increase in stress applied across joint surfaces not specialized to sustain such loads.
- It shortens the moment arm of the hip abductors, placing them in a position of mechanical disadvantage.[25] This causes the abductors to contract more vigorously to stabilize the pelvis, producing an increase in the joint reaction force.[19]
- It increases the overall length of the lower extremity, affecting other components in the kinetic chain (genu varum).

If the collum angle is reduced, it is known as coxa vara. The mechanical effects of coxa vara are,

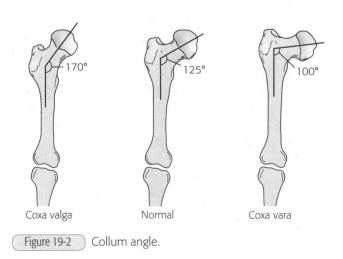

Figure 19-2 Collum angle.

for the most part, the opposite of those found in coxa valga:[26]

- It changes the orientation of the joint reaction force. The more horizontal position of the proximal femoral physis increases not only the resultant shear force component of the hip articulation, but also the net medial compressive force on the metaphyseal bone of the femoral neck.
- It lengthens the movement arm of the hip abductors, placing them in a position of mechanical disadvantage.[25]
- It decreases the overall length of the lower extremity, affecting other components in the kinetic chain (genu valgum).

Anteversion/Retroversion

Femoral alignment in the transverse plane also influences the mechanics of the hip joint.

> ● **Key Point** Version is the normal angular difference between the transverse axis of each end of a long bone. The terms *femoral anteversion* and *femoral retroversion* refer to the relationship between the neck of the femur and the femoral shaft, ending in the femoral condyles, that dictates the position of the femoral head when the knee is pointing straight ahead.

Anteversion (Figure 19-3) is defined as the anterior position of the axis through the femoral condyles.[27,28] Retroversion is defined as a femoral neck axis that is parallel or posterior to the condylar axis.[19] The normal range for femoral alignment in the transverse plane in adults is 15 degrees of anteversion.[28,29]

Excessive anteversion directs the femoral head toward the anterior aspect of the acetabulum when the femoral condyles are aligned in their normal orientation, producing a relatively shorter leg. Subjects with excessive anteversion usually have more hip internal rotation range of motion than external rotation, and they gravitate to the typical "frog-sitting" (W-sitting) posture as a position of comfort. There is also associated genu valgum and in-toeing while weight bearing.[19]

Excessive retroversion directs the femoral head toward the posterior aspect of the acetabulum when the femoral condyles are aligned in their normal orientation, producing a relatively longer leg. Subjects with excessive anteversion usually have more hip external rotation range of motion than internal rotation. There is also associated out-toeing while weight bearing.[19]

Examination

Given that the hip region is also a common source of symptom referral from other regions, the physical therapists' examination of the hip rarely occurs in isolation, and almost always involves an assessment of the lumbar spine, pelvis, and knee joint complex. The physical therapist's examination of the hip typically follows the outline in **Table 19-3**. The evidence-based special tests of the hip are outlined in **Table 19-4**.

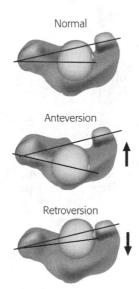

Normal

Anteversion

Retroversion

Figure 19-3) Femoral version.

TABLE 19-3	**Examination of the Hip Joint**

I. History.
II. Observation and inspection.
III. Upper quarter scan as appropriate.
IV. Examination of movements. Active range of motion with passive overpressure of the following movements:
   a. Hip flexion, extension, abduction, adduction, internal rotation, and external rotation
   b. Knee flexion and extension
V. Resisted isometric movements:
   a. Hip flexion, extension, abduction, adduction, internal rotation, and external rotation
   b. Knee flexion and extension
VI. Palpation.
VII. Neurological tests as appropriate (reflexes, sensory scan, peripheral nerve assessment).
VIII. Joint mobility tests:
   a. Lateral distraction
   b. Quadrant (scour) test
IX. Special tests (refer to Table 19-4).
X. Diagnostic imaging.

TABLE
19-4

Evidence-Based Special Tests of the Hip Joint Complex

Name of Test	Brief Description	Positive Findings	Evidence-Based.
Internal rotation-flexion-axial compression maneuver[a]	Patient is supine. Clinician flexes and internally rotates the hip, then applies an axial compression force through the femur.	Provocation of pain is considered positive for acetabular labrum tear.	Sensitivity: 0.75 Specificity: 0.43
Thomas test (acetabular labrum tear)[a]	Patient is supine. Clinician extends involved extremity from the flexed position.	Provocation of pain is considered positive for acetabular labrum tear.	Sensitivity: 0.25 Specificity: not provided
Flexion-adduction test[b]	Patient is supine with hip flexed to 90 degrees and in neutral rotation. The hip is then allowed to adduct.	Provocation of pain is considered positive for hip disease.	Demonstrated that the test possessed diagnostic utility (sensitivity) for detecting the involved extremity but should not be used in isolation
Positive Trendelenburg test[c]	The patient is standing. The patient lifts one foot off the ground at a time.	Positive if the patient is unable to elevate his or her pelvis on the nonstance side and hold the position for at least 30 seconds.	Sensitivity: 0.23 Specificity: 0.94
Patrick's test[d] (FABER, figure-4 test)	With the patient supine, the clinician flexes, abducts, and externally rotates the involved hip so the lateral ankle is placed just proximal to the contralateral knee. While stabilizing the anterior superior iliac spine, the involved leg is lowered toward the table to end range.	Positive for hip dysfunction if it reproduces the patient's symptoms.	Sensitivity: 0.60 Specificity: 0.18
Scour test[e]	With the patient supine, the clinician passively flexes the symptomatic hip to 90 degrees and then moves the knee toward the opposite shoulder and applies an axial load to the femur.	Positive test if it causes lateral hip pain or groin pain.	Sensitivity: 0.62 Specificity: 0.75
Patellar pubic percussion test[f]	With the patient supine, the clinician percusses (taps) one patella at a time while auscultating the pubic symphysis with a stethoscope.	A positive test for suspected hip fracture is a diminution of the percussion note on the involved side.	Sensitivity: 0.94 Specificity: 0.96

Data from (a) Narvani AA, Tsiridis E, Kendall S, et al: A preliminary report on prevalence of acetabular labrum tears in sports patients with groin pain. Knee Surg Sports Traumatol Arthrosc 11:403–408, 2003; (b) Woods D, Macnicol M: The flexion-adduction test: An early sign of hip disease. J Pediatr Orthop B 10:180–185, 2001; (c) Woodley SJ, Nicholson HD, Livingstone V, et al: Lateral hip pain: Findings from magnetic resonance imaging and clinical examination. J Orthop Sports Phys Ther 38:313–328, 2008; (d) Martin RL, Irrgang JJ, Sekiya JK: The diagnostic accuracy of a clinical examination in determining intra-articular hip pain for potential hip arthroscopy candidates. Arthroscopy 24:1013–1018, 2008; (e) Sutlive TG, Lopez HP, Schnitker DE, et al: Development of a clinical prediction rule for diagnosing hip osteoarthritis in individuals with unilateral hip pain. J Orthop Sports Phys Ther 38:542–550, 2008; and (f) Adams SL, Yarnold PR: Clinical use of the patellar-pubic percussion sign in hip trauma. Am J Emerg Med 15:173–175, 1997

General Intervention Strategies

The hip joint and surrounding tissues are prone to soft tissue injuries, impingement syndromes, muscle imbalances of strength and flexibility, and joint dysfunctions. These are also an area of symptom referral from other regions. The intervention of the hip joint must take into account the influences that the lumbar spine, pelvis, and lower extremities can have on this area. It is imperative that the clinician views the hip as part of a kinetic chain extending from the foot to the lumbar spine. A dysfunction in any part of this kinetic chain can have either a direct or an indirect effect on hip function and symptoms.

Acute Phase

The goals of the acute phase include:

- *Protection of the injury site and promotion of healing:* The promotion and progression of healing may involve decreasing the weight-bearing function of the hip through rest and modification of activity, or by using an assistive device. Assistive devices such as crutches or canes may be necessary to offset the load through the hip joint and promote a symmetric gait pattern.[21,30] Some patients may need to use a walker for maximum functional ambulation and safety.[21]
- *Promotion of pain-free ROM in the entire kinetic chain:* According to patient tolerance, the PT may attempt to remove any other stresses to the hip joint, such as joint restrictions in the lumbar spine or sacroiliac joint, by using joint mobilizations.
- *Improvement of patient comfort by decreasing pain and inflammation:* During the acute phase, the principles of PRICEMEM (protection, rest, ice, compression, elevation, manual therapy, early motion, and medication) are applied as appropriate. Elevation of the hip joint is usually not applicable or possible.
- *Maintaining general fitness:* Cardiovascular fitness can be maintained during this phase using an upper body ergonometer. If tolerated, a stationary bicycle can be used.
- *Retardation of muscle atrophy and minimization of detrimental effects of immobilization and activity restriction:*[31–36] The approach during this phase may depend on the specific tissue involved:
  - ❑ Contractile tissue lesions are treated with rest, gentle friction massage, gentle isometric exercises, pain-free range-of-motion exercises, and appropriate modalities.
  - ❑ Articular lesions are best treated with positioning in the open-packed position (flexion, abduction, and external rotation) and grades I and II joint mobilizations.

Functional Phase

The patient progresses to the functional stage once there is no pain and when the ROM is equal to that of the uninvolved limb. The goals of the functional phase include:

- *Attaining full range of pain-free motion and restoring normal joint kinematics:* A progressive stretching program is initiated for those muscles that are prone to adaptive shortening. These include the hip flexors (Figure 19-4 and Figure 19-5) and rectus femoris (Figure 19-6),

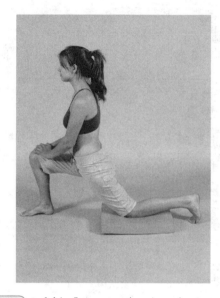

Figure 19-4 Left hip flexor stretch using a lunge.

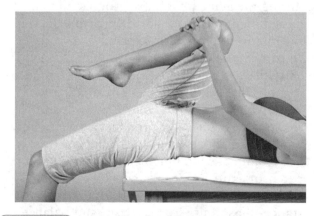

Figure 19-5 Left hip flexor stretch in supine.

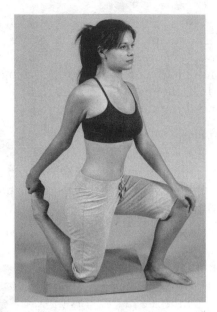

Figure 19-6 Right hip flexor and rectus femoris stretch.

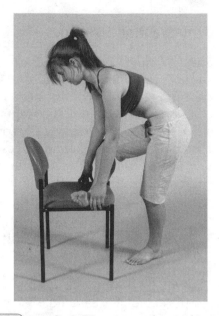

Figure 19-8 Standing piriformis stretch on right.

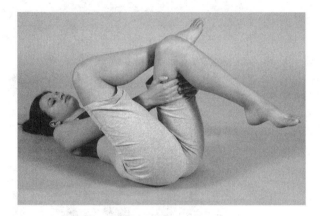

Figure 19-7 Supine piriformis stretch on right.

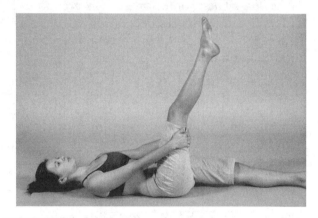

Figure 19-9 Supine hamstring stretch.

piriformis (Figure 19-7 and Figure 19-8), hamstrings (Figure 19-9 and Figure 19-10), and TFL and ITB (Figure 19-11). Self-stretching is taught to the patient. The AROM exercises, initiated during the acute phase, are progressed until the patient demonstrates that they have achieved the maximum range anticipated.

- *Improving neuromuscular control:* These activities are usually performed in weight bearing, provided there are no contraindications (pain or instability) to weight bearing and resistance.[21] Wherever possible, active exercises are performed within a functional context. For example, simultaneous contraction of hip extensors and abductors in weight bearing is the normal co-activation pattern used in early stance-phase gait.[21,37] Exercises and balance training in standing can be used to reinforce

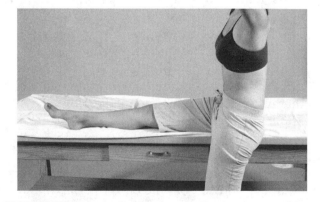

Figure 19-10 Standing hamstring stretch.

this pattern. Initially, the balance exercises are performed with double limb support and then progressed to single leg support.

- *Restoration of normal gait mechanics as appropriate:* Once the static weight-bearing exercises

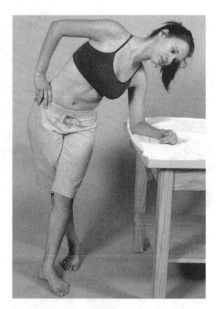

Figure 19-11   Right ITB and TFL stretch.

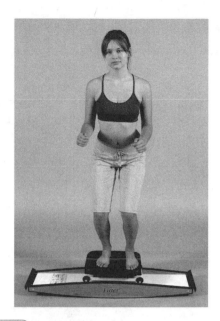

Figure 19-12   Weight shifting.

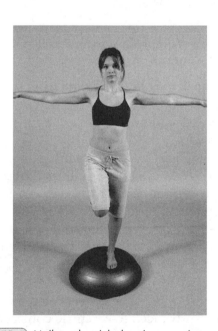

Figure 19-13   Unilateral weight-bearing exercise.

in double limb support can be performed, gait activities are introduced. Gait involves the integration of the entire lower kinetic chain. Dysfunctions of gait (see Chapter 25) are typically related to biomechanical alterations occurring during the swing and/or stance phases of gait.[21] Such dysfunctions include pain on weight bearing or movement, joint range restrictions, functional muscle weakness, leg length discrepancy, or deformity.[21] Gait-training procedures[38,39] for the stance phase involve the use of manual contacts at the pelvis to guide and stretch and to apply joint approximation or resistance. These exercises promote the development of appropriate patterns of neuromuscular control. Variable surfaces can be used for weight-shift practice (Figure 19-12). Unilateral stance activities may also be performed (Figure 19-13) and (Figure 19-14).

The essential components of normal swing-phase gait[37,39] to develop are:

- Forward rotation of the pelvis on swing-phase flexion of the hip
- Pelvic dip (drop) of approximately 5 degrees on the side of the swing limb
- Flexion of the hip to a maximum of 30 degrees (activation of hip flexors) with kinematic knee flexion and dorsiflexion

Active hip flexion with adduction, knee flexion, and dorsiflexion in standing simulates the normal swing phase of gait and promotes balance control in weight bearing on the contralateral stance leg.[21] Neuromuscular re-education exercises for the hip are prescribed to emphasize specific movement patterns and sequencing of muscle contractions. These exercises demand a high level of control and coordination.[40–43] Ambulation activities can be used initially, progressing to more difficult unilateral extremity exercises.

One can improve muscle strength to within normal limits and restore normal muscle force couple

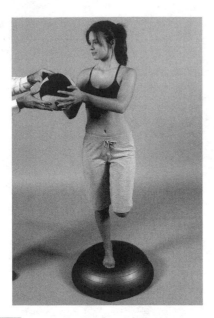

Figure 19-14 Unilateral weight-bearing exercise.

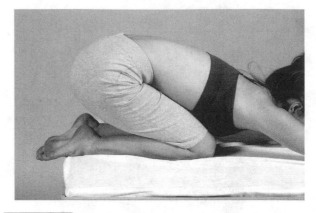

Figure 19-15 Quadruped exercise with backward rocking.

relationships. The following exercises are recommended during this phase:

- Quadruped exercises incorporating rocking forward and backward (Figure 19-15) help to stretch the joint capsule and apply joint compression.
- Lunging (Figure 19-16), squatting (Figure 19-17), and hip straddles (Figure 19-18) simulate weight bearing while increasing ROM and stretching the capsule.
- Open-chain exercises using cuff weights or tubing may be used to develop strength and endurance of all of the hip musculature (Figure 19-19 through Figure 19-24). The exercises are initially performed using concentric contractions and then advanced to eccentric contractions.
- Bridging utilizes body weight as a resistance force to the hip extensors and abductors.[21] A variety of bridging exercises exist, from the traditional (where the patient lies supine with the hips and knees flexed and the feet resting on the table and then raises the trunk until it is parallel with the thighs) (Figure 19-25) to the more difficult unilateral bridging exercises (Figure 19-26). Manually applied resistance can be superimposed on the pelvis or thighs to generate maximal muscular tension in the contracting muscles.
- Strengthening of the gluteus medius muscle is often an important component of the hip

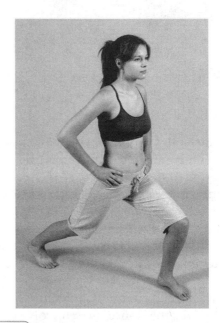

Figure 19-16 Lunge.

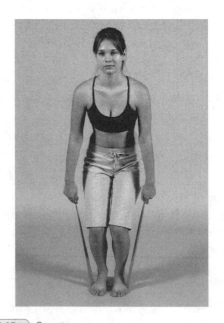

Figure 19-17 Squat.

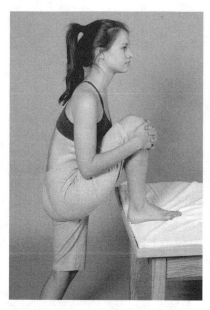

Figure 19-18   Straddle.

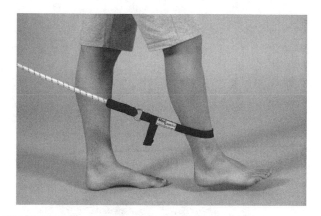

Figure 19-21   Resisted hip flexion.

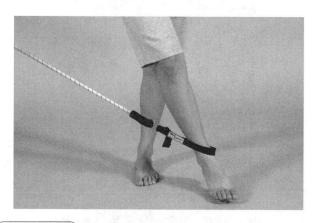

Figure 19-19   Resisted hip adduction.

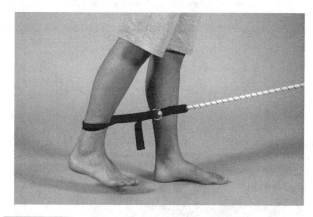

Figure 19-22   Resisted hip extension.

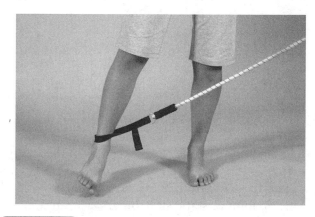

Figure 19-20   Resisted hip abduction.

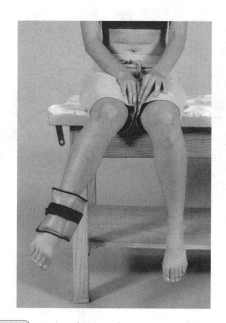

Figure 19-23   Resisted internal rotation in sitting.

General Intervention Strategies   **491**

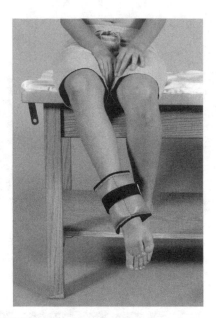

Figure 19-24   Resisted external rotation in sitting.

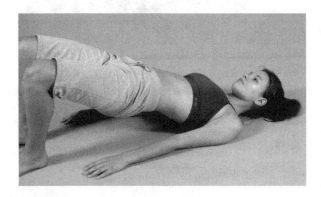

Figure 19-25   Bridging.

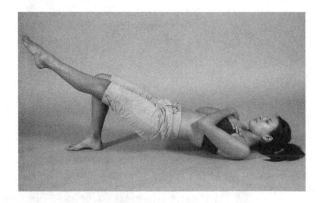

Figure 19-26   Unilateral bridging.

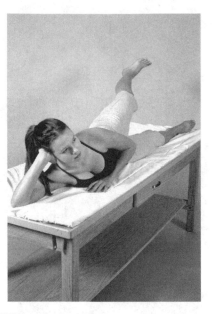

Figure 19-27   Gluteus medius strengthening.

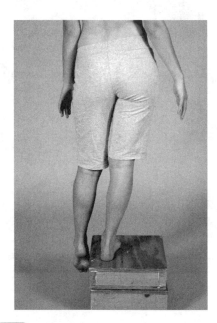

Figure 19-28   Pelvic drop exercise for right gluteus medius.

rehabilitation program. The gluteus medius can be strengthened in side lying, with the upper leg in slight hip extension and external rotation (Figure 19-27), or in standing with the pelvic drop exercise (Figure 19-28). The pelvic drop exercise involves standing on a step with the involved leg and lowering the uninvolved leg off the step while keeping both knees locked.

- The stationary bicycle is used to increase lower extremity strength, endurance, and range during repetitive reciprocal movements of the lower extremities.[21] Stationary bicycling also has been found to be as effective for increasing ROM at the hip joint as static stretching.[44] The stationary bicycle is a convenient mode of exercise for home use; however, the use of vigorous protocols should be carefully monitored for cardiac effects, especially in light of the fact that both blood pressure and heart rates have been found to increase markedly during this type of exercise.[21,45]

- Pool walking, swimming, and kicking also may be incorporated.

A multihip machine can be introduced as the hip muscles become stronger. Likewise, task-oriented exercise programs (work hardening) should be instituted for the patient who intends to resume a type of employment that requires a predetermined level of work performance.

Common Conditions

The common conditions that can affect the hip joint complex include those that relate to poor biomechanics due to weakness or adaptive shortening, trauma, repetitive activities, or overuse.

Hip Flexion Contracture

A hip flexion contracture is a limitation of passive hip extension caused by a lack of extensibility of the muscles or ligaments of the hip. Whether mild or severe, hip flexion contractures are relatively common impairments in persons with compromised mobility, particularly those who spend a great deal of time sitting or in an otherwise hip-flexed position. A hip-flexed position produces a relative anterior pelvic tilt. Over time, a slackened ligament or muscle will adapt to its shortened position and eventually remain shortened, and the long-term effects of the hip flexion contracture can destabilize the hip and have a negative impact on the lumbar spine and the lower kinetic chain. For example, when a person with a hip flexion contracture attempts to stand upright, the line of gravity shifts anterior to the medial lateral axis of rotation, which in turn disables the passive standing mechanism, and results in the need for continuous activation of the hip and back extensor muscles to maintain an upright position. In addition, the compression forces from weight bearing are directed to regions of the hip that are not anatomically designed to dissipate these large forces, creating increased wear and tear on the joint. In an attempt to maintain an upright posture, one of three mechanisms can occur:

- The lower spine must compensate through overextension, resulting in increased lordosis of the lumbar spine, adaptive shortening of the

low back extensor muscles, and an increase in the wear and tear on the lumbar facet joints.
- The trunk must flex. Instead of increasing the lordosis, the patient adopts a stooped position (round back).
- The knee joint must flex. When the knees are slightly flexed, the compensation at the lumbar spine is less noticeable.

In addition to disturbing posture, hip flexion contractures can have an adverse effect on gait. If the contracture is severe enough, the patient can adopt a knee-flexed, ankle-plantarflexed, and trunk-flexed gait, in which velocity is slowed and high energy costs are imposed.

Intervention

The intervention is based on the severity. If the physician determines that the contracture is amenable to physical therapy, a progressive stretching program is initiated, emphasizing a low load prolonged stretch. Almost all hip flexion contractures include the rectus femoris, sartorius, tensor fascia latae (iliotibial band), and the soft tissues of the anterior compartment of the hip. Of these, the tensor fascia latae, the rectus femoris, and the sartorius muscles are the joint muscles particularly responsible for the hip flexion contracture. Prevention is the key and can include:

- Prone lying, placing the hips in a neutral or extended position
- Strengthening of the hip extensors to move the hip out of the flexed position into extension and to shift the muscular strength bias of the hip toward extension
- Patient education: encourage standing versus sitting, lying flat, and avoidance of sleeping with pillows under the knees
- Regular stretching of the hip flexors through a home exercise program

Osteoarthritis

Osteoarthritis (OA) is defined as focal loss of articular cartilage with variable subchondral bone reaction. The prevalence of hip OA ranges from 7 to 25 percent in adults age 55 years or older in the white European population.[46] The two clinical sequelae of OA that are most relevant to epidemiological studies are joint pain and functional impairment. The start of symptomatic hip OA is usually insidious, although in a few cases pain starts abruptly. Individual risk factors, which may be associated with a generalized susceptibility to the disorder, include obesity, a family history, and hypermobility.[47] The pain may be felt in the area of the buttock, groin, thigh, or knee and varies in character from a dull ache to sharp stabbing pains. The discomfort is generally related to activity, and exercise may induce bouts of pain that last for several hours.[48] As the disease process progresses, the patient begins to have difficulty climbing stairs with the involved leg and may have difficulty putting on socks or stockings.[49] In advanced disease, a decline in the participation of even mild recreational activities occurs and the patient may complain of severe pain that is present at night or during rest. Stiffness of the hip is usual, particularly after inactivity, and can be the presenting feature.

Conservative Approach

Systematic reviews have concluded that exercise reduces pain and disability in patients with hip OA. Weigl et al.[50] showed that strengthening exercises, flexibility, relaxation, and endurance training decreased pain and improved physical function in patients with osteoarthritis.[51] In addition, van Baar and colleagues[52] showed that exercise improved function and reduced pain in patients with hip osteoarthritis, but later found that the beneficial effect of exercise declined over time.[51,53] Based on the above research, the intervention goals for hip OA include relieving symptoms, minimizing disability and handicap, and reducing the risk of disease progression.[48] Interventions in the earlier stages include:

- *Education and empowerment:* Giving advice about what patients can do for themselves is of immense value.
  - ❑ Joint protection strategies, including assistive devices for ambulation and modifying chairs and toilet seats to provide an elevated surface. A simple cane can reduce loading on a hip by 20–30 percent. In most cases, it will be most beneficial if the cane is held on the unaffected side of the body.[48] Many people with arthritis of the spine or legs are more comfortable wearing athletic shoes or other shoes with good shock-absorbing properties than they are in regular footwear. Shock-absorbing insoles, which are available in sports and shoe shops, may be helpful.[48]
  - ❑ Activities to avoid, including those activities associated with high stress through the hip joint (kneeling, squatting). Contact sports and activities such as jogging, which can cause repetitive high impact loading of the hip, are probably best avoided.[54] Patients

need to learn an appropriate balance, and intersperse periods of activity with rest.
  - ❑ Promotion of a healthy lifestyle (e.g., weight reduction). Although there is no evidence for the involvement of any dietary factor in the etiopathogenesis of hip OA,[48] it is possible that obesity may accelerate progression or cause more pain. A reduction in weight can significantly improve a patient's symptoms, increase mobility, and improve health status.[55]
- *Modalities for muscle relaxation, pain relief, and anti-inflammation.* Depending on the cause, a variety of modalities can be employed. Thermotherapy is typically used to enhance muscle relaxation and decrease chronic pain whereas acute pain and inflammation responds better to crytpherapy.
- *Modification of activities of daily living and self-care.* This is one of the most important components. Patients are often frightened that use will "wear out" a damaged hip joint and need "permission" to use it.[48] Evidence suggests that although the affected joint will benefit from regular loading to help maintain its integrity, prolonged or heavy activity may cause further damage.[54]
- *Maintaining full range of hip movement, if possible.* In addition to specific frequent exercises for hip ROM, recreations such as swimming or cycling may help. Aquatic therapy can be particularly beneficial for this group of patients.

The patient should be advised to engage in adequate warm-ups before exercising and to pay attention to and respect the limitations of their body and not exercise if in discomfort.

Other measures include the following:

- Manual techniques to mobilize the joint and passive stretches of the capsule, particularly distractive techniques, are helpful to maintain mobility.[56] Following these distractions, a fairly vigorous stretching program into flexion, abduction, and external rotation should be initiated. The FABER position, or cross-legged sitting, is ideal for this, and patients should be encouraged to adopt this position regularly.
- Strengthening exercises are performed for the trunk stabilizers and the major muscle groups of the hip region, especially the gluteus medius.

Medical Intervention

The medical intervention for OA includes:

- Nonsteroidal anti-inflammatory drugs (NSAIDs)
- Corticosteroid injections
- Topical analgesics
- Surgical joint replacement (total hip arthroplasty and hemiarthroplasty are described later in the chapter)

Muscle Strains

Muscle strains at the hip can occur insidiously or be incurred traumatically. First- and second-degree muscle strains are frequent injuries.[21] The adductors, iliopsoas, rectus abdominis, gluteus medius, and hamstring muscles are commonly involved.

Adductors

The hip adductor muscles, including the gracilis; pectineus; and adductor longus, brevis, and magnus, are the most frequent cause of groin region pain, with the adductor longus being the most commonly injured.[16,57] There are a number of causative factors for an adductor strain, including a muscular imbalance of the combined action of the muscles stabilizing the hip joint resulting from fatigue or an abduction overload.[58] Adductor strains are associated with jumping, running, and twisting activities, particularly when external rotation of the affected leg is an added component of the activity.[59] Soccer players involved with forceful kicking that is stopped by an opponent's foot or by a sliding tackle with an abducted leg are particularly vulnerable to an adductor strain. In fact, the incidence of groin pain among male soccer players is 10–18 percent per year.[60-62] The signs and symptoms of an adductor strain are easily recognizable:[63]

- Twinging or stabbing pain in the groin area with quick starts and stops
- Edema or ecchymosis several days postinjury
- Pain with passive abduction or manual resistance to hip adduction when tested in different degrees of hip flexion (0 degrees [gracilis], 45 degrees [adductor longus and brevis], and 90 degrees [if combined with adduction, pectineus])
- Possibly a palpable defect in severe ruptures
- Muscle guarding

Intervention

Conservative intervention involves the principles of PRICEMEM in the acute stage. This is followed by heat applications, hip adductor isometrics, and gentle stretching during the subacute stage, progressing to a graded resistive program, including concentric and eccentric exercises, PNF diagonal motions to promote balance, strength, and flexibility around the joint, and then a gradual return to full activity. In addition, the clinician should examine the patient's technique in the required activity, because poor technique can overload and fatigue the adductors.

Iliopsoas

As the strongest flexor of the hip, the iliopsoas is one of the more frequently strained muscles of this region.[64] The mechanism of injury is forced extension of the hip while it is being actively flexed. Clinical findings include:

- Complaints of pain with attempts at acceleration and high-stepping activities
- Increased pain with resisted flexion, adduction, and external rotation[65]

Intervention

Conservative intervention involves rest and ice during the acute phase, progressing to prone lying, heat, a graded resistive exercise program, and specific instructions on proper warm-up and cool-down. Recovery from this condition can be lengthy, and recurrences are frequent.

Quadriceps

Strains of the quadriceps most commonly involve the rectus femoris and occur during sports involving sprinting, jumping, or kicking. Typically, the patient complains of local pain and tenderness in the anterior thigh, which may be gradual in onset or experienced suddenly during an explosive muscle contraction. Grade I strains result in pain with resisted active contraction and with passive stretching. Grade II strains cause significant pain with passive and unopposed active stretching. Complete tears of the rectus femoris are rare and are usually associated with a palpable defect when the muscle is contracted.

Intervention

During the initial period following injury, the principles of PRICEMEM are applied. Pain-free stretching and soft tissue mobilization are instituted early to preserve ROM. Straight-leg raises are initiated in the supine position and are progressed to long sitting. Short arc quad sets in pain-free ranges are expanded to full range as tolerated. Closed-kinetic-chain exercises at submaximal weight are initiated in short arcs and progressed to full range. Both concentric and eccentric exercises are performed. Attention must be given to hip flexor and hamstring strength and flexibility to ensure correct muscular balance.

Hamstrings

The hamstrings are the most commonly strained muscles of the hip, especially in running sports.[59] A hamstring tear is typically partial and commonly takes place during the eccentric phase of muscle usage, when the muscle develops tension while lengthening. Most strain injuries of a muscle/tendon occur near the musculotendinous junction. The most commonly injured hamstring muscle is the biceps femoris. Strain is most likely to occur in the hamstrings during two stages of the running cycle: late forward swing and takeoff (toe-off).[21,66,67] A hamstring strain has a varied list of potential causes, including:[68]

- *A prior hamstring injury:* There is a strong correlation between a history of prior hamstring injury and recurrence. This is likely due to the fact that the initial injury results in a loss of extensibility and a loss of eccentric strength.
- *Lumbar degenerative joint disease:* Lumbar (LB) pain and injury result in restricted ROM and decreased hamstring extensibility. In addition, LB pain has been shown to decrease proprioception and neuromuscular control of the lower extremities. It is presumed that muscles and tendons are more susceptible to injury as they age, but it is not clear why injuries to soft tissues with an L5 and S1 nerve supply have such a strong correlation with advancing age, whereas there is little or no correlation between age and the soft tissue injuries with an L2–L4 nerve supply. Anecdotally, it would appear that the lumbar nerve roots of L5 and S1, which supply the hamstring and calf muscles, are more likely to be affected by age-related spinal degeneration than the nerve supply of the quadriceps muscles (L2, L3, and L4).[69]
- *Biomechanical inadequacies:* This can include excessive anterior pelvic tilt, leg length inequality, and anatomical arrangement:
  - *Anterior pelvic tilt:* A common finding is anterior tilt of the innominate bone on the injured side that increases tension in the hamstrings and causes a lengthened position of their origin and insertion. This altered pelvic position also can contribute to decreased hamstring strength.

  - *Leg length inequality:* The shorter leg can develop overly tight hamstrings.
  - *Anatomical arrangement:* One factor that makes hamstring muscles so susceptible to injury is their anatomical arrangement. Being a biarticular muscle group means they are more susceptible to adaptive shortening[70] and can also be subjected to large length changes during certain activities. During everyday movements, such as walking, squatting, and sitting, flexion of the hip and knee occur together, with opposing effects on hamstring length. However, in running and kicking, in particular, the knee is extended and the hip flexed, bringing hamstrings to long lengths where risk of muscle tears becomes significant. Antagonists to prime movers, muscles that are used to control or resist motion, are also at a greater risk of injury than the prime movers themselves. While decelerating the body, these muscles will contract while being rapidly lengthened (eccentric contraction).
- *Poor posture:* Adaptive shortening of the hip flexors and the erector spinae, weak/inhibited gluteal and abdominal muscles, an increased anterior pelvic tilt, and a hyperlordosis of the spine all place the hamstrings in a more lengthened resting position.
- *Muscle imbalance:* Muscle balance is a term used to describe either:
  - The relationship between agonist and antagonist muscle groups. The hamstrings are directly antagonistic to the quadriceps during the first 160–165 degrees of leg extension but assume a paradoxical extensor action concurrent with foot strike.
  - The relationship of agonist muscle groups between limbs (inhibited gluteus maximus).
  - Eccentric to concentric muscle ratios.
  - Hamstring to trunk stabilizer ratios.
- *Decreased flexibility:* This has long been cited as the primary cause of hamstring injuries, although there is little to no evidence to support this theory. A differentiation must be made between active flexibility (the absolute range of movement in a joint or series of joints that is attainable in a momentary effort with the help of a partner or a piece of equipment) and passive flexibility (the ability to assume and maintain extended positions using only the tension of the agonists and synergists,

while the antagonists are being stretched). Research has shown that active flexibility, which requires a combination of passive flexibility and muscle strength, is more closely related to the level of sports achievement than is passive flexibility.

- *Hamstring strength:* The overall relationship between strength and the risk of hamstring injuries is not made clear by reviewing the studies available. More recently, it has been suggested that poor eccentric strength in the hamstring muscle group might be a causative factor in hamstring strains.
- *Fatigue:* An exhausted muscle from overtraining or overexertion is easily damaged. In a study of professional soccer players, nearly half (47 percent) of the hamstring injuries sustained during matches occurred during the last third of the first and second halves of the match.

It is likely that a combination of the aforementioned factors plays a role in hamstring injuries. Some of these factors are modifiable; others are not. The modifiable factors include muscle imbalances between flexibility and strength, overall conditioning, and playing surface.

Clinical findings associated with hamstring injury include:

- Patient reports a distinctive mechanism of injury with immediate pain during full stride running or while decelerating quickly.[65] In acute cases, the patient may report a "pop" or a tearing sensation.
- Tenderness is reported with passive stretching of the hamstrings.
- Posterior thigh pain, often approximately near the buttock, is reported, which is worsened with resisted knee flexion.
- Tenderness to palpation is present. It is generally located at the muscle origin at the ischial tuberosity but may also be present in the muscle belly and distal insertions.

With grade I strains, gait appears normal and there is only pain with extreme range of a straight-leg raise. A patient with a grade II strain normally ambulates with an antalgic gait or may ambulate with a flexed knee. Resisted knee flexion and hip extension are both painful and weak. A grade III strain usually requires the use of crutches for ambulation. In severe cases, ecchymosis, hemorrhage, and a muscle defect may be visible several days postinjury.[65]

Intervention

Patients with a grade I strain may continue activities as much as possible. A grade II strain typically requires 5–21 days for rehabilitation, whereas a patient with a grade III strain might require 3–12 weeks of rehabilitation. Muscle imbalances of strength and flexibility must be addressed, and proper techniques to stretch and strengthen the hamstrings should be taught. Special emphasis should be placed on eccentric loading. Where possible the biomechanical factors, including excessive anterior tilt of the pelvis, lumbar spine and sacroiliac joint dysfunction, and leg length discrepancies, should be corrected. Because there is a great deal of variability in the rehabilitation time, anywhere from 2–3 weeks to 2–6 months, an athlete should not be permitted to return to full participation in sports until flexibility and strength ratios have been restored, and plyometric and functional exercises are able to be performed pain free.[65,68]

Iliotibial Band Friction Syndrome

As its name suggests, iliotibial band friction syndrome (ITBFS) is a repetitive stress injury that results from friction of the iliotibial band as it slides over the prominent lateral femoral condyle at approximately 30 degrees of knee flexion[71] (Figure 19-29). The friction has been found to occur at the posterior edge of the band, which is felt to be tighter against the lateral femoral condyle than the anterior fibers.[71,72] The friction causes a gradual development

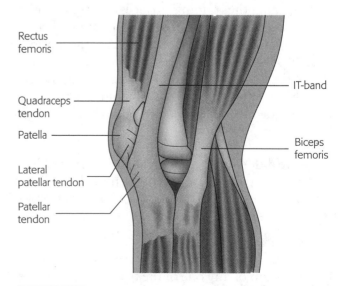

Figure 19-29 Iliotibial band friction syndrome.

Rectus femoris
Quadraceps tendon
Patella
Lateral patellar tendon
Patellar tendon
IT-band
Biceps femoris

of a reddish-brown bursal thickening at the lateral femoral condyle. ITBFS is particularly common in long-distance runners (20–40 miles/week) and in cyclists.[73–75] To control coronal plane movement during stance phase, the gluteus medius and TFL must exert a continuous hip abductor movement. Fatigued runners or those with weak gluteus medius muscles are prone to increased thigh adduction and internal rotation at midstance. This, in turn, leads to an increased valgus vector at the knee and increased tension on the iliotibial band, making it more prone to impingement.[76]

Subjectively, the patient reports pain with repetitive motions of the knee. There is rarely a history of trauma. Although walking on level surfaces does not generally reproduce symptoms, especially if a stiff-legged gait is used,[72,77] climbing or descending stairs often aggravates the pain.[78] Patients do not usually complain of pain during sprinting, squatting, or during such stop-and-go activities as tennis, racquetball, or squash.[72] The progression of symptoms is often associated with changes in training surfaces, increased mileage, or training on crowned roads. The lateral knee pain is described as diffuse and hard to localize.

Objectively, there is localized tenderness to palpation at the lateral femoral condyle or Gerdy's tubercle on the anterolateral portion of the proximal tibia. The resisted tests are likely to be negative for pain.

Intervention

Conservative intervention for ITBFS consists of activity modification to reduce the irritating stress (decreasing mileage, changing the bike seat position, and changing the training surfaces), using new running shoes,[79] heat or ice applications, strengthening of the hip abductors, and stretching of the iliotibial band.[80] Surgical intervention, consisting of a resection of the posterior half of the iliotibial band at the level that passes over the lateral femoral condyle, is reserved for the more recalcitrant cases.[75]

Bursitis

There are different types of hip bursitis. Types include trochanteric (pain on the side of the hip), iliopectineal bursitis (pain in the groin), and ischial/gluteal bursitis (pain at the base of the hips/buttocks).

Trochanteric

Trochanteric bursitis is the collective name given to inflammation of any one of the trochanteric bursae. The bursae become inflamed through either friction (compression and friction of the bursa from an adaptively shortened TFL) or direct trauma, such as a fall on the side of the hip.

Intervention

There is very little research evidence on physical therapy intervention for trochanteric bursitis.[81] The intervention usually consists of the removal of the causative factors by stretching the soft tissues of the lateral thigh, especially the TFL and ITB, and focusing on the flexibility of the external rotators, quadriceps, and hip flexors. Strengthening of the hip abductors and establishment of muscular balance between the adductors and abductors is also important. Other interventions include heat and ultrasound. Transverse frictional massage (TFM) has also been advocated.[82] Orthotics may be prescribed if there is a biomechanical fault in the kinetic chain due to an ankle/foot dysfunction.

Iliopectineal

The iliopectineal bursa is located between the anterior side of the joint capsule of the hip and the musculotendinous junction of the iliopsoas. Major causes of iliopsoas tendinitis are acute trauma and overuse resulting from repetitive hip flexion. The usual complaint is one of anterior hip or groin pain, which is aggravated by lumbar or hip hyperextension or power walking.

Intervention

Conservative intervention consists of a stretching and strengthening program of the hip rotators and hip flexors. The following protocol is recommended:[83]

- Seated hip internal and external resisted exercises using elastic resistance
- Side-lying abduction/external rotation resisted exercises using elastic resistance
- Mini-squats, weight bearing on the affected leg
- Stretching of the hip flexor, quadriceps, lateral hip/piriformis, and hamstring muscles

Ischial/Gluteal

An ischial bursitis (Weaver's bottom) involves two different bursae, one between the ischial tuberosity and the inferior part of the gluteus maximus belly, and the other between the tendons of the biceps femoris and semimembranosus. Inflammation of these bursae usually results from chronic compression or direct trauma. With ischial bursitis, the patient typically reports pain with sitting in a firm chair, almost as soon as the buttocks touch the chair.

Ischial bursitis tends to affect thinner people more than obese individuals and women more than men. It is also common in cyclists.

Intervention

Conservative intervention should be causal. This involves relative rest, the use of a padded seat cushion, soft tissue massage, correction of hamstring strength and flexibility deficits, anti-inflammatory measures such as ice massage, and ultrasound.

Gluteal

Inflammation of the gluteal bursa (located above and behind the greater trochanter, underneath the gluteus maximus and medius) is one of the most frequent causes of pseudoradicular pain in the lower limb. The patient is usually in their fourth or fifth decade and complains of pain in the gluteal or trochanteric area. The pain may spread to the outer or posterior thigh, and down to the calf muscles and the malleolus.

Intervention

Conservative intervention should be causal. This involves the use of a padded seat cushion, anti-inflammatory measures such as ice massage, and ultrasound.

Fractures of the Pelvis

A pelvic fracture is a disruption of the bony structures of the pelvis. This type of fracture is common in the geriatric population secondary to a fall, and has a high mortality rate. Pelvic fractures can occur to any combination of the pelvic bones resulting in either a stable or an unstable fracture. The stability of the fracture is judged by the integrity of the pelvic ring. Unstable fractures require surgical fixation. Pubic rami fractures are the most commonly seen pubic fractures, with the superior ramus more commonly involved than the inferior ramus. Pubic rami and pubic bone fractures account for more than 70 percent of all pelvic fractures.[84]

Intervention

The rehabilitation protocol for a patient with a fracture of the pelvis must include early mobilization in terms of getting the patient out of bed, because prolonged immobilization can lead to a number of complications including respiratory or circulatory compromise. The intensity of the rehabilitation depends on whether the fracture was stable or unstable. The goals of the physical therapy program should be to provide the patient with an optimal return of function by improving functional skills, self-care skills, and safety awareness.

Stable

Stable pelvic fractures are managed conservatively, and the patient normally progresses well without severe complications and with only pain as the major limiting factor. The patient is encouraged to get out of bed as quickly as possible, and weight bearing as tolerated using a walker is normally permitted during the first week. Treatment during this period focuses on functional activities including bed mobility, transfers, and gait training. Bilateral upper extremity exercises and bilateral ankle pumps can begin early in the rehabilitation process. Strength training begins in the second week using isometric exercises. Open chain exercises such as the straight leg raise are avoided due to the forces that can be placed on the pelvis. The most important muscle group to strengthen is the hip abductors because they provide dynamic stabilization of the pelvis during gait. By the fourth to sixth week, the patient is typically full weight bearing and is able to return to most activities as tolerated. Use of an assisted device for gait continues until no gait deviations are present.

Unstable

Typically, patients who have undergone surgical fixation for an unstable fracture have limited weight bearing for as long as 3 months after surgery. (Patients who sustained a vertically and rotationally unstable fracture may not begin weight bearing until 6 to 8 weeks after surgery, making the focus of the rehabilitation program on independent wheelchair mobility and bed-to-chair transfers.) This delay in weight bearing is likely responsible for the high mortality rate associated with this type of fracture.

● **Key Point** The postsurgical rehabilitation program is specific to the type and severity of fracture and the methods used to stabilize the fracture.

Based on the physician's orders, the patient is typically introduced to the vertical position using a tilt table, during which pulse, blood pressure, and respiration are carefully monitored for signs of postural hypotension (see Chapter 1) or other complications. Bilateral upper extremity exercises and bilateral ankle pumps can begin early in the rehabilitation process. Based on physician orders, gentle hip and knee motion can be progressed within the limits imposed. Once the physician has determined that the fracture site is stable, the rehabilitation progression mirrors that of the stable fracture.

Fractures of the Acetabulum

Fractures of the acetabulum occur primarily in young adults as a result of high-velocity trauma. The position of the femur at the time of impact and the direction of the force determine the type and displacement of the fracture.

Intervention

Table 19-5 outlines the postsurgical rehabilitation program following the open reduction and internal fixation (ORIF).

Hip Fractures

Hip fractures are associated with substantial morbidity and mortality in the elderly. A number of types of hip fractures exist. Intertrochanteric fractures occur on the proximal, upper part of the femur or thigh bone between the greater trochanter, where the gluteus medius and minimus muscles attach, and the lesser trochanter, where the iliopsoas muscle attaches. Fractures of the femoral neck are proximal to intertrochanteric fractures, and subtrochanteric fractures are distal to or below the trochanters.

Intertrochanteric

The intertrochanteric area of the femur is distal to the femoral neck and proximal to the femoral shaft. It is the area of the femoral trochanters, the lesser and greater trochanters. The intertrochanteric area can also be seen as the area where the femur changes from an essentially vertical bone to a bone angling at a 45-degree angle from the near-vertical to the acetabulum or pelvis. The etiology of intertrochanteric fractures is the combination of increased bone fragility of the intertrochanteric area of the femur associated with decreased agility and decreased muscle tone of the muscles in the area secondary to the aging process.

Intervention

The current treatment of intertrochanteric fractures is surgical intervention. Currently, with a few exceptions, ORIF is used to treat essentially all intertrochanteric fractures. The procedure is designed to maintain the nondisplaced, minimally displaced, or postreduction fracture fragments in their anatomic, near-anatomic, or acceptable postreduction position. Following the procedure, preventive protocol is followed with an appropriate combination or selection of antiembolism stockings and anticoagulants. Physical therapy involves functional and gait training according to the weight-bearing status, and a progressive exercise program of range of motion and strengthening exercises.

> ● **Key Point** Hip fractures are associated with a high risk of deep vein thrombosis (DVT) due to the accompanying vessel trauma, venous stasis, coagulation activation, and older age of most patients (see Chapter 1). Although changes in surgical and anesthetic techniques, and early mobilization, may reduce the risk of venous thromboembolism, routine thromboprophylaxis remains extremely important and is the standard of care.

TABLE 19-5	Postsurgical Rehabilitation Following Acetabular ORIF
Time Frame	**Intervention**
Day 1	Static quadriceps exercises are started.
Day 2 or 3	Continuous passive motion (CPM) is started, limiting the range to about 60 degrees for the first 3 days to avoid tension on the wound.
Days 3–7	Dynamic quadriceps exercises are performed.
	Once pain has subsided, the patient may begin gait training on a walker or axillary crutches. Toe-touch weight bearing is permitted. The patient is encouraged to ambulate with a step-through gait and a heel-to-toe motion.
	Active flexion, extension, and abduction exercises while standing are encouraged.
Weeks 8–12	Weight bearing is limited for 8–12 weeks postoperatively.
Week 12	Full weight-bearing ambulation is permitted only after the fracture unites, usually by about 12 weeks, with gradual discarding of walking aids as tolerated.
One year	Return to sporting activity may be advised after about a year, in the absence of complications.

Subtrochanteric

The subtrochanteric region of the femur consists primarily of cortical bone, so healing in this region is predominantly through a primary cortical healing, making fracture consolidation quite slow to occur. In addition, this region is exposed to high stresses during activities of daily living. During normal activities of daily living, up to 6 times the body weight is transmitted across the subtrochanteric region of the femur.[85] Subtrochanteric fractures account for approximately 10–30 percent of all hip fractures, and they affect persons of all ages. Most frequently, these fractures are seen in two patient populations, namely older osteopenic patients after a low-energy fall and younger patients involved in high-energy trauma. Surgical treatment can be divided into three main techniques: external fixation, open reduction with plates and screws, and intramedullary fixation. External fixation is rarely used but is indicated in severe open fractures. For most patients, external fixation is temporary, and conversion to internal fixation can be made if and when the soft tissues have healed sufficiently.

Intervention

Following intramedullary nailing, if the bone quality and cortical contact is adequate, 50 percent partial weight bearing can be allowed immediately. With less stability, patients can perform touch-down weight bearing. Following ORIF and plate fixation, minimal protected weight bearing can begin immediately but is advanced slowly beginning approximately 4 weeks after surgery, with full weight bearing anticipated at 8–12 weeks. Elderly patients may have difficulty with compliance with weight-bearing restrictions. Such patients are slow to progress and generally avoid aggressive weight bearing on the injured extremity. As a result, most elderly patients can be safely permitted to progress to full postoperative weight-bearing status.

Femoral Neck Fracture

Femoral neck fractures in young patients are usually caused by high-energy trauma. These fractures are often associated with multiple injuries and high rates of avascular necrosis and nonunion. A number of factors predispose the elderly population to fractures, including osteoporosis, malnutrition, decreased physical activity, impaired vision, neurologic disease, poor balance, and muscle atrophy. Hip fractures are common and are often devastating in the geriatric population. Femoral neck fractures can be divided into the following four grades based on the degree of displacement of the fracture fragment:

- Grade I is an incomplete or valgus impacted fracture.
- Grade II is a complete fracture without bone displacement.
- Grade III is a complete fracture with partial displacement of the fracture fragments.
- Grade IV is a complete fracture with total displacement of the fracture fragments.

The prognosis for this injury depend on (1) the extent of injury (i.e., amount of displacement, amount of comminution, whether circulation has been disturbed), (2) the adequacy of the reduction, and (3) the adequacy of fixation. Recognition of the disabling complications of femoral neck fractures requires meticulous attention to detail in their management.

Intervention

The decision for operative or nonoperative treatment of femoral neck fractures and the decision regarding the type of surgical intervention are based on many factors. Tension fractures are potentially unstable and may require operative stabilization. Nondisplaced femoral neck fractures may need to be stabilized with multiple parallel screws or pins. The treatment of a displaced fracture is based on the person's age and activity level. In the elderly population, premorbid cognitive function, walking ability, and independence in activities of daily living should be considered when determining the optimal method of surgical repair.

Compression fractures are more stable than tension-type fractures, and they can be treated nonoperatively. Treatment for nondisplaced fractures is bed rest and/or the use of crutches until passive hip movement is pain free and x-ray films show evidence of callus formation. Patients are monitored closely with serial x-ray films because the risk of displacement of the fracture is high and immediate open reduction and internal fixation is indicated if the fracture widens. Postoperatively, the patient rests until pain resolves and then progresses to full activity as healing occurs. Once the plate is removed, further rehabilitation is needed. Removal of the plate depends on the age and activity level of the patient.

> ● **Key Point** Femoral neck fractures are frequently treated using a prosthesis or replacement device to substitute for the proximal femoral fragment, including the residual neck fragment with the devitalized femoral head (i.e., total hip arthroplasty or hemiarthroplasty).

Therapeutic Progression Following Surgery

The weight-bearing status depends on the stability of reduction, bone, and method of fixation (see above). The exercises performed initially include quadriceps sets, gluteal sets, heel slides, active-assisted hip abduction and adduction, and supine internal and external hip rotation. Once full weight bearing is achieved, exercises begin to address functional strengthening using the principles of closed kinetic chain progressions. Strengthening of the gluteus medius is important for postoperative stability. Other important muscles include the iliopsoas, gluteus maximus, adductors (magnus, longus, and brevis), quadriceps, and hamstrings.

Functional goals include normalizing the patient's gait pattern. Once partial weight-bearing ambulation is allowed, aquatic training may be used, such as swimming or deep-water running.

Maintaining aerobic conditioning throughout the rehabilitation process is important. If protected or non–weight-bearing ambulation is necessary, then upper body exercise, such as an upper body ergometer, can be used.

Legg-Calvé-Perthes Disease

Legg-Calvé-Perthes disease (LCPD) is the name given to idiopathic osteonecrosis of the capital femoral epiphysis of the femoral head (see Chapter 22).

Slipped Capital Femoral Epiphysis

Slipped capital femoral epiphysis (SCFE) is classified as a disorder of epiphyseal growth (see Chapter 22).

Total Hip Arthroplasty

The total hip arthroplasty (THA), a common procedure performed in many acute care hospitals, is used in cases of severe joint damage resulting from osteoarthritis, rheumatoid arthritis, hip fracture, and avascular necrosis.[86] Arthroplasty of the hip may be categorized as a total hip arthroplasty or a hemiarthroplasty (see the next section). In a total hip arthroplasty, the articular surfaces of both the acetabulum and femur are replaced. This involves either replacement of the femoral head and neck (conventional total hip arthroplasty) or replacement of the surface of the femoral head (resurfacing total hip arthroplasty); both procedures also replace the acetabulum (Figure 19-30).

The most common indications for a THA are as follows:[87]

- *Pain:* Pain is the principal indication for hip replacement. This includes pain with movement and pain at rest. A significant amount of pain

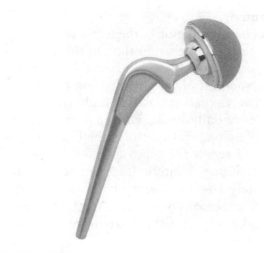

Figure 19-30 Total hip replacement components.

may be reliably relieved as early as 1 week after surgery.[88]
- *Functional limitations:* Capsular contractions and joint deformity cause a decreased ROM in the hip with subsequent functional restrictions.
- *Loss of mobility:* There are certain patient subgroups in which joint stiffness, without hip pain, is an indication for surgery. These groups include patients with ankylosing spondylitis.
- *Post-hip fracture, when the risk of avascular necrosis is high:* Arthroplasty of the hip is also considered in the presence of aseptic necrosis, congenital abnormalities, rheumatoid arthritis, and Paget's disease, among other conditions.[89]
- *Radiographic indications of intra-articular disease:* Although radiographic changes are considered in the decision to operate, the more significant determinant is the severity of symptoms.

> ● **Key Point** Although most THAs are performed in patients between 60 and 80 years of age, hip replacement is occasionally performed in younger patients including those in their teens and early 20s, due to severe trauma.[90,91]

The first successful THA used a transtrochanteric lateral approach. Three other approaches have evolved since: the anterolateral approach, the direct lateral approach, and the posterolateral approach.[92] Controversy remains as to which approach results in the lowest complication rate.[87,88,90,93–95]

- *Anterolateral approach:* There are numerous variations of the anterolateral approach.

All variations approach the hip through the interval between the tensor fascia lata and the gluteus medius muscle. Some portion of the hip abductor is released from the greater trochanter, and the hip is dislocated anteriorly.[91]

- *Direct lateral approach:* The direct lateral approach leaves the posterior portion of the gluteus medius attached to the greater trochanter. Because the posterior soft tissues and capsule are left intact, this approach is preferred in the more noncompliant patients to prevent postsurgical dislocation.[91]
- *Posterolateral approach:* The posterolateral approach, the most commonly used approach, gains access to the hip joint by splitting the gluteus maximus muscle. The short external rotators are then released, and the hip abductors are retracted anteriorly. The femur is then dislocated posteriorly.

● **Key Point** During the surgical approach to the hip joint, a trochanteric osteotomy may be necessary, especially in revision surgery. This procedure involves detaching the hip abductor mechanism. After this mechanism is repaired, the patient should avoid abduction exercises.

More recently, the *minimally invasive anterior approach* has become more popular. Despite being classed as an open approach, this procedure occurs through one or two small incisions. The rationale for minimally invasive procedures is that compared with traditional procedures, the use of small incisions potentially lessens soft tissue trauma during surgery and therefore should improve and accelerate a patient's postoperative recovery.[96] Other benefits are reduced blood loss, reduced postoperative pain, shorter length of hospital stay and lower cost of hospitalization, more rapid recovery of functional mobility, and a better cosmetic appearance of the surgical scar.[96]

The hip joint may be replaced with a variety of materials, including metal, polyethylene, and ceramic. There also are various methods of arthroplasty fixation, such as polymethylmethacrylate (PMMA) cement and screw fixation, although cementless press fit and porous ingrowth arthroplasties may also be used. The most common materials used for a total hip replacement articulation are a metal femoral head (cobalt-chromium), which articulates with an acetabular cup (polyethylene with metal backing).

The PTA must be aware of several complications associated with THA. These include, but are not limited to, the following:

- *Deep vein thrombosis (DVT):* DVT remains the most common and potentially lethal complication following either elective or emergency surgery of the hip in adults.[89] Peak incidence, which is probably between 40 and 60 percent for distal (calf) vein thrombosis, and 20 percent for proximal (popliteal, femoral, and iliac) thrombosis, occurs most commonly during the second or third week postsurgery.[97] However, the period of increased risk can be up to 3 months after surgery.[98] Even with prophylaxis, the incidence of angiographically proven asymptomatic pulmonary embolism has been reported to be approximately 20 percent.[99–103]
- *Heterotopic ossification:* Heterotopic ossification (HO) is a well-known complication of surgical approaches to the hip that involve dissection of the gluteal muscles, and is the most common complication following THA.[104,105] The exact mechanism for heterotopic bone formation has not been thoroughly determined, although trauma to the muscles during surgery appears to be a major contributing factor in provoking pluripotent mesenchymal cell differentiation into osteoprogenitor cells.[106,107] This process begins as soon as 16 hours after injury and is maximal at 36–48 hours.[107,108] HO and DVT have been positively associated, perhaps because the mass effect and local inflammation of HO encourage adjacent thrombus formation by venous compression and phlebitis.[109] HO often begins as a painful palpable mass that gradually becomes nontender and smaller but firmer to palpation. Bone scan is the method of choice for earliest detection.[109]
- *Femoral fractures:* Fracture of the femur in association with THA is a challenging complication that has been well described.[110–114] The prevalence of these fractures has ranged from 0.1 percent (7 of 5400)[112] to 20 percent (16 of 79).[113] Risk factors include female gender, rheumatoid arthritis, cortical perforation, osteopenia, osteoporosis, preoperative femoral deformity, a revision operation, osteolysis, and loosening of the stem.[112,114]
- *Dislocation:* Dislocation of the total hip replacement remains a common and potentially

extremely problematic complication. As many as 85 percent of dislocations are reported to occur within 2 months after THA.[115] Dislocation is more common in elderly people, particularly those with impaired cognition and balance and vibration sensitivity.[116] It occurs more commonly in women.[117] There is also a correlation with history of trauma or developmental dysplasia of the hip.[90] Patients with cerebral dysfunction or excessive alcohol use are also at higher risk.[118] Dislocation rate is a factor of many other requirements including component position, technical errors, imbalance of tissues, surgical approach, and patient compliance.[119]

> **● Key Point** Standard precautions given to patients who underwent a lateral or posterolateral approach to prevent posterior hip dislocation include the following:
>
> - Do not cross your legs (avoid hip adduction). Typically an abduction wedge or pillow is prescribed.
> - Put a pillow between your legs if you lie on your side.
> - Do not turn your leg inward (avoid hip internal rotation).
> - Do not bend forward at the hip.
> - Sit only on elevated chairs or toilet seats and do not bend over from the hips to reach objects or tie your shoes (avoid hip flexion greater than 90 degrees).
> - An assistive device or reacher is necessary to safely perform activities of daily living (ADLs).
> - Combinations of hip flexion, internal rotation, and adduction must be avoided for up to 4 months after surgery or until physician clearance.
>
> Precautions for a patient who underwent an anterior/anterior lateral or direct lateral approach, with or without trochanteric osteotomy, include:
>
> - Avoid hip flexion greater than 90 degrees.
> - Avoid hip extension, adduction, and external rotation past neutral.
> - Avoid the combined motions of flexion, abduction, and external rotation.
> - If a trochanteric osteotomy was performed, or if the gluteus medius was incised and repaired, do not perform active, anti-gravity hip abduction for at least 6–8 weeks or until approved by the surgeon.

■ *Neurovascular injury:* A review of the literature reveals that the prevalence of nerve palsy following THA varies from 0.08 to 7.5 percent, depending on the study, with an overall prevalence of 1 percent.[120] The fibular division of the sciatic nerve is involved in almost 80 percent of cases, with the femoral nerve and the obturator nerve involved less frequently.[120] There are many proposed causes for neuropathy associated with THA, including direct trauma; excessive tension because of an increase in limb length, or offset, or both; bleeding, or compression, or both, by a hematoma; and unknown.[120–122]

Following the surgery, thromboembolic disease (TED) hose are placed on the patient. For patients who have undergone either a posterolateral approach or a transtrochanteric approach, a triangular foam cushion (abduction pillow) is strapped between the legs to keep the hip in an abducted position. Patients at a high risk of dislocation, such as those who have undergone a postrevision arthroplasty or those with cognitive impairments, may need to wear a hip abduction orthosis that maintains the hip in abduction for 6–12 weeks. These orthoses may make ambulation difficult if the abduction is more than 5–10 degrees.

> **● Key Point** Patients with cemented joint replacements can weight bear as tolerated (WBAT) unless the operative procedure involved a soft-tissue repair or internal fixation of bone. Patients with cementless, or ingrowth, joint replacements are put on partial weight bearing (PWB) or toe-touch weight bearing (TTWB) to allow maximum bony ingrowth to take place but may also be non-weight-bearing (NWB).

Intervention

Following the postsurgical examination performed by the physical therapist on postoperative day 1, exercises are initiated. The postsurgical rehabilitation protocol for an arthroplasty of the hip is outlined in **Table 19-6**.

On the first day after the surgery, the clinician begins transfer training and instructs the patient with regard to bed mobility. Training includes transfers from supine to sitting on the bed, and then from sitting to standing, while observing all of the necessary hip precautions.[123] If permitted by the surgeon, the patient can be shown how to transfer to an appropriate bedside chair. The patient is encouraged to sit on the chair for about 30–60 minutes, depending on tolerance, which can be measured using the vital signs of pulse and blood pressure, as well as subjective complaints such as light-headedness or dizziness.

Gait training with crutches (younger more active patients) or a walker (more elderly patients) is usually begun on the second day following surgery.[123] The patient's assistive device is adjusted to the correct height. Close attention must be paid to these patients during gait training because of the potential balance deficiencies and the possibility of temporary postural (orthostatic) hypotension (see Chapter 1).

The weight-bearing status of the patient with a noncemented THA is decided by the surgeon. It can vary from non-weight bearing, to toe-touch weight bearing, to partial weight bearing (20–25 pounds of pressure). Toe-touch weight bearing is used for

TABLE 19-6 Total Hip Replacement Protocol

Time Frame	Intervention	Description
Pre-op or immediately post-op	Patient education	*Posterior approach:* • No hip flexion beyond 90 degrees • No crossing of the legs (hip adduction beyond neutral) • No hip internal rotation past neutral *Anterior approach:* • Avoid extremes of hip extension and external rotation • Weight-bearing status
Postoperative (day 1)	Bedside exercises	Ankle pumps, quadriceps sets, and gluteal sets
	Bed mobility and transfer training	Bed to/from chair
Postoperative (day 2)	Gait training	Crutches or walker instruction
Postoperative (days 3–5 or on discharge to the rehabilitation unit)	Therapeutic exercises	Progression of ROM and strengthening exercises to the patient's tolerance
	Gait training	Progression of ambulation on level surfaces and stairs (if applicable) with the least restrictive device
Postoperative (day 5 to 4 weeks)	Therapeutic exercises	Seated leg extensions, side-lying/standing hip abduction, standing hip extension and hip abduction, knee bends, bridging (depending on weight-bearing status) Stretching exercises to increase the flexibility of hip muscles
	Gait training	Progression of ambulation distance

balance only. It has been described as analogous to walking on eggshells. Partial weight bearing is a difficult concept for most patients to grasp. Using a bathroom scale, or a description such as "one-tenth of body weight" (depending on the patient's weight) usually helps. Force platforms are also available to measure these forces directly and can provide beneficial feedback for the patient.

The weight-bearing status for the patient with a cemented THA is usually weight bearing as tolerated with a walker for 6 weeks prior to full weight bearing.

Normalization of the gait pattern should be taught early. Stand-step transfers should also be taught to prevent the patient from rotating at the involved hip.

Stair negotiation, based on the patient's home situation, is typically taught on day 3.[123]

The outpatient phase of treatment, if appropriate, involves a continued progression of the therapeutic exercise program developed in the inpatient phase with an emphasis on a return to normal activities of daily living and recreational pursuits allowed by the surgeon.

Hemiarthroplasty

In contrast to a total hip arthroplasty, a hemiarthroplasty involves replacement of the articular surface of the femoral head without surgical alteration to the acetabular articular surface. This may involve replacement of the femoral head and neck (unipolar hemiarthroplasty), replacement of the femoral head and neck with an additional acetabular cup that is not attached to the pelvis (bipolar hemiarthroplasty), or replacement of the surface of the femoral head (resurfacing hemiarthroplasty). With a bipolar hemiarthroplasty, there is normal motion between the femoral head and acetabular cup, and between the acetabular cup and native acetabulum.

● **Key Point** Proximal femoral osteotomy is a joint-sparing procedure that relies on maintaining the biological integrity of the femoral head. Preserving the blood supply to the femoral head is of the utmost importance. Proximal femoral osteotomy is currently commonly used for adults in the treatment of hip fracture nonunions and malunions and in cases of congenital and acquired hip deformities. Partial weight bearing is typically allowed immediately and continued for 8 to 12 weeks. The postsurgical rehabilitation protocol is similar to that of the total joint replacement.

Therapeutic Techniques

A number of therapeutic techniques can be used to assist the patient. These include self-stretches and selective manual techniques.

Self-Stretching

Anterior–Inferior Capsule
The patient places one foot on a chair or table in the front (refer to Figure 19-18). While maintaining the spine in a functional neutral position, the patient slowly leans toward the chair, thereby stretching the anterior–inferior aspect of the hip joint of the standing leg. The position is held for about 30 seconds.

Posterior Capsule and Piriformis Stretch
The patient is positioned in the quadruped position. The stretch is performed by the patient by having them perform oscillatory sit back motions in the direction of the hip joint to be mobilized (refer to Figure 19-15).

Alternatively, the hip internal rotators can be stretched by placing the lateral aspect of the foot and lower leg on a chair or hi-lo table. In order to stretch the internal rotators and to increase external rotation, the patient leans forward at the waist (refer to Figure 19-8).

Iliopsoas and Rectus Femoris
A number of exercises to stretch these muscle groups have already been described for this area, including the lunge (refer to Figure 19-4), supine (refer to Figure 19-5), and kneeling (refer to Figure 19-6). The stretch also can be performed in standing (Figure 19-31).

Hamstrings
A number of techniques have evolved over the years to stretch the hamstrings. The problem with most of these techniques is that they do not afford the lumbar spine much protection while performing the stretch.

The hamstring stretch should be taught with the patient in a supine position. The lumbar spine can be protected by placing a small towel roll under the lumbar spine to maintain a slight lordosis, or by having the patient sustain a pelvic tilt opposite to the lordosis during the stretch. The uninvolved leg is kept straight while the patient flexes the hip of the side to be stretched to about 90 degrees and holds onto the back of the thigh for support. From this position, the patient extends the knee on the tested leg until a stretch is felt on the posterior aspect of the thigh (Figure 19-9). This position is maintained for about 30 seconds before allowing the knee to flex slightly.

Hip Adductors
The patient sits in the cross-legged position, with the soles of the feet touching (Figure 19-32). The pelvis is tilted to adopt a functional neutral position of the spine. The patient can then allow gravity to move the thighs towards the floor or can apply manual pressure using the elbows.

Gluteus Maximus and Short Hip Extensors
This stretch is performed in supine by pulling one or both knees to the chest (Figure 19-33), or in the lunge position, depending on the patient's ability and tolerance.

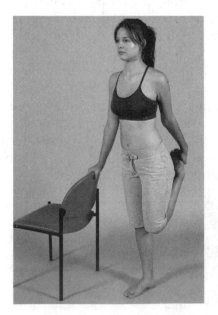

Figure 19-31 Standing hip flexor stretch.

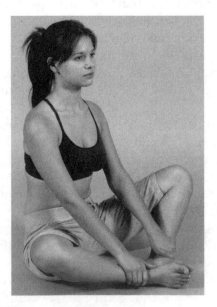

Figure 19-32 Hip adductor stretch.

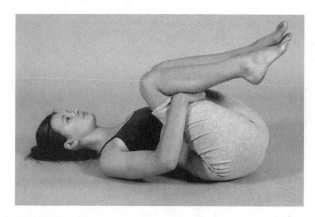

Figure 19-33 Stretch for gluteus maximus and short hip extensors.

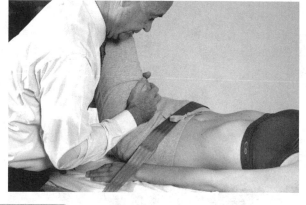

Figure 19-34 Hip distraction.

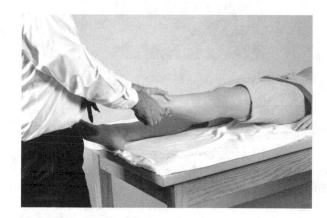

Figure 19-35 Leg traction.

Tensor Fascia Latae/Iliotibial Band

The patient stands close to a bed, with the uninvolved side being closer to the bed and the balance supported. Both legs are crossed, and the hip is translated away from the bed while the trunk is leaned toward the bed, until a stretch is felt on the outside of the hip and thigh (refer to Figure 19-11).[124]

Selective Joint Mobilizations

Mobilizations of this joint are typically performed using a sustained stretch to decrease a hip joint capsular restriction, with the stretch being governed by the direction of the restriction, rather than by the concave–convex rule. For example, if hip joint extension is restricted, the distal femur is moved into the direction of hip extension.[125] The joint is initially positioned in its neutral position and is progressively moved closer to the end of range. Rotations can be combined with any sustained stretch performed in a cardinal plane. Distraction or compression techniques can be used alone or combined with rotations.

Distraction

Joint distractions are indicated for pain and any hypomobility at the hip joint. The patient is positioned in supine, and the hip is placed in its resting position. The patient's thigh is grasped by the clinician as proximal as possible, and a distraction force is applied along the line of the femoral neck (Figure 19-34). A belt can also be used for this technique.

Leg Traction (Inferior Glide)

The patient is positioned in supine. The clinician grasps the patient's ankle and applies a series of oscillations along the length of the leg (Figure 19-35). An assistant or a belt may be necessary to provide stabilization at the hip.

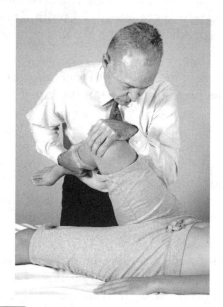

Figure 19-36 Quadrant mobilization.

Quadrant (Scouring) Mobilizations

Quadrant mobilizations involve flexion and adduction of the hip, combined with simultaneous joint compression through the femur (Figure 19-36).[21,125–127] The flexed and adducted thigh is swept through a

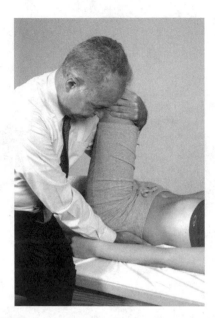

Figure 19-37   Posterior glide.

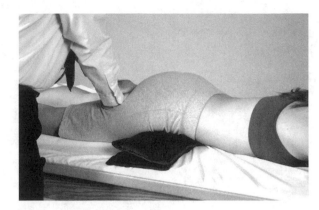

Figure 19-38   Anterior glide.

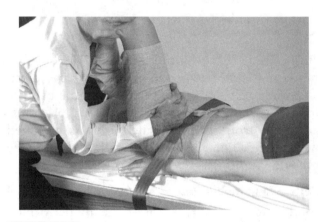

Figure 19-39   Inferior glide.

90- to 140-degree arc of flexion, while maintaining joint compression. This arc of motion should feel smooth and should be pain free. In an abnormal joint, pain or an obstruction to the arc occurs during the movement. In selected nonacute cases, the procedure may be used as an effective mobilizing procedure, where grade II to III mobilizations are applied perpendicular to the arc throughout.[21,126]

Posterior Glide

The posterior glide is used to increase flexion and to increase internal rotation of the hip. The patient is positioned in supine with the hip at 90 degrees of flexion. The clinician stands on the medial side of the patient's thigh. The clinician places a hand under the pelvis of the patient and the proximal hand on the anterior surface of the patient's knee. The clinician applies a force through the patient's knee in a posterior direction (Figure 19-37).

Anterior Glide

The anterior glide is used to increase extension and to increase external rotation of the hip. The patient is positioned prone, with the trunk resting on the table and his or her pelvis over firm support (Figure 19-38). The clinician stands next to the patient's thigh and places both hands posteriorly on the proximal thigh of the patient, just below the buttock. Keeping the elbows extended and flexing the knees, the clinician applies a force through the hands in a downward direction toward the table.

Inferior Glide

The inferior glide is used to increase flexion of the hip. The patient is positioned in supine with the hip and knee each flexed to 90 degrees and the lower leg placed over the clinician's shoulder (Figure 19-39). The patient's upper body can be stabilized using a belt. The clinician grasps the anterior aspect of the proximal femur as far proximally as possible and interlocks the fingers. An inferior glide is imparted using the hands, while simultaneously rocking the patient's thigh into flexion.

Summary

The hip is anatomically designed with a deep socket and an extensive ligamentous network to withstand the large and potentially dislocating forces that can routinely occur during walking and more vigorous activities. The failure of any of these protective mechanisms, due to disease, injury, or even advanced age, may lead to deterioration and weakening of the joint structure.

REVIEW Questions

1. When manually testing the sartorius muscle, in which three planes of motion at the hip should your resistance be?
2. In which position is the hip in its most stable position?
3. What is the close-packed position of the hip?
4. How many degrees of freedom are available at the hip joint?
5. In which direction does the pelvis tilt in order to increase the lumbar lordosis?
6. Which two muscles originate from the anterior superior iliac spine?
7. In a patient with excessive lumbar lordosis, which muscle(s) will not need stretching?
   a. Hip flexors
   b. Hamstrings
   c. Back extensors
   d. Pectoralis major
8. A coxa valga deformity is:
   a. An increase in the angle of inclination between the neck of the femur and the shaft
   b. A lengthening of the extremity on the involved side
   c. A deformity of the knee
   d. None of the above
9. You are planning an intervention for a 73-year-old inpatient who received a cemented total hip replacement 2 days ago. Your plan of care should focus on:
   a. Patient education regarding positions and movements to avoid
   b. Active range of motion exercises and early ambulation using a walker
   c. Passive range of motion exercises
   d. Tilt table
10. A patient who is substituting with the sartorius muscle during testing of the iliopsoas muscle for a fair grade (grade 3) muscle test would demonstrate:
    a. Internal rotation and abduction of the hip
    b. Flexion of the hip and extension of the knee
    c. External rotation and abduction of the hip
    d. Extension of the hip and knee
11. A 72-year-old patient is unable to bring her right foot up on the stair during stair climbing training. The most functional method to develop this skill is to:
    a. Have the patient practice marching in place
    b. Passively place the foot on the next step
    c. Strengthen the patient's hip flexors using an isokinetic training device before attempting stair climbing
    d. Practice stair climbing inside the parallel bars using a 3-inch step
12. You are treating a patient who has been admitted to a skilled nursing facility following an ORIF to the right hip for a femoral neck fracture. The PT plan of care includes gait training, strengthening of the lower extremities, transfer training, and patient education. Which of the following complications would you least likely have to be concerned with?
    a. Dislocation of the hip joint
    b. Avascular necrosis
    c. Deep vein thrombosis
    d. Respiratory compromise

References

1. Crowninshield RD, Johnston RC, Andrews JG, et al: A biomechanical investigation of the human hip. J Biomech 11:75–85, 1978
2. Takahashi M, Sugiuchi Y, Shinoda Y: Commissural mirror-symmetric excitation and reciprocal inhibition between the two superior colliculi and their roles in vertical and horizontal eye movements. J Neurophysiol 98:2664–2682, 2007
3. Jackson-Manfield P, Neumann DA: Structure and function of the hip, in Jackson-Manfield P, Neumann DA (eds): Essentials of Kinesiology for the Physical Therapist Assistant. St Louis, MO, Mosby Elsevier, 2009, pp 227–271
4. Hall SJ: The biomechanics of the human lower extremity, in Hall SJ (ed): Basic Biomechanics (ed 3). New York, McGraw-Hill, 1999, pp 234–281
5. Pick TP, Howden R: Gray's Anatomy (ed 15). New York, Barnes & Noble Books, 1995
6. Johnson CE, Basmajian JV, Dasher W: Electromyography of the sartorius muscle. Anat Rec 173:127–130, 1972
7. Janda V: On the concept of postural muscles and posture in man. Aust J Physiother 29:83–84, 1983
8. Kapandji IA: The Physiology of the Joints, Lower Limb. New York, Churchill Livingstone, 1991
9. Durrani Z, Winnie AP: Piriformis muscle syndrome: An underdiagnosed cause of sciatica. J Pain Symptom Manage 6:374–379, 1991
10. Julsrud ME: Piriformis syndrome. J Am Podiat Med Assoc 79:128–131, 1989
11. Pace JB, Nagle D: Piriformis syndrome. Western J Med 124:435–439, 1976
12. Steiner C, Staubs C, Ganon M, et al: Piriformis syndrome: Pathogenesis, diagnosis, and treatment. J Am Osteopath Assoc 87:318–323, 1987
13. Harvey G, Bell S: Obturator neuropathy. An anatomic perspective. Clin Orthop Rel Res 363:203–211, 1999
14. Williams PL, Warwick R, Dyson M, et al: Gray's Anatomy (ed 37). London, Churchill Livingstone, 1989

15. Holmich P: Adductor related groin pain in athletes. Sports Med Arth Rev 5:285–291, 1998

16. Hasselman CT, Best TM, Garrett WE: When groin pain signals an adductor strain. Phys Sports Med 23:53–60, 1995

17. Cibulka MT, Sinacore DR, Cromer GS, et al: Unilateral hip rotation range of motion asymmetry in patients with sacroiliac joint regional pain. Spine 23:1009–1015, 1998

18. Afoke NYP, Byers PD, Hutton WC: Contact pressures in the human hip joint. J Bone Joint Surg [Am] 69B:536, 1987

19. Oatis CA: Biomechanics of the hip, in Echternach J (ed): Clinics in Physical Therapy: Physical Therapy of the Hip. New York, Churchill Livingstone, 1990, pp 37–50

20. Kaltenborn FM: Manual Mobilization of the Extremity Joints: Basic Examination and Treatment Techniques (ed 4). Oslo, Norway, Olaf Norlis Bokhandel, Universitetsgaten, 1989

21. Yoder E: Physical therapy management of nonsurgical hip problems in adults, in Echternach JL (ed): Physical Therapy of the Hip. New York, Churchill Livingstone, 1990, pp 103–137

22. Cyriax J: Textbook of Orthopaedic Medicine, Diagnosis of Soft Tissue Lesions (ed 8). London, Bailliere Tindall, 1982

23. Cyriax JH, Cyriax PJ: Illustrated Manual of Orthopaedic Medicine. London, Butterworth, 1983

24. Pauwels F: Biomechanics of the Normal and Diseased Hip. Berlin, Springer-Verlag, 1976

25. Maquet PGJ: Biomechanics of the Hip as Applied to Osteoarthritis and Related Conditions. Berlin, Springer-Verlag, 1985

26. Menke W, Schmitz B, Schild H, et al: Transversale Skelettachsen der unteren Extremitat bei Coxarthrose. Zeitschr Orthop 129:255–259, 1991

27. Pizzutillo PT, MacEwen GD, Shands AR: Anteversion of the femur, in Tronzo RG (ed): Surgery of the Hip Joint. New York, Springer-Verlag, 1984, pp 22–41

28. Lausten GS, Jorgensen F, Boesen J: Measurement of anteversion of the femoral neck, ultrasound and CT compared. J Bone Joint Surg [Am] 71B:237, 1989

29. Gross MT: Lower quarter screening for skeletal malalignment—suggestions for orthotics and shoewear. J Orthop Sports Phys Ther 21:389–405, 1995

30. Mennet P, Egger B: Hüftdisziplin. Rheinfelden, Switzerland, Solbadklink Rheinfelden, 1986

31. Booth FW: Physiologic and biochemical effects of immobilization on muscle. Clin Orthop Relat Res 219:15–21, 1987

32. Eiff MP, Smith AT, Smith GE: Early mobilization versus immobilization in the treatment of lateral ankle sprains. Am J Sports Med 22:83–88, 1994

33. Akeson WH, Amiel D, Mechanic GL, et al: Collagen cross-linking alterations in the joint contractures: Changes in the reducible cross-links in periarticular connective tissue after 9 weeks immobilization. Connect Tissue Res 5:15, 1977

34. Akeson WH, Amiel D, Abel MF, et al: Effects of immobilization on joints. Clin Orthop 219:28–37, 1987

35. Akeson WH, Amiel D, Woo SL-Y: Immobility effects on synovial joints: The pathomechanics of joint contracture. Biorheology 17:95–110, 1980

36. Woo SL-Y, Matthews J, Akeson WH, et al: Connective tissue response to immobility: A correlative study of biochemical and biomechanical measurements of normal and immobilized rabbit knee. Arthritis Rheum 18:257–264, 1975

37. Inman VT, Ralston HJ, Todd F: Human Walking. Baltimore, Williams & Wilkins, 1981

38. Rothstein JM: Muscle biology: Clinical considerations. Phys Ther 62:1823, 1982

39. Carr JH: A Motor Relearning Programme for Stroke. Rockville, MD, Aspen, 1987

40. Knott M, Voss DE: Proprioceptive Neuromuscular Facilitation (ed 2). New York, Harper & Row, 1968

41. Malone T, Nitz AJ, Kuperstein J, et al: Neuromuscular concepts, in Ellenbecker TS (ed): Knee Ligament Rehabilitation. Philadelphia, Churchill Livingstone, 2000, pp 399–411

42. Risberg MA, Mork M, Krogstad-Jenssen H, et al: Design and implementation of a neuromuscular training program following anterior cruciate ligament reconstruction. J Orthop Sports Phys Ther 31:620–631, 2001

43. Saliba V, Johnson G, Wardlaw C: Proprioceptive neuromuscular facilitation, in Basmajian JV, Nyberg R (eds): Rational Manual Therapies. Baltimore, Williams & Wilkins, 1993

44. Hubley CL, Kozey JW, Stanish WD: The effects of static stretching exercises and stationary cycling on range of motion at the hip joint. J Orthop Sports Phys Ther 6:104, 1984

45. Negus RA, Rippe JM, Freedson P, et al: Heart rate, blood pressure, and oxygen consumption during orthopaedic rehabilitation exercise. J Orthop Sports Phys Ther 8:346, 1987

46. Tepper S, Hochberg MC: Factors associated with hip osteoarthritis: Data from the first National Health and Nutrition Examination Survey (NHANES-I). Am J Epidemiol 137:1081–1088, 1993

47. Cooper C, Campbell L, Byng P, et al: Occupational activity and the risk of hip osteoarthritis. Ann Rheum Dis 55:680–682, 1996

48. Dieppe P: Management of hip osteoarthritis. BMJ 311:853–857, 1995

49. Spear CV: Common pathological problems of the hip, in Echternach JL (ed): Physical Therapy of the Hip. New York, Churchill Livingstone, 1990, pp 51–69

50. Weigl M, Angst F, Stucki G, et al: Inpatient rehabilitation for hip or knee osteoarthritis: 2 year follow up study. Ann Rheum Dis 63:360–368, 2004

51. Cibulka MT, Threlkeld J: The early clinical diagnosis of osteoarthritis of the hip. J Orthop Sports Phys Ther 34:461–467, 2004

52. van Baar ME, Dekker J, Oostendorp RA, et al: The effectiveness of exercise therapy in patients with osteoarthritis of the hip or knee: A randomized clinical trial. J Rheumatol 25:2432–2439, 1998

53. van Baar ME, Dekker J, Oostendorp RA, et al: Effectiveness of exercise in patients with osteoarthritis of hip or knee: Nine months' follow up. Ann Rheum Dis 60:1123–1130, 2001

54. Minor MA, Hewett JE, Webel RR, et al: Efficacy of physical conditioning exercise in patients with rheumatoid arthritis and osteoarthritis. Arthritis Rheum 32:1396–1405, 1989

55. Felson DT: The epidemiology of osteoarthritis: Prevalence and risk factors, in Keuttner KE, Goldberg VM (eds): Osteoarthritic Disorders. Rosemont, IL, American Academy of Orthopaedic Surgeons, 1995, pp 13–24

56. MacDonald CW, Whitman JM, Cleland JA, et al: Clinical outcomes following manual physical therapy and exercise for hip osteoarthritis: A case series. J Orthop Sports Phys Ther 36:588–599, 2006

57. Lovell G: The diagnosis of chronic groin pain in athletes: A review of 189 cases. Aust J Sci Med Sport 27:76–79, 1995

58. Holmich P, Uhrskou P, Ulnits L, et al: Effectiveness of active physical training as treatment for long-standing adductor-related groin pain in athletes: Randomised trial. Lancet 353:439–443, 1999

59. Klaffs CE, Arnheim DD: Modern Principles of Athletic Training. St Louis, CV Mosby, 1989

60. Ekstrand J, Gillquist J: Soccer injuries and their mechanisms: A prospective study. Med Sci Sports Exerc 15:267–270, 1983

61. Nielsen AB, Yde J: Epidemiology and traumatology of injuries in soccer. Am J Sports Med 17:803–807, 1989

62. Engstrom B, Forssblad M, Johansson C, et al: Does a major knee injury definitely sideline an elite soccer player? Am J Sports Med 18:101–105, 1990

63. Casperson PC, Kauerman D: Groin and hamstring injuries. Athl Train 17:43, 1982

64. Peterson L, Renstrom P: Sports Injuries—Their Prevention and Treatment. Chicago, Year Book Medical Publishers, 1986

65. Lambert SD: Athletic injuries to the hip, in Echternach J (ed): Physical Therapy of the Hip. New York, Churchill Livingstone, 1990, pp 143–164

66. Sutton G: Hamstrung by hamstring strains: A review of the literature. J Orthop Sports Phys Ther 5:184–195, 1984

67. Stanton PE: Hamstring injuries in sprinting—the role of eccentric exercise. J Orthop Sports Phys Ther 10:343, 1989

68. Ellison AE, Boland AL, Jr., DeHaven KE, et al: Athletic Training and Sports Medicine. Chicago, American Academy of Orthopaedic Surgery, 1984

69. Orchard JW, Farhart P, Leopold C: Lumbar spine region pathology and hamstring and calf injuries in athletes: Is there a connection? Br J Sports Med 38:502–504, 2004

70. Janda V: Muscle strength in relation to muscle length, pain and muscle imbalance, in Harms-Ringdahl K (ed): Muscle Strength. New York, Churchill Livingstone, 1993, pp 83–91

71. Noble CA: The treatment of iliotibial band friction syndrome. Br J Sports Med 13:51–54, 1979

72. Noble CA: Iliotibial band friction syndrome in runners. Am J Sports Med 8:232–234, 1980

73. Sutker AN, Jackson DW, Pagliano JW: Iliotibial band syndrome in distance runners. Phys Sportsmed 9:69–73, 1981

74. Holmes JC, Pruitt AL, Whalen NJ: Iliotibial band syndrome in cyclists. Am J Sports Med 21:419–424, 1993

75. Biundo JJ, Jr., Irwin RW, Umpierre E: Sports and other soft tissue injuries, tendinitis, bursitis, and occupation-related syndromes. Curr Opin Rheum 13:146–149, 2001

76. Fredericson M, Cookingham CL, Chaudhari AM, et al: Hip abductor weakness in distance runners with iliotibial band syndrome. Clin J Sport Med 10:169–175, 2000

77. Renne JW: The iliotibial band friction syndrome. J Bone Joint Surg 57:1110–1111, 1975

78. Barber FA, Sutker AN: Iliotibial band syndrome. Sports Med 14:144–148, 1992

79. Pinshaw R, Atlas V, Noakes TD: The nature and response to therapy of 196 consecutive injuries seen at a runners' clinic. S Afr Med J 65:291–298, 1984

80. Cox JS: Patellofemoral problems in runners. Clin J Sports Med 4:699–715, 1985

81. Cibulka MT, Delitto A: A comparison of two different methods to treat hip pain in runners. J Orthop Sports Phys Ther 17:172–176, 1993

82. Hammer WI: Friction massage, in Hammer WI (ed): Functional Soft Tissue Examination and Treatment by Manual Methods. Gaithersburg, MD, Aspen, 1991, pp 235–249

83. Johnston CAM, Kindsay DM, Wiley JP: Treatment of iliopsoas syndrome with a hip rotation strengthening program: A retrospective case series. J Orthop Sports Phys Ther 29:218–224, 1999

84. Connolly WB, Hedburg EA: Observations on fractures of the pelvis. J Trauma 9:104, 1969

85. Bergmann G, Graichen F, Rohlmann A: Hip joint loading during walking and running, measured in two patients. J Biomech 26:969, 1993

86. Harris WH: Traumatic arthritis of the hip after dislocation and acetabular fractures. Treatment by mold arthroplasty: An end-result study using a new method of result evaluation. J Bone Joint Surg 51:737–755, 1969

87. Mulliken BD, Rorabeck CH, Bourne RB, et al: A modified direct lateral approach in total hip arthroplasty: A comprehensive review. J Arthroplasty 13:737–747, 1998

88. Hedlundh U, Ahnfelt L, Hybbinette CH, et al: Surgical experience related to dislocation after total hip arthroplasty. J Bone Joint Surg 78B:206–209, 1996

89. Garden FH: Rehabilitation following total hip arthroplasty. J Back Musculoskel Rehabil 4:185–192, 1994

90. Mallory TH, Lombardi AV, Fada RA, et al: Dislocation after total hip arthroplasty using the anterolateral abductor split approach. Clin Orthop 358:166–172, 1999

91. Dee R, DiMaio F, Pae R: Inflammatory and degenerative disorders of the hip joint, in Dee R, Hurst LC, Gruber MA, et al (eds): Principles of Orthopaedic Practice (ed 2). New York, McGraw-Hill, 1997, pp 839–893

92. Ritter MA, Harty LD, Keating ME, et al: A clinical comparison of the anterolateral and posterolateral approaches to the hip. Clin Orthop Rel Res 385:95–99, 2001

93. Baker AS, Bitounis VC: Abductor function after total hip arthroplasty: An electromyographical and clinical review. J Bone Joint Surg 71B:47–50, 1989

94. Frndak PA, Mallory TH, Lombardi AV: Translateral surgical approach to the hip: The abductor muscle "split." Clin Orthop 295:135–141, 1993

95. Roberts JM, Fu FH, McClain EJ, et al: A comparison of the posterolateral and anterolateral approaches to total hip arthroplasty. Clin Orthop 187:205–210, 1984

96. Baerga-Varela L, Malanga GA: Rehabilitation and minimally invasive surgery, in Hozack WJ, Krismer M, Nogler M, et al (eds): Minimally invasive total joint arthroplasty. Heidelberg, Springer Verlag, 2004, pp 2–5

97. Anderson FA, Wheeler HB: Natural history and epidemiology of venous thromboembolism. Orthop Rev 23:5–9, 1994

98. Lotke P, Steinberg ME, Ecker ML: Significance of deep venous thrombosis in the lower extremity after total joint arthroplasty. Clin Orth Rel Res 299:25–30, 1994

99. Takagi H, Umemoto T: An algorithm for managing suspected pulmonary embolism. JAMA 295:2603–2604, 2006

100. Skaf E, Stein PD, Beemath A, et al: Fatal pulmonary embolism and stroke. Am J Cardiol 97:1776–1777, 2006

101. Subramaniam RM, Blair D, Gilbert K, et al: Computed tomography pulmonary angiogram diagnosis of pulmonary embolism. Australas Radiol 50:193–200, 2006

102. Weiss CR, Scatarige JC, Diette GB, et al: CT pulmonary angiography is the first-line imaging test for acute pulmonary embolism: A survey of US clinicians. Acad Radiol 13:434–446, 2006

103. Hogg K, Brown G, Dunning J, et al: Diagnosis of pulmonary embolism with CT pulmonary angiography: A systematic review. Emerg Med J 23:172–178, 2006

104. Brooker AF, Bowerman JW, Robinson RA, et al: Ectopic ossification following total hip replacement. Incidence and a method of classification. J Bone Joint Surg 55A:1629–1632, 1973

105. Morrey BF, Adams RA, Cabanela ME: Comparison of heterotopic bone after anterolateral, transtrochanteric, and posterior approaches for total hip arthroplasty. Clin Orthop 188:160–167, 1984

106. Sawyer JR, Myers MA, Rosier RN, et al: Heterotopic ossification: Clinical and cellular aspects. Calcif Tissue Int 49:208–215, 1991

107. Ayers DC, Pellegrini VD, Jr., Evarts CM: Prevention of heterotopic ossification in high-risk patients by radiation therapy. Clin Orthop 263:87–93, 1991

108. Bosse MJ, Poka A, Reinert CM, et al: Heterotopic ossification as a complication of acetabular fracture. Prophylaxis with low-dose irradiation. J Bone Joint Surg 70A:1231–1237, 1988

109. Moore DS, Cho G: Heterotopic ossification, 2005. http://www.emedicine.com/radio/topic336.htm

110. Bethea JS, III, DeAndrade JR, Fleming LL, et al: Proximal femoral fractures following total hip arthroplasty. Clin Orthop 170:95–106, 1982

111. Johansson JE, McBroom R, Barrington TW, et al: Fracture of the ipsilateral femur in patients with total hip replacement. J Bone Joint Surg 63-A:1435–1442, 1981

112. McElfresh EC, Coventry MB: Femoral and pelvic fractures after total hip arthroplasty. J Bone Joint Surg 56A:483–492, 1974

113. Stuchin SA: Femoral shaft fracture in porous and press-fit total hip arthroplasty. Orthop Rev 19:153–159, 1990

114. Crockarell JR, Jr., Berry DJ, Lewallen DG: Nonunion after periprosthetic femoral fracture associated with total hip arthroplasty. J Bone Joint Surg 81:1073–1079, 1999

115. Li E, Meding JB, Ritter MA, et al: The natural history of a posteriorly dislocated total hip replacement. J Arthroplasty 14:964–968, 1999

116. Hedlundh U, Karlsson M, Ringsberg K, et al: Muscular and neurologic function in patients with recurrent dislocation after total hip arthroplasty: A matched controlled study of 65 patients using dual-energy x-ray absorptiometry and postural stability tests. J Arthroplasty 14:319–325, 1999

117. Woo RY, Morrey BF: Dislocations after total hip arthroplasty. J Bone Joint Surg 64A:1295–1306, 1982

118. Paterno SA, Lachiewicz PF, Kelley SS: The influence of patient-related factors and the position of the acetabular component on the rate of dislocation after total hip replacement. J Bone Joint Surg 79A:1202–1210, 1997

119. Demos HA, Rorabeck CH, Bourne RB, et al: Instability in primary total hip arthroplasty with the direct lateral approach. Clin Orthop Rel Res 393:168–180, 2001

120. Schmalzried TP, Noordin S, Amstutz HC: Update on nerve palsy associated with total hip replacement. Clin Orthop 344:188–206, 1997

121. Edwards BN, Tullos HS, Noble PC: Contributory factors and etiology of sciatic nerve palsy in total hip replacement. Clin Orthop 218:136–141, 1987

122. Cohen B, Bhamra M, Ferris BD: Delayed sciatic nerve palsy following total hip replacement. Br J Clin Pract 45:292–293, 1991

123. Enloe LJ, et al: Total hip and knee replacement treatment programs: A report using consensus. J Orthop Sports Phys Ther 23:3–11, 1996

124. Kisner C, Colby LA: Therapeutic Exercise. Foundations and Techniques. Philadelphia, FA Davis, 1997

125. Maitland G: Peripheral Manipulation (ed 3). London, Butterworth, 1991

126. Grieve GP: The hip. Physiotherapy 69:196, 1983

127. Maitland GD: The hypothesis of adding compression when examining and treating synovial joints. J Orthop Sports Phys Ther 2:7, 1980

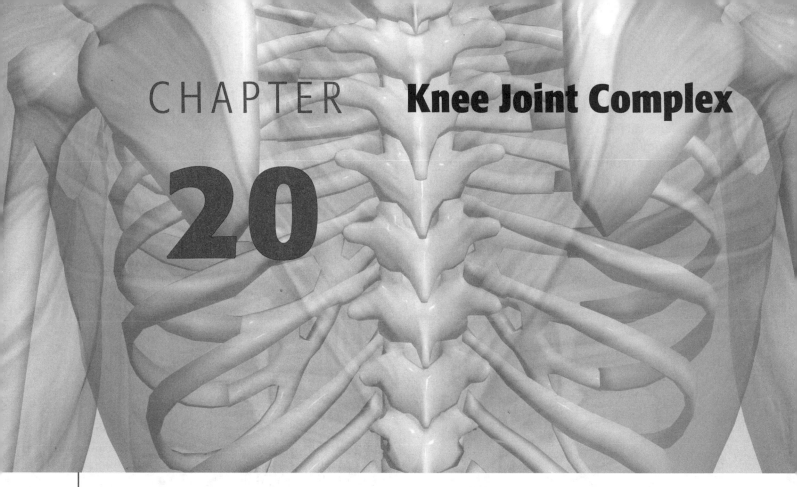

CHAPTER 20   Knee Joint Complex

Chapter Objectives

At the completion of this chapter, the reader will be able to:

1. Describe the anatomy of the joints, ligaments, muscles, blood, and nerve supply that comprise the region.
2. Describe the biomechanics of the knee complex, including the open- and close-packed positions, muscle force couples, and static and dynamic stabilizers.
3. Describe the relationship between muscle imbalance and functional performance of the knee.
4. Summarize the various causes of knee dysfunction.
5. Describe and demonstrate intervention strategies and techniques based on clinical findings and established goals by the physical therapist.
6. Evaluate the intervention effectiveness in order to determine progress and suggest modifications to the intervention as needed.

Overview

The knee, consisting of the tibiofemoral joint and the patellofemoral joint, is the largest and most complex joint in the body. The tibiofemoral joint is formed between the large condyles of the distal femur and the relatively plane proximal tibia. The patellofemoral joint is formed between the patella and the distal femur

Despite its proximity to the tibiofemoral joint, the patellofemoral joint can be considered as its own entity, in much the same way as the cranioverlebral joints are when compared to the rest of the cervical spine.[1,2] The motions about the knee occur in two planes: flexion and extension in the sagittal plane and internal and external rotation in the horizontal (transverse) plane. Motions about the knee rarely occur in isolation and typically involve movement at the hip and ankle.

Anatomy

The tibiofemoral joint, or knee joint, is a ginglymoid or hinge joint (Figure 20-1). The bony configuration of the knee joint complex is geometrically incongruous and lacks a deep concave socket, which lends little inherent stability to the joint. Joint stability is therefore dependent upon the static restraints of the joint capsule, ligaments (Figure 20-2 and **Table 20-1**), and menisci (**Table 20-2**), and the dynamic restraints of the surrounding musculature (**Table 20-3**).[3,4] In the standing position, the articulation between the angled femur and the relatively upright tibia does not typically form a straight line. In fact, the femur usually meets the tibia to form a lateral angle of 170–175 degrees (a medial angulation of 5–10 degrees) (Figure 20-3). This alignment is referred to as normal genu valgum. A lateral angle of less than 170 degrees is considered excessive genu valgum (knock-kneed). A lateral angle greater than 180 degrees is called genu varum (bow-legged). The patella, the largest sesamoid bone in the body, possesses the thickest articular cartilage in the body.

Osteokinematics of the Tibiofemoral Joint

The tibiofemoral joint allows two degrees of freedom, flexion and extension, as well as internal and external rotation. Normal ROM is from about 5 degrees of hyperextension to about 130–140 degrees of flexion. With the knee flexed, the knee joint permits 40–50 degrees of total rotation (internal and external); however, with the knee fully extended, essentially no rotation occurs.

Arthrokinematics of the Tibiofemoral Joint

All of the motions about the tibiofemoral joint consist of a rolling, gliding, and rotation between the femoral condyles and the tibial plateaus. The

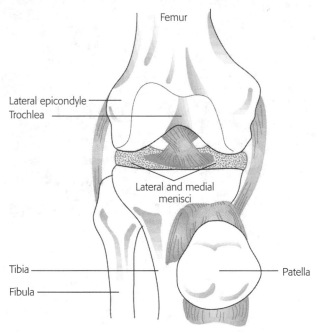

Femur

Lateral epicondyle

Trochlea

Lateral and medial
menisci

Tibia

Fibula

Patella

Figure 20-1   Bony anatomy of the knee complex.

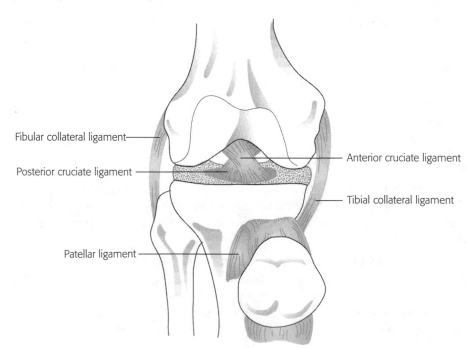

Fibular collateral ligament

Posterior cruciate ligament

Patellar ligament

Anterior cruciate ligament

Tibial collateral ligament

Figure 20-2   Major ligaments of the knee.

TABLE 20-1	Ligaments of the Knee Joint Complex
Ligament	**Function**
Anterior cruciate ligament (ACL)	Resists anterior translation of the tibia relative to a fixed femur
	Resists the extremes of knee extension
	Resists valgus and varus deformations and excessive horizontal plane rotations
Posterior cruciate ligament (PCL)	Resists posterior translation of the tibia relative to a fixed femur
	Resists the extremes of knee flexion
	Resists valgus and varus deformations and excessive horizontal plane rotations
Lateral collateral ligament (LCL)	The primary restraint to a varus force of the knee and a secondary restraint to excessive knee extension
Medial collateral ligament (MCL)	The primary restraint to valgus force of the knee and a secondary restraint to excessive knee extension

TABLE 20-2	The Medial and Lateral Menisci
Medial meniscus	Semilunar or *U*-shaped
	Larger and thicker than its lateral counterpart
	Wider posteriorly than anteriorly
Lateral meniscus	Forms a *C*-shaped incomplete circle
	Smaller, thinner, and more mobile than its medial counterpart
Medial and lateral menisci	Act as shock absorbers for the knee, reducing friction and dissipating compressive force
	Improve joint congruency
	Increase surface area of joint contact, thereby reducing joint pressure
	Enable normal joint arthrokinematics
	The blood supply of the meniscus, which is key to successful meniscal repair, comes from the perimeniscal capsular arteries, which are branches of the lateral, medial, and middle genicular arteries

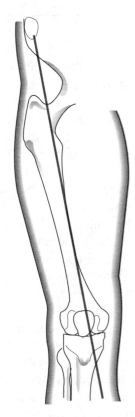

Figure 20-3 Normal genu valgum.

TABLE
20-3   Muscles of the Knee

Action	Muscles Acting	Nerve Supply	Nerve Root Derivation
Flexion of knee	Biceps femoris	Sciatic	L5, S1–S2
	Semimembranosus	Sciatic	L5, S2–S2
	Semitendinosus	Sciatic	L5, S1–S2
	Gracilis	Obturator	L2–L3
	Sartorius	Femoral	L2–L3
	Popliteus	Tibial	L4–L5, S1
	Gastrocnemius	Tibial	S1–S2
	Tensor fascia latae	Superior gluteal	L4–L5
Extension of knee	Rectus femoris	Femoral	L2–L4
	Vastus medialis	Femoral	L2–L4
	Vastus intermedius	Femoral	L2–L4
	Vastus lateralis	Femoral	L2–L4
	Tensor fascia latae	Superior gluteal	L4–L5
Internal rotation of flexed leg (non–weight bearing)	Popliteus	Tibial	L4–L5
	Semimembranosus	Sciatic	L5, S1–S2
	Semitendinosus	Sciatic	L5, S1–S2
	Sartorius	Femoral	L2–L3
	Gracilis	Obturator	L2–L3
External rotation of flexed leg (non–weight bearing)	Biceps femoris	Sciatic	L5, S1–S2

rolling, gliding, and rotation occur almost simultaneously and serve to maintain joint congruency. The direction of the roll and glide between the convex condyles of the femur and the concave tibial condyles depends on whether the knee is involved in an open-chain or closed-chain activity (see Chapter 4). During an open-chain activity, the rolling and sliding occur in the same direction, as the concave tibia moves on the convex femur. During closed-chain extension, however, the rolling and sliding occur in opposite directions, as the convex femur moves on the concave tibia. The shape of the articular surfaces of the tibiofemoral joint necessitates a flexion and extension arc accompanied by slight automatic rotational movements. In the last 30 degrees to 5 degrees of closed-chain knee extension, the lateral condyle of the femur, together with the lateral meniscus, becomes congruent and moves the axis of movement more laterally. Because the medial condyle is larger, and because the sliding stops on the lateral condyle sooner than on the medial condyle, the tibia glides more on the medial side, producing internal

rotation of the femur. In addition, the ligaments, both extrinsic and intrinsic, start to become taut near terminal extension. At this point, the cruciate ligaments become crossed and are tightened. In the last 5 degrees of extension, rotation is the only movement accompanying the extension. This rotation is referred to as the *screw-home* mechanism, and is a characteristic motion in the normal knee, in which the tibia externally rotates and the femur internally rotates as the knee approaches extension. During knee hyperextension, the femur does not continue to roll anteriorly but instead tilts forward. This creates anterior compression between the femur and tibia.[5] In the normal knee, bony contact does not limit hyperextension as it does at the elbow; rather, hyperextension is checked by the soft tissue structures. When the knee is fully extended, the tibia is slightly externally rotated on the femur (femur slightly medially rotated on the tibia). This, in essence, "locks" the knee. For flexion to be initiated from a position of full extension in a closed-chain activity, the knee joint must first be "unlocked." The service of locksmith is provided by the popliteus muscle, which contracts to internally rotate the tibia (if in an open chain—or externally rotate the femur if in a closed chain) with respect to the femur, enabling the flexion to occur.

The normal capsular pattern of the tibiofemoral joint is gross limitation of flexion and slight limitation of extension. The ratio of flexion to extension is roughly 1:10, thus 5 degrees of limited extension corresponds to a 45- to 60-degree limitation of flexion.

The Patellofemoral Joint

The patellofemoral joint is the articulation between the smooth, posterior surface of the patella and the intercondylar groove of the femur. The patella enhances the torque-producing capability of the quadriceps by about 25 percent. The patella is divided into seven facets. On the medial and lateral sides, there are superior, middle, and inferior facets. The "odd" facet, medial to the medial facet, is frequently the first part of the patella to be affected in premature degeneration of articular cartilage.

Muscles of the Knee Joint Complex

The major muscles that act on the knee joint complex are the quadriceps, the hamstrings (semimembranosus, semitendinosus, and biceps femoris), the gastrocnemius, the popliteus, the gracilis, and the hip adductors (refer to Table 20-3).

Quadriceps

The quadriceps muscles can act to extend the knee when the foot is off the ground, although more commonly they work as decelerators, preventing the knee from buckling when the foot strikes the ground.

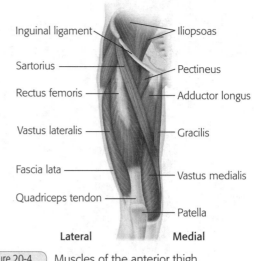

Figure 20-4 Muscles of the anterior thigh.

The four muscles that make up the quadriceps are the rectus femoris, the vastus intermedius, the vastus lateralis, and the vastus medialis (Figure 20-4). The quadriceps tendon represents the convergence of all four muscles tendon units, and it inserts at the anterior aspect of the superior pole of the patella. The quadriceps muscle group is innervated by the femoral nerve.

Rectus Femoris

The rectus femoris is the only quadriceps muscle that crosses the hip joint. It originates at the anterior inferior iliac spine. The other quadriceps muscles originate on the femoral shaft. This gives the hip joint considerable importance with respect to the knee extensor mechanism in the examination and intervention.[6] The line of pull of the rectus femoris, with respect to the patella, is at an angle of about 5 degrees with the femoral shaft (Figure 20-5).

Vastus Intermedius

The vastus intermedius has its origin on the proximal part of the femur, and its line of action is directly in line with the femur.

Vastus Lateralis

The vastus lateralis (VL) is composed of two functional parts: the VL and the vastus lateralis oblique (VLO).[7] The VL has a line of pull of about 12–15 degrees to the long axis of the femur in the frontal plane, whereas the VLO has a pull of 38–48 degrees.[6]

Vastus Medialis

The vastus medialis is composed of two functional parts that are anatomically distinct:[7] the vastus medialis obliquus (VMO) and the vastus medialis proper, or longus (VML).[8]

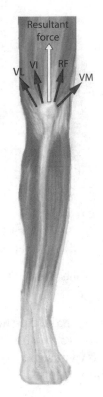

Figure 20-5 Quadriceps muscle forces.

The VMO arises from the adductor magnus tendon.[9] The insertion site of the normal VMO is the medial border of the patella, approximately one-third to one-half of the way down from the proximal pole. If the VMO remains proximal to the proximal pole of the patella and does not reach the patella, there is an increased potential for malalignment.[10]

The vector of the VMO is medially directed, and it forms an angle of 50–55 degrees with the mechanical axis of the leg.[7,9,11,12] The VMO is least active in the fully extended position[13–15] and plays little role in extending the knee, acting instead to realign the patella medially during the extension maneuver. It is active in this function throughout the whole range of extension.

According to Fox,[16] the vastus medialis is the weakest of the quadriceps group and appears to be the first muscle of the quadriceps group to atrophy and the last to rehabilitate.[17] The normal VMO/VL ratio of electromyographic (EMG) activity in standing knee extension from 30 to 0 degrees is 1:1,[18] but in patients who have patellofemoral pain, the activity in the VMO decreases significantly; instead of being tonically active, it becomes phasic in action.[19] The presence of swelling also inhibits the VMO, and it requires almost half of the volume of effusion

to inhibit the VMO as it does to inhibit the rectus femoris and VL muscles.[20]

The VMO is frequently innervated independently from the rest of the quadriceps by a separate branch from the femoral nerve.[7] The VMO originates from the medial aspect of the upper femur and inserts anteriorly into the quadriceps tendon, giving it a line of action of approximately 15–17 degrees off the long axis of the femur in the frontal plane.[6]

Because the quadriceps group is aligned anatomically with the shaft of the femur and not with the mechanical axis of the lower extremity, a dynamic lateral force is applied to the patella during extension of the knee.[21]

Hamstrings

As a group, the hamstrings primarily function to extend the hip and to flex the knee. The hamstrings are innervated by branches of the sciatic nerve.

Semimembranosus

The semimembranosus muscle (Figure 20-6) originates from the lateral facet of the ischial tuberosity and receives slips from the ischial ramus. This muscle inserts on the posterior medial aspect of the medial condyle of the tibia and has an important expansion that reinforces the posteromedial corner of the knee capsule. The semimembranosus pulls the meniscus posteriorly, and internally rotates the tibia on the femur during knee flexion, although its primary function is to extend the hip and flex the knee.

Semitendinosus

The semitendinosus originates from the upper portion of the ischial tuberosity via a shared tendon with the long head of the biceps femoris. It travels

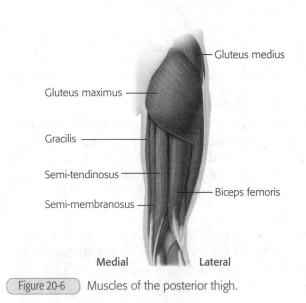

Figure 20-6   Muscles of the posterior thigh.

distally, becoming cordlike about two-thirds of the way down the posteromedial thigh. Passing over the MCL, it inserts into the medial surface of the tibia and deep fascia of the lower leg, distal to the attachment of the gracilis and posterior to the attachment of the sartorius. These three structures are collectively called the *pes anserinus* ("goose's foot") at this point. Like the semimembranosus, the semitendinosus functions to extend the hip, flex the knee, and internally rotate the tibia.

Biceps Femoris
The biceps femoris muscle is a two-headed muscle. The longer of the two heads originates from the inferomedial facet of the ischial tuberosity, whereas the shorter head arises from the lateral lip of the linea aspera of the femur. The muscle inserts on the lateral condyle of the tibia and the head of the fibula. The biceps femoris functions to extend the hip, flex the knee, and externally rotate the tibia. The superficial layer of the common tendon has been identified as the major force creating external tibial rotation and controlling internal rotation of the femur.[22] The pull of the biceps femoris on the tibia retracts the joint capsule and pulls the iliotibial tract posteriorly, keeping it taut throughout flexion.

Gastrocnemius
The gastrocnemius has two heads that originate above the knee; each head is connected to a femoral condyle and to the joint capsule ((Figure 20-7)). Approximately halfway down the leg the gastrocnemius muscles blend to form an aponeurosis. As the aponeurosis progressively contracts, it accepts the tendon of the soleus, a flat broad muscle deep to the gastrocnemius. The aponeurosis and the soleus tendon end in a flat tendon, called the *Achilles tendon*, which attaches to the posterior aspect of the calcaneus. The two heads of the gastrocnemius and the soleus are collectively known as the *triceps surae* (see Chapter 21).

Although the primary function of the gastrocnemius–soleus complex is to plantarflex the ankle and supinate the subtalar joint, the gastrocnemius also functions to flex or extend the knee, depending on whether the lower extremity is weight bearing or not. Kendall and colleagues[5] have proposed that a weakness of the gastrocnemius may cause knee hyperextension.

In addition, it has been proposed that the gastrocnemius acts as an antagonist of the anterior cruciate ligament (ACL), exerting a posteriorly directed pull throughout the range of knee flexion–extension motion, particularly when the knee is near extension.[23,24]

Hip Adductors
Although some of the hip adductors play an indirect role in the medial stability of the knee, they are primarily movers of the hip, and thus are described in Chapter 19. The exception to this is the two-joint gracilis muscle, which in addition to adducting and flexing the hip, assists in flexion of the knee and internal rotation of the lower leg.

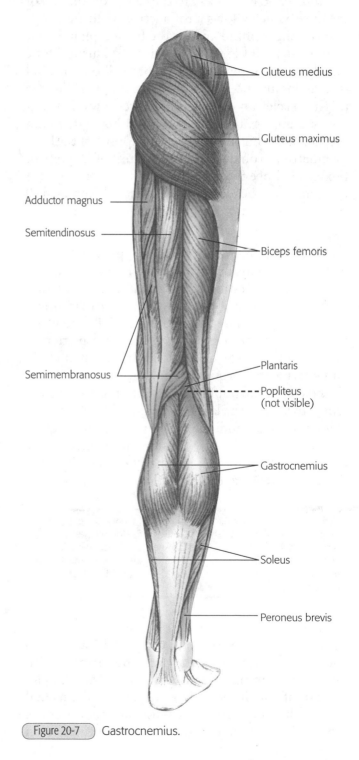

Figure 20-7 Gastrocnemius.

Iliotibial Band (Tract)

Laterally, the iliotibial band supports the extensor mechanism and is an important lateral stabilizer of the patellofemoral joint. It originates above the hip joint as a wide fascial band, originating from the gluteal muscles, tensor fascia lata (see Chapter 19), and vastus lateralis. Distally, the iliotibial band consists of two tracts. The iliotibial tract inserts on Gerdy's tubercle (a lateral tubercle of the tibial plateau). The iliotibial band is adjacent to the center of rotation of the knee, which allows it to function as an anterolateral stabilizer of the knee in the frontal plane[25] and to both flex and extend the knee.[6,26] During static standing, the primary function of the iliotibial band is to maintain knee and hip extension, providing the thigh muscles an opportunity to rest. While walking or running, the iliotibial band helps maintain flexion of the hip and is a major support of the knee in squatting from full extension until 30 degrees of flexion. In knee flexion greater than 30 degrees, the iliotibial tract becomes a weak knee flexor, as well as an external rotator of the tibia.

Popliteus

As described previously in this chapter, the knee is locked into extension by the screw-home mechanism (i.e., external rotation of the tibia/internal rotation of the femur). The popliteus muscle, due to its origin on the posterior lateral femoral condyle and insertion on the posterior medial tibia, can function as an internal rotator of the tibia in an open chain and provide the torque that unlocks the knee. In the closed chain, the popliteus can externally rotate the femur to unlock the knee. For example, as one transitions from a standing position to a partial squat, the popliteus externally rotates the femur slightly and, in a relative sense, internally rotates the tibia, thereby allowing the knee to flex.

● **Key Point** The internal rotator muscles of the tibia far outweigh the number and the strength of the external rotator muscles. This is based on the functional need at the knee during activities such as "cutting" motions to either accelerate the knee into internal rotation (by concentric contraction), or decelerate external rotation of the knee (by eccentric contraction).[27]

Sartorius

The sartorius is described in Chapter 19 with reference to its functions at the hip. The sartorius also flexes and internally rotates the tibia and plays an important role in providing stability to the medial side of the knee. Together with the tendon of the semitendinosus and the gracilis, the sartorius tendon conjoins to form one common tendon, commonly referred to as the pes anserinus.

Patellar Tracking

The patella is a passive component of the knee extensor mechanism, in which the dynamic and static relationships of the underlying tibia and femur determine the patellar-tracking pattern. The primary dynamic mechanisms of the knee are the quadriceps group. The quadriceps tendon represents the confluence of the four muscle tendon units and inserts on the superior pole of the patella. The primary static restraints for this joint are the medial and lateral retinacula and the contact of the patella with the lateral edge of the patellar groove. The thicker lateral retinaculum comprises a distinct, thick deep layer and a thin superficial layer. Deep to the medial patellar retinaculum are three focal capsular thickenings. These occasionally are referred to as the medial patellofemoral, patellomeniscal, and patellotibial ligaments.

The patella produces a concave, lateral, C-shaped curve as it moves from approximately 120 degrees of knee flexion toward approximately 30 degrees of knee extension. The lateral curve produces a gradual medial glide of the patella in the frontal plane and a medial tilt in the sagittal plane.[28,29] Further extension of the knee (between 30 and 0 degrees) produces a lateral glide of the patella in the frontal plane and a lateral tilt in the sagittal plane.[28,29] There is a natural tendency for the patella to be pulled laterally during these patellar movements due to the pull of the static restraints. For example, inappropriate tension within the iliotibial band and lateral retinaculum may result in excessive pressure on the lateral patellofemoral joint surfaces (lateral patellofemoral pressure syndrome) or lateral subluxation of the patella from the trochlear groove. In addition, weakness of the hip abductors and external rotators may result in adduction of the femur and valgus at the knee under loaded weight bearing. The quadriceps muscles, particularly the VMO, are considered critical in counteracting this lateral pull by stabilizing the patella medially.

● **Key Point** The VMO muscle has been noted to provide a medially directed dynamic stabilizing force on the patella during knee extension.

The Quadriceps Angle

The quadriceps (Q) angle, the overall line of force of the quadriceps that determines the pressure distributions on the patella, can be described as the

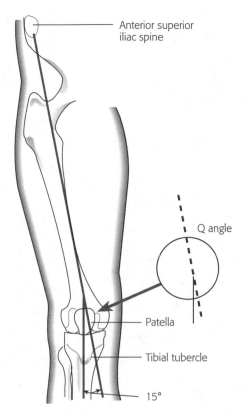

Figure 20-8 The Q-angle.

angle formed by the bisection of two lines, one line drawn from the anterior superior iliac spine (ASIS) to the center of the patella, and the other line drawn from the center of the patella to the tibial tubercle (Figure 20-8). Various normal values for the Q-angle have been reported in the literature. The most common ranges cited are 8–14 degrees for males and 15–17 degrees for females. The discrepancy between males and females is supposedly due to the wider pelvis of the female, although this has yet to be proven. Whatever the reason, females have a greater incidence of lateral dislocation of the patella and a higher frequency of patellofemoral joint pain. An increased Q-angle can result in increased pressure of the lateral facet against the lateral femoral condyle when the knee flexes during weight bearing.

> ● **Key Point** The Q-angle can vary significantly with the degree of foot pronation and supination, and when compared with measurements made in the supine position.[30,31] For example, the Q-angle will be increased if the foot is pronated, but decreased if the foot is supinated. Similarly, if the patient is non–weight bearing the compressive forces through the legs will be removed, often resulting in a decreased/increased Q-angle when compared to standing.

Lower extremity motions that can increase the Q-angle include external tibial rotation, internal femoral rotation, and functional knee valgus during dynamic activities.

> ● **Key Point** The vector force placed on the patella may be affected by the Q-angle, resulting in increased peak patellofemoral contact pressures.

The Patellofemoral Joint Reaction Forces

The patellofemoral joint reaction forces (PJRF) cause compression of the patellofemoral joint. The PJRF are due to a number of variables including the acuity of the Q-angle, the angle of knee flexion (which can increase tension in the patellar and quadriceps tendons), the location of patella contact, and the surface area of contact. (As the knee flexes from 0–60 degrees, the surface area of the patella contacting the femur progressively enlarges, providing a larger contact surface area over which to distribute the load as the load is increasing.)[32]

> ● **Key Point** Using the knowledge of the compressive forces at the patellofemoral joint:
> • Open-chain exercises (e.g., short-arc quadriceps, multiple-angle isometrics) should be performed from 0 to 5 degrees of flexion and from 90 degrees to full flexion.[33,34]
> • Closed-chain exercises (e.g., squats, lunges) should be performed in the range of 0–45 degrees of flexion.

Examination

The physical therapist's examination of the knee joint complex typically follows the outline in **Table 20-4**. The evidence-based special tests of the knee are outlined in **Table 20-5**.

General Intervention Strategies

Most knee pain of nontraumatic origin diminishes with conservative intervention.[35] Different approaches have been emphasized over the years, including patient education,[36–38] modification of activity,[17,37,39,40] progressive muscle stretching and strengthening (particularly the vastus medialis for the patellofemoral joint),[17,36,38–44] functional lower extremity training,[45] external patellar supports and braces,[17,36,38,46,47] foot orthotics,[47,48] and taping to improve patella tracking.[36,39,42,49,50] Whatever the cause of the knee injury, the goal of the rehabilitation program is to return the patient to the optimum level of function. Emphasis during knee rehabilitation must focus on achieving a balance among permitting the

TABLE 20-4	Examination of the Knee Joint Complex

I. History.

II. Observation and inspection.

III. Upper quarter scan as appropriate.

IV. Examination of movements. Active range of motion with passive overpressure of the following movements:

    a. Hip flexion, extension, abduction, adduction, internal rotation, and external rotation

    b. Knee flexion and extension

    c. Ankle dorsiflexion and plantarflexion

    d. Internal and external rotation of the tibia on the femur

V. Resisted isometric movements:

    a. Hip flexion, extension, abduction, adduction, internal rotation, and external rotation

    b. Knee flexion and extension

    c. Ankle dorsiflexion and plantarflexion

VI. Ligament stability tests:

    a. One plane medial instability

    b. One plane lateral instability

    c. One plane anterior and posterior instability

    d. Anteromedial and anterolateral rotary instability

    e. Posteromedial and posterolateral rotary instability

VII. Palpation.

VIII. Neurological tests as appropriate (reflexes, sensory scan, peripheral nerve assessment).

IX. Joint mobility tests:

    a. Anterior and posterior glides of the tibia on the femur

    b. Medial and lateral translation of the tibia on the femur

    c. Patellar glides

    d. Anteroposterior glides of the proximal tibiofibular joint

X. Special tests (refer to Table 20-5) and diagnostic imaging as appropriate.

---

healing of damaged structures, improving the strength of the controlling musculature, and increasing the efficiency of the static restraints. In addition, consideration must be given to the various forces placed on the knee during closed- and open-chain exercises so the healing process is allowed to proceed.

Acute Phase

During the acute phase, every attempt is made to protect the joint to promote and progress the healing. The goals during the acute phase are the following:

- *Reduce pain and swelling and control inflammation.* The reduction of pain and the control of swelling are extremely important. Pain and swelling can both inhibit normal muscle function and control. Pain, swelling, and inflammation are minimized by using the principles of PRICEMEM (protection, rest, ice, compression, elevation, manual therapy, early motion, and medication). Icing for 20–30 minutes, three to four times a day, concurrent with nonsteroidal anti-inflammatory drugs (NSAIDs) or aspirin prescribed by the physician, can aid in reducing pain and swelling.

- *Regain ROM.* Once the pain, swelling, and inflammation are under control, early controlled ROM exercises are initiated. In the acute phase of healing, the interventions focus on decreased loading of the joint complex, which might include postural correction, activity modification, or the use of an assistive device. Bracing may be needed to provide adequate protection and support.

- *Maintain or improve the patient's general fitness.* It is important with any injury to ensure that the patient's general level of fitness does

TABLE
20-5

Evidence-Based Special Tests of the Knee Joint Complex

Name of Test	Brief Description	Positive Findings	Evidence-Based
Lachman	Patient is supine. Knee joint is flexed between 10 and 20 degrees, and femur is stabilized with one hand.	Lack of end feel for tibial translation or subluxation is positive for ACL deficiency.	Sensitivity: 0.82[a] 0.65[b] 0.78[c] Specificity: 0.97[a] 0.42[b] 1.0[c]
Anterior drawer	Patient is supine. Knee is flexed between 60 and 90 degrees with the foot on the examination table. The clinician draws the tibia anteriorly.	Increased anterior tibial displacement compared with the opposite side is positive for ACL deficiency.	Sensitivity: 0.41[a] 0.78[c] Specificity: 0.95[a] 1.0[c]
Pivot shift test[a]	Patient is supine. Knee is placed in 10 to 20 degrees of flexion, and the tibia is rotated internally while the clinician applies a valgus force.	Positive for ACL deficiency if lateral tibial plateau subluxes anteriorly.	Sensitivity: 0.82 Specificity: 0.98
Posterior sag sign[d]	Patient is supine. Knee and hip are flexed to 90 degrees.	Increased posterior tibial displacement is positive for PCL injury.	Sensitivity: 0.79 Specificity: 1.0
Varus test[e]	Patient is supine. Clinician places patient's knee in 20 degrees of flexion and applies a varus stress to the knee.	Positive for LCL injury if pain or laxity is present.	Sensitivity: 0.25 Specificity: not provided
Valgus stress test[e]	Patient is supine. Clinician places patient's knee in 20 degrees of flexion and applies a valgus stress to the knee.	Positive for MCL injury if pain or laxity is present.	Sensitivity: 0.86 Specificity: not provided
McMurray test[f]	Patient is supine. Clinician brings the leg from extension into 90 degrees of flexion while the foot is held first in internal rotation, and then in external rotation.	Positive for meniscal tear if there is a palpable clunk.	Sensitivity: 0.16 Specificity: 0.98
Apley grind test[g]	Patient is prone with knee flexed to 90 degrees. Clinician places downward pressure on the foot, compressing the knee while internally and externally rotating the tibia.	Positive for meniscal tear if tibial rotation reproduces the patient's pain.	Sensitivity: 0.97 Specificity: 0.87
Ballottement test[h]	Patient is supine. Clinician quickly pushes the patient's patella posteriorly with two or three fingers.	Positive for knee swelling if the patella bounces off the trochlea with a distinct impact.	Sensitivity: 0.83 Specificity: 0.49

(continued)

TABLE 20-5	Evidence-Based Special Tests of the Knee Joint Complex (continued)		
Name of Test	Brief Description	Positive Findings	Evidence-Based
Thessaly test	The patient stands on the symptomatic leg while holding the clinician's hands. The patient then rotates the body and leg internally and externally with the knee flexed to 20 degrees.	Positive for meniscal tear when the patient feels pain and/or a click in the joint line.	Sensitivity: 0.90[i] 0.79[j] Specificity: 0.98[i] 0.40[j]

Data from (a) Katz JW, Fingeroth RJ: The diagnostic accuracy of ruptures of the anterior cruciate ligament comparing the Lachman test, the anterior drawer sign, and the pivot shift test in acute and chronic knee injuries. Am J Sports Med 14:88–91, 1986; (b) Cooperman JM, Riddle DL, Rothstein JM: Reliability and validity of judgments of the integrity of the anterior cruciate ligament of the knee using the Lachman's test. Phys Ther 70:225–233, 1990; (c) Lee JK, Yao L, Phelps CT, et al: Anterior cruciate ligament tears: MR imaging compared with arthroscopy and clinical tests. Radiology 166:861–864, 1988; (d) Rubinstein RA, Jr., Shelbourne KD, McCarroll JR, et al: The accuracy of the clinical examination in the setting of posterior cruciate ligament injuries. Am J Sports Med 22:550–557, 1994; (e) Harilainen A: Evaluation of knee instability in acute ligamentous injuries. Ann Chir Gynaecol 76:269–273, 1987; (f) Evans PJ, Bell GD, Frank C: Prospective evaluation of the McMurray test. Am J Sports Med 21:604–608, 1993; (g) Fowler PJ, Lubliner JA: The predictive value of five clinical signs in the evaluation of meniscal pathology. Arthroscopy 5:184–186, 1989; (h) Kastelein M, Luijsterburg PA, Wagemakers HP, et al: Diagnostic value of history taking and physical examination to assess effusion of the knee in traumatic knee patients in general practice. Arch Phys Med Rehabil 90:82–86, 2009; (i) Harrison BK, Abell BE, Gibson TW: The Thessaly test for detection of meniscal tears: Validation of a new physical examination technique for primary care medicine. Clin J Sport Med 19:9–12, 2009; and (j) Mirzatolooei F, Yekta Z, Bayazidchi M, et al: Validation of the Thessaly test for detecting meniscal tears in anterior cruciate deficient knees. Knee 17:221–223, 2010

not deteriorate due to a decrease in activity or function. An upper body ergonometer can be used in these cases.

- *Minimize muscle atrophy and weakness and attain early neuromuscular control.* Exercises prescribed for the knee joint complex must include those that promote neuromuscular control, timing, balance, and proprioception. Exercises recommended for this phase include isometric muscle setting (quadriceps sets, hamstring sets, gluteal sets), active knee flexion (heel slides) (Figure 20-9), and straight leg raises (if appropriate). Proprioceptive neuromuscular facilitation (PNF) activities may be initiated with slow-speed, low-force, controlled exercises. Electrical stimulation can be used to facilitate muscle activity and to promote muscle re-education.[51] The training of the VMO to decrease patellofemoral dysfunction should be regarded as a motor skill acquisition rather than a strengthening procedure,[20,52] with the goal of the training to produce a modification of the length–tension relationship between the VMO and its antagonist, the VL.

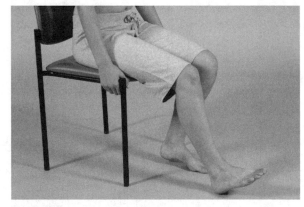

Figure 20-9   Heel slide.

This may result in a change of the equilibrium point, which will enable the appropriate alignment of the patella.[53] If the muscle control of the VMO is poor, biofeedback can be used to augment the hip adductor training.[54] Once the muscle control is achieved, gentle closed-chain exercises are initiated. Contractions of the quadriceps should be encouraged in the functional knee positions that provoke pain, such as sitting and stair negotiation. The benefit of closed-chain exercises is that they decrease shear forces and emphasize co-contractions.[55,56] All the exercises performed in the clinic should be performed by the patient at home whenever possible.

Functional Phase

The functional or chronic phase of the knee rehabilitation program addresses any tissue overload problems and functional biomechanical deficits. Once the painful symptoms have improved, the patient may gradually and incrementally increase joint-loading activities. As an approximation, patients typically progress to this phase when terminal knee extension exercises can be done with 25- to 30-pound weights.[57] Among the goals for this phase are the following:

- *Attain full range of pain-free motion.* ROM exercises during this phase include flexion and extension exercises; stationary cycling, progressing to moderate resistance; and standing wall slides. The stationary bike exercises are initially performed with a high seat (providing about 15 degrees of knee flexion in the extended leg), progressing to a lower seat to increase knee flexion ROM as tolerated.
- *Restore normal joint arthrokinematics.* Normal joint arthrokinematics are restored as the PT performs joint mobilization techniques.
- *Improve muscle strength and neuromuscular control, and restore normal muscle force–couple relationships.* There is controversy about whether knee exercises should be performed in an open-chain or closed-chain manner.[33] Closed kinetic chain exercises (CKCEs), such as the squat, leg press, dead lift, and power-clean, have long been used as core exercises by athletes to enhance performance in sport.[58,59] These multijoint exercises develop the largest and most powerful muscles of the body and have biomechanical and neuromuscular similarities to many athletic movements, such as running and jumping.[60] Open kinetic chain exercises (OKCEs) appear to be less functional in terms of many athletic movements and primarily serve a supportive role in strength and conditioning programs. However, it is advised that a combination of the open- and closed-chain exercises be used.

Closed Kinetic Chain Exercises

CKCEs during this phase include a progression of those exercises introduced during the acute phase. In addition, other exercises are introduced including one-quarter step-ups (Figure 20-10) and step-downs (Figure 20-11), single leg toe raises (Figure 20-12), partial to full squats with added resistance (see Chapter 19),[36] the seated leg press, front lunges (see Chapter 19) and side lunges (Figure 20-13), plyometric exercises (Figure 20-14 and Figure 20-15), slide-board exercises (see Chapter 21), weight-bearing

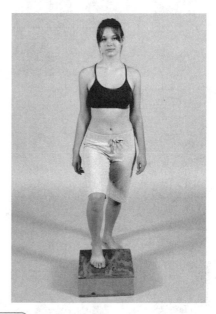

Figure 20-10   Step-ups.

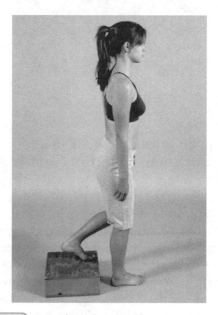

Figure 20-11   Step-downs.

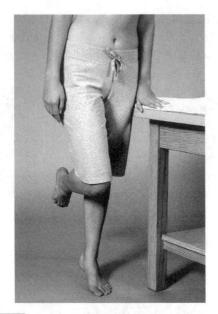

Figure 20-12   Single leg toe raises.

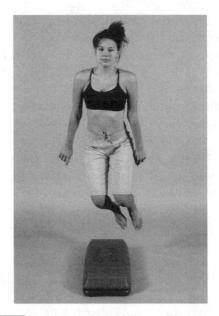

Figure 20-14   Plyometric exercise.

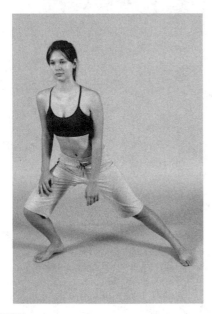

Figure 20-13   Side lunges.

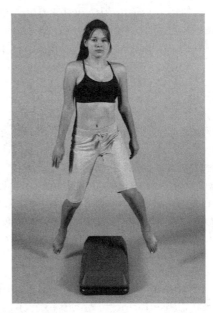

Figure 20-15   Plyometric exercise.

resisted walking with leg pulls in all four planes (flexion, extension, abduction, and adduction) using elastic tubing (Figure 20-16 and Figure 20-17), balance activities, and agility/balance drills[61] (Figure 20-18 and Figure 20-19).

CKCEs to strengthen the hamstrings, gastrocnemii, and quadriceps in a functional manner include a variety of exercises on a stair climber. The patient stands on the machine backward for the quadriceps and forward for the hamstrings. An inclined treadmill can also be used to selectively exercise the hamstrings, gastrocnemii, and quadriceps as follows:

- Walking or running downhill works the quadriceps eccentrically.
- Walking or running uphill works the gastrocnemii and hamstrings concentrically.
- Walking or running downhill backward works the gastrocnemii and hamstrings eccentrically.
- Walking uphill backward uses the quadriceps concentrically.

● **Key Point**   Uphill and retrotreadmill walking have been found to produce less patellofemoral joint restrictive forces than forward walking.[62]

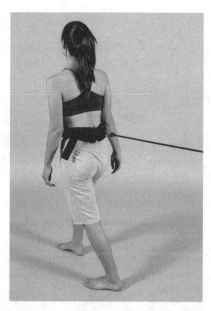

Figure 20-16   Resisted walking.

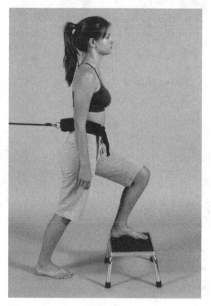

Figure 20-17   Resisted walking.

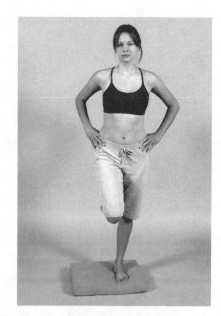

Figure 20-18   Agility and balance drills.

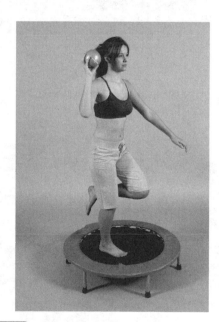

Figure 20-19   Agility and balance drills.

Open Kinetic Chain Exercises

OKCEs during this phase include seated knee extension and knee flexion exercises and are viewed as single-joint, single-muscle-group exercises.[60] Other exercises include:

- Resisted straight leg raises in the planes of flexion (Figure 20-20), extension (Figure 20-21), abduction (Figure 20-22), and adduction (Figure 20-23)
- Short-arc quadriceps progression (Figure 20-24) to about 10 percent of body weight in resistance

- Standing (Figure 20-25) and prone (Figure 20-26) hamstring curls
- Stool sweeps (Figure 20-27 and Figure 20-28)

Common Conditions

The common conditions that can affect the knee joint complex are typically traumatically induced, but also can include those that relate to poor biomechanics due to weakness or adaptive shortening, repetitive activities, or overuse.

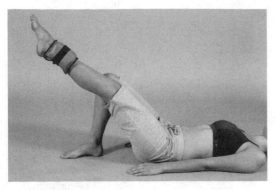

Figure 20-20   Straight leg raise into flexion.

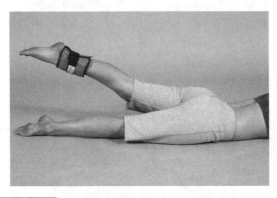

Figure 20-21   Straight leg raise into extension.

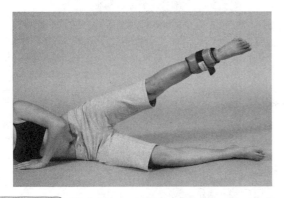

Figure 20-22   Straight leg raise into abduction.

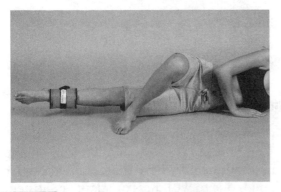

Figure 20-23   Straight leg raise into adduction.

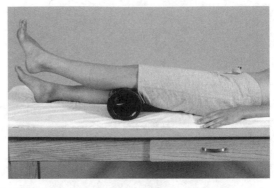

Figure 20-24   Short arc quadriceps progression.

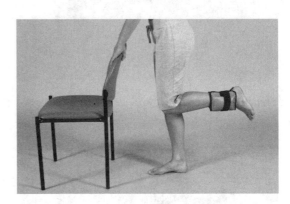

Figure 20-25   Standing hamstring curls.

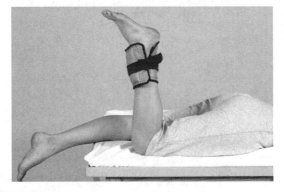

Figure 20-26   Prone hamstring curls.

Anterior Cruciate Ligament Tear

ACL injury factors have been divided into intrinsic and extrinsic factors:[63]

- Intrinsic factors include a narrow intercondylar notch, weak ACL, generalized overall joint laxity, and lower-extremity malalignment.
- Extrinsic factors include abnormal quadriceps and hamstring interactions, altered neuromuscular control, shoe-to-surface interface, playing surface, and athlete's playing style.

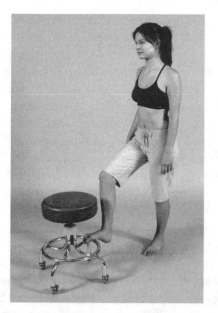

Figure 20-27   Stool sweep.

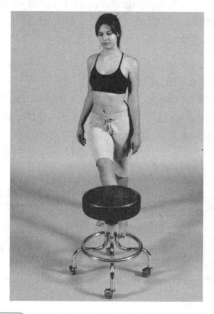

Figure 20-28   Stool sweep.

Gender also has been implicated. ACL injury rates are two to eight times higher in women than in men participating in the same sports.[63,64] Speculation about the possible etiology of ACL injuries in women has centered on the following:[65]

- *Differences in pelvic width and tibiofemoral angle between males and females, which can alter the Q-angle:*[66] Theoretically, larger Q-angles increase the lateral pull of the quadriceps femoris muscle on the patella and put medial stress on the knee.[66] This increased Q-angle also decreases the functional effectiveness of the quadriceps

as a knee extensor and of the hamstrings—the antagonist muscle group responsible for exerting a posterior force on the proximal tibia to protect the ACL.

- *Femoral notch:* A narrow intercondylar notch may be a predictive factor for ACL ruptures.[67]
- *Joint laxity:* Several studies have shown that joint laxity tends to be greater in women than in men,[68–70] although the relationship between ligamentous laxity and injury is not clear.
- *Hormonal influence:* Hormones, especially estrogen, estradiol, and relaxin, may be involved indirectly in increased ACL injury in females.[71,72]
- *ACL size:* Females typically have a smaller ACL than males, which would tend to increase the risk of tissue failure.[73]
- *Muscular strength and muscular activation patterns:* Several researchers have documented that women have significantly less muscle strength in the quadriceps and hamstrings compared with men, even when muscle strength is normalized for body weight.[70,74–77]

All ACL sprains are categorized by degree of injury as grades I, II, or III (see Chapter 5), that is mild, moderate, or complete tears of the ligament, respectively.

● Key Point   The term *midsubstance tear* refers to the site of the ACL injury and indicates a central ligament tear as opposed to a tear at one of the ligament's bony attachment sites. Almost all ACL tears are complete midsubstance tears.[78,79] Young athletes may sustain growth plate injuries (e.g., avulsion fractures) rather than midsubstance tears because the epiphyseal cartilage in their growth plates is structurally weaker than their ligaments, collagen, or bones.

Mechanism of Injury

Sudden deceleration, an abrupt change of direction, and a fixed foot have all been cited as key elements of an ACL injury.[80] The knee undergoes a combination of external rotation, valgus stress, and internal tibial rotation. A less common mechanism of injury to the ACL occurs with extreme hyperflexion or hyperextension of the knee joint.[81]

Unlike the LCL and MCL, which are extracapsular structures, the ACL is an intracapsular structure. A classic sign of ACL injuries is acute hemarthrosis (i.e., extravasation of blood into a joint or synovial cavity).[82] Atrophy of the quadriceps is an almost constant finding with patients who have a torn ACL.[83–87] Common manual tests used by the PT to assess the ACL include the anterior drawer and the Lachman (refer to Table 20-5).

Arthrometer

An arthrometer, such as the KT1000 and KT2000, is a mechanical testing device for measuring antero-posterior knee ligament instability. The patient is positioned in supine with both knees flexed approximately 20 to 25 degrees over a bolster. The arthrometer is attached to the tibia with Velcro straps while stabilizing the patella using the patella reference pad. The patient is asked to relax. Using the handle of the arthrometer, the PT directs an anterior and posterior force to the proximal tibia. A needle on the surface of the device deflects in a positive or negative direction based on the degree of tibial translation relative to the stable femur at a given force in millimeters.

Associated Knee Injuries

Isolated ACL injuries are rare, because the ACL functions in conjunction with other structures of the knee (**Table 20-6**). When the outer aspect of the knee receives a direct blow that causes valgus stress, the MCL is often torn first, followed by the ACL, which becomes the second component of a sports-related ACL injury.[81] Meniscal injuries also can occur in conjunction with ACL tears. Approximately 49 percent of patients with sports-related ACL injuries have meniscal tears.[88]

Treatment options or surgical indications are based on the following:[89,90]

- *Amount of knee instability:* Surgical treatment is usually recommended for young adult athletes because they have more years to develop degenerative joint conditions from chronic rotary knee instabilities caused by ACL deficiencies.
- *Presence of meniscal tears:* It is becoming clear that a torn ACL that is associated with a meniscal injury needs particular attention because the menisci contribute to stability of the knee.[91,92] The loss of the stabilizing effect of the meniscus appears to predispose patients who have a torn ACL to osteoarthrosis.[4,93–97]
- *Skeletal maturity of patients:* The decision to perform surgery on children with open growth plates who are diagnosed with complete ACL disruption remains questionable. This is because of the potential damage to the growth plates that may result in growth arrest.[98,99] The risk of growth disturbance appears to be low if young athletes are within 1 year of skeletal maturity at the time of surgery.[100]
- *Expected levels of patients' participation in future sports activities:* The expected future activity levels and participation in sports activities for the younger patient are often more vigorous than those for middle-aged adult athletes.[101] Nonoperative treatment of the ACL-deficient knee may be indicated in older, sedentary people.

Surgical treatment for patients undergoing ACL reconstruction procedures involves the use of grafts to replace their damaged cruciate ligament. The graft is placed through drilled femoral and tibial tunnels, and anchored in place at the proximal and distal attachment sites with a fixation device. Graft options include the use of the following:

- Autologous grafts are harvested from tissue from the body of the patient. They consist of tendons, or tendons with attached bone blocks. Bone-patella-bone autografts are currently popular because they yield a significantly higher percentage of stable knees with a higher rate

TABLE 20-6	Common Ligamentous and Meniscal Injuries	
Structure	**Mechanism of Injury**	**Subjective Complaints**
MCL	Most commonly involves external valgus or rotational force while the leg is firmly planted. Often associated with ACL injury.	Localized swelling and tenderness over injured area
Meniscus	Usually caused by noncontact injury; a rotational/torsional force is applied to a flexed knee with the foot firmly planted.	Reports of swelling developing within 12 hours of injury; localized swelling and tenderness over injured area; history of popping, clicking, or locking with knee motions

of return to preinjury sports. These grafts are usually taken from the involved extremity. The two most common autologous grafts harvested for ACL reconstruction procedures are the hamstring and patellar tendons. These grafts are used frequently because they are easy to harvest. Autologous grafts also allow return of the patient's proprioceptive response, a proven stabilizing mechanism for ACL-deficient knee joints.[102] When the semitendonosus and gracilis tendons are used together, the strength of the hamstring graft far exceeds that of the ACL. Patellar tendons are also reliable autologous grafts for ACL-deficient knee joints[103] and are used frequently because they maintain their inherent strength. They consist of bone-tendon-bone contacts.

- Allogenous grafts involve the use of biologic tissue taken from another human body. These types of grafts are less favorable due to the risk of disease transmission and problems with effective sterilization procedures. Allografts tend to be used in revisions.

- Synthetic grafts and ligament augmentation devices have been used in the past. However, synthetic grafts are no longer acceptable, because of their high rate of complications, including failure and aseptic effusions.

> ● **Key Point** Double-tunnel ACL reconstructions attempt to reproduce stability in internal rotation and valgus torque applied to the knee. Investigations into the benefits of such surgical treatment versus the increased level of difficulty and operative time are currently ongoing.

Tibiofemoral Bracing

Functional knee braces are commonly prescribed following an ACL injury or reconstruction to promote healing by reducing anterior translation of the tibia with respect to the femur and thereby restoring normal joint kinematics.[104–106]

> ● **Key Point** The efficacy of tibiofemoral bracing with regard to providing adequate protection is controversial, because the compliance of the soft tissues around the thigh decreases the ability of the brace to function correctly, particularly at high loads.[106,107]

> ● **Key Point** Interestingly, bandaging of the knee, or the use of a neoprene brace, has been shown to improve proprioception in both normal individuals and those with different types of knee disorders, including knee OA and an ACL tear.[105,108]

Intervention

The goal of the preoperative period is to maintain full range of motion. Following the surgery, care must be taken to progressively work the knee through the safe ranges of motion. During the hospital stay, the patient is fitted with a hinged knee brace locked in full extension. The brace remains locked in full extension during ambulation for the first 2 to 6 weeks after surgery, depending on surgeon preference. In general, weight bearing with crutches is allowed as tolerated as soon as possible after surgery. The typical initial postsurgical protocol (maximum-protection phase) may be divided into the following phases:

- *Phase I (0–2 weeks):* The goal is to minimize pain and swelling, achieve full extension, recover quadriceps control, and achieve knee flexion to 90 degrees. Modalities to control pain and swelling, such as cryotherapy, elevation, compression, and anti-inflammatory medication, are helpful. The efficacy of continuous passive movement (CPM) after ACL reconstruction is controversial. Quadriceps setting (at 60 and 90 degrees) and straight leg raises (flexion, extension, abduction, and adduction performed in the brace) are useful to reactivate the lower extremity musculature and to help regain full extension. In addition, activities such as prone hangs, supine wall slides, and extension boards can be used to gain the last few degrees of extension. Hamstring setting exercises (at 15, 30, 60, and 90 degrees) and glute sets are also used to initiate a strengthening of these muscles. Co-contraction of the quadriceps and hamstring muscles are performed at 30, 60, and 90 degrees of knee flexion. Patellar mobilizations may be delegated by the supervising physical therapist to prevent patellar tendon shortening or retinacular contracture. The patient is instructed on how to perform the stretches two to three times daily.

- *Phase II (3–5 weeks):* Maintain full extension and increase knee flexion up to full ROM. Stair-climbers and bicycles may be used. Active flexion-extension motions of the knee from 35 degrees to full flexion are emphasized, as are passive flexion-extension motions of the knee without muscle contraction.

- *Phase III (6 weeks):* Increase range of motion and strength in preparation for the moderate-protection phase. In order to progress to this phase, the patient must be able to demonstrate quadriceps and hamstring control, full weight bearing, and a knee range of motion of 0 degrees extension to 120 degrees of flexion.

> **● Key Point** In the first 6 to 12 weeks of rehabilitation, the fixation of the graft rather than the graft itself is the limiting factor for strength in the graft complex. The graft gradually loses strength and is quite fragile during the first 2 months after surgery; at 3 months the tensile strength is less than 50 percent of its original strength. Although graft strength never reaches preoperative levels, full maturation may take as long as a year.

The moderate-protection phase (6–12 weeks) is characterized by proprioceptive and closed-chain activities. Closed-chain activities begin with standing and weight-shifting activities, and leg press exercises performed in a short arc. All exercises are performed while wearing the brace, until permission is given by the physician or supervising physical therapist to remove it. Other exercises introduced at this time are standing wall slides, step ups, stair-steppers, and stationary cycling with the seat height adjusted to accommodate any limitation in knee flexion range of motion. In order to progress to the next phase the patient must demonstrate full range of motion, normalized gait without the brace, and continued improvement of hamstring and quadriceps strength.

The final phase, often referred to as the minimum-protection or functional phase, indicates the patient's return to more challenging functional activities and a gradual resumption of sport as appropriate. During this phase the physician may request isokinetic testing or instrumented stability examinations (arthrometer) of the involved knee.

> **● Key Point** Return to all sports or heavy duty occupations may take 6–9 months and should be closely monitored by the surgeon and physical therapist.

Posterior Cruciate Ligament Tear

Because of its inherent strength, damage to the PCL usually occurs only with significant trauma such as a motor vehicle accident,[109] when landing in a hyperflexed knee position from a jump, or with hyperextension of the knee with the foot planted.[110]

Clinical findings for a PCL tear include pain in the posterior aspect of the knee joint that may be aggravated with kneeling, and minimal swelling. Instability may or may not be present, depending on the severity of the tear.

Many isolated PCL grade I–II injuries heal with conservative intervention because many PCL-deficient patients do not experience functional instability.[111] However, due to the forces needed to rupture the PCL, isolated PCL tears are rare, and most occur with simultaneous injuries to other structures around the knee. The management of patients who have PCL injuries combined with other ligament or capsular injuries is less definitive. In general, rehabilitation after a grade III PCL injury tends to be more conservative than that after ACL injury.

Conservative Intervention

Following a short period of immobilization, the focus of conservative intervention for an isolated PCL injury is to restore ROM and to strengthen the quadriceps, while avoiding positions that encourage posterior displacement of the tibia. Quadriceps strengthening, the foundation of PCL rehabilitation, is performed to help reduce posterior tibial translation.[112] Hamstring strengthening is delayed for approximately 6–8 weeks following the injury to decrease the potential for PCL stress. OKCEs have the potential to exert significant forces on the PCL during flexion exercises in the 60- to 90-degree range. In addition, heavy resistance OKC knee extension exercises through a range of 45–20 degrees place significant stress on the patellofemoral joint.[113,114] Even though throughout the 0- to 60-degree range, minimal or no force appears to be generated in the PCL, the performance of OKCEs should be avoided.

> **● Key Point** During PCL rehabilitation, CKCEs should be performed in the 0- to 45-degree range to help protect both the PCL and the patellofemoral joint, whereas OKC flexion exercises should be avoided.

Important CKCEs used in rehabilitation of the PCL include squats, lunges, and CKC knee extensions. It is important to remember that active CKCEs of any kind, in any ROM, should be used cautiously and should only be carried out in a ROM that limits flexion of the knee to about 45 degrees or less. Balance and proprioceptive exercises also are performed. Plyometrics are introduced for appropriate patients such as athletes. Return to sport may occur in as little as 6–8 weeks, but on average takes 12–16 weeks, provided there are no complicating factors such as significant varus or valgus alignment or damage to additional tissues.

Surgical Intervention

A postoperative knee immobilizer or hinged range-limiting brace is worn until the patient demonstrates quadriceps control, full extension, and full weight bearing. The weight-bearing status is usually weight bearing as tolerated with crutches and the brace locked in extension. Therapeutic exercises during the early postsurgical period include patellar mobilizations, prone passive flexion and extension, quad sets, ankle pumps, calf exercises, standing hip extension from neutral, and straight leg raising (in the locked brace). The next phase begins at around 4 weeks and lasts for a further 8 weeks (12 weeks postsurgery). Criteria for progression to this phase include good quadriceps control, approximately 60 degrees of knee flexion, full knee extension, and no signs of active inflammation. The rehabilitation progression for phases 2 and 3 are outlined in **Table 20-7**. Criteria for progression to phase 2 include full, pain-free range of motion; normal gait; good to normal quadriceps strength; no patellofemoral complaints;

and clearance by physician to begin a more concentrated CKC progression.

Medial Collateral Ligament Injuries

Injury to the medial collateral ligament (MCL) is the most common ligamentous knee injury. The superficial MCL fibers attach proximally to the medial femoral epicondyle and distally to the medial aspect of the tibia, approximately 4 centimeters distal to the joint line. The deep MCL fibers originate from the medial joint capsule and are attached to the medial meniscus. Consequently, the medial meniscus may become injured with a severe MCL sprain. Medial collateral ligament injuries are caused primarily by valgus stress to the knee joint. Injuries also can occur to the MCL with excessive external rotation of the tibia. Noncontact, or indirect, injuries are

TABLE 20-7	Postsurgical PCL Repair Rehabilitation Progression for Phases 2 and 3
Phase 2	**Intervention**
Bracing and weight bearing	Braces unlocked: • At 4 to 6 weeks for control gait training only • At 6 to 8 weeks for all activities • At 8 weeks brace use is discontinued Weight bearing: • At 4 to 8 weeks: As tolerated with crutches • At 8 weeks: Crutches discontinued if patient exhibits full knee extension, knee flexion at 90 to 100 degrees, no quadriceps lag with SLR
Therapeutic exercises	Weeks 4–8: • Wall slides (0–45 degrees) • Mini-squats (0–45 degrees) • Leg press (0– 60 degrees) • SLR in all four planes Weeks 8–12: • Stationary bike (without use of toe clips and seat height slightly higher than normal to minimize hamstring activity) • Balance and proprioception exercises • Seated calf raises • Leg press (0–90 degrees) • Stairmaster/elliptical stepper
Phase 3 (months 3–6)	**Intervention**
Therapeutic exercises	Continuation of closed kinetic chain exercises progression Treadmill walking Swimming (no breaststroke)

Data from D'Amato, M, Bach BR: Knee injuries, in Brotzman SB, Wilk KE (eds): Clinical Orthopaedic Rehabilitation. Philadelphia, Mosby, 2003, pp 251–370

observed with deceleration, cutting, and pivoting motions. Overuse injuries of the MCL have been described in swimmers: the whip-kick technique of the breaststroke involves repetitive valgus loads across the knee. Other structures within the knee may be injured in association with the MCL. These include the ACL, medial meniscus, and extensor mechanism, including the vastus medialis obliquus and retinacular fibers. The most common symptom following an MCL injury is pain directly over the ligament. Swelling over the torn ligament may appear, and bruising and generalized joint swelling are common 1 to 2 days after the injury. In more severe injuries, patients may complain that the knee is unstable. In addition to the history and physical examination results, the PT may use the valgus stress test of the knee (Table 20-5) to help confirm the diagnosis. MCL injuries are graded according to severity (see Chapter 5).

Intervention

The type of physical therapy treatment indicated for an MCL injury depends on the severity of the injury:

- *Grade I:* Compression, elevation, and cryotherapy are recommended. Short-term use of crutches may be indicated, with weight-bearing-as-tolerated (WBAT) ambulation. Early ambulation is recommended.
- *Grade II:* A knee immobilizer or a short-hinged brace that blocks 20 degrees of terminal extension but allows full flexion is typically used. The patient may ambulate, WBAT with crutches. The crutches are discontinued as pain lessens and quadriceps strength increases.
- *Grade III:* The patient initially should be non–weight bearing (NWB) on the affected lower extremity. A hinged brace should be used, with gradual progression to full weight bearing (FWB) over 4 weeks. Grade III injuries may require 8–12 weeks to heal.

All MCL injuries should be treated with early range of motion (ROM) and strengthening of musculature that stabilizes the knee joint (semi-membranosus, vastus medialis, and pes anserine muscles—sartorius, gracilis, and semitendinosus) as tolerated. Ankle pumps are initiated immediately, together with quadriceps strengthening (quad sets, straight leg raises), and progressed to closed-chain exercises as tolerated. The knee immobilizer or brace is removed several times a day for active and passive knee flexion and extension exercises (seated assisted knee flexion and supine wall slides). For the athlete, running is allowed when weight bearing is comfortable, and is progressed to more narrow S-shaped patterns until pivoting is comfortable. At this point, sport-specific exercises and drills are added and advanced until the athlete is ready to return to the sport. Return to play is allowed when sport-specific agility testing is performed comfortably. People with grade I and II injuries usually return to play within 2–3 weeks. People with grade III injuries frequently require 6 or more weeks before a return to play.

Meniscus Injuries

The peripheral, convex borders of the menisci are thick and attach to the joint capsule; the opposite border tapers inward to a thin, free edge centrally. Therefore, menisci have a triangular shape in cross-section. Each covers approximately two-thirds of the corresponding articular surface of the tibia. Studies have demonstrated that 10–30 percent of the periphery of the medial meniscus and 10–25 percent of the lateral meniscus receive a vascular supply; the remainder receives its nutrition from the synovial fluid from passive diffusion and mechanical pumping. The menisci assist in a number of functions, including load transmission, shock absorption, joint lubrication and nutrition, secondary mechanical stability (particularly the posterior horn of the medial meniscus, which blocks anterior translation of the tibia on the femur),[115] and the guiding of movements.[116] Meniscus tears are sometimes related to trauma (twisting or change of position of the weight-bearing knee in varying degrees of flexion or extension), but significant trauma is not necessary— a sudden twist or repeated squatting can tear the meniscus. The classification of meniscal tears provides a description of pathoanatomy. Five types of meniscus tears are recognized: (1) longitudinal tears, (2) radial tears, (3) parrot-beak or oblique flap tears, (4) horizontal tears, and (5) complex tears that combine variants of these (Figure 20-29).

The physical therapist may use a number of special tests (refer to Table 20-5) to help confirm the diagnosis.

The injured meniscus may or may not heal or repair itself, depending on the location of the tear. The natural history of a short (less than 1 centimeter), vascular, longitudinal tear is often one of healing or resolution of symptoms.[95] Meniscus repair is recommended for tears that occur in the vascular region (red zone or red-white zone), are longer than

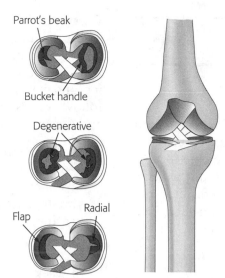

Figure 20-29 Types of meniscus tears.

Parrot's beak

Bucket handle

Degenerative

Flap   Radial

1 centimeter, involve greater than 50 percent of the meniscal thickness, or are unstable to arthroscopic probing.[95]

> **Key Point** The location of a meniscal tear is of paramount importance because tears in the vascular portion of the meniscus, termed the "red zone" (zone I: vascular on both sides of the meniscus), are far more likely to heal than tears in the middle portion of the meniscus, or "red–white zone" (zone II: vascular supply on only one side of the meniscus). The nonvascular, central body of the meniscus, termed the "white zone," does not have the potential to heal.

Conservative Approach

The physical therapy program goals in the acute phase are to minimize the effusion, normalize gait, normalize pain-free range of motion, prevent muscular atrophy, maintain proprioception, and maintain cardiovascular fitness. The rehabilitation program must include consideration of the patient's age, activity level, duration of symptoms, type of meniscus tear, and associated injuries such as ligamentous pathology.

Surgical Intervention

Surgical options include partial meniscectomy or meniscus repair. Arthroscopy, a minimally invasive outpatient procedure with lower morbidity, improved visualization, faster rehabilitation, and better outcomes than open meniscal surgery, is now the standard of care.

> **Key Point** In cases of previous total or subtotal meniscectomy, meniscus transplantation may be used. Human allograft meniscal transplantation is a relatively new procedure but is being performed increasingly frequently.

A stable knee is important for successful meniscus repair and healing. Thus, associated ligamentous injuries must be addressed. The most commonly associated ligamentous disruption is complete tear of the ACL, which must be reconstructed to prevent recurrent meniscal tears.

For partial meniscectomy, patients may return to low-impact or nonimpact workouts such as stationary cycling or straight-leg raising on the first postoperative day, and may advance rapidly to preoperative activities. Many different rehabilitation protocols for meniscal repair are described in the literature. The major difference between a meniscectomy and a meniscus repair is that the surgically repaired meniscus must be allowed to heal by avoiding loads and stresses that compromise the surgical site. A common protocol is avoidance of weight bearing for 4–6 weeks (to avoid axial compressive loads), with knee flexion limited to approximately 90–100 degrees. More aggressive approaches allow full weight bearing with the knee braced and locked in full extension for 6 weeks, while encouraging full motion when the knee is not bearing weight. The following exercises are initiated immediately after surgery: ankle pumps, quadriceps sets, hamstring sets, short arc knee extensions, and straight leg raising in all four planes (flexion, extension, abduction, and adduction). The range of motion exercises, which can include prone knee flexion and supine wall slides, are progressed as tolerated. At 3 to 4 weeks, concentric exercises for the quadriceps and hamstrings are initiated in addition to stationary cycling. CKC exercises are not typically introduced until at least 8 weeks after repair.

Articular Cartilage Defects

Articular cartilage defects of the knee are a common cause of pain and functional disability. Because nonoperative rehabilitation and palliative care for this condition are frequently unsuccessful, many patients opt for surgical procedures designed to facilitate the repair or transplantation of autogenous cartilage tissue.[117] Reparative techniques include:

- *Arthroscopic lavage and debridement:* This procedure is performed to reduce the inflammation and mechanical irritation within a given joint. Debridement can include smoothing of the fibrillated articular or meniscal surfaces, shaving of motion-limiting osteophytes, and removal of inflamed synovium.[118]
- *Microfracture:* A microfracture creates small holes in the subchondral bone, which lacks good blood flow. By penetrating this layer, a microfracture allows the deeper, more vascular bone to access the surface layer. This deeper bone has more blood supply, and the cells can then get to the surface layer and stimulate cartilage growth.[118]
- *Autologous chondrocyte implantation (ACI):* This is a cartilage restorative procedure in which a concentrated solution of autologous chondrocytes is implanted into a defect with the goal of restoring hyaline cartilage to the injured area.[118]
- *Osteochondral autograft transfer (OAT):* Osteochondral autograft is most clearly indicated for a symptomatic, unipolar lesion of the distal femoral condyle in a nondegenerative joint that has proper limb alignment, as well as ligamentous stability and meniscal competence.[118]
- *Osteochondral allograft transplantation:* In contrast to OAT, osteochondral allograft transplantation relies upon tissue taken from cadaveric donors rather than from the patient's own knee. The benefits of allografting include elimination of donor site morbidity and the ability to provide fully formed articular cartilage without specific limitation with respect to defect size. The drawbacks to the procedure are graft availability, cell viability, immunogenicity, and risk of disease transmission.[118]

Intervention

The postsurgical rehabilitation progression is designed based on the four biological phases of cartilage maturation: proliferation, transition, remodeling, and maturation. The duration of each phase that follows varies depending on the lesion, the patient, and the specifics of the surgery:[117]

- *Proliferation phase:* This phase generally lasts 4–6 weeks following surgery. The goals during this phase are to protect the repair, decrease swelling, gradually restore PROM and weight bearing, and enhance volitional control of the quadriceps.
- *Transition phase:* This phase typically consists of weeks 4 through 12 postsurgery. During this phase, the patient progresses from partial to full weight bearing while full ROM and soft tissue flexibility is achieved.[117] It is during this phase in which patients typically resume most normal activities of daily living.
- *Remodeling phase:* This phase generally takes place from 3 to 6 months postoperatively. At this point, the patient typically notes improvement of symptoms and has normal ROM. Low to moderate impact activities, such as bicycle riding, golfing, and recreational walking, are gradually incorporated.
- *Maturation phase:* This phase begins in a range of 4–6 months and can last up to 15–18 months postsurgery. The duration of this phase varies based on lesion size and location, and the specific surgical procedure performed.

Tibiofemoral Osteoarthritis

Osteoarthritis (OA) has been identified as the most common cause of disability in the United States, and often limits a person's ability to rise from a chair, stand comfortably, walk, and use stairs.[119,120]

For many years, OA has been regarded as a "wear-and-tear" or "degenerative" condition, a view supported by epidemiologic surveys that demonstrated associations with certain occupations and life choices, and its increased prevalence with advancing age.[121] Established risk factors include physically demanding occupations, particularly in jobs that involve kneeling or squatting,[122–126] certain sports,[127,128] older age, female sex, evidence of OA in other joints, obesity,[129] and previous injury or surgery of the knee.[130]

Usually, the patient complains of pain with weight-bearing activities and, occasionally, pain at rest. The loss of motion, if present, is typically in a capsular pattern. Muscle weakness is probably the longest recognized and best established correlate of functional limitation in individuals with OA, particularly of the knee OA.[122,131–133]

Conservative Approach

Regular participation in physical activity has been recognized for several years as being beneficial in the management of knee OA.[134–140] Exercises to strengthen the quadriceps are becoming accepted as useful conservative treatment for OA of the knee.[141] Although there is agreement exercise therapy can be helpful, the effect of exercise therapy on pain, quadriceps strength, and physical function appears to be small to moderate in most clinical trials.

In addition to exercises that improve lower extremity strength, ROM, and cardiovascular endurance, it is now being recommended that exercise therapy programs also include techniques to improve balance and coordination, and provide patients with an opportunity to practice various skills that they will likely encounter during normal daily activities.[142]

The conservative intervention for OA of the knee also includes NSAIDs prescribed by the physician, cortisone injections performed by the physician, patient education, weight loss, thermal modalities, and shoe inserts.[141,143] The use of shoes with a well-cushioned sole is recommended, as are frequent rest periods during the day. Wedged insoles with an outward angle of 5–10 degrees on a frontal section have been shown to be helpful for OA of the medial compartment knee.[144,145] The patient is instructed in principles of joint protection, and advised to seek alternatives to prolonged standing, kneeling, and squatting.[141]

Surgical Intervention

There are two common surgical approaches: high tibial osteotomy and total knee arthroplasty.

High Tibial Osteotomy

Because total knee arthroplasty (TKA) is generally contraindicated in younger and more active patients, those with unicompartmental osteoarthritis of the knee may be considered candidates for a high tibial osteotomy or a distal femoral osteotomy. The osteotomy is a mechanical load shifting procedure, whereby the axis of the knee is transferred from the worn compartment to the healthier compartment by surgically creating a wedge into the tibia or femur. The high tibial osteotomy is used with isolated medial compartment arthritis (more common). The distal femoral osteotomy is used in lateral compartment arthritis. The short-term results for these procedures have been very successful,[146,147] even to the point where the need for TKA is eliminated.[148] However, permanent pain relief with high tibial osteotomy is as yet unlikely. Following the procedure, the knee is usually placed in an immobilizer in full extension. The weight-bearing status is guided by the mechanism, type of fixation, and time constraints of bone healing. A typical rehabilitation protocol is outlined in **Table 20-8**.

Total Knee Arthroplasty

Total knee arthroplasty (TKA) has been shown to be an effective long-term intervention for the elderly population to relieve knee pain, improve function, increase social mobility and interaction, and contribute to psychological well-being.[149–151] Although pain and loss of function are the primary reasons for a TKA, the procedure can also be used to correct knee instability and lower extremity alignment and for the treatment of isolated but severe patellofemoral disease.[152,153] The term *tricompartmental* is used to describe the replacement of the degenerated articular surfaces of the tibia, the femur, and the patella. Tricompartmental knee implants (Figure 20-30) can be classified as follows:

- *Unconstrained:* This type of implant, which is rarely used, relies heavily on soft tissue integrity to provide joint stability.
- *Semi-constrained:* Used with the vast majority of patients.
- *Fully constrained:* Provides inhibited motion in one or more planes, which can increase the amount of stress imparted through the implant, resulting in a higher incidence of loosening.

The fate of the PCL in primary TKA is controversial. Retaining the PCL has the potential to restore more normal knee kinematics and better stair climbing ability. If the PCL is sacrificed, a posterior stabilizer is used; however, the long-term results of PCL-retaining and posterior-stabilized TKAs are similar.[154,155]

TABLE 20-8 High Tibial Osteotomy Rehabilitation Protocol

Phase 1 (0–4 weeks)	Intervention
Weight bearing	0–2 weeks: Partial weight bearing (25 percent) with crutches and brace locked in extension
	2–4 weeks: Advanced to full weight bearing with crutches and brace locked in extension
Brace	Locked in full extension for all activities (except when exercising), including sleeping
ROM	Possible use of CPM: performed twice daily (out of brace) for 2 hours from 0 to 90 degrees of flexion
Therapeutic exercises	Heel slides, quad sets, ankle pumps, non–weight-bearing calf/hamstring stretches, straight leg raise (SLR) with brace locked in full extension, resisted plantarflexion
Phase 2 (4–6 weeks)	**Intervention**
Weight bearing	As tolerated with crutches; initiate progression to a normalized gait pattern without crutches
Brace	Unlocked for ambulation and removed for sleeping
ROM	CPM discontinued if knee flexion is at least 90 degrees
Therapeutic exercises	Progression of phase 1 exercises
	SLR without brace if able to maintain full knee extension
	Stationary bike with no resistance and appropriate seat height
Phase 3 (6 weeks to 3 months)	**Intervention**
Weight bearing	Full weight bearing without use of crutches and with normalized gait pattern
Brace	Discontinue use of per physician
ROM	Full and pain-free
Therapeutic exercises	Mini-squats (0 to 45 degrees), progressing to step ups, leg press (0 to 60 degrees), closed-chain terminal knee extensions, toe raises, balance activities, and hamstring curls
	Increase to moderate resistance on stationary bike

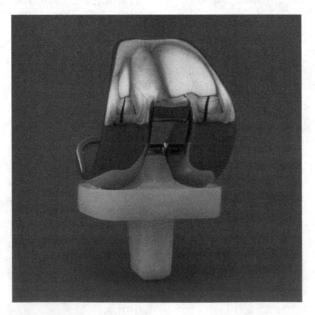

Figure 20-30 Tricompartmental knee implants.

Many early designs of TKA replaced only the tibiofemoral joint and did not address the patellofemoral articulation. The posterior stabilizer was developed to increase the arc of motion of these earlier models and thereby improve the functional results of TKA. Although the ROM improved substantially with these components, patellofemoral complications emerged as a major problem after knee replacement. Errors in sizing, alignment, and rotation of the tibial and femoral component were eventually appreciated as contributing factors to many of these patellofemoral problems. In addition, many of these complications appear to be secondary to patellar resurfacing, which may be a part of the procedure. Whether to resurface the patella remains among the most controversial topics in TKA. Surprisingly high loads are transmitted across the patellofemoral articulation. Following a knee replacement, there is a decrease in the contact area and consequent increase in the contract stress.[156] A study by Matsuda and colleagues[156] showed that resurfacing the patella decreased the contact area to a greater degree compared with not resurfacing the patella. In addition, kinematic studies of motion of the patellofemoral joint after knee replacement have consistently shown some degree of altered kinematics.[157] The success of the rehabilitation program for this patient population is dependent on component design; fixation methods; bone quality; knowledge of the surgical procedure; communication with the surgeon, physical therapist, and patient; and above all, the ability of the rehabilitation team to educate the patient to participate actively in the treatment program.[158]

Complications associated with TKA include the following:[159]

- Thromboembolic disease
- Fat embolism
- Poor wound healing
- Infection
- Periprosthetic fractures

- Neurologic problems; peroneal nerve palsy is the most common neurologic complication of TKA
- Vascular problems; injuries to the superficial femoral, popliteal, and genicular vessels have all been reported following TKA
- Arthrofibrosis
- Disruption of the extensor mechanism

Postoperative rehabilitation for primary TKA continues to be studied in an effort to decrease the cost while still providing the quality of clinical results expected by the surgeon and the patient.[160]

Intervention

A review of the literature reveals inconsistent practice patterns in the physical therapy management of TKA patients.[161] A typical program consists of the following (an accelerated postoperative rehabilitation protocol is outlined in **Table 20-9**):

- Resistive exercises to the uninvolved extremities.
- Deep breathing exercises.
- Proper elevation and positioning of the involved lower extremity.
- Active assisted knee flexion and extension to the involved knee. If CPM is ordered, it is typically applied immediately after surgery in the recovery room to patient's tolerance, so as not to irritate the soft tissue response to the surgery. The patient is encouraged to remain on the unit for 10–12 hours each day, with gradual increases in both extension and flexion ranges as tolerated.
- Ankle pumps, quadriceps sets, gluteal sets, hamstring sets, and heel slides.
- Straight leg raising.[161] During the early days postoperatively, leg raises are limited to the supine and prone positions to prevent the varus and valgus forces associated with hip abduction and adduction in the initial healing phase.[158] Cemented fixation allows for these movements at 2 weeks postsurgery. However, in uncemented knee replacements, hip abduction and adduction are not permitted until 4–6 weeks, pending sufficient bony ingrowth on radiographic examination.[158]
- Seated knee extension.[161]
- Standing knee flexion of the involved leg.

Functional training includes the following:

- Transfer training in and out of bed, from bed to and from a chair, and to and from a commode or elevated toilet seat.

TABLE 20-9 Accelerated Rehabilitation Protocol Following a TKA

Phase 1 (day 1 to 2 weeks)	Intervention
Control of inflammation	Ice, compression, and electrical stimulation
Therapeutic exercise	Initiate isometric and concentric exercises (quad sets, active-assisted SLR, glut sets, short-arc terminal knee extensions)
Ambulation	Knee immobilizer may be used during ambulation until patient is able to perform three to five SLRs in succession out of the immobilizer
	Cemented prosthesis: weight bearing as tolerated with walker
	Noncemented prosthesis: TDWB with walker
Range of motion	Continuous passive motion (if used): Progress 5–10 degrees a day as tolerated
	Initiate active-assisted and active range of motion; ninety degrees of knee flexion is generally considered the minimal requirement for activities of daily living
	Gentle passive range of motion exercises (knee flexion/extension, heel slides, and wall slides)
	Patella mobilizations (3 to 5 days postop)
Phase 2 (10 days to 3 weeks)	**Intervention**
Therapeutic exercise	Continue progression of previous exercises
	General conditioning program as tolerated and as appropriate
Ambulation	Continue use of walker (unless instructed otherwise by physician), emphasizing enhanced gait mechanics
	Driving is not permitted for 4 to 6 weeks postop
Phase 3 (6 weeks)	**Intervention**
Therapeutic exercise	Introduce wall slides and progress to lunges
	Initiate step ups and begin closed-chain knee exercise progression
	Stool walking exercises (if permitted)
	Cone-walking progression from 4- to 6- to 8-inch cones
Ambulation	Begin weight bearing as tolerated with assistive device and progress as appropriate
Range of motion	Stationary bicycle progression

Data from Cameron H, Brotzman, SB: The arthritic lower extremity, in Brotzman SB, Wilk KE (eds): Clinical Orthopaedic Rehabilitation. Philadelphia, Mosby, 2003, pp 441–474

- Gait training, including instruction on weight-bearing status, use of an assistive device, and stair negotiation. Ambulation on different levels can occur by the second or third day, if appropriate.[161] The correct progression of weight bearing is crucial to the overall success of the joint replacement, and depends on the type of fixation and alignment.[158] In patients with porous-coated prostheses, limited weight bearing is essential to allow for sufficient bony ingrowth into the prosthesis, and to prevent loosening of the appliance and premature failure of the surgical alignment.[158] Full weight bearing is generally allowed at 6 weeks, based on a radiographic examination and the patient's body weight.[158]

Manual therapy techniques can include patellar mobilization and soft tissue techniques. Because unrestricted patellofemoral mobility is essential for normal knee motion, mediolateral and superior patellofemoral mobilizations are initiated as early as the second postoperative day.[158]

The patient is discharged from the hospital to home or an extended care facility when medically stable. To be discharged to home, the patient should be able to demonstrate 80–90 degrees of active or active assisted knee motion,[161] transfer supine to sit and sit to stand, ambulate 100 feet, and ascend and descend three steps[162] or more, as the home environment dictates.[161]

If functional independence is required before a patient returns home, the patient is typically transferred to an acute or subacute care setting. If adequate home care and safe transport are available, the patient is allowed to return home.

The outpatient phase of treatment, if appropriate, involves a continued progression of the therapeutic exercise program developed in the inpatient phase with an emphasis on a return to normal activities of daily living and recreational pursuits.

Patellofemoral Pain Syndrome

Patellofemoral pain syndrome is a commonly recognized symptom complex characterized by pain in the vicinity of the patella that is worsened by positions of the knee that result in increased or misdirected mechanical forces between the patella and femur. A number of activities have been identified that increase patellofemoral compression, including inclined walking, jumping, stair climbing, squatting, prolonged sitting with the knee flexed beyond 40 degrees, prolonged kneeling, arising from chairs, prone lying, or standing in genu recurvatum.[17,57]

> ● **Key Point** The *miserable malalignment syndrome* involves a combination of malalignments of the lower kinetic chain that include excess femoral anteversion with internal rotation of the hip, genu valgus, squinting patellae (inward facing), external tibial torsion, and foot pronation.

The patella is a passive component of the knee extensor mechanism, in which the static and dynamic relationships of the underlying tibia and femur determine the patellar-tracking pattern. As the knee flexes, the compression forces between the patella and the femur increase as the contact surface area increases, in an attempt to normalize the contact stress unit load. Lateral tracking of the patella can be caused by intrinsic and extrinsic factors:

- *Intrinsic:* These include an imbalance of forces between the VMO and the vastus lateralis, an adaptively shortened iliotibial band, a tight lateral patella retinaculum, or a decreased slope of the lateral facet on the intercondylar groove of the femur. For example, adaptively shortened hamstrings can antagonize the quadriceps function and increase patellofemoral joint loading.

> ● **Key Point** A medial glide of the patella of less than 5 millimeters (1 quadrant) can indicate a tight retinaculum.

- *Extrinsic:* These include a large Q-angle, weakness of the external rotators or abductors of the hip, and excessive pronation of the foot.

Conservative Intervention

Rehabilitation that includes a combination of painless muscle strengthening, stretching, and patellofemoral taping often is beneficial in creating an internal biomechanical environment that encourages maximal tissue healing.[163] A number of classification systems have been used to categorize individuals with patellofemoral disorders. During the early stages of healing, the patient must try to avoid those activities that are associated with high joint compressive forces, or at least minimize exposure. In the presence of biomechanical dysfunctions of the foot, including pronation, correct footwear must be worn. If the malalignment of the lower extremity is severe, a foot orthosis can be recommended.[46,53] The type of orthosis used is dependent on the diagnosis. Most commonly, an orthosis is used to correct a flat foot so that the patella no longer squints. Foot pronation imparts internal torsion to the tibia and a valgus moment (force) at the knee. In the presence of genu recurvatum, a heel raise can be issued for use during exercise.[164,165]

> ● **Key Point** Klingman and colleagues[166] have shown that medial rearfoot-posted orthoses result in a more medial (aligned) position of the patella during static weight-bearing radiographs.

It remains unclear to what extent there are specific exercises to strengthen the VMO.[10,16,167] In actuality, what may be occurring is that, by changing the mechanics of an exercise, the VMO is placed in a position of enhanced biomechanical advantage rather than becoming stronger. Wilk and colleagues[168] believe that a focus on strengthening of the VMO should occur only if the fibers of the VMO attach onto the patella in a position that can prevent lateralization of the patella dynamically (50–55 degrees). The VMO does not extend the knee and is not, therefore, activated by traditional straight leg raises,[34] even with the addition of adduction.[169] However, because of the relationship of the VMO to the adductor magnus, and its separate nerve supply in most cases,[7] the clinician should still promote adduction of the thigh, while minimizing internal rotation of the hip, to facilitate a VMO contraction.[54]

> **● Key Point** According to Hodges and Richardson,[170] activation of the adductor magnus significantly improves the VMO contraction in weight bearing, but maximum contraction of adductor magnus in non–weight bearing is required before facilitating VMO activity.

The hip external rotators and abductors affect lower limb control, and a strengthening program that addresses these muscle groups should be gradually integrated into the overall progression. For example, weakness of the hip external rotators may allow uncontrolled and excessive pronation of the foot to occur along with excessive femoral internal rotation, both contributing to an increase in the valgus alignment of the knee, thereby increasing the Q-angle.[26] Strengthening of the hip rotators may need to be initiated in the open kinetic chain, but should be advanced to strengthening in the closed kinetic chain as soon as functional muscular control is present.[26]

Exercises during this early phase include:

- Isometric quadriceps sets at 20 degrees of flexion, progressing to multiple angle isometrics.
- Heel slides with the tibia positioned in internal and then external rotation.
- Straight leg raises performed with the thigh externally rotated and the knee flexed to 20 degrees. Performing the exercise in this fashion is reported to allow the least amount of patellofemoral contact force while maximally stressing the vastus medialis component of the quadriceps muscle.[113,171,172] The resistance is progressed from 0 to 5 pounds.
- Straight leg raises performed into abduction with the thigh externally rotated to help isolate the gluteus medius.
- Low-resistance terminal knee extension (short-arc quadriceps) exercises performed with the leg externally rotated from 50 to 20 degrees (Figure 20-31). The resistance is progressed from 0 to 5 pounds.
- Hip adduction exercises performed in the side-lying position on the involved side, with the hip internally rotated and the knee flexed to 20 degrees.[9,173] This position of knee flexion places the patella midway between the two femoral condyles.

Functional exercises that incorporate the entire lower kinetic chain are implemented as soon as tolerated. Kibler[174] advocates the following protocol:

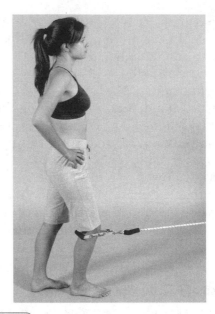

Figure 20-31   Terminal knee extensions.

- Active hip extension and quadriceps activation with the foot flat on the floor or stepping on or off a flat step. This reactivates the normal sequencing pattern for the entire leg.
- Isolation and maximal activation of the quadriceps in a closed-chain position by working with the foot on a slant board, effectively removing the hip and ankle from full activation, but placing maximal load on the slightly flexed knee. Care must be taken not to exercise through pain because this may indicate that muscle control is insufficient.[20]
- Unilateral stance with hip extension, slight knee flexion, and hip and trunk rotation.

The correction of muscle inflexibilities is very important in the rehabilitative process. This activity can be made more challenging using softer surfaces (refer to Figure 20-18).

Stretching of the quadriceps, hip flexors, iliotibial band, lateral retinaculum, hamstrings, and gastrocnemius (**Table 20-10**) are usually initiated during this phase. The rationale for stretching the iliotibial band and lateral retinaculum is well recognized due to their effect on patella position.[36,175,176] Adaptive shortening in the hamstrings and gastrocnemii has been associated with a compensatory pronation.[177] In addition, adaptively shortened hamstrings may cause increased flexion of the knee and increased patellofemoral compression forces, especially during the stance phase of gait.[178]

TABLE 20-10	Muscle Stretching: Positions of Maximal Elongation and Stretch	
Muscle	**Maximal Elongation**	**Stretch**
Gastrocnemius	Subtalar joint neutral, knee extension	Ankle dorsiflexion
Soleus	Subtalar joint neutral, knee flexion	Ankle dorsiflexion
Medial hamstrings	Hip external rotation, abduction, and flexion	Knee extension
Lateral hamstrings	Hip internal rotation and flexion	Knee extension
Rectus femoris	Hip extension	Knee flexion
Tensor fascia lata	Knee flexion, hip extension and external rotation	Hip adduction
Iliotibial band	Hip extension, neutral hip rotation, slight knee flexion	Hip adduction

Taping

The use of tape in the management of patellofemoral disorders was originally proposed by McConnell, whose initial success rate in an uncontrolled study was 96 percent.[36]

The primary goal of taping[179,180] is to pull the patella away from a painful area, thereby unloading it and reducing pain, rather than correcting patellofemoral malalignment.[36,181,182] The extent to which this is possible and the amount of displacement required to provide pain relief varies from patient to patient and from study to study.[10]

A secondary goal of taping is to increase the beneficial proprioceptive characteristics of the patellofemoral joint.[183,184] Grabiner and colleagues[185] have postulated that the VMO needs time to develop force, relative to the VL, to optimally track the patella. This lag time can cause the patella to track laterally. By applying tape across an overly powerful VL, the clinician may be able to change the relative excitation of the VMO and VL, diminishing the pull of the VL,[10,179,180] although the mechanisms by which this works are unknown.

The final goal of taping for malalignment of the patella is to position the patella optimally so that the area of contact between the patella and femur is maximized.[186] This position places the patella parallel to the femur in the frontal and sagittal planes, and the patella is midway between the two condyles when the knee is flexed to 20 degrees.[186]

Once the tape is applied, the clinician assesses:

- The overall limb alignment, including an assessment of the dynamic alignments when walking normally, on the heels, and with the feet in the inverted and everted positions; stair climbing; and squatting
- The effect on functional painful and pain-free ranges

From this information, the patellar position is adjusted by taping. The more obvious deviation is always corrected first. Often, repositioning of the patella involves positioning the patella so that it is approximately midway between the two femoral condyles and parallel with the long axis of the femur. The glide component can be corrected by firmly gliding the patella medially and taping the lateral patellar border (Figure 20-32). The tilt component can be corrected by firm taping from the middle of the patella medially, which lifts the lateral border and provides a passive stretch to the lateral structures. To correct external rotation of the patella, firm taping from the middle inferior pole upward and medially is required. For correction of internal rotation, firm taping from the middle superior pole downward and medially is needed.

In addition to the taping, biofeedback, stretching of the lateral structures, and a home exercise program are recommended. For a more detailed description of the application of the tape, the reader is referred to an excellent book, *The Patella: A Team Approach*.[165]

> ● **Key Point** Taping can also be used with patients who have patellar OA. A controlled clinical trial[187] found that patients achieved significant reduction in pain after medial knee taping to realign the patella.

Patellofemoral Bracing

External patellar supports, which range in complexity from simple straps across the patellar tendon to

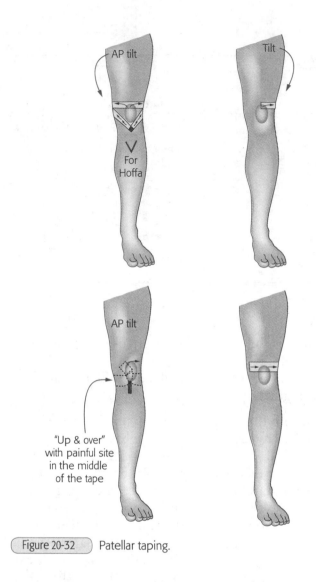

AP tilt

For Hoffa

Tilt

AP tilt

"Up & over" with painful site in the middle of the tape

Figure 20-32 Patellar taping.

complex supports, are commonly employed in the management of patellofemoral pain as an adjunct to other intervention methods. Theoretically, the purpose of the brace is to centralize the patella within the patellar groove, thereby reducing symptoms and improving function.[46,188] Although they relieve symptoms in many patients, their mode of action remains speculative and their effectiveness is unpredictable.[189]

Despite the wide use of patellofemoral bracing, only a few studies have attempted to document its effectiveness in correcting patellar alignment. Although it can be debated whether bracing can influence patellar tracking, it appears that external supports must, in some way, interact mechanically with the patellofemoral joint because many patients report significant clinical improvements.

Surgical Intervention

Surgical intervention may be appropriate in three different patient populations: (1) those with normal anatomy who experience recurrent dislocation or pain, (2) those with an anatomic abnormality, and (3) active young adult patients who have not been helped by 12 months of nonoperative treatment and who have patellar tilt and/or subluxation. Operative choices may be classified into distal (tibial tubercle transfers), proximal (medial repair, lateral release), and combined procedures.

● **Key Point** Rigid, distal procedures are associated with increased rates of progressive retropatellar arthrosis but lower rates of redislocation, whereas dynamic proximal procedures are associated with a lower incidence of arthrosis but a higher risk of redislocation.

The rehabilitation protocol following proximal procedures is essential the same as for the conservative approach following a period of immobilization. However, the rehabilitation protocol for distal procedures is modified based on bone and soft tissue healing, and a period of immobilization in plaster or a hinged range-limiting brace for 4 to 6 weeks. The weight-bearing status is typically non–weight bearing, then touchdown weight bearing, then partial weight bearing, and then weight bearing as tolerated over the weeks of immobilization, so that by 6 weeks the patient is at full weight bearing. Also during this period of immobilization, range of motion exercises, quadriceps, straight leg raises, and short arc quadriceps exercises are introduced as tolerated or by physician preference.

Tendonitis

Patellar tendonitis (jumper's knee) and quadriceps tendonitis are overuse conditions that are frequently associated with eccentric overloading during deceleration activities (e.g., repeated jumping and landing, downhill running).[190]

● **Key Point** The patellar "tendon," which connects two bones, is in fact a ligament, although in clinic practice it is referred to as a tendon—hence *patellar tendonitis*.[191,192]

Overuse is simply a mismatch between stress on a given structure and the ability of that structure to dissipate the forces, resulting in inflammatory changes.[193]

Pain on palpation near the patellar insertion is present in both patellar and quadriceps tendonitis. With patellar tendonitis pain is the first symptom. The pain usually is located in the tendon between the patella and tibial tuberosity. During physical activity, the pain may feel sharp—especially when running or jumping. After a workout or practice, the pain may persist as a dull ache. Quadriceps tendonitis occurs most often as a result of stresses placed on the supporting structures of the knee. Running, jumping, and quick starts and stops contribute to this condition. Pain from quadriceps tendonitis is felt in the area at the distal thigh, just above the patella. The pain is most noticeable during active or resisted knee motions.

Conservative Approach

Reid[194] proposes a protocol based on the severity of the lesion. Grade I lesions, which are characterized by no undue functional impairment and pain only after the activity, are addressed with adequate warm-up before training and ice massage after training. With grade II to III strains, activity modification, localized heating of the area, a detailed flexibility assessment, and an evaluation of athletic techniques are recommended. In addition, a concentric–eccentric program for the anterior tibialis muscle group is prescribed, which progresses into a purely eccentric program as the pain decreases.[195] The patient starts with the foot in full plantarflexion. The clinician applies overpressure on the posterior aspect of the foot, placing the foot into further plantarflexion and stretching the anterior tibialis. The patient is asked to perform a concentric contraction into full dorsiflexion, which is resisted by the clinician. An eccentric contraction is then performed by the patient as the clinician resists the motion from full dorsiflexion to full plantarflexion. This maneuver is repeated to the point of fatigue of the anterior tibialis.[195] As soon as possible, the eccentric loading program is added.

It is not clear why a program initially directed at the anterior tibialis muscle group should be therapeutic for the infrapatellar tendon and ligament, but it is theorized that the program may stretch the infrapatellar ligament, change the quadriceps-to-foreleg strength ratio, or alter the biomechanics of take-off and landing.[194]

Surgical Intervention

Surgical intervention is usually required only if significant tendonosis develops; it is successful in the majority of patients.[196]

Patellar Fractures

Fractures of the patella occur as a result of a compressive force such as a direct blow, a sudden tensile force as occurs with hyperflexion of the knee, or from a combination of these. A variety of fracture patterns result, depending on the mechanism of injury. The primary types include transverse (most common), vertical, marginal, and osteochondral fractures. Fractures can be displaced or nondisplaced. A fracture of the patella should be considered when the patient presents with persistent patellar tenderness and pain or a joint effusion and a history of a direct injury to the kneecap.

Intervention

Patella fractures can become problematic if the extensor mechanism of the knee is nonfunctional, articular congruity is lost, or stiffness of the knee joint ensues. To avoid these problems, anatomic restoration of the joint that allows early motion must be achieved.

Nondisplaced

If the fracture is not displaced and the extensor mechanism is intact, the fracture may be treated with immobilization. This usually involves placing the affected extremity in a cylinder cast for 4–6 weeks. The patient is allowed to bear weight in the cast. Once radiographic evidence indicates union and once clinical signs of healing (nontender to palpation) are present, the patient is prescribed a removable brace. A hinged knee brace is used while ambulating. A program emphasizing range of motion and strengthening is then implemented. Once the patient is able to perform a straight leg raise without extensor lag and has greater than 90 degrees of knee flexion, brace use may be discontinued.

Displaced

Displaced patellar fractures warrant surgical treatment to maximize the potential for successful outcomes. In rare cases, a partial patellectomy or total patellectomy must be performed. Postoperative rehabilitation is dependent on the fracture pattern, stability of fixation, and status of the soft tissue. Early range of motion may be initiated if the fracture pattern allowed for stable fixation and no wound problems exist. However, comminuted fractures with less than optimal fixation should be monitored closely for stability and progressive signs of radiographic healing. Direct communication between the surgeon and the PT by the PTA is essential to ensure proper rehabilitation. It is essential that the patient understands the importance of attaining and maintaining full knee extension. The patient should avoid using pillows under the knee; rather, a heel roll or towel should be placed to allow gravity to act on the knee when in supine.

Supracondylar Femur Fractures

The distal femur is funnel shaped, and the area where the stronger diaphyseal bone meets the thinner and weaker metaphyseal bone is more prone to fracture. Supracondylar femur fractures usually occur as a result of low-energy trauma in osteoporotic bone in elderly persons or high-energy trauma in young patients. Supracondylar femur fractures may also occur after total knee replacement. Surgical therapy requires reduction followed by fixation to maintain alignment. Options include external fixation or internal fixation. Internal fixation is with intramedullary devices (e.g., flexible rods, more rigid retrograde or antegrade rods) or extramedullary plates and screws.

Intervention

If the fixation is solid and bone quality is good, some patients can be allowed early weight bearing and motion, especially when intramedullary fixation is used. If bone quality is good but not enough to allow early weight bearing, the patient may be placed in a hinged knee brace to allow early motion but kept off full weight bearing until radiographs show bone healing (at about 12 weeks). If bone quality is poor, more rigid splinting may be required for about 6 weeks and then the patient may be switched to a hinged brace.

Tibial Plateau Fractures

The tibial plateau is one of the most critical load-bearing areas in the human body. The most common mechanism resulting in a tibial plateau fracture is a valgus force with axial loading, or a twisting injury. Soft tissue injuries (e.g., to cruciate and collateral ligaments) occur in approximately 10 percent of patients. In addition, medial plateau injuries may result in fracture of the fibular head, which may injure the peroneal nerve or may be associated with popliteal artery occlusion. Not all tibial plateau fractures require surgery. Treatment of these fractures is governed by the vascularity (local tissue and distal), the condition of soft tissues, and the presence or absence of compartment syndrome.

Intervention

Recovering range of motion is a challenge for patients who are unable to actively participate in rehabilitation, have soft-tissue injuries that preclude immediate range of motion, and have had external-fixation pins inserted near their quadriceps. Every effort should be made to avoid a chronic knee flexion contracture after surgery. Typically, these patients are placed in a hinged knee brace that is locked in extension. Motion is restricted until surgical and traumatic wounds are dry. Continuous passive motion is typically prescribed when wounds are dry, with the goal of full extension and 90 degrees of flexion within 5–7 days. If other injuries allow, the patient is mobilized with a hinged brace locked in extension for 6 weeks. Non–weight-bearing precautions generally continue for 12 weeks. Active flexion and passive extension are encouraged for 6 weeks, after which active knee extension is started. Active knee extension is delayed if open reduction and internal fixation of a tibial tubercle avulsion was required.

Osgood Schlatter Disease

Osgood Schlatter disease is described in Chapter 22.

Therapeutic Techniques

A number of therapeutic techniques can be used to assist the patient. These include self-stretches, soft tissue techniques, and selective manual techniques.

Self-Stretching

To increase extension:

- *Towel hyperextensions:* A towel of sufficient height to elevate the calf and thigh off the table is placed under the heel (Figure 20-33). A weight can be added to the anterior tibia or femur to assist in regaining hyperextension at the knee.
- *Prone hangs:* See Figure 20-34 .
- *Quadriceps setting:* These exercises are done repeatedly during the day and can also be performed during the towel extension exercise.

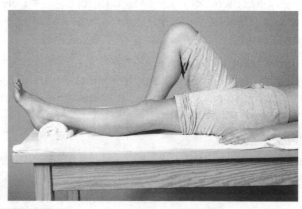

Figure 20-33   Towel hyperextensions.

To increase flexion:

- Wall slides in supine are performed until 90 degrees of flexion is obtained, and then seated heel slides with passive overpressure are initiated.
- Heel slides (refer to Figure 20-9) with a belt or sheet around the ankle are performed.

Techniques to Increase Soft Tissue Extensibility

Stretching

Increasing soft tissue extensibility is the hallmark of the functional knee rehabilitation protocol and includes stretching of the iliotibial band, hamstring muscles, quadriceps, hip flexors (see Chapter 19 for all four), and Achilles-soleus complex[168,179] (Figure 20-35).

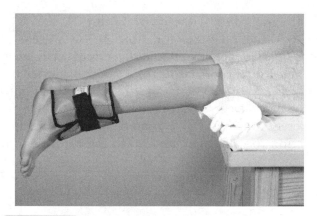

Figure 20-34 Prone hangs.

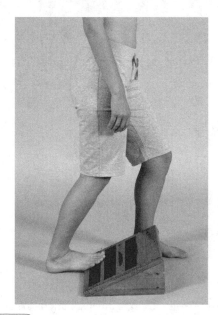

Figure 20-35 Soleus stretch.

Deep Massage of the Iliotibial Band

The patient is placed in the side-lying position, with the uppermost leg flexed at the hip to approximately 80 degrees, facing away from the clinician (Figure 20-36). Using the thumbs of both hands, the clinician places them at the distal end of the ITB and then applies deep pressure in a superior direction, following the path of the ITB. The deep stroke is repeated several times, and the flexibility of the ITB is reassessed. The clinician can also use the knuckle of the middle finger or the point of the elbow to apply the deep pressure, although care should be taken to avoid applying too much force.

Deep Massage of the Hamstring Area

The patient is positioned prone, with the leg supported. Using one elbow, the clinician applies a series of vertical strokes along the hamstrings (Figure 20-37). The clinician can also use the knuckle of the middle finger to apply the deep pressure.

Selective Joint Mobilizations

The various joint mobilizations techniques are described in Chapter 6.

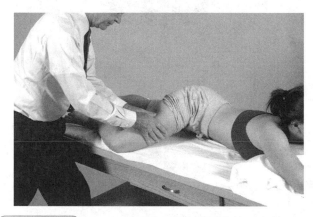

Figure 20-36 Deep massage of the iliotibial band.

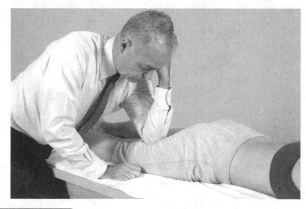

Figure 20-37 Deep massage of the hamstrings.

Patellar

Patellar mobilizations are advocated to be performed in a variety of directions to increase the mobility of the patella, presumably to allow it to track better. These include superior, inferior, and medial and lateral glides (Figure 20-38). The knee is placed in the open-packed position for the patellofemoral joint (extension) and the patella is moved in the desired direction. However, from an evidence-based perspective, at present there is not one randomized study supporting the efficacy of patellofemoral mobilizations in the treatment of patellofemoral disorders.

Posterior Glide of the Tibia on the Femur

The patient is positioned in supine with the knee flexed and the foot resting on the table. Grasping the proximal tibia, the clinician applies a posterior force (Figure 20-39). This technique is used to increase the joint glide associated with flexion of the tibiofemoral joint. In the midranges of flexion, the posterior glide of the tibia is applied along the plane of the joint, whereas in the last few degrees of flexion, the posterior glide is applied with the congruent rotation of internal rotation of the tibia. Active mobilization can also be employed by positioning the patient's foot and leg into internal rotation, and asking the patient to pull isometrically with the hamstrings.

Anterior Glide of the Tibia on the Femur

The patient is positioned in supine with the knee flexed and the foot resting on the table. Grasping the proximal tibia, the clinician pulls the tibia in an anterior direction. This technique is used to increase the joint glide associated with extension of the tibiofemoral joint. If the clinician is attempting to regain the last 10–30 degrees of extension, the emphasis is placed on positioning the tibia in external rotation and applying a posterior glide of the femur, thereby addressing the conjunct rotation.

Distraction of the Tibiofemoral Joint

Joint distraction is used for pain control and general mobility. Distraction at this joint tends to occur when moving into flexion. Using the resting position of the joint as a starting point, and the tibia rotated into either neutral, external rotation, or internal rotation, different ranges of flexion can be used. A long-axis traction force is then applied to the tibiofemoral joint (Figure 20-40).

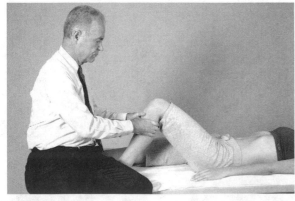

Figure 20-38   Patellar glides.

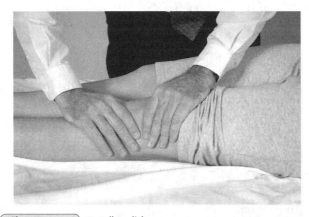

Figure 20-39   Anterior/posterior glide of the tibia on the femur.

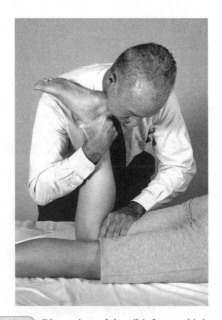

Figure 20-40   Distraction of the tibiofemoral joint.

Summary

The knee joint complex is extremely elaborate and includes three articulating surfaces, which form two distinct joints contained within a single joint capsule: the patellofemoral and tibiofemoral joint. The knee is one of the most commonly injured joints in the body. The types of knee injuries seen clinically can be generalized into the following categories:

- Unspecified sprains or strains, and other minor injuries, including overuse injuries
- Contusions
- Meniscal or ligamentous injuries

It is important that the PTA be familiar with the anatomy and kinesiology of this joint complex, to be able to apply the therapeutic procedures appropriate for all of the categories of injury. It is also important that the PTA has an awareness that thigh, knee, and calf pain can result from a broad spectrum of conditions.

REVIEW Questions

1. Which three tendons form the pes anserine?
2. Which muscle unlocks the fully extended knee?
3. In the knee, which of the two menisci is more prone to injury?
4. What is the primary function of the posterior cruciate ligament?
5. Which muscles act as the secondary restraint for the anterior cruciate ligament?
6. Which gender and age range tend to suffer more from patellofemoral dysfunction?
7. Strengthening of which muscle is used to help with patellofemoral dysfunction?
8. Which of the following structures of the knee joint is primarily responsible for preventing anterior movement of the tibia on the femur?
   a. Medial collateral ligaments
   b. Posterior cruciate ligament
   c. Anterior cruciate ligament
   d. Quadriceps tendon
9. An osteotomy is:
   a. Operative sectioning of a bone
   b. Fusion of a joint
   c. A bag that collects fluid from the surgical site
   d. A form of debridement

10. You are treating a patient with a history of knee trauma. There is marked swelling of the knee joint, the tibia can be displaced forward on the femur, and there is pain and marked instability of the knee joint. Which of the following structures are likely to be involved?
    a. Medial collateral ligament
    b. Lateral collateral ligament
    c. Anterior cruciate ligament
    d. Posterior cruciate ligament
11. During your assessment you notice that the patient cannot fully extend his knee while positioned in supine with the foot dorsiflexed and the hip flexed first to 60 degrees and then 90 degrees. The tightness is most likely caused by the:
    a. Hamstrings
    b. Gastrocnemius
    c. Hip flexors
    d. None of the above
12. The patient has complained of pain and discomfort with knee flexion greater than 80 degrees. The most appropriate treatment program for this patient would include moist heat for 20 minutes followed by:
    a. Immediate static, progressive stretching just beyond tissue resistance with a 30- to 60-second stretch
    b. Immediate static stretching at end range with a 10- to 20-second stretch
    c. Immediate ballistic stretching with 10 passive stretches to end range, repeat two sets
    d. Three repetitions of hold/relax with a 30-second hold and 10-second relax with stretch at end range
13. An 18-year-old basketball player is undergoing rehabilitation status post left knee anterior cruciate reconstruction. The orthopedic surgeon utilized a bone-patellar tendon-bone graft and has ordered that an accelerated rehabilitation protocol be utilized to restore function to the athlete's lower extremities. The best description regarding the positive impact of utilizing closed kinetic chain exercises as part of an accelerated rehabilitation protocol is that it:
    a. Promotes the functional recruitment of motor units
    b. Facilitates long axis distraction of the joint
    c. Enhances functional movement in the transverse plane
    d. Creates shear forces at the articular level

14. A physical therapist assistant is preparing to treat a patient with an injury to the posterior knee that crushed the tibial nerve. The PT evaluation identifies both motor and sensory involvement. The PTA would expect the patient to present with:

a. Decreased muscle tone of the knee flexors, as well as paresthesia of the posterior thigh and knee

b. Increased muscle tone and spasticity of the knee flexors, as well as absent sensation over the posterior thigh area

c. Increased muscle tone and spasticity of the plantarflexors and invertors of the ankle, as well as absent sensation over the posterior calf and plantar surface of the foot

d. Decreased muscle tone of the plantarflexors and invertors of the ankle, as well as paresthesia of the posterior calf and plantar surface of the foot.

15. A 56-year-old male has just undergone a total knee replacement secondary to severe degenerative joint disease. In the recovery room, a continuous passive movement (CPM) machine has been applied. All of the following are benefits of CPM, except:

a. Increase strength

b. Increase range of motion

c. Decrease risk of a deep vein thrombosis

d. Decrease postoperative pain

References

1. Dye SF: An evolutionary perspective of the knee. J Bone Joint Surg 69A:976–983, 1987
2. Davids JR: Pediatric knee. Clinical assessment and common disorders. Pediatr Clin North Am 43:1067–1090, 1996
3. Wojtys EM, Huston LJ: Neuromuscular performance in normal and anterior cruciate ligament-deficient lower extremities. Am J Sports Med 22:89–104, 1994
4. Frank CB, Jackson DW: The science of reconstruction of the anterior cruciate ligament. J Bone Joint Surg 79:1556–1576, 1997
5. Kendall FP, McCreary EK, Provance PG: Muscles: Testing and Function. Baltimore, Williams & Wilkins, 1993
6. Grelsamer RP, McConnell J: Normal and abnormal anatomy of the extensor mechanism, in Grelsamer RP, McConnell J (eds): The Patella: A Team Approach. Gaithersburg, MD, Aspen, 1998, pp 11–24
7. Lieb F, Perry J: Quadriceps function. J Bone Joint Surg [Am] 50:1535, 1968
8. Hallisey MJ, Doherty N, Bennett WF, et al: Anatomy of the junction of the vastus lateralis tendon and the patella. J Bone Joint Surg [Am] 69, 1987
9. Bose K, Kanagasuntheram R, Osman MBH: Vastus medialis oblique: An anatomic and physiologic study. Orthopedics 3:880–883, 1980
10. Grelsamer RP: Patellar malalignment. J Bone Joint Surg [Am] 82A:1639–1650, 2000
11. Koskinen SK, Kujala UM: Patellofemoral relationships and distal insertion of the vastus medialis muscle: A magnetic resonance imaging study in nonsymptomatic subjects and in patients with patellar dislocation. Arthroscopy 8:465–468, 1992
12. Raimondo RA, Ahmad CS, Blankevoort L, et al: Patellar stabilization: A quantitative evaluation of the vastus medialis obliquus muscle. Orthopedics 21:791–795, 1998
13. Nakamura Y, Ohmichi H, Miyashita M: EMG relationship during maximum voluntary contraction of the quadriceps, IX Congress of the International Society of Biomechanics. Waterloo, Ontario, 1983
14. Knight KL, Martin JA, Londerdee BR: EMG comparison of quadriceps femoris activity during knee extensions and straight leg raises. Am J Phys Med 58:57–69, 1979
15. Brownstein BA, Lamb RL, Mangine RE: Quadriceps torque and integrated electromyography. J Orthop Sports Phys Ther 6:309–314, 1985
16. Fox TA: Dysplasia of the quadriceps mechanism: Hypoplasia of the vastus medialis muscle as related to the hypermobile patella syndrome. Surg Clin North Am 55:199–226, 1975
17. Tria AJ, Palumbo RC, Alicia JA: Conservative care for patellofemoral pain. Orthop Clin North Am 23:545–554, 1992
18. Reynolds L, Levin TA, Medeiros JM, et al: EMG activity of the vastus medialis oblique and the vastus lateralis in their role in patellar alignment. Am J Sports Med 62:62–70, 1983
19. Moller BN, Krebs B, Tideman-Dal C, et al: Isometric contractions in the patellofemoral pain syndrome. Arch Orthop Trauma Surg 105:24, 1986
20. Reid DC: Anterior knee pain and the patellofemoral pain syndrome, in Reid DC (ed): Sports Injury Assessment and Rehabilitation. New York, Churchill Livingstone, 1992, pp 345–398
21. Larson RL, Jones DC: Dislocations and ligamentous injuries of the knee, in Rockwood CA, Green DP (eds): Fractures in Adults (ed 2). Philadelphia, JB Lippincott, 1984, pp 1480–1591
22. Gill DM, Corbacio EJ, Lauchle LE: Anatomy of the knee, in Engle RP (ed): Knee Ligament Rehabilitation. New York, Churchill Livingstone, 1991, pp 1–15
23. O'Connor JJ: Can muscle co-contraction protect knee ligaments after injury or repair? J Bone Joint Surg 75B:41–48, 1993
24. Fleming BC, Renstrom PA, Goran O, et al: The gastrocnemius muscle is an antagonist of the anterior cruciate ligament. J Orthop Res 19:1178–1184, 2001
25. Evans P: The postural function of the iliotibial tract. Ann Royal Coll Surg Engl 61:271–280, 1979
26. Pease BJ, Cortese M: Anterior knee pain: Differential diagnosis and physical therapy management, Orthopaedic Physical Therapy Home Study Course 92-1. La Crosse, WI, Orthopaedic Section, American Physical Therapy Association, 1992

27. Jackson-Manfield P, Neumann DA: Structure and function of the knee, in Jackson-Manfield P, Neumann DA (eds): Essentials of Kinesiology for the Physical Therapist Assistant. St Louis, MO, Mosby Elsevier, 2009, pp 273–304

28. Ahmed AM, Burke DL, Hyder A: Force analysis of the patellar mechanism. J Orthop Res 5:69–85, 1987

29. van Kampen A, Huiskes R: The three-dimensional tracking pattern of the human patella. J Orthop Res 8:372–382, 1990

30. Woodland LH, Francis RS: Parameters and comparisons of the quadriceps angle of college aged men and women in the supine and standing positions. Am J Sports Med 20:208–211, 1992

31. Olerud C, Berg P: The variation of the quadriceps angle with different positions of the foot. Clin Orthop 191:162–165, 1984

32. Rand JA: The patellofemoral joint in total knee arthroplasty. J Bone Joint Surg [Am] 76:612–620, 1994

33. Steinkamp LA, Dilligham MF, Markel MD, et al: Biomechanical considerations in patellofemoral joint rehabilitation. Am J Sports Med 21:438–444, 1993

34. Soderberg G, Cook T: An electromyographic analysis of quadriceps femoris muscle settings and straight leg raising. Phys Ther 63:1434, 1983

35. Henry JH, Crosland JW: Conservative treatment of patellofemoral subluxation. Am J Sports Med 7:12–14, 1979

36. McConnell J: The management of chondromalacia patellae: A long-term solution. Austr J Physiother 32:215–223, 1986

37. Reid DC: The myth, mystic and frustration of anterior knee pain [editorial]. Clin J Sports Med 3:139–143, 1993

38. Shelton GL: Conservative management of patellofemoral dysfunction. Prim Care 19:331–350, 1992

39. Hilyard A: Recent advances in the management of patellofemoral pain: The McConnell programme. Physiotherapy 76:559–565, 1990

40. Kujala UM: Patellofemoral problems in sports medicine. Ann Chir Gynaecol 80:219–223, 1991

41. Garrick JG: Anterior knee pain (chondromalacia patella). Phys Sportsmed 17:75–84, 1989

42. Fulkerson JP, Shea KP: Current concepts review: Disorders of patellofemoral alignment. J Bone Joint Surg Am 72:1424–1429, 1990

43. Levine J: Chondromalacia patellae. Phys Sportsmed 7:41–49, 1979

44. Paulos L, Rusche K, Johnson C, et al: Patellar malalignment: A treatment rationale. Phys Ther 60:1624–1632, 1980

45. O'Neill DB: Arthroscopically assisted reconstruction of the anterior cruciate ligament. J Bone Joint Surg 78A:803–813, 1996

46. Palumbo PM: Dynamic patellar brace: A new orthosis in the management of patellofemoral pain. Am J Sports Med 9:45–49, 1981

47. Walsh WM, Helzer-Julin M: Patellar tracking problems in athletes. Prim Care 19:303–330, 1992

48. Whitelaw GP, Rullo DJ, Markowitz HD, et al: A conservative approach to anterior knee pain. Clin Orthop 246:234–237, 1989

49. Gerrard B: The patello-femoral pain syndrome: A clinical trial of the McConnell programme. Austral J Physiother 35:71–80, 1989

50. Gilleard W, McConnell J, Parsons D: The effect of patella taping on the onset of vastus medialis obliquus and vastus lateralis muscle activity in persons with patellofemoral pain. Phys Ther 78:25–32, 1998

51. Bohannon RW: The effect of electrical stimulation to the vastus medialis muscle in a patient with chronically dislocating patella. Phys Ther 63:1445–1447, 1983

52. Mariani P, Caruso I: An electromyographic investigation of subluxation of the patella. J Bone Joint Surg [Br] 61:169, 1979

53. Villar RN: Patellofemoral pain and the infrapatellar brace: A military view. Am J Sports Med 13:313, 1985

54. Grelsamer RP, McConnell J: Conservative management of patellofemoral problems, in Grelsamer RP, McConnell J (eds): The Patella: A Team Approach. Gaithersburg, MD, Aspen, 1998, pp 109–118

55. Chu DA: Rehabilitation of the lower extremity. Clin Sports Med 14:205–222, 1995

56. Lehman RC, Host JV, Craig R: Patellofemoral dysfunction in tennis players. A dynamic problem. Clin J Sports Med 14:177–205, 1995

57. Bourne MH, Hazel WA, Scott SG, et al: Anterior knee pain. Mayo Clinic Proc 63:482–491, 1988

58. Cahill BR, Griffith EH: Effect of preseason conditioning on the incidence and severity of high school football knee injuries. Am J Sports Med 6:180–184, 1978

59. Klein W, Shah N, Gassen A: Arthroscopic management of postoperative arthrofibrosis of the knee joint: Indication, technique, and results. Arthroscopy 10:591–597, 1994

60. Escamilla RF, Fleisig GS, Zheng N, et al: Biomechanics of the knee during closed kinetic chain and open kinetic chain exercises. Med Sci Sports Exerc 30:556–569, 1998

61. Thomeé R: A comprehensive treatment approach for patellofemoral pain syndrome in young women. Phys Ther 77:1690–1703, 1997

62. Flynn TW, Soutas-Little RW: Patellofemoral joint compressive forces in forward and backward running. J Orthop Sports Phys Ther 21:277–282, 1995

63. Arendt E, Dick R: Knee injury patterns among men and women in collegiate basketball and soccer. NCAA data and review of literature. Am J Sports Med 23:694–701, 1995

64. Bjordal JM, Arnly F, Hannestad B, et al: Epidemiology of anterior cruciate ligament injuries in soccer. Am J Sports Med 25:341–345, 1997

65. Huston LJ, Greenfield ML, Wojtys EM: Anterior cruciate ligament injuries in the female athlete. Potential risk factors. Clin Orthop Relat Res 372:50–63, 2000

66. Shambaugh JP, Klein A, Herbert JH: Structural measures as predictors of injury in basketball players. Med Sci Sports Exerc 23:522–527, 1991

67. Muneta T, Takakuda K, Yamomoto H: Intercondylar notch width and its relation to the configuration of cross-sectional area of the anterior cruciate ligament. Am J Sports Med 25:69–72, 1997

68. Grana WA, Moretz JA: Ligamentous laxity in secondary school athletes. JAMA 240:1975–1976, 1978

69. Hutchinson MR, Ireland ML: Knee injuries in female athletes. Sports Med 19:288–302, 1995

70. Huston LJ, Wojtys EM: Neuromuscular performance characteristics in elite female athletes. Am J Sports Med 24:427–436, 1996

71. Liu SH, Al-Shaikh RA, Panossian V, et al: Estrogen affects the cellular metabolism of the anterior cruciate ligament. A potential explanation for female athletic injury. Am J Sports Med 25:704–709, 1997

72. Slauterbeck JR, Narayan RS, Clevenger C, et al: Effects of estrogen level on the tensile properties of the rabbit anterior cruciate ligament. J Orthop Res 17:405–408, 1999

73. Ireland ML: The female ACL: Why is it more prone to injury? Orthop Clin North Am 33:637–651, 2002

74. Griffin JW, Tooms RE, Zwaag RV, et al: Eccentric muscle performance of elbow and knee muscle groups in untrained men and women. Med Sci Sports Exerc 25:936–944, 1993

75. Hakkinen K, Kraemer WJ, Newton RU: Muscle activation and force production during bilateral and unilateral concentric and isometric contractions of the knee extensors in men and women at different ages. Electromyogr Clin Neurophysiol 37:131–142, 1997

76. Kanehisa H, Okuyama H, Ikegawa S, et al: Sex difference in force generation capacity during repeated maximal knee extensions. Eur J Appl Physiol 73:557–562, 1996

77. Miller AEJ, MacDougall JD, Tarnopolsky MA, et al: Gender differences in strength and muscle fiber characteristics. Eur J Appl Physiol 66:254–262, 1993

78. Arnoczky SP: Anatomy of the anterior cruciate ligament, in Urist MR (ed): Clinical Orthopedics and Related Research. Philadelphia, JB Lippincott, 1983, pp 19–20

79. Cabaud HE: Biomechanics of the anterior cruciate ligament, in Urist MR (ed): Clinical Orthopedics and Related Research. Philadelphia, JB Lippincott, 1983, pp 26–30

80. Feagin J, J.A., Lambert KL: Mechanism of injury and pathology of anterior cruciate ligament injuries. Orthop Clin North Am 16:41–45, 1985

81. Stanish WD, Lai A: New concepts of rehabilitation following anterior cruciate reconstruction. Clin Sports Med 12:25–58, 1993

82. Liu SH, Osti L, Henry M, et al: The diagnosis of acute complete tears of the anterior cruciate ligament. J Bone Joint Surg 77:586, 1995

83. Gerber C, Hoppeler H, Claassen H, et al: The lower-extremity musculature in chronic symptomatic instability of the anterior cruciate ligament. J Bone Joint Surg 67A:1034–1043, 1985

84. Kariya Y, Itoh M, Nakamura T, et al: Magnetic resonance imaging and spectroscopy of thigh muscles in cruciate ligament insufficiency. Acta Orthop Scand 60:322–325, 1989

85. Lorentzon R, Elmqvist LG, Sjostrom M, et al: Thigh musculature in relation to chronic anterior cruciate ligament tear: Muscle size, morphology, and mechanical output before reconstruction. Am J Sports Med 17:423–429, 1989

86. Noyes FR, Mangine RE, Barber S: Early knee motion after open and arthroscopic anterior cruciate ligament reconstruction. Am J Sports Med 15:149–160, 1987

87. Yasuda K, Ohkoshi Y, Tanabe Y, et al: Quantitative evaluation of knee instability and muscle strength after anterior cruciate ligament reconstruction using patellar and quadriceps tendon. Am J Sports Med 20:471–475, 1992

88. Daniel DM, et al: Fate of the ACL-injured patient. Am J Sports Med 22:642, 1994

89. Williams JS, Bernard RB: Operative and nonoperative rehabilitation of the ACL-injured knee. Sports Med Arth Rev 4:69–82, 1996

90. Keays SL, Bullock-Saxton J, Keays AC: Strength and function before and after anterior cruciate ligament reconstruction. Clin Orthop Relat Res 373:174–183, 2000

91. Hefzy MS, Grood ES: Ligament restraints in anterior cruciate ligament-deficient knees, in Jackson DW, Arnoczky SP, Woo SL-Y, et al (eds): The Anterior Cruciate Ligament. Current and Future Concepts. New York, Raven Press, 1993, pp 141–151

92. Levy IM, Torzilli PA, Warren RF: The effect of medial meniscectomy on anterior-posterior motion of the knee. J Bone Joint Surg [Am] 64A:883–888, 1982

93. Daniel DM, Stone ML, Dobson BE, et al: Fate of the ACL-injured patient. A prospective outcome study. Am J Sports Med 22: 632–644, 1994

94. Ferretti A, Conteduca F, De Carli A, et al: Osteoarthritis of the knee after ACL reconstruction. Int Orthop 15: 367–371, 1991

95. Henning CE: Current status of meniscal salvage. Clin Sports Med 9:567–576, 1990

96. Shirakura K, Terauchi M, Kizuki S, et al: The natural history of untreated anterior cruciate tears in recreational ahtletes. Clin Orthop 317:227–236, 1995

97. Sommerlath K, Lysholm J, Gillquist J: The long-term course after treatment of acute anterior cruciate ligament ruptures. A 9 to 16 year followup. Am J Sports Med 19:156–162, 1991

98. Janarv PM, Nystrom A, Werner S, et al: Anterior cruciate ligament injuries in skeletally immature patients. J Pediatr Orthop 16:673, 1996

99. Parker AW, Drez D, Cooper JL: Anterior cruciate injuries in patients with open physes. Am J Sports Med 22:47, 1994

100. Busch MT: Sports medicine, in Morrissey RT, Weinstein SL (eds): Lovell and Winter's Pediatric Orthopedics (ed 4). Philadelphia, JB Lippincott, 1996, pp 886, 889

101. Micheli LJ, Jenkins M: Knee injuries, in Micheli LJ (ed): The Sports Medicine Bible. Scranton, PA, Harper Row, 1995, pp 118–151

102. Koenig VS, Barrett GR: Endoscopic anterior cruciate ligament reconstruction. Todays OR Nurse 18:6, 1995

103. Moyen B, Lerat JL: Artificial ligaments for anterior cruciate replacement. J Bone Joint Surg 76:173, 1994

104. Branch TP, Hunter R, Donath M: Dynamic EMG analysis of anterior cruciate deficient legs with and without bracing during cutting. Am J Sports Med 17:35–41, 1989

105. Beynnon BD, Good L, Risberg MA: The effect of bracing on proprioception of knees with anterior cruciate ligament injury. J Orthop Sports Phys Ther 32:11–15, 2002

106. Fleming BC, Renstrom PA, Beynnon BD, et al: The influence of functional knee bracing on the anterior cruciate ligament strain biomechanics in weightbearing and nonweightbearing knees. Am J Sports Med 28:815–824, 2000

107. Liu SH, Daluiski A, Kabo JM: The effects of thigh soft tissue stiffness on the control of anterior tibial displacement by functional knee orthoses. J Rehabil Res Dev 32:135–140, 1995

108. Barrett DS, Cobb AG, Bentley G: Joint proprioception in normal, osteoarthritic and replaced knees. J Bone Joint Surg 73B:53–56, 1991

109. Trickey EL: Injuries to the PCL: Diagnosis and treatment of early injuries and reconstruction of late instability. Clin Orthop 147:76–81, 1980

110. Insall JN, Hood RW: Bone block transfer of the medial head of the gastrocnemius for posterior cruciate insufficiency. J Bone Joint Surg 65A:691–699, 1982

111. Harner CD, Hoher J: Evaluation and treatment of posterior cruciate ligament injuries. Am J Sports Med 26:471–482, 1998

112. Tibone JE, Antich TJ, Perry J, et al: Functional analysis of untreated and reconstructed posterior cruciate ligament injuries. Am J Sports Med 16:217–223, 1988

113. Hungerford DS, Barry M: Biomechanics of the patellofemoral joint. Clin Orthop 144:9–15, 1979

114. Reilly DT, Martens M: Experimental analysis of the quadriceps muscle force and patello-femoral joint reaction force for various activities. Acta Orthop Scand 43:126–137, 1972

115. Alford W, Cole BJ: The indications and technique for meniscal transplant. Orthop Clin North Am 36:469–484, 2005

116. Fritz JM, Irrgang JJ, Harner CD: Rehabilitation following allograft meniscal transplantation: A review of the literature and case study. J Orthop Sports Phys Ther 24:98–106, 1996

117. Reinold MM, Wilk KE, Macrina LC, et al: Current concepts in the rehabilitation following articular cartilage repair procedures in the knee. J Orthop Sports Phys Ther 36:774–794, 2006

118. Lewis PB, McCarty LP, III, Kang RW, et al: Basic science and treatment options for articular cartilage injuries. J Orthop Sports Phys Ther 36:717–727, 2006

119. Felson DT, Naimark A, Anderson JJ, et al: The prevalence of knee osteoarthritis in the elderly. The Framingham Osteoarthritis Study. Arthritis Rheum 30:914–918, 1987

120. Felson DT: The epidemiology of knee osteoarthritis: Results from the Framingham Osteoarthritis Study. Sem Arthritis Rheum 20:42–50, 1990

121. Peyron JG, Altman RD: The epidemiology of osteoarthritis, in Moskowitz RW, Howell DS, Goldberg VM, et al (eds): Osteoarthritis: Diagnosis and Medical/Surgical Management. Philadelphia, WB Saunders, 1992, pp 15–37

122. Anderson JJ, Felson DT: Factors associated with osteoarthritis of the knee in the first National Health and Nutrition Examination Survey. Am J Epidemiol 128:179–189, 1988

123. Felson DT, Hannan MT, Naimark A: Occupational physical demands, knee bending and knee osteoarthritis: Results from the Framingham study. J Rheumatol 18:1587–1592, 1991

124. Cooper C, McAlindon T, Coggon D, et al: Occupational activity and osteoarthritis of the knee. Ann Rheum Dis 53:90–93, 1994

125. Jensen LK, Eenberg W: Occupation as a risk factor for knee disorders. Scand J Work Environ Health 22:165–175, 1996

126. Maetzel A, Makela M, Hawker G, et al: Osteoarthritis of the hip and knee and mechanical occupational exposure: A systematic overview of the evidence. J Rheum 24:1599–1607, 1997

127. Kujala UM, Kaprio J, Sarna S: Osteoarthritis of weight bearing joints of lower limbs in former elite male athletes. BMJ 308:231–234, 1994

128. Kujala UM, Kettunen J, Paananen H, et al: Knee osteoarthritis in former runners, soccer players, weight lifters, and shooters. Arthritis Rheum 38:539–546, 1995

129. Felson DT, Zhang Y, Hannan MT, et al: Risk factors for incident radiographic knee osteoarthritis in the elderly: The Framingham Study. Arthritis Rheum 40:728–733, 1997

130. Felson DT: Epidemiology of hip and knee osteoarthritis. Epidemiol Rev 10:1–28, 1988

131. Baker K, McAlindon T: Exercise for knee osteoarthritis. Curr Opin Rheumatol 12:456–463, 2000

132. Wessel J: Isometric strength measurements of knee extensors in women with osteoarthritis of the knee. J Rheumatol 23:328–331, 1996

133. Slemenda C, Heilman DK, Brandt KD, et al: Quadriceps weakness and osteoarthritis of the knee. Ann Intern Med 127:97–104, 1998

134. Puett DW, Griffin MR: Published trials of nonmedicinal and noninvasive therapies for hip and knee osteoarthritis. Ann Intern Med 121:133–140, 1994

135. Fisher NM, Pendergast DR, Gresham GE, et al: Muscle rehabilitation: Its effect on muscular and functional performance of patients with knee osteoarthritis. Arch Phys Med Rehabil 72:367–374, 1991

136. Fisher NM, Gresham GE, Pendergast DR: Effects of a quantitative progressive rehabilitation program applied unilaterally to the osteoarthritic knee. Arch Phys Med Rehabil 74:1319–1326, 1993

137. Fisher NM, Gresham GE, Abrams M, et al: Quantitative effects of physical therapy on muscular and functional performance in subjects with osteoarthritis of the knees. Arch Phys Med Rehabil 74:840–847, 1993

138. Kovar PA, Allegrante JP, MacKenzie CR, et al: Supervised fitness walking in patients with osteoarthritis of the knee. A randomized, controlled trial. Ann Intern Med 116:529–534, 1992

139. Ettinger WH, Jr, Burns R, Messier SP, et al: A randomized trial comparing aerobic exercise and resistance exercise with a health education program in older adults with knee osteoarthritis. The Fitness Arthritis and Seniors Trial. JAMA 277:25–31, 1997

140. Lane NE, Buckwalter JA: Exercise: A cause of osteoarthritis? Rheum Dis Clin North Am 19:617–633, 1993

141. Brandt KD: Nonsurgical management of osteoarthritis, with an emphasis on nonpharmacologic measures. Arch Fam Med 4:1057–1064, 1995

142. Fitzgerald GK, Childs JD, Ridge TM, et al: Agility and perturbation training for a physically active individual with knee osteoarthritis. Phys Ther 82:372–382, 2002

143. Deyle GD, Henderson NE, Matekel RL, et al: Effectiveness of manual physical therapy and exercise in osteoarthritis of the knee. A randomized, controlled trial. Ann Intern Med 132:173–181, 2000

144. Yasuda K, Sasaki T: The mechanics of treatment of the osteoarthritic knee with a wedged insole. Clin Orthop 215:162–172, 1985

145. Yasuda K, Sasaki T: Clinical evaluation of the treatment of osteoarthritic knees using a newly designed wedged insole. Clin Orthop 221:181–187, 1985

146. Aglietti P, Rinonapoli E, Stringa G, et al: Tibial osteotomy for the varus osteoarthritic knee. Clin Orthop 176:239–251, 1983

147. Insall JN, Shoji H, Mayer V: High tibial osteotomy: A five year evaluation. J Bone Joint Surg 56A:1397–1405, 1974

148. Windsor RE, Insall JN, Vince KG: Technical considerations of total knee arthroplasty after proximal tibial osteotomy. J Bone Joint Surg 70A:547–555, 1988

149. Rorabeck CH, Murray P: The benefit of total knee arthroplasty. Orthopedics 19:777–779, 1996

150. Diduch DR, Insall JN, Scott WN, et al: Total knee replacement in young, active patients. Long-term follow-up and functional outcome. J Bone Joint Surg 79A:575–582, 1997

151. Ritter MA, Herbst SA, Keating EM, et al: Long-term survival analysis of a posterior cruciate-retaining total condylar total knee arthroplasty. Clin Orthop 309:136–145, 1994

152. Greenfield B, Tovin BJ, Bennett JG: Knee, in Wadsworth C (ed): Current Concepts of Orthopedic Physical Therapy. La Crosse, WI, Orthopaedic Section, American Physical Therapy Association, 2001, pp 1–8

153. Kolettis GT, Stern SH: Patellar resurfacing for patellofemoral arthritis. Orthop Clin North Am 23:665–673, 1992

154. Aglietti P, Buzzi R, De Felice R, et al: The Insall-Burstein total knee replacement in osteoarthritis: A 10-year minimum follow-up. J Arthroplasty 14:560–565, 1999

155. Banks SA, Markovich GD, Hodge WA: In vivo kinematics of cruciate-retaining and substituting knee arthroplasties. J Arthroplasty 12:297–304, 1997

156. Matsuda S, Ishinishi T, White SE, et al: Patellofemoral joint after total knee arthroplasty: Effect on contact area and contact stress. J Arthroplasty 12:790–797, 1997

157. Chew JTH, Stewart NJ, Hanssen AD, et al: Differences in patellar tracking and knee kinematics among three different total knee designs. Clin Orthop 345:87–98, 1997

158. Auberger SS, Mangine RE: Innovative Approaches to Surgery and Rehabilitation, Physical Therapy of the Knee. New York, Churchill Livingstone, 1988, pp 233–262

159. Ecker ML, Lotke PA: Postoperative care of the total knee patient. Orthop Clin North Am 20:55–62, 1989

160. Kumar PJ, McPherson EJ, Dorr LD, et al: Rehabilitation after total knee arthroplasty: A comparison of 2 rehabilitation techniques. Clin Orthop Relat Res 331:93–101, 1996

161. Enloe LJ, Shields RK, Smith K, et al: Total hip and knee replacement treatment programs: A report using consensus. J Orthop Sports Phys Ther 23:3, 1996

162. Shields RK, Enloe LJ, Evans RE, et al: Reliability, validity, and responsiveness of functional tests in patients with total joint replacement. Phys Ther 75:169, 1995

163. Dye S: Patellofemoral pain without malalignment: A tissue homeostasis perspective, in Fulkerson JP (ed): Common Patellofemoral Problems. Rosemont, IL, American Academy of Orthopaedic Surgeons, 2005, pp 1–9

164. Grelsamer RP, McConnell J: The Patella: A Team Approach. Gaithersburg, MD, Aspen, 1998

165. Pedowitz WJ, Kovatis P: Flatfoot in the adult. J Am Acad Orthop Surg 3:293–302, 1995

166. Klingman RE, Liaos SM, Hardin KM: The effect of subtalar joint posting on patellar glide position in subjects with excessive rearfoot pronation. J Orthop Sports Phys Ther 25:185–191, 1997

167. LeVeau BF, Rogers C: Selective training of the vastus medialis muscle using EMG biofeedback. Phys Ther 60:1410–1415, 1980

168. Wilk KE, Davies GJ, Mangine RE, et al: Patellofemoral disorders: A classification system and clinical guidelines for nonoperative rehabilitation. J Orthop Sports Phys Ther 28:307–322, 1998

169. Karst GM, Jewett PD: Electromyographic analysis of exercises proposed for differential activation of medial and lateral quadriceps femoris muscle components. Phys Ther 73:286–295, 1993

170. Hodges P, Richardson C: An investigation into the effectiveness of hip adduction in the optimization of the vastus medialis oblique contraction. Scand J Rehabil Med 25:57–62, 1993

171. Huberti HH, Hayes WC: Patellofemoral contact pressures. The influence of Q-angle and tendofemoral contact. J. Bone Joint Surg 66A:715–724, 1984

172. Doucette SA, Goble EM: The effect of exercise on patellar tracking in lateral patellar compression syndrome. Am J Sports Med 20:434–440, 1992

173. Hanten WP, Schulthies SS: Exercise effect on electromyographic activity of the vastus medialis oblique and the vastus lateralis muscles. Phys Ther 70:561–565, 1990

174. Kibler BW: Closed kinetic chain rehabilitation for sports injuries. Phys Med Rehab Clin N Am 11:369–384, 2000

175. McNicol K, Taunton JE, Clement DB: Iliotibial band friction syndrome in athletes. Can J Appl Sport Sci 6:76–80, 1981

176. Fulkerson JP, Gossling HR: Anatomy of the knee joint lateral retinaculum. Clin Orthop 153:183–188, 1980

177. Root M, Orien W, Weed J: Clinical Biomechanics. Los Angeles, Clinical Biomechanics Corp, 1977

178. Winter DA: Biomechanical motor patterns in normal walking. J Motor Behav 15:302–329, 1983

179. McConnell J: Conservative management of patellofemoral problems, in Grelsamer RP, McConnell J (eds): The Patella. A Team Approach. Gaithersburg, MD, Aspen, 1998, pp 119–136

180. McConnell J: Promoting effective segmental alignment, in Crosbie J, McConnell J (eds): Key Issues in Musculoskeletal Physiotherapy. Boston, Butterworth Heinemann, 1993, pp 172–194

181. Bockrath K, Wooden C, Worrell T, et al: Effects of patella taping on patella position and perceived pain. Med Sci Sports Exerc 25:989–992, 1993

182. Gerrard B: The patello-femoral pain syndrome in young, active patients: A prospective study. Clin Orthop 179:129–133, 1989

183. Marumoto JM, Jordan C, Akins R: A biomechanical comparison of lateral retinacular releases. Am J Sports Med 23:151–155, 1995

184. Masse Y: "La trochléoplastie." Restauration de la gouttière trochléene dans les subluxations et luxations de la rotule. Rev Chir Orthop 64:3–17, 1978

185. Grabiner M, Koh T, Draganich L: Neuromechanics of the patellofemoral joint. Med Sci Sports Exerc 26:10–21, 1994

186. Grelsamer RP, McConnell J: Examination of the patellofemoral joint, in Grelsamer RP, McConnell J (eds): The Patella: A Team Approach. Gaithersburg, MD, Aspen, 1998, pp 109–118

187. Cushnaghan J, McCarthy C, Dieppe P: Taping the patella medially: A new treatment for osteoarthritis of the knee joint? BMJ 308:753–755, 1994

188. Hunter LY: Braces and taping. Clin Sports Med 4:439–454, 1985

189. Shellock FG, Mink JH, Deutsch AL, et al: Patellofemoral joint: Identification of abnormalities using active movement, "unloaded" vs "loaded" kinematic MR imaging techniques. Radiology 188:575–578, 1993

190. Blazina ME, Kerlan RK, Jobe F, et al: Jumper's knee. Orthop Clin North Am 4:665–678, 1973

191. Anderson JE: Grant's Atlas of Anatomy (ed 7). Baltimore, Williams & Wilkins, 1980

192. Hollinshead WH, Rosse C: Textbook of Anatomy. Philadelphia, Harper & Row, 1985

193. Fredberg U, Bolvig L: Jumper's knee. Scand J Med Sci Sports 9:66–73, 1999

194. Reid DC: Bursitis and knee extensor mechanism pain syndromes, in Reid DC (ed): Sports Injury Assessment and Rehabilitation. New York, Churchill Livingstone, 1992, pp 399–437

195. Black JE, Alten SR: How I manage infrapatellar tendinitis. Physician Sports Med 12:86–90, 1984

196. Popp JE, Yu SS, Kaeding CC: Recalcitrant patellar tendinitis, magnetic resonance imaging, histologic evaluation, and surgical treatment. Am J Sports Med 25:218–222, 1997

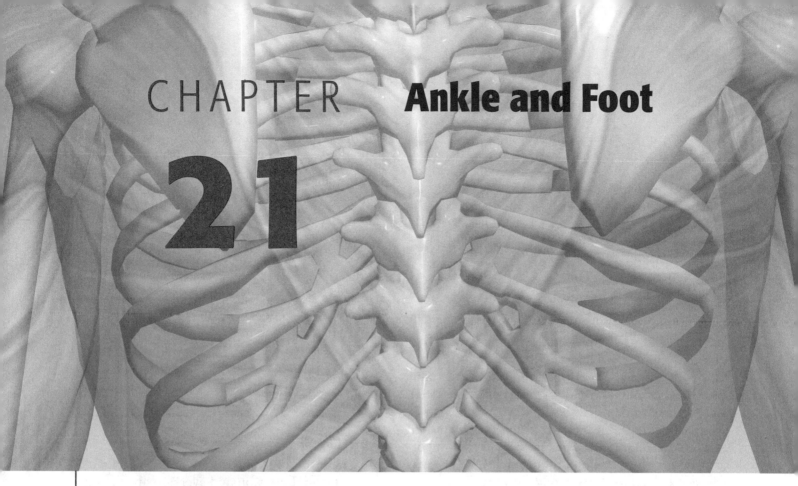

CHAPTER 21   Ankle and Foot

Chapter Objectives

At the completion of this chapter, the reader will be able to:

1. Describe the anatomy of the joints, ligaments, muscles, blood, and nerve supply that comprise the region.
2. Describe the biomechanics of the ankle and foot complex, including the open- and close-packed positions, muscle force couples, and the static and dynamic stabilizers.
3. Describe the relationship between muscle imbalance and functional performance of the ankle and foot.
4. Summarize the various causes of ankle and foot dysfunction.
5. Describe and demonstrate intervention strategies and techniques based on clinical findings and established goals by the physical therapist.
6. Evaluate an intervention's effectiveness in order to determine progress and modify an intervention as needed.
7. Teach an effective home program, and instruct the patient in its use.

Overview

The tibia and fibula bones, bound together by an interosseous membrane along the shaft of the bones and by strong anterior and posterior inferior tibiofibular ligament, make up the leg. Unlike the radius and ulna in the upper extremity, the tibia and fibula do not rotate around each other during functional movement. The ankle and foot is a complex structure of 28 bones (including two sesamoid bones) and 55 articulations (including 30 synovial joints), interconnected by ligaments and muscles. Even with a remarkable level of protection through joint congruency and a network of ligaments, the foot and ankle complex is at the mercy of truly impressive forces that act upon it. Peak vertical forces reach 120 percent of body weight during walking, and approach 275 percent during running.[1]

Five times the body weight is placed across the talocrural joint during initial contact while running.[1] As a consequence, it is estimated that an average 150-pound man absorbs 63.5 tons on each foot while walking 1 mile, and that the same man absorbs 110 tons per foot while running 1 mile.[2] About 60 percent of this weight-bearing load is carried out by the rearfoot, 8 percent by the midfoot, and 28 percent by the metatarsal heads,[3] with the second and third metatarsal heads bearing the greatest forefoot pressures.[4]

Anatomy and Kinesiology

The anatomy and kinematics of the ankle and foot may be the most complex in the human body. Anatomically and biomechanically, the foot is often subdivided into the rearfoot or hindfoot (the talus and calcaneus), the midfoot (the navicular, cuboid, and the three cuneiforms), and the forefoot (the 14 bones of the toes, the 5 metatarsals, and the medial and lateral sesamoids). The majority of the support provided to the ankle and foot joints (**Table 21-1** and Figure 21-1) comes by way of the arrangement of the ankle mortise and by the numerous ligaments found here (**Table 21-2**). Further stabilization is afforded by an abundant number of tendons that cross this joint complex (**Table 21-3**). These tendons are also involved in producing foot and ankle movements and are held in place by retinaculae. Some foot stability is provided by the intrinsic muscles (**Table 21-4**).

Terminology

The plantar aspect of the foot refers to the sole or its bottom, whereas the dorsal aspect refers to the top, or superior aspect, of the foot. Motions of the leg, foot, and ankle consist of single plane and multiplane movements.

● **Key Point**

- Plantarflexion refers to the motion of pushing the foot downward.
- Dorsiflexion refers to the motion of bringing the foot upward so the toes approximate the shin.
- Inversion refers to the motion of the foot resulting in the sole of the foot facing medially.
- Eversion refers to the motion of the foot resulting in the sole of the foot facing laterally.

The single plane motions include:

- The frontal plane motions of inversion and eversion. Inversion and eversion are single plane motions that occur in the frontal plane at the subtalar joint around a sagittal axis.

TABLE 21-1	The Joints of the Foot and Ankle		
	Open-Packed Position	**Close-Packed Position**	**Capsular Pattern**
Joints of the Hindfoot			
Tibiofibular joint	Plantarflexion	Maximum dorsiflexion	Pain on stress
Talocrural joint	10 degrees plantarflexion and midway between inversion and eversion	Maximum dorsiflexion	Plantarflexion, dorsiflexion
Subtalar joint	Midway between extremes of range of motion	Supination	Varus, valgus
Joints of the Midfoot			
Midtarsal joints	Midway between extremes of range of motion	Supination	Dorsiflexion, plantarflexion, adduction, medial rotation
Joints of the Forefoot			
Tarsometatarsal joints	Midway between extremes of range of motion	Supination	None
Metatarsophalangeal joints	10 degrees extension	Full extension	Great toe: extension, flexion Second to fifth toes: variable
Interphalangeal joints	Slight flexion	Full extension	Flexion, extension

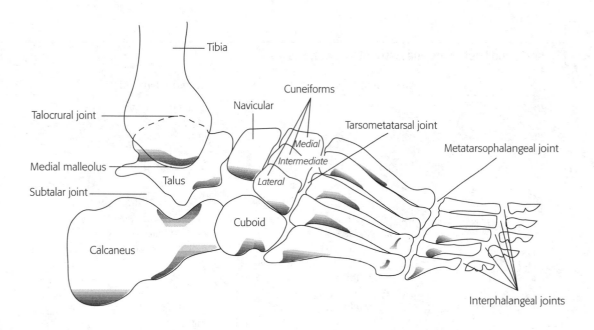

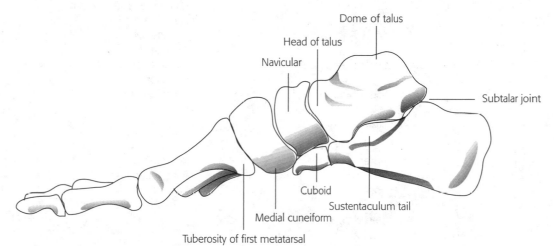

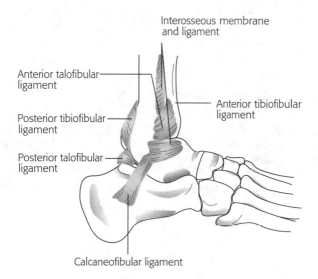

Figure 21-1 Major bones, joints, and lateral ligaments of the foot and ankle.

TABLE
21-2

Ankle and Foot Joints and Associated Ligaments

Joint	Associated Ligament	Motions Limited
Distal tibiofibular	Anterior tibiofibular	Distal glide of fibula Plantarflexion
	Posterior tibiofibular	Distal glide of fibula Plantarflexion
	Interosseous	Separation of tibia and fibula
Ankle	Deltoid (medial collateral) Superficial	
	Tibionavicular	Plantarflexion, abduction
	Tibiocalcaneal	Eversion, abduction
	Posterior tibiotalar	Dorsiflexion, abduction
	Deep	
	Anterior tibiotalar	Eversion, abduction, plantarflexion
	Lateral or fibular collateral	
	Anterior talofibular	Plantarflexion Inversion
	Calcaneofibular	Anterior displacement of foot Inversion
	Posterior talofibular	Dorsiflexion Dorsiflexion
	Lateral talocalcaneal	Posterior displacement of foot Inversion
	Anterior capsule	Dorsiflexion Plantarflexion
	Posterior capsule	Dorsiflexion
Subtalar	Interosseous talocalcaneal	
	Anterior band	Inversion Joint separation
	Posterior band	Inversion Joint separation
	Lateral talocalcaneal Deltoid Lateral collateral	
	Posterior talocalcaneal	Dorsiflexion
	Medial talocalcaneal	Eversion
	Anterior talocalcaneal (cervical ligaments)	Inversion
Main ligamentous support of longitudinal arches	Long plantar	Eversion
	Short plantar	Eversion
	Plantar calcaneonavicular	Eversion
	Plantar aponeurosis	Eversion
Midtarsal or transverse	Bifurcated	Joint separation
	Medial band	Plantarflexion
	Lateral band	Inversion
	Dorsal talonavicular	Plantarflexion of talus on navicular
	Dorsal calcaneocuboid	Inversion, plantarflexion

TABLE 21-3

Extrinsic Muscle Attachments and Innervation

Muscle	Proximal	Distal	Innervation	Function
Gastrocnemius	Medial and lateral condyle of femur	Posterior surface of calcaneus through Achilles tendon	Tibial S2 (S1)	Plantarflexion Flexion of the knee
Plantaris	Lateral supracondylar line of femur	Posterior surface of calcaneus through Achilles tendon	Tibial S2 (S1)	Plantarflexion Flexion of the knee
Soleus	Head of fibula, proximal third of shaft, soleal line and midshaft of posterior tibia	Posterior surface of calcaneus through Achilles tendon	Tibial S2 (S1)	Plantarflexion
Tibialis anterior	Distal to lateral tibial condyle, proximal half of lateral tibial shaft, and interosseous membrane	First cuneiform bone, medial and plantar surfaces and base of first metatarsal	Deep fibular (peroneal) L4 (L5)	Dorsiflexion Inversion
Tibialis posterior	Posterior surface of tibia, proximal two-thirds of the posterior of the fibula, and interosseous membrane	Tuberosity of navicular bone, tendinous expansion to other tarsals and metatarsals	Tibial L4 and L5	Plantarflexion Inversion
Fibularis (peroneus) longus	Lateral condyle of tibia, head and proximal two-thirds of fibula	Base of first metatarsal and first cuneiform, lateral side	Superficial fibular (peroneal) L5 and S1 (S2)	Eversion Plantarflexion
Fibularis (peroneus) brevis	Distal two-thirds of lateral fibular shaft	Tuberosity of fifth metatarsal	Superficial fibular (peroneal) L5 and S1 (S2)	Plantarflexion Eversion
Fibularis (peroneus) tertius	Lateral slip from extensor digitorum longus	Tuberosity of fifth metatarsal	Deep fibular (peroneal) L5 and S1	Dorsiflexion Eversion
Flexor hallucis longus	Posterior distal two-thirds of fibula	Base of distal phalanx of great toe	Tibial S2 (S3)	Flexion of the great toe Plantarflexion Inversion
Flexor digitorum longus	Middle three-fifths of posterior tibia	Base of distal phalanx of lateral four toes	Tibial S2 (S3)	Flexion of toes 2 to 5 Plantarflexion Inversion
Extensor hallucis longus	Middle half of anterior shaft of fibula	Base of distal phalanx of great toe	Deep fibular (peroneal) L5 and S1	Extension of the great toe Dorsiflexion
Extensor digitorum longus	Lateral condyle of tibia, proximal anterior surface of shaft of fibula	One tendon to each lateral four toes, to middle phalanx and extending to distal phalanges	Deep fibular (peroneal) L5 and S1	Extension of toes 2–5 (MTP, PIP, and DIP joints) Dorsiflexion Eversion

MTP, metatarsophalangeal; PIP, proximal interphalangeal; DIP, distal interphalangeal.

TABLE 21-4 Intrinsic Muscles of the Foot

Muscle	Proximal	Distal	Innervation	Function
Extensor digitorum brevis	Distal superior surface of calcaneus	Dorsal surface of second through fourth toes, base of proximal phalanx	Deep fibularis (peroneal) S1 and S2	Extension of the first four toes
Flexor digitorum brevis	Tuberosity of calcaneus	One tendon slips into base of middle phalanx of each of the lateral four toes	Medial and lateral plantar S3 (S2)	Flexion of the MTP and PIP joints of the lesser four toes
Extensor hallucis brevis	Distal superior and lateral surfaces of calcaneus	Dorsal surface of proximal phalanx	Deep fibular (peroneal) S1 and S2	
Flexor hallucis brevis	Plantar surface of cuboid and third cuneiform bones	Base of proximal phalanx of great toe	Medial plantar S3 (S2)	MTP flexion of the great toe
Quadratus plantae	By two heads to the plantar aspect of the calcaneus	Lateral border of the flexor digitorum longus tendon	Lateral plantar S1 and S2	Helps to stabilize the tendon of the flexor digitorumlongus, preventing it from migrating medially when under force
Abductor hallucis	Tuberosity of calcaneus and plantar aponeurosis	Base of proximal phalanx, medial side	Medial plantar L5 and S1 (L4)	Abduction of the great toe
Adductor hallucis	Base of second, third, and fourth metatarsals and deep plantar ligaments	Proximal phalanx of first digit lateral side	Medial and lateral plantar S1 and S2	Flexion and abduction of the MTP joint of the great toe
Lumbricals	Medial and adjacent sides of flexor digitorum longus tendon to each lateral digit	Medial side of proximal phalanx and extensor hood	Medial and lateral plantar L5, S1, and S2 (L4)	Flexion of the MTP joints, simultaneously extending the IP joints
Plantar interossei			Medial and lateral plantar S1 and S2	Adduction of toes
First	Base and medial side of third metatarsal	Base of proximal phalanx and extensor hood of third digit		
Second	Base and medial side of fourth metatarsal	Base of proximal phalanx and extensor hood of fourth digit		
Third	Base and medial side of fifth metatarsal	Base of proximal phalanx and extensor hood of fifth digit		
Dorsal interossei			Medial and lateral plantar S1 and S2	Abduction of toes 2–4
First	First and second metatarsal bones	Proximal phalanx and extensor hood of second digit medially		
Second	Second and third metatarsal bones	Proximal phalanx and extensor hood of second digit laterally		
Third	Third and fourth metatarsal bones	Proximal phalanx and extensor hood of third digit laterally		
Fourth	Fourth and fifth metatarsal bones	Proximal phalanx and extensor hood of fourth digit laterally		
Abductor digitiminimi	Lateral side of fifth metatarsal bone	Proximal phalanx of fifth digit	Lateral plantar S1 and S2	Abduction of the fifth toe
Flexor digitiminimi	Plantar aspect of the base of the fifth metatarsal	Lateral base of the proximal phalanx of the fifth toe	Lateral plantar S1 and S2	MTP flexion of the fifth toe

MTP, metatarsophalangeal; PIP, proximal interphalangeal; DIP, distal interphalangeal.

- The sagittal plane motions of dorsiflexion and plantarflexion. These terms describe movement at the ankle and the mid-tarsal joint.
- The horizontal plane motions of adduction and abduction. These terms describe motions of the forefoot in the horizontal plane about a superior-inferior axis. Abduction moves the forefoot laterally, whereas adduction moves the forefoot medially on the midfoot.

A triplane motion describes a movement about an obliquely oriented axis through all three body planes. Triplanar motions occur at the talocrural, subtalar, and midtarsal joints, and at the first and fifth rays.

> ● **Key Point** In pronation, the forefoot rotates the big toe downward and little toe upwards, whereas in supination, the reverse occurs.

Joints of the Ankle and Foot
The ankle of the foot is comprised of numerous joints, all of which together to provide both mobility and stability to this area.

Proximal Tibiofibular Joint
The proximal tibiofibular joint is stabilized by four ligaments, collectively known as the syndesmotic ligaments. These include the inferior interosseous ligament, the anterior inferior tibiofibular ligament, the posterior inferior tibiofibular ligament, and the inferior transverse ligament. Of these ligaments, the inferior interosseous ligament is the primary stabilizer.

The Talocrural Joint
The major ligaments of the talocrural joint can be divided into two main groups: lateral collaterals and medial (deltoid) collaterals.

- *Lateral collaterals:* The lateral collateral ligament complex consists of the anterior talofibular ligament (ATFL), which resists ankle inversion in plantarflexion; the calcaneofibular ligament (CFL), which resists inversion with the posterior talofibular ligament (PTFL), the strongest of the lateral ligament complex.
- *Medial collaterals:* Collectively, the medial collateral ligaments form a triangular-shaped ligamentous structure known as the medial (deltoid) ligament of the ankle. Wide variations have been noted in the anatomic description of the medial (deltoid) ligament of the ankle, but it is generally agreed that it consists of both superficial and deep fibers.

  ◻ *Superficial fibers:* These consist of the tibionavicular, which resists lateral translation and external rotation of the talus; the posterior talotibial, which resists ankle dorsiflexion and lateral translation and external rotation of the talus; and the calcaneotibial, which resists abduction of the talus, calcaneus, and navicular when the foot and ankle are positioned in plantarflexion and eversion.
  ◻ *Deep fibers:* These consist of the anterior talotibial and the calcaneotibial ligament. Rasmussen and colleagues[5,6] found that the superficial fibers of the medial (deltoid) ligament of the ankle specifically limited talar abduction or negative talar tilt but that the deep layers of the medial (deltoid) ligament of the ankle ruptured with external rotation of the leg, without the superficial portion being involved.

> ● **Key Point** The strength of the ankle ligaments from weakest to strongest is the ATFL, CFL, PTFL, and deltoid complex.[7]

Distal Tibiofibular Joint
The two tibiofibular joints (proximal and distal) are described as individual articulations, but in fact, they function as a pair. The movements that occur at these joints are primarily a result of the ankle's influence.

> ● **Key Point** The ligaments of the distal tibiofibular joint (refer to Table 21-2) are more commonly injured than the anterior talofibular ligament. Injuries to the ankle syndesmosis most often occur as a result of forced external rotation of the foot or during internal rotation of the tibia on a planted foot. Hyperdorsiflexion may also be a contributing mechanism.

Talocrural Joint
The talocrural joint is formed between the talus and the distal tibia. The saddle-shaped talus is considered to be the mechanical keystone of the ankle, because it distributes the body weight backward toward the heel and forward to the midfoot. This ability to distribute forces is due to the massive articulating surface of the talus that both spreads and focuses forces. The talus is divided into a head (anteriorly) and a neck and body (posteriorly). The orientation of the talocrural joint axis is, on average, 20–30 degrees posterior to the frontal plane as it passes posteriorly from the medial malleolus to the lateral

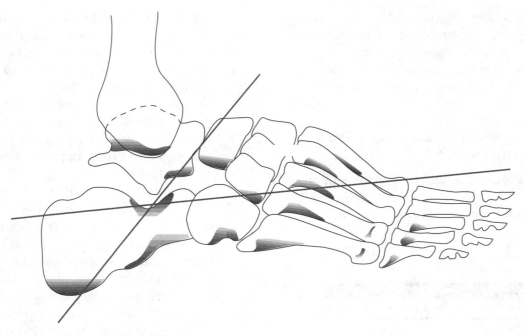

Figure 21-2 The orientation of the talocrural joint axis.

malleolus (Figure 21-2). The primary motions at this joint are dorsiflexion and plantarflexion, with a total range of 70 degrees (0 to 20 degrees of dorsiflexion and 0 to 50 degrees of plantarflexion). Although talocrural motion occurs primarily in the sagittal plane, an appreciable amount of horizontal motion appears to occur in the horizontal plane, especially during internal rotation of the tibia or pronation of the foot. The tibia follows the talus during weight bearing so that the talocrural joint externally rotates with supination and internally rotates with pronation.[8] Therefore, the tibia internally rotates during pronation and externally rotates during supination.[9] Stability for this joint in weight bearing is provided by the articular surfaces, whereas in non–weight bearing, the ligaments appear to provide the majority of stability.

● **Key Point** During the gait cycle, maximal dorsiflexion occurs late in the stance phase (see Chapter 25), which corresponds with the close-packed position of the ankle. The least stable position of the talocrural joint is full plantarflexion.

Subtalar Joint

The subtalar joint is a synovial, bicondylar compound joint consisting of two separate, modified ovoid surfaces with their own joint cavities (one male and one female). The two surfaces, consisting of anterior and posterior articulations, are connected by an interosseous membrane. The anterior

component is situated more medial than the posterior, giving the plane of the joint an average 42 degrees (± 9 degrees) superior from the transverse foot plane and 23 degrees (± 11 degrees) medial from the sagittal foot plane (refer to Figure 21-2).

The subtalar joint is responsible for inversion and eversion of the hindfoot. Approximately 50 percent of apparent ankle inversion observed actually comes from the subtalar joint. The axis of motion for the subtalar joint is approximately 45 degrees from horizontal and 20 degrees medial to the mid-sagittal plane. This axis, which moves during subtalar joint motion, allows the subtalar joint to also produce triplanar (pronation/supination) motions in close conjunction with the transverse tarsal joints of the midfoot. Pronation and supination motions at the subtalar joint vary according to whether the joint is weight bearing (closed-chain), or non–weight bearing (open-chain).[10]

- During weight-bearing activities, pronation involves a combination of calcaneal eversion, adduction and plantarflexion of the talus, and internal rotation of the tibia (Figure 21-3), whereas supination involves a combination of calcaneal inversion, abduction and dorsiflexion of the talus, and external rotation of the tibia (Figure 21-4).
- During non–weight-bearing activities, pronation involves a combination of calcaneal eversion, and abduction and dorsiflexion of the

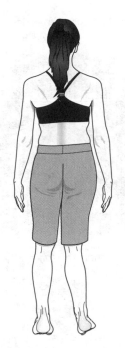

Figure 21-3   Non–weight-bearing pronation.

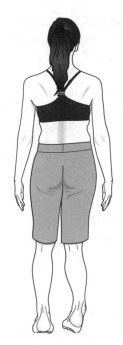

Figure 21-4   Non–weight-bearing supination.

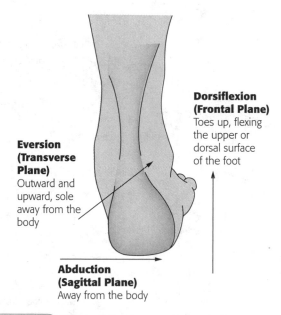

Eversion (Transverse Plane)
Outward and upward, sole away from the body

Dorsiflexion (Frontal Plane)
Toes up, flexing the upper or dorsal surface of the foot

Abduction (Sagittal Plane)
Away from the body

Figure 21-5   Weight-bearing pronation.

Inversion (Transverse Plane)
Inward and upward, sole toward the body

Adduction (Sagittal Plane)
Toward the body

Plantarflexion (Frontal Plane)
Toes down, flexing the lower, or plantar surface of the foot

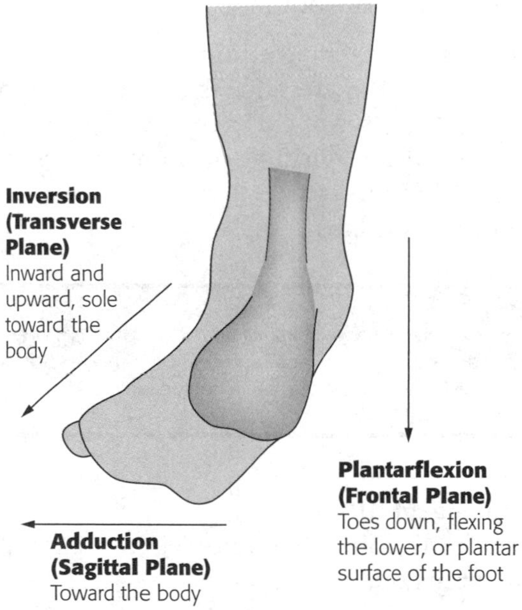

Figure 21-6   Weight-bearing supination.

talus (Figure 21-5), whereas supination involves a combination of calcaneal inversion, and adduction and plantarflexion of the talus (Figure 21-6).

The "righting" mechanism of the foot provided by eversion and inversion allows the leg to remain vertical, even while standing or walking on uneven surfaces.[11]

● **Key Point**   In normal individuals, there is an inversion to eversion ratio of 2:1, which amounts to approximately 20 degrees of inversion and 10 degrees of eversion.

● **Key Point**   For normal gait on a level surface, a minimum of 4–6 degrees of eversion and 8–12 degrees of inversion are required.[12]

Midtarsal (Transverse Tarsal) Joint Complex

The midtarsal joint complex consists of the talonavicular and calcaneocuboid articulations. The function of the midtarsal joint complex, which separates the rearfoot from the midfoot, is to provide the foot with an additional mechanism for raising and lowering the arch, and to absorb some of the horizontal plane tibial motion that is transmitted to the foot during stance.[8,13] This joint complex works in conjunction with the subtalar joint during activities involving pronation and supination.

Cuneonavicular Joint

The cuneonavicular joint has one to two degrees of freedom: plantar/dorsiflexion and inversion/eversion.

Metatarsophalangeal Joints

The metatarsophalangeal (MTP) joints have two degrees of freedom: flexion/extension and abduction/adduction. Range of motion of these joint varies, ranging from 40 to 100 degrees of extension, 3 to 43 degrees of flexion, and 5 to 20 degrees of abduction and adduction.

First Metatarsophalangeal Joint

The function of the great toe is to provide stability to the medial aspect of the foot and to provide for normal propulsion during gait. Normal alignment of the first MTP joint varies between 5 degrees varus and 15 degrees valgus.

> **● Key Point** The great toe is characterized by having a remarkable discrepancy between active and passive motion. Approximately 30 degrees of active flexion is present, and at least 50 degrees of active extension, the latter of which frequently can be increased passively to between 70 and 90 degrees.

Interphalangeal (IP) Joints

Each of the IP joints has one degree of freedom: flexion/extension.

Medial Longitudinal Arch of the Foot

The medial longitudinal arch plays an important role in foot function during weight-bearing activities. The arch is composed of the calcaneus, talus, navicular, medial cuneiform, and first metatarsals (two sesamoids) (Figure 21-7). Although some of the integrity of the arch depends on the bony architecture, support is also provided by the ligaments and muscles, including the plantar calcaneonavicular (spring) ligament, plantar fascia, tibialis posterior, flexor digitorum longus, flexor hallucis longus, and fibularis (peroneus) longus.[14–16] The soleus and gastrocnemius

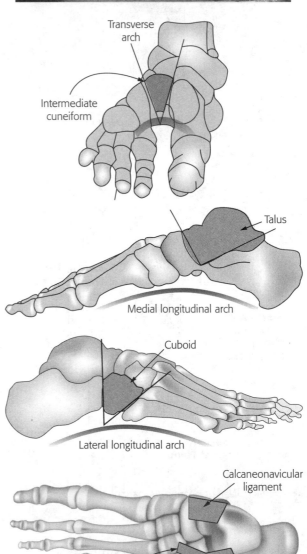

Figure 21-7   Arches of the foot.

muscle group has also been noted to have an effect on the arch and can flatten it with adaptive shortening.[16] The arch is not only a major source of frontal plane motion of the foot, but also is a major load-bearing structure.[17] Analysis of the medial longitudinal arch has long been used by clinicians to make determinations about foot abnormalities, with a high arch indicating a supinated foot and a low or collapsed arch being associated with a pronated or flatfoot, respectively.[18] Studies have found a higher incidence of stress fractures, plantar heel pain, metatarsalgia, and lower extremity injuries, including knee strains and iliotibial band syndrome, in individuals with high arches, compared with those who have low arches.[19-21]

Examination

The examination of the foot and ankle by the physical therapist typically follows the outline in **Table 21-5**. The evidence-based special tests of the foot and ankle are outlined in **Table 21-6**. Selection for their use is at the discretion of the clinician and is based on a complete patient history and clinical findings.

General Intervention Strategies

Due to the integrated nature of the foot and ankle in functional activities, the rehabilitation is organized around a common framework for most foot and ankle pathologies.[22]

TABLE 21-5	Examination of the Lower Leg, Ankle, and Foot

  I. History.

 II. Observation and inspection.

III. Upper quarter scan as appropriate.

IV. Examination of movements. Active range of motion with passive overpressure of the following movements:
   a. Plantarflexion and dorsiflexion in weight bearing and non–weight bearing
   b. Supination and pronation in weight bearing and non–weight bearing
   c. Toe extension and flexion in weight bearing and non–weight bearing

 V. Resisted isometric movements:
   a. Knee flexion and extension
   b. Plantarflexion and dorsiflexion
   c. Supination and pronation
   d. Toe extension and flexion

VI. Palpation.

VII. Neurological tests as appropriate (reflexes, sensory scan, peripheral nerve assessment).

VIII. Joint mobility tests:
   a. Inversion and eversion at the subtalar joint
   b. Adduction and abduction at the midtarsal joints
   c. Anteroposterior glide at the talocrural joint
   d. Tarsal bone mobility

 IX. Special tests (refer to Table 21-6).

  X. Diagnostic imaging.

TABLE 21-6	Evidence-Based Special Tests for the Foot and Ankle

Name of Test	Brief Description	Positive Findings	Evidence-Based
Anterior drawer[a]	Patient is supine. Clinician maintains the ankle in 10 to 15 degrees of plantarflexion while drawing the heel gently forward.	Test is positive for anterior talofibular ligament tear if talus rotates out of the ankle mortise anteriorly.	Sensitivity: 0.71 (<48 hours after injury), 0.96 (5 days after injury) Specificity: 0.33 (<48 hours after injury), 0.84 (5 days after injury)
Impingement sign[b]	Patient is seated. Clinician grasps calcaneus with one hand and uses other hand to grasp forefoot and bring it into plantarflexion. Clinician uses thumb to place pressure over anterolateral ankle. Foot is then brought from plantarflexion to dorsiflexion while thumb pressure is maintained.	Positive for anterolateral ankle impingement if pain is provoked with pressure from clinician's thumb is greater in dorsiflexion than in plantarflexion.	Sensitivity: 0.95 Specificity: 0.88

(continued)

TABLE
21-6

Evidence-Based Special Tests for the Foot and Ankle (continued)

Name of Test	Brief Description	Positive Findings	Evidence-Based
Gap test[c]	Patient is prone. Clinician palpates the course of the Achilles tendon.	Positive for Achilles tendon tear if gap in Achilles tendon is noted.	Sensitivity: 0.73 Specificity: not provided
Windlass test[d]	Patient is standing on a stepstool with toes over the stool's edge. The clinician extends the MTP joint of the great toe while allowing the IP joint to flex.	Positive for plantar fasciitis if pain is reproduced at the end range of MTP extension.	Sensitivity: 0.32 Specificity: 1.0
Paper grip test[e]	The patient is positioned in sitting with the hips, knees, and ankles at 90 degrees and toes placed on a piece of cardboard. The clinician stabilizes the feet while attempting to slide cardboard away from the toes.	Positive for toe plantarflexion weakness if participant cannot maintain cardboard under the toes.	Sensitivity: 0.80 Specificity: 0.79

Data from (a) van Dijk CN, Mol BW, Lim LS, et al: Diagnosis of ligament rupture of the ankle joint. Physical examination, arthrography, stress radiography and sonography compared in 160 patients after inversion trauma. Acta Orthop Scand 67:566–570, 1996; (b) Molloy S, Solan MC, Bendall SP: Synovial impingement in the ankle. A new physical sign. J Bone Joint Surg Br 85:330–333, 2003; (c) Maffulli N: The clinical diagnosis of subcutaneous tear of the Achilles tendon. A prospective study in 174 patients. Am J Sports Med 26:266–270, 1998; (d) De Garceau D, Dean D, Requejo SM, et al: The association between diagnosis of plantar fasciitis and Windlass test results. Foot Ankle Int 24:251–255, 2003; and (e) Menz HB, Zammit GV, Munteanu SE, et al: Plantarflexion strength of the toes: Age and gender differences and evaluation of a clinical screening test. Foot Ankle Int 27:1103–1108, 2006

Acute Phase

The general goals during the acute phase include:

- *Decrease pain, inflammation, and swelling.* The control of pain, inflammation, and swelling is accomplished by applying the principles of PRICEMEM (protection, rest, ice, compression, elevation, manual therapy, early motion, and medication). Icing for 20–30 minutes three to four times a day, concurrent with nonsteroidal anti-inflammatory drugs (NSAIDs) or aspirin prescribed by the physician can aid in reducing pain and swelling.
- *Protect the healing area from reinjury.* The means by which to support or protect the ankle and foot during this phase will vary depending on the type and severity of the injury, the individual patient's requirements, and the anticipated compliance of the patient to any restrictions placed on them by the physician.[23,24]
- *Begin to re-establish pain-free ROM.* To increase ROM, the therapist may perform gentle capsular stretches and grades I–II joint mobilizations. Exercises in this phase include towel stretches (Figure 21-8); ankle circles and pumps; low-level (seated) biomechanical ankle platform system (BAPS) or wobble board exercises (Figure 21-9); and active and active assisted exercises into plantarflexion (Figure 21-10), dorsiflexion, inversion, and eversion, and combined planes (e.g., plantarflexion and inversion). Active motion and exercise may also be used to effectively increase local circulation and further promote the resorption of any lingering edema.[25,26]

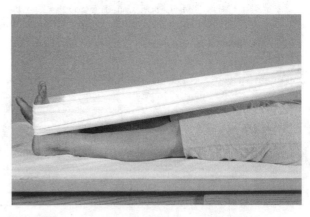

Figure 21-8   Towel/sheet stretch into dorsiflexion.

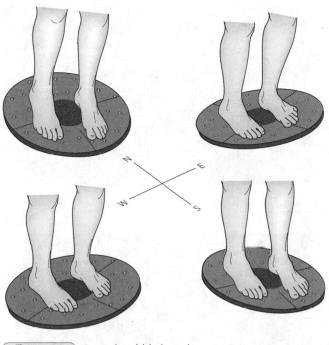

Figure 21-9   Seated wobble board.

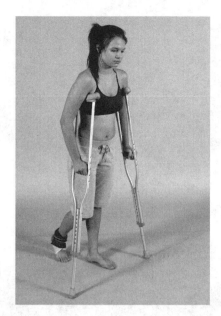

Figure 21-11   Crutch walking.

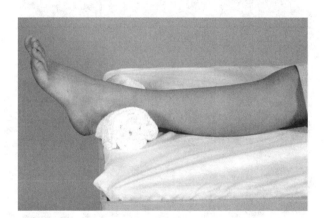

Figure 21-10   Active plantarflexion.

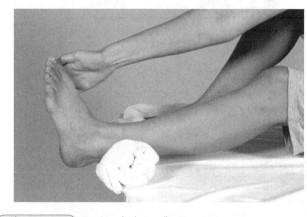

Figure 21-12   Resisted plantarflexion.

- *Increase weight-bearing tolerance.* Pain-free weight bearing as tolerated is encouraged with the use of any appropriate assistive devices such as a cane or crutches (Figure 21-11). During ambulation, joint protection and positioning are continued as needed using taping techniques, thermoplastic stirrups, or functional walking orthosis.[27,28] The use of crutches or other assistive devices is usually continued until the patient has a pain-free uncompensated gait. While the patient uses crutches, pain-free ankle motion during the normal gait cycle continues to be encouraged. Patients should be encouraged to walk with as normal a gait as possible,

given the limitations on ankle and knee motion. The application of ice is continued after therapeutic activities or after prolonged weight bearing to prevent or minimize any recurrence of swelling.

- *Maintain fitness levels as appropriate.* Stationary cycling can also be performed (at a comfortable intensity for up to 30 minutes) to provide cardiovascular endurance training and controlled ankle ROM.[29]

- *Prevent muscle atrophy and increase neuromuscular control.* Isometric exercises within the patient's pain tolerance (Figure 21-12 through Figure 21-15) and pain-free ROM are initiated

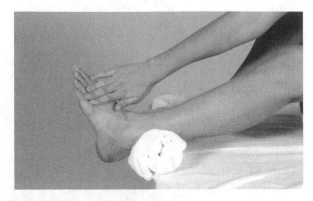

Figure 21-13   Resisted dorsiflexion.

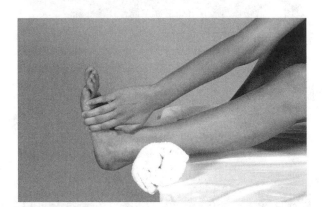

Figure 21-14   Resisted eversion.

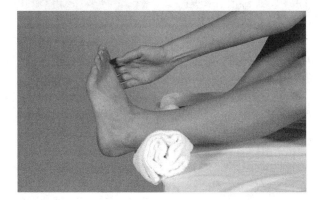

Figure 21-15   Resisted inversion.

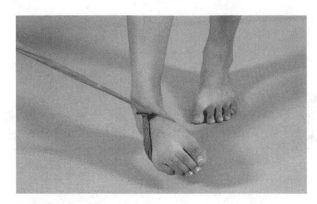

Figure 21-16   Theraband PREs: inversion.

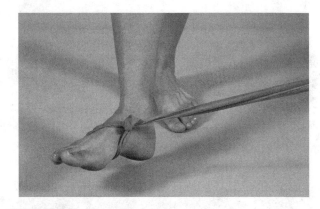

Figure 21-17   Theraband PREs: eversion.

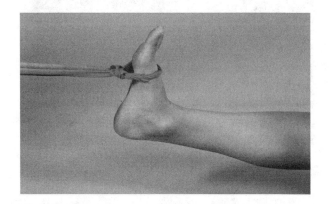

Figure 21-18   Theraband PREs: dorsiflexion.

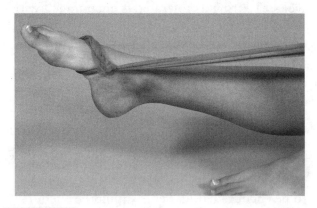

Figure 21-19   Theraband PREs: plantarflexion.

for all motions. These exercises are initially performed submaximally, progressing to maximal isometric contractions as tolerated. Mild manual resistive isometrics in all planes may also be started throughout the pain-free range. Exercises are progressed to include concentric and eccentric exercises (Figure 21-16) through (Figure 21-19)), once the isometric exercises are pain-free. Exercises for the foot intrinsics may include toe curl exercises with a towel (Figure 21-20) and (Figure 21-21)) or having the

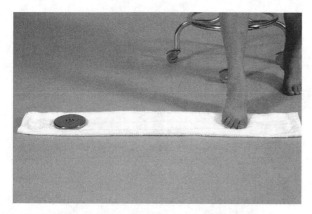

Figure 21-20   Lateral to medial towel curls.

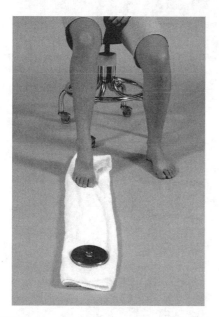

Figure 21-21   Anterior to posterior towel curls.

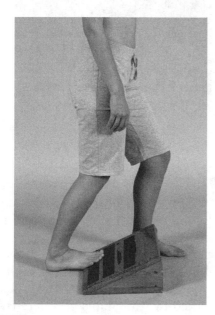

Figure 21-22   Heel cord stretching box.

patient pick up marbles from the floor with their toes and place the marbles in a small container or bowl. Each muscle or muscle group should be strengthened with a specific exercise that isolates the muscle or group. Resistance (rubber tubing/bands, weights, isokinetic devices, body weight exercises, etc.) is increased as tolerated. Emphasis should initially be on low resistance and endurance in all pain-free positions. As the program progresses, the joint range is increased from a stress-free position to a more stressful position. As with all exercises, the patient should become an active participant at the earliest opportunity. The exercises learned in the clinic need to be integrated appropriately into a home-exercise regimen.

Progression to the functional phase occurs when there is minimal pain and tenderness, full passive range of motion (PROM), strength rated at 4/5 to 5/5 with manual muscle testing as compared to the uninvolved side, and pain-free weight bearing and an uncompensated gait pattern present. At this time, crutches or other assistive devices are discontinued. However, pain may still be felt with activities more vigorous than walking.

Functional/Chronic Phase

A recurrence of symptoms should not be provoked. The goals of this phase are the following:

- *Restore normal joint arthrokinematics.* Specific joint mobilization techniques may be performed by the PT.[30]
- *Attain full range of pain-free motion.* Muscle stretching is initiated to begin to increase ROM. Emphasis should also be placed on regaining any dorsiflexion that was lost. Dorsiflexion can be regained through gastrocnemius and soleus stretches, and can also be assisted by the use of a tilt board (see Chapter 20) or heel cord stretching box (Figure 21-22).[28,31]
- *Improve neuromuscular control of the lower extremity in a full-weight-bearing posture on both level and uneven surfaces.* Closed chain exercises are introduced with a graduated increase in weight bearing. Specific exercises include, but are not limited to, chair/Swiss ball seated marching (hip flexion) on the floor (Figure 21-23) or on a pillow (Figure 21-24), standing bilateral (Figure 21-25) to unilateral (Figure 21-26) heel raises, and wall

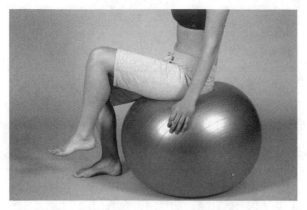

Figure 21-23   Seated marching on a Swiss ball.

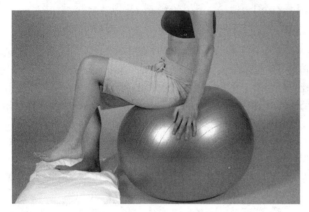

Figure 21-24   Seated marching on a Swiss ball, on a pillow.

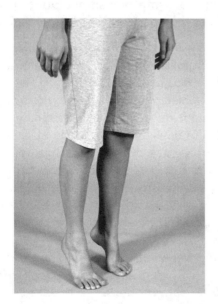

Figure 21-25   Bilateral heel raises.

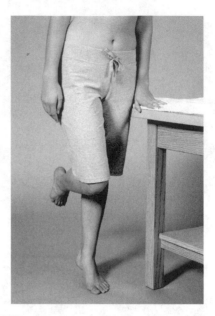

Figure 21-26   Unilateral heel raises.

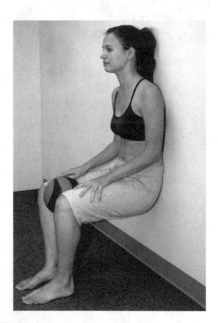

Figure 21-27   Wall slide.

slides (Figure 21-27). The neuromuscular progression begins with a unilateral stance on the floor (Figure 21-28), and progresses to increasingly softer surfaces (Figure 21-29 and Figure 21-30), and then perturbations (Figure 21-31). Proprioceptive exercises are especially important for full functional return and injury prevention.[23,24] Using a balance board, the patient balances on the involved limb, while playing "catch" with the clinician (see Chapter 20). The intensity of this exercise can be varied by using balls of different sizes and weights. The clinician may also make the

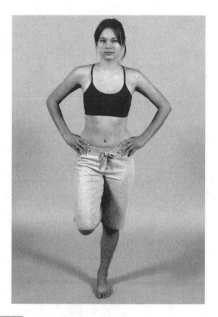

Figure 21-28 Unilateral stance on floor.

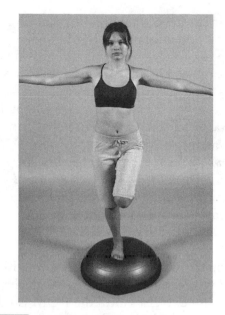

Figure 21-30 Unilateral stance on BOSU.

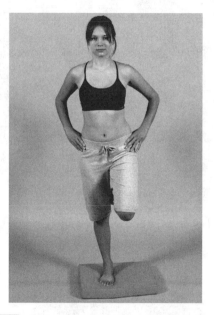

Figure 21-29 Unilateral stance on soft surface.

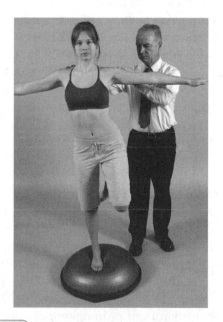

Figure 21-31 Unilateral stance with perturbations.

exercises more challenging by throwing the ball to a variety of locations. This will require a shift in the center of gravity and an instantaneous adjustment of balance from the patient. One of the all-too-common consequences of an ankle injury is an alteration of the motor conduction velocity of the fibular (peroneal) nerve and the protective function of the fibular muscles on the ankle joint.[32–34] A decrease in

fibular reaction time has been demonstrated to continue for up to 12 weeks after injury,[32,33] despite a nearly full return of strength (96 percent) in comparison with the contralateral side.[32] It has also been demonstrated in normal subjects that there is an increase in the latency response of the fibular muscles with an increase in plantarflexion, indicating a loss of protective reflexes when in this position.[35]

The patient must train and be rehabilitated in all potential positions of injury.[23,24] Examples of exercises to perform to enhance proprioception include side (lateral) step-ups (Figure 21-32), front step-ups (Figure 21-33), lunges onto or over a pillow (see Chapter 20), backward step-ups (see Chapter 18), and cross-over walking (Figure 21-34).

- *Improve or regain lower extremity strength and endurance through integration of local and kinetic chain exercises.* Exercises during this phase include weight-bearing activities of increasing difficulty.[36]

- *Return to previous level of function or recreation.* Multidirectional balance activities should progress from the non–weight-bearing, open-chain exercises until the ROM is full and painless, at which time closed-chain exercises are introduced with a progression to full weight bearing.[23,24] The greater the severity of injury, the more critical the need for multidirectional balance board activities and weight-bearing rehabilitation activities.[37–44] The progression begins with a phase of walking or jogging on flat surfaces and ascending and descending stairs forward and backward, with a progression to turning, changing directions, and lateral movements while running, and eccentric loading with stair running.[45] Activities to help achieve these goals include heel-to-toe anterior–posterior walking (10 meters for 20 reps), and mini-trampoline balancing exercises (unilateral stance with eyes open and then closed, and catching and passing activities with a medicine ball—see Chapter 11). For some patients, the goal may be to return to sport. Progression to this level occurs when there is:[22]

  □ Full pain-free active and passive ROM
  □ No complaints of pain or tenderness
  □ A return of 75–80 percent strength of the plantarflexors, dorsiflexors, invertors, and evertors compared to the uninvolved side
  □ Adequate unilateral stance balance (30 seconds with eyes closed)

Before being allowed to return to a strenuous occupation or sport, the patient should be put through a functional test that simulates all requirements of his or her occupation or sport.[23,24] The PT should analyze the patient's quality of movement and whether they are favoring the injured extremity in any way.[23,24] Activities during this phase involve

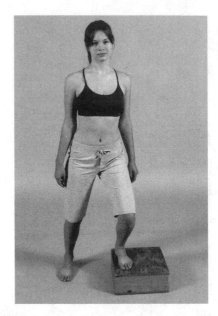

Figure 21-32   Side step-up.

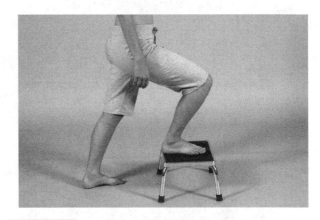

Figure 21-33   Front step-up.

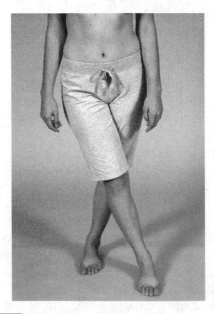

Figure 21-34   Cross-over walking.

cutting drills, shuttle runs, carioca crossover drills, and sports-specific activities such as lay-ups and dribbling.[45] Plyometric activities are introduced during this activity phase. These can include two-foot ankle hopping, single ankle hops, and then multi-direction single ankle hops. If appropriate, barrier jumps or hops may be introduced.

> **● Key Point** A study by Rozzi et al.[46] demonstrated that a 4-week course of single-leg balance training showed an improvement in balance ability in both the trained and the untrained limbs.

Common Conditions

Due to the significant forces placed on this region and its importance in the lower kinematic chain, there are a number of biomechanical conditions that warrant mention. In addition, other conditions due to trauma or disease are included.

Deformities of the Arch

The Pronated Foot

Pronation of the foot and ankle during the stance phase of gait is essentially a temporary collapse of the ankle, rearfoot, and midfoot. Some pronation of the foot is necessary during functional activities; however, excessive pronation has been linked to lower limb overuse injuries, as maintenance of the equilibrium becomes the function of the muscles, specifically the fibularis (peroneus) brevis and the posterior tibialis.[47–51] Excessive pronation can occur as the result of a number of different factors including congenital, developmental, equinus at the ankle, subtalar varus, and rearfoot varus.[52] These deformities produce a rotation of the lower limb, which can have the following consequences:

- *Excessive external rotation of the lower limb:* This may shift the center of gravity in weight bearing to the medial aspect of the foot. Ideally, the center of gravity during weight bearing should pass through the center of the foot. This increase in medial stress causes the talus to plantarflex and adduct, while the calcaneus tilts laterally (into valgus).
- *Excessive internal rotation of the lower limb:* This produces excessive weight bearing on the lateral aspect of the foot. In an attempt to shift the center of gravity more medially, the forefoot abducts on the rearfoot or the foot abducts on the leg. These compensations produce excessive pronation of the subtalar joint.

Intervention

The intervention for an abnormally and symptomatic pronated foot depends on the type, but typically involves the following:

- Alleviation of the abnormal tissue stress
- Stretching of the gastrocnemius–soleus complex
- Activity and shoe modification: Shoes that have rearfoot control, a high lacing pattern, and a straighter last may be enough to control excessive motion, particularly if it is not severe;[53,54] a straighter last is more desirable for a person with excessive pronation
- Taping or arch strapping to limit excessive pronation[55,56]
- Orthotics

The Flatfoot

A patient with little or no longitudinal arch with full weight bearing is said to have a flatfoot or pes planus. Flatfeet and a minimal longitudinal arch are standard in infants and common in children up to the age of 6 years.[57] A flatfoot is said to be flexible if the arch can be re-created with the patient standing up on their toes. Flexible pes planus has been reported to occur in 15 percent of the general population,[58] with the majority being asymptomatic.[59]

> **● Key Point** A rigid flatfoot, a relatively rare condition, positions the calcaneus in a valgus position and the midtarsal region in pronation, resulting in a displaced navicular (posteriorly [dorsally]) and a talus that faces medially and inferiorly.

Adult-acquired flatfoot deformity (AAFD) involves some physiologic or structural change that causes deformity in a foot that was structurally normal at one time. A mismatch between active (posterior tibials tendon) and passive arch stabilizers (the spring-ligament complex and the talocalcaneal interosseous ligament) is the most likely cause.

Intervention

Management of the painful posterior tibials tendon (PTT)–deficient foot continues to be controversial. Treatment options range from conservative management with the use of medication and orthotics to various surgical procedures. If the patient is evaluated in an acute state, a short period of immobilization is recommended with or without a trial of nonsteroidal anti-inflammatory drugs (NSAIDs) prescribed by the physician. Often, the casting trial must be for as long as one month before a significant clinical effect is noted. Once the acute symptoms have diminished, the patient can begin a course of stretching and strengthening of the PTT. In addition, a custom-fabricated orthotic may be indicated.

The Stiff Foot

Normal supination is designed to allow the foot to function as a rigid lever during push-off, torque conversion, and a lengthening mechanism of the leg.[18] An abnormally supinated foot is described as pes cavus. Pes cavus is characterized by a high arch, increased external rotation of the tibia, increased forefoot varus, and an inability to pronate during the stance phase. Without the normal amount of pronation needed to allow the dissipation of stresses, the foot loses its ability to absorb shock. This produces increased pressure on the heel and on the metatarsal heads.[60]

Intervention

The intervention for a symptomatic cavus foot is supportive and involves having the patient wear a soft shoe with adequate padding to provide more midsole cushion for the plantar aspect of the foot.[60] Total-contact foot orthoses increase the weight-bearing surface of the foot and are recommended with this foot type.[61]

Sprains

A sprain of a ligament is defined as an injury that stretches the fibers of the ligament. Greater than 40 percent of ankle sprains can potentially progress to chronic problems.[62-72]

> ● **Key Point** Dynamic stability is provided to the lateral ankle by the strength of the fibularis (peroneus) longus and brevis tendons.

The most common mechanism of an ankle sprain is one of inversion and plantarflexion with subsequent damage to the lateral ligaments.[24,73] With eversion and external rotation, the deltoid and/or ligaments of the distal tibiofibular joint can be injured, producing the so-called medial and central sprains, respectively.

> ● **Key Point** Eversion injuries to the medial (deltoid) ligament of the ankles account for only 5 percent of ankle sprains.[74-76]

The prognosis for ankle sprains is inversely proportional to the severity and grade of the injury (**Table 21-7**),[77] the age of the patient, and the recurrence rate.[23,24]

> ● **Key Point** The prognosis for ankle injuries is worse when the ankle has been sprained previously.[65] The prognosis is also diminished when sprains occur in younger patients,[65] presumably relating to a greater mechanistic energy of injury.[23,24]

> ● **Key Point** Three factors are thought to cause functional instability of the ankle joint:[78]
> • Anatomic or mechanical instability
> • Muscle weakness
> • Deficits in joint proprioception

Lateral Ankle (Inversion) Sprain

The ATFL, which is the least elastic of the lateral ligaments,[79] is involved in 60–70 percent of all ankle sprains; 20 percent of sprains involve both the ATFL and the CFL.[74-76] The sequence of ligament tears in an inversion injury is first the ATFL, then the anterolateral capsule (which is in close proximity to the ATFL and results in hemarthrosis when torn), and then the distal tibiofibular ligament. Progressive

TABLE 21-7	The West Point Ankle Sprain Grading System		
Criterion	**Grade I**	**Grade II**	**Grade III**
Location of tenderness	ATFL	ATFL and CFL	ATFL, CFL, and PTFL
Edema and ecchymosis	Slight and local	Moderate and local	Significant and diffuse
Weight-bearing ability	Full or partial	Difficult without crutches	Impossible without significant pain
Ligament damage	Stretched	Partial tear	Complete tear
Instability	None	None or slight	Definite

ATFL, anterior talofibular ligament; CFL, calcaneofibular ligament; PTFL, posterior talofibular ligament.

Data from Gerber JP, Williams GN, Scoville CR, et al: Persistent disability associated with ankle sprains: A prospective examination of an athletic population. Foot Ankle Int 19:653–660, 1998

inversion strain results in a CFL tear. As the inversion force continues, the PTFL, the strongest of the lateral ligaments, ruptures.[80,81] High ankle sprains, or syndesmotic sprains, which involve disruption of the ligamentous structures between the distal fibula and tibia, just proximal to the ankle joint, occur less frequently than lateral ankle sprains. Lateral ligament sprains are more common than medial ligament sprains for two major reasons:[7]

- The lateral malleolus projects more distally than the medial malleolus, producing less bony obstruction to inversion than eversion.
- The medial (deltoid) ligament of the ankle is much stronger than the lateral ligaments.

No single symptom or test can provide a completely accurate diagnosis of a lateral ankle ligament rupture. One study[82] demonstrated that a combination of tenderness at the level of the ATFL, a lateral hematoma, discoloration, and a positive drawer test (refer to Table 21-6) indicated a ligament rupture in 95 percent of cases, whereas the absence of these findings always indicated an intact ligament.

Lateral ankle sprains can be categorized as follows using the West Point Ankle Sprain Grading (WPASG) system:

- Grade I sprains are characterized by minimal to no swelling and localized tenderness over the ATFL. These sprains require, on average, 11.7 days before the full resumption of athletic activities.[83]
- Grade II sprains are characterized by localized swelling and more diffuse lateral tenderness. These sprains require approximately 2–6 weeks for return to full athletic function.[84,85]
- Grade III sprains are characterized by significant swelling, pain, and ecchymosis and should be referred to a specialist.[86] Grade III injuries may require greater than 6 weeks to return to full function. For acute grade III ankle sprains, the average duration of disability has been reported to be anywhere from 4.5 to 26 weeks, and only 25–60 percent of patients are symptom free 1–4 years after injury.[87] Some controversy exists regarding the appropriate treatment of grade III injuries, particularly in high-level athletes.[23,24] In a summary of all prospective and controlled studies on grade III sprains, it was concluded that the long-term prognosis is good to excellent in 80–90 percent of patients with this injury, regardless of the type of intervention chosen.[88]

Intervention

Conservative intervention has been found to be uniformly effective in treating grades I and II ankle sprains[89] and high ankle sprains (**Table 21-8**), and generally patients are completely asymptomatic and functionally stable at follow-up. Although conservative treatment may be appropriate, the time required to return to full function in any conservative program will increase as the severity of injury increases. Although early motion and mobility rather than immobilization have demonstrated the stimulation of collagen bundle orientation and the promotion of healing,[90] it must be remembered that full ligamentous strength is not gained for a period of months.[91–94] The injured ankle should be positioned

TABLE 21-8	Summary of Conservative Treatment for Ankle Sprains
Phase	**Intervention**
I	Pain and swelling control: rest, ice, compression, elevation, electrical stimulation, toe curls, ankle pump, and cryotherapy
	Temporary immobilization/stabilization (cast, splint, brace)
	Non–weight-bearing with crutches
II	Patient can ambulate using partial weight bearing with assistive device without pain
	Lower-level balance training (while being careful to avoid plantarflexion/inversion)
	Lower-level strengthening of hip and lower leg using Theraband
III	Ambulation with full weight bearing without pain
	Unilateral balance training
	Progress from double-heel raises to single-heel raises
	Treadmill walking or over ground walking
	Progress to fast walking without heel lift
IV	Jog to run progression
	Shuttle runs and cutting maneuvers
	Sport-specific training

The timeline for progression of an individual patient depends on the severity of the injury, the ability of the patient, and the criteria listed in the table for progression to each phase.

Data from Lin CF, Gross ML, Weinhold P: Ankle syndesmosis injuries: Anatomy, biomechanics, mechanism of injury, and clinical guidelines for diagnosis and intervention. J Orthop Sports Phys Ther 36:372–384, 2006

and supported in the maximum amount of dorsiflexion allowed by pain and effusion as appropriate. Maximal dorsiflexion places the joint in its close-packed position or position of greatest congruency.[95] This allows for the least capsular distention and resultant joint effusion. With ankle sprains, this position produces an approximation of the torn ligament ends in grade III injuries to reduce the amount of gap scarring, and reduces the tension in the grades I and II injured ligaments.[23,24]

Braces can play an important role in both the initial intervention and the prevention of ankle sprains. Acutely, their role is to compress, protect, and support the ankle. They also function to limit range of motion of the injured ankle, most importantly plantarflexion, which is a precarious position for the sprained ankle.[45] Mild-to-moderate ankle sprains (grades I and II sprains) can be readily supported by the use of an elastic bandage, open Gibney strapping (with or without felt-pad incorporation), taping,[31,81,96–99] or the use of some type of thermoplastic stirrup such as an Air Cast.[33,100] One of the main advantages of these types of immobilization is that pain-free protected plantarflexion and dorsiflexion are allowed whereas inversion and eversion are minimized. Protected weight bearing with an orthosis is permitted, with weight bearing to tolerance as soon as possible following injury.[101] Patients who suffer a grade III ligament injury may require more protection and support than can be afforded by a thermoplastic device. In cases such as this, consideration should be given to recommending a functional walking orthosis, either with a fixed ankle or a hinged ankle (which can be motion restricted) that allows only plantarflexion and dorsiflexion.[23,24] The advantage of the orthosis is that it is removable, which allows the patient to continue to ice to minimize inflammation.

> ● **Key Point** In the presence of instability, the ankle joint is best supported by a commercial brace, with or without taping, depending on the stress of the sport.[23,24]

Historically, ankle taping was the athletic trainer's method of choice to attempt to prevent ankle sprains. Ankle taping is effective in restricting the motion of the ankle and has also been proven to decrease the incidence of ankle sprains.[102–107] However, although taping initially restricts motion, the tape loses 50 percent of its net support after as little as 10 minutes of exercise.[107–116] Because of this deterioration of support, and the cost of tape, removable and reusable ankle braces were designed as an alternative to taping.[23,24] The use of tape for increased proprioception remains controversial. It is hypothesized that the tape can either provide additional cutaneous cues or provide a general facilitation at spinal or higher levels, thereby enhancing the perception of movement signals from other proprioceptive sources,[117–120] although this has yet to be proved conclusively.[118,121,122] The more common instabilities treated with taping include splaying of the mortise, inversion instability of the ankle, plantar instability of the talonavicular joint, and inversion or eversion instability of the talocalcaneal joint.[23,24]

- For a splayed mortise, the tape is wrapped circumferentially around the lateral and medial malleolus.
- Talocalcaneal instabilities are taped around the neck of the talus and the heel.

The decision as to whether to utilize some type of protective taping or bracing upon the return to activity to prevent reinjury is based upon the individual and his or her case. No type of taping or bracing will prevent all injuries.[23,24]

> ● **Key Point**
> - Often a player may argue that their performance will be adversely affected by the use of taping or bracing.[23,24] A review of the literature demonstrates that for normal athletic movement and function there does not appear to be an adverse impact on function or performance.[114,123–128] Indeed, one study involving soccer players demonstrated a fivefold decrease in the incidence of recurrent ankle sprains when using semi-rigid orthoses, without significantly affecting sports performance.[129] However, it was not clear what impact there was on the incidence of other injuries at nearby joints.
> - The type of sneaker worn during basketball, high top versus low top, has been studied and shown to have no relationship to the incidence of injury.[103] However, it does appear that increased shoe height can enhance the passive resistance to inversion when the foot is in plantarflexion, and can also increase the passive resistance afforded by tape and orthoses.[116]

As the healing progresses and the patient is able to bear more weight on his or her ankle, there is a corresponding increase in the use of weight-bearing (closed-chain) exercises. A useful activity during this phase is the "cross drill." The patient stands independently or with minimal external assistance on the involved limb only. The patient then moves the uninvolved limb into hip flexion, hip extension, hip abduction, and hip adduction. The exercise is performed initially on a firm surface with the eyes open. As the patient improves, the exercise is performed on a foam surface or balance board, first with the eyes open and then with the eyes closed.

External support may still be required during the subacute stages of the rehabilitation process (4–14 days).

Medial Ankle (Eversion) Sprain

The ligaments of the medial ankle, collectively known as the deltoid ligament complex, form a broad, strong, thick ligamentous stability to prevent eversion and provide medial ankle stability. A medial ligament sprain is rare but can occur, and is often associated with a fracture.

Intervention

Medial ligament sprains without an associated fracture are treated in the same way as lateral ligament sprains, although recovery can take twice as long.

Recurrent Ankle Sprains

The patient who suffers from recurrent sprains and functional instability poses a problem to the clinician and other members of the sports medicine team. Functional instability and loss of normal ankle kinematics as a complication of ankle sprains may lead to early degenerative changes.[67,130] Talar displacement of greater than 1 millimeter reduces the ankle's weight-bearing surface by 42.3 percent,[131–133] thus creating asymmetric load bearing of the articular surface. Thus, degenerative change may be due to small amounts of articular displacement or the abnormal shearing forces of instability.

> ● **Key Point** Chronic lateral ankle instability is manifested by recurrent injuries with pain, tenderness, and sometimes bruising over the lateral ligaments.[65,71,134–137]

Intervention

The intervention for all recurrent ankle sprains should begin with a trial of conservative management for 2–3 months.[62,63,72,138,139] Any or all of the following have been shown to help in some patients: a lateral heel wedge, fibular (peroneal) muscle strengthening, proprioceptive/coordination exercises, taping, elastic or thermoplastic ankle supports, and/or a short leg brace. Many patients with ankle instability can be treated satisfactorily with late repair or reconstruction of the lateral ligaments.[65,140–145] However, in spite of surgery, some patients will be left with persistent disability including subjective or objective instability, persistent talar tilt, stretching of the ligaments, pain, stiffness, or range-of-motion limitations.[136,146]

Hallux Valgus

Hallux valgus is the term used to describe a lateral or valgus deformity of the great toe (medial deviation of the first metatarsal and lateral deviation and/or rotation of the hallux). The term has been expanded to include varying degrees of metatarsus primus varus/valgus deviation of the proximal phalanx, medial deviation of the first metatarsal head, and bunion formation.

Hallux valgus has been observed to occur almost exclusively in populations that wear shoes, although some predisposing anatomic factors make some feet more vulnerable than others to the effects of extrinsic factors. Women have been observed to have hallux valgus at a rate of 9:1 compared with men.[147] Hallux valgus also has been reported to affect 22–36 percent of adolescents.[148–153]

Intervention

The intervention for hallux valgus should be conservative if possible. The intervention with any associated bunion includes wider shoes and orthotics.[148,149,151] The supervising PT may prescribe Achilles stretching in cases of Achilles contracture, a simple toe spacer between the first and second toes, or a silicone bunion pad placed over the bunion to alleviate direct pressure on the prominence.[154] In cases of pes planus associated with hallux valgus, the PT may ask for a medial longitudinal arch support with Morton's extension to be placed under the first MTP joint to alleviate symptoms.[154] Functional orthotic therapy may be implemented to control foot biomechanics. This approach can relieve symptomatic bunions, though the foot and first metatarsophalangeal joint must maintain some degree of flexibility.

If pain persists, however, structural realignment of the first metatarsal varus through surgery is usually necessary as the bunion deformity becomes more severe and decompensated. The goals of surgical treatment are to relieve symptoms, restore function, and correct the deformity. The specific procedures vary depending on the surgeon's preference, the nature of the deformity, and the particular needs of the patient. The type of procedure performed and its inherent stability determine postoperative management. The dressings applied at the time of the surgery are designed to apply corrective forces (e.g., derotation, plantarflexion, adduction) while the soft tissue remodels, with mild compression to control postoperative edema. The patient's weight-bearing status is determined on the basis of the procedure performed, but generally is limited during the first 2 weeks to prevent deviation or displacement and to minimize edema. The patient may begin ROM exercises on a daily basis after the sutures are removed,

TABLE 21-9	Lesser Toe Deformities			

Deformity	MTP Joint	PIP Joint	DIP Joint
Claw toe	Dorsiflexed	Plantarflexed	Plantarflexed
Hammer toe	Dorsiflexed or neutral	Plantarflexed	Neutral, hyperextended, or plantarflexed
Mallet toe	Neutral	Neutral	Plantarflexed

and weight bearing is advocated to prevent limitation of joint motion from excessive scarring.

Turf Toe

The term *turf toe* refers to a sprain of the first MTP joint.[154] Turf toe primarily affects football, baseball, and soccer players. Soccer players tend to develop the problem in the nonkicking foot due to the forced dorsiflexion during kicking. The MTP sprain can result in hypermobility of the first ray, which in turn can lead to biomechanical problems including lesser metatarsalgia, acquired flatfoot, posterior tibialis tendinitis, plantar fasciitis, and shin splints.[155,156]

Clinically, patients with turf toe present with a red, swollen, stiff first MTP joint. Clanton and Ford[157] have classified the severity of turf toe injuries from grades I to III:

- A grade I sprain is a minor stretch injury to the soft tissue restraints with little pain, swelling, or disability.
- A grade II sprain is a partial tear of the capsuloligamentous structures with moderate pain, swelling, ecchymosis, and disability.
- A grade III sprain is a complete tear of the plantar plate with severe swelling, pain, ecchymosis, and inability to bear weight normally. Radiographs of the foot should be obtained to rule out fracture of the sesamoids or metatarsal head articular surface and to check joint congruity.

Intervention

The initial intervention for turf toe is rest, ice, a compressive dressing, and elevation.

An NSAID may be prescribed by the physician. The toe should be taped to limit dorsiflexion, with multiple loops of tape placed over the posterior (dorsal) aspect of the hallucal proximal phalanx and criss-crossed under the ball of the foot plantarly,[158] or a forefoot steel plate can be used.[73] PROM and progressive resistance exercises are begun as soon as symptoms allow.[158,159] Patients with grade I sprains are usually allowed to return to regular activities as soon as symptoms allow, sometimes immediately. Patients with grade II sprains usually require 3–14 days' rest. Grade III sprains usually require crutches for a few days and up to 6 weeks' rest.

Lesser Toe Deformities

Three common lesser toe deformities (**Table 21-9**) worth noting are claw toe, hammer toe, and mallet toe.

Claw Toe

The term *claw toe* (Figure 21-35) is most likely derived from the affected toe's similarity in appearance to the claw of an animal: dorsiflexion of the proximal phalanx on the lesser metatarsophalangeal

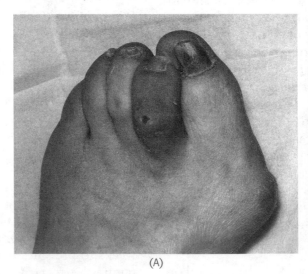
(A)

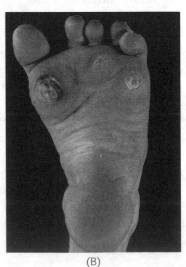
(B)

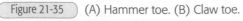
Figure 21-35   (A) Hammer toe. (B) Claw toe.

(MTP) joint and concurrent flexion of the proximal interphalangeal (PIP) and distal interphalangeal (DIP) joints. Claw toe deformity results from altered anatomy and/or neurologic deficit, resulting in an imbalance between the intrinsic and extrinsic musculature to the toes.

> **● Key Point** All lesser-toe procedures result in stiffness of the MTP and interphalangeal joints. Because some stiffness is intentional to maintain lasting correction of the deformity, exercises to improve range of motion should be used judiciously. Some stretching may be necessary to improve mobility, but general mobilization through everyday use, as tolerated, is usually sufficient.

Intervention

Conservative intervention for flexible deformities includes avoiding wearing high-heeled and/or narrow-toed shoes, which increase dorsal ground reactive forces on the toe and crowd the toes against each other, producing impingement. Shoes with a wide toe box, soft upper shoe, and stiff sole to absorb dorsally directed forces against the plantar plate are appropriate. A metatarsal bar can be added to the shoe to avoid metatarsal pressure, but patients more easily accept metatarsal pads. Cushioning sleeves or stocking caps with silicon linings can relieve pressure points at the PIP joint and tip of the toe. A longitudinal pad beneath the toes can prevent point pressure at the tip of the toes. Because the MTP joint is always dorsiflexed by definition, surgical correction of its position is necessary to restore a more neutral angle at the MTP joint. Forefoot surgery is typically performed in an outpatient setting. A fresh dressing is applied the next day, and stitches are removed after 2 weeks. Arthrodesis pins are removed after 4 weeks, and the other types of pins are removed after 2 weeks. Patients may shower with pins protruding from the toes.

Hammer Toe

This is the most common deformity of the lesser toes (Figure 21-35). It primarily comprises flexion deformity of the PIP joint of the toe, with hyperextension of the MTP and DIP joints. The hyperextension of the MTP joint and flexion of the PIP joint make the PIP joint prominent dorsally. This prominence rubs against the patient's shoe, causing pain. The deformity is flexible and passively correctable early in its natural history, but typically becomes fixed with time.

Intervention

Although no reliably effective physical therapy program for hammer toe deformity has been described,

it may be of use for the patient with a flexible deformity to perform passive stretching exercises. The indication for surgical treatment of hammer toe deformity is disabling pain that does not improve with conservative treatment, including taping (for flexible deformity) and the use of accommodative footwear featuring a toe box of adequate depth (for fixed deformity). Pin fixation is necessary for 4–6 weeks after surgery. The pin is cut to length outside the skin. A pin cap protects the sharp end of the cut pin so that it does not catch on the patient's bed sheets. A compression dressing is applied. Plaster immobilization is rarely, if ever, necessary. A hard-soled postoperative shoe is provided. Elevation of the foot with the toes above the heart is essential to minimize swelling, which can cause pain and delay wound healing. Weight bearing as tolerated in a hard-soled shoe occurs once the pin does not cross the MTP joint. Once the pin is removed (typically 4–6 weeks postsurgery), footwear may be advanced as tolerated. The patient should be advised that mild to moderate swelling may persist for many months after surgery, and this limits footwear options until it has resolved. Patients should also be advised to continue wearing shoes of adequate length and depth, with a rounded or squared toe area to minimize the risk of recurrence.

Mallet Toe

Mallet toe is a fixed or flexible flexion deformity of the DIP joint of the toe.

Intervention

Conservative treatment focuses on relieving the pressure under the tip of the toe. This can be accomplished with extra-depth toe-box footwear. Surgical therapy includes flexor tenotomy; condylectomy and fusion of the middle to distal phalanx; and, occasionally, partial or complete amputation of the distal phalanx. Sutures are removed after 10–14 days. Pins are usually removed at 4 weeks.

Tendon Injuries

Overuse tendonitis in the tendons spanning the ankle can be seen with training errors, sudden changes in training patterns, muscle–tendon imbalance, anatomic malalignment, improper footwear, or a sudden growth spurt.[160] Tendonitis can also be seen in the adolescent who resumes play after a period of decreased training.[161]

Fibular (Peroneal) Tendon Tendonitis

Fibular (peroneal) tendonitis is particularly common in young dancers and ice skaters but can be seen in any running athlete. After repeated inversion strain, the sheaths of the fibularis (peroneus) longus and brevis tendons may be stretched and become inflamed (runner's foot). Instability between the fourth and fifth metatarsals is also associated with this disorder.

Intervention

The intervention for fibular tendonitis includes a program of stretching, strengthening, icing, and sometimes ankle bracing[161] during contact sports.

Fibular (Peroneal) Tendon Subluxation

Subluxation of the fibular tendons is an uncommon but potentially disabling condition that can affect young athletes,[162] and it is often difficult to distinguish from lateral ankle sprain acutely.[163] Acute symptoms are pain at the posterior distal fibula, swelling, ecchymosis, and apprehension or inability to evert the foot against resistance.[73] Chronic symptoms are lateral ankle pain, popping or snapping, and instability.[73] A chronic fibular tendon subluxation can both mimic and coexist with chronic ankle instability.

In some young patients, there may be an anatomic predisposition to fibular tendon subluxation. These include an absent or shallow fibula groove,[160,164–166] possibly combined with pes planus, hindfoot valgus, or lax/absent fibular retinaculum.[161,164,165,167,168] The retinaculum can also traumatically rupture from a violent forced dorsiflexion of the ankle with reflex contraction of the fibular muscles and dislocation.[160,164,167–171]

Intervention

Many different surgical procedures have been described for chronic fibular tendon subluxation, including acute repair of the superior peroneal retinaculum, tissue transfer (using the Achilles tendon, as well as the plantaris and peroneus brevis tendons) to reinforce the superior peroneal retinaculum, tendon rerouting (beneath the calcaneofibular ligament), and groove-deepening procedures.[162,164,168,170,172]

Tibialis Posterior Tendonitis

The tibialis posterior tendon lies just posterior to the medial malleolus and supports the medial arch of the foot. The tendon is lined with a tenosynovial sheath that can become inflamed, producing a tenosynovitis. If left untreated, the condition can progress to an eventual rupture.[173]

The pain is usually felt in one of three locations:

- Distal to the medial malleoli in the area of the navicular
- Proximal to the medial malleoli

- At the musculotendinous origin (medial shin splints), which often refers symptoms to the anterior shin or at the insertion

Posterior tibialis tendonitis is seen relatively frequently in dancers, joggers, and ice skaters, especially in those participants with a pronated foot and flattened longitudinal arch.[174] Running sports that require rapid changes in direction (basketball, tennis, soccer, and ice hockey) place increased stress across the tendon as well.[175] Contributing factors include adaptive shortening of the gastrocnemius–soleus complex and weakness of the posterior tibialis.

Intervention

The intervention for posterior tibialis dysfunction depends on the cause, but the overall approach includes tibialis posterior stretching and strengthening, orthotics, occasional casting, and icing.[175]

Tibialis Anterior Tendonitis

Patients with tibialis anterior tendonitis usually experience pain at the front of the shin (anterior shin splints) during activities placing large amounts of stress on the tibialis anterior tendon (or after these activities with rest, especially upon waking in the morning). These activities may include walking or running excessively (especially up or down hills or on hard or uneven surfaces), kicking an object with toes pointed (e.g., a football), wearing excessively tight shoes, or kneeling. The pain associated with this condition tends to be of gradual onset that progressively worsens over weeks or months with continuation of aggravating activities. Patients with this condition may also experience pain on firmly touching the tibialis anterior tendon.

Intervention

Conservative intervention includes tibialis anterior stretching, strengthening, orthotics, and occasional casting and icing.

Flexor Hallucis Longus Tendonitis

The flexor hallucis longus (FHL) is lined by a tenosynovial sheath, which can become inflamed. FHL tendonitis is characterized by pain posterior to the medial malleolus, which is most often confused with posterior tibialis tendonitis.[176] Dancers who assume the repeated plantarflexion posture of demipointe or pointe are particularly susceptible to FHL tendonitis, with the tendon actually locking in demipointe in the latter group.[177–179] It can also be seen in runners and gymnasts. Clinical findings with FHL tendonitis usually include tenderness on the medial aspect of the ankle along a course that travels from just posterior to the medial malleolus to just under the medial malleolus. Passive motion of the great toe and ankle may induce symptoms of tendinitis when palpating along the FHL.

Intervention

Conservative intervention includes icing, stretching, strengthening, decreased activity, correcting improper techniques, orthotics, a hard-soled shoe, and NSAIDs.[180] Operative intervention typically involves releasing the tendon sheath.

Achilles Tendonitis

Achilles tendonitis is the most common overuse syndrome of the lower leg,[181] accounting for 5–18 percent of the total number of running injuries. The underlying mechanism of Achilles tendonitis in runners is not well understood, but a number of mechanisms have been proposed:

- *Stretching:* In a study by McCrory and colleagues,[182] whether a runner incorporated stretching of the gastrocnemius into his or her training routine appeared to be a significant discriminator between the injured and uninjured cohorts. Specifically, injured runners were less likely to incorporate stretching into their regular training routines. Whether stretching habits can be related to the incidence of overuse injuries remains undetermined.[183–186]

- *Training variables:* The incidence of overuse injuries has been strongly associated with a faster training pace, with injured runners running at a significantly faster training pace than uninjured runners.[183,187,188] Hill training has also been suggested as an etiological factor in the onset of Achilles tendonitis.[189–191]

- *Fatigue: Overtraining* has been found to correlate to calf muscle fatigue and microtears of the tendon.[49,192]

- *Isokinetic variables:* Muscular insufficiency has been cited as a significant factor in the inability to eccentrically restrain dorsiflexion during the beginning of the support phase of running.[182,188,189,193]

- *Anthropometric variables:* In one study, 20 percent of the injured runners with Achilles tendonitis had cavus feet.[192] Clement and coworkers,[189] after having found cavus feet to be rigid, suggested that the compensatory overpronation resulting from the inflexibility of the cavus foot is a precursor to Achilles tendonitis. Other studies also have related a high-arched

foot to the incidence of various overuse syndromes.[50,187,194,195]

- *Age:* The role that age plays in Achilles tendonitis is inconclusive, with some studies finding a correlation[182,196] and others[185,195,197–199] finding no associations between age and the pathogenesis of running injuries.

- *Shoe type:* Spike shoes lock the feet on the surface during the single support phase in running and increase the athlete's foot grip but also transfer lateral and torque shear forces directly to the foot and ankle and through to the Achilles tendon.[200] The soles of spike shoes have minimal shock absorption, transferring the vertical force directly to the Achilles tendon.[201] This may increase the overloading of the tendon, causing microtrauma and inflammation of the Achilles tendon.

- *Sacroiliac joint dysfunction:* Changes in sacroiliac joint mechanics as compared with the contralateral side have also been associated with Achilles tendonitis.[200]

Clinical symptoms consist of a gradual onset of pain and swelling in the Achilles tendon, which is exacerbated by activity.

> ● **Key Point** An inability to dorsiflex 20 degrees with knee extension signifies gastrocnemius tightness; an inability to dorsiflex 30 degrees with knee flexion implicates the soleus as well.[202]

Intervention

A literature review by Goodnite[203] that investigated the current evidence-based practice, in order to determine the best intervention for a patient with recurrent Achilles tendonitis, based on the intervention's validity and strength, recommended the 12-week eccentric program as outlined by Alfredson et al.[204] In brief, the program consists of two types of eccentric exercises—eccentrically loading the calf muscles with the knee bent and eccentrically loading the calf with the knee straight. He recommends three sets of 15 repetitions using body weight to start, with the patient being instructed to continue unless the pain becomes disabling. The exercises are performed two times per day, every day, for 12 weeks. If only minor pain or discomfort is experienced, the patient is instructed to increase the load by using a backpack loaded with weight.

Rupture of the Achilles Tendon

The etiology of a spontaneous rupture of the Achilles tendon remains incompletely understood.

Three activities have been implicated in rupturing an Achilles' tendon:[205]

- Pushing off (plantarflexion) with weight bearing on the forefoot while extending the knee
- Sudden dorsiflexion with full weight bearing, as might occur with a slip or fall
- Violent dorsiflexion, such as occurs when jumping or falling from a height and landing on a plantarflexed foot

The classic history is a report of sudden pain in the calf area, often associated with an audible snap, followed by difficulty in stepping off on the foot.[206] Physical examination reveals swelling of the calf as well as a palpable defect in the tendon (sometimes called a hatchet strike) and ecchymosis around the malleoli.[207]

Intervention

The intervention for Achilles tendon ruptures can be conservative or surgical.

- *Conservative:* The conservative intervention for Achilles tendon rupture is best for small partial ruptures, because this approach appears to result in a high incidence of rerupture (10–30 percent)[208-211] and a decrease in maximal muscle function if used with complete ruptures.[212-214] This approach consists of placing the patient in short- or long-leg cast immobilization in the gravity equinus position (10–20 degrees of plantarflexion) for approximately 8 weeks of non–weight bearing. At 6 to 8 weeks, plantarflexion of the cast is slowly decreased and, when progressive weight bearing is initiated, a heel lift of 2 to 2.5 centimeters is worn for approximately 1 month. The height of the heel lift is decreased at 10 to 12 weeks to 1 centimeter, and over the next month is progressively decreased so that the patient is walking without a heel lift by 3 months. Maximal plantarflexion power may not return for 12 months or more. The exercise progression is outlined in **Table 21-10**.

Once the cast is removed, gentle active dorsiflexion and plantarflexion exercises are initiated immediately and proprioception exercises can begin with the patient in a seated position. As the motion increases, closed chain resistive exercises can be initiated based on the surgeon's preference. Bilateral heel raises are introduced as strength improves, progressing to unilateral heel raises based on patient tolerance.

- *Surgical:* Surgical repair often is advocated for high-level and competitive athletes—surgically repaired tendons have a rerupture rate of 0 to 5 percent.[215-217] Other indications for surgical intervention appear to be for better restoration of the continuity of the tendon, to facilitate healing, and to restore maximum muscle function. During the surgical procedure, the severed ends of the tendon are brought together and then sutured with the ankle positioned in a neutral position. A cast is applied. The length of time the cast remains on the patient varies according to the surgical technique. A study[218] that involved early active motion of the ankle and weight bearing, without casting, demonstrated remarkable functional recovery without serious complications. If casting is used, it incorporates varying degrees of plantarflexion (typically 10–20 degrees) to protect the repair site from stress. Long-term immobilization impairs the recovery of the injured tendon and delays remodeling of newly formed collagen fibrils,[219] so long-term casting has become less popular. After the cast is removed, the patient can be fitted with a short walking cast for about 4 weeks with partial weight bearing. If early weight bearing is the aim, the patient is issued either a specially designed shoe that has a 3-centimeter heel lift or a removable ankle–foot orthosis with a rocking sole.[220] The postoperative rehabilitation follows a similar rehabilitation program as that described for the conservative approach.

TABLE 21-10	Exercise Progression for Conservative or Surgical Treatment of an Achilles Tendon Rupture	
6 Weeks	**8–10 Weeks**	**4–6 Months**
Stationary bicycling (no resistance) and swimming	Progressive resistance exercises for the calf muscles	Resumption of running (if strength is 70 percent of the uninvolved leg)

Plantar Heel Pain

Plantar heel pain, which is defined as pain arising from the insertion of the plantar fascia with or without heel spur, has been experienced at one time or another by 10 percent of the population.[221–223] Although often referred to as plantar fasciitis, Waugh[224] has recently proposed that accepted inflammatory conditions, such as epicondylitis, may be more accurately referred to as chronic pain syndromes. Therefore, individuals suffering from what has traditionally been referred to as plantar fasciitis may be more accurately described as suffering from plantar heel pain.[225]

The etiology of plantar heel pain is poorly understood, although a number of factors have been proposed including obesity,[226] occupations involving prolonged standing or walking, acute injury to the heel,[227] loss of elasticity of the heel pad, biomechanics (pes cavus or pes planus), and adaptive shortening of the calf muscles and Achilles tendon. The role of the heel spur in plantar heel pain is controversial.[227] Half of patients with plantar heel pain have heel spurs,[228] whereas 16–27 percent of the population have heel spurs without symptoms.[229,230]

Common findings include a history of pain and tenderness on the plantar medial aspect of the heel, especially during initial weight bearing in the morning. The heel pain often decreases during the day but worsens with increased activity (such as jogging, climbing stairs, or going up on the toes) or upon arising after a period of sitting. The main area of tenderness is typically just over and distal to the medial calcaneal tubercle, and usually there is one small exquisitely painful area.

It is worth noting that almost 90 percent of patients with plantar heel pain who undergo a conservative intervention improve significantly within 12 months, although approximately 10 percent can develop persistent and often disabling symptoms.[231]

Intervention

Based on studies, the intervention for plantar heel pain should include the following:

- Rest, or at least elimination of any activity that continually provides axial loading of the heel and tensile stresses on the fascia.
- Shoes that provide good shock absorption at the heel and support to the medial longitudinal arch and plantar fascia band. The clinician must identify any tissue overloading that is occurring, as well as any functional biomechanical deficits (plantarflexor inflexibility and weakness) and functional adaptations (running on toes, shortened stride length, and foot inversion).
- Strengthening exercises. A number of strengthening exercises have been devised for plantar heel pain:
  - *Towel curls:* A towel is placed on a smooth surface with a small weight placed at one end. The foot is placed on the other end of the towel. The patient is instructed to pull the towel toward the body by curling up the toes (refer to Figure 21-21). The same exercise can be performed from the side direction (refer to Figure 21-20).
  - *Marble pick-ups:* A few marbles are placed on the floor near a cup. While keeping the heel on the floor, the patient uses the toes to pick up the marbles and drop them in the cup (Figure 21-36).
- A regimen of stretching of the gastrocnemius and the plantar fascia is especially important before arising in the morning and after sedentary periods during the day as well as before and after exercise.[232]
  - *Gastrocnemius and soleus:* Patients are taught how to stretch the gastrocnemius and soleus components of the triceps surae independently. The stretching must be performed in such a way as to minimize stress on the plantar fascia.
  - *Plantar fascia stretch:* The plantar fascia stretch is performed with the patient sitting with their legs crossed, with the involved leg over the contralateral leg. Then, while using the hand on the affected side, the patient places his or her fingers across the base of

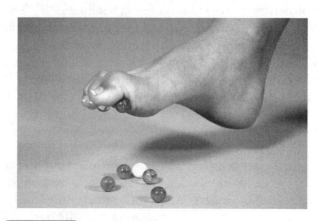

Figure 21-36) Marble pick-ups.

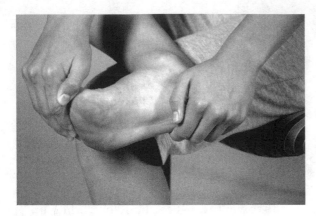

Figure 21-37 Fascia stretch.

the toes on the bottom of the foot (distal to the MTP joints) and pulls the toes back toward the shin until a stretch is felt in the arch of the foot (Figure 21-37). The correct stretch is confirmed by palpating the tension in the plantar fascia with the contralateral hand while performing the stretching.

The stretches are performed twice a day, beginning with a sustained stretch for 1 minute and progressing to 3 minutes as tolerated.[233] The rest period should entail gentle dorsiflexion and plantarflexion, while resting the Achilles tendon and calf on a hot pack to enhance the subsequent stretch and utilize an active rest period.[227] Massage to the foot in the area of the arch and heel over a tennis ball or a 15-ounce can, or rolling a tennis ball or a bottle of frozen water back and forth across the floor from the calcaneus to the metatarsal heads also may be helpful.

Night splinting of the ankle in dorsiflexion has been postulated to prevent nocturnal contracture of the gastrocnemius–soleus complex, which is thought to be detrimental to plantar fascia healing.[234–236] The splint holds the ankle fixed in 5 degrees of dorsiflexion and the toes slightly stretched into extension (i.e., at a functional length).[237] For most patients, this orthosis reduces morning pain considerably.[236] Powell et al.[235] performed a crossover study using splinting with the ankle in dorsiflexion as the sole method of treatment in 47 patients. This study also showed improvement in 80 percent of involved feet.

Orthotics may have a role in the intervention for plantar heel pain. A wide variety of rigid, semirigid, and soft shoe inserts are available commercially, although rigid plastic orthoses rarely alleviate the symptoms and often aggravate the heel pain.[228]

Metatarsalgia

Metatarsalgia is a common overuse symptom described as pain in the forefoot that is associated with increased stress over the metatarsal head region. The foot is frequently injured during activities that typically involve repetitive high-pressure loading on the forefoot. As in many other overuse syndromes, the condition may also be the result of an alteration in normal biomechanics that has caused an abnormal weight distribution among the metatarsal heads.

Intervention

The initial treatment includes PRICE (protection, rest, icing, compression, and elevation). Non–weight-bearing ambulation is recommended for the first 24 hours, after which PROM and ultrasound treatments can be initiated if delegated by the supervising physical therapist. The use of metatarsal pads and other orthotic devices may provide relief, even in the early phases of treatment. The metatarsal pad is placed proximal to the painful metatarsal heads. Adhesive-backed metatarsal pads of different shapes and sizes are available to unload one or several metatarsal heads. Custom orthotics may also be molded specifically for the cavus foot to decrease load on the plantarflexed first and second rays, in order to distribute weight evenly across the forefoot. A trial of Achilles stretching is helpful in the initial treatment of metatarsalgia. The wearing of high heels should be discouraged in patients with metatarsalgia.

If unresponsive to conservative intervention, surgical plantar condylectomy may be required for resolution of a discrete plantar keratosis. More generalized diffuse painful calluses, such as those seen under the first and second metatarsal heads in the cavus foot, may require posterior (dorsal) closing wedge osteotomies of the metatarsal bases to achieve pain relief.[238]

Tarsal Tunnel Syndrome

Tarsal tunnel syndrome (TTS) is an entrapment neuropathy of the tibial nerve as it passes through the anatomic tunnel between the flexor retinaculum and the medial malleolus (Figure 21-38). In addition, the terminal branches of the tibial, medial, and lateral plantar nerves may be involved. These latter nerves are often called the *posterior tibial nerve*. The onset of TTS may be acute or insidious. Etiologic factors for TTS can be classified as internal or external. Internal factors include anatomical variations such as an accessory flexor digitorum longus muscle. External factors include excessive pronation, which

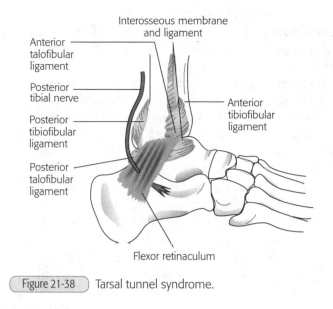

Anterior talofibular ligament

Interosseous membrane and ligament

Posterior tibial nerve

Posterior tibiofibular ligament

Posterior talofibular ligament

Anterior tibiofibular ligament

Flexor retinaculum

Figure 21-38 Tarsal tunnel syndrome.

can tighten the flexor retinaculum and the calcaneo-navicular ligament.

Intervention

Conservative intervention for TTS includes the use of orthotics to correct biomechanical gait abnormalities. Specifically, a foot orthosis with a rearfoot varus post can limit excessive pronation. In cases of early excessive rearfoot pronation and subtalar joint pronation at heel strike, an orthosis with a deepened heel cup can help to control rearfoot motion. In cases of severe hyperpronation, a rearfoot wedge may be helpful. The stretches employed for plantar fasciitis can also be used with this condition.

Interdigital Neuroma

Interdigital neuroma, or Morton's neuroma, is a common condition that involves enlargement of the interdigital nerve of the foot. The name of the condition is a misnomer, because this is not a true neuroma; rather, there is a thickening of the tissues around the nerve due to perineural fibrosis, fibrinoid degeneration, demyelination, and endoneural fibrosis.[154,239]

> ● **Key Point** In a study of 91 patients with "interdigital neuromas," the male:female ratio was 1:9.[240]

Although a common cause of this condition is chronic compression of the interdigital nerve, it can also arise due to an acute dorsiflexion injury to the toes, with an associated injury to the collateral ligaments of the MTP joint.[154,241]

Symptoms are usually exacerbated with weight bearing and somewhat relieved by removing the shoe and massaging the forefoot.[154,241] Poor shoe selection, such as wearing a firm cross-training or racket shoe for long-distance running, may increase the impact forces on the forefoot and contribute to the symptoms.[154] Narrow shoes and high-heeled shoes have also been implicated.

Squeezing the forefoot with one hand, while carefully palpating the involved interspace with the thumb and index fingers of the other hand, is usually successful in eliciting marked discomfort.[154] This compression may produce a painful audible click, known as Mulder's sign.[242]

Intervention

The intervention initially entails avoiding the offending activity, cross-training in lower-impact sports, and modification of footwear.[154] A switch to wider, more accommodating shoes with soft soles and better shock absorption will often improve symptoms.[154] A metatarsal pad, such as an adhesive-backed felt pad, placed proximal to the symptomatic interspace is helpful.[154] When the patient steps down, the pad is designed to separate the metatarsal heads to prevent rubbing or irritating the affected area.[154] The physician may prescribe a trial of NSAIDs to decrease inflammation around the interdigital nerve.[154] Recalcitrant cases that fail to respond to 2–3 months of these conservative measures may benefit from an injection of corticosteroids into the involved interspace.[154] Surgery, the intervention of last resort, is usually performed from a dorsal approach to prevent scar formation on the plantar aspect of the foot and to allow for early weight bearing.

Acute Compartment Syndrome

Acute compartment syndrome is a condition of pain associated with sudden compression of nerves, blood vessels, and muscle inside a closed space (compartment) within the body. Because the connective tissue that defines the compartment is not pliable, a small amount of bleeding into the compartment, or swelling of the muscles within the compartment, can cause the intracompartmental pressure to rise greatly. Common causes of compartment syndrome include tibial fractures, hemorrhage, intravenous drug injection, casts, prolonged limb compression, crush injuries, and burns. When compartment syndrome is caused by repetitive use of the muscles, it is known as chronic compartment syndrome. This is usually not an emergency, but the loss of circulation can cause temporary or permanent damage to nearby nerves and muscles. The clinical signs of compartment syndrome can be remembered using the mnemonic of the five Ps: pain, paralysis, paresthesia, pallor, and pulses. Pain, especially disproportionate pain, is often the earliest sign, but the loss of normal neurologic sensation is the most reliable sign.[243,244]

There are four compartments within the lower leg:

- *Anterior:* Contains the dorsiflexors (extensors) of the foot. These include the tibialis anterior, extensor digitorum longus, extensor hallucis longus, and fibularis tertius.
- *Lateral:* Contains the fibularis longus and brevis. The fibular tendons lie behind the lateral malleolus in a fibro-osseous tunnel formed by a groove in the fibula and the superficial fibular retinaculum. The fibular retinaculum and the CFL form the posterior wall of this tunnel.
- *Superficial posterior:* Contains the calf muscles that plantarflex the foot. These include the gastrocnemius, soleus, and plantaris muscles.
- *Deep posterior:* Contains the flexors of the foot. These muscles course behind the medial malleolus. They include the posterior tibialis, flexor digitorum longus, and FHL.

Palpation of the compartment in question may demonstrate swelling or tenseness.[245] Decrease or loss of two-point discrimination also can be an early finding of compartment syndrome.[243,244] Clinical findings may also include shiny, erythematous skin overlying the involved compartment (described as a "woody" feeling) and excessive swelling.

Intervention

Acute compartment syndrome is a medical emergency requiring immediate medical attention to prevent potential loss of limb.

> ● **Key Point** An acute compartment syndrome is considered a medical emergency, requiring an open fasciotomy to prevent severe and irreversible damage. The PTA should immediately contact the emergency services and then notify the PT.

Medial Tibial Stress Syndrome

Over the past 30 years, a number of generic terms such as *medial tibial syndrome, tibial stress syndrome, shin splints, posterior tibial syndrome, soleus syndrome,* and *periostitis* have evolved to describe exercise-related leg pain. Despite all these terms, *medial tibial stress syndrome (MTSS)* is the most appropriate term to describe this condition.

Neither the precise pathophysiologic mechanism nor the specific pathologic lesion in MTSS is known, although it appears to involve periosteal irritation indicated by a diffuse linear uptake on a bone scan along the length of the tibia.[246] The anatomic site of the abnormality has been fairly well localized. Initially, it was thought that the tibialis posterior muscle was the source. However, recent information has identified the fascial insertion of the medial soleus as the more probable source.

The most common complaint in these patients is a dull aching pain along the middle or distal posteromedial tibia. However, symptoms can also refer to the anterior tibia, just lateral to the tibial crest. Early in this process, the pain may occur at the beginning of a run, resolve with continued exertion, only to recur toward the end or after a workout.[247] Alternatively, the pain may be noted only toward the end of a run. At this early stage, the pain typically subsides promptly with rest.[247] With continued training the pain may become more severe, sharp, and persistent.[247] Patients may attempt trials of complete rest only to have the pain recur with resumption of training. With increasing chronicity, the pain may be present with ambulation or at rest.[247]

In contrast, with anterior shin splints, overuse or weakness of the tibialis anterior, extensor digitorum longus, or extensor digitorum brevis may be the causative factors in anterior shin splints, as are excessive or abnormal pronation, restricted ankle joint dorsiflexion, training errors, and inadequate footwear.[53] The physician and/or physical therapist will make that determination.

Intervention

As with most overuse injuries, the intervention for shin splints involves physician-prescribed NSAIDs or analgesics and activity modification, followed by a gradual return to sports, having corrected any training errors or abnormal foot biomechanics. The patient should be instructed to apply ice to the involved area for 20 minutes twice daily, and to reduce running activities, run on softer surfaces, and wear appropriate anti-pronation shoes. Custom foot orthoses are recommended for the vast majority of these individuals unless their symptoms are mild or resolve quickly.

Stress Fractures

A stress or fatigue fracture is a break that develops in bone after cyclical, submaximal loading. Extrinsic factors that may result in stress fractures of the leg and foot are running on hard surfaces, improper running shoes, or sudden increases in jogging or running distance. Intrinsic factors include malalignment of the lower extremity, particularly excessive pronation.

Metatarsal Stress Fracture

Patients who abruptly increase their training, whether it be training mileage, time spent in high-impact activities (marching, jumping, and landing), or training intensity, are susceptible to stress fractures.[154] The second and third metatarsals are the most frequently injured.[249] Military studies have found stress fractures to be more common in women, older individuals, and Caucasians.[250,251] Amenorrhea is present in up to 20 percent of vigorously exercising women and may be as high as 50 percent in elite runners and dancers.[252] Female long-distance runners, ballet dancers, and gymnasts are notorious for dieting to achieve low body fat despite rigorous training schedules. Patients with amenorrhea for more than 6 months experience the same bone loss as postmenopausal women.[253] Whole-body bone-mineral density is significantly lower in amenorrheic athletes, which predisposes them to stress fracture.[253] A recent study found that the simulation of fatigue of the toe plantarflexors resulted in an increase in second metatarsal strain. Therefore, muscular fatigue of the foot may play a role in the etiology of metatarsal stress fractures.[254]

The patient with a metatarsal stress fracture usually reports mild forefoot discomfort, which may be relieved by rest, but as the stress fracture worsens, pain is experienced while walking and even at rest.[154] Occasionally, there is local point tenderness of the involved metatarsal, induration, swelling, and palpable mass.[249,259] Symptoms usually present 4–5 weeks after a change in training regimen.[249]

Proximal Second Metatarsal Stress Fracture

The proximal second metatarsal stress fracture differs from other metatarsal stress fractures because it can be difficult to heal and may result in chronic nonunion. The anatomy in this area is such that the base of the shaft is countersunk into the bony arch of the foot and is therefore rigid (Lisfranc's joint). This tends to place an abnormal amount of stress across this area. The patient typically reports pain in the first web space, usually accompanied by proximal second metatarsal pain.[260]

Navicular Stress Fracture

Although navicular stress fractures are uncommon, they are the most common midfoot fracture and typically present with an insidious onset or with a history of repeated cyclic loading, which results in fatigue failure through the relatively avascular central portion of the tarsal navicular.[73,171,261] The cyclic loading across the navicular may be exacerbated due to a short first metatarsal, metatarsus adductus, or limited dorsiflexion or subtalar motion.[73] Complaints include chronic pain that is vague in nature but tender to palpation on the posterior aspect of the foot and/or the medial aspect of the midfoot.[249]

Sesamoid Stress Fracture

The sesamoid bones act as a pulley for tendons, help the big toe move normally and provide leverage when the big toe "pushes off" during walking and running. In addition, the sesamoids also serve as a weight-bearing surface for the first metatarsal bone. A sesamoid stress fracture produces long-standing pain in the ball of the foot beneath the big toe joint. The pain, which tends to fluctuate and be intermitent, generally is aggravated with activity and relieved with rest. Complaints include chronic pain that is vague in nature but tender to palpation on the inferior aspect of the ball of the foot at the proximal aspect of the great toe.

Interventions

To create an environment conducive for healing, interrupting the cycle of repetitive overload is essential. For most stress fractures, the period of relative rest may be expected to last from 4–12 weeks. Factors influencing the duration of the activity restriction include the anatomic site and extent of the fracture, and the anticipated demands on the individual upon return to work or play. The rehabilitation program should include a gradual resumption of active range of motion (AROM) and a program of muscle strengthening and generalized conditioning. Closed-chain activities must be deferred until there is radiographic evidence of complete bone healing.

Metatarsal Stress Fracture

The intervention for metatarsal stress fractures includes rest from the offending activity and cross-training in a low-impact sport.[154] Weight bearing to tolerance may be allowed in comfortable shoes of choice or a wooden shoe. If weight bearing is painful, or the fracture is diagnosed after a long delay, a short leg cast or hard-soled shoe is worn for 4–6 weeks until a healing callus is seen radiographically.[249,259]

Proximal Second Metatarsal Stress Fracture
The intervention for second metatarsal stress fracture usually consists of 6–8 weeks of rest in a hard shoe or cast,[260,262] with gradual return to activities when the tenderness resolves.

Navicular Stress Fracture
The intervention varies according to the type of fracture. Nondisplaced fractures are treated with a short-leg non–weight-bearing cast for 6–8 weeks.[160,261] If the fracture fails to heal or is displaced, operative intervention of fixation with compression screw and additional bone grafting where necessary, is used.[160,261] Return to sport may take as long as 16–20 weeks.[249]

Sesamoid Stress Fracture
The intervention for a sesamoid fracture is initially rest from the offending high-impact activity and a wooden-soled shoe or a short-leg cast for 6–8 weeks. If cast, a CT scan is performed at 8 weeks to detect signs of avascular necrosis. If avascular necrosis is present and the young patient has persistent symptoms, resection may be necessary.[263] Surgical choices include excision of the involved sesamoid or bone grafting, in an attempt to achieve union and preserve the sesamoid.

An alternative treatment is the use of a "C" or "J" pad, which unloads the injured sesamoid. Pads with adhesive backing may be fixed to the insole of the shoe or may be incorporated into a custom-molded orthotic to unload the sesamoid.

Pilon Fractures
Pilon fractures in the distal tibia result from axial forces, where the tibia is driven down into the talus, producing a spectrum of articular and metaphyseal injuries and resulting in long-term morbidity in the majority of cases.[264]

Intervention
Surgery is undertaken when the condition of soft tissues is optimized. Many surgery options are available and include the following:

- Open reduction and internal fixation
- External fixation (either spanning the ankle or not)
- Limited internal fixation with external fixation
- Percutaneous plating

Ankle Fractures
Ankle fractures can be classified as single malleolar, bimalleolar, and trimalleolar if the posterior part of the tibial plafond (posterior margin) is involved.

Intervention
Fractures without medial-sided injury involving only the fibula are typically symptomatically treated with a walking cast or stirrup brace and weight bearing as tolerated. The patient is instructed to apply ice to the injured area over a compressive dressing for 20 minutes every 2–3 hours for the first 24 hours and every 4–6 hours thereafter. After the acute phase, cast immobilization is accomplished with either a short leg walking cast or a walking cast fracture boot (for a reliable patient with a stable ankle fracture). Bimalleolar or trimalleolar injuries are always unstable and are treated with open reduction and internal fixation. All displaced medial malleolar fractures are openly reduced and fixed to restore normal ankle congruency and deltoid integrity. Generally, 4–6 weeks of immobilization is required for healing. Cast boots are generally preferred after swelling dissipates so that intermittent motion can commence. If the fracture site is not tender, gradual ankle rehabilitation can begin because clinical healing is present. After the immobilization period, range of motion and then strengthening exercises are initiated. Particular attention should be made to acquiring dorsiflexion.

Talar Fractures
Fractures of the talus can be divided into types based on the three main anatomic divisions of the talus: body, neck, and head. Fractures of the body of the talus are further subdivided based on whether they traverse the main portion of the body or involve the talar dome, lateral process, or posterior process.

> ● **Key Point** Major fractures of the talar head, neck, and body are associated with high-energy mechanisms, with 50 percent of major talar injuries involving fractures of the talar neck, 15–20 percent involving talar body fractures, and the remainder involving talar head fractures.[265]

The mechanism of injury usually involves an axial load with the foot in plantarflexion or excessive dorsiflexion, resulting in compression of the talar head against the anterior aspect of the tibia.[266]

Intervention
The intervention varies according to location and severity, with nondisplaced fractures treated

with a short-leg non–weight-bearing cast for 6–8 weeks and displaced fractures involving emergency reduction.[265]

Calcaneus Fractures

The calcaneus is the largest and most frequently fractured tarsal, accounting for over 60 percent of foot fractures.[267] Calcaneus fractures may occur as a result of falls from heights, from torsional injuries, or through a pathologic process such as osteoporosis. Calcaneus fractures can be classified as extra-articular (25–30 percent) or intra-articular (70–75 percent) fractures.

Intervention

Conservative intervention for calcaneal fractures has shown poor long-term clinical results with significant loss of ankle function.[268,269] Most extra-articular calcaneus fractures are managed non-operatively, provided that the injury does not change the weight-bearing surface of the foot and does not alter hindfoot biomechanics. Open reduction and internal fixation (ORIF) with a lateral plate and without joint transfixation is the standard surgical intervention for displaced intra-articular fractures. Following an ORIF, the foot is elevated with the ankle positioned in the standard neutral position of a 90-degree angle between the foot and the tibia. This position is maintained for up to 72 hours to reduce postoperative swelling. Early range-of-motion exercises are encouraged after the surgical incision has begun healing, usually 10–12 days after surgery. A well-fitting orthosis is provided for comfort and to prevent gastrocnemius–soleus contracture. Sutures are removed at 2–3 weeks, but weight bearing is delayed for up to 12 weeks, depending on the original degree of comminution and the subsequent rigidity of the fixation.

Metatarsal Fractures

All fractures of the proximal fifth metatarsal have been indiscriminately labeled a "Jones fracture." A true Jones fracture is an acute fracture of the proximal fifth metatarsal caused by forefoot adduction, which occurs at the diametaphyseal junction involving the fourth to fifth metatarsal articulation. The most common fifth metatarsal base fracture is an avulsion fracture of the tuberosity caused by traction of the fibularis brevis and lateral band of the plantar fascia during hindfoot inversion.[270]

> ● **Key Point** The proximal fifth metatarsal has a poor blood supply and is at significant risk for delayed union or nonunion.

Intervention

These fractures should be treated with non–weight-bearing short-leg cast immobilization for 6–8 weeks or until healing is seen radiographically. If an established nonunion develops, screw fixation and/or bone grafting may be required.[271]

Therapeutic Techniques

A number of therapeutic techniques can be used to assist the patient. These include self-stretches, strengthening exercises, and manual techniques.

Techniques to Increase Soft Tissue Extensibility

The following are self-stretching exercises for the specified muscles:

- Gastrocnemius stretch (Figure 21-39)
- Soleus stretch (Figure 21-40)
- Stretch into plantarflexion to stretch the dorsiflexors (Figure 21-41) and (Figure 21-42)

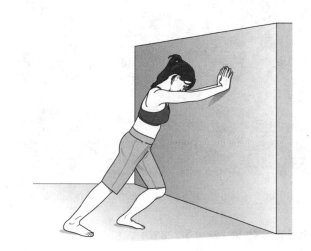

Figure 21-39 Gastrocnemius stretch.

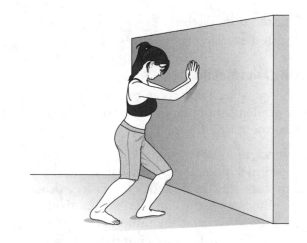

Figure 21-40 Soleus stretch.

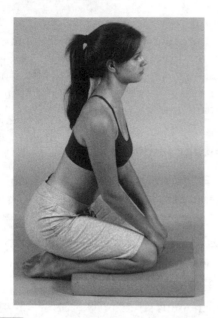

Figure 21-41   Stretch into plantarflexion: start position.

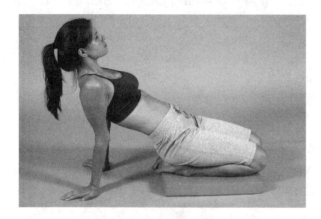

Figure 21-42   Stretch into plantarflexion: end position.

Techniques to Increase Strength

The following are home exercises that use elastic resistance:

- Resisted dorsiflexion (Figure 21-43)
- Resisted eversion (Figure 21-44)

Selective Joint Mobilizations

The following techniques can be used with the appropriate grade of mobilization based on the intent of the treatment (see Chapter 6).

- *Talocrural joint traction:* The patient is positioned in supine. Using one hand, the clinician stabilizes the patient's lower leg. Using the other hand, the clinician grasps around the patient's foot at the talocrural junction (Figure 21-45). The clinician then applies a traction force. This technique can be used to

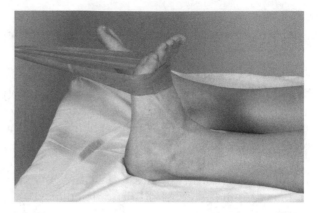

Figure 21-43   Resisted dorsiflexion.

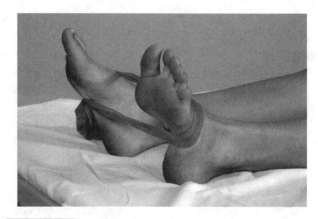

Figure 21-44   Resisted eversion.

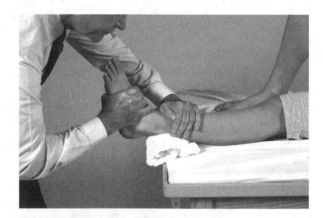

Figure 21-45   Talocrural joint distraction.

reduce pain and to increase dorsiflexion and plantarflexion.

- *Anterior talar glide:* The patient is positioned in prone, with the tibia stabilized on the table. Pressure is applied to the posterior aspect of the talus to glide anteriorly (Figure 21-46). This technique can be used to increase plantarflexion.
- *Subtalar joint distraction:* The lower leg is stabilized on the table, and traction is applied by

grasping the posterior aspect of the calcaneus (Figure 21-47). This technique can be used to reduce pain and to increase inversion and eversion.

- *Posterior talar glide:* The patient is positioned in supine and the lower leg is stabilized. Pressure is applied to the anterior aspect of the talus to glide it posteriorly (Figure 21-48). This technique can be used to increase dorsiflexion.

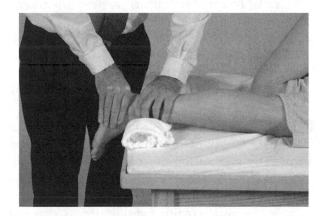

Figure 21-46 Anterior talar glide.

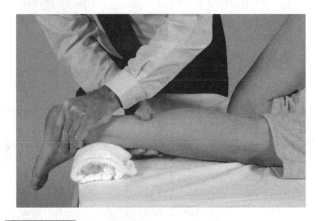

Figure 21-47 Subtalar joint distraction.

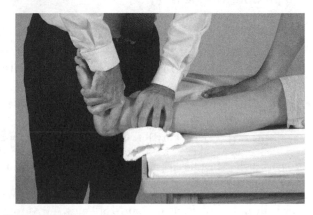

Figure 21-48 Posterior talar glide.

Summary

The key to developing a successful intervention for the ankle and foot is to understand the interactions among the lower extremity joints. The ankle joint sustains the greatest load per surface area of any joint of the body.[272] The joints and ligaments of the ankle and foot complex act as stabilizers and constantly adapt during weight-bearing activities. This is particularly true on uneven surfaces. Although the ankle and foot complex normally adapts well to the stresses of everyday life, sudden or unanticipated stresses to this region have the potential to produce dysfunction. The early phase of treatment uses ice, compression, elevation, rest, and protection, all of which are critical components in controlling inflammation and preventing swelling. At the earliest opportunity, controlled weight bearing is introduced.

REVIEW Questions

1. Which three muscles attach to the first cuneiform bone?
   a. The anterior tibialis, the posterior tibialis, and the fibularis (peroneus) longus
   b. The extensor digitorum, the flexor hallucis, and the fibularis (peroneus) longus
   c. The anterior tibialis, the peroneus brevis, and the fibularis (peroneus) longus
   d. The anterior tibialis, the posterior tibialis, and the fibularis (peroneus) brevis
2. What is the close-packed position of the ankle?
3. Which is the most commonly injured ankle ligament with a mechanism of plantarflexion and inversion?
4. The subtalar joint of the foot is an articulation between which two bones?
5. The "spring" ligament, which provides some elasticity to the arch of the foot, is also known by which name?
6. Which structure serves as the apex of the medial longitudinal arch of the foot?
   a. The base of the first metatarsal
   b. The head of the first metatarsal
   c. The midshaft of the first metatarsal
   d. The navicular tuberosity
7. A 17-year-old high school basketball player sprained his left ankle 2 days ago. He complains of moderate pain (6/10), and there is moderate swelling that seems to be worsening, causing him

to ambulate with an antalgic gait. In this case, the *best* intervention would be:
a. Cold/intermittent compression followed by elevation
b. Cold whirlpool, followed by elastic compression and elevation
c. Contrast baths and elastic compression
d. None of the above

8. Which of the following muscles is/are *not* considered part of the triceps surae?
a. Gastrocnemius
b. Flexor digitorum longus
c. Soleus
d. A and C

9. Which of the following nerves innervates most of the muscles that dorsiflex the foot?
a. Tibial nerve
b. Superficial fibularis (peroneal) nerve
c. Deep fibularis (peroneal) nerve
d. Lateral plantar nerve

10. Which of the following muscles has the potential to plantarflex the ankle and flex the knee?
a. Fibularis (peroneus) brevis
b. Gastrocnemius
c. Soleus
d. Popliteus

11. You are treating a 15-year-old male soccer player who sustained a grade II inversion ankle sprain 2 weeks ago. You determine that the patient is now in the early subacute phase of rehabilitation. Which of the following interventions should the patient be performing?
a. Closed-chain lower extremity strengthening, proprioceptive exercises, and wearing an orthosis
b. Weaning off crutches to a cane
c. Protection, rest, ice, compression, and elevation (PRICE)
d. Open-chain lower extremity exercises only

12. A patient presents with a grade II lateral ankle sprain incurred during a volleyball game the previous night. Today, the patient ambulates into the clinic non–weight bearing using bilateral axillary crutches and has a compression wrap on her involved ankle. During the early maximum-protection phase of rehabilitation, an appropriate treatment intervention would be to:
a. Incorporate muscle setting exercises.
b. Encourage full range of motion exercises.
c. Perform isotonic exercise at 60 percent maximum strength.
d. Use plyometric activities.

13. You have discovered an individual who apparently fell on ice in the parking lot outside the clinic. She is calling for help. Visual inspection reveals her ankle is swollen and resting at an extreme range of inversion. The appropriate first aid intervention is to call for help and/or call 911, then:
a. Cover the patient for warmth and implement the steps for assessment until help arrives.
b. Encourage the patient, with verbal cueing only, to come into a sitting position and assess her heart rate.
c. Straighten the ankle and fabricate and apply a splint from available material.
d. Attempt to transfer her from the ground into an available vehicle and apply ice to their ankle until help arrives.

14. Following a complex fracture of the tibia at mid-shaft, a patient's tibia is immobilized with an external fixation device. While the external fixator is in place a rehabilitation program for the affected limb would include:
a. Increasing cardiovascular fitness through aerobic exercises
b. Maintaining or increasing muscle strength of the affected limb using cuff weights at the ankle
c. Isometric exercises of the distal limb and resisted exercises of the hip and knee musculature
d. Increasing muscle strength using closed-chain activities

15. Your patient has progressed through a range of motion program for rehabilitating a grade II lateral ankle sprain. The available range of motion is now equal to that of the opposite extremity and the patient is free from pain with active range of motion. The next phase of rehabilitation will focus on:
a. Joint mobilization
b. Strengthening and proprioception
c. Strengthening for power
d. Proprioception for return to sport or activity

References

1. Sammarco GJ, Hockenbury RT: Biomechanics of the foot and ankle, in Frankel VH, Nordin M (eds): Basic Biomechanics of the Musculoskeletal System. Baltimore, Williams and Wilkins, 2000
2. Mann RA: Biomechanics of running, AAOS Symposium on the Foot and Leg in Running Sports. St Louis, CV Mosby, 1982, pp 30–44

3. Cavanagh PR, Rodgers MM, Iiboshi A: Pressure distribution under symptom-free feet during barefoot standing. Foot Ankle Int 7:262–276, 1987

4. Gieve DW, Rashi T: Pressures under normal feet in standing and walking as measured by foil pedobarography. Ann Rheum Dis 43:816, 1984

5. Rasmussen O, Kroman-Andersen C, Boe S: Deltoid ligament: Functional analysis of the medial collateral ligamentous apparatus of the ankle joint. Acta Orthop Scand 54:36–44, 1983

6. Rasmussen O, Tovberg-Jensen I: Mobility of the ankle joint: Recording of rotatory movements in the talocrural joint in vitro with and without the lateral collateral ligaments of the ankle. Acta Orthop Scand 53:155–160, 1982

7. Attarian DE, McCracken HJ, Devito DP, et al: Biomechanical characteristics of human ankle ligaments. Foot Ankle 6:54–58, 1985

8. Lundberg A, Goldie I, Kalin B, et al: Kinematics of the ankle/foot complex: Plantar flexion and dorsiflexion. Foot Ankle 9:194–200, 1989

9. Levens AS, Inman VT, Blosser JA: Transverse rotations of the lower extremity in locomotion. J Bone Joint Surg 30A:859–872, 1948

10. Oatis CA: Biomechanics of the foot and ankle under static conditions. Phys Ther 68:1815–1821, 1988

11. Jackson-Manfield P, Neumann DA: Structure and function of the ankle and foot, in Jackson-Manfield P, Neumann DA (eds): Essentials of Kinesiology for the Physical Therapist Assistant. St Louis, Mosby Elsevier, 2009, pp 305–338

12. Subotnick SI: Biomechanics of the subtalar and midtarsal joints. J Am Podiatry Assoc 65:756–764, 1975

13. Elftman H: The transverse tarsal joint and its control. Clin Orth Rel Res 16:41–45, 1960

14. Huang C, Kitaoka HB, An K, et al: Biomechanical evaluation of longitudinal arch stability. Foot Ankle 14:352–357, 1993

15. Hicks JH: Mechanics of the foot. J Anat 87:345–357, 1953

16. Thordarson DB, Schotzer H, Chon J, et al: Dynamic support of the human longitudinal arch. Clin Orthop 316:165–172, 1995

17. Saltzman CL, Nawoczenski DA: Complexities of foot architecture as a base of support. J Orthop Sports Phys Ther 21:354–360, 1995

18. Donatelli R: Normal anatomy and pathophysiology of the foot and ankle, in Wadsworth C (ed): Contemporary Topics on the Foot and Ankle. La Crosse, WI, Orthopedic Section, American Physical Therapy Association, 2000

19. Simkin A, Leichter I, Giladi M, et al: Combined effect of foot structure and an orthotic device on stress fractures. Foot Ankle 10:25–29, 1989

20. Giladi M, Milgrom C, Stein M, et al: The low arch, a protective factor in stress fractures: A prospective study of 295 military recruits. Orthop Review 14:709–712, 1985

21. Cowan DN, Jones BH, Robinson JR: Foot morphological characteristics and risk of exercise-related injury. Arch Fam Med 2:773–777, 1993

22. Kibler BW: Rehabilitation of the ankle and foot, in Kibler BW, Herring JA, Press JM (eds): Functional Rehabilitation of Sports and Musculoskeletal Injuries. Gaithersburg, MD, Aspen, 1998, pp 273–283

23. Safran MR, Zachazewski JE, Benedetti RS, et al: Lateral ankle sprains: A comprehensive review: Part 2: Treatment and rehabilitation with an emphasis on the athlete. Med Sci Sports Exerc 31:S438–S447, 1999

24. Safran MR, Benedetti RS, Bartolozzi AR, III., et al: Lateral ankle sprains: A comprehensive review: Part 1: Etiology, pathoanatomy, histopathogenesis, and diagnosis. Med Sci Sports Exerc 31:S429–S437, 1999

25. Knight KL, Aquino J, Johannes SM, et al: A re-examination of Lewis' cold induced vasodilation in the finger and ankle. Athl Training 15:248–250, 1980

26. Knight KL, Londeree BR: Comparison of blood flow in the ankle of uninjured subjects during therapeutic applications of heat, cold, and exercise. Med Sci Sports Exerc 12:76–80, 1980

27. Knue J, Hitchings C: The use of a rigid stirrup for prophylactic ankle support. Athl Training 18:121, 1982

28. Quillen WS: An alternative management protocol for lateral ankle sprains. J Orthop Sports Phys Ther 2:187–190, 1981

29. Roy S, Irvin R: Sports Medicine—Prevention, Evaluation, Management, and Rehabilitation. Englewood Cliffs, NJ, Prentice-Hall, 1983

30. Kaltenborn FM: Manual Mobilization of the Extremity Joints: Basic Examination and Treatment Techniques (ed 4). Oslo, Norway, Olaf Norlis Bokhandel, 1989

31. McClusky GM, Blackburn TA, Lewis TA: A treatment for ankle sprains. Am J Sports Med 4:158–161, 1976

32. Kleinrensink GJ, Stoeckart R, Meulstee J, et al: Lowered motor conduction velocity of the peroneal nerve after inversion moments. Am J Sports Med 24:362–369, 1996

33. Konradsen L, Olesen S, Hansen HM: Ankle sensorimotor control and eversion strength after acute ankle inversion injuries. Am J Sports Med 26:72–78, 1998

34. Nawoczenski DA, Owen MG, Ecker ML, et al: Objective evaluation of peroneal response to sudden inversion stress. J Orthop Sports Phys Ther 7:107–109, 1985

35. Lynch SA, Edlund U, Gottlieb D, et al: Electromyographic latency changes in the ankle musculature during inversion moments. Am J Sports Med 24:362–369, 1996

36. Voss DE, Ionta MK, Myers DJ: Proprioceptive Neuromuscular Facilitation: Patterns and Techniques (ed 3). Philadelphia, Harper and Row, 1985

37. Docherty CL, Moore JH, Arnold BL: Effects of strength training on strength development and joint position sense in functionally unstable ankles. J Athl Training 33:310–314, 1998

38. Fiore RD, Leard JS: A functional approach in the rehabilitation of the ankle and rear foot. Athl Training 16:231–235, 1980

39. Hoffman M, Payne VG: The effects of proprioceptive ankle disk training on healthy subjects. J Orthop Sports Phys Ther. 21:90–93, 1995

40. Keggereis S: The construction and implementation of functional progressions as a component of athletic rehabilitation. J Orthop Sports Phys Ther 5:14–19, 1985

41. Mattacola CG, Lloyd JW: Effects of a 6 week strength and proprioception training program on measures of dynamic balance: A single case design. J Athl Training 32:127–135, 1997

42. Sheth P, Yu B, Laskowski ER, et al: Ankle disk training influences reaction times of selected muscles in a simulated sprain. Am J Sports Med 25:538–543, 1997

43. Tropp H, Askling C, Gillquist J: Prevention of ankle sprains. Am J Sports Med 13:259–262, 1985

44. Wester JU, Jespersen SM, Nielsen DK, et al: Wobble board training after partial sprains of the lateral ligaments of the ankle: A prospective randomized study. J Orthop Sports Phys Ther 23:332–336, 1996

45. Adamson C, Cymet T: Ankle sprains: Evaluation, treatment, rehabilitation. Maryland Med J 46:530–537, 1997

46. Rozzi SL, Lephart SM, Sterner R, et al: Balance training for persons with functionally unstable ankles. J Orthop Sports Phys Ther 29:478–486, 1999

47. Lutter L: Injuries in the runner and jogger. Minn Med 63:45–52, 1980

48. Viitasalo JT, Kvist M: Some biomechanical aspects of the foot and ankle in athletes with and without shin splints. Am J Sports Med 11:125–130, 1983

49. Clement DB, Taunton JE, Smart GW: Achilles tendinitis and peritendinitis: Etiology and treatment. Am J Sports Med 12:179–183, 1984

50. Messier SP, Pittala KA: Etiologic factors associated with selected running injuries. Med Sci Sports Exerc 20:501–505, 1988

51. DeLacerda FG: A study of anatomical factors involved in shin splints. J Orthop Sports Phys Ther 2:55–59, 1980

52. Subotnick SI: Clinical biomechanics, in Subotnick SI (ed): Sports Medicine of the Lower Extremity. Philadelphia, Churchill Livingstone, 1999, pp 127–156

53. Appling SA, Kasser RJ: Foot and ankle, in Wadsworth C (ed): Current Concepts of Orthopedic Physical Therapy—Home Study Course. La Crosse, WI, Orthopaedic Section, American Physical Therapy Association, 2001

54. Johanson MA, Donatelli R, Wooden MJ, et al: Effects of three different posting methods on controlling abnormal subtalar pronation. Phys Ther 74:149–161, 1994

55. Hadley A, Griffiths S, Griffiths L, et al: Antipronation taping and temporary orthoses: Effects on tibial rotation position after exercise. J Am Podiatr Med Assoc 89:118–123, 1999

56. Keenan AM, Tanner CM: The effect of high-dye and low-dye taping on rearfoot motion. J Am Podiatr Med Assoc 91:255–261, 2001

57. Staheli LT: Evaluation of planovalgus foot deformities with special reference to the natural history. J Am Podiatr Med Assoc 77:2–6, 1987

58. Barry RJ, Scranton PE, Jr.: Flatfeet in children. Clin Orthop 181:68–75, 1983

59. Griffin LY: Common sports injuries of the foot and ankle seen in children and adolescents. Orthop Clin North Am 25:83–93, 1994

60. Mann RA: Pain in the foot. Postgrad Med 82:154–162, 1987

61. McPoil TG: The foot and ankle, in Malone TR, McPoil TG, Nitz AJ (eds): Orthopaedic and Sports Physical Therapy (ed 3). St Louis, Mosby-Year-Book, 1997, pp 261–293

62. Anderson KJ, Lecocq JF, Lecocq EA: Recurrent anterior subluxation of the ankle joint: A report of two cases and an experimental study. J Bone Joint Surg 34A:853–860, 1952

63. Brand RL, Black HM, Cox JS: The natural history of inadequately treated ankle sprains. Am J Sports Med 5:248–249, 1977

64. Brostrom L, Sundelin P: Sprained ankles: IV. Histologic changes in recent and "chronic" ligament ruptures. Acta Chir Scand 132:248–253, 1966

65. Brostrom L: Sprained ankles: V. Treatment and prognosis in recent ligament ruptures. Acta Chir Scand 132:537–550, 1966

66. Brostrom L: Sprained ankles: VI. Surgical treatment of "chronic" ligament ruptures. Acta Chir Scand 132:551–565, 1966

67. Harrington KD: Degenerative arthritis of the ankle secondary to long standing lateral ligament instability. J Bone Joint Surg 61A:354–361, 1979

68. Javors JR, Violet JT: Correction of chronic lateral ligament instability of the ankle by use of the Brostrom procedure. Clin Orthop 198:201–207, 1985

69. Lauttamus L, Korkala O, Tanskanen P: Lateral ligament injuries of the ankle: Surgical treatment of the late cases. Ann Chir Gynaecol 71:164–167, 1982

70. Riegler HF: Reconstruction for lateral instability of the ankle. J Bone Joint Surg 66A:336–339, 1984

71. Staples OS: Rupture of the fibular collateral ligaments of the ankle. J Bone Joint Surg 57A:101–107, 1975

72. Stewart MJ, Hutchings WC: Repair of the lateral ligament of the ankle. Am J Sports Med 6:272–275, 1978

73. Omey ML, Micheli LJ: Foot and ankle problems in the young athlete. Med Sci Sports Exerc 31:S470–S486, 1999

74. Brostrom L: Sprained ankles: III. Clinical observations in recent ligament ruptures. Acta Chir Scand 130:560–569, 1965

75. Brostrom L: Sprained ankles: I. Anatomic lesions on recent sprains. Acta Chir Scand 128:483–495, 1964

76. Brostrom L, Liljedahl S-O, Lindvall N: Sprained ankles: II. Arthrographic diagnosis of recent ligament ruptures. Acta Chir Scand 129:485–499, 1965

77. Gerber JP, Williams GN, Scoville CR, et al: Persistent disability associated with ankle sprains: A prospective examination of an athletic population. Foot Ankle Int 19:653–660, 1998

78. Lentell GL, Katzman LL, Walters MR: The relationship between muscle function and ankle stability. J Orthop Sports Phys Ther 11:605–611, 1990

79. Reid DC: Sports Injury Assessment and Rehabilitation. New York, Churchill Livingstone, 1992

80. Cox JS: Surgical and nonsurgical treatment of acute ankle sprains. Clin Orthop 198:118–126, 1985

81. O'Donoghue DH: Treatment of ankle injuries. Northwest Med 57:1277–1286, 1958

82. van Dijk CN, Lim LSL, Bossuyt PMM, et al: Physical examination is sufficient for the diagnosis of sprained ankles. J Bone Joint Surg [Br] 78B:958–962, 1996

83. Thorndike A: Athletic Injuries: Prevention, Diagnosis and Treatment. Philadelphia, Lea and Febiger, 1962

84. Inman VT: Sprains of the ankle, in Chapman MW (ed): AAOS Instructional Course Lectures. Rosemont, Il, AAOS, 1975, pp 294–308

85. O'Donoghue DH: Treatment of Injuries to Athletes. Philadelphia, WB Saunders, 1976, pp 698–746

86. Gronmark T, Johnson O, Kogstad O: Rupture of the lateral ligaments of the ankle. Foot Ankle 1:84–89, 1980

87. Iversen LD, Clawson DK: Manual of Acute Orthopaedics. Boston, Little, Brown, and Company, 1982

88. Kannus P, Renstrom P: Current concepts review: Treatment of acute tears of the lateral ligaments of the ankle. J Bone Joint Surg 73A:305–312, 1991

89. Balduini FC, Tetzelaff J: Historical perspectives on injuries of the ligaments of the ankle. Clin Sports Med 1:3–12, 1982

90. Eiff MP, Smith AT, Smith GE: Early mobilization versus immobilization in the treatment of lateral ankle sprains. Am J Sports Med 22:83–88, 1994

91. Noyes FR, Torvik PJ, Hyde WB, et al: Biomechanics of ligament failure: II. An analysis of immobilization, exercise, and reconditioning effects in primates. J Bone Joint Surg 56A:1406–1418, 1974

92. Tipton CM, James SL, Mergner W, et al: Influence of exercise in strength of medial collateral knee ligaments of dogs. Am J Physiol 218:894–902, 1970

93. Tipton CM, Matthes RD, Maynard JA, et al: The influence of physical activity on ligaments and tendons. Med Sci Sports Exerc 7:165–175, 1975

94. Vailas AC, Tipton CM, Mathes RD, et al: Physical activity and its influence on the repair process of medial collateral ligaments. Connect Tissue Res 9:25–31, 1981

95. Kessler RM, Hertling D: Management of Common Musculoskeletal Disorders. Philadelphia, Harper and Row, 1983, pp 379–443

96. Hettinga DL: Inflammatory response of synovial joint structures, in Gould JA, Davies GJ (eds): Orthopaedic and Sports Physical Therapy. St Louis, CV Mosby, 1985, pp 87–117

97. Maadalo A, Waller JF: Rehabilitation of the foot and ankle linkage system, in Nicholas JA, Hershman EB (eds): The Lower Extremity and Spine in Sports Medicine. St Louis, CV Mosby, 1986, pp 560–583

98. Vegso JJ, Harmon LE: Non-operative management of athletic ankle injuries. Clin Sports Med 1:85–98, 1982

99. Wilkerson GB: Treatment of ankle sprains with external compression and early mobilization. Phys Sports Med 13:83–90, 1985

100. Korkala O, Rusanen M, Jokipii P, et al: A prospective study of the treatment of severe tears of the lateral ligament of the ankle. Int Orthop 11:13–17, 1987

101. Hockenbury RT, Sammarco GJ: Evaluation and treatment of ankle sprains—clinical recommendations for a positive outcome. Phys Sports Med 24:57–64, 2001

102. Abdenour TE, Saville WA, White RC, et al: The effect of ankle taping upon torque and range of motion. Athl Training 14:227–228, 1979

103. Barnett JR, Tanji JL, Drake C, et al: High versus low top shoes for the prevention of ankle sprains in basketball players: A prospective randomized study. Am J Sports Med 21:582–596, 1993

104. Delacerde FG: Effect of underwrap conditions on the supportive effectiveness of ankle strapping with tape. J Sports Med Phys Fitness 18:77–81, 1978

105. Garrick JG, Requa RK: Role of external support in the prevention of ankle sprains. Med Sci Sports Exerc 5:200–203, 1973

106. Metcalfe RC, Schlabach GE, Looney MA, et al: A comparison of moleskin tape, linen tape and lace up brace on joint restriction and movement performance. J Athl Training 32:136–140, 1997

107. Pederson TS, Richard MD, Merrill G, et al: The effects of spatting and ankle taping on inversion before and after exercise. J Athl Training 32:29–33, 1997

108. Bunch RP, Dednarski K, Holland D, et al: Ankle joint support: A comparison of reusable lace on braces with taping and wrapping. Physician Sportsmed 13:59–62, 1985

109. Fumich RM, Ellison AE, Guerin GJ, et al: The measured effect of taping on combined foot and ankle motion before and after exercise. Am J Sports Med 9:165–170, 1981

110. Glick JM, Gordon RB, Nishimoto D: The prevention and treatment of ankle injuries. Am J Sports Med 4:136–141, 1976

111. Laughman RK, Carr TA, Chao EY, et al: Three-dimensional kinematics of the taped ankle before and after exercise. Am J Sports Med 8:425–431, 1980

112. Malina RM, Plagenz LB, Rarick GL: Effect of exercise upon measurable supporting strength of cloth and tape on ankle wraps. Res Q 34:158–165, 1963

113. Manfroy PP, Ashton-Miller JA, Wojtys EM: The effect of exercise, pre-wrap and athletic tape on the maximal active and passive ankle resistance to ankle inversion. Am J Sports Med 25:156–163, 1997

114. Paris DL, Vardaxis V, Kokkaliaris J: Ankle ranges of motion during extended activity periods while taped and braced. J Athl Training 30:223–228, 1995

115. Rarick GL, Bigley G, Karst R, et al: The measurable support of the ankle joint by conventional methods of taping. J Bone Joint Surg 44A:1183–1190, 1962

116. Shapiro MS, Kabo JM, Mitchell PW, et al: Ankle sprain prophylaxis: An analysis of the stabilizing effects of braces and tapes. Am J Sports Med 22:78–82, 1994

117. Karlsson J, Andreasson GO: The effect of external ankle support in chronic lateral ankle joint instability. Am J Sports Med 20:257–261, 1992

118. Refshauge KM, Kilbreath SL, Raymond J: The effect of recurrent ankle inversion sprain and taping on proprioception at the ankle. Med Sci Sports Exerc 32:10–15, 2000

119. Gandevia SC, McCloskey DI: Joint sense, muscle sense, and their combination as position sense, measured at the distal interphalangeal joint of the middle finger. J Physiol 260:387–407, 1976

120. Provins KA: The effect of peripheral nerve block on the appreciation and execution of finger movements. J Physiol 143:55–67, 1958

121. Jerosch J, Hoffstetter I, Bork H, et al: The influence of orthoses on the proprioception of the ankle joint. Knee Surg Sports Traumatol Arthrosc 3:39–46, 1995

122. Robbins S, Waked E, Rappel R: Ankle taping improves proprioception before and after exercise in young men. Br J Sports Med 29:242–247, 1995

123. Gross MT, Clemence LM, Cox BD, et al: Effect of ankle orthosis on functional performance for individuals with recurrent ankle sprains. J Orthop Sports Phys Ther 25:245–252, 1997

124. Lindley TR, Kernozed TW: Taping and semirigid bracing may not affect ankle functional range of motion. J Athl Training 30:109–112, 1995

125. MacKean LC, Bell G, Burnham RS: Prophylactic ankle bracing versus taping: Effects of functional performance

in female basketball players. J Orthop Sports Phys Ther 22:77–82, 1995

126. MacPherson K, Sitler M, Kimura I, et al: Effects of a semi-rigid and soft shell prophylactic ankle stabilizer on selected performance tests among high school football players. J Orthop Sports Phys Ther 21:147–152, 1995

127. Verbrugge JD: The effects of semirigid air stirrup bracing versus adhesive ankle taping on motor performance. J Sports Orthop Phys Ther 23:320–325, 1996

128. Wiley JP, Nigg BM: The effect of an ankle orthosis on ankle range of motion and performance. J Orthop Sports Phys Ther 23:362–369, 1996

129. Surve I, Schwellnus MP, Noakes T, et al: A fivefold reduction in the incidence of recurrent ankle sprains in soccer players using the sport-stirrup orthosis. Am J Sports Med 22:601–606, 1994

130. Landeros O, Frost HM, Higgins CC: Post traumatic anterior ankle instability. Clin Orthop 56:169–178, 1968

131. Dias LS: The lateral ankle sprain: An experimental study. J Trauma 19:266–269, 1977

132. Johnson EE, Markolf K: The contribution of the anterior talofibular ligament to ankle laxity. J Bone Joint Surg 65A:81–88, 1983

133. Ramsey PL, Hamilton WC: Lateral talar subluxation: The effect of tibiotalar contact surfaces. J Bone Joint Surg 57A:567–568, 1975

134. Brand RL, Collins MDF, Templeton T: Surgical repair of ruptured lateral ankle ligaments. Am J Sports Med 9:40–44, 1981

135. Freeman MAR, Dean MRE, Hanham IWF: The etiology and prevention of functional instability of the foot. J Bone Joint Surg 47B:678–685, 1965

136. Karlsson J, Bergstern T, Peterson L: Reconstruction of the lateral ligaments of the ankle for chronic lateral instability. J Bone Joint Surg 70A:581–588, 1988

137. Ruth CJ: The surgical treatment of injuries of the fibular collateral ligaments of the ankle. J Bone Joint Surg 43A:229–239, 1961

138. Nicholas JA: Ankle injuries in athletes. Orthop Clin North Am 15:153–175, 1974

139. Tropp H: Functional Instability of the Ankle Joint. Linkoping, Sweden, Linkoping University, 1985

140. Elmslie RC: Recurrent subluxation of the ankle joint. Ann Surg 100:364–367, 1934

141. Hintermann B: Die anatomische Rekonstruktion des Aussenbandapparates mit der Plantarissehne. [Anatomical reconstruction of the lateral ligament complex of the ankle.] Operat Orthop Traumatol 10:210–218, 1998

142. Karlsson J, Bergsten T, Lansinger O, et al: Surgical treatment of chronic lateral instability of the ankle joint: A new procedure. Am J Sports Med 17:268–274, 1989

143. Karlsson J, Eriksson BI, Bergsten T, et al: Comparison of two anatomic reconstructions for chronic lateral instability of the ankle joint. Am J Sports Med 25:48–53, 1997

144. Rudert M, Wülker N, Wirth CJ: Reconstruction of the lateral ligaments of the ankle using a regional periosteal flap. J Bone Joint Surg 79B:446–451, 1997

145. Sammarco GJ, Diraimondo CV: Surgical treatment of lateral ankle instability syndrome. Am J Sports Med 16:501–511, 1988

146. Rosenbaum D, Becker HP, Sterk J, et al: Functional evaluation of the 10-year outcome after modified Evans repair for chronic ankle instability. Foot Ankle Int 18:765–771, 1997

147. Frey C: Foot health and shoewear for women. Clin Orthop Relat Res 372:32–44, 2000

148. Geissele AE, Stanton RP: Surgical treatment of adolescent hallux valgus. J Pediatr Orthop 10:642–648, 1990

149. McDonald MD, Stevens. DB: Modified Mitchell bunionectomy for management of adolescent hallux valgus. Clin Orthop 332:163–169, 1996

150. Cole S: Foot inspection of the school child. J Am Podiatr Assoc 49:446–454, 1959

151. Coughlin MJ: Juvenile bunions, in Mann RA, Coughlin MJ (eds): Surgery of the Foot and Ankle (ed 6). St Louis, Mosby-Year Book, 1993, pp 297–339

152. Craigmile DA: Incidence, origin, and prevention of certain foot defects. BMJ 2:749–752, 1953

153. Scranton PE, Jr., Zuckerman JD: Bunion surgery in adolescents: Results of surgical treatment. J Pediatr Orthop 4:39–43, 1984

154. Hockenbury RT: Forefoot problems in athletes. Med Sci Sports Exerc 31:S448–S458, 1999

155. Glasoe WM, Yack HJ, Saltzman CL: Anatomy and biomechanics of the first ray. Phys Ther 79:854–859, 1999

156. Cornwall MW, Fishco WD, McPoil TG, et al: Reliability and validity of clinically assessing first-ray mobility of the foot. J Am Podiatr Med Assoc 94:470–476, 2004

157. Clanton TO, Ford JJ: Turf toe injury. Clin Sports Med 13:731–741, 1984

158. Sammarco GJ: Turf toe. Instr Course Lect 42:207–212, 1993

159. Katcherian DA: Pathology of the first ray, in Mizel MS, Miller RA, Scioli MW (eds): Orthopaedic Knowledge Update, Foot and Ankle. Rosemont, IL, American Academy of Orthopaedic Surgeons, 1998, pp 157–159

160. McManama GB, Jr.: Ankle injuries in the young athlete. Clin Sports Med 7:547, 1988

161. Sammarco GJ: Peroneal tendon injuries. Orthop Clin North Am 25:135–145, 1994

162. Micheli LJ, Waters PM, Sanders DP: Sliding fibular graft repair for chronic dislocation of the peroneal tendons. Am J Sports Med 17:68–71, 1989

163. Clanton TO, Schon LC: Athletic injuries to the soft tissues of the foot and ankle, in Mann RA, Coughlin MJ (eds): Surgery of the Foot and Ankle (ed 6). St Louis, Mosby-Year Book, 1993, pp 1167–1177

164. Clarke HD, Kitaoka HB, Ehman RL: Peroneal tendon injuries. Foot Ankle 19:280–288, 1998

165. Frey CC, Shereff MJ: Tendon injuries about the ankle in athletes. Clin Sports Med 7:103–118, 1988

166. Niemi WJ, Savidakis J, Dejesus JM: Peroneal subluxation: A comprehensive review of the literature with case presentations. J Foot Ankle Surg 36:141–145, 1997

167. Brage ME, Hansen ST: Traumatic subluxation/dislocation of the peroneal tendons. Foot Ankle 13:423–431, 1992

168. Stover CN, Bryan DR: Traumatic dislocation of the peroneal tendons. Am J Surg 103:180–186, 1962

169. Arrowsmith SR, Fleming LL, Allman FL: Traumatic dislocations of the peroneal tendons. Am J Sports Med 11:142–146, 1983

170. Eckert WR, Davis FA: Acute rupture of the peroneal retinaculum. J Bone Joint Surg 58A:670–673, 1976

171. Keene JS, Lange RH: Diagnostic dilemmas in foot and ankle injuries. JAMA 256:247–251, 1986

172. Slatis P, Santavirta S, Sandelin J: Surgical treatment of chronic dislocation of the peroneal tendons. Br J Sports Med 22:16–18, 1988

173. Kettlecamp D, Alexander H: Spontaneous rupture of the posterior tibialis tendon. J Bone Joint Surg 51A:759, 1969

174. Leach RE, Dizorio E, Harvey RA: Pathologic hindfoot conditions in the athlete. Clin Orthop 177:116–121, 1983

175. Conti SF: Posterior tibial tendon problems in athletes. Orthop Clin North Am 25:109–121, 1994

176. Hamilton WG, Geppert MJ, Thompson FM: Pain in the posterior aspect of the ankle in dancers. J Bone Joint Surg 78A:1491–1500, 1996

177. Khan K, Brown J, Way S, et al: Overuse injuries in classical ballet. Sports Med 19:341–357, 1995

178. Garth WP: Flexor hallucis tendonitis in a ballet dancer. J Bone Joint Surg 63A:1489, 1981

179. Koleitis GJ, Micheli LJ, Klein JD: Release of the flexor hallucis longus tendon in ballet dancers. J Bone Joint Surg 78A:1386–1390, 1996

180. Teitz CC: Sports medicine concerns in dance and gymnastics. Pediatr Clin North Am 29:1399–1421, 1982

181. Nelen G, Martens M, Bursens A: Surgical treatment of chronic Achilles tendinitis. Am J Sports Med 17:754–759, 1989

182. McCrory JL, Martin DF, Lowery RB, et al: Etiologic factors associated with Achilles tendinitis in runners. Med Sci Sports Exerc 31:1374–1381, 1999

183. Jacobs SJ, Berson BJ: Injuries to runners: A study of entrants to a 10,000 meter race. Am J Sports Med 14:151–155, 1986

184. Pinshaw R, Atlas V, Noakes TD: The nature and response to therapy of 196 consecutive injuries seen at a runners' clinic. S Afr Med J 65:291–298, 1984

185. Brunet ME, Cook SD, Brinker MR, et al: A survey of running injuries in 1505 competitive and recreational runners. J Sports Med Phys Fitness 30:307–315, 1990

186. van Mechelen W, Hlobil H, Kemper HCG, et al: Prevention of running injuries by warm-up, cool-down and stretching exercises. Am J Sports Med 21:711–719, 1993

187. Soma CA, Mandelbaum BR: Achilles tendon disorders. Clin Sports Med 13:811–823, 1994

188. Hess GP, Cappiello WL, Poole RM, et al: Prevention and treatment of overuse tendon injuries. Sports Med 8:371–384, 1989

189. Clement DB, Taunton JE, Smart GW, et al: A survey of overuse running injuries. Phys Sportsmed 9:47–58, 1981

190. Reynolds NL, Worrell TW: Chronic Achilles peritendinitis: Etiology, pathophysiology, and treatment. J Orthop Sports Phys Ther 13:171–176, 1991

191. Smart GW, Taunton JE, Clement DB: Achilles tendon disorders in runners: A review. Med Sci Sport Exerc 12:231–243, 1980

192. James SL, Bates BT, Osternig LR: Injuries to runners. Am J Sports Med 6:40–49, 1978

193. Renstrom P, Johnson RJ: Overuse injuries in sports: A review. Sports Med 2:316–333, 1985

194. Lyshold J, Wiklander J: Injuries in runners. Am J Sports Med 15:168–171, 1987

195. Sheehan GA: An overview of overuse syndromes in distance runners. Ann NY Acad Sci 301:877–880, 1977

196. Barry NN, McGuire JL: Overuse syndromes in adult athletes. Rheum Dis Clin North Am 22:515–530, 1996

197. Gudas CJ: Patterns of lower extremity injury in 224 runners. Exerc Sports Med 12:50–59, 1980

198. Hogan DG, Cape RD: Marathoners over sixty years of age: Results of a survey. J Am Geriatr Soc 32:121–123, 1984

199. Janis LR: Results of the Ohio runners sports medicine survey. J Am Podiatr Med Assoc 10:586–589, 1986

200. Voorn R: Case report: Can sacroiliac joint dysfunction cause chronic Achilles tendinitis? J Orthop Sports Phys Ther 27:436–443, 1998

201. Sarrafian SK: Functional anatomy: Anatomy of the Ankle and Foot. Philadelphia, JB Lippincott, 1992, pp 559–590

202. Reid DC: Heel pain and problems of the hindfoot, in Reid DC (ed): Sports Injury Assessment and Rehabilitation. New York, Churchill Livingstone, 1992, pp 437–493

203. Goodnite EA: The practical use of evidence-based practice in determining the best treatment for a patient with recurrent Achilles tendinitis. Orthop Pract 17:12–14, 2005

204. Alfredson H, Pietila T, Jonsson P, et al: Heavy-load eccentric calf muscle training for the treatment of chronic Achilles tendinosis. Am J Sports Med 26:360–366, 1998

205. Arner O, Lindholm A, Orell SR: Histologic changes in subcutaneous rupture of the Achilles tendon. Acta Chir Scand 116:484, 1958/1959

206. Popovic N, Lemaire R: Diagnosis and treatment of acute ruptures of the Achilles tendon: Current concepts review. Acta Orthop Belg 65:458–471, 1999

207. Wills CA, Washburn S, Caiozzo V, et al: Achilles tendon rupture: A review of the literature comparing surgical versus nonsurgical treatment. Clin Orthop 207:156–163, 1986

208. Cetti A, Christensen SE, Ejsted R, et al: Operative versus non-operative treatment of Achilles tendon rupture. Am J Sports Med 21:791–799, 1993

209. Jacobs D, Martens M, Van Audekercke R, et al: Comparison of conservative and operative treatment of Achilles tendon rupture. Am J Sports Med 6:107–111, 1978

210. Lea RB, Smith L: Non-surgical treatment of tendo Achilles rupture. J Bone Joint Surg 54A:1398–1407, 1972

211. Leppilahti J, Orava S: Total Achilles tendon rupture. Sports Med 25:79–100, 1998

212. Soma CA, Mandelbaum BR: Repair of acute Achilles tendon ruptures. Orthop Clin North Am 26:241–246, 1995

213. Nistor L: Surgical and non-surgical treatment of Achilles tendon rupture. J Bone Joint Surg 63A:394–399, 1981

214. Inglis AE, Scott WN, Sculco TP, et al: Surgical repair of ruptures of the tendo Achilles. J Bone Joint Surg 58A:990–993, 1976

215. Edna TH: Non-operative treatment of Achilles tendon ruptures. Acta Orthop Scand 51:991–993, 1980

216. Haggmark T, Liedberg H, Eriksson E, et al: Calf muscle atrophy and muscle function after non-operative vs

operative treatment of Achilles tendon ruptures. Orthopedics 9:160–164, 1986

217. Hart TJ, Napoli RC, Wolf JA, et al: Diagnosis and treatment of the ruptured Achilles tendon. J Foot Surg 27:30–39, 1988

218. Aoki M, Ogiwara N, Ohta T, et al: Early active motion and weightbearing after cross-stitch Achilles tendon repair. Am J Sports Med 26:794–800, 1998

219. Gelberman RH, Woo SL-Y, Lothringer K, et al: Effects of early intermittent passive mobilization on healing canine flexor tendons. J Hand Surg 7A:170–175, 1982

220. Speck M, Klaue K: Early full weightbearing and functional treatment after surgical repair of acute Achilles tendon rupture. Am J Sports Med 26:789–793, 1998

221. Crawford F: Plantar heel pain and fasciitis. Clin Evid 11:1589–1602, 2004

222. Crawford F, Thomson C: Interventions for treating plantar heel pain. Cochrane Database Syst Rev 3, 2003

223. Crawford F, Atkins D, Edwards J: Interventions for treating plantar heel pain. Cochrane Database Syst Rev 3, 2000

224. Waugh EJ: Lateral epicondylalgia or epicondylitis: What's in a name? J Orthop Sports Phys Ther 35:200–202, 2005

225. Hyland MR, Webber-Gaffney A, Cohen L, et al: Randomized controlled trial of calcaneal taping, sham taping, and plantar fascia stretching for the short-term management of plantar heel pain. J Orthop Sports Phys Ther 36:364–371, 2006

226. Warren BL, Jones CJ: Predicting plantar fasciitis in runners. Med Sci Sports Exerc 19:71–73, 1987

227. Charles LM: Why does my foot hurt? Plantar fasciitis. Lippincotts Prim Care Pract 3:408–409, 1999

228. DeMaio M, Paine R, Mangine RE, et al: Plantar fasciitis. Orthopedics 16:1153–1163, 1993

229. Baxter DE: The heel in sport. Clin Sports Med 13:683–693, 1994

230. Barrett SL, Day SV, Pugnetti TT, et al: Endoscopic heel anatomy: Analysis of 200 fresh frozen specimens. J Foot Ankle Surg 34:51–56, 1995

231. Davis PF, Severud E, Baxter DE: Painful heel syndrome: Results of nonoperative treatment. Foot Ankle Int 15:531–535, 1994

232. Van Wyngarden TM: The painful foot, part II: Common rearfoot deformities. Am Fam Phys 55:2207–2212, 1997

233. Pfeffer GB: Planter heel pain, in Baxter DE (ed): The Foot and Ankle in Sport. St Louis, Mosby, 1995, pp 195–206

234. Mizel MD, Marymont JV, Trapman E: Treatment of plantar fasciitis with a night splint and shoe modification consisting of a steel shank and anterior rocker bottom. Foot Ankle Int 17:732–735, 1997

235. Powell MW, Post WR, Keener JK: Effective treatment of chronic plantar fasciitis with dorsiflexion night splints: A cross-over prospective randomized study. Foot Ankle Int 19:10–18, 1998

236. Wapner KL, Sharkey PF: The use of night splints for treatment of recalcitrant plantar fasciitis. Foot Ankle 1:135–137, 1991

237. Singh D, Angel J, Bentley G, et al: Fortnightly review. Plantar fasciitis. BMJ 315:172–175, 1997

238. Baxter DE, Zingas C: The foot in running. J Am Acad Orthop Surg 3:136–145, 1995

239. Graham CE, Graham DM: Morton's neuroma: A microscopic evaluation. Foot Ankle 5:150, 1984

240. Wu KK: Morton's interdigital neuroma: A clinical review of its etiology, treatment, and results. J Foot Ankle Surg 35:112–119, 1996

241. Schon LC: Nerve entrapment, neuropathy, and nerve dysfunction in athletes. Orthop Clin North Am 25:47–59, 1994

242. Mulder JD: The causative mechanism in Morton's metatarsalgia. J Bone Joint Surg 33B:94–95, 1951

243. Mars M, Hadley GP: Raised intracompartmental pressure and compartment syndromes. Injury 29:403–411, 1998

244. Matsen FA, Winquist RA, Krugmire RB: Diagnosis and management of compartment syndromes. J Bone Joint Surg 62A:286–291, 1980

245. Perron AD, Brady WJ, Keats TE: Orthopedic pitfalls in the ED: Acute compartment syndrome. Am J Emerg Med 19:413–416, 2001

246. Blue JM, Mathews LS: Leg injuries. Clin Sports Med 16:467–478, 1997

247. Andrish JT: Leg pain, in DeLee JC, Drez D (eds): Orthopedic Sports Medicine. Philadelphia, WB Saunders, 1994, pp 1603–1607

248. McBryde AM, Jr.: Stress fractures in athletes. J Sports Med 3:212–217, 1975

249. Monteleone GP: Stress fractures in the athlete. Orthop Clin North Am 26:423, 1995

250. Brudvig TJ, Gudger TD, Obermeyer L: Stress fractures in 295 trainees: A one-year study of incidence as related to age, sex, and race. Mil Med 148:666–667, 1983

251. Protzman PR: Physiologic performance of women compared to men at the U.S. Military Academy. Am J Sports Med 7:191–196, 1979

252. Marshall LA: Clinical evaluation of amenorrhea, in Agostini R, Titus S (eds): Medical and Orthopedic Issues of Active and Athletic Women. Philadelphia, Hanley and Belfus, 1994, pp 152–163

253. Myburgh KH, Bachrach LK, Lewis B, et al: Low bone mineral density at axial and appendicular sites in amenorrheic athletes. Med Sci Sports Exerc 25:1197–1202, 1993

254. Sharkey NA, Ferris L, Smith TS, et al: Strain and loading of the second metatarsal during heel life. J Bone Joint Surg 77A:1050–1057, 1995

255. Pester S, Smith PC: Stress fractures in the lower extremities of soldiers in basic training. Orthop Rev 21:297–303, 1992

256. Gardner LI, Dziados JE, Jones BH, et al: Prevention of lower extremity stress fractures: A controlled trial of a shock absorbent insole. Am J Public Health 78:1563, 1988

257. Milgrom C, Giladi M, Kashton H, et al: A prospective study of the effect of a shock-absorbing orthotic device on the incidence of stress fractures in military recruits. Foot Ankle 6:101–104, 1985

258. Schwellnus MP, Jordaan G, Noakes TD: Prevention of common overuse injuries by the use of shock absorbing insoles: A prospective study. Am J Sports Med 18:636–641, 1990

259. Gross RH: Fractures and dislocations of the foot, in Rockwood CA, Wilkins KE, King RE (eds): Fractures

in Children (ed 3). Philadelphia, Lippincott, 1991, pp 1383–1453

260. O'Malley MJ, Hamilton WG, Munyak J, et al: Stress fractures at the base of the second metatarsal in ballet dancers. Foot Ankle 17:89–94, 1996

261. Torg JS, Pavlov H, Cooley LH, et al: Stress fractures of the tarsal navicular: A retrospective review of twenty-one cases. J Bone Joint Surg 64A:700–712, 1982

262. Harrington T, Crichton KJ, Anderson IF: Overuse ballet injury of the base of the second metatarsal: A diagnostic problem. Am J Sports Med 21:591–598, 1993

263. Richardson EG: Injuries to the hallucal sesamoids in the athlete. Foot Ankle 7:229–244, 1987

264. Bourne RB, Rorabeck CH, MacNab J: Intra-articular fractures of the distal tibia: The pilon fracture. J Trauma 23:591–595, 1983

265. Wedmore IS, Charette J: Emergency department evaluation and treatment of ankle and foot injuries. Emerg Med Clin North Am 18:86–114, 2000

266. Tomaro JE: Injuries of the leg, foot, and ankle, in Wadsworth C (ed): Contemporary Topics on the Foot and Ankle—Home Study Course. La Crosse, WI, Orthopaedic Section, American Physical Therapy Association, 2000

267. Starosta D, Sacceti A, Sharkey P, et al: Calcaneal fracture with compartment syndrome of the foot. Ann Emerg Med 17:144, 1988

268. Kitaoka HB, Schaap EJ, Chao EYS, et al: Displaced intra-articular fractures of the calcaneus treated non-operatively. J Bone Joint Surg 76A:1531–1540, 1994

269. Thoradson DB, Kreiger LE: Operative vs. non-operative treatment of intra-articular fractures of the calcaneus: A prospective randomized trial. Foot Ankle Int 17:2–9, 1996

270. Lawrence SJ, Botte MJ: Jones' fractures and related fractures of the proximal fifth metatarsal. Foot Ankle 14:358–365, 1993

271. Torg JS, Balduini FC, Zelko RR, et al: Fractures of the fifth metatarsal distal to the tuberosity. J Bone Joint Surg 66A:209–214, 1984

272. Sartoris DJ: Diagnosis of ankle injuries: The essentials. J Foot Ankle Surg 33:101–107, 1994

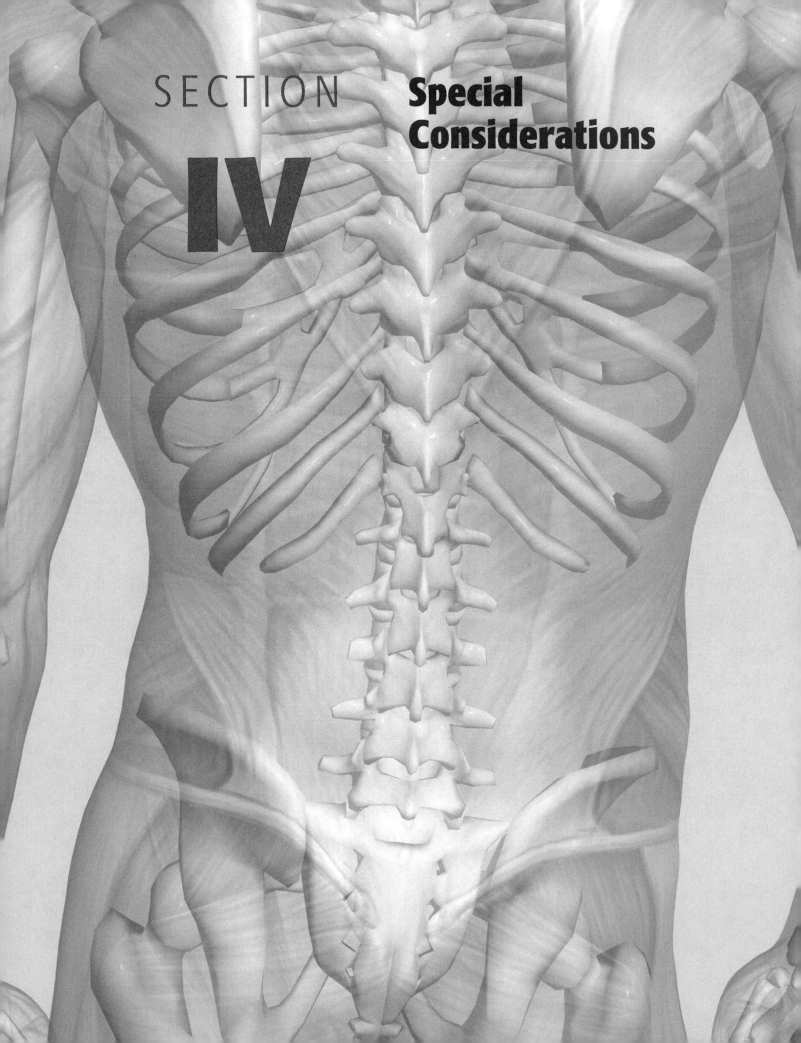

SECTION

IV

**Special
Considerations**

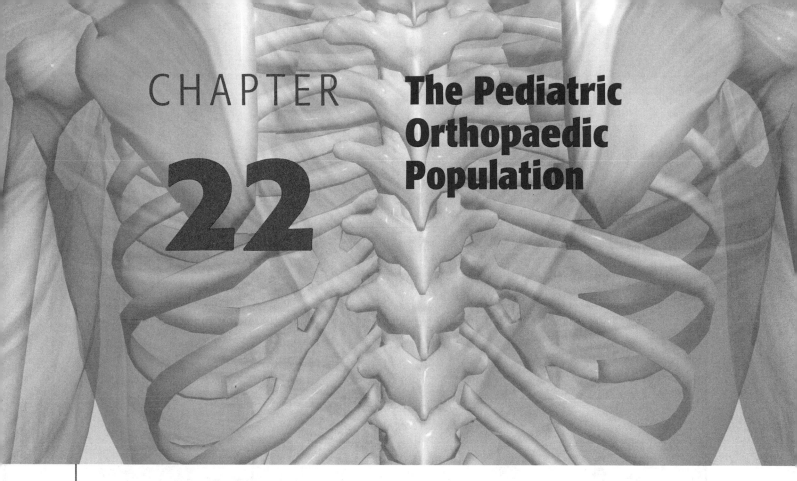

The Pediatric Orthopaedic Population

Chapter Objectives

At the completion of this chapter, the reader will be able to:

1. Discuss the physical therapy role in interventions for the pediatric population.
2. Describe the various pediatric pathologies in terms of their presentation and the role that physical therapy plays in treating them.
3. Outline the differences between a congenital condition and an acquired condition.

Overview

Pediatric physical therapy relates to the period during which an individual ages, changes, evolves and matures (0–21 years). Motor development is a complex process that starts in utero and has psycho-motor, physiological, biochemical, biomechanical, psychosocial, and even gender considerations.[1] Factors to be considered when treating a pediatric patient include, but are not limited to:[2]

- *Current life circumstances:* The pediatric patient's current health, the attitudes and values of the child's immediate family, and acculturation of the patient.
- *Health history:* Health and nutrition history, repeated hospitalizations, and so on.
- *Developmental history:* The pediatric patient's past rate of achievement of developmental milestones (**Table 22-1** and **Table 22-2**), and events that might have had profound effects on the patient either physically or psychologically.
- *Extrapersonal interactions:* The reaction of the pediatric patient to the treating clinician and the conditions under which the pediatric patient is observed.
- *Age-related changes in muscle and muscle performance:* The pediatric patient is continually developing and the musculoskeletal system undergoes numerous changes with growth (**Table 22-3**).

TABLE 22-1	Development Milestones According to Position			
Age	**Prone**	**Supine**	**Sitting**	**Standing**	**Comments**

Age	Prone	Supine	Sitting	Standing	Comments
Newborn (0–1 month)	• Physiological flexor activity—arms and hands tucked in close to the body, rounded shoulders, elbows flexed, and hands closed loosely and positioned close to mouth. • Lifts head briefly. • Head to side.	• No control of neck flexion in supine is present, so the baby cannot maintain the head in midline but keeps it rotated to one side.	• Lack of trunk muscular control—the back is round and the head flops forward. • Sacral sitting if supported.	• Demonstrates the remarkable capabilities of primary standing—automatic walking when supported.	• Grasp is a reflex in which the hand automatically closes on objects the baby touches due to tactile stimulation of the palm of the hand. • No organized response to postural perturbations. • Poor head control. • Very active when awake. • Random wide ranging movements primarily in supine. • The baby touches and feels, and is soon sucking and learning about the hands. • Regards objects in direct line of sight—vision limited to 8–9 feet. Follows moving objects midline. • Skeletal characteristics include coxa valgus, genu varum, tibial varum and torsion, calcaneal varus, and occasionally metatarsus adductus.
1 month	• Head lifting in prone may appear to be improved. • Increased cervical rotation mobility. • Elbows moving forward with arms away from body.	• Head to one side resulting in lateral vision becoming dominant. • Eye hand regard and uncontrolled swiping at toys at the baby's side is frequently observed. • Wider ranges of movement. • Heels hit surface.	N/A	• Positive support and primary walking reflexes in supported standing.	• Decreasing physiologic flexion (less "recoil"). • Increasing level of arousal. • Neonatal reaching. • Able to visually track a moving object horizontally.
2 months	• Able to hold the head steady in all positions and to raise it about 45 degrees due to increased activity of active shoulder abduction. • Arms and hands begin to work to support the actions of the head and trunk. • Hand movements more goal directed.	• Increased asymmetry with more visual interaction.	• Head lag occurs with pull to sit. • Begins to develop head and trunk control and more attempts at sustained extension. • Head bobs in supported sitting.	• May not accept weight on lower extremities (astasia-abasia). • No more neonatal stepping.	• Increasing asymmetry/decreased tone. • Increased head and trunk control lets the baby use the arms for reaching and playing rather than for support. • Holds objects placed in the hand.

(continued)

3 months	• Change occurs in the general position of the arms, from a position where the arms are tucked in close to the body with the elbows near the ribs, to one in which the elbows are almost in line with the shoulders, which allows for forearm weight bearing. • Legs abducted and externally rotated. • Head/face can be raised 45–90 degrees when prone.	• Beginning of symmetry is evident—the head is in midline with chin tucking and the hands are in midline on the chest/to mouth.	• Attempts pull to sit but falls forward.	• Minimal weight through extended legs.
				• Period of controlled symmetry. • The grasp becomes more controlled and voluntary and the hands can adjust to the shape of objects. • Symmetry is very obvious in the lower extremities as they assume their "frog legged" position of hip abduction, external rotation and flexion, and knee flexion. The feet come together and the baby is able to take some weight with toes curled in supported standing.
4 months	• Able to prop up on the forearms and look around. The head and chest are lifted and maintained in midline. • Prone pivots.	• Can roll from prone to side and from supine to side, although these are usually accidental occurrences. • Able to bring the hands together in the space above the body due to increased shoulder girdle control. • Hands to knees. • Active anterior and posterior pelvic tilt.	• Assists in pull to sit by flexing elbows. • Very minimal head bobbing—stabilized through shoulder elevation. • Tends to sit in a slumped position. • Protective reactions develop, first laterally, then forward, and then backward.	• Because of the increased head-neck-trunk control, the baby is able to take more of his or her weight when placed in standing, and can now be held by the hands instead of at the chest. • Legs are extended and the toes are clawed.
				• Ulnar palmar grasp develops. • Able to perform bilateral reaching with the forearm pronated when the trunk is supported. • Sidelying. • Starts hand to mouth activities. • Emerging righting and equilibrium reactions. • Findings of concern include poor midline orientation (persistent asymmetrical tonic neck reflex [ATNR]), imbalance between flexors and extensors, poor visual attention/tracking, persistent wide base of support in standing, and poor anti-gravity strength.
5 months	• Equilibrium reactions begin in prone position. • Can roll from prone to supine. • Able to assume and maintain a position of extended arm weight bearing in prone and can weight shift from one forearm to the other to reach out with one arm.	• Chin tuck, downward gaze. • Feet to mouth. • Anterior and posterior pelvic tilt more active. • Active roll to sidelying. • Manipulation and transfer of toys.	• No head lag when pulled from supine to sit. • Assists during pull to sit with chin tuck and head lift. • Able to control head in supported sitting although still leans forward from the hips.	• Tends to be able to bear almost all weight.
				Findings of concern include: • Poor antigravity flexion. • Poor tolerance for prone/inability to bear weight to extended arms/poor weight shifting.

TABLE
22-1

Development Milestones According to Position (continued)

Age	Prone	Supine	Sitting	Standing	Comments
6 months	• Completes turning and can roll from prone to supine. • Can lay prone on hands with the elbows extended and is able to weight shift on extended arms from hand to hand and to reach forward due to sufficient shoulder girdle control.	• Active hip extension. • Transfers toys. • Flexes head independently.	• Can sit independently, although initially uses the arms and hands for support.	• In standing, is able to bear weight on both legs and bounce and can independently hold onto the support of a person due to sufficient trunk and hip control.	• Uses rolling for locomotion. • Findings of concern include: • Poor tolerance for prone position. • Paucity of movement patterns. • Inability to sit independently. • Inability to roll or rolling with neck hyperextension.
7 months	• Trunk and arms free. • Able to achieve and maintain the quadruped position, although prone is usually the preferred position. • Can pivot on belly, often moving body in a circle.	• Tends to avoid except for playing.	• Protective reactions more consistent. • Able to perform trunk rotation in sitting. • Can assume the sitting position from the quadruped position.	• Can often pull to stand from the quadruped position. • Able to actively flex and extend both legs simultaneously while standing and supporting independently.	• Very active with large variety of movements and positions available. • May show fear of strangers. • Findings of concern include: • Lack of weight shifting in prone. • Reliance on more primitive movement patterns as compensations in order to explore. • Inability to assume or maintain quadruped. • Poor weight bearing in supported stance.
8 months	• Minimal time spent in prone—able to creep/crawl in the quadruped position at 9 months as the primary means of locomotion.	N/A	• Full equilibrium reactions in sitting, and the beginning of equilibrium reactions in quadruped. • Able to side-sit and also able to go from sitting to quadruped. • May also kneel.	• Can stand by leaning on supporting surfaces. • Able to pull to stand. • Early walking, cruising.	• Can reach out for objects and reach across the midline of the body without losing balance. • The thumb can wrap around objects—now the baby can hold two small objects, such as cubes, in one hand. • Findings of concern include: • Poor sitting ability. • Unable to use hand for play. • Overall reliance on upper extremities.
9 months	N/A	N/A	• Large variety of sitting positions and movement. • Pivoting/long sitting. • Sitting often used as a transitional position.	• Uses arms, hands, and body together while pulling up to standing through half-kneel position (9 months). • Immature stepping. • The sequence in rising to standing is kneeling, half kneeling, weight shift forward, squat, then upright.	• The index finger starts to move separately from the rest of the hand when poking at objects. This leads to the pincer grasp, with the tips of the thumb and index finger meeting in a precise pattern. • The baby's ability to let go of an object smoothly has also improved. • Findings of concern include: • Poor standing control. • Poor/inadequate sitting. • Inability to assume quadruped.

Age				
10 months	N/A	• Arms reach above shoulders. • Active site sitting. • Rarely stationary.	• Creeping/climbing. • Legs very active. "High guard." • Cruising with wide base of support.	N/A
11 months	N/A	• Able to play across midline.	• Mostly using legs. • Very symmetrical standing with a wide base of support.	N/A
12 to 15 months	N/A	N/A	• Many babies are walking unassisted.	• Able to self-feed. • Can build a tower of two cubes.
Two years	N/A	N/A	Runs well. Goes up stairs using reciprocal pattern (reciprocal stair climbing).	N/A

Data from van Blankenstein M, Welbergen UR, de Haas JH: Le Developpement du Nourrisson: Sa Premiere Annee en 130 Photographies. Paris, Presses Universitaires de France, 1962; and Prechtl HF: New perspectives in early human development. Eur J Obstet Gynecol Reprod Biol 21:347–355, 1986

TABLE 22-2	Locomotion Checklist: Ages 2–5	
Year	**Milestone**	
Two years	Walks up/down stairs one at a time holding rail	
	Walks with heel-toe gait	
	Runs forward well	
Three years	Pedals and steers tricycle well	
	Jumps forward on both feet	
	Alternates feet going up stairs	
	Walks backward easily	
Four years	Walks down stairs with alternating feet, holding rail	
	Gallops	
Five years	Able to walk long distances on toes	
	Skips	
	Hops forward on 1 foot	
	Smooth reciprocal movements in walking and running	

Data from Ratliffe KT: Clinical Pediatric Physical Therapy: A Guide for the Physical Therapy Team. Philadelphia, Mosby, 1998; and Kahn-D'Angel L: Pediatric physical therapy, in O'Sullivan SB, Siegelman RP (eds): National Physical Therapy Examination: Review and Study Guide (ed 9). Evanston, IL, International Educational Resources, 2006

TABLE 22-3	Age-Related Changes in Muscle and Muscle Performance in the Pediatric Population
Infancy, early childhood, and preadolescence	At birth, muscle accounts for about 25 percent of body weight.
	Total number of muscle fibers is established prior to or early during infancy.
	Postnatal changes in the distribution of type I and type II fibers in muscle are relatively complete by the end of the first year of life.
	Muscle fiber size and muscle mass increase linearly from infancy to puberty.
	Muscle strength and muscle endurance increase linearly with chronological age in boys and girls throughout childhood until puberty.
	Muscle mass (absolute and relative) and muscle strength are just slightly greater (approximately 10 percent) in boys than girls from early childhood to puberty.
	Training-induced strength gains occur equally in both sexes during childhood without evidence of hypertrophy until puberty.
Puberty	Rapid acceleration in muscle fiber size and muscle mass, especially in boys. During puberty, muscle mass increases more than 30 percent per year.
	Rapid increase in muscle strength in both sexes.
	Marked difference in strength levels develops between boys and girls.
	In boys, muscle mass and body weight peak before muscle strength; in girls, strength peaks before body weight.
	Relative strength gains as a result of resistance training are comparable between the sexes, with significantly greater muscle hypertrophy in boys.

Data from Kisner C, Colby LA: Resistance exercise for impaired muscle performance, in Kisner C, Colby LA (eds): Therapeutic Exercise. Foundations and Techniques (ed 5). Philadelphia, FA Davis, 2002, pp 147–152

- *Cardiovascular differences:* The pediatric heart is smaller than that of the mature adult, so its capacity as a reservoir for blood is also smaller, which results in a lower stroke volume at all levels of exercise. This is compensated for with an increased heart rate. Although systolic blood pressure rises during exercise in the pediatric patient, the elevation is less than that seen in the adult. Finally, because the thoracic cavity is smaller than that of the mature adult, the pediatric patient demonstrates a smaller vital capacity than an adult, which results in an elevated respiration rate as compared to the mature adult.

- *Physiologic differences:* A child has a greater surface area–to-mass ratio than the typical adult, resulting in a greater transfer of heat into their young bodies. The child also has a higher metabolic rate as compared to adult counterparts, which serves to further challenge the young thermoregulatory system.

● **Key Point** The main goals of a physical therapy intervention in pediatric rehabilitation are to reduce barriers limiting the performance of daily routines and to facilitate the successful integration of children into the home, play, and school environments.

Pediatric Orthopaedic Conditions

A child differs from an adult in many ways, particularly because the tissues and joints of the child are in the process of development. The childhood years from birth to skeletal maturity bring physiological and anatomical changes to bones and joints. Pediatric orthopaedic conditions usually fall into one of two categories: congenital or acquired (**Table 22-4**).

Acquired Conditions

Acquired conditions are those that occur during life. Examples include aging changes, infection, and trauma.

Skeletal Fracture

The mechanical properties and healing qualities of skeletal bone are described in Chapter 2 and Chapter 4, respectively. Fractures of bone in pediatric patients may be due to direct trauma such as a blow, or indirect trauma such as a fall on an outstretched hand (FOOSH injury) or a twisting injury. The point on a bone at which the metaphysis connects to the physis is an anatomic point of weakness. The various types of fractures are described in Chapter 5. Three

TABLE 22-4	Congenital and Acquired Conditions
Condition	**Examples**
Acquired	Skeletal fracture
	Juvenile rheumatoid arthritis (JRA)
	Idiopathic scoliosis
	Slipped capital femoral epiphysis (SCFE)
	Legg-Calvé-Perthes disease
	Scheuermann's disease
	Osteochondritis dissecans
	Osgood-Schlatter disease
	Pulled elbow
Congenital	Amputation
	Developmental dysplasia of the hip (DDH)
	Equinovarus

types of fractures are worth noting in the pediatric population:

- *Avulsion:* Occurs when a piece of bone attached to a tendon or ligament is torn away. In the younger population, ligaments and tendons are stronger than bone.
- *Growth plate (physeal):* A disruption in the cartilaginous physis of long bones that may or may not involve epiphyseal or metaphyseal bone (Figure 22-1). Injuries to the physes are more likely to occur in the pediatric population, in part due to the greater structural strength and integrity of the ligaments and joint capsules than of the growth plates, and the fact that the physes of an adult have ossified. Growth plate fractures can have severe consequences because of the potential for growth plate closure, which inhibits future growth resulting in limb length discrepancies. Conversely, an injury near, but not at, the physis can stimulate increased bone growth.
- *Greenstick:* A type of simple fracture in which only one side of the bone is fractured while the opposite side is bent (Figure 22-2). Because the bones in a pediatric patient have not fully developed, they are less rigid and brittle than adult bones. This type of fracture tends to heal faster than other types.

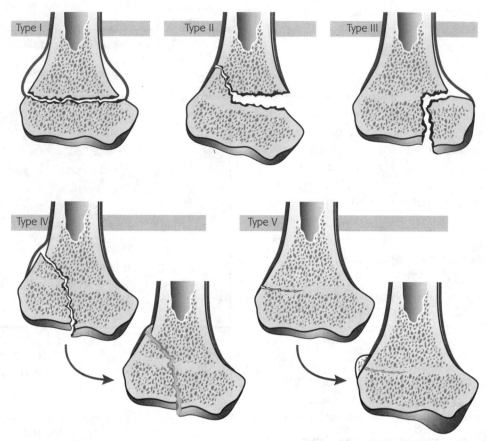

Figure 22-1   Salter-Harris classification of growth plate fractures.

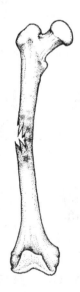

Figure 22-2   Greenstick fracture.

The most common clinical presentation with a pediatric fracture is pain, weakness, and functional loss of the involved area. The most common areas for pediatric fracture include the distal radius, the elbow, the clavicle, and the tibia. The Salter-Harris classification is the preferred and accepted standard in North America for diagnosing physeal fracture patterns (**Table 22-5**). The most common of the Salter-Harris fractures is II, followed by I, III, IV, and V.

TABLE 22-5	Salter-Harris Classification of Physeal Fractures

Type	Description
I	This fracture typically traverses through the hypertrophic zone of the cartilaginous physis, splitting it longitudinally and separating the epiphysis from the metaphysis. When these fractures are undisplaced, they may not be readily evident on radiographs due to the lack of bony involvement. In many instances, only mild-to-moderate soft tissue swelling is noted radiographically.

In general, the prognosis for this type of fracture is excellent. Usually, only closed reduction is necessary for displaced fractures; however, open reduction and internal fixation may be necessary if a stable satisfactory reduction cannot be maintained. |
II	This fracture splits partially through the physis and includes a variably sized triangular bone fragment of metaphysis. This particular fracture pattern occurs in an estimated 75 percent of all physeal fractures, and it is the most common physeal fracture.
III	This fracture pattern combines physeal injury with an articular discontinuity. This fracture partially involves the physis and then extends through the epiphysis into the joint. It has the potential to disrupt the joint surface. This injury is less common and often requires open reduction and internal fixation to ensure proper anatomical realignment of both the physis and the joint surface.
IV	This fracture runs obliquely through the metaphysis, traverses the physis and epiphysis, and enters the joint. Good treatment results for this fracture are considered to be related to the amount of energy associated with the injury and the adequacy of reduction.
V	This lesion involves a compression or crush injury to the physis and is virtually impossible to diagnose definitively at the time of injury. Knowledge of the injury mechanism simply makes one more or less suspicious of this injury. No fracture lines are evident on initial radiographs, but they may be associated with diaphyseal fractures. This fracture is generally very rare; however, family members should be warned of the potential disturbance in growth, and that if growth disturbance occurs, treatment is still available (depending upon the child's age and remaining growth potential).
VI	This is an additional classification of physeal fractures not considered in the original classification but now occasionally included. It describes an injury to the peripheral portion of the physis and a resultant bony bridge formation that may produce considerable angular deformity.

Intervention

In most cases, the medical management of a fracture involves immobilization through casting, splints, or surgical fixation to allow full healing to occur. Pediatric fractures tend to heal faster than an equivalent one in an adult. This can be advantageous: Children typically require shorter immobilization times. A disadvantage, however, is that any malpositioned fragments become immovable or fixed much earlier than in adults (3 to 5 days in a young child, 5 to 7 days in an older child, as opposed to 8 to 10 days in an adult). However, the normal process of bone remodeling in a child may correct malalignment, making near-anatomic reductions less important in children than in adults. Remodeling can be expected if the patient has two or more years of bone growth remaining. Rotational deformity remodels poorly, if at all, and is therefore corrected by surgical reduction. A further complication is that pediatric fractures may stimulate longitudinal growth of the bone, making the bone longer than it would have been had it not been injured. This is particularly true for fractures of the femoral or tibial shaft.

Children tolerate prolonged immobilization much better than adults, and disabling stiffness or loss of range of motion is distinctly unusual after pediatric fractures. Physical therapy, if needed, typically begins after this immobilization period, and depending on the type of fracture, can involve any or all of the following depending on the location of the fracture:

- Pain management techniques including the use of noncontraindicated electrotherapeutic modalities (see Chapter 7) and manual techniques, including joint mobilizations by the physical therapist

- Range of motion exercises, following the hierarchy of progression outlined in Chapter 9
- Strengthening exercises, beginning with isometrics and progressing using the hierarchy of progression outlined in Chapter 10
- Gait and/or crutch training with an appropriate assistive device and following the prescribed prescription for weight bearing (see Chapter 25)
- Proprioception exercises for balance and coordination (see Chapter 11)
- Functional training including adaptive, supportive, or protective devices and activities of daily living and self-care
- Patient and family education to decrease the risk of re-injury and to promote healing

Juvenile Rheumatoid Arthritis

Juvenile rheumatoid arthritis[3,4] (JRA) is a group of diseases that are manifested by chronic joint inflammation. The exact etiology of JRA is unclear, but the current theory is that it is an autoimmune inflammatory disorder, activated by an external trigger, in a genetically predisposed host. JRA is defined as persistent arthritis, lasting at least 6 weeks, in one or more joints in a child younger than 16 years of age, when all other causes of arthritis have been excluded.

JRA can be classified as systemic, oligoarthritis (pauciarticular disease), or polyarticular disease according to onset within the first 6 months.

- Systemic-onset JRA is characterized by spiking fevers, typically occurring several times each day, with temperature returning to the reference range or below the reference range. The fever may also be accompanied by an evanescent rash, which is typically linear, affecting the trunk and extremities. Arthralgia is often present. Frank joint swelling is atypical; arthritis may not occur for months following onset, making diagnosis difficult.
- Pauciarticular disease is characterized by arthritis affecting four or fewer joints (typically larger ones such as knees, ankles, or wrists).
- Polyarticular disease affects at least five joints. Both large and small joints can be involved, often in symmetric bilateral distribution. Severe limitations in motion are usually accompanied by weakness and decreased physical function.

In addition to those already mentioned, the general history and observation of JRA includes the following:

- Morning stiffness
- A school history of absences and an inability to participate in physical education classes may reflect the severity of the disease
- Gait deviations

A detailed physical examination by a physician is a critical tool in diagnosing JRA to help rule out other causes. Medical care of children with JRA must be provided in the context of a team-based approach, considering all aspects of their illness (e.g., physical functioning in school, psychological adjustment to disease).

Intervention

Physical therapists and physical therapist assistants are essential members of the pediatric rheumatology team that includes the rheumatologist, nurse, occupational therapist, ophthalmologist, orthopaedist, and pediatrician.[5] Other specialists, including cardiologists, dermatologists, orthotists, psychologists, and social workers, provide occasional consultation as needed. Following the comprehensive examination by the PT to identify impairments caused by the disease, a determination is made as to the relationship between the impairments and observed or reported activity restrictions. The PT develops a prioritized problem list and an intervention plan to reduce current impairments, maintain or improve function, prevent or minimize secondary problems, and provide education and support to the child and family. Specific interventions can include any or all of the following:

- *Range of motion and stretching exercises*
  - *Acute stage:* Passive and active assisted exercises to avoid joint compression
  - *Subacute/chronic stages:* Active exercises
- *Strengthening:* Avoid substitutions; minimize instability, atrophy, deformity, pain, and injury
  - *Acute and subacute stages:* Isometric exercises progressing cautiously to resistive exercises
  - *Chronic stage:* Judicious use of concentrics/eccentrics
- *Endurance exercises:* Encouragement to exercise—fun and recreational activities, swimming
- *Joint protection strategies and body mechanics education*
  - Mobility assistive devices.
  - Rest, as needed—balance rest with activity by using splinting (articular resting).

- ❑ Posture and positioning to maintain joint range of motion.
- ❑ Patients should spend 20 minutes/day in prone to stretch the hip and knee flexors.
- ❑ Avoid high impact activities.
- Assessing leg length discrepancy in standing and avoiding scoliosis
- Therapeutic modalities for pain control
  - ❑ Instructions on the wearing of warm pajamas, using a sleeping bag, or using an electric blanket

Idiopathic Scoliosis[6–19]

The overall contour of the normal vertebral column in the coronal plane is straight. In contrast, the contour of the sagittal plane changes with development. At birth, a series of primary curves give a kyphotic posture to the whole spine. With development of the erect posture, secondary curves develop in the cervical and lumbar spines, producing a lordosis in these regions. The curves in the spinal column provide it with increased flexibility and shock-absorbing capabilities.[2] Scoliosis represents a progressive disturbance of the intercalated series of spinal segments that produces a three-dimensional deformity (lateral curvature and vertebral rotation) of the spine. Despite an extensive amount of research devoted to discovering the cause of idiopathic scoliosis, the mechanics and specific etiology are not clearly understood, hence the name. It is known, however, that there is a familial prevalence of idiopathic scoliosis. Using the James classification system, scoliosis has three age distinctions. These distinctions, though seemingly arbitrary, have prognostic significance.

- *Infantile idiopathic:* Children diagnosed when they are younger than 3 years, usually manifesting shortly after birth. Although 80–90 percent of these curves spontaneously resolve, many of the remainder of cases will progress throughout childhood, resulting in severe deformity. In the most common curve pattern (right thoracic), the right shoulder is consistently rotated forward and the medial border of the right scapula protrudes posteriorly.
- *Juvenile idiopathic:* Children diagnosed when they are aged 3–9 years.
- *Adolescent idiopathic:* Manifesting at or around the onset of puberty and accounting for approximately 80 percent of all cases of idiopathic scoliosis.

The following are the main factors that influence the probability of progression in the skeleton of the immature patient:

- The younger the patient at diagnosis, the greater the risk of progression.
- Double-curve patterns have a greater risk for progression than single-curve patterns.
- Curves with greater magnitude are at a greater risk to progress.
- Risk of progression in females is approximately 10 times that of males with curves of comparable magnitude.
- In females, greater risk of progression is present when curves develop before menarche.

Scoliosis is generally described by the location of the curve or curves. One should also describe whether the convexity of the curve points to the right or left. If there is a double curve, each curve must be described and measured. As the disease progresses, the spinous processes of the vertebrae in the area of the major curve rotate toward the concavity of the curve. On the concave side of the curve, the ribs are close together (Figure 22-3). On the convex side, they are widely separated. As the vertebral bodies rotate, the spinous processes deviate more and more to the concave side and the ribs follow the rotation of the vertebrae. The ribs on the convex side are rotated more posteriorly, causing the characteristic rib hump seen in thoracic scoliosis. The ribs on the concave side are rotated more anteriorly. Because the onset and progression of scoliosis (until skeletal

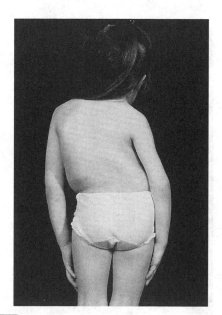

Figure 22-3 Scoliosis.

maturity) are generally asymptomatic, it can develop undetected without close examination.

The significant incidence of scoliosis in the adolescent population has prompted the creation of school screening programs in all 50 states. Visual observation is used during the Adam's forward bending test. The Adam's forward bending test involves asking the patient to bend forward at the waist as though touching his or her toes while the clinician, who is standing behind the patient, looks along the line at the back and determines whether one side is higher than the other. If scoliosis is suspected, the magnitude of a rib hump is quantified using a scoliometer (an inclinometer) during the Adam's forward bending test (Figure 22-4). The scoliometer is placed over the spinous process at the apex of the curve to measure the angle of trunk rotation as the patient bends forward. During the physical examination by the patient's physician, a determination is made as to whether the deformity is structural (cannot be corrected with active or passive movement and there is rotation toward the convexity of the curve) or nonstructural (fully corrects clinically and radiographically on lateral bending toward the apex of the curve, and lacks vertebral rotation). Nonstructural scoliotic curves can result from leg-length discrepancies, muscle disuse/overuse, habitual postures, and muscle guarding.

Height measurements are taken in sitting and standing. Changes in sitting height can be less than changes in standing height and give a better estimate of truncal growth rate. Trunk compensation is typically assessed using a plumb-line, and a radiographic leg length measurement is also obtained.

● **Key Point** Radiographs, which are usually considered only when a patient has a curve that might require treatment or could progress to a stage requiring treatment, can be used to determine location, type, and magnitude of the curve (using the Cobb method) as well as skeletal age. Alternatively, a noninvasive technique (which reduces radiation exposure) called Moiré topography can be used, in which light is projected through grids onto the back of the patient to assess topographical asymmetry.

Skeletal maturity is determined using the Risser sign, which is defined by the amount of calcification present in the iliac apophysis. The Risser sign measures the progressive ossification from anterolaterally to posteromedially (**Table 22-6**). When children reach a grade 5 on the Risser scale, their scoliotic curves will stabilize. Children with idiopathic scoliosis usually progress from a Risser grade 1 to a grade 5 over a 2-year period.

● **Key Point** If scoliosis is neglected, the curves may progress dramatically, creating significant physical deformity and even cardiopulmonary problems with especially severe curves. Pulmonary function tests are warranted in the presence of severe curves due to the resultant rib cage restrictions and decreased chest wall expansion.

Most curves can be treated nonoperatively through observation with appropriate intermittent radiographs to check for the presence or absence of curve progression. However, 60 percent of curvatures in rapidly growing prepubertal children will

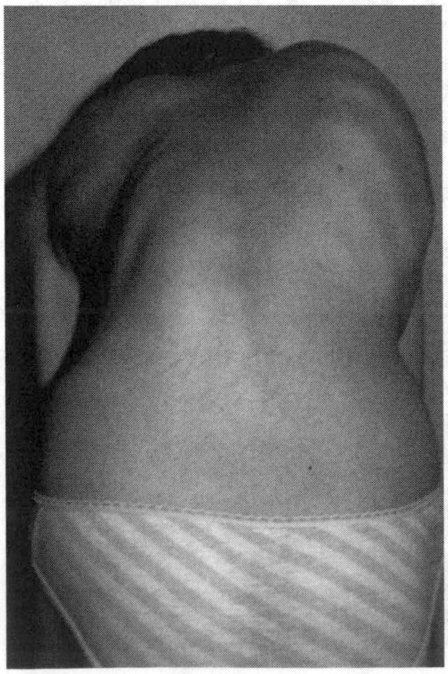

Figure 22-4 Adam's forward bending test.

TABLE 22-6	Risser Grades
Grade	**Interpretation**
0	Absence of ossification
1	25 percent ossification of the iliac apophysis
2	50 percent ossification of the iliac apophysis
3	75 percent ossification of the iliac apophysis
4	100 percent ossification of the iliac apophysis
5	The iliac apophysis has fused to the iliac crest after 100 percent ossification

Data from Biondi J, Weiner DS, Bethem D, et al: Correlation of Risser sign and bone age determination in adolescent idiopathic scoliosis. J Pediatr Orthop 5:697–701, 1985; and Little DG, Sussman MD: The Risser sign: A critical analysis. J Pediatr Orthop 14:569–575, 1994

progress and may require bracing (Boston, or custom thoracolumbosacral orthosis [TLSO]) or surgery.

> **● Key Point** Orthoses are typically prescribed for children with idiopathic scoliosis who are skeletally immature (with a Risser sign of 0, 1, or 2) and have a curve from 25 to 45 degrees. The active theory of orthotics is that curve progression is prevented by muscle contractions responding to the brace wear. Exercises to be performed while wearing a brace, such as pelvic tilts, thoracic flexion, and lateral shifts, are often taught to patients to improve the active forces, although there is little evidence to support this.

Intervention

Physical therapy intervention for scoliosis is based on skeletal maturity of the child, growth potential of the child, and curve magnitude. At the time of writing, the primary benefits of exercise in a nonsurgical patient with mild scoliosis are the following:[20]

- Help with correct postural alignment following the bracing program. It is important to correct any asymmetrical postural habits to help prevent further development.
- Maintain proper respiration and chest mobility.
- Help reduce back pain.
- Improve overall posture and spinal mobility.
- Help the patient resume prebracing functional skills.
- Maintain muscle strength, particularly in the abdominals.
- Maintain or improve range of motion and spinal flexibility through promotion of proper length and strength relationships of the spinal and extremity musculature. The general rule is to stretch the muscles on the concave side and to strengthen the muscles on the convex side. Asymmetric exercise is used to promote symmetry. For example, in a patient with a right thoracic, left lumbar curve, typical findings may include weakness of the right iliopsoas and right external oblique. Exercises that could be prescribed for this patient would include resisted right hip flexion at the end range with the patient in sitting to address the weakness of the right iliopsoas. Weakness of the right external oblique can be addressed using a left upper extremity diagonal reaching movement pattern emphasizing right thoracic sidebending (Figure 22-5). Other functional exercises for scoliosis include:
  - ❑ The patient is positioned in prone and is asked to place both hands behind his or her head while deviating the thorax

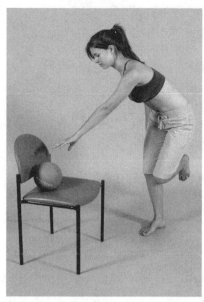

Figure 22-5   Upper extremity diagonal reaching.

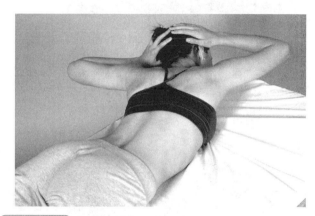

Figure 22-6   Prone sidebending.

away from the concave side of the curve (Figure 22-6).
  - ❑ The patient is positioned in prone and is asked to reach overhead and extend the arm on the concave side (Figure 22-7).
  - ❑ The patient is positioned in heel-sitting and is asked to place both hands forward and flat while emphasizing trunk axial elongation. The patient is then asked to stretch both arms laterally away from the concave side of the curve (Figure 22-8).
  - ❑ The patient is positioned in sidelying (convex side down) over the end of the table while the clinician stabilizes the patient. A pillow is placed directly under the apex of the thoracic convex curve. Using the arm that is closest to the ceiling, the patient reaches overhead and

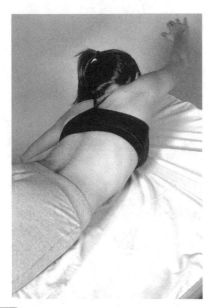

Figure 22-7   Prone reach.

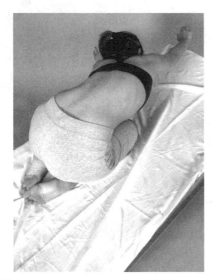

Figure 22-8   Heel-sitting stretch.

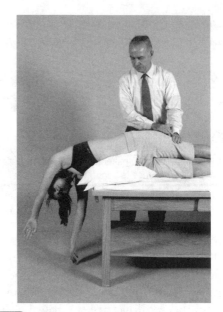

Figure 22-9   Sidelying stretch.

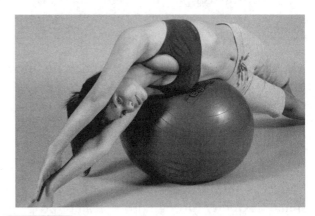

Figure 22-10   Swiss ball stretch.

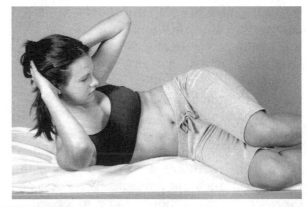

Figure 22-11   Sidelying sit-up.

then down toward the floor to enhance the stretch (Figure 22-9).

❑ Swiss ball exercises can also be used, focusing on gaining increased thoracic extension while stretching the concave side (Figure 22-10).

❑ Any of the strengthening exercises described in the intervention strategy section of Chapter 14 can be used to increase strength in the extensor muscle groups. Sidelying techniques (lying on the concave side) can be incorporated to strengthen the lateral muscle groups. The sidelying sit-up exercise is particularly effective (Figure 22-11).

If surgery is considered, the primary goal of scoliosis surgery is to achieve a solid bony fusion. Even in the setting of adequate correction and solid fusion, up to 38 percent of patients still have occasional back pain. If surgery is warranted, the postsurgical management can include the previously mentioned strategies and the following:[21]

- Breathing exercises to promote rib cage expansion, pulmonary hygiene, and effective coughing
- Patient and family education

Slipped Capital Femoral Epiphysis

The hip is the largest joint in the body and is important for postural stability as well as mobility (see Chapter 19). Disorders of the developing hip can cause delays or deficiencies in gross motor development with resultant developmental lag in other areas. Slipped capital femoral epiphysis (SCFE) is classified as a disorder of epiphyseal growth and represents a unique type of instability of the proximal femoral growth plate due to a Salter-Harris type I fracture through the proximal femoral physis.[22–28] The cause of SCFE is unclear. Stress around the hip causes a shear force to be applied at the growth plate and causes the epiphysis to move posteriorly and medially. In addition, the position of the proximal physis normally changes from horizontal to oblique during preadolescence and adolescence, redirecting hip forces from compression forces to shear forces. The severity of SCFE is measured in grades of slippage (Figure 22-12).

The patient usually presents with an antalgic limp and pain in the groin. The leg is usually held in external rotation, both when supine and when standing. With attempts to flex the hip, the leg moves into external rotation to avoid impingement of the metaphysis on the anterior lip of the acetabulum.

Consequently, there is reduced hip flexion, internal rotation, and abduction.

> **● Key Point** Knowledge of SCFE and its manifestations will facilitate prompt referral by the PTA to the supervising physical therapist and ultimately to an orthopaedic surgeon.

Intervention

The PTA may be involved in the treatment of these patients as inpatients or outpatients, in home care, or in a school-based setting. Functions of the PTA with this population include ordering equipment, providing mobility training, teaching and monitoring range of motion and strengthening exercises, and consulting about environmental adaptations. The goals of treatment are to:[26]

- Avoid further damage or remodeling of the affected hip joint to keep the displacement to a minimum
- Maintain motion
- Delay or prevent premature degenerative arthritis

Following surgical fixation, using one or two pins or screws, usually in situ, the PT completes a careful and thorough examination of the motion of the hip joint, and subsequent measurements should be taken after every operation and removal of the cast. The weight-bearing status can vary but is usually non–weight-bearing or touch down weight bearing. Full weight bearing is permitted when the growth plate has fused (within approximately 3 to 4 months).

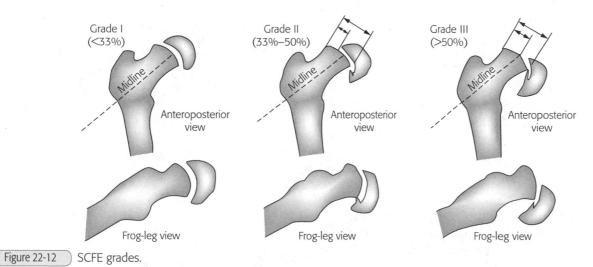

Figure 22-12 SCFE grades.

Reproduced from Douglas Katz, *Brain Injury Medicine: Principles and Practice* (New York: Demos Medical Publishing LLC, 2007).

Range of motion exercises for the hip should be done in all planes, with particular emphasis on hip flexion, internal rotation, and abduction. Strengthening of the involved extremity is introduced when sufficient healing has occurred. Gait training post-surgery is initiated once lower extremity strength and range of motion are adequate for ambulation skills.

Legg-Calvé-Perthes Disease

Legg-Calvé-Perthes disease (LCPD) is an idiopathic osteonecrosis of the capital femoral epiphysis of the femoral head. LCPD has an unconfirmed etiology, but may involve an interruption of the blood supply to the capital femoral epiphysis—osteochondrosis (avascular necrosis of the epiphysis).[29–35] As with those patients with an SCFE, knowledge of this disease and its manifestations will facilitate early recognition and referral by the PTA to the supervising physical therapist. Patients tend to have a limp and frequently have a positive Trendelenburg sign resulting from pain or hip abduction weakness.[26] Limited hip range of motion is noted, especially in hip abduction and internal rotation. The child complains of pain in the groin, hip, or knee (referred pain).[26] The disease process takes from 2 to 4 years to complete.[32] Controversy exists regarding the appropriate treatment, or whether treatment is even necessary.[26] The goals of treatment are to relieve pain, to maintain the spherical shape of the femoral head, and to prevent extrusion of the enlarged femoral head from the joint. Physical therapy may be provided at home, at school, or in the clinic.

Intervention

The various approaches to SCFE include:

- Observation only
- Range of motion exercises in all planes of hip motion (especially internal rotation and abduction)
- Bracing
- Casting
- Surgery

Specific procedural interventions (e.g., crutch training, aquatic therapy) can be used to relieve the forces incurred during weight bearing. Gait training may be initiated with an orthosis or with bracing.

The specific gait pattern and assistive devices depend on the type of orthosis. Patient and family education is necessary to teach hip protection strategies, thereby minimizing degenerative changes as the child ages.

Scheuermann's Disease

Scheuermann's disease, which is found in approximately 10 percent of the population and in males and females equally, typically is seen in pubescent athletes.[36] The disease involves a defect to the ring apophysis of the vertebral body and anterior wedging of the affected vertebrae, as a result of a flexion overload of the anterior vertebral body (Figure 22-13).[37] The end plate can crack, thus making it possible for disk material to bulge into the vertebral body (Schmorl's node). The initial onset is typically asymptomatic but as the condition progresses, the patient may complain of an aching sensation in the upper spine. In addition there may be observational

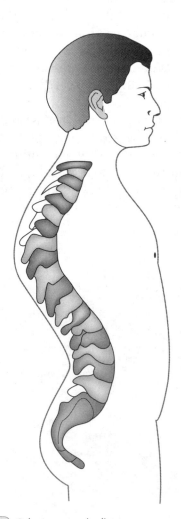

Figure 22-13 Scheuermann's disease.

evidence of an increased thoracic kyphosis and pain with thoracic extension and rotation, usually detected during a school physical or noted by the parents.

Intervention

The intervention depends on the severity, but typically involves postural education, a modification of the aggravating activity, exercise, or bracing. The exercise program involves stretching of the pectoralis major and minor muscles, and muscle strengthening exercises for the thoracic spine extensors (seated rotation, and extension in lying exercises) and the scapular adductors.[38]

Osteochondritis Dissecans

Osteochondritis dissecans (OCD) is a rare cause of anterior knee or elbow pain in the young athlete. OCD is a joint disorder in which cracks form in the articular cartilage and the underlying subchondral bone due to vascular deprivation (avascular necrosis). The result is fragmentation (dissection) of both cartilage and bone, and the free movement of these osteochondral fragments within the joint space, causing pain and further damage. If it occurs in the knee, it involves the weight-bearing portions of the medial and lateral femoral condyles.

Occasionally, pain may not be the most prominent symptom, but a catching sensation with joint motion may be the primary complaint if there is a loose body within the joint space. If the lesion is small, a painful arc is present during active and passive movement. Nonsurgical treatment is rarely an option because the capacity for articular cartilage to heal is limited. As a result, even moderate cases require some form of surgery. When possible, nonoperative forms of management such as protected weight bearing (partial or non–weight-bearing) and immobilization are used. Surgical treatment varies widely and includes arthroscopic drilling of intact lesions, securing of cartilage flap lesions with pins or screws, drilling and replacement of cartilage plugs, stem cell transplantation, and joint replacement.

Intervention

Postoperative rehabilitation usually involves immobilization and then physical therapy. During the immobilization period, isometric exercises are commonly used to restore muscle lost to atrophy without disturbing the cartilage of the affected joint. Once the immobilization period has ended, physical therapy involves protection of the joint's cartilage surface and underlying subchondral bone with maintenance

of muscle strength and range of motion and low impact activities, such as walking or swimming.

Osgood-Schlatter Disease

Osgood-Schlatter (OS) disease (traction apophysitis) is a benign, self-limiting knee condition that is one of the most common causes of knee pain in the adolescent.[39] The condition occurs in active boys and girls ages 11–18 coinciding with periods of growth spurts. OS occurs more frequently in boys than in girls, with reports of a male-to-female ratio ranging from 3:1 to as high as 7:1. During periods of rapid growth, stress from contraction of the quadriceps is transmitted through the patellar tendon onto a small portion of the partially developed tibial tuberosity. This may result in a partial avulsion fracture through the ossification center. Eventually, secondary heterotopic bone formation occurs in the tendon near its insertion, producing a visible lump. Pain over the tibial tuberosity is mild and intermittent initially. In the acute phase the pain is severe and continuous in nature. The pain occurs during activities such as running, jumping, squatting, and especially ascending or descending stairs and during kneeling. The pain is worse with acute knee impact. The pain can be reproduced by extending the knee against resistance or stressing the quadriceps. Bilateral symptoms are observed in 20–30 percent of patients.

Intervention

The intervention for this condition is usually symptomatic, including anti-inflammatory measures. Specific procedural interventions include bracing (neoprene knee brace); progressive quadriceps stretching exercises, including hip extension for a complete stretch of the extensor mechanism; and stretching exercises for the hamstrings. The traditional approach of activity limitations is no longer considered necessary, although the more persistent cases may require cast immobilization for 6–8 weeks. Rarely, individuals will require surgical excision of symptomatic ossicles or degenerated tendons for persistent symptoms at skeletal maturity.

Little Leaguer's Elbow

Little leaguer's elbow is a common term for an avulsion lesion to the medial apophysis as a result of repetitive valgus stress.[40] The repetitive motions involved in the various phases of throwing place enormous strains on the elbow, particularly during the late cocking and acceleration phases, which can result in inflammation, scar formation, loose bodies, ligament sprains or ruptures, and the more serious conditions of osteochondritis or an avulsion fracture.[41,42] Little leaguer's elbow may start insidiously or suddenly. Usually, a sudden onset of pain is secondary to fracture at the site of the lesion.

Intervention
Management is conservative, involving rest and elimination of the offending activity. Lesions involving less than 0.5–1 centimeter of apophyseal separation are initially treated with rest. This is followed by a rehabilitation program similar to that described for medial epicondylitis; however, resistance exercises are avoided until active range of motion can be performed to full motion without pain (generally 2–3 weeks). Throwing is avoided for 6–12 weeks. If osteochondritis dissecans is present, the joint needs protection for several months.[43] Separation greater than 0.5–1 centimeter, failure to respond to conservative measures, or sudden traumatic avulsions are indications for surgery. The patient cannot return to pitching until full and normal motion and strength has returned.

Pulled Elbow
The term *pulled elbow*, also referred to as "nursemaid's elbow," refers to a common minor soft-tissue injury of the radiohumeral joint in children of preschool age, caused by a sudden longitudinal traction force on the pronated forearm and extended elbow.[44,45] A pulled elbow results from the radial head slipping through the annular ligament, causing the fibers of the annular ligament to become interposed between the radius and the capitellum of the humerus.[46,47]

The incidence of pulled elbow is 3 percent in children under the age of 8 years,[48] and it comprises 5.6 percent of all injuries involving the upper extremity in children under the age of 10 years.[47,49] The disorder is more common in boys than in girls, and the left elbow is more commonly affected than the right.[50] These are the common causes of pulled elbow:[47]

- The child's forearm or hand is being held firmly by a parent as the child attempts to walk away.
- The child is lifted by an adult from the ground by the child's hands.
- A parent snatches the hand of a child to prevent a fall as the child wanders toward the edge of the pavement.
- The young child may be lifted by the hand from a lying or sitting position or may even be swung around by the hands several times during the course of play.

- The child actually does the pulling, either as he or she stumbles and falls or while trying to escape the grasping hand of an adult.

The child presents with a painful and dangling arm, which hangs limply with the elbow extended and the forearm pronated.[47] There is usually no obvious swelling or deformity. The common sites of pain are (in order of occurrence) the forearm and wrist, the wrist alone, and the elbow alone.[46] In all cases the child resists attempted supination of the forearm.

Intervention
The intervention of choice is manipulation by either the physical therapist or physician.[47] Soon after the manipulation, the child usually begins to use the arm again, but sometimes there is a delay of a day or two. In such cases, a sling can be used to both give comfort and protect the arm from being pulled again.

An important aspect in the management is to advise the parents to avoid longitudinal traction strain on the child's arm—the parents should not pull on the hands or wrists of the child.[47]

Sever's Disease (Calcaneal Apophysitis)
Sever's disease is a traction apophysitis at the insertion of the Achilles tendon and is a common cause of heel pain in the athletically active child, with 61 percent of cases occurring bilaterally.[51]

The calcaneal apophysis serves as the attachment for the Achilles tendon superiorly and for the plantar fascia and the short muscles of the sole of the foot inferiorly.[52] Young gymnasts and dancers are particularly susceptible to this condition because of their repetitive jumping or landing from a height.[53]

Intervention
The intervention for Sever's disease begins with shortening the heel cord using heel cups or heel wedges, and avoiding barefoot walking until becoming asymptomatic.[54] Stretching of the heel cord is initiated only after symptoms have subsided.

Congenital
Congenital conditions are conditions an individual is born with but are not necessarily inherited. Congenital conditions can be caused by any number of "problems" during pregnancy (e.g., infection, poor positioning in the uterus, toxins, unknown causes) whereas inherited conditions refer to a trait (dominant, recessive, or polygenic) that is linked to a gene passed on from one generation to another.

Developmental Dysplasia of the Hip

Developmental dysplasia of the hip (DDH), formerly referred to as congenital hip dysplasia (CHD), involves an abnormal growth/development of the hip including the osseous structures, such as the acetabulum and the proximal femur, and the labrum, capsule, and other soft tissues, which results in a failure of the femoral head to rest in the acetabulum of the pelvis. The condition may occur at any time during fetal growth, from conception to skeletal maturity, but usually develops in the last trimester of pregnancy. The various types of developmental dysplasia of the hip in infancy are outlined in **Table 22-7**.

> ● **Key Point** Early detection is key with this condition. Evidence suggests that early detection within the first 3 months of life is critical in preventing the development of any secondary complications.[55] Diagnosis by x-ray examination is difficult or impossible in infants younger than 6 to 8 months of age because of the lack of ossification of the joint. Ultrasound is the diagnostic modality of choice.[55]

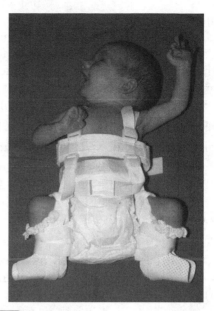

Figure 22-14   Pavlik harness.

Intervention

The treatment of this condition depends on the child's age and the severity of the condition. Although surgical intervention is an option in severe cases, the conservative approach is discussed here. Conservative treatment will be most effective for infants whose subluxation or dislocation has been discovered and treated early, within the first 6 months of life. The conservative approach involves maintaining the hip in flexion and abduction through bracing, splinting, or diapering until it is adequately remodeled.

- *Diapering:* The child is placed in two or three diapers holding the legs in abduction, and parents are instructed to position the infant in hip flexion as well.

- *Pavlik harness* (Figure 22-14): This is used if symptoms persist after several weeks. The harness, which is initially worn 24 hours a day for 6 to 12 weeks, restricts hip extension and adduction and allows the hip to be maintained in flexion and abduction, the "protective position."[26] The position of flexion and abduction enhances normal acetabular development, and the kicking motion allowed in this position stretches the contracted hip adductors and promotes spontaneous reduction of the dislocated hip.[26] After the initial period, the harness is worn 12 hours per day for 3 to 6 additional months, or until both clinical and radiographic signs are normal. In infants older than 9 months of age who are beginning to

TABLE 22-7	Types of Developmental Dysplasia of the Hip in Infancy
Type	**Definition**
Dysplasia	Acetabulum may be shallow or small with diminished lateral borders.
	May occur alone or with any level of femoral deformity or displacement.
Subluxation	The femoral head is displaced to the rim of the acetabulum, sliding laterally.
Dislocated	The femoral head is displaced completely outside the acetabulum but can be reduced with manual pressure.
Tetraologic	The femoral head lies completely outside the hip socket and cannot be reduced with manual pressure.

walk independently, an abduction orthosis can be used as an alternative to the Pavlik harness.[26] If the Pavlik harness is used, it is important to teach the parents to place the hips in the correct position—too much flexion or abduction can cause excessive pressure through the femoral heads, resulting in possible avascular necrosis.

The PTA may provide strengthening and range of motion activities; progressive gait training; caregiver training for transfers, mobility, and exercise; or consult for adaptive equipment and functional access for the child.

Equinovarus

Clubfoot, or talipes equinovarus, is a congenital deformity consisting of hindfoot equinus (i.e., plantarflexion), hindfoot varus, and forefoot varus (the forefoot is curved inward in relation to the heel, the heel is bent inward in relation to the leg, and the ankle is fixed in plantarflexion with toes pointed down), which can be classified as:

- *Postural or positional:* Not true clubfoot
- *Fixed or rigid:* This type of equinovarus can be either flexible (i.e., correctable without surgery) or resistant (i.e., require surgical release)

Intervention

Treatment consists of manipulation (reducing the talonavicular joint by moving the navicular laterally and the head of the talus medially) by the PT, taping, stretching, bracing, and serial casting, which is most effective if started immediately after birth. The role of the PTA involves monitoring of the casts, providing developmental intervention to promote typical functional skills, and assisting in stretching and splinting.

Congenital Limb Deficiencies

Children with congenital limb deficiencies (CLDs) or amputations need to make substantial adaptations to achieve effective function as growth and maturation occur. A variety of genetic syndromes have been implicated in patterns of skeletal abnormalities in children, but the cause is unknown in approximately 60 to 70 percent of cases. Congenital limb deficiencies can be classified into two major groups:

- *Transverse deficiencies:* A limb that has developed normally to a certain point, with structures beyond that point absent. For example, a child's lower extremity has a fully developed femur, but no tibia, fibula, tarsal, metatarsals, or phalanges.

- *Longitudinal deficiencies:* A limb that has elements in the long axis of the limb that are absent. For example, a child who is missing the radius and thumb in one upper extremity, with the ulna, carpals, and other digits present.

The clinical presentation varies according to the type of CLD, the level of the deficiency, and the number of deficiencies or limbs involved.

Intervention

The intervention for this population is directed toward helping the child develop appropriate functional and developmental skills while reducing any secondary impairments, such as soft tissue contractures. The PTA may be involved in problem solving, checking prosthetic fit, and communicating with team members.

Summary

The pediatric patient has many physical and physiologic characteristics that constitute unique challenges for assessing and treating injuries. Growing musculoskeletal tissue is innately predisposed to specific injuries that vary greatly from injuries sustained by skeletally mature adults. Most of this growth occurs in two phases. There is a rapid gain in growth in infancy and early childhood that slows down during middle childhood. The second rapid increase in growth occurs during adolescence. A significant injury during one of these phases that interrupts the growth process can present serious challenges. When therapeutic exercise is prescribed for the pediatric patient, the PTA must be creative and try to make exercise fun in order to increase compliance.

REVIEW Questions

1. At approximately what age (in months) would you expect a normally developing child to be able to perform rolling?
2. At approximately what age (in months) would you expect a normally developing child to be able to perform independent sitting?
3. At approximately what age (in months) would you expect a normally developing child to be able to perform creeping (quadruped)?
4. At approximately what age (in months) would you expect a normally developing child to be able to walk?

5. All of the following are pathologies of the skeletal system that are present at birth in the neonate, except:
   a. Talipes equinovarus
   b. Scoliosis
   c. Sickle cell
   d. Osteogenesis imperfecta

6. While observing a patient's foot you notice the following deformity: foot inversion, forefoot adduction, and plantarflexion. What is the name of this deformity?
   a. Talipes equinovarus
   b. Talipes calcaneovalgus
   c. Talipes valgus
   d. Talipes calcaneus

7. The most common and serious deformities as far as congenital dislocations are concerned affect the:
   a. Spine
   b. Hip
   c. Shoulder
   d. Knee

8. The clinical picture of idiopathic scoliosis includes:
   a. Inequality of leg length
   b. Lateral curvature of the spine
   c. Rotation of the spine
   d. All of the above

9. You are treating an overweight teenage male who has symptoms of moderate groin and knee pain. His leg abducts and externally rotates during hip flexion. The most likely diagnosis is:
   a. Congenital dislocated hip
   b. Legg-Calvé-Perthes disease
   c. Slipped capital femoral epiphysis
   d. None of the above

10. You are beginning an intervention of a 6-year-old boy with his mother. The mother reports that she pulled the child from a seated position by grasping the boy's right wrist. The child then experienced immediate pain at the right elbow. Which of the following is the most likely diagnosis?
    a. Pulled elbow
    b. Little leaguer's elbow
    c. Radial head fracture
    d. Muscle strain

11. While treating an infant, you observe that there is limitation of abduction of the flexed right hip and an asymmetry of the gluteal folds. What deformity would you suspect?
    a. Osgood-Schlatter's disease
    b. Osteogenesis imperfecta
    c. Acetabular dysplasia
    d. Osteochondritis dissecans

12. You are treating a child with a diagnosis of Sever's disease. What joint will be the focus of your treatment?
    a. Shoulder
    b. Knee
    c. Ankle
    d. Hip

13. Which of the following is characterized by tendinitis of the patella tendon and osteochondroses of its tibial attachment?
    a. Legg-Calvé-Perthes disease
    b. Rickets
    c. Paget's disease
    d. Osgood-Schlatter disease

References

1. Lewis C: Physiological response to exercise in the child: Considerations for the typically and atypically developing youngster. Proceedings from the American Physical Therapy Association combined sections meeting. San Antonio, Texas, 2001
2. Connolly BH, Lupinnaci NS, Bush AJ: Changes in attitudes and perceptions about research in physical therapy among professional physical therapist students and new graduates. Phys Ther 81:1127–1134, 2001
3. Duffy CM, Arsenault L, Duffy KN, et al: The Juvenile Arthritis Quality of Life Questionnaire—development of a new responsive index for juvenile rheumatoid arthritis and juvenile spondyloarthritides. J Rheumatol 24:738–746, 1997
4. Brewer EJ, Jr, Bass J, Baum J, et al: Current proposed revision of JRA criteria. JRA Criteria Subcommittee of the Diagnostic and Therapeutic Criteria Committee of the American Rheumatism Section of the Arthritis Foundation. Arthritis Rheum 20:195–199, 1977
5. Klepper SE: Juvenile rheumatoid arthritis, in Campbell SK, Vander Linden DW, Palisano RJ (eds): Physical Therapy for Children. St Louis, Saunders, 2006, pp 291–323
6. Patrick C: Spinal conditions, in Campbell SK, Vander Linden DW, Palisano RJ (eds): Physical Therapy for Children. St Louis, Saunders, 2006, pp 337–358
7. McKenzie RA: Manual correction of sciatic scoliosis. N Z Med J 76:194–199, 1972
8. Blum CL: Chiropractic and pilates therapy for the treatment of adult scoliosis. J Manip Physiol Ther 25:E3, 2002
9. Miller NH: Genetics of familial idiopathic scoliosis. Clin Orthop Relat Res 401:60–64, 2002
10. Kane WJ: Scoliosis prevalence: A call for a statement of terms. Clin Orthop 126:43–46, 1977
11. Miller NH: Cause and natural history of adolescent idiopathic scoliosis. Orthop Clin North Am 30:343–352, vii, 1999
12. Dobbs MB, Weinstein SL: Infantile and juvenile scoliosis. Orthop Clin North Am 30:331–341, vii, 1999
13. Greiner KA: Adolescent idiopathic scoliosis: Radiologic decision-making. Am Fam Physician 65:1817–1822, 2002

14. Lonstein JE, Winter RB: Adolescent idiopathic scoliosis. Nonoperative treatment. Orthop Clin North Am 19:239–246, 1988

15. Lenke LG: Lenke classification system of adolescent idiopathic scoliosis: Treatment recommendations. Instr Course Lect 54:537–542, 2005

16. Lenke LG, Edwards CC, 2nd, Bridwell KH: The Lenke classification of adolescent idiopathic scoliosis: How it organizes curve patterns as a template to perform selective fusions of the spine. Spine 28:S199–S207, 2003

17. Weinstein SL, Ponseti IV: Curve progression in idiopathic scoliosis. J Bone Joint Surg Am 65:447-455, 1983

18. Ponseti IV, Pedrini V, Wynne-Davies R, et al: Pathogenesis of scoliosis. Clin Orthop Relat Res 120:268–280, 1976

19. Ponseti IV, Friedman B: Prognosis in idiopathic scoliosis. J Bone Joint Surg Am 32:381–395, 1950

20. Hundozi-Hysenaj H, Dallku IB, Murtezani A, et al: Treatment of the idiopathic scoliosis with brace and physiotherapy. Niger J Med 18:256–259, 2009

21. Cassella MC, Hall JE: Current treatment approach in the non-operative and operative management of adolescent idiopathic scoliosis. Phys Ther 71:897, 1991

22. Kalogrianitis S, Tan CK, Kemp GJ, et al: Does unstable slipped capital femoral epiphysis require urgent stabilization? J Pediatr Orthop B 16:6–9, 2007

23. Kamarulzaman MA, Abdul Halim AR, Ibrahim S: Slipped capital femoral epiphysis (SCFE): A 12-year review. Med J Malaysia 61:71–78, 2006 (Suppl A)

24. Flores M, Satish SG, Key T: Slipped capital femoral epiphysis in identical twins: Is there an HLA predisposition? Report of a case and review of the literature. Bull Hosp Jt Dis 63:158–160, 2006

25. Aronsson DD, Loder RT, Breur GJ, et al: Slipped capital femoral epiphysis: Current concepts. J Am Acad Orthop Surg 14:666–679, 2006

26. Leach J: Orthopedic conditions, in Campbell SK, Vander Linden DW, Palisano RJ (eds): Physical Therapy for Children (ed 3). St Louis, Saunders, 2006, pp 481–515

27. Umans H, Liebling MS, Moy L, et al: Slipped capital femoral epiphysis: A physeal lesion diagnosed by MRI, with radiographic and CT correlation. Skeletal Radiol 27:139–144, 1998

28. Busch MT, Morrissy RT: Slipped capital femoral epiphysis. Orthop Clin North Am 18:637–647, 1987

29. Herring JA, Kim HT, Browne R: Legg-Calve-Perthes disease. Part II: Prospective multicenter study of the effect of treatment on outcome. J Bone Joint Surg Am 86-A:2121–2134, 2004

30. Herring JA, Kim HT, Browne R: Legg-Calve-Perthes disease. Part I: Classification of radiographs with use of the modified lateral pillar and Stulberg classifications. J Bone Joint Surg Am 86A:2103–2120, 2004

31. Moens P, Fabry G: Legg-Calve-Perthes disease: One century later. Acta Orthop Belg 69:97–103, 2003

32. Thompson GH, Price CT, Roy D, et al: Legg-Calve-Perthes disease: Current concepts. Instr Course Lect 51:367–384, 2002

33. Gross GW, Articolo GA, Bowen JR: Legg-Calve-Perthes disease: Imaging evaluation and management. Semin Musculoskelet Radiol 3:379–391, 1999

34. Roy DR: Current concepts in Legg-Calve-Perthes disease. Pediatr Ann 28:748–752, 1999

35. Townsend DJ: Legg-Calve-Perthes disease. Orthopedics 22:381, 1999

36. Bradford DS, Loustein JE, Moe JH, et al: Moe's Textbook of Scoliosis and Other Spinal Deformities (ed 2). Philadelphia, WB Saunders, 1987

37. Benson MK, Byrnes DP: The clinical syndromes and surgical treatment of thoracic intervertebral disc prolapse. J Bone Joint Surg 57B:471–477, 1975

38. Winkel D, Matthijs O, Phelps V: Thoracic spine, in Winkel D, Matthijs O, Phelps V (eds): Diagnosis and Treatment of the Spine. Gaithersburg, MD, Aspen, 1997, pp 389–541

39. Mital MA, Matza RA: Osgood-Schlatter's disease: The painful puzzler. Physician Sports Med 5:60, 1977

40. Brogden BG, Cros NW: Little leaguer's elbow. Am J Rad 83:671, 1960

41. Jobe FW, Nuber G: Throwing injuries of the elbow. Clin Sports Med 5:621, 1986

42. Cabrera JM, McCue FC: Nonosseous athletic injuries of the elbow, forearm, and hand. Clin Sports Med 5:681–700, 1986

43. Onieal M-E: Common wrist and elbow unjuries in primary care. Lippincotts Prim Care Pract Musculoskel Cond 3:441–450, 1999

44. Salter RB, Zaltz C: Anatomic investigations of the mechanism of injury and pathologic anatomy of pulled elbow in young children. Clin Orthop 77:134–143, 1971

45. Dee R, Carrion W: Pulled elbow, in Dee R, Hurst LC, Gruber MA, et al (eds): Principles of Orthopaedic Practice. New York, McGraw-Hill, 1997, pp 579–596

46. Hagroo GA, Zaki HM, Choudhary MT, et al: Pulled elbow—not the effect of hypermobility of joints. Injury 26:687–690, 1995

47. Sai N: Pulled elbow. J Royal Soc Med 92:462–464, 1999

48. Corrigan AB: The pulled elbow. Med J Aust 2:1, 1965

49. Amir D, Frankl U, Pogrund H: Pulled elbow and hypermobility of joints. Clin Orthop 257:94, 1990

50. Matles AL, Eliopoulous K: Internal derangement of the elbow in children. Int Surg 48:259–263, 1967

51. Micheli LJ, Ireland ML: Prevention and management of calcaneal apophysitis in children: An overuse syndrome. J Pediatr Orthop 7:34–38, 1987

52. Mafulli N: Intensive training in young athletes. Sports Med 9:229–243, 1990

53. Meeusen R, Borms J: Gymnastic injuries. Sports Med 13:337–356, 1992

54. McManama GB, Jr: Ankle injuries in the young athlete. Clin Sports Med 7:547, 1988

55. Graf R: Hip Sonography: Diagnosis and Management of Infant Hip Dysplasia (ed 2). New York, Springer, 2006

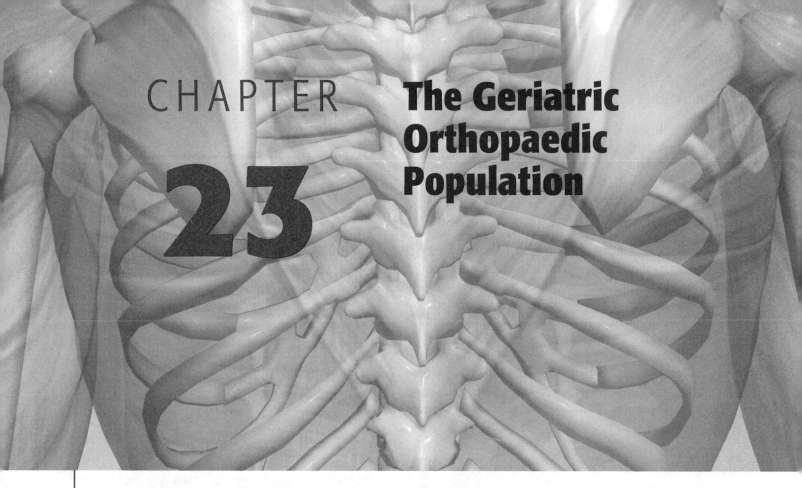

CHAPTER 23

The Geriatric Orthopaedic Population

Chapter Objectives

At the completion of this chapter, the reader will be able to:

1. Describe the normal aging process as it relates to orthopaedics.
2. Describe the various theories of aging.
3. Discuss and describe the physiologic factors that contribute to disease, impairment, functional limitation, and disability.
4. Discuss the various pathological conditions associated with the elderly.
5. Describe the common functional limitations associated with the geriatric population.
6. Differentiate the principles of rehabilitation as they relate to the aging patient.

Overview

The purpose of this chapter is to provide an overview of the aging process in multiple systems and the impact of aging on the rehabilitation of acute and chronic musculoskeletal conditions that are common in the elderly. Aging is the accumulation of diverse adverse changes that increase the risk of death.[1] The rate of aging, that is, the rate at which aging changes occur, normally varies from individual to individual, resulting in differences in the age of death, the onset of various diseases, and the impact of aging on function.[1]

The Aging Process

Aging changes can be attributed to a combination of development, genetic defects, the environment, disease, and an inborn factor, the aging process. These aging changes are responsible for both the commonly recognized sequential alterations that accompany advancing age beyond the early period of life and the progressive increases in the probability of experiencing a chronic debilitating disease.[1] The incidence of chronic conditions has been shown to increase with advancing age and, because aging is often accompanied by a deterioration of general health, the geriatric population is especially vulnerable to loss of function and independence. In addition, because elderly individuals often suffer from several diseases at the same time (comorbidities), such as cardiovascular disorders, osteoporosis, arthritis, and diabetes, the interaction of these diseases produces a cumulative effect.

> **● Key Point**
>
> - *Geriatrics* is the branch of medicine that focuses on health promotion and the prevention and treatment of disease and disability in later life.
> - *Gerontology* is the study of the aging process and the science related to the care of the elderly.
> - *Ageism* can be defined as any attitude or action that subordinates a person, group, or perception purely on the basis of age. When that bias is the primary motivation behind acts of discrimination against that person or group, then those acts constitute age discrimination.
> - *Senescence* can be defined as the combination of processes of deterioration that follow the period of development of an organism.

Aging is a heterogeneous process and therefore differs greatly among individuals, producing a great variability in health and functional status in the older population. Many changes are associated with aging throughout adulthood and into old age. **Table 23-1** summarizes these system changes. Musculoskeletal impairments are among the most prevalent and symptomatic health problems of middle and old age.[2] The subsequent loss of strength, motion, and increasing pain prevent elderly individuals from making full use of their abilities and from participating in the regular physical activity necessary to maintain optimum mobility, general health, and, in some cases, independence.[3] Although some elderly adults succumb to the functional limitations and disability associated with aging, disease, or injury, many elderly adults retain high levels of activity and functional abilities well into advanced age.

> **● Key Point** Normal aging can be defined as age-related changes that are the result of the passage of time rather than the result of pathologic conditions. Chronologic age should not be used to determine potential for recovery or the appropriateness of referral for rehabilitation.

Coexisting pathologic processes can exacerbate the effects of other conditions and result in greater functional limitations and disability. Throughout youth and early adulthood, the body has reserve physiologic capacities and system redundancies that enable it to adapt to physical challenges and injury without a loss of functional abilities. The gradual decline of health and increased incidence of injury and disease experienced by older individuals can be partially attributed to the gradual loss of this physiologic reserve.[3] Without this physiologic reserve, an older individual is more susceptible to functional limitations and disability, resulting in frailty. Frailty is viewed as usual aging, and the opposite end of the spectrum from successful aging.[3] It is important to remember that frailty is not a natural consequence of aging and that the performance of physical activity throughout the aging years can produce a number of physiologic benefits:

- Substantial improvements can be made in almost all aspects of cardiovascular functioning.
- Individuals of all ages can benefit from muscle strengthening exercises. In particular, resistance training can have a significant impact on the maintenance of independence in old age.
- Regular activity helps prevent and/or postpone age-associated declines in flexibility, balance, and coordination.

Conversely, disuse exacerbates the aging process and negatively impacts the physiologic reserve in the face of disease and injury.

Theories of Aging

A wide array of theories exist as to why aging occurs, why species have the life spans they do, and what kinds of factors are likely to influence the aging process.

- Genetic theories focus on the mechanisms for aging located in the nucleus of the cell, implicating mutations and chromosomal anomalies that accumulate with age.
- Neuroendocrine-immuno theories focus on the decline in the system's ability to produce necessary antibodies that fight disease with aging, and a decrease in its ability to distinguish

TABLE 23-1	Summary of Multisystem Changes in the Elderly

System	Changes
Musculoskeletal	Muscle mass and strength decrease at a rate of about 30 percent between the ages of 60 and 90.
	Change in muscle fiber type (white and red). Type II fibers (fast twitch) decrease by about 50 percent.
	The recruitment of motor units decreases.
	Bone tensile strength decreases. (More than 30 percent of women over the age of 65 have osteoporosis.)
	Joint flexibility is reduced by 25 to 30 percent over the age of 70.
Neuromuscular	Atrophy of neurons; nerve fibers decrease and change in structure.
	The myoneural junction decreases in transmission speed.
	Nerve conduction velocity decreases by about 0.4 percent a year after age 70.
	Motor neuron conduction slows, which contributes to alterations in the autonomic system.
	Decreasing reflexes result from a decrease in nerve conduction. Ankle jerk is absent in about 70 percent, and knee and biceps jerk are absent in about 15 percent of geriatric population.
	Overall slow and decreased responsiveness in reaction time (simple reflexes less than complex).
	Increased postural sway (less in women than in men, with linear increase with age).
Neurosensory	Decrease in sweating (implications for modalities and exercise).
	Ten to twenty percent decrease in brain weight by age 90.
	Decrease in mechanoreceptors.
	Decrease in visual acuity and ability to accommodate to lighting changes resulting from increased density of lens.
	Decrease in hearing capabilities.
Cardiovascular and pulmonary	Decrease in cardiac output by about 0.7 percent a year after 20 years of age.
	Increased vascular resistance.
	Decreased arterial elasticity.
	Decreased cardiac reserve, and decreased physical and psychological response to stress.
	Increased irritation of myocardium contributes to increased risk of atrial fibrillation and arrhythmias.
	Decrease in lung function. (From age 25 to age 85 there is as much as a 50 percent decrease in maximal voluntary ventilation due to an increase in air resistance; this results in about a 40 percent decrease in vital capacity.)
	Respiratory gas exchange surface decreases at a rate of about 0.27 m^2 a year. (Maximum oxygen consumption for sedentary individuals of any age is 0.62 to 0.7 mL per minute.)
	Decrease in elastin in the lungs (increased rigidity) and chest wall soft tissues results in decrease in chest wall compliance.
	Decrease in vital capacity and decrease in pulmonary blood flow contribute to lower oxygen saturation levels.
	Decreased cough reflex.
Urogenital/renal	Gradual overall structure changes in all renal components.
	Decreased glomerular filtration rate and creatinine clearance.
	Change in response to sodium intake.
	Muscle hypertrophy in the urethra and bladder.
Gastrointestinal	Decreased peristalsis.
	Diminished secretions of pepsin and acid in the stomach.
	Decreasing hepatic and pancreatic enzymes.
Immunologic	Decrease in overall function with respect to infection.
	Decreased temperature regulation.
	Decrease in T cells.

Data from Bottomley JM: The geriatric population, in Boissonnault WG (ed): Primary Care for the Physical Therapist: Examination and Triage. St Louis, Elsevier Saunders, 2005, pp 288–306; and Bottomley JM: Summary of system changes. Comparing and contrasting age-related changes, in Bottomley JM, Lewis CB (eds): Geriatric Rehabilitation: A Clinical Approach (ed 2). Upper Saddle River, NJ, Prentice-Hall, 2003, pp 50–75

between antibodies and proteins. In essence, the immune system becomes self-destructive and reacts against itself. Examples of such autoimmune diseases are lupus, scleroderma, and adult-onset diabetes.

- Environmental theories focus on the cumulative damage caused by free-radical reactions.[4] A free radical is any molecule that has a free electron. Theoretically, the free radical reacts with healthy molecules in a destructive way. It is known that diet, lifestyle, some drugs (e.g., tobacco, alcohol), and radiation are all accelerators of free radical production within the body. However, there is also natural production of free radicals within the body as a byproduct of energy production, particularly from the mitochondria.

- Planned obsolescence theories focus on the genetic programming of senescence genes in the DNA.[1] According to these theories, individuals are born with a unique code and a preprogrammed lifespan of physical and mental functioning, and certain genes regulate the rate at which we age.

- Telomeres are DNA–protein complexes that cap the ends of chromosomes and promote genetic stability. Telomere shortening theories focus on scientific findings that telomeres play a critical role in determining the number of times a cell divides, its health, and its life span.

Pathological Conditions Associated with the Elderly

Many changes are associated with aging throughout adulthood and into old age, of which some are part of the normal aging process while others are pathological. Complicating matters is the fact that comorbidities are more common in the elderly, which results in secondary complications associated with the primary pathology.

Musculoskeletal Disorders and Diseases

The musculoskeletal changes associated with aging (refer to Table 23-1) affect all of the soft tissues, including skeletal muscle, articular cartilage, and intervertebral disks. Many of these changes are associated with a decrease in physical activity and the subsequent loss of strength. Muscle size can decrease an average of 30 to 40 percent over one's lifetime and affects the lower extremities more than the upper extremities.[5] Fiber loss appears to be more

accelerated in type II muscle fibers, which decrease from an average of 60 percent of total muscle fiber type in sedentary young men to below 30 percent after the age of 80.[6] Type II fibers are used primarily in activities requiring more power, such as sprinting or strength training, and are not stimulated by normal activities of daily living.[3] Therefore, resistive exercise for this age group should be directed toward increasing power, not just strength.

● **Key Point** The decrease in muscle performance with advancing age affects men and women differently—women experience a less steep absolute decline in strength than men.

A number of musculoskeletal disorders are associated more with the elderly population than with any other age group, for example osteoarthritis. A description of osteoarthritis, its related signs and symptoms, and associated impairments is included in Chapter 5. Osteoarthritis of the hip is described in Chapter 19 and tibiofemoral osteoarthritis is described in Chapter 20. The general goals of a physical therapy intervention for patients with osteoarthritis include:

- Reduce pain and muscle spasm through the use of modalities and relaxation training
- Maintain or improve range of motion
- Correct muscle imbalances
- Strengthen weak muscles
- Improve flexibility
- Improve balance and ambulation
- Improve aerobic conditioning using low- to no-impact exercises (e.g., walking program, pool exercises)
- Train patient in the use of appropriate assistive devices, as needed (e.g., canes, walkers, orthotics, reachers)
- Provide patient education and empowerment in joint protection strategies, energy conservation techniques, activities to avoid, and how to maintain a healthy lifestyle (e.g., weight reduction)

Osteoporosis

Osteoporosis is a systemic skeletal disorder characterized by decreased bone mass and deterioration of bony microarchitecture (see Chapter 5).

Fractures

Fractures commonly occur among seniors and can have a significant impact on the morbidity, mortality, and functional dependence of this population. Most commonly, such fractures include pathologic fractures, stress fractures, distal radius fractures, proximal humerus fractures, proximal femur fractures, and compression fractures of the spine. These fractures are described in the relevant chapters throughout this book. Fractures in the elderly have their own set of problems because the fractures heal more slowly than for younger adults. Also, older adults are prone to secondary complications, including:

- Pneumonia, if the fracture causes a period of immobility or bed rest
- Changes in mental status secondary to anesthesia from surgery or pain medications utilized
- Decubiti from immobility
- Comorbidities that may make healing and/or rehabilitation more difficult
- Decreased vision, placing patients at increased risk of falls and reinjury
- Poor balance worsened by limited weight-bearing status after a lower extremity fracture

Neurologic Disorders and Diseases

A wide variety of neurologic disorders and diseases can affect the aging population. Age-related changes in the brain start at around age 60. Normal, nonprogressive, and negligible declines among the aged do not dramatically impact daily functioning until the early 80s, but the more serious disorders/diseases can significantly affect cognitive function in old age. Not all cognitive disorders are irreversible, but many require timely identification and intercession to offset permanent dysfunction.

Delirium and Dementia

Delirium, dementia, and certain other alterations in cognition are often referred to as mental status change (MSC), acute confusional state (ACS), or organic brain syndrome (OBS).

Delirium presents with acute onset of impaired awareness, easy distraction, confusion, and disturbances of perception (e.g., illusions, misinterpretations, visual hallucinations). Recent memory is usually deficient, and the patient often is disoriented to time and place. The patient may be agitated or obtunded (have a depressed level of consciousness), and the level of awareness may fluctuate over brief periods. Speech may be incoherent, nonsensical, perseverating, or rambling, which may make the taking of an accurate history from the patient impossible. Delirium is often caused by medications, anesthetics, or infection and is reversible if treated early. If not, delirium can lead to dementia.

Primarily a disease of the elderly, *dementia* is a generic term most often applied to geropsychological problems applying broadly to a progressive, persistent loss of cognitive and intellectual functions. Dementia presents with a history of chronic, steady decline in short- and long-term memory and is associated with difficulties in social relationships, work, and activities of daily life. In contrast to delirium, the patient's perception is clear. However, delirium can be superimposed on an underlying dementing process. Earlier stages of dementia may present subtly, and patients may minimize or attempt to hide their impairments. Patients at this stage often have associated depression.

● **Key Point** Any serious infection can lead to mental status changes.

Regardless of the definition, the end result of these dysfunctions is impairment of cognition that affects some or all of the following: alertness, orientation, emotion, behavior, memory, perception, language, praxis (applying knowledge), problem solving, judgment, and psychomotor activity.

● **Key Point** In the elderly, the combined effects of visual and auditory impairments; dementia or other chronic brain dysfunction; medication side effects, particularly polypharmacy; and/or an unfamiliar environment or nighttime darkness can lead to acute confusion or psychosis, which is known as *sundowning*. As the name implies, this condition usually occurs in the evening hours.

Intervention
The physical therapy intervention for delerium or dementia will depend on the extent of the disease; the treatment approach must be modified based on the level of cognitive impairment of the patient. For example, it may be necessary to speak slowly and clearly and have the patient repeat back or demonstrate back. Visual reminders that provide reorienting information (handouts, calendars, signs, memory aids, or notes on items to be utilized by patient) may be required. It is often important to have the patient repeat activities multiple times, and to elicit help from family members/caregivers. The major areas to cover include:

- Improve self-care abilities to carry out activities of daily living (e.g., grooming, hygiene, continence)
- Provide a safe environment to prevent falls, injury, or further dysfunction
- Provide a soothing environment by reducing environmental distractions, which will help to decrease agitation and to increase attention

Depression

The multiple possible causes for depression in the elderly have many different sources. Examples include:

- Unresolved, repressed traumatic experiences from childhood or later life that may surface when a senior slows down
- Previous history of depression
- Damage to body image (from amputation, cancer surgery, or heart attack) ·
- Fear of death or dying
- Frustration with memory loss
- Difficulty adjusting to stressful or changing conditions (e.g., housing and living conditions, loss of loved ones or friends, loss of capabilities)
- Substance abuse (alcohol)
- Loneliness, isolation
- Impact of retirement (whether the individual has chosen to stop working, been laid off, or been forced to stop because of chronic health problems or a disability)
- Being unmarried (especially if widowed), or recent bereavement
- Lack of a supportive social network
- Decreased mobility due to illness or loss of driving privileges
- Extreme dependency

Intervention

Depression often requires professional help, but the PTA can play an important role by demonstrating empathy and support, helping the patient to find support groups, and, in some cases, referring the patient to an appropriate resource (e.g., psychotherapy, social service).

Cardiovascular Disorders and Diseases

Age-related anatomic and physiologic changes of the heart and blood vessels result in reduced capacity for oxygen transport at rest and in response to situations imposing an increase in metabolic demand for oxygen.[3] In addition, maximal oxygen consumption (PO_2 max), an index of maximal cardiovascular function, decreases 5 to 15 percent per decade after the age of 25 years.[7] As a result, at submaximal exercise, heart rate responses such as cardiac output and stroke volume are lower in older adults than younger ones at the same absolute work rates, while blood pressure tends to be higher.[7]

Hypertension

Regulation of normal blood pressure is a complex process. Although a function of cardiac output and peripheral vascular resistance, both of these variables are influenced by multiple factors.

Hypertension may be either essential or secondary:

- *Essential:*[8–17] A possible pathogenesis of essential hypertension has been proposed in which multiple factors, including genetic predisposition, excess dietary salt intake, and adrenergic tone, may interact to produce hypertension. The progression begins with prehypertension in persons ages 10–30 years (by increased cardiac output), moving on to early hypertension in persons ages 20–40 years (in which increased peripheral resistance is prominent), then established hypertension in persons ages 30–50 years, and, finally, complicated hypertension in persons ages 40–60 years.
- *Secondary:* The historical and physical findings that suggest the possibility of secondary hypertension are a history of known renal disease, parathyroid dysfunction, adrenal dysfunction, various prescription medications, and obesity.

Hypertension can have a number of negative consequences that can impact rehabilitation including:

- Left ventricular hypertrophy (LVH), left atrial enlargement, aortic root dilatation, atrial and ventricular arrhythmias, systolic and diastolic heart failure, and ischemic heart disease
- Hemorrhagic and atheroembolic stroke or encephalopathy
- A reduction in renal blood flow in conjunction with elevated afferent glomerular arteriolar resistance, causing increased glomerular hydrostatic pressure secondary to efferent glomerular arteriolar constriction

● Key Point A number of medications prescribed for cardiovascular conditions can have significant implications for the exercising patient (see Chapter 1).

Intervention

No consensus exists regarding optimal drug therapy for treatment of hypertension. Most intervention approaches address lifestyle modifications:

- Lose weight if overweight
- Limit alcohol intake
- Increase aerobic activity (30–45 minutes most days of the week)
- Reduce sodium intake

- Maintain adequate intake of dietary potassium, calcium, and magnesium for general health
- Stop smoking and reduce intake of dietary saturated fat and cholesterol for overall cardiovascular health

Cardiac Disease

The patient admitted to a rehabilitation program may not have been physically active for some time, and his or her level of fitness may have declined considerably. Two diseases of the cardiovascular system are worth noting:

- Coronary artery disease (CAD) is a complex disease involving a narrowing of the lumen of one or more of the arteries that encircle and supply the heart, resulting in ischemia to the myocardium. Injury to the endothelial lining of arteries (an inflammatory reaction), thrombosis, calcification, and hemorrhage all contribute to arteriosclerosis or scarring of an artery wall. The clinical symptoms of CAD include any symptoms that may represent cardiac ischemia, including angina (which may be reported as an ache, pressure, pain, or other discomfort in the chest, arms, back, or neck), or simply a decreased activity tolerance due to fatigue, shortness of breath, or palpitations.
- Myocardial infarction (MI) is the rapid development of myocardial necrosis caused by a critical imbalance between the oxygen supply and demand of the myocardium. This usually results from plaque rupture with thrombus formation in a coronary vessel, resulting in an acute reduction of blood supply to a portion of the myocardium.

> **● Key Point** It is very important that elderly patients have a physician's evaluation of their cardiovascular status before engaging in a rehabilitation program. In addition, the patient should be carefully monitored for their cardiovascular response and tolerance to exercise during their rehabilitation sessions. Heart rate (HR), blood pressure (BP), and rate of perceived exertion (RPE) should be assessed before, during, and after exercise, and the PT should be notified of any abnormal or unusual findings.

Intervention

The specific interventions for cardiovascular disease are outlined in Chapter 6. Although the contraindications to exercise training for older adults are the same as for young adults, older adults have an increased prevalence of comorbidities that can affect cardiovascular function, such as diabetes, hypertension, obesity, and left ventricular dysfunction. The absolute contraindications for exercising in all adults—but in particular the elderly—include but are not limited to:

- Severe coronary artery disease with unstable angina pectoris
- Acute myocardial infarction (less than 2 days after infarction)
- Severe valvular heart disease
- Rapid or prolonged atrial or ventricular arrhythmias/tachycardias
- Uncontrolled hypertension
- Profound orthostatic hypotension
- Acute thrombophlebitis
- Acute pulmonary embolism (less than 2 days after event)
- Known or suspected dissecting aneurysm

Multi-System Dysfunction

Immobility/Disability

Immobility is a common pathway by which a host of diseases and problems in the elderly produce further disability. Persons who are chronically ill, aged, or disabled are particularly susceptible to the adverse effects of prolonged bed rest, immobilization, and inactivity. The effects of immobility are rarely confined to only one body system (**Table 23-2**). Common causes for immobility in the elderly include:

- *Musculoskeletal system:* Arthritis, osteoporosis, fractures (especially hip and femur), and podiatric problems
- *Cardiopulmonary system:* Chronic coronary heart disease, chronic obstructive lung disease, severe heart failure, and peripheral vascular disease
- *Neurologic system:* Cerebrovascular accident; Parkinson's disease; cerebellar dysfunction; neuropathies; cognitive, psychological, and sensory problems (dementia, depression, fear, and anxiety); pain; and impaired vision
- *Environmental factors:* Forced immobilization (restraint use), inadequate aids for mobility
- *Malnutrition:* Malnutrition and poor nutritional status in the elderly contribute to progressive decline in health, reduced physical and cognitive functional status, increased utilization of health care services, premature institutionalization, and increased mortality

TABLE 23-2	Pathophysiologic Alterations Due to Immobility
Body System	**Effects**
Musculoskeletal	Decreased range of motion
	Decreased joint flexibility
	Development of contractures
	Loss of muscular strength (muscular atrophy)
	Loss of muscular endurance (deconditioning)
	Loss of bone mass
	Loss of bone strength
Integumentary	Development of pressure sores
	Skin atrophy and breakdown
Psychological/ neurological	Depression
	Decreased perceptual ability
	Social isolation
	Learned helplessness
	Altered sleep patterns
	Anxiety, irritability, hostility
Cardiopulmonary	Decreased ventilation
	Atelectasis
	Aspiration pneumonia
	Deterioration of respiratory system
	Increased cardiac output
	Increased resting heart rate
	Orthostatic hypotension
Genitourinary	Urinary infection
	Urinary retention
	Bladder calculi
Metabolic	Negative balance
	Loss of calcium

Data from Gillette PD: Exercise in aging and disease, in Placzek JD, Boyce DA (eds): Orthopaedic Physical Therapy Secrets. Philadelphia, Hanley & Belfus, 2001, pp 235–242; and Thompson LV: Iatrogenic effects, in Kaufmann TL (ed): Geriatric Rehabilitation Manual. New York, Churchill Livingstone, 1999, pp 318–324

diminished muscle mass, decreases of muscle strength by 2% to 5% per day, muscle shortening, changes in periarticular and cartilaginous joint structure and marked loss of leg strength that seriously limit mobility. The aforementioned decline in muscle mass and strength has been linked to falls, functional decline, increased frailty and immobility.

Intervention
Intervention strategies to prevent disability from immobility should include the following, while monitoring vital signs:

- Minimize duration of bed rest. Avoid strict bed rest unless absolutely necessary.
- Be aware of possible adverse effects of medications.
- Encourage the continuation of daily activities that the patient is able to perform as tolerated while avoiding overexertion.
- Provide bathroom privileges or a bedside commode.
- Let patient stand 30–60 seconds during transfers (bed to chair).
- Encourage sitting up at a table for meals.
- Encourage getting dressed in street clothes each day.
- Encourage daily exercises as a basis of good care. Exercises should emphasize:
  - ❏ Balance and proprioception
  - ❏ Strength and endurance
  - ❏ Coordination and equilibrium
  - ❏ Aerobic capacity
  - ❏ Posture
  - ❏ Gait and gait deviations
  - ❏ Cadence
  - ❏ Base of support
- Design possible ways to enhance mobility through the use of assistive devices (e.g., walking aids, wheelchairs) and making the home accessible.
- Ensure that a sufficient fluid intake is being maintained (1.5–2 liters of fluid intake per day as possible) as well as adequate nutritional levels.
- Encourage socialization with family, friends, or caregivers.
- If the patient is bed-bound, maintain proper body alignment and change positions every few hours. Pressure padding and heel protectors may be used to provide comfort and prevent pressure sores. It is very

- *Deconditioning*: Deconditioning is a complex physiological process following a period of inactivity, bedrest or sedentary lifestyle, which can result in functional losses in such areas as mental status, degree of continence, and ability to accomplish activities of daily living. The most common effects of deconditioning include

important that an assessment is made with regard to:

- Skin integrity
- Protective sensations
- Discriminatory sensations

Impaired Balance

Age-related balance dysfunctions can occur through a loss of sensory elements such as degenerative changes in the vestibular apparatus of the inner ear, an inability to integrate sensory information, and muscle weakness. Diseases common in aging populations (e.g, Ménière's disease, benign paroxysmal positional vertigo [BPPV], cerebrovascular disease, vertebrobasilar artery insufficiency, cerebellar dysfunction, cardiac disease) lead to further deterioration in balance function in some patients. Balance disorders can be associated with a number of other causes including:

- Cardiac abnormalities
- Medications; classes of medications that may predispose a person to balance disorders include:
  - Tricyclic antidepressants—may cause hypotension
  - Antihypertensives
  - Anticonvulsants
  - Antianxiety drugs—may cause confusion
  - Antipsychotics—may cause hypotension
  - Sedatives
- Postural hypotension
- Sensory loss
- Joint stiffness
- Cognitive issues
- Visual/auditory deficits
- Postural impairments

The clinical implications of impaired balance include:

- Diminished perception
- Delayed reaction times, particularly in the ankle, hip, and stepping strategies (see Chapter 11)
- Altered sensory organization—higher dependence upon somatosensory inputs
- Disorganized postural response patterns—diminished ankle torque, increased hip torque, and increased postural sway

Falls can be markers of poor health and declining function, and they are often associated with significant morbidity.[18] More than 90 percent of hip fractures occur as a result of falls, with most of these fractures occurring in persons over 70 years of age. One-third of community-dwelling elderly persons and 60 percent of nursing home residents fall each year. Elderly persons who survive a fall experience significant morbidity. Hospital stays are almost twice as long for elderly patients who are hospitalized after a fall than for elderly patients who are admitted for another reason. Elderly patients with known risk factors for falling should be questioned about falls on a periodic basis. A single fall is not always a sign of a major problem and an increased risk for subsequent falls. The fall may simply be an isolated event. However, recurrent falls, defined as more than two falls in a 6-month period, should be assessed by qualified personnel for treatable causes.

A mnemonic (I HATE FALLING) can be used to remind the clinician of key physical findings in patients who fall or nearly fall (**Table 23-3**).[19]

A home visit is invaluable for assessing modifiable risk factors and determining appropriate interventions. A home safety checklist can guide the visit and ensure a thorough evaluation (**Table 23-4**). It is particularly important to assess caregiver and housing arrangements, environmental hazards, alcohol use, and compliance with medications.

TABLE 23-3	A Mnemonic for Key Physical Findings in the Elderly Patient Who Falls or Nearly Falls
I	Inflammation of joints (or joint deformity)
H	Hypotension (orthostatic blood pressure changes)
A	Auditory and visual abnormalities
T	Tremor (Parkinson's disease or other causes of tremor)
E	Equilibrium (balance) problems
F	Foot problems
A	Arrhythmia, heart block, or valvular disease
L	Leg-length discrepancy
L	Lack of conditioning (generalized weakness)
I	Illness
N	Nutritional status (poor, weight loss)
G	Gait disturbance

Data from Sloan JP: Mobility failure, in Sloan JP (ed): Protocols in Primary Care Geriatrics. New York, Springer, 1997, pp 33–38

TABLE 23-4	Home Safety Checklist		

All Living Spaces	Bathrooms	Outdoors
_____ Remove throw rugs	_____ Install grab bars in the bathtub or shower and by the toilet	_____ Repair cracked sidewalks
_____ Secure carpet edges	_____ Use rubber mats in the bathtub or shower	_____ Install handrails on stairs and steps
_____ Remove low furniture and objects on the floor	_____ Take up floor mats when the bathtub or shower is not in use	_____ Trim shrubbery along the pathway to the home
_____ Reduce clutter	_____ Install a raised toilet seat	_____ Install adequate lighting by doorways and along walkways leading to doors
_____ Remove cords and wires on the floor		
_____ Check lighting for adequate illumination at night (especially in the pathway to the bathroom)		
_____ Secure carpet or treads on stairs		
_____ Install handrails on staircases		
_____ Eliminate chairs that are too low to sit in and get out of easily		
_____ Avoid floor wax (or use nonskid wax)		
_____ Ensure that the telephone can be reached from the floor		

Data from Rubenstein LZ: Falls, in Yoshikawa TT, Cobbs EL, Brummel-Smith K (eds): Ambulatory Geriatric Care. St Louis: Mosby, 1993, pp 296–304

Several simple tests have exhibited a strong correlation with a history of falling. These functional balance measures are quantifiable and correlate well with the ability of older adults to ambulate safely in their environment. The tests can also be used to measure changes in mobility after interventions have been applied.

- *One-leg balance:* Tested by having the patient stand unassisted on one leg for 30 seconds. The patient chooses which leg to stand on (based on personal comfort), flexes the opposite knee to allow the foot to clear the floor, and then balances on one leg. The clinician uses a watch to time the patient's one-leg balance.
- *The timed "Up and Go" test:* This test (**Table 23-5**) evaluates gait and balance. The patient gets up out of a standard armchair (seat height of approximately 46 centimeters [18.4 inches]), walks a distance of 3 meters (10 feet), turns, walks back to the chair, and sits down again. A simpler alternative is the "Get Up and Go" test. In this test, the patient is seated in an armless chair placed 3 meters (10 feet) from a wall. The patient stands, walks toward the wall (using a walking aid if one is typically employed), turns without touching the wall, returns to the chair, turns, and sits down. This activity does not need to be timed. Instead, the clinician observes the patient for any balance or gait problems.

Overall physical function should also be assessed. This is accomplished by evaluating the patient's ADLs and instrumental activities of daily living (IADLs).

Intervention
With patients who have a history of falling, the intervention is directed at the underlying cause of the fall and preventing recurrence. The supervising PT determines the presence of any disease states that can contribute to balance disorders. Fall-risk questionnaires can be used to help identify fall risk. The PT assesses the patient's static and dynamic balance and the need for an appropriate and safe assistive device/adaptive equipment. Functional training should include:

- Sit to stand transitions
- Turning, walking, and stair negotiation

TABLE 23-5	Timed "Up and Go" Test	
Task	Get up out of a standard armchair (seat height of approximately 46 cm [18.4 in.]), walk a distance of 3 m (10 ft.), turn, walk back to the chair, and sit down again.	
Requirement	Ambulate with or without assistive device and follow a three-step command.	
Trials	One practice trial and then three actual trials. The times from the three actual trials are averaged.	
Time	1 to 2 minutes	
Equipment	Armchair, stopwatch (or wristwatch with a second hand), and a measured path	
Predictive Results	**Seconds**	**Rating**
	≤10	Freely mobile
	10 to 20	Mostly independent
	21 to 29	Variable mobility
	≥30	Impaired mobility

Data from Podsiadlo D, Richardson S: The timed "Up & Go:" A test of basic functional mobility for frail elderly persons. J Am Geriatr Soc 39: 142–148, 1991.

- Patient and family/caregiver education, including identification of risks, safety issues and education, adequate lighting at home, using contrasting colors, reduction of clutter, and advice about modifying the living environment, as appropriate (refer to Table 22-4)

Therapeutic exercises should focus on:

- Strengthening and flexibility exercises
- Weight-bearing exercises to help prevent osteoporosis
- Balance and gait exercises

Impaired Coordination

The most salient age-related changes impacting coordinated movement include:

- Decreased strength
- Slowed reaction time
- Decreased range of motion
- Postural changes
- Impaired balance

These changes may be accentuated further by alterations in sensation, perceptual impairments, and diminished vision and hearing acuity.

Nutritional Deficiency[20–25]

Nutritional status is a "vital sign" of health. Nutrition takes on greater importance in the context of chronic illness. With increase in age, there is an increased risk of developing nutritional deficiencies that can lead to such debilitating consequences as functional dependency, morbidity, and mortality. Some older persons are at increased risk for nutritional deficiency because of multiple drug therapies, dental problems, economic hardship, and reduced social contacts. These problems arise from many varied environmental, social, and economic factors that are compounded by physiological changes of aging.

Intervention

Although not directly involved with the patient's nutritional status, the PTA should attempt to:

- Maintain or improve the patient's physical function.
- Assist in monitoring the patient's nutritional intake by observing any physical or mental changes that could be nutritionally related.
- Speak with the PT about requesting a nutritional consultation as necessary.
- Communicate with social services about the potential need for elderly food programs (Meals on Wheels, federal food stamp programs).
- Discuss with the PT recommendations for home health aides, including:
  - Assistance in grocery shopping
  - Meal preparation

Ethical and Legal Issues

The health care industry is subject to numerous ethical and legal regulations, which throughout the years have brought changes to the actions of medical care providers and insurers to protect patients.

The Living Will (Advanced Care and Medical Directive)

Sometimes a patient may desire a treatment because it is a temporary measure potentially leading to the restoration of health. At other times, a treatment may be undesirable because it may only prolong the process of dying rather than restore the patient to an acceptable quality of life. The advanced care medical directive (ACMD), established by the federal Patient Self-Determination Act of 1990, was designed to address such issues. Advance directives are documents signed by a competent person giving direction to healthcare providers about treatment choices in certain circumstances. There are two types of advance directives:

- A durable power of attorney for health care ("durable power") allows a patient to name a patient advocate to act on behalf of the patient and carry out his or her wishes (see the "Healthcare Proxy" section later in this chapter).
- A living will allows a patient to state his or her wishes in writing, but does not name a patient advocate.

The regulations for ACMDs vary by state; however, in order to be deemed a legal document the ACMD must be signed by the principal and witnessed by two adults. There are generally two broad types of situations in which the directive may apply:

- Terminal illness, where death is expected in a relatively short time.
- Permanent disability in an intolerable situation. This is a highly individualized decision.
- Many standard healthcare declarations instruct physicians to withhold "extraordinary care" or "life-sustaining or life-prolonging" treatments.

Refusal of Treatment

If deemed mentally competent (the patient understands his or her condition and the consequences any decision may have), the patient has the right to decide to accept or refuse any medical treatment.

There are basically three broad reasons to refuse a certain treatment:

- The benefit of the treatment is not great enough to justify its risk or discomfort. This is the basis for most treatment decisions, and involves the individual attitudes each patient will bring to the decision. Some people will endure unpleasant and risky treatments for a chance to live longer; others prefer a more comfortable, shorter life, using the least possible medical intervention.
- The treatment will prolong life under intolerable conditions. Even an easily tolerated treatment with minimal discomfort might be unacceptable if it prolongs life in the face of unwanted circumstances. A feeding tube may be simple, safe, comfortable, and highly effective in preventing death from starvation and dehydration. Nevertheless, some may not want it used if another irreversible condition exists (for example, a persistent vegetative state).
- Religious or cultural concerns. A patient's religious and cultural beliefs can play an important role in the type of healthcare delivery.

"Do Not Resuscitate" (DNR) Orders

These orders apply only to cardiopulmonary resuscitation. There are specific rules concerning how they are to be written and who may authorize them.

Healthcare Proxy

A healthcare proxy is an agent who makes healthcare decisions for the patient when he or she has been determined to be incapable of making such decisions.

Informed Consent

Informed consent is the process by which a competent and fully informed patient can participate in choices about his or her health care. It is generally accepted that complete informed consent includes a discussion of the following elements:

- The nature and purpose of the decision/ procedure.
- Reasonable alternatives to the proposed intervention.
- The relevant risks, benefits, consequences, and uncertainties related to each alternative.

- The likelihood of success or failure of the intervention.
- An assessment of patient understanding. In order for the patient's consent to be valid, he or she must be considered competent to make the decision at hand and his or her consent must be voluntary. If the patient is not deemed competent, consent must be obtained from a legal guardian or healthcare proxy.
- The acceptance of the intervention by the patient.

Summary

The field of geriatrics continues to gain attention due to the rapid growth of this segment of the population and its predicted future socioeconomic impact. It is therefore inevitable that future rehabilitation professionals will see an increase in the number of elderly individuals seeking services for the management of both acute and chronic conditions that can negatively impact active life expectancy or the number of years that an individual may expect to be independent in activities of daily living.[26,27] Therefore, rehabilitation, with its potential to restore function, prolong independence, and improve quality of life, can be extremely important in this population.

REVIEW Questions

1. What is the name given to the study of the aging process and the science related to the care of the elderly?
2. The degenerative changes associated with osteoarthritis are most pronounced on the articular cartilage of which type of joints?
3. When evaluating risk of falling in an elderly patient, all of the following factors are known to increase risk, except:
   a. Using a walker
   b. Taking three prescription medications
   c. Fear of falling
   d. History of falls
4. Which of these interventions would NOT help reduce risk of falling in a 70-year-old man who lives in a nursing home?
   a. Gait training
   b. An exercise program
   c. Educating the staff about ways to prevent falls
   d. Evaluating whether assistive devices are being used appropriately
5. An 80-year-old woman who lives at home says she has never fallen but would like to reduce her risk of falling. All of the following interventions would be appropriate, except:
   a. A multifactorial program that includes exercise with balance training
   b. A multifactorial program that includes a review of medications
   c. A single intervention that consists of education on risk factor modification
   d. A single intervention that consists of gait training
6. You are advising a 72-year-old individual who wants to take part in a graduated conditioning program. Which of the following would be appropriate when prescribing exercise for the healthy elderly?
   a. Intensity prescribed using maximal age-related HR
   b. An initial conservative approach to reduce characteristic muscle fatigability
   c. An emphasis on low intensity and increased duration of exercise to avoid injury
   d. All of the above
7. While walking around a nursing home, you come across a patient who is lying on the ground and who complains of pain in the right groin and gluteal area. The right hip is flexed, abducted, and internally rotated. The most likely diagnosis is:
   a. Dislocated tibia
   b. Fractured femoral head
   c. Dislocated hip
   d. Fractured acetabulum
8. Which of the following is not a neurological change associated with aging?
   a. Reduction in blood flow
   b. Reduction in muscle mass
   c. Increase in ventricular size
   d. Reduction of nerve conduction velocity
9. What is the earliest clinical symptom associated with dementia?
10. What are the two types of advance directives?
11. The process by which a competent and fully informed patient can participate in choices about his or her health care is called what?

12. You are working with a 72-year-old patient who has middle stage Alzheimer's disease and a recent total hip replacement. The patient is having difficulty following directions for ambulation activities using a walker. To best facilitate ambulation using the walker you should:
   a. First demonstrate the activity, and then provide physical guidance.
   b. Use single-step verbal directions.
   c. Physically assist the patient to perform the activities.
   d. Perform ambulation activities on the treadmill.

13. A 75-year-old is coming to physical therapy following a Colles' fracture and the subsequent diagnosis of osteoporosis. The fracture is now well healed and the plan of care includes the development of a home exercise program. At a minimum the exercise program should include:
   a. Wall push-ups and upper extremity Theraband exercises
   b. Aerobic activity and exercises using eccentric muscle contractions
   c. Active upper extremity diagonals and core stability exercises
   d. Submaximal upper extremity active exercise and bike riding

14. An 89-year-old resident in a nursing home constantly delays treatment because he insists on relating stories about his involvement in World War II. Your best response in this situation would be to:
   a. Indicate the stories are delaying treatment but that you would come back in your spare time to listen to them.
   b. Suggest it would be more beneficial if the resident talked with people his own age about World War II.
   c. Try to change the subject when the patient begins telling the stories.
   d. Indicate, in a tactful manner, that the stories are distracting to you.

References

1. Harman D: Aging: Phenomena and theories. Ann N Y Acad Sci 854:1–7, 1998
2. Jette AM, Branch LG, Berlin J: Musculoskeletal impairments and physical disablement among the aged. J Gerontol 45:M203–M208, 1990
3. Voight C: Rehabilitation considerations with the geriatric patient, in Prentice WE, Jr, Voight ML (eds): Techniques in Musculoskeletal Rehabilitation. New York, McGraw-Hill, 2001, pp 679–696
4. Harman D: Free radical involvement in aging. Pathophysiology and therapeutic implications. Drugs Aging 3:60–80, 1993
5. Gallagher D, Visser M, De Meersman RE, et al: Appendicular skeletal muscle mass: Effects of age, gender, and ethnicity. J Appl Physiol 83:229–239, 1997
6. Larsson L, Sjodin B, Karlsson J: Histochemical and biochemical changes in human skeletal muscle with age in sedentary males, age 22–65 years. Acta Physiol Scand 103:31–39, 1978
7. Heath GW, Hagberg JM, Ehsani AA, et al: A physiological comparison of young and older endurance athletes. J Appl Physiol 51:634–640, 1981
8. Avdic S, Mujcinovic Z, Asceric M, et al: Left ventricular diastolic dysfunction in essential hypertension. Bosn J Basic Med Sci 7:15–20, 2007
9. Binder A: A review of the genetics of essential hypertension. Curr Opin Cardiol 22:176–184, 2007
10. Cuspidi C, Meani S, Valerio C, et al: Age and target organ damage in essential hypertension: Role of the metabolic syndrome. Am J Hypertens 20:296–303, 2007
11. El-Shafei SA, Bassili A, Hassanien NM, et al: Genetic determinants of essential hypertension. J Egypt Public Health Assoc 77:231–246, 2002
12. Hollenberg NK, Williams GH: Nonmodulation and essential hypertension. Curr Hypertens Rep 8:127–131, 2006
13. Kennedy S: Essential hypertension 2: Treatment and monitoring update. Community Pract 79:64–66, 2006
14. Kennedy S: Essential hypertension: Recent changes in management. Community Pract 79:23–24, 2006
15. Krzych LJ: Blood pressure variability in children with essential hypertension. J Hum Hypertens 21:494–500, 2007
16. Parrilli G, Manguso F, Orsini L, et al: Essential hypertension and chronic viral hepatitis. Dig Liver Dis 39:466–472, 2007
17. Pierdomenico SD: Blood pressure variability and cardiovascular outcome in essential hypertension. Am J Hypertens 20:162–163, 2007
18. Fuller GF: Falls in the elderly. Am Fam Physician 61:2159–2168, 2173–2174, 2000
19. Sloan JP: Mobility failure, in Sloan JP (ed): Protocols in Primary Care Geriatrics. New York, Springer, 1997, pp 33–38
20. Baxter J: Screening and treating those at risk of nutritional deficiency. Community Nurse 6:S1–S2, S5, 2000
21. Callen BL, Wells TJ: Screening for nutritional risk in community-dwelling old-old. Public Health Nurs 22:138–146, 2005
22. Corish CA, Flood P, Kennedy NP: Comparison of nutritional risk screening tools in patients on admission to hospital. J Hum Nutr Diet 17:133–139; quiz 141–143, 2004
23. Hedberg AM, Garcia N, Trejus IJ, et al: Nutritional risk screening: Development of a standardized protocol using dietetic technicians. J Am Diet Assoc 88:1553–1556, 1988

24. Melnik TA, Helferd SJ, Firmery LA, et al: Screening elderly in the community: The relationship between dietary adequacy and nutritional risk. J Am Diet Assoc 94:1425–1427, 1994

25. Reilly HM: Screening for nutritional risk. Proc Nutr Soc 55:841–853, 1996

26. Katz S, Branch LG, Branson MH, et al: Active life expectancy. N Engl J Med 309:1218–1224, 1983

27. Branch LG, Guralnik JM, Foley DJ, et al: Active life expectancy for 10,000 Caucasian men and women in three communities. J Gerontol 46:M145–M150, 1991

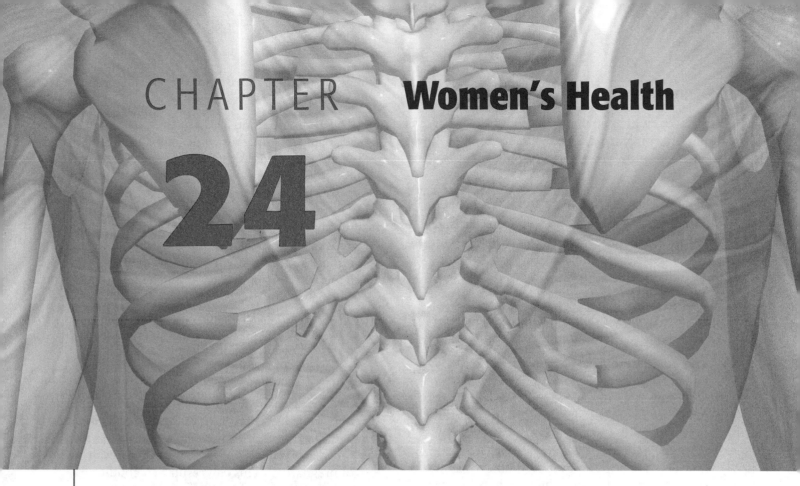

CHAPTER 24   Women's Health

Chapter Objectives

At the completion of this chapter, the reader will be able to:

1. Describe some of the conditions that can affect women's health.
2. Describe the physiologic changes that occur during pregnancy within the various bodily systems.
3. Outline some of the complications that can occur during pregnancy.
4. Describe the physical therapy interventions for pregnancy-related dysfunctions.
5. Outline the various types of stress incontinence.
6. Describe the various interventions for stress incontinence.
7. List the muscles involved in the pelvic floor and their various functions.
8. Describe the complications surrounding breast cancer–related lymphedema.

Overview

Research has demonstrated that women have distinct physiological differences and are more prone to certain conditions than men, such as myocardial infarction and ovarian and breast cancer. Pregnancy, which is clearly gender-based; urinary incontinence; and breast cancer–related lymphatic dysfunction provide a number of challenges for the PTA.

Pregnancy

Pregnancy, which spans approximately 40 weeks from conception to delivery, is a state of wellness despite the number of physiologic changes that occur.

Physiologic Changes That Occur During Pregnancy

A number of physiologic changes occur during pregnancy and the postpartum period within the various body systems. These can present the PTA with some unique challenges.

Endocrine System

Changes that occur in the endocrine system include, but are not limited to, the following:

- The adrenal, thyroid, parathyroid, and pituitary glands enlarge.
- Hormone levels increase to support the pregnancy and the placenta, and to prepare the mother's body for labor. During pregnancy, a female hormone (relaxin) is released that assists in the softening of the pubic symphysis so that during delivery, the female pelvis can expand sufficiently to allow birth. However, these hormonal changes are also thought to induce a greater laxity in all joints.[1,2] This can result in:
    - Joint hypermobility, especially throughout the pelvic ring, which relies heavily on ligamentous support[3]
    - Symphysis pubic dysfunction (SPD) (see "Complications Associated with Pregnancy" later in this chapter)
    - SIJ dysfunction (see "Complications Associated with Pregnancy")
    - Increased susceptibility to musculoskeletal injury

Musculoskeletal System

The recommended weight gain during pregnancy is based on the patient's body mass index (BMI):

- If the BMI is 30+, the recommended weight gain is 11–20 lbs.
- If the BMI is 25–29.9, the recommended weight gain is 15–25 lbs.
- If the BMI is 18.6–24.9, the recommended weight gain is 25–35 lbs.
- If the BMI is 18.5 and lower, the recommended weight gain is 28–40 lbs.

Pregnancy can produce a number of changes within the musculoskeletal system:

- The abdominal muscles are stretched and weakened as pregnancy develops (see "Complications Associated with Pregnancy").
- Relative ligamentous laxity, both capsular and extracapsular, develops.
- The rib cage circumference increases, increasing the subcostal angle and the transverse diameter. This results in an increase in tidal volume and minute ventilation, a natural state of hyperventilation to meet oxygen demands.
- The pelvic floor weakens. The term *pelvic floor muscles* primarily refers to the levator ani, a muscle group composed of the pubococcygeus, puborectalis, and iliococcygeus. The levator ani muscles join the coccygeus muscles to complete the pelvic floor. Pelvic floor weakness can develop with advanced pregnancy and childbirth due to the increased weight and pressure directly over these muscles—the pelvic floor drops as much as 2.5 centimeters (1 inch) as a result of pregnancy.[5] This can result in a condition called *stress incontinence* (refer to the "Urinary Incontinence" section later in this chapter). The pelvic floor muscles can also become stretched or torn during childbirth, producing an even greater risk of urinary incontinence.
- Postural changes related to the weight of growing breasts, and the uterus and fetus, result in a shift in the woman's center of gravity in an anterior and superior direction, resulting in the need for postural compensations to maintain stability and balance. In advanced pregnancy, the patient develops a wider base of support and increased external rotation at the hips, and has increased difficulty with walking, stair climbing, and rapid changes in position. Specific postural changes include:[6]
    - Increased thoracic kyphosis with scapular retraction
    - Increased cervical lordosis and forward head
    - Increased lumbar lordosis

These changes in posture do not automatically correct postpartum and can become habitual.

> ● **Key Point** Pregnant females should be taught correct body mechanics and postural exercises to stretch, strengthen, and train postural muscles.

Neurologic

Swelling and increased fluid volume can cause symptoms of thoracic outlet syndrome due to compression of the brachial plexus, carpal tunnel syndrome due to median nerve compression, or meralgia paresthetica, which is compression of the lateral femoral cutaneous nerve of the thigh.[7-9]

Gastrointestinal

Nausea and vomiting may occur in early pregnancy, and are generally confined to the first 16 weeks of pregnancy but occasionally remain throughout the entire 10 lunar months (see "Complications Associated with Pregnancy").[10-14] Other changes related to the gastrointestinal system include:[11-14]

- A slowing of intestinal motility
- The development of constipation, abdominal bloating, and hemorrhoids
- Esophageal reflux
- Heartburn (pyrosis); fifty to eighty percent of women report heartburn during pregnancy, with its incidence peaking in the third trimester[10]
- An increase in the incidence and symptoms of gallbladder disease

Respiratory System

Adaptive changes that occur in the pulmonary system during pregnancy include:

- The diaphragm elevates with a widening of the thoracic cage. This results in a predominance of costal versus abdominal breathing.
- There is a mild increase in oxygen consumption, which is caused by increased respiratory center sensitivity and drive due to the increased oxygen requirement of the fetus.[15] With mild exercise, pregnant women have a greater increase in respiratory frequency and oxygen consumption to meet their greater oxygen demand.[15] As exercise increases to moderate and maximal levels, however, pregnant women demonstrate decreased respiratory frequency and maximal oxygen consumption.[15]
- A compensated respiratory alkalosis.[16]
- A low expiratory reserve volume. The vital capacity and measures of forced expiration are well preserved.[15,17]

Cardiovascular System

The pregnancy-induced changes in the cardiovascular system develop primarily to meet the increased metabolic demands of the mother and fetus. These include the following:

- Blood volume increases progressively from 6–8 weeks' gestation (pregnancy) and reaches a maximum at approximately 32–34 weeks with little change thereafter.[18] The increased blood volume serves two purposes:[19,20]
  - ❏ It facilitates maternal and fetal exchanges of respiratory gases, nutrients, and metabolites.
  - ❏ It reduces the impact of maternal blood loss at delivery. Typical losses of 300–500 milliliters for vaginal births and 750–1000 milliliters for Caesarean sections are thus compensated for by the so-called "autotransfusion" of blood from the contracting uterus.
- Increased plasma volume (40–50 percent) is relatively greater than that of red cell mass (20–30 percent), resulting in hemodilution and a decrease in hemoglobin concentration. (Intake of supplemental iron and folic acid is necessary to restore hemoglobin levels to normal [12 g/dL]).[19,21,22]
- Cardiac output increases to a similar degree as the blood volume.[19,20] During the first trimester cardiac output is 30–40 percent higher than in the nonpregnant state.[21] During labor, further increases are seen. The heart is enlarged by both chamber dilation and hypertrophy.

> **● Key Point** The effects of blood pressure during pregnancy include:
> - Systemic arterial pressure should not increase during normal gestation.
> - Pulmonary arterial pressure also maintains a constant level.
> - Vascular tone is more dependent upon sympathetic control than in the nonpregnant state, so hypotension develops more readily and more markedly.
> - Central venous and brachial venous pressures remain unchanged during pregnancy, but femoral venous pressure is progressively increased due to mechanical factors.

Metabolic System

Because of the increased demand for tissue growth, insulin is elevated from plasma expansion, and blood glucose is reduced for a given insulin load. Fats and minerals are stored for maternal use. The metabolic rate increases during both exercise and pregnancy, resulting in greater heat production. Fetoplacental metabolism generates additional heat, which maintains fetal temperature at 0.5 to 1.0°C (0.9 to 1.8°F) above maternal levels.[23-25]

Renal and Urologic Systems

During pregnancy, the renal threshold for glucose drops because of an increase in the glomerular filtration rate, and there is an increase in sodium and water retention.[10] Anatomic and hormonal changes during pregnancy place the pregnant woman at risk for both lower and upper urinary tract infections and for urinary incontinence.[10] As the fetus grows, stress on the mother's bladder can occur. This can result in urinary incontinence (refer to "Urinary Incontinence" later in this chapter).

Complications Associated with Pregnancy

Hypertension

Hypertensive disorders complicating pregnancy are the most common medical risk factor responsible for maternal morbidity and death related to pregnancy.[10] Hypertensive disorders complicating pregnancy have been divided into five types (**Table 24-1**).

Symphysis Pubis Dysfunction and Diastasis Symphysis Pubis

Symphysis pubis dysfunction (SPD) and diastasis symphysis pubis (DSP)[26–29] can occur in a pregnant woman or, more commonly, as a result of trauma during vaginal delivery. The symptoms of SPD and DSP vary from person to person. On examination, the patient typically demonstrates an antalgic, waddling gait. Subjectively, the patient reports pain with any activity that involves lifting one leg at a time or parting the legs. Lifting the leg to put on clothes, getting out of a car, bending over, turning over in bed, sitting down or getting up, walking up stairs, standing on one leg, lifting heavy objects, and walking in general are all painful. Patients may also report that the hip joint seems stuck in place or they describe having to wait for it to "pop into place" before being able to walk.

Palpation reveals anterior pubic symphyseal tenderness. Occasional clicking can be felt or heard. The findings on the physical examination include range of hip movements limited by pain, and an inability to stand on one leg. Characteristic pain can often be evoked by bilateral pressure on the trochanters or by hip flexion with the legs in extension. However, such maneuvers may result in severe pain or muscle spasm and are not necessary for diagnosis. Radiological evaluation may occasionally be useful in confirming the diagnosis.[30] The amount of symphyseal separation does not always correlate with the severity of symptoms or the degree of disability. Therefore, the intervention is based on the severity of symptoms rather than the degree of separation as measured by imaging studies.[30]

> **● Key Point** Symphysis pubis dysfunction (SPD) should always be considered when treating patients in the postpartum period who are experiencing suprapubic, sacroiliac, or thigh pain.

Although the symptoms can be dramatically severe in presentation for SPD and DSP, a conservative management approach is often effective in cases of SPD and DSP. In more severe cases, the interventions can include bed rest in the lateral decubitus position, pelvic support with a brace or girdle, ambulation with assistance or with devices such as walkers, and graded exercise protocols.[30] PTs may

TABLE 24-1	Summary of Types of Hypertension During Pregnancy
Disorder	**Signs/Symptoms**
Gestational hypertension	Epigastric pain, thrombocytopenia, headache.
Preeclampsia	The more severe the hypertension or proteinuria, the more certain is the severity of preeclampsia; symptoms of eclampsia, such as headache, cerebral visual disturbance, and epigastric pain, can occur.
Eclampsia	Mother may develop abruptio placentae, neurological deficits, aspiration pneumonia, pulmonary edema, cardiopulmonary arrest, or acute renal failure; may cause maternal death.
Superimposed preeclampsia on chronic hypertension	The risk of abruptio placentae; fetus at risk for growth restriction and death.
Chronic hypertension	Risk of abruptio placentae; fetus is at risk for growth restriction and death; pulmonary edema; hypertensive encephalopathy; renal failure.

Data from Boissonnault JS, Stephenson R: The obstetric patient, in Boissonnault WG (ed): Primary Care for the Physical Therapist: Examination and Triage. St Louis, Elsevier Saunders, 2005, pp 239–270

perform mobilization techniques as well. In all cases, patient education is extremely important in terms of providing advice on how to avoid stress to the area. Some of the suggestions to provide include:

- Use a pillow between the legs when sleeping.
- Move slowly and without sudden movements. Keep the legs and hips parallel and as symmetrical as possible when moving or turning in standing and in bed. Silk/satin sheets and night garments may make it easier to turn over in bed.
- A waterbed mattress may be helpful.
- When standing, stand symmetrically, with the weight evenly distributed through both legs. Avoid "straddle" movements.
- Sit down to get dressed, especially when putting on underwear or pants.
- An ice pack may feel soothing and help reduce inflammation in the pubic area.
- Swimming may help relieve pressure on the joint (the breaststroke may prove aggravating). Deep-water aerobics or deep-water running using floatation devices may also be helpful.

Resolution of symptoms in approximately 6 to 8 weeks with no lasting sequela is the most common outcome in SDP and DSP.[30] Occasionally, patients report residual pain requiring several months of physical therapy, but long-term impairment is unusual. Surgical intervention is rarely required but may be utilized in cases of inadequate reduction, recurrent diastasis, or persistent symptoms.

Low Back Pain

Low back pain[6,31–38] is said to occur in 50–70 percent of pregnant women.[39] However, it is not clear whether the low back pain is the result of the shift in the center of gravity and concomitant postural changes in the spinal curvature. Because the annulus is a ligamentous structure, and therefore softens with the release of relaxin, it could be postulated that the low back pain may be related to structural changes in the intervertebral disk. However, frank disk herniations are no more common during pregnancy than at other times. Thus, the pain is likely mechanical in nature.

● **Key Point** It is worth remembering that complaints of low back pain in this population may be because of a kidney or urinary tract infection.

Peripartum Posterior Pelvic Pain

More than 50 percent of women experience peripartum posterior pelvic pain (PPPP) during pregnancy, with one-third of these women experiencing severe pain.[35,40,41] The etiology of PPPP has been linked to the physiological adaptation of the pelvis in preparation for childbirth, which is accomplished through softening of connective tissue structures around the pelvis, pubic symphysis, and sacroiliac joint.[42] Patients with PPPP typically complain of weight-bearing low back pain with symptoms referred below the level of the buttocks (with no findings suggesting nerve root involvement) and with the first episode of pain occurring during pregnancy. Stuge and colleagues[43] performed a systematic review of the literature investigating the effectiveness of physical therapy interventions in the treatment of PPPP and LBP and found scant evidence to support the use of exercise or mobilization in this patient population. However, exercise is thought to be beneficial (see the "Specific Exercises" section later in this chapter). In addition, patient education should be given about posture/body mechanics and equal weight bearing through both lower extremities (avoiding one-legged standing).

Coccydynia

Coccygeal pain,[44–48] pain in and around the region of the coccyx, is relatively common postpartum. Symptoms include pain with sitting. The patient should be provided with a seating adaptation (donut cushion) to lessen the weight on the coccyx and to support the lumbar lordosis.

If symptoms persist for more than a few weeks, the displaced coccyx can often be corrected manually by the PT or physician.

Gestational Diabetes

Gestational diabetes is defined as carbohydrate intolerance of variable severity, with onset or first recognition during pregnancy. After the birth, blood sugars usually return to normal levels; however, frank diabetes often develops later in life. Typical causes include:

- Genetic predisposition
- Being a member of a high-risk population, such as being of aboriginal, Hispanic, Asian, or African descent
- Family history of diabetes, gestational diabetes, or glucose intolerance
- Increased tissue resistance to insulin during pregnancy, due to increased levels of estrogen and progesterone

Current risk factors include:

- Maternal obesity (more than 20 percent above ideal weight)
- Excessive weight gain during pregnancy

- Low level of high-density-lipoprotein (HDL) cholesterol (less than 0.9 mmol/L) or elevated fasting level of triglycerides (greater than 2.8 mmol/L)
- Hypertension or preeclampsia (risk for gestational diabetes is increased to 10 to 15 percent when hypertension is diagnosed)
- Maternal age older than 35 years

Most individuals with gestational diabetes are asymptomatic. However, subjectively the patient may complain of:

- Polydipsia
- Polyuria
- Polyphagia
- Weight loss

Diastasis Recti Abdominis

Diastasis recti abdominis (DRA) is defined as a lateral separation of greater than two fingertip widths of the two bellies of the rectus abdominis at the linea alba (or linea nigra, in pregnancy) that can occur during pregnancy or delivery. DRA can result in a decreased ability of the abdominal musculature to stabilize the pelvis and lumbar spine with subsequent functional limitations, decreased fetal protection, and an increased potential for herniation of abdominal viscera. All pregnant patients should be tested for DRA prior to performing any abdominal exercises. To check for diastasis recti, the patient is asked to lie supine with her knees bent and feet flat on the floor. The clinician places his or her fingertips in the center of the abdomen just above the navel. The patient is then asked to perform a posterior pelvic tilt, and then exhale as she lifts the head off the floor. If a diastasis recti is present the clinician will be able to press the fingertips into the gap between the two sides of the muscle (Figure 24-1). This assessment

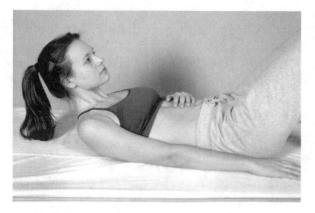

Figure 24-1   Diastasis recti check.

should be done below the umbilicus, as well. If diastasis recti abdominis is confirmed, corrective exercises need to be performed to prevent further muscle trauma (see the "Specific Exercises" section later in this chapter).

Cesarean Childbirth

Cesarean delivery, also known as cesarean section, is a major abdominal surgery involving two incisions:

- An incision through the abdominal wall
- An incision involving the uterus to deliver the baby

Although the PTA is not involved in the surgical procedure, he or she can play an important role postoperatively:

- TENS can be used to decrease incisional pain. (Electrodes are placed parallel to the incision.)
- Patient education:
  - Correct breathing and coughing to prevent postsurgical pulmonary complications
  - Heavy lifting precautions (4 to 6 weeks), use of pillow for incisional support
  - Instruction on transverse fictional massage to prevent incisional adhesions
- Ambulation. Progressive ambulation is encouraged after 24 hours.
- Exercise:
  - Postural exercises
  - Pelvic floor exercises
  - Gentle abdominal exercises

Hyperemesis Gravidarum

The causes of this condition are largely unknown. Indications that the patient may have this condition include persistent and excessive nausea and vomiting throughout the day and an inability to keep down any solids or liquids. If the condition is prolonged, the patient may also report fatigue or lethargy, headache, and faintness.[11,14]

Various degrees of dehydration may be present: skin may be pale, there may be dark circles under the eyes, the eyes may appear sunken, the mucous membranes may be dry, and skin flexibility may be poor.[11,14]

Supine Hypotension

Supine hypotension (also known as inferior vena cava syndrome) may develop in the supine position, especially after the first trimester. The decrease in blood pressure is thought to be caused by the occlusion of the aorta and inferior vena cava by the increased weight and size of the uterus. Spontaneous recovery usually occurs upon change of maternal position. However, patients should not be allowed to stand up quickly because of the potential for orthostatic hypotension. Signs and symptoms of this condition include:

- Bradycardia
- Shortness of breath
- Syncope (fainting)
- Dizziness
- Nausea and vomiting
- Sweating or cold, clammy skin
- Headache
- Numbness in extremities
- Weakness
- Restlessness

In general, limiting the time the patient spends in supine to approximately 5 minutes helps to minimize the effects of this problem. Alternative positions include left sidelying (best position for minimizing compression), right sidelying, supine reclined, or supine with a small wedge under the right hip.

Psychiatric Changes

Pregnancy-related depression and postpartum depression may occur. Postnatal depression has been documented to occur in 5 to 20 percent of all postpartum mothers,[49–51] but can also occur in fathers.[52] Depressive postpartum disorders range from "postpartum blues," which occurs from 1 to 5 days after birth and lasts for only a few days, to postpartum depression and postpartum psychosis, the latter two of which are more serious conditions and require medical or social intervention to avoid serious ramifications to the family unit.[10,53,54]

Exercise Prescription

Both exercise and pregnancy are associated with a high demand for energy. Caloric demands with exercise during pregnancy are very high. The competing energy demands of the exercising mother and the growing fetus raise the theoretic concern that excessive exercise might adversely affect fetal development.[10] Contraindications to exercise include an incompetent cervix (early dilation of the cervix before pregnancy is full term), vaginal bleeding (especially in the second or third trimester), placenta previa (the placenta is located on the uterus in a position where it may detach before the baby is delivered), multiple gestation with risk of premature labor, pregnancy-induced hypertension, premature labor (labor beginning before the thirty-seventh week of pregnancy), maternal heart disease, maternal type I diabetes, and intrauterine growth retardation.[55] Even without these conditions, the patient should obtain permission from her physician before embarking on an exercise program. Theoretically, because of the physiologic changes associated with pregnancy, as well as the hemodynamic response to exercise, some precautions should be observed during exercise:[56–63]

- Although it is strongly recommended for all women to participate in mild to moderate exercise, based on prepregnancy fitness level, for both strength and cardiopulmonary benefits, exercise activity should occur at a moderate rate during a low-risk pregnancy. Exercise programs for high-risk pregnancies should be individually established based on diagnosis, limitations, physical therapy examination, and evaluation, in consultation with the physician. Guidelines for a low-risk pregnancy permit women to remain at 50 to 60 percent (12–14 on the Borg scale of perceived exertion) of their maximal heart rate (monitored intermittently) for approximately 15–30 minutes per session. Exercise acts in concert with pregnancy to increase heart rate, stroke volume, and cardiac output; however, during exercise, blood is diverted from abdominal viscera, including the uterus, to supply exercising muscle. The decrease in splanchnic blood flow can reach 50 percent and raises theoretic concerns about fetal hypoxemia. Recommended activities include stationary cycling, swimming, or water aerobics.
- Increases in joint laxity due to changes in hormonal levels may lead to a higher risk of strains or sprains, so weight-bearing exercises should be prescribed judiciously. Abdominal and pelvic discomfort from weight-bearing exercise is most likely secondary to tension on the round ligaments, increased uterine mobility, or pelvic instability.
- Women should avoid becoming overtired and should not exercise in the supine position for more than 5 minutes after the first trimester (see the "Supine Hypotension" section earlier in this chapter). To prevent inferior vena cava compression when the patient is lying supine, a folded towel can be placed under the right side of the pelvis so that the patient is tipped slightly to the left.
- Positions that involve abdominal compression (such as flat prone lying) should be avoided in mid-to-late pregnancy.

- Adequate hydration and appropriate ventilation are important in preventing the possible teratogenic effects of overheating. Theoretically, when exercise and pregnancy are combined, a rise in maternal core temperature could decrease fetal heat dissipation to the mother. Some data suggest a teratogenic potential when maternal temperatures rise above 39.2°C (102.6°F), especially in the first trimester.

> **● Key Point** Warning signs associated with exercise during pregnancy include:
> - Pain
> - Vaginal bleeding
> - Dizziness, feeling faint
> - Tachycardia
> - Dyspnea
> - Chest pain
> - Uterine contractions

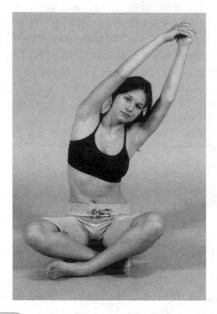

Figure 24-2 Lumbar stabilization in sitting.

Specific Exercises

The following guidelines are for a normal pregnancy. Exercise programs for high-risk pregnancies should be individually established based on diagnosis, limitations, physical therapy examination, and evaluation, in consultation with the physician. The goals of therapeutic exercise during pregnancy are to improve muscle balance and posture, help provide support of the growing uterus, stabilize the trunk and pelvis, and maintain function for more rapid recovery after delivery.[64] Lumbar stabilization exercises (see Chapter 15) can be performed in supine with frequent position changes. If the supine position is contraindicated, exercises can be performed in sidelying, the quadruped position (see Chapter 15), or sitting (Figure 24-2).

Modifications to exercise for the abdominal muscles must be made for a woman with diastasis recti, because the presence of this condition potentially reduces the ability of the abdominal wall muscles to contribute to their role in trunk and pelvic girdle alignment, motion, and stability; support of pelvic viscera; and prevention of increasing intra-abdominal pressure, forced expiration, defecation, urination, vomiting, and the second stage of labor (i.e., pushing).[64,65] A diastasis correction exercise can be performed to maintain alignment and encourage further separation. The exercise is performed in the supine hooklying position (if tolerated and not contraindicated). With the arms crisscrossed over the abdomen, the patient manually approximates the recti muscles toward midline, performs a posterior pelvic tilt, and slowly exhales while lifting her head so that the scapulae clear the surface.[64,66] In addition, the patient can perform any exercise that does not stress the sacroiliac joint or increase intra-abdominal pressure, including leg sliding (see Chapter 15), supine bridging (see Chapter 15), quadruped leg raising (see Chapter 15), modified squats (see Chapter 15), and posterior pelvic tilts (see Chapter 15) while using her hands to support the abdominal wall. Traditional abdominal exercises, such as full sit-ups or bilateral straight leg raises, are not recommended because they may encourage further separation; however, these exercises can be resumed when the separation is less than 2 centimeters. Exercises for the pelvic floor are described in the "Urinary Incontinence" section.

Adjunctive Interventions

On occasion, the patient may require the use of modalities as part of the intervention. However, modalities that increase body heat (e.g., hot packs, ultrasound, shortwave or microwave diathermy) should be used with caution, especially over the abdomen or uterus. Electrical stimulation is contraindicated during pregnancy, except for the use of transcutaneous electrical stimulation (TENS) during labor and delivery.

Cesarean Delivery

Exercise may begin within 24 hours after delivery but should be graded and based on the patient's comfort level.[66] Postpartum precautions in exercises apply, but exercise must be progressed more

Urinary Incontinence

Incontinence is defined as the complaint of any involuntary leakage of urine, feces, or gas.[67] Urinary incontinence may be defined as an involuntary loss of urine that is sufficient to be a problem, and occurs most often when bladder pressure exceeds sphincter resistance. The following four categories can be used to classify urinary incontinence:[68]

- *Functional incontinence:* Includes people who have normal urine control but are unwilling to use a toilet (impaired cognition) or who have difficulty reaching a toilet in time because of muscle or joint dysfunction or environmental barriers.
- *Stress incontinence:* The loss of urine during activities that increase intra-abdominal pressure, such as coughing, lifting, or laughing.
- *Overflow incontinence:* The constant leaking of urine from a bladder that is full but unable to empty due to anatomic obstruction (e.g., pregnancy) or neurogenic bladder (e.g., spinal cord injury).
- *Urge incontinence:* The sudden unexpected urge to urinate and the uncontrolled loss of urine; often related to reduced bladder capacity, detrusor instability, or hypersensitive bladder.

Medical management of urinary incontinence is aimed at prevention, and may include:

- Nutritional counseling to help prevent constipation and to encourage adequate hydration
- Medications to relieve urge incontinence, such as estrogen replacement therapy (ERT), anticholinergics, alpha-adrenergic blockers to increase bladder outlet/sphincteric tone, antispasmodics, and combination therapy with tricyclic antidepressant agents and antidiuretic hormone[69–73]
- Surgical intervention can include catheterization, and surgically implanted artificial sphincters and bladder generators (sends impulses to the nerves that control the bladder function)

Intervention

Physical therapy has an important direct role in the assessment and treatment of urge and stress urinary incontinence, particularly in pelvic floor muscle rehabilitation. The pelvic floor muscles (Figure 24-3) can be divided into four layers, from superficial to deep:

- Anal sphincter
- Superficial perineal muscles
- Urogenital diaphragm
- Pelvic diaphragm

The pelvic diaphragm (the coccygeus muscle and the levator ani muscles) is the largest muscle group

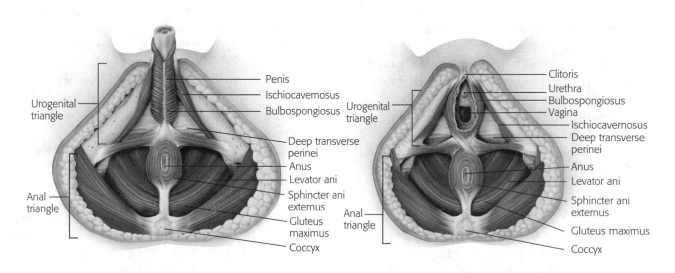

Figure 24-3   Pelvic floor muscles.

in the pelvic floor and is responsible for most of the function or dysfunction of this area.[74]

Coccygeus

This muscle arises from the pelvic surface of the ischial spine and sacrospinous ligament and inserts on the coccyx margin and side of the lowest segment of the sacrum. Supplied by the muscular branches of the pudendal plexus, the coccygeus pulls forward and supports the coccyx. In addition, the coccygeus muscle provides support for the pelvic contents and the sacroiliac joint.

Levator Ani

The levator ani originates anteriorly from the pelvic surface of the pubis, posteriorly from the inner surface of the ischial spine, and from the obturator fascia. It inserts on the front and sides of the coccyx, to the sides of the rectum, and into the perineal body. The levator ani forms the floor of the pelvic cavity and constricts the lower end of the rectum and vagina; it can also be activated during forced expiration. The muscle, which consists of anterior, intermediate, and posterior fibers (refer to Figure 24-3), is innervated by the muscular branches of the pudendal plexus (anterior divisions of S2–S4 of the sacral plexus; see Chapter 3).

- *Anterior fibers:* The anterior fibers insert into the perineal body, comprise the levator prostate or sphincter vaginae, and form a sling around the prostate or vagina.
- *Intermediate fibers:* The intermediate fibers consist of:
  - *Puborectalis:* The puborectalis originates at the pubis and forms a sling around the junction of the rectum and the anal canal. The muscle pulls the anorectal junction anteriorly, assisting the external sphincter in anal closure.
  - *Pubococcygeus:* The pubococcygeal muscle arises from the pubis and its superior ramus, and passes posteriorly to insert into the anococcygeal body between the coccyx and the anal canal. The muscle functions to pull the coccyx forward. It also serves to elevate the pelvic organs and compress the rectum and vagina.
- *Posterior fibers:* The iliococcygeal muscle arises from the arcus tendineus and ischial spine and inserts onto the last segment of the coccyx and anococcygeal body. The muscle functions to pull the coccyx from side to side and to elevate the rectum.

The pubococcygeal muscle and the iliococcygeal muscle unite posterior to the anorectal junction to form the levator plate, which inserts into the coccyx.

The pelvic floor muscles work in a coordinated manner to increase intra-abdominal pressure, provide rectal support during defecation, inhibit bladder activity, help support the pelvic organs, and assist in lumbopelvic stability.[75] Many factors contribute to normal function of the pelvic floor muscles. The two major causes of anatomic impairment are birth injury and neurologic dysfunction. A complete pelvic floor muscle evaluation by the PT is necessary to prescribe an appropriate exercise program. A typical physical therapy intervention for pelvic floor dysfunction includes:

- Patient education, which should include:
  - Visual aids, with emphasis placed on both the sling/hammock (anterior-posterior) orientation of the fibers and the figure of eight (circumferential) orientation
  - Advising the patient to avoid the Valsalva maneuver
  - Advising the patient to avoid activities that strain the pelvic floor and abdominal muscles
  - Education to preserve acceptable skin condition[76]
  - Education with regard to adequate protection—adult diapers, underpads
  - Maintenance of toileting schedule
  - The importance of psychological and emotional support
- Exercise to improve control of the pelvic floor and to maintain abdominal function. This includes pelvic floor muscle exercises, emphasizing exercises that address both fast-twitch and slow-twitch muscle fibers so there is a significant increase in the force of the urethral closure without an appreciable Valsalva effort.[77-79] These exercises include two types of Kegel exercises:
  - *Type 1:* Works on holding contractions, progressing to 10-second holds, and resting 10 seconds between contractions.
  - *Type 2:* Works on quick contractions to shut off urine flow. Patient should perform 10–80 repetitions per day, while avoiding buttock squeezing or contracting the abdominals.
  The patient should be encouraged to incorporate Kegel exercises into everyday life,

especially with lifting, coughing, laughing, changing positions, and the like. Exercises should also include progressive strengthening of the pelvic floor musculature with weighted vaginal cones and pelvic floor exerciser.

- Biofeedback to reinforce active contraction and relaxation of the bladder.[80]
- Functional electrical stimulation for muscle re-education of the bladder and pelvic floor muscles.[80]
- Noninvasive pulsed magnetic fields (extracorporeal magnetic innervation) for pelvic floor muscle strengthening.[76]

Breast Cancer–Related Lymphedema

The lymphatic system is a network of strategically placed lymph nodes connected by a substantial network of lymphatic vessels, which act as the circulatory system for the immune system.

> ● **Key Point** The lymphatic system has four major purposes:
> - To return proteins, lipids, and water from the interstitium to the intravascular space
> - To act as a safety valve for fluid overload and to help keep edema from forming
> - To maintain the homeostasis of the extracellular environment
> - To cleanse the interstitial fluid and provide a blockade to the spread of infection or malignant cells in the lymph nodes

As lymph fluid moves more centrally, the diameter of lymph vessels increases. Larger lymph collectors, known as trunks or ducts, handle these larger volumes of lymph fluid. The major lymph nodes are the submaxillary, cervical, maxillary, mesenteric, iliac, inguinal, popliteal, and cubital nodes. The majority of the lymph produced by the body in a 24-hour period (2 to 4 liters) returns to the heart. Interstitial fluid normally contributes to the nourishment of tissues, and about 90 percent of the fluid returns to the circulation via entry into venous capillaries. The remaining 10 percent is composed of high molecular weight proteins and their oncotically associated water, which are too large to readily pass through venous capillary walls. This leads to flow into the lymphatic capillaries where pressures are typically subatmospheric and can accommodate the large size of the proteins and their accompanying water. The proteins then travel as lymph through numerous filtering lymph nodes on their way to join the venous circulation. Immune responses to infections cause the lymph nodes to swell.

> ● **Key Point** Lymph nodes, in conjunction with the spleen, tonsils, adenoids, and Peyer's patches, are highly organized centers of immune cells that filter antigen from the extracellular fluid. Lymph nodes also are one of the first places to which cancer cells can spread. Cancer cells in a lymph node can cause the node to swell.

> ● **Key Point** Edema is an increase of water in the interstitial space, which results from immobility, chronic venous insufficiency, hypoproteinuria, cardiac insufficiencies, or pregnancy. Lymphedema arises from a mechanical insufficiency in an area when lymph collectors sustain functional and structural damage resulting in the accumulation of hydrophilic proteins in the tissues.

Breast cancer–related dysfunction of the lymphatic system and subsequent lymphedema of the upper extremity can occur as a complication of the treatment for breast cancer. Current treatment for breast cancer usually involves removing a portion or all of the breast accompanied by excision or radiation of the adjacent axillary lymph nodes, the principal site of regional metastasis.[81] Axillary dissection places a patient at risk not only for upper extremity lymphedema, but also for loss of shoulder mobility and limited function of the arm and hand.[82]

The following impairments and complications may occur in association with the treatment of breast cancer:[81]

- Incisional pain.
- Posterior cervical and shoulder girdle pain.
- Vascular and pulmonary complications including pneumonia and deep vein thrombosis.
- Lymphedema. Clinicians use a variety of strategies to diagnose upper extremity (UE) lymphedema. The most widely used strategy is circumferential UE measurements using specific anatomical landmarks. Arm circumference measurements are used to estimate volume differences between the affected and unaffected UEs. A more accurate measure of volume difference is the water displacement technique.
- Chest wall adhesions.
- Decreased shoulder mobility.
- Weakness of the involved upper extremity.
- Postural malalignment.
- Fatigue and decreased endurance.

Intervention

The intervention for breast cancer–related lymphatic dysfunction includes the following:[81]

- Exercise, massage, and use of compression devices. Exercise encourages skeletal muscle contractions to provide the primary pumping mechanism for lymphatic and venous drainage, and therefore should stimulate the contraction of lymph vessels because these vessels are innervated by the sympathetic nervous system. Progressive resistance training (using light weights initially and progressing as tolerated) while wearing fitted compression sleeves should include the following exercises: seated row, bench press, latissimus dorsi muscle pull-down, one-arm bent-over rowing, triceps muscle extension, and biceps curl.[83] After 2 weeks, additional progressive upper-body aerobic exercise can be implemented on an arm ergometer.

- Individualized shoulder (Chapter 16) and cervical (Chapter 13) range of motion exercises to address any muscle imbalances listed in the plan of care.
- Moderate-intensity aerobic conditioning exercises.

> **● Key Point** Traditional pneumatic compression devices are generally contraindicated for lymphedema because the natural drainage system has been damaged, and these devices can potentially cause more damage to the system. Instead, various types of specialized wrapping, taping, and lymphedema massage are advocated, followed by pressure garment wear.

Summary

A number of physiologic changes occur within the various body systems during pregnancy and the postpartum period, which can present the PTA with some unique challenges. Given the number of physiologic changes that occur during pregnancy and the postpartum period, the extent of the physical therapy intervention will depend on the findings of the examination. Therapeutic exercise plays a key role with this patient population. Breast cancer lymphedema and urinary incontinence present their own set of challenges, both physical and psychological. The intervention for these patient populations is highly individualized.

REVIEW **Questions**

1. You have been asked to develop an exercise plan for a pregnant woman. The strengthening of which of the following muscles should be the focus to maintain a strong pelvic floor?
   a. Rectus abdominis, iliococcygeus, and piriformis
   b. Piriformis, obturator internus, and pubococcygeus
   c. Iliococcygeus, pubococcygeus, and coccygeus
   d. Obturator internus, piriformis, and external obliques
2. What is the name given to the type of exercises designed to improve control of the pelvic floor and to maintain abdominal function used to help prevent urinary incontinence?
3. During pregnancy, which female hormone is released that assists in the softening of the pubic symphysis so that during delivery, the female pelvis can stretch enough to allow birth?
4. True or false: Thoracic kyphosis with scapular retraction, increased cervical lordosis and forward head, and increased lumbar lordosis are all postural changes associated with pregnancy.
5. True or false: Diabetes can occur during pregnancy.
6. What is diastasis recti?
7. True or false: Supine hypotension rarely occurs after the first trimester of pregnancy.
8. What term is used to describe the constant leaking of urine from a bladder that is full but unable to empty?
9. What is lymphedema?
10. True or false: Breast cancer surgery is associated with chest wall adhesions, decreased shoulder mobility, and weakness of the involved upper extremity.
11. A patient in the third trimester of pregnancy needs prenatal exercises. In the hooklying position you note a one-finger gap on the abdomen near the umbilicus when the patient attempts a partial sit-up. You immediately stop and modify the exercise due to the possibility of:
    a. Diastasis recti
    b. Preeclampsia
    c. Low back pain
    d. Varicose veins

References

1. Lee HY, Zhao S, Fields PA, et al: Clinical use of relaxin to facilitate birth: Reasons for investigating the premise. Ann N Y Acad Sci 1041:351–366, 2005
2. Lubahn J, Ivance D, Konieczko E, et al: Immunohistochemical detection of relaxin binding to the volar oblique ligament. J Hand Surg [Am] 31:80–84, 2006

3. Goldsmith LT, Weiss G, Steinetz BG: Relaxin and its role in pregnancy. Endocrinol Metab Clin North Am 24:171–186, 1995

4. Wiles R: The views of women of above average weight about appropriate weight gain in pregnancy. Midwifery 14:254–260, 1998

5. Stephenson R, O'Connor L: Obstetric and Gynecologic Care in Physical Therapy (ed 2). Thorofare, NJ, Charles B Slack, 2000

6. Moore K, Dumas GA, Reid JG: Postural changes associated with pregnancy and their relationship with low back pain. Clin Biomech 5:169–174, 1990

7. Noronha A: Neurologic disorders during pregnancy and the puerperium. Clin Perinatol 12:695–713, 1985

8. Godfrey CM: Carpal tunnel syndrome in pregnancy. Can Med Assoc J 129:928, 1983

9. Graham JG: Neurological complications of pregnancy and anaesthesia. Clin Obstet Gynaecol 9:333–350, 1982

10. Boissonnault JS, Stephenson R: The obstetric patient, in Boissonnault WG (ed): Primary Care for the Physical Therapist: Examination and Triage. St Louis, Elsevier Saunders, 2005, pp 239–270

11. Lamondy AM: Managing hyperemesis gravidarum. Nursing 37:66–68, 2007

12. Dodds L, Fell DB, Joseph KS, et al: Outcomes of pregnancies complicated by hyperemesis gravidarum. Obstet Gynecol 107:285–292, 2006

13. Fell DB, Dodds L, Joseph KS, et al: Risk factors for hyperemesis gravidarum requiring hospital admission during pregnancy. Obstet Gynecol 107:277–284, 2006

14. Loh KY, Sivalingam N: Understanding hyperemesis gravidarum. Med J Malaysia 60:394–399; quiz 400, 2005

15. Wise RA, Polito AJ, Krishnan V: Respiratory physiologic changes in pregnancy. Immunol Allergy Clin North Am 26:1–12, 2006

16. Prowse CM, Gaensler EA: Respiratory and acid-base changes during pregnancy. Anesthesiology 26:381–392, 1965

17. Bonica JJ: Maternal respiratory changes during pregnancy and parturition. Clin Anesth 10:1–19, 1974

18. Sadaniantz A, Kocheril AG, Emaus SP, et al: Cardiovascular changes in pregnancy evaluated by two-dimensional and Doppler echocardiography. J Am Soc Echocardiogr 5:253–258, 1992

19. Atkins AF, Watt JM, Milan P, et al: A longitudinal study of cardiovascular dynamic changes throughout pregnancy. Eur J Obstet Gynecol Reprod Biol 12:215–224, 1981

20. Chesley LC: Cardiovascular changes in pregnancy. Obstet Gynecol Annu 4:71–97, 1975

21. Capeless EL, Clapp JF: Cardiovascular changes in early phase of pregnancy. Am J Obstet Gynecol 161:1449–1453, 1989

22. Walters WA, Lim YL: Changes in the maternal cardiovascular system during human pregnancy. Surg Gynecol Obstet 131:765–784, 1970

23. Urman BC, McComb PF: A biphasic basal body temperature record during pregnancy. Acta Eur Fertil 20:371–372, 1989

24. Grant A, Mc BW: The 100 day basal body temperature graph in early pregnancy. Med J Aust 46:458–460, 1959

25. Siegler AM: Basal body temperature in pregnancy. Obstet Gynecol 5:830–832, 1955

26. Depledge J, McNair PJ, Keal-Smith C, et al: Management of symphysis pubis dysfunction during pregnancy using exercise and pelvic support belts. Phys Ther 85:1290–1300, 2005

27. Leadbetter RE, Mawer D, Lindow SW: Symphysis pubis dysfunction: A review of the literature. J Matern Fetal Neonatal Med 16:349–354, 2004

28. Owens K, Pearson A, Mason G: Symphysis pubis dysfunction: A cause of significant obstetric morbidity. Eur J Obstet Gynecol Reprod Biol 105:143–146, 2002

29. Allsop JR: Symphysis pubis dysfunction. Br J Gen Pract 47:256, 1997

30. Snow RE, Neubert AG: Peripartum pubic symphysis separation: A case series and review of the literature. Obstet Gynecol Surv 52:438–443, 1997

31. Whitman JM: Pregnancy, low back pain, and manual physical therapy interventions. J Orthop Sports Phys Ther 32:314–317, 2002

32. Mogren IM, Pohjanen AI: Low back pain and pelvic pain during pregnancy: Prevalence and risk factors. Spine 30:983–991, 2005

33. Pool-Goudzwaard AL, Slieker ten Hove MC, Vierhout ME, et al: Relations between pregnancy-related low back pain, pelvic floor activity and pelvic floor dysfunction. Int Urogynecol J Pelvic Floor Dysfunct 16:468–474, 2005

34. Wang SM, Dezinno P, Maranets I, et al: Low back pain during pregnancy: Prevalence, risk factors, and outcomes. Obstet Gynecol 104:65–70, 2004

35. Fast A, Weiss L, Ducommun EJ, et al: Low back pain in pregnancy. Abdominal muscles, sit-up performance and back pain. Spine 15:28–30, 1990

36. Berg G, Hammar M, Moller-Nielsen J, et al: Low back pain during pregnancy. Obstet Gynecol 71:71–75, 1988

37. Bullock JE, Jull GA, Bullock MI: The relationship of low back pain to postural changes during pregnancy. Aust J Physiother 33:10–17, 1987

38. Ostgaard HC, Andersson GBJ, Schultz AB, et al: Influence of some biomechanical factors on low back pain in pregnancy. Spine 18:61–65, 1993

39. Nilsson-Wikmar L, Holm K, Oijerstedt R, et al: Effect of three different physical therapy treatments on pain and activity in pregnant women with pelvic girdle pain: A randomized clinical trial with 3, 6, and 12 months follow-up postpartum. Spine 30:850–856, 2005

40. Hall J, Cleland JA, Palmer JA: The effects of manual physical therapy and therapeutic exercise on peripartum posterior pelvic pain: Two case reports. J Man Manip Ther 13:94–102, 2005

41. Fast A, Shapiro D, Ducommun EJ, et al: Low-back pain in pregnancy. Spine 12:368–371, 1987

42. Hainline B: Low-back pain in pregnancy. Adv Neurol 64:65–76, 1994

43. Stuge B, Hilde G, Vollestad N: Physical therapy for pregnancy-related low back and pelvic pain: A systematic review. Acta Obstet Gynecol Scand 82:983–990, 2003

44. Hodges SD, Eck JC, Humphreys SC: A treatment and outcomes analysis of patients with coccydynia. Spine 4:138–140, 2004

45. Ryder I, Alexander J: Coccydynia: A woman's tail. Midwifery 16:155–160, 2000

46. Maigne JY, Lagauche D, Doursounian L: Instability of the coccyx in coccydynia. J Bone Joint Surg Br 82:1038–1041, 2000

47. Boeglin ER, Jr.: Coccydynia. J Bone Joint Surg Br 73:1009, 1991

48. Wray CC, Easom S, Hoskinson J: Coccydynia. Aetiology and treatment. J Bone Joint Surg Br 73:335–338, 1991

49. Lee DT, Chung TK: Postnatal depression: An update. Best Pract Res Clin Obstet Gynaecol 21:183–191, 2006

50. Howard L: Postnatal depression. Clin Evid 14:1919–1931, 2006

51. Howard L: Postnatal depression. Am Fam Physician 72(7):1294–1296, 2005

52. Cox J: Postnatal depression in fathers. Lancet 366:982, 2005

53. Hanley J: The assessment and treatment of postnatal depression. Nurs Times 102:24–26, 2006

54. Mallikarjun PK, Oyebode F: Prevention of postnatal depression. J R Soc Health 125:221–226, 2005

55. Settles-Huge B: Women's health: Obstetrics and pelvic floor, in Kisner C, Colby LA (eds): Therapeutic Exercise. Foundations and Techniques (ed 5). Philadelphia, FA Davis, 2002, pp 797–824

56. Parker KM, Smith SA: Aquatic-aerobic exercise as a means of stress reduction during pregnancy. J Perinat Educ 12:6–17, 2003

57. Kramer MS, McDonald SW: Aerobic exercise for women during pregnancy. Cochrane Database Syst Rev 3:CD000180, 2006

58. Morris SN, Johnson NR: Exercise during pregnancy: A critical appraisal of the literature. J Reprod Med 50:181–188, 2005

59. Larsson L, Lindqvist PG: Low-impact exercise during pregnancy—a study of safety. Acta Obstet Gynecol Scand 84:34–38, 2005

60. Fazlani SA: Protocols for exercise during pregnancy. J Pak Med Assoc 54:226–229, 2004

61. Snyder S, Pendergraph B: Exercise during pregnancy: What do we really know? Am Fam Physician 69:1053, 1056, 2004

62. Paisley TS, Joy EA, Price RJ, Jr.: Exercise during pregnancy: A practical approach. Curr Sports Med Rep 2:325–330, 2003

63. Information from your family doctor. Pregnancy and exercise. Am Fam Physician 68:1168, 2003

64. Strauhal MJ: Therapeutic exercise in obstetrics, in Hall C, Thein-Brody L (eds): Therapeutic Exercise: Moving Toward Function (ed 2). Baltimore, Lippincott Williams & Wilkins, 2005, pp 259–281

65. Wilder E: Obstetric and gynecologic physical therapy, in Wilder E (ed): Clinics in Physical Therapy. New York, Churchill Livingstone, 1988, pp 63–82

66. Noble E: Essential exercises for the childbearing years (ed 4). Harwich, MA, New Life Images, 1995

67. Abrams P, Cardozo L, Fall M, et al: The standardisation of terminology of lower urinary tract function: Report from the Standardisation Sub-committee of the International Continence Society. Am J Obstet Gynecol 187:116–126, 2002

68. Boissonnault WG, Goodman CC: The renal and urologic systems, in Goodman CC, Boissonnault WG, Fuller KS (eds): Pathology: Implications for the Physical Therapist (ed 2). Philadelphia, Saunders, 2003, pp 704–728

69. Urinary incontinence. Know your drug options. Mayo Clin Health Lett 23:6, 2005

70. Blackwell RE: Estrogen, progestin, and urinary incontinence. JAMA 294:2696–2697; author reply 2697–2698, 2005

71. Bren L: Controlling urinary incontinence. FDA Consum 39:10–15, 2005

72. Castro-Diaz D, Amoros MA: Pharmacotherapy for stress urinary incontinence. Curr Opin Urol 15:227–230, 2005

73. Kelleher C, Cardozo L, Kobashi K, et al: Solifenacin: As effective in mixed urinary incontinence as in urge urinary incontinence. Int Urogynecol J Pelvic Floor Dysfunct 17:382–388, 2006

74. Shelly E: The pelvic floor, in Hall C, Thein-Brody L (eds): Therapeutic Exercise: Moving Toward Function (ed 2). Baltimore, Lippincott Williams & Wilkins, 2005, pp 402–435

75. Markwell SJ: Physical therapy management of pelvi/perineal and perianal pain syndromes. World J Urol 19:194–199, 2001

76. Wilson MM: Urinary incontinence: Selected current concepts. Med Clin North Am 90:825–836, 2006

77. Borello-France DF, Zyczynski HM, Downey PA, et al: Effect of pelvic-floor muscle exercise position on continence and quality-of-life outcomes in women with stress urinary incontinence. Phys Ther 86:974–986, 2006

78. Neumann PB, Grimmer KA, Deenadayalan Y: Pelvic floor muscle training and adjunctive therapies for the treatment of stress urinary incontinence in women: A systematic review. BMC Womens Health 6:11, 2006

79. Hay-Smith EJ, Dumoulin C: Pelvic floor muscle training versus no treatment, or inactive control treatments, for urinary incontinence in women. Cochrane Database Syst Rev:CD005654, 2006

80. Anders K: Treatments for stress urinary incontinence. Nurs Times 102:55–57, 2006

81. Kisner C, Colby LA: Management of vascular disorders of the extremities, in Kisner C, Colby LA (eds): Therapeutic Exercise. Foundations and Techniques (ed 5). Philadelphia, FA Davis, 2002, pp 825–849

82. Bicego D, Brown K, Ruddick M, et al: Exercise for women with or at risk for breast cancer-related lymphedema. Phys Ther 86:1398–1405, 2006

83. Johansson K, Tibe K, Weibull A, et al: Low intensity resistance exercise for breast cancer patients with arm lymphedema with or without compression sleeve. Lymphology 38:167–180, 2005

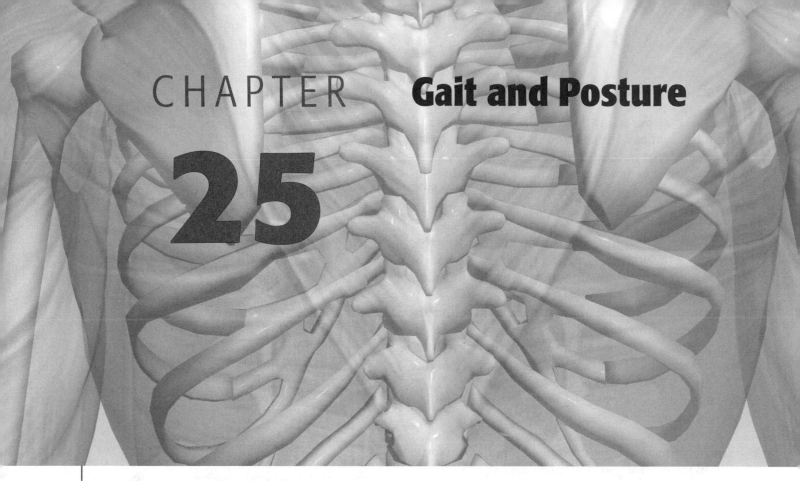

CHAPTER 25 — Gait and Posture

Chapter Objectives

At the completion of this chapter, the reader will be able to:

1. Summarize the various components of the gait cycle.
2. Apply the knowledge of gait components to a rehabilitation program.
3. Categorize the various compensations of the body and their influences on gait.
4. Describe the characteristics of a number of abnormal gait syndromes.
5. Describe and demonstrate the various gait patterns used with assistive devices.
6. Recognize the most common manifestations of abnormal posture.

Overview

Gait involves the displacement of body weight in a desired direction, utilizing a coordinated effort between the joints of the trunk and extremities and the muscles that control or produce these motions. Any interference that alters this relationship may result in a deviation or disturbance of the normal gait pattern. This, in turn, may result in increased energy expenditure or functional impairment. The PTA requires an understanding of what constitutes normal human gait and must be able to recognize the deviations from normal that can occur with this functional activity. For example, the PTA is frequently delegated the responsibility of teaching patients how to use assistive devices in an appropriate manner and using a specific gait pattern with the appropriate weight-bearing status. In addition, the PTA frequently educates patients on how to perform functional activities and exercises while maintaining correct posture.

Gait

The fall that occurs at the initiation of gait so that an individual can lift one foot off the ground and take the first step is controlled by the central nervous system.[1] The central nervous system computes in advance the required size and direction of this fall of the body toward the supporting foot. It is not clear whether gait is learned or is preprogrammed at the spinal cord level, but it is clear that gait relies on the control of the limb movements by reflexes. Two such reflexes are the stretch reflex and the extensor thrust. The stretch reflex is involved in the extremes of joint motion. The extensor thrust, present in a human in the first 2 months of life, is an exaggeration of the positive support reflex. The reflex consists of an uncontrolled extension of a flexed leg when the sole of the foot is stimulated, which may facilitate the extensor muscles of the lower extremity during weight bearing.[2]

In patients who have developed dysfunctional gait patterns, physical therapy can help to restore this exquisite evolutionary gift.[3] Pain, weakness, and disease can all cause a disturbance in the normal rhythm of gait (see "Influences on Normal Gait" later in this chapter); however, except in obvious cases, abnormal gait does not always equate with impairment.

Terminology

The following terminology is commonly used when discussing gait:

- *Base of support:* The base of support, defined as the distance between an individual's feet while standing and during ambulation, includes the part of the body in contact with the supporting surface and the intervening area.[4] The normal base of support is considered to be between 5 and 10 centimeters.

> **● Key Point**   Larger than normal bases of support are observed in individuals who have muscle imbalances of the lower limbs and trunk, as well as those who have problems with overall static and dynamic balance.[5]

- *Center of gravity:* The center of gravity (COG), which changes both vertically and horizontally during gait (see The Kinematics of Gait), may be defined as the point at which the three planes of the body intersect (see Chapter 4). In the human, that point is approximately 2 inches (5 centimeters) anterior to the second

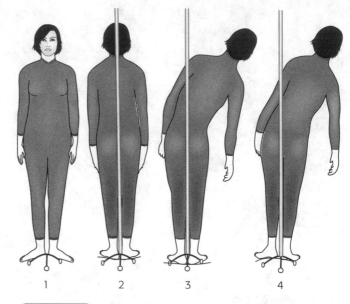

Figure 25-1   Center of gravity.

sacral vertebra (Figure 25-1). As the COG moves forward with each step, it briefly passes beyond the anterior margin of the base of support, resulting in a temporary loss of balance.[4] This temporary loss of equilibrium is counteracted by the advancing foot at initial contact, which establishes a new base of support.

- *Step length:* Step length is defined as the linear distance between the right and left foot during gait (Figure 25-2). Step length is measured as the distance between the same point on each foot with successive footprints (ipsilateral to the contralateral foot fall).
- *Stride length:* Stride length is the distance between successive points of foot-to-floor contact of the same foot. A stride is one full lower extremity cycle. Two step lengths added together make up the stride length (**Table 25-1**). Stride length can be estimated based on height (females: height × 0.413; males: height × 0.415). The average length of the female stride is 2 feet. The average length of the male stride is 2.5 feet.[6] Typically, the stride length does not vary more than a few inches between tall and short individuals.
- *Cadence:* Cadence is defined as the number of separate steps taken in a certain time period. Normal cadence is between 90 and 120 steps per minute.[7,8] The cadence of women is usually six to nine steps per minute slower than that of men. Cadence is also affected by age, decreasing

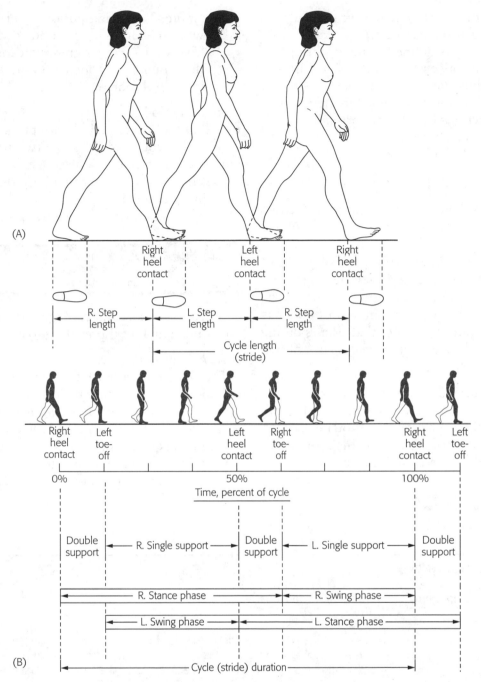

Figure 25-2   The gait cycle.

Source: Inman VT, Ralston H, Todd F: Human Walking. Baltimore, Lippincott, Williams & Wilkins, 1981.

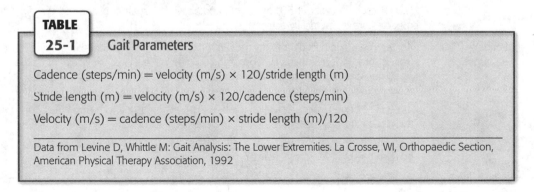

TABLE 25-1   Gait Parameters

Cadence (steps/min) = velocity (m/s) × 120/stride length (m)

Stride length (m) = velocity (m/s) × 120/cadence (steps/min)

Velocity (m/s) = cadence (steps/min) × stride length (m)/120

Data from Levine D, Whittle M: Gait Analysis: The Lower Extremities. La Crosse, WI, Orthopaedic Section, American Physical Therapy Association, 1992

from the age of 4 to the age of 7 years, and then again in advancing years.[9]

- *Velocity:* Velocity is defined as the distance a body moves in a given time and is thus calculated by dividing the distance traveled by the time taken. Velocity is expressed in meters per second. Reductions in velocity correlate with joint impairments, amputation levels, and many acute pathologies due to pain.

Gait Cycle

Walking involves the alternating action of the two lower extremities. The walking pattern is studied as a gait cycle. A gait cycle is defined as the interval of time between any of the repetitive events of walking. Such an event could include everything from the point when the foot initially contacts the ground to the point when the same foot contacts the ground again, or all activity that occurs during one stride length.[10] The gait cycle consists of two periods (**Table 25-2**):

1. *Stance:* This period describes the entire time the foot is in contact with the ground and the limb is bearing weight. The stance period begins with the initial contact of the foot on the ground and concludes when the ipsilateral foot leaves the ground.

2. *Swing:* The swing period describes the period when the foot is not in contact with the ground. The swing period begins as the foot is lifted from the ground and ends with initial contact of the ipsilateral foot.[10]

Stance Period

Within the stance period, two tasks and four intervals are recognized.[11-13] The two tasks are weight acceptance and single limb support. According to the Rancho Los Amigos terminology, the four intervals are initial contact, loading response, midstance, and terminal stance (refer to Figure 25-2).[13]

> ● **Key Point** For the stance phase, standard terminology uses the terms *heelstrike* (initial contact), *foot flat* (loading response), *midstance*, *heel off* (terminal stance), and *toe off* (preswing).

As the initial contact of one foot is occurring, the contralateral foot is preparing to come off the floor.

Task 1: Weight Acceptance
The weight acceptance task occurs during the first 10 percent of the stance period (refer to Figure 25-2). This consists of intervals of *initial contact* (when the heel first hits the ground) and *loading response*. The loading response interval begins as the foot comes flat with the floor and one limb bears weight while the other leg begins to go through its swing period.

TABLE 25-2	**The Gait Cycle**	
Period	**Component**	**Biomechanics and Muscle Actions**
Stance phase	Initial contact	The center of gravity is at its lowest point.
		Ankle: The ankle is held in neutral dorsiflexion through isometric activation of the dorsiflexor muscles (e.g., tibialis anterior). As the ankle transitions toward the loading response, the dorsiflexor muscles are eccentrically active to lower the ankle into plantarflexion.
		Knee: The knee is slightly flexed as a way to absorb the shock of initial weight bearing. The quadriceps are eccentrically active to allow a slight give to the flexed knee and to prevent the knee from buckling as weight is transferred onto the stance limb.
		Hip: The hip is in about 30° of flexion, and as weight-bearing continues, the hip extensor muscles are isometrically active.
	Loading response	*Ankle:* The ankle has just rapidly moved into 5° to 10° of plantarflexion. This motion is controlled through eccentric activation of the dorsiflexor muscles. Immediately following this point, the ankle begins to move toward dorsiflexion as the lower leg advances forward over the fixed foot.
		Knee: The knee continues to flex to about 15°, acting as a shock-absorbing spring; the knee extensor muscles continue to be active eccentrically.
		Hip: The hip extensor muscles shift from isometric to slight concentric activation, guiding the hip toward extension.

| TABLE 25-2 | The Gait Cycle (continued) |

Period	Component	Biomechanics and Muscle Actions
	Midstance	*Ankle:* The ankle approaches about 5° of dorsiflexion, during which time the dorsiflexor muscles are inactive and the plantarflexor muscles are eccentrically active, controlling the rate at which the lower leg advances forward over the foot.
		Knee: The knee reaches near full extension. Because the line of gravity falls just anterior to the medial-lateral axis of rotation of the knee, the knee is mechanically locked into extension, requiring little activation from the quadriceps at this time.
		Hip: The hip approaches 0° of extension, and the hip extensors such as the gluteus maximus are only slightly active to help stabilize the hip as the body is propelled forward. This activation is minimal during slow walking on level surfaces, but it increases significantly with increasing speed and slope of the walking surface. During midstance, the stance leg is in single limb support as the other leg is freely swinging toward the next step. The hip abductor muscles (e.g., gluteus medius) of the stance leg therefore are active to stabilize the hip in the frontal plane, preventing the opposite side of the pelvis from dropping excessively.
	Preswing	*Ankle:* At the beginning of preswing, the heel breaks contact with the ground and the ankle continues to dorsiflex to about 10°, stretching the Achilles tendon, which prepares the calf muscles for propulsion. As the heel lift continues, the plantarflexor muscles switch their activation from eccentric (to control forward motion of the leg) to concentric. This concentric action produces plantarflexion for propulsion or push-off.
		Knee: The extended knee prepares to flex, often driven by a short burst of activity from the hamstring muscles.
		Hip: The hip continues to extend to about 10° of extension with eccentric activation of the hip flexors, in particular the iliopsoas, helping to control the rate and amount of extension. Tight ligaments of the hip or tight hip flexor muscles will reduce the amount of extension at this point in the gait cycle, thereby reducing stride length.
	Toe-off	*Ankle:* The ankle continues plantarflexing (to about 15°) through concentric activation of the plantarflexor muscles. The muscular force for push-off is typically shared between the plantarflexors and the hip extensor muscles. Activation of the gastrocnemius and soleus is usually minimal while walking on level surfaces and at slow speed, but it increases significantly with increasing speed and incline.
		Knee: The knee is flexed 30°.
		Hip: The slightly extended hip starts to flex due to concentric activation of the hip flexor muscles.
Swing phase	Initial swing	*Ankle:* The plantarflexed ankle begins to dorsiflex by concentric activation of the dorsiflexor muscles. The dorsiflexing ankle allows the foot to clear the ground as it is advanced forward.
		Knee: The knee continues to flex, largely driven by indirect action of the flexing hip.
		Hip: The hip flexor muscles continue to contract, pulling the extended thigh forward.
	Midswing	*Ankle:* The ankle is held in neutral dorsiflexion via isometric activation of the dorsiflexor muscles.
		Knee: The knee is flexed about 45° to 55°, which helps shorten the functional length of the lower limb to facilitate its advance.
		Hip: The hip approaches about 30° of flexion through concentric activation of the hip flexor muscles.
	Terminal swing	*Ankle:* The ankle dorsiflexors continue their isometric activation, holding the ankle in neutral dorsiflexion and preparing for initial contact.
		Knee: The knee has moved from a flexed position in midswing to almost full extension.
		Hip: The hip flexor muscles, which have powered the leg in to nearly 35° of hip flexion, become inactive in terminal swing, but the hip extensor muscles are active eccentrically to decelerate the forward progression of the thigh.

This interval may be referred to as the initial double stance period, and consists of the first 0–10 percent of the gait cycle.[13]

Task 2: Single Leg Support

The middle 40 percent of the stance period is divided equally into midstance and terminal stance.

The midstance interval (refer to Figure 25-2), representing the first half of the single limb support task, begins as one foot is lifted and continues until the body weight is aligned over the forefoot.[13]

The terminal stance interval is the second half of the single limb support task. It begins when the heel of the weight-bearing foot lifts off the ground and continues until the contralateral foot strikes the ground. Terminal stance comprises the 30–50 percent phase of the gait cycle.[13]

Swing Period

Gravity and momentum are the primary sources of motion for the swing period.[2] Within the swing period, one task (limb advancement) and three to four intervals are recognized (preswing, initial swing, midswing, and terminal swing).[11–13]

> **● Key Point** In addition to representing the final portion of the stance period and single limb support task, the preswing interval is considered in some texts as part of the swing period.

Limb Advancement

The swing period involves the forward motion of the non-weight-bearing foot. The three intervals of the swing period are:[13]

1. *Initial swing:* This interval (referred to as *acceleration* in traditional terminology) begins with lifting of the foot from the floor and ends when the swinging foot is opposite the stance foot. It represents the 60–73 percent phase of the gait cycle.[13]
2. *Midswing:* This interval begins as the swinging limb is opposite the stance limb and ends when the swinging limb is forward and the tibia is vertical. It represents the 73–87 percent phase of the gait cycle.[13]
3. *Terminal swing:* This interval (referred to as *deceleration* in traditional terminology) begins with a vertical tibia of the swing leg with respect to the floor and ends the moment the foot strikes the floor. It represents the last 87–100 percent of the gait cycle.

> **● Key Point** For the swing phase, standard terminology uses the following terms: acceleration (initial swing), midswing, and deceleration (terminal swing).

> **● Key Point** The precise duration of the gait cycle intervals depends on a number of factors, including age, impairment, and the patient's walking velocity. As gait speed increases, it develops into jogging and then running, with changes in each of the intervals. For example, as speed increases, the stance period decreases and the terminal double stance phase disappears altogether. This produces a double unsupported phase.[14]

Characteristics of Normal Gait

Much has been written about the criteria for normal and abnormal gait.[10,15–23] Although the presence of symmetry in gait appears to be important, asymmetry in itself does not guarantee impairment. It must be remembered that the definition of what constitutes the so-called normal gait is elusive. Five prerequisites are required for normal gait:[7]

1. Stability of the weight-bearing foot throughout the stance period
2. Clearance of the non-weight-bearing foot during the swing period
3. Appropriate prepositioning (during terminal swing) of the foot for the next gait cycle
4. Adequate step length
5. Energy conservation

The Six Determinants of Gait

During gait, as the upper body moves forward, the trunk rotates about a vertical axis. The thoracic spine and the pelvis rotate in opposite directions to each other to enhance stability and balance. In contrast, the lumbar spine tends to rotate with the pelvis. The shoulders and trunk rotate out of phase with each other during the gait cycle.[24] Unless they are restrained, the arms tend to swing in opposition to the legs—the left arm swinging forward as the right leg swings forward, and vice versa.[2] When the arm swing is prevented, the upper trunk tends to rotate in the same direction as the pelvis, producing an inefficient gait. For gait to be efficient and to conserve energy, the center of gravity (COG) must undergo minimal displacement. To minimize the energy costs of walking, the body uses a number of biomechanical mechanisms. In 1953, Saunders, Inman, and Eberhart[25] proposed that six kinematic features—the Six Determinants—were employed to reduce the energetic cost of human walking. These determinants of gait are based on two principles: (1) Any displacement that elevates, depresses, or moves the COG beyond normal maximum excursion limits wastes energy, and (2) Any abrupt or irregular movement will waste energy even when that movement does not exceed the normal maximum displacement limits of the COG. The six determinants are:[26]

- *Pelvic rotation:* The rotation of the pelvis normally occurs about a vertical axis in the transverse plane toward the weight-bearing limb. The total pelvic rotation is approximately 4 degrees to each side.[9] Forward rotation of the pelvis on the swing side prevents an excessive drop in the body's center of gravity. The pelvic rotation also results in a relative lengthening of the femur, and thus step length, during the termination of the swing period.[13] If the pelvis does not rotate, the COG's position is somewhat lower during periods of double limb support, and the COG's total vertical displacement increases.

- *Pelvic tilt:* Lateral pelvic tilting (dropping on the unsupported side) during midstance prevents an excessive rise in the body's center of gravity. If the pelvis does not drop, the COG's position is somewhat higher during midstance, and the COG's total vertical displacement is greater.

> **● Key Point** The amount of lateral tilting of the pelvis may be accentuated in the presence of a leg length discrepancy or hip abductor weakness, the latter of which results in a Trendelenburg sign. The Trendelenburg sign is said to be positive if, when standing on one leg, the pelvis drops on the side opposite to the stance leg. The weakness is present on the side of the stance leg—the gluteus medius is not able to maintain the center of gravity on the side of the stance leg.

- *Displacement of the pelvis:* To avoid significant muscular and balancing demands, the pelvis shifts over the support point of the stance limb. If the lower extremities dropped directly vertical from the hip joint, the center of mass would have to shift 3 to 4 inches to each side to be positioned effectively over the supporting foot. The combination of femoral varus and anatomical valgum at the knee permits a vertical tibial posture with both tibias in close proximity to each other. This narrows the walking base to 5–10 centimeters (2–4 inches) from heel center to heel center, thereby reducing the lateral shift required of the COG to 2.5 centimeters (1 inch) toward either side.

- *Knee flexion in stance:* Knee motion is intrinsically associated with foot and ankle motion. At initial contact before the ankle moves into a plantarflexed position, and thus is relatively more elevated, the knee is in relative extension. Responding to a plantarflexed posture at loading response, the knee flexes. Midstance knee flexion prevents an excessive rise in the body's

COG during that period of the gait cycle. If not for the midstance knee flexion, the COG's rise during midstance would be larger, as would its total vertical displacement. Passing through midstance as the ankle remains stationary with the foot flat on the floor, the knee again reverses its direction to one of extension. As the heel comes off the floor in terminal stance, the heel begins to rise as the ankle plantarflexes, and the knee flexes. In preswing, as the forefoot rolls over the metatarsal heads, the heel elevates even more as further plantarflexion occurs and flexion of the knee increases.

> **● Key Point** The movements of the thigh and lower leg occur in conjunction with the rotation of the pelvis. The pelvis, thigh, and lower leg normally rotate toward the weight-bearing limb at the beginning of the swing period. Hip motion occurs in all three planes during the gait cycle.
> - Hip rotation occurs in the transverse plane. The hip begins in internal rotation during the loading response. Maximum internal rotation is reached near midstance and then the hip externally rotates during the swing period, with maximal external rotation occurring in terminal swing.[19]
> - The hip flexes and extends once during the gait cycle, with the limit of flexion occurring at the middle of the swing period, and the limit of extension being achieved before the end of the stance period.
> - In the frontal plane, hip adduction occurs throughout early stance and reaches a maximum at 40 percent of the cycle. Hip adduction occurs in early swing period, which is followed by slight hip abduction at the end of the swing phase, especially if a long stride is taken.[19,27,28]

- *Ankle mechanism:* For normal foot function and human ambulation, the amount of ankle joint motion required is approximately 10 degrees of dorsiflexion (to complete midstance and begin terminal stance) and 20 degrees of plantarflexion (for full push-off in preswing). At initial contact, the foot is in relative dorsiflexion due to the muscle action of the pretibial muscles and the triceps surae. This muscle action produces a relative lengthening of the leg, resulting in a smoothing of the pathway of the COG during stance phase.

> **● Key Point** In normal walking, about 60 degrees of knee motion is required for adequate clearance of the foot in the swing period. A loss of knee extension, which can occur with a flexion deformity, results in the hip being unable to extend fully, which can alter the gait mechanics.

- *Foot mechanism:* The controlled lever arm of the forefoot at preswing is particularly helpful as it rounds out the sharp downward reversal of the COG. Thus, it does not reduce a peak displacement period of the COG as the earlier determinants did, but rather smoothes the pathway.

> **● Key Point** An adaptively shortened gastrocnemius muscle may produce movement impairment by restricting normal dorsiflexion of the ankle from occurring during the midstance to heel raise portion of the gait cycle. This motion is compensated for by increased pronation of the subtalar joint, increased internal rotation of the tibia, and resultant stresses to the knee joint complex.

The Kinematics of Gait

Forces in walking can be internal or external:

- *Internal:* The ankle and hip muscles are responsible for the majority of positive (concentric) work performed during walking (54 percent of the hip and 36 percent of the ankle).[29] The knee contributes the majority of the negative (eccentric) work (56 percent).[29] The internal joint moment is the net result of all of the internal forces acting about the joint, including moments due to muscles, ligaments, joint friction, and structural constraints. The joint moment usually is calculated around a joint center; for example, a net knee extensor moment means the knee extensors (quadriceps) are dominant at the knee joint, and the knee extensors are creating a greater moment than the knee flexors (hamstrings and gastrocnemius). The units used to express moments or torques are newton meters (Nm). The term *joint power* is used to describe the product of a joint moment and the joint angular velocity. Joint power is said to be generated when the moment and the angular velocity are in the same direction and is said to be absorbed when they are in opposite directions. The units used to measure joint power are watts (W).
- *External:* Gravity and inertia are two external forces that produce the force that the foot exerts on the floor during stance phase. This is opposed by another external force: the *ground reaction force.*

> **● Key Point** Ground reaction force is any force exerted by the ground on a body in contact with it. It is composed of three components:
>
> 1. *Vertical force:* During gait, vertical ground reaction forces are created by a combination of gravity, body weight, and the firmness of the ground. Vertical ground reaction force begins with an impact peak of less than body weight and then exceeds body weight at the end of the initial contact interval, dropping during midstance, and rising again to exceed body weight, reaching its highest peak during the terminal stance interval.
> 2. *Anteroposterior shear:* Anteroposterior shear forces in walking gait begin with an anterior shear force at initial contact and the loading response intervals, and a posterior shear at the end of the terminal stance interval.
> 3. *Mediolateral shear:* Mediolateral shear in walking gait begins with an initial medial shear (occasionally lateral) after initial contact, followed by lateral shear for the remainder of the stance period.[19,28] At the end of the stance period, the shear shifts to a medial direction because of propulsion forces.

An appreciation of the six determinants of gait and the direction of the ground reaction force vector during the gait cycle leads to an understanding of muscle activity during gait.[30]

Initial Contact

At the moment the foot strikes the ground, the ankle is at the neutral position and the knee is close to full extension. In the sagittal plane, the alignment of the ground reaction force vector at initial contact is posterior to the ankle joint, creating a plantarflexion moment (Figure 25-3). The three pretibial muscles

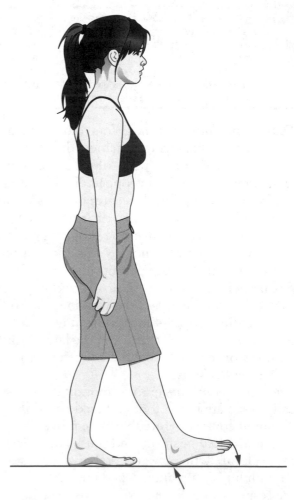

Figure 25-3   Ground reaction force at initial contact.

(tibialis anterior, extensor digitorum longus, and extensor hallucis longus), whose line of pull is anterior to the ankle joint, maintain the ankle and subtalar joint in neutral through eccentric contraction. The function of the peroneus tertius is considered identical to the extensor digitorum longus—they share the identical lateral tendon, and their muscle bellies blend into each other. At the knee, the vector is anterior to the joint axis, creating a passive extensor torque (refer to Figure 25-3). Activity of the quadriceps and hamstring muscle groups continues from the previous terminal swing to preserve and stabilize the neutral position of the knee joint. The hip and pelvis are emerging from a function of swing limb advancement with significant flexion, about 30 degrees. In normal gait, maximum hip flexion occurs during terminal swing and initial contact. A rapid high-intensity flexion moment thus is created at the hip as the vector falls anterior to the joint, placing great demand on the hip extensors. To restrain this impending flexion torque created by the anterior position of the vector, both the gluteus maximus and the hamstrings are activated. In the coronal plane, the gluteus medius is active preparing to stabilize the pelvis.

Loading Response

To absorb the impact force of loading and to maintain forward momentum, the eccentric action of the pretibial muscles regulates the rate of ankle plantarflexion. A heel rocker action occurs as the pretibials begin to pull the tibia forward over the fulcrum of the os calcis even as the foot is moving into a plantargrade position. This movement enables forward momentum of the tibia relative to the foot, but it also flexes the knee. During the peak of loading response, the magnitude of the vertical ground reaction force exceeds body weight. The pretibials (tibialis anterior, extensor halucis longus, and extensor digitorum longus) act as a shock absorber during loading response. As a shock-absorbing mechanism and for energy efficiency, the knee flexes under the eccentric action of the quadriceps to about 15 to 18 degrees. During the stance phase of gait, the maximum knee-flexion angle usually is reached at foot flat. The quadriceps muscle group following this plantargrade posture controls the degree of knee flexion. Just as the pretibials advance the tibia forward over the foot in the rocker mechanism described, the quadriceps assist in advancing the femur over the tibia. This integrated action provides controlled forward movement of the entire lower-extremity unit.

The hip maintains its posture of about 30 degrees of flexion, creating a rapid, high-intensity flexion torque, the second-highest joint torque in normal gait after the dorsiflexion torque, which occurs at the talocrural joint during terminal stance. During loading response the hip extensors (gluteus maximus, hamstrings) act as a shock absorber around the hip joint. The hamstrings also limit forward flexion of the pelvis and trunk. The function of the hamstrings when the hip is in flexion during stance is taken over by the gluteus maximus as stance progresses. Hip extensors prevent further flexion at the hip, and shock absorption is provided by the gluteus maximus, hamstrings, and adductor magnus. The medial-lateral control function of the hip adductors occurs as body weight is assumed by the stance leg.

Midstance

The momentum of forward progression over a stable foot with tibial stability maintained is referred to as the ankle rocker (Figure 25-4). The ankle rocker movement that progresses the tibia over a stationary foot is controlled early in midstance by the eccentric contraction of the soleus and is assisted by the gastrocnemius as the knee nears extension. At the beginning of midstance, the ankle is in a posture of 10 degrees of plantarflexion and moves through a range of more than 15 degrees to arrive at 5 to 7 degrees of dorsiflexion by the end of this phase. As the lower limb rolls forward over the stance foot, the body weight vector becomes anterior to the ankle joint, creating an increasing dorsiflexion moment (refer to Figure 25-4). Activity of the soleus assisted by the gastrocnemius controls the rate of dorsiflexion. Action of the plantarflexors is crucial in providing limb stability as the contralateral toe off transfers the body weight onto the stance foot.

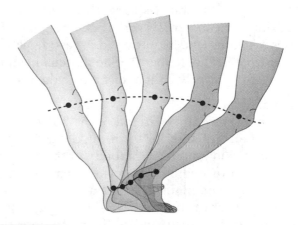

Figure 25-4   Midstance ankle rocker mechanism.

At the beginning of midstance, the vector is posterior to the knee joint but moves anterior as midstance progresses. The knee extends from 15 degrees of flexion to a neutral position. This is particularly mechanically efficient because plantarflexion of the ankle is most forceful with the knee in extension. The quads are active as knee extensors in early midstance only. Momentum of the contralateral swing leg creates an extension torque on the ipsilateral knee that decreases demand on the quadriceps and extends the knee without muscle action. By the end of midstance, the vector is anterior to the knee, creating passive stability. In the coronal plane, the ground reaction force line is medial to the anatomical knee joint on the stance side, creating a varus moment. The moment is restrained by the capsular structures of the knee, especially the lateral collateral ligaments. The hip joint is in a flexed posture of 30 degrees, which is reduced to 10 degrees as midstance progresses (with the gluteus maximus contracting to produce the progression toward hip extension). The vector is anterior to the hip in early midstance and moves increasingly posterior to the hip, gradually reducing the flexion torque and diminishing the demand on the hip extensors. The vertical ground reaction force is reduced in magnitude at midstance due to the upward momentum of the contralateral swing limb. This upward momentum improves stability at the ipsilateral hip. The gluteus maximus, at this point not needed for sagittal stability, is active as an abductor rather than a hip extensor. In the coronal plane, activity of hip abductors during midstance is essential to provide hip stability and avoid excessive pelvic tilt. In the frontal view the body mass and the ground reaction force are quite medial to the structural support point at the head of the femur. At the time of midstance during gait it has been estimated that the vertical loading on the head of the femur on the stance side reaches a magnitude approximately equal to 2½ times body weight. This creates a strong tendency toward excessive pelvic tilt (positive Trendelenberg). The gluteus medius responds to limit pelvic tilt and stabilize the pelvis.

Terminal Stance

In terminal stance, forward fall of the body moves the vector further anterior to the ankle, creating a large dorsiflexion moment. Stability of the tibia on the ankle is provided by the eccentric action of the calf muscles. The plantarflexors are more active during this heel-off period than during any other period of gait. The soleus and gastrocnemius prevent forward tibial collapse and allow the heel to rise over the metatarsal heads as the center of mass of the HAT (head, arms, and trunk) advances over the foot. This is referred to as the forefoot rocker. The forefoot rocker is composed of two components, and some believe there are two distinct forefoot rockers. The initial forefoot rocker (third rocker) begins at heel off and ends when the contralateral limb contacts the ground. The mechanics are much different in the terminal forefoot rocker (fourth rocker), which occurs in preswing as body weight rapidly is unloading the ipsilateral limb and shifting to the contralateral side. The initial forefoot rocker (third rocker) serves as an axis around which progression of the body vector advances beyond the area of foot support, creating the highest demand of the entire gait cycle on the calf muscles. Minimal ankle movement of 5 degrees is required to reach 10 degrees of dorsiflexion, which then is maintained. The maximum amount of dorsiflexion of the anatomical ankle joint occurs during heel off. The knee achieves an angular position of full extension accompanied by a mild extension torque (Figure 25-5) that diminishes in the latter part of terminal stance. Joint stability and forward progression at the knee are achieved without muscle action. Although it once was believed the hip underwent up to 10 degrees of hyperextension during this period, it actually is likely to be less—hip extension combined with 5 degrees of pelvic rotation provides a smooth progression and facilitates an increased step length. The posture of the trailing limb and the presence of the vector posterior to the hip provide passive stability at the hip joint. The tensor fascia lata serves to restrain the posterior vector at the hip. At the end of terminal stance, the magnitude of the vertical force reaches a second peak greater than body

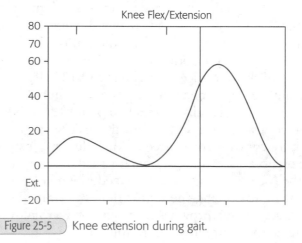

Figure 25-5 Knee extension during gait.

weight, similar to that which occurred at the end of loading response.

Preswing

During preswing, the ankle moves rapidly from its dorsiflexion position at terminal stance to 20 degrees of plantarflexion. Although the ankle reaches its angular peak of plantarflexion during this period, actual plantarflexor activity is decreased in intensity as the limb is unloaded. In late preswing, the vertical force is diminished, and the plantarflexors are quiescent. There is no "push off" in normal reciprocal free walk bipedal gait. The dorsiflexion torque present at the beginning of preswing diminishes rapidly as the metatarsophalangeal joints extend to 60 degrees. Passive knee flexion is created by planted hyperextended toes, advancement of the body past the metatarsal heads, and contralateral loading. An early extension torque at the knee quickly gives way to a flexion torque. With the vector posterior to the knee, the knee flexes rapidly to achieve 35 degrees of flexion by the end of preswing, more than half the requirement for toe clearance in swing phase. The hip flexes to a neutral position initiated by the rectus femoris, sartorius, and adductor longus and assisted by momentum. The sagittal vector extends through the hip as the hip returns to a neutral posture. The adductor longus also decelerates the passive abduction created by contralateral body weight transfer. The continuing backward rotation of the pelvis effectively lengthens the trailing limb and counteracts hip flexion.

Initial Swing

Action of the pretibial muscles and long toe extensors begins to lift the foot and the ankle, which initially are at approximately 20 degrees of plantarflexion, the maximum achieved at any period in the gait cycle (Figure 25-6). By the end of initial swing, however,

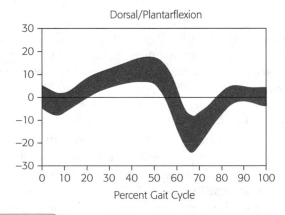

Dorsal/Plantarflexion

Figure 25-6   Action of the pretibial muscles.

the plantarflexion position is reduced to about 5 to 10 degrees, providing foot clearance for the midswing phase. Although the knee began initial swing in only 30 degrees of flexion, the momentum from hip flexion assisted by the short head of the biceps femoris, sartorius, and gracilis creates further rapid knee flexion to 60 degrees with the goal of providing limb advancement and foot clearance. The hip is flexed 20 degrees, initiated not only by the iliacus but also by activity of both the gracilis and sartorius, which contribute to flexion of both the hip and knee joints.

Midswing

The knee extends as the ankle dorsiflexes, contributing to foot clearance while advancing the tibia. Pretibial muscle activity continues to preserve foot clearance as the ankle moves further toward dorsiflexion to reach a neutral position. Movement from plantarflexion toward dorsiflexion during the swing phase is referred to as dorsiflexion recovery. Rapid knee extension, a passive event created by momentum, moves the knee from 60 to 30 degrees of flexion. Half of the knee extension needed for subsequent step length is achieved. The tibia assumes a relatively vertical position. The hip flexors continue to preserve 30 degrees of hip flexion with mild EMG activity. The foot achieves ground clearance by 1 centimeter. The gracilis, sartorius, and iliacus cut off in early midswing, and the hamstrings begin midway to decelerate the thigh. Additional limb advancement is created largely by momentum. Pelvic rotation is now neutral. The gluteus medius is quiescent on the ipsilateral side.

Terminal Swing

During terminal swing, the function of pretibial activity changes from one of foot clearance in swing to more appropriate limb placement and positioning for initial contact. A neutral position prepares the foot for the heel rocker function, assuring a heel first posture. In the second half of terminal swing, the quadriceps extend the knee concentrically in a shortening contraction to facilitate full knee extension, which, assisted by pelvic rotation, accomplishes a full step length. Eccentric contraction of both the hamstrings and the gluteus maximus is critical to accomplish deceleration of the thigh segment and restrain further hip flexion, which remains at 30 degrees. The long hamstrings have multiple roles—decelerating the leg, stabilizing the knee, and limiting hip flexion in an eccentric or lengthening contraction. The gluteus maximus prepares for the impending forces of loading.

Influences on Normal Gait

Although gait on a level surface typically occurs at the subconscious level, requiring little or no thought, there are a number of important influences that can impact the quality of gait.

Endurance: Economy of Mobility

It has been proposed that the type of gait selected is based on metabolic energy considerations.[31] Age-related declines in economy of mobility have been reported in the literature, with differing results. Some researchers reported that older adults were less economical than younger adults while walking at various speeds.[32–34] Conversely, economy of mobility appears to be unaffected by aging for individuals who maintain higher levels of physical activity.[35–37]

> ● **Key Point** The cardiovascular benefits derived from increases in gait speed may be acceptable for a normal population or advanced rehabilitation but should be used cautiously with postsurgical patients.[38]

Base of Support

The size of the base of support and its relation to the COG are important factors in the maintenance of balance and, thus, the stability of an object. The COG must be maintained over the base of support, if equilibrium is to be maintained.

> ● **Key Point** Assistive devices, such as crutches or walkers, can be prescribed to increase the base of support and, therefore, enhance stability.

Gender

On average, women walk at a higher cadence than men (6 to 9 steps higher), but at lower speeds.[23,39–42] Because leg length in women is 51.2 percent of total body height, compared with 56 percent in men, women must strike the ground more often to cover the same distance.[43] Furthermore, because their feet are shorter, women complete the heel-to-toe gait in a shorter time than men do.

Pregnancy

Substantial hormonal and anatomic changes occur during pregnancy that dramatically alter body mass, body mass distribution, and joint laxity. It is widely presumed that pregnant women exhibit marked gait deviations. However, one study[44] showed only small deviations in pelvic tilt and hip flexion, extension, and adduction occur during pregnancy.[44] It was unclear from this study whether the women

examined had gained normal amounts of weight associated with pregnancy. It would seem obvious that obesity associated with pregnancy may have differing effects on gait.

Obesity

The gait used by the obese patient is often described as a waddling gait. Depending on the degree of obesity, the waddling gait is characterized by increased lateral displacement, pelvic obliquity, hip circumduction, increased knee valgus, external foot progression angle, overpronation, and increases in the normalized dynamic base of support. The changes in the natural alignment of the weight-bearing segments may result in musculoskeletal dysfunction, including overuse injuries such as tendonitis and bursitis and eventual osteoarthritis of the hip or knee, or both.

Age

Age may be a factor in gait variations. As the body ages, there may be some decrease in both strength and flexibility. Balance strategies during gait are task specific and vary according to age and visual acuity. Consequently, older people tend not to increase their speed and stride length to the same extent as younger adults.[45] In addition, the width of the base of support tends to be wider, and the time spent in the double support phase is increased in the older adult to maintain stability.[45]

Lateral and Vertical Displacement of the COG

Rotation of the trunk may be excessive or lacking. Excessive trunk rotation may result from a restricted or exaggerated arm swing. A pelvic hike (excessive elevation of the ipsilateral side of the pelvis) may result during the swing period to help with foot clearance in the presence of inadequate hip or knee flexion, or excessive plantarflexion of the ankle.[46] Weakness of the hip abductors is noted during the single support phase of stance, because the hip abductors are required to prevent collapse of the pelvis toward the unsupported side. As previously discussed, an increase in lateral displacement may also occur with obesity.

Abnormal Gait Syndromes[47]

Each of the attributes of normal gait described earlier under "Characteristics of Normal Gait" are subject to compromise by disease states, particularly neuromuscular conditions.[29] A summary of the common gait deviations and their causes is provided in **Table 25-3**.

TABLE
25-3

Some Gait Deviations and Their Causes

Deviation	Possible Reasons
Slower cadence than expected for person's age	Generalized weakness Poor endurance Pain Joint motion restrictions Poor voluntary motor control
Shorter stance phase on involved side and decreased swing phase on uninvolved side	Pain in lower limb and/or pelvic region Decreased joint motion
Stance phase longer on one side	Pain Lack of trunk and pelvic rotation Weakness of lower limb muscles Restrictions in lower limb joints Poor muscle control Increased muscle tone
Lateral trunk lean	Ipsilateral lean—hip abductor weakness (gluteus medius/Trendelenburg gait) Contralateral lean—decreased hip flexion in swing limb Painful hip Abnormal hip joint (due to congenital dysplasia, coxa vara, etc.) Wide walking base Unequal leg length
Anterior trunk leaning at initial contact	Weak or paralyzed knee extensors or gluteus maximus Decreased ankle dorsiflexion Hip flexion contracture
Posterior trunk leaning at initial contact	Weak or paralyzed hip extensors, especially gluteus maximus (gluteus maximus gait) Hip pain Hip flexion contracture Inadequate hip flexion in swing Decreased knee range of motion
Increased lumbar lordosis at end of stance	Inability to extend hip, usually due to flexion contracture or ankylosis
Pelvic drop during stance	Contralateral gluteus medius weakness Adaptive shortening of quadratus lumborum on swing side Contralateral hip adductor spasticity
Excessive pelvic rotation	Adaptively shortened/spasticity of hip flexors on same side Limited hip joint flexion
Circumducting hip	Functional leg-length discrepancy Arthrogenic stiff hip or knee
Hip hiking	Functional leg-length discrepancy Inadequate hip flexion, knee flexion, or ankle dorsiflexion Hamstring weakness Quadratus lumborum shortening
Vaulting	Functional leg-length discrepancy Vaulting occurs on shorter limb side

(continued)

| TABLE 25-3 | Some Gait Deviations and Their Causes (continued) |

Deviation	Possible Reasons
Abnormal internal hip rotation (toe-in)	Adaptive shortening of iliotibial band
	Weakness of hip external rotators
	Femoral anteversion
	Adaptive shortening of hip internal rotators
Abnormal external hip rotation (toe-out)	Adaptive shortening of hip external rotators
	Femoral retroversion
	Weakness of hip internal rotators
Increased hip adduction (scissors gait)	Spasticity or contracture of ipsilateral hip adductors
	Ipsilateral hip adductor weakness
	Coxa vara
Inadequate hip extension (mid- and late stance)/ excessive hip flexion (swing)	Hip flexion contracture
	Iliotibial band contracture
	Hip flexor spasticity
	Pain
	Arthrodesis (surgical or spontaneous ankylosis)
	Loss of ankle dorsiflexion
Inadequate hip flexion	Hip flexor weakness
	Hip joint arthrodesis
Decreased hip swing through (psoatic limp)	Legg–Calvé–Perthes disease
	Weakness or reflex inhibition of psoas major muscle
Excessive knee extension/inadequate knee flexion at initial contact and loading response: increased knee extension during stance, and decreased knee flexion during swing	Pain
	Anterior trunk deviation/bending
	Weakness of quadriceps; hyperextension is a compensation and places body weight vector anterior to knee
	Spasticity of the quadriceps; noted more during the loading response and during initial swing intervals
	Joint deformity
Excessive knee flexion/inadequate knee extension at initial contact or around midstance: increased knee flexion in early stance, decreased knee extension in midstance and terminal stance, and decreased knee extension during swing	Knee flexion contracture, resulting in decreased step length and decreased knee extension in stance
	Increased tone/spasticity of hamstrings or hip flexors
	Decreased range of motion of ankle dorsiflexion in swing period
	Weakness of plantarflexors, resulting in increased dorsiflexion in stance
	Lengthened limb
Inadequate dorsiflexion control ("foot slap") during initial contact to midstance Steppage gait during the acceleration through deceleration of the swing phase	Weak or paralyzed dorsiflexors
	Lack of lower limb proprioception
	Weak or paralyzed dorsiflexor muscles
	Functional leg-length discrepancy
Increased walking base (>20 cm)	Deformity such as hip abductor muscle contracture
	Genu valgus
	Fear of losing balance
	Leg-length discrepancy
Decreased walking base (<10 cm)	Hip adductor muscle contracture
	Genu varum

| TABLE 25-3 | Some Gait Deviations and Their Causes (continued) |

Deviation	Possible Reasons
Excessive eversion of calcaneus during initial contact through midstance	Excessive tibia vara (refers to frontal plane position of the distal one-third of leg as it relates to supporting surface)
	Forefoot varus
	Weakness of tibialis posterior
	Excessive lower extremity internal rotation (due to muscle imbalances, femoral anteversion)
Excessive pronation during midstance through terminal stance	Insufficient ankle dorsiflexion (<10°)
	Increased tibial varum
	Compensated forefoot or rearfoot varus deformity
	Uncompensated forefoot valgus deformity
	Pes planus
	Long limb
	Uncompensated medial rotation of tibia or femur
	Weak tibialis anterior
Excessive supination during initial contact through midstance	Limited calcaneal eversion
	Rigid forefoot valgus
	Pes cavus
	Uncompensated lateral rotation of tibia or femur
	Short limb
	Plantarflexed first ray
	Upper motor neuron muscle imbalance
Excessive dorsiflexion	Compensation for knee flexion contracture
	Inadequate plantarflexor strength
	Adaptive shortening of dorsiflexors
	Increased muscle tone of dorsiflexors
	Pes calcaneus deformity
Excessive plantarflexion	Increased plantarflexor activity
	Plantarflexor contracture
Excessive varus	Contracture
	Overactivity of muscles on medial aspect of foot
Excessive valgus	Weak invertors
	Foot hypermobility
Decreased or absence of propulsion (plantarflexor gait)	Inability of plantarflexors to perform function, resulting in a shorter step length on involved side

Data from Perry J: Hip gait deviations, in Perry J (ed): Gait Analysis: Normal and Pathological Function. Thorofare, NJ, Slack, 1992, pp 245–263; Perry J: Knee abnormal gait, in Perry J (ed): Gait Analysis: Normal and Pathological Function. Thorofare, NJ, Slack, 1992, pp 223–243; Perry J: Ankle and foot gait deviations, in Perry J (ed): Gait Analysis: Normal and Pathological Function. Thorofare, NJ, Slack, 1992, pp 185–220; Perry J: Pelvis and trunk pathological gait, in Perry J (ed): Gait Analysis: Normal and Pathological Function. Thorofare, NJ, Slack, 1992, pp 265–279; Perry J: Gait analysis: Normal and pathological dunction. Thorofare, NJ, Slack, 1992; Levine D, Whittle M: Gait Analysis: The Lower Extremities. La Crosse, WI, Orthopaedic Section, APTA, 1992; and Dutton M: McGraw-Hill's NPTE (National Physical Therapy Examination). New York, McGraw-Hill, 2009

Antalgic Gait

The antalgic gait pattern can result from pain caused by disease, a joint inflammation, or an injury to the muscles, tendons, and ligaments of the lower extremity. The antalgic gait is characterized by a decrease in the stance period on the involved side in an attempt to eliminate the weight from the involved leg and use of the injured body part as much as possible. In the case of joint inflammation, attempts may be made to avoid positions of maximal intra-articular pressure and to seek the position of minimum articular pressure.[48]

Gluteus Maximus Gait

The gluteus maximus gait, which results from weakness of the gluteus maximus, is characterized by a posterior thrusting of the trunk at initial contact in an attempt to maintain hip extension of the stance leg and prevent the trunk from moving forward. Leaning the trunk posteriorly during the stance phase shifts the body's line of gravity posterior to the hip, reducing the demands of the hip extensor muscles.

Quadriceps Gait

This type of gait occurs if there is weakness of the quadriceps. Quadriceps weakness can result from a peripheral nerve lesion (femoral), spinal nerve root lesion, trauma, or disease (muscular dystrophy). To prevent buckling of the knee or excessive flexion of the knee during stance, particularly midstance, the patient compensates by maintaining the knee in extension during stance by bending forward at the waist and/or by pushing back on the thigh with the hand. The bending forward at the waist shifts the line of gravity anterior to the medial-lateral axis of the knee, thereby mechanically locking the knee in extension, which reduces the need for activation of the quadriceps muscle.

Steppage (Foot Slap) Gait

This type of gait occurs in patients with a foot drop. A foot drop is the result of weakness or paralysis of the dorsiflexor muscles resulting from an injury to the muscles, their peripheral nerve supply, or the nerve roots supplying the muscles.[49] Depending on the severity of the weakness, the patient's foot will either slap the ground at initial contact (the dorsiflexors are too weak to eccentrically control the plantarflexion), or, in severe cases, the patient has to lift the leg high enough to clear the flail foot off the floor (as though stepping over an imaginary obstacle), by flexing excessively at the hip and knee, and then slaps the foot on the floor, producing a reverse loading from the toes to the heel.

Vaulting Gait

This type of gait occurs when there is an impairment of the lower extremity that reduces the ability to functionally reduce the length of the advancing limb (e.g., an inability to flex the hip or knee). To compensate, the patient raises up on the toes of the uninvolved extremity during stance to provide extra clearance for the involved leg to swing through.

Hip Hiking Gait

This type of gait occurs when there is an inability to functionally shorten the swing leg. To compensate, there is excessive elevation of the pelvis on the side of the swing leg to provide extra clearance for the advancing leg. Alternatively, the patient may circumduct the swing leg, moving it forward in a semicircular arc to create extra clearance. However, this maneuver may place additional demands on the hip abductor muscles to help advance the swing limb.

Trendelenburg Gait

This type of gait results from weakness of the hip abductors (gluteus medius and minimus). It can be characterized in one of two ways:

- *Uncompensated:* During single-limb support the pelvis leans to the side opposite the weak hip abductor muscles. The pelvic lean lasts until initial contact on the uninvolved side and is accompanied by an apparent lateral protrusion of the affected hip. This deviation occurs because the hip abductors of the stance leg are unable to produce enough force to hold the pelvis level.
- *Compensated:* During single-limb support, the trunk and pelvis lean to the side of the weak hip abductors. This deviation occurs because by purposely leaning the pelvis and trunk to the same side as the weak hip abductors, the line of gravity shifts closer to the axis of rotation of the stance hip, reducing the external torque demands, and thereby reducing the demand on the weak hip abductors.

Gait Training with Assistive Devices

Assistive devices function to reduce ground reaction forces and increase the base of support, with the size of the base of support that they provide being proportional to the amount of reduction in these forces. Assistive devices, in order of the stability they provide, from most to least, include a walker, crutches, walker cane (hemi-walker), quad cane, straight cane, and bent cane.

Correct fitting of an assistive device is important to ensure the safety of the patient and to allow for minimal energy expenditure. Once fitted, the patient should be taught the correct walking technique with the device. The fitting depends on the device chosen:

- *Walkers, hemiwalker canes, quad canes, and standard canes:* The height of the device handle should be adjusted to the level of the greater trochanter of the patient's hip to a point 6 inches to the side of the toes and/or at the level of the ulnar styloid process with the elbow flexed to 20–25 degrees.
- *Standard crutches:* A number of methods can be used for determining the correct crutch length for axillary crutches. The crutch tip should be vertical to the ground and positioned approximately 15 centimeters (6 inches) lateral and 5 centimeters (2 inches) anterior to the patient's foot. The handgrips of the crutch are adjusted to the height of the greater trochanter of the hip of the patient and/or at the level of the ulnar styloid process with the elbow flexed to 20–25 degrees. There should be a 5- to 8-centimeter (2- to 3-inch) gap between the tops of the axillary pads and the patient's axilla. Bauer and colleagues[50] found that the best calculation of ideal crutch length was either 77 percent of the patient's height or the height minus 40.6 centimeters (16 inches).
- *Forearm/Loftstrand crutches:* The crutch is adjusted so that the handgrip is level with the greater trochanter of the patient's hip and the top of the forearm cuff 1–1.5 inches distal to the olecranon process, and/or at the level of the ulnar styloid process with the elbow flexed to 20–25 degrees.

- *Canes:* Canes are used to provide support and protection, to reduce pain in the lower extremities, and to improve balance during ambulation.[51] It is common practice to instruct patients with lower extremity pain to use the cane in the hand contralateral to the symptomatic side.[52] The use of a cane in the contralateral hand helps preserve reciprocal motion and a more normal pathway for the COG.[53] Use of a cane can transmit 20–25 percent of body weight away from the lower extremities.[54,55] The cane also allows the subject to increase the effective base of support, thereby decreasing the hip abductor force exerted.

The clinician must always provide adequate physical support and instruction while working with a patient using an assistive gait device. The clinician positions him- or herself posterolaterally on the involved side of the patient, to be able to assist the patient on the side where the patient will most likely have difficulty. In addition, a gait belt should be fitted around the patient's waist to enable the clinician to assist the patient.

The selection of the proper gait pattern to instruct the patient is dependent on the patient's balance, strength, cardiovascular status, coordination, functional needs, and weight-bearing status (**Table 25-4**). In addition to observing the weight-bearing status, the patient may be prescribed an appropriate gait pattern. Several gait patterns are recognized.

Two-Point Pattern

The two-point gait pattern, which closely approximates the normal gait pattern, requires the use of an assistive gait device (canes or crutches) on each

TABLE 25-4	Types of Weight-Bearing Status	
Weight-Bearing Status	**Description**
Non–weight bearing (NWB)	Patient not permitted to bear any weight through the injured limb.
Partial weight bearing (PWB)	Patient permitted to bear a portion (e.g., 25%, 50%) of his or her weight through the injured limb.
Touch-down weight-bearing (TDWB)/ toe-touch weight-bearing (TTWB)	Patient permitted minimal contact of the injured limb with the ground for balance. The expression "as though walking on eggshells" can be used to help the patient understand.
Weight bearing as tolerated (WBAT)	The patient is permitted to bear as much weight through the injured limb as is comfortable.
Full weight bearing	Patient no longer medically requires an assistive device.

side of the body. This pattern requires the patient to move the assistive gait device and the contralateral lower extremity at the same time (Figure 25-7). This pattern requires some coordination and is used when there are no weight-bearing restrictions in the presence of bilateral weakness or when there is a need to enhance balance.

Two-Point Modified

The two-point modified pattern is the same as the two-point except that it requires only one assistive device, positioned on the opposite side of the involved lower extremity. This pattern cannot be used if there are any weight-bearing restrictions (i.e., PWB, NWB), but is appropriate for a patient with unilateral weakness

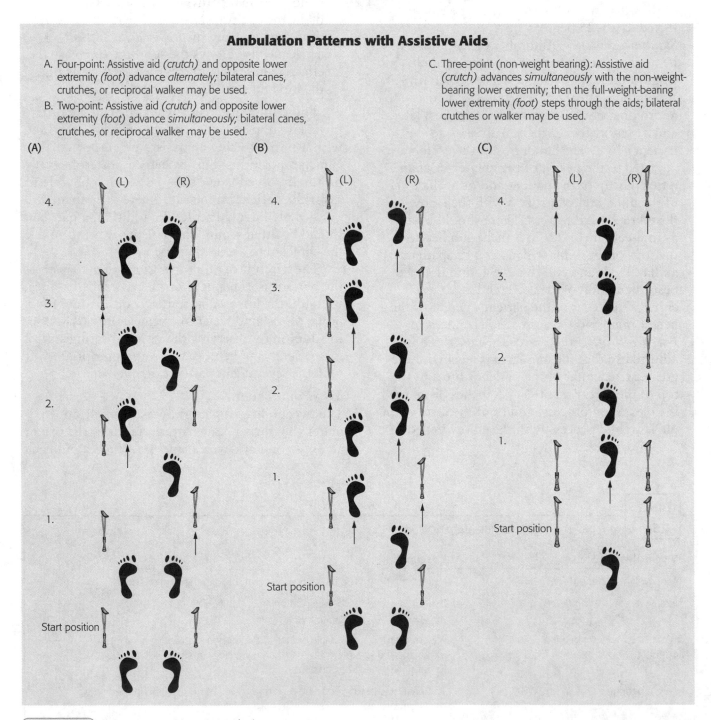

Ambulation Patterns with Assistive Aids

A. Four-point: Assistive aid *(crutch)* and opposite lower extremity *(foot)* advance *alternately;* bilateral canes, crutches, or reciprocal walker may be used.

B. Two-point: Assistive aid *(crutch)* and opposite lower extremity *(foot)* advance *simultaneously;* bilateral canes, crutches, or reciprocal walker may be used.

C. Three-point (non-weight bearing): Assistive aid *(crutch)* advances *simultaneously* with the non-weight-bearing lower extremity; then the full-weight-bearing lower extremity *(foot)* steps through the aids; bilateral crutches or walker may be used.

Figure 25-7   Gait patterns with assistive devices.

Adapted from Frank M. Pierson and Sheryl L. Fairchild, *Principles and Techniques of Patient Care Philadelphia:* W. B. Saunders Company, 1994.

D. Three-one-point (partial weight bearing): Assistive aid *(crutch)* and partial-weight-bearing lower extremity *(foot)* advance *simultaneously;* then the full-weight-bearing lower extremity steps through the aids; bilateral cane, crutches, or walker may be used.

E. Modified four-point: Only one assistive aid *(crutch)* is used; the assistive aid and the opposite lower extremity *(foot)* advance *alternately;* the assistive aid is held in the hand a

opposite the affected lower extremity; one cane or crutch may be used.

F. Modified two-point: Only one assistive aid *(crutch)* is used; the assistive aid and the opposite lower extremity *(foot)* advance *simultaneously;* the assistive aid is held in the hand opposite the affected lower extremity; one cane or crutch may be used.

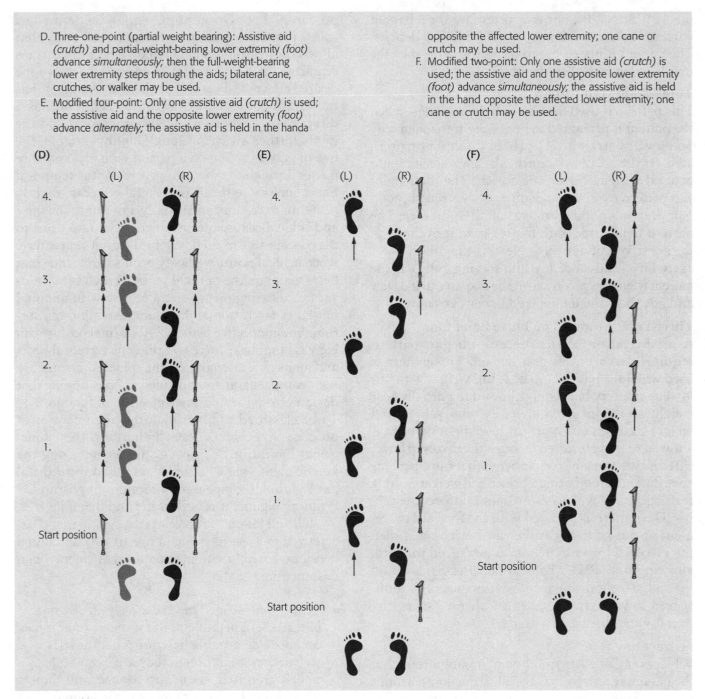

Figure 25-7   *(Continued)*

or mild balance deficits. The patient is instructed to move the cane and the involved leg simultaneously, and then the uninvolved leg (refer to Figure 25-7).

Four-Point Pattern

The four-point gait pattern, which requires the use of an assistive gait device (canes or crutches) on each side of the body, is used when the patient requires maximum assistance with balance and stability. The pattern is initiated with the forward movement of one of the assistive gait devices, and then

the contralateral lower extremity, the other assistive gait device, and finally the opposite lower extremity (e.g., right crutch, then left foot; left crutch, then right foot).

Four-Point Modified

The four-point modified pattern is the same as the four-point except that it requires only one assistive device, positioned on the opposite side of the involved lower extremity. This pattern cannot be used if there are any weight-bearing restrictions (i.e., PWB, NWB), but is appropriate for a patient with unilateral weakness or mild balance deficits. The patient is instructed to move the cane, then the involved leg, and then the uninvolved leg.

Three-Point Gait Pattern

This pattern is used for non–weight bearing—when the patient is permitted to bear weight through only one lower extremity. The three-point gait pattern involves the use of two crutches or a walker. It cannot be used with a cane or one crutch. The three-point gait pattern requires good upper body strength, good balance, and good cardiovascular endurance. The pattern is initiated with the forward movement of the assistive gait device(s). Next, the involved lower extremity is advanced, while staying NWB as the patient then presses down on the assistive gait device and advances the uninvolved lower extremity.

Three-Point Modified or Three Point One

A modification of the three-point gait pattern requires two crutches or a walker. This pattern is used when the patient can bear full weight with one lower extremity but is only allowed to partially bear weight on the involved lower extremity. In partial weight bearing, only part of the patient's weight is allowed to be transferred through the involved lower extremity. It must be remembered that most patients have difficulty replicating a prescribed weight-bearing restriction and will need constant reinforcement.[56]

The pattern is initiated with the forward movement of one of the assistive gait devices, and then the involved lower extremity is advanced forward, allowing only PWB. The patient presses down on the assistive gait device and advances the uninvolved lower extremity, using either a "swing-to" or a "swing-through" pattern.

Instructions

Whichever gait pattern is chosen, it is important that the patient receive verbal and illustrated instructions for use of the assistive gait device to negotiate stairs, curbs, ramps, doors, and transfers. These instructions should include any weight-bearing precautions pertinent to the patient, the appropriate gait sequence, and a contact number at which to reach the clinician if questions arise.

Posture

As with the so-called good movement, good posture is a subjective term reflecting what the clinician believes to be correct based on ideal models. Various attempts have been made to define and interpret posture.[27,57–60] Good posture may be defined as "the optimal alignment of the patient's body that allows the neuromuscular system to perform actions requiring the least amount of energy to achieve the desired effect."[61] Postural or skeletal alignment has important consequences because each joint has a direct effect on both its neighboring joint and the joints further away. Although highly variable, the line of gravity acting on a person with ideal posture passes through the mastoid process of the temporal bone, anterior to the second sacral vertebra, slightly posterior to the hip, and slightly anterior to the knee and ankle. Because the line of gravity courses just to the concave side of each vertebral region's curvature, when in ideal posture, gravity produces a torque that helps maintain the optimal shape of each spinal curvature, allowing one to stand at ease with minimal muscular activation and minimal stress on the surrounding connective tissues.[61] Abnormal posture can increase the shear forces on the intervertebral disks and joints that interconnect the spine. Abnormal, or *nonneutral*, alignment is defined as "positioning that deviates from the midrange position of function."[62] To be classified as abnormal, the alignment must produce physical functional limitations. These functional limitations can occur anywhere along the kinetic chain (see Chapter 4), at adjacent or distal joints through compensatory motions or postures.[63] Postural alignment is both static and dynamic.

Jull and Janda[64–66] developed a system that characterized muscles as being in one of two functional divisions, based on common patterns of kinetic chain dysfunction:

- *Postural muscles:* These relatively strong muscles are designed to counter gravitational forces and provide a stable base for other muscles to work from, although they are likely to be poorly recruited, lax in appearance, and show an inability to perform inner range contractions over time (e.g., rotator cuff, rhomboids, mid and lower trapezius).
- *Phasic muscles:* These muscles tend to function in a dynamically antagonistic manner to the postural muscles. Phasic muscles tend to become relatively weak compared to the postural muscles, are more prone to atrophy and adaptive shortening, and show preferential recruitment in synergistic activities. In addition, these muscles will tend to dominate movements and may alter posture by restricting movement (e.g., upper trapezius, deltoid, latissimus dorsi).

The pain from any sustained position is thought to result from ischemia of the isometrically contracting muscles, localized fatigue, or an excessive mechanical strain on the structures. Intramuscular pressure can compress the blood vessels and prevent the removal of metabolites and the supply of oxygen, either of which can cause temporary pain.[70,71] Although most clinicians can appreciate that repeated movement patterns performed in a therapeutic manner may be beneficial, it must also be remembered that repeated motions performed erroneously can produce changes in muscle tension, strength, length, and stiffness.[72]

It is quite normal for muscles to frequently change their lengths during movements; however, this change in resting length may become pathologic when it is sustained through incorrect habituation or as a response to pain.

Muscles maintained in a shortened or lengthened position eventually will adapt to their new positions. These muscles initially are incapable of producing a maximal contraction in the newly acquired positions;[74] however, changes at the sarcomere level eventually allow the muscle to produce maximal tension at this new length.[72] Although this may appear to be a satisfactory adaptation, the changes in length produce changes in tension development, as well as changes in the angle of pull.[75]

The ability to maintain correct posture appears to be related to a number of factors including disease, energy cost, strength and flexibility, age, pregnancy, and habit:[76,77]

- *Disease:* The adult spine is divided into four curves: two primary, or posterior, curves, and two compensatory, or anterior, curves. The posterior curves are in the thoracic and sacral regions. *Kyphosis* is a term used to denote a posterior curve. The anterior curves are in the cervical and lumbar region. *Lordosis* is a term used to describe an anterior curve. Together, the curves function to withstand the effects of gravity and other external forces. The normal coronal alignment of the spine can be altered by many conditions, including joint degeneration and scoliosis. Scoliosis, which is a descriptive term for lateral curvature, is usually accompanied by a rotational abnormality. Scoliosis (see Chapter 22) can be idiopathic; a result of congenital deformity, pain, or degeneration; or be associated with numerous neuromuscular conditions, such as leg-length inequality. Sagittal plane alignment can also be altered by disease and injury, and is manifested clinically with areas of excessive kyphosis or lordosis, or a loss of the normal curves. Respiratory conditions (e.g., emphysema), general weakness, excess weight, loss of proprioception, or muscle spasm (as seen in cerebral palsy or with trauma) may also lead to poor posture.[78]
- *Energy cost:*[77] The increase in metabolic rate over the basal rate when standing is so small compared with the metabolic cost of moving and exercising, as to be negligible. The abnormal type of posture that involves a minimum of metabolic increase over the basal rate is one in which the knees are hyperextended, the hips are pushed forward to the limit of extension, the thoracic curve is increased, the head is projected forward, and the upper trunk is inclined backward in a posterior lean (also known as slouched or sway-back posture—see later in this chapter).
- *Strength and flexibility:* Pathological changes to the neuromuscular system (e.g., excessive wearing of the articular surfaces of joints, the development of osteophytes and traction spurs, and maladaptive changes in the length-tension development and angle of pull of muscles and tendons) may be the result of the cumulative effect of repeated small stresses (microtrauma) over a long period of time or of constant abnormal stresses (macrotrauma) over a short period of time. Strong, flexible muscles are able to resist the detrimental effects of faulty postures for longer periods and provide the ability to unload the structures through a change of position. However, these changes in

position are not possible if the joints are stiff (hypomobile) or too mobile (hypermobile), or the muscles are weak, shortened, or lengthened.

- *Age:* As the human body develops from infancy to old age, several physical and neurological factors may affect posture. At birth, a series of primary curves cause the entire vertebral column to be concave forward, or flexed, giving a kyphotic posture to the whole spine, although the overall contour in the coronal plane is straight. At the other end of the lifespan, there may be numerous causes for age-related postural changes. With increasing age there is an increased probability for developing specific pathologies that lead to accelerated degeneration in neural and/or musculoskeletal systems.[79] A relatively inactive lifestyle also may result in disuse-related changes in the neuromuscular system, including muscle weakness and slowed response time. In elderly persons, weaker muscles impose a relatively higher demand during muscular activity, leading to early fatigue and postural imbalance.[80] Reduced sensation, leg muscle weakness, and increased reaction time appear to be important factors associated with postural instability in the elderly.[81]
- *Pregnancy:* Although not yet substantiated, postural changes have often been implicated as a major cause of back pain in pregnant women.[82,83] The relationship between posture and the back pain experienced during pregnancy is unclear. This may be because significant skeletal alignment changes that are related to back pain are occurring at the pelvis during pregnancy, but may not be directly measured by postural assessments, such as lumbar lordosis, sacral base angle (the angle that the superior border of the first sacral vertebral body makes with the horizontal, which optimally is 30 degrees), and pelvic tilt. The results from a study by Franklin and Conner-Kerr[84] suggest that from the first to the third trimester of pregnancy, lumbar lordosis, posterior head position, lumbar angle, and pelvic tilt increase; however, the magnitudes and the changes of these posture variables are not related to back pain (see Chapter 24).
- *Habit:* The most common postural problem is poor postural habit and its associated adaptive changes. Poor posture, and, in particular, poor sitting posture, is considered to be a major contributing factor in the development and perpetuation of shoulder, neck, and back pain. Two of the

manifestations of poor sitting posture are a forward head (increased flexion of the lower cervical and upper thoracic regions, increased extension of the upper cervical vertebrae, and extension of the occiput on C1) and forward rounded shoulders. Dynamic postural habits can also result in dysfunction. For example, loads carried in a backpack shift the COG behind the body. In order to compensate, the COG of the body plus the load is moved back over the base of support: the feet. This is accomplished by either leaning forward at the ankle or the hip or inclining the head; the rigidity of postural muscles controlling these adjustments increases to support the load.[85] As individuals fatigue and these changes become more pronounced, there is potential for injury to the load carrier.[85]

- *Pain:* The motor system tends to prioritize its response in relation to incoming sensory information or demands placed upon it. Nociception appears to occupy high priority in this relative system. Pain can cause the body to unconsciously adopt a posture that decreases the pain. For example, pressure on a nerve root in the lumbar spine can lead to pain in the back and result in a sciatic scoliosis.

Postural Examination

To assess posture accurately, the patient must be adequately undressed. Standard protocols for patient attire vary with respect to, among other factors, regional, societal, religious, legal, healthcare specialty, gender, and age-related issues.[86] Ideally, male patients should be in shorts, and female patients should be in a bra and shorts, and the patient should not wear shoes or stockings. The patient should assume a comfortable and relaxed posture, looking straight ahead, with feet approximately 4–6 inches apart.

> **● Key Point** A simple and commonly applied parameter of global balance is the plumbline offset taken from a full-length standing radiograph. The center of C2 (or C7) is drawn vertically downward, and the distance from the center of the sacrum is noted on the coronal projection, while the offset from the anterior–superior edge or posterior–superior edge of S1 is noted on the lateral projection.

When observing a patient for abnormalities in posture, the clinician looks for asymmetry.[78] Regional asymmetry should trigger further evaluation of that area, but asymmetry alone does not confirm or rule out the presence of dysfunction. A summary of the most common findings and faults are outlined in Figure 25-8 and listed in **Table 25-5.**

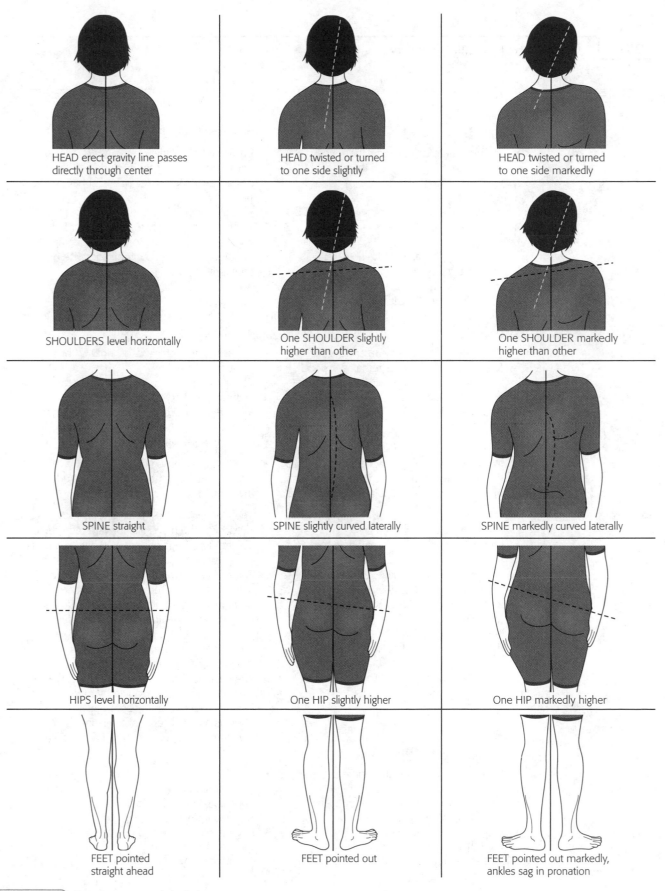

HEAD erect gravity line passes
directly through center

HEAD twisted or turned
to one side slightly

HEAD twisted or turned
to one side markedly

SHOULDERS level horizontally

One SHOULDER slightly
higher than other

One SHOULDER markedly
higher than other

SPINE straight

SPINE slightly curved laterally

SPINE markedly curved laterally

HIPS level horizontally

One HIP slightly higher

One HIP markedly higher

FEET pointed
straight ahead

FEET pointed out

FEET pointed out markedly,
ankles sag in pronation

Figure 25-8 Common postural deviations.

TABLE
25-5
Good and Faulty Posture Summary

	Good Posture	Faulty Posture
Head	• Head is held erect in a position of good balance.	• Chin is up too high. • Head is protruding forward. Head is tilted or rotated to one side.
Shoulder and arms	• Shoulders are level, and neither one is more forward or backward than the other when seen from the side. • Arms hang relaxed at the sides with palms of the hands facing toward the body. • Elbows are slightly bent, so forearms hang slightly forward. • Scapulae lie flat against the rib cage. • Scapulae are neither too close together nor too wide apart (in adults; a separation of approximately 10 centimeters (4 inches) is average).	• Arms are held stiffly in any position forward, backward, or out from the body. • Arms are turned so that palms of hands face backward. • One shoulder is higher than the other. Both shoulders are hiked up. One or both shoulders is drooping forward or sloping. • Shoulders are rotated either clockwise or counterclockwise. • Scapulae are pulled back too hard. Scapulae are too far apart. • Scapulae are too prominent, standing out from the rib cage ("winged scapulae").
Chest	• Chest should be slightly up and slightly forward (while the back remains in good alignment) and in a position about halfway between that of a full inspiration and a forced expiration.	• Chest is in a depressed, or "hollow-chest," position. • Chest is lifted and held up too high, caused by arching the back. • Ribs are more prominent on one side than on the other. • Lower ribs are flaring out or protruding.
Abdomen	• In young children up to about the age of 10, the abdomen normally protrudes somewhat. • In older children and adults, it should be flat.	• The entire abdomen protrudes. • The lower part of the abdomen protrudes while the upper part is pulled in.
Spine and pelvis (side view)	• The front of the pelvis and the thighs are in a straight line. • The buttocks are not prominent in back but instead slope slightly downward. • The spine has four natural curves. In the neck and lower back, the curve is forward, and in the upper back and lowest part of the spine (sacral region), it is backward. • The sacral curve is a fixed curve, whereas the other three are flexible.	• The low back arches forward too much (lordosis). The pelvis tilts forward too much. The front of the thigh forms an angle with the pelvis when this tilt is present. • The normal forward curve in the low back has straightened out. The pelvis tips backward, and there is a slightly backward slant to the line of the pelvis in relation to the front of the hips (flat back). • There is an increased backward curve in the upper back (kyphosis or round upper back). • The neck has an increased forward curve, almost always accompanied by round upper back and seen as a forward head. • There is a lateral curve of the spine (scoliosis), toward one side (C-curve) or toward both sides (S-curve).
Hips, pelvis, and spine (back view)	• Ideally, the body weight is borne evenly by both feet, and the hips are level. • One side is not more prominent than the other as seen from front or back, nor is one hip more forward or backward than the other as seen from the side. • The spine does not curve to the left or the right side.	• One hip is higher than the other (lateral pelvic tilt). Sometimes it is not really much higher but appears so because a sideways sway of the body has made it more prominent. • The hips are rotated so that one is farther forward than the other (clockwise or counterclockwise rotation).

**TABLE
25-5**   Good and Faulty Posture Summary (continued)

	Good Posture	Faulty Posture
Knees and legs	• Legs are straight up and down. • Patellae face straight ahead when feet are in good position. Looking at the knees from the side, the knees are straight (i.e., neither bent forward nor "locked" backward).	• Knees touch when feet are apart (genu valgum). • Knees are apart when feet touch (genu varum). • Knee curves slightly backward (hyperextended knee) (genu recurvatum). • Knee bends slightly forward—that is, it is not as straight as it should be (flexed knee). Patellae face slightly toward each other (medially rotated femurs). • Patellae face slightly outward (laterally rotated femurs).
Foot	• In standing, the longitudinal arch has the shape of a half dome. • Barefoot, the feet toe-out slightly.	• There is a low longitudinal arch or flatfoot. • There is a low metatarsal arch, usually indicated by calluses under the ball of the foot. • Weight is borne on the inner side of the foot (pronation; "Ankle rolls in"). • Weight is borne on the outer border of the foot (supination; "Ankle rolls out"). • Toeing-out occurs while walking or while standing in shoes with heels ("outflared" or "slue-footed"). • Toeing-in occurs while walking or standing ("pigeon-toed").
Toes	• Toes should be straight—that is, neither curled downward nor bent upward. They should extend forward in line with the foot and not be squeezed together or overlap.	• Toes bend up at the first joint and down at middle and end joints so that the weight rests on the tips of the toes (hammer toes). This fault is often associated with wearing shoes that are too short. • The big toe slants inward toward the midline of the foot (hallus valgus). This fault is often associated with wearing shoes that are too narrow and pointed at the toes.

Data from Magee DJ: Assessment of posture, in Magee DJ (ed): Orthopedic Physical Assessment. Philadelphia, WB Saunders, 2002, pp 873–903; Kendall FP, McCreary EK, Provance PG: Muscles: Testing and Function. Baltimore, Williams & Wilkins, 1993; and Dutton M: Orthopaedic Examination, Evaluation, and Intervention (ed 2). New York, McGraw Hill, 2008

Common Faulty Postures

Due to the relationships among the head, neck, thorax, lumbar spine, and pelvis, any deviation in one region can affect the other areas.

Pelvic and Lumbar Region

The more common faulty postures of the pelvic and lumbar region include lordotic posture, slouched posture, and flat low back posture.[87]

Lordotic Posture

This is characterized by an increase in the lumbosacral angle, an increase in lumbar lordosis, and an increase in the anterior pelvic tilt and hip flexion (Figure 25-9).[88] This posture is commonly seen in pregnancy, obesity, and those individuals with weakened abdominal muscles. Potential muscle impairments include:

- Decreased mobility in the hip flexor muscles (iliopsoas, tensor fascia latae, rectus femoris) and lumbar extensor muscles (erector spinae)
- Impaired muscle performance due to stretched and weakened abdominal muscles (rectus abdominis, internal and external obliques, and transversus abdominis)

This posture places stress throughout the lumbar spine on the anterior longitudinal ligament and the zygapophyseal (facet) joints, and narrows the

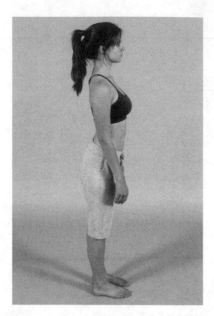

Figure 25-9 Lordotic posture.

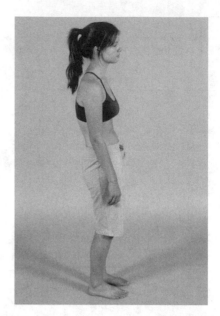

Figure 25-11 Flat low back posture.

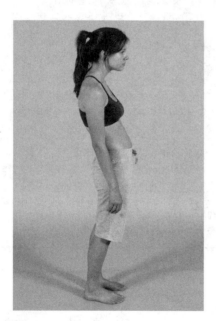

Figure 25-10 Slouched posture.

posterior disk space and the intervertebral foramen, all of which are potential sources of symptoms.

Slouched Posture

This posture, also referred to as the swayback,[57] is characterized by a shifting of the entire pelvic segment anteriorly, resulting in relative hip extension, and a shifting of the thoracic segment posteriorly, resulting in a relative flexion of the thorax on the upper lumbar spine (Figure 25-10). As a result, there

is an increased lordosis in the lower lumbar region, increased kyphosis in the thoracic region, and usually a forward (protracted) head. This posture is commonly seen throughout most age groups and is typically the result of fatigue or muscle weakness. Potential muscle impairments include:

- Decreased mobility in the upper abdominal muscles (upper segments of the rectus abdominis and obliques), internal intercostal, hip extensor, and lower lumbar extensor muscles and related fascia
- Impaired muscle performance due to stretched and weakened lower abdominal muscles (lower segments of the rectus abdominis and obliques), extensor muscles of the lower thoracic region, and hip flexor muscles.

This posture places stress on the iliofemoral ligaments, the anterior longitudinal ligament of the lower lumbar spine, and the posterior longitudinal ligament of the upper lumbar or thoracic spine. In addition, there is narrowing of the intervertebral foramen in the lower lumbar spine and approximation of the zygapophyseal (facet) joints in the lower lumbar spine.

Flat Low Back Posture

This is characterized by a decreased lumbosacral angle, decreased lumbar lordosis/extension, and posterior tilting of the pelvis (Figure 25-11). This posture is commonly seen in those individuals who spend long periods slouching, or flexing in the sitting or standing positions. The potential muscle impairments include:

- Decreased mobility in the trunk flexor (rectus abdominis, intercostals) and hip extensor muscles
- Impaired muscle performance due to stretched and weak lumbar extensor and possibly hip flexor muscles

This posture can apply stress on the posterior longitudinal ligament, the posterior disk space, and the normal physiological lumbar curve, which reduces the shock absorbing effects of the lumbar region and predisposes the patient to injury.

Cervical and Thoracic Region

The more common faulty postures of the cervical and thoracic region include round back with forward head and flat upper back and neck.[87]

Round Back with Forward Head

This is characterized by an increased kyphotic thoracic curve, protracted scapulae (round shoulders), and forward head (excessive flexion of the lower cervical spine and hyperextension of the upper cervical spine). The causes for this posture are similar to those found with the flat low back posture. The potential muscle impairments include:

- Decreased mobility in the muscles of the anterior thorax (intercostal muscles), muscles of the upper extremity originating on the thorax (pectoralis major and minor, latissimus dorsi, serratus anterior), muscles of the cervical spine and head that attach to the scapular and upper thorax (levator scapulae, sternocleidomastoid, scalene, upper trapezius), and muscles of the suboccipital region (rectus capitis posterior major and minor, obliquus capitis inferior and superior)
- Impaired muscle performance due to stretched and weak lower cervical and upper thoracic erector spinae and scapular retractor muscles (rhomboids, middle trapezius), anterior throat muscles (suprahyoid and infrahyoid), and capital flexors (rectus capitis anterior and lateralis, superior oblique longus colli, longus capitis)

This posture can cause the following problems:

- Excessive stress on the anterior longitudinal ligament in the upper cervical spine and posterior longitudinal ligament in the lower cervical and thoracic spine
- Irritation of the zygapophyseal (facet) joints in the upper cervical spine

- Impingement on the neurovascular bundle due to anterior scalene or pectoralis minor muscle tightness (thoracic outlet syndrome)
- Impingement of the cervical plexus from levator scapulae muscle tightness
- Temporomandibular joint dysfunction
- Lower cervical disk lesions

Flat Upper Back and Neck Posture

This is characterized by a decrease in the thoracic curve, depressed scapulae, depressed clavicles, and decreased cervical lordosis with increased flexion of the occiput on the atlas. Although not common, this posture occurs primarily with exaggeration of the military posture. The potential muscle impairments include:

- Decreased mobility in the anterior neck muscles, thoracic erector spinae, and scapular retractors, with potentially restricted scapular movement, which can interfere with shoulder elevation
- Impaired muscle performance in the scapular protractor and intercostal muscles of the anterior thorax

This posture can place stress on the neurovascular bundle in the thoracic outlet between the clavicle and ribs, and can decrease the shock absorbing function of the kyphotic curvature, thereby predisposing the neck to injury.

Intervention

The methods for postural correction involve appropriate strengthening of weak muscles, stretching of adaptively shortened structures, and educating the patient on the importance of maintaining a correct posture while standing, sitting, or performing other activities of daily living. The focus of therapeutic intervention for posture and movement impairment syndromes is to alleviate symptoms and to play a significant role in educating the patient against habitual abuse. Interestingly, despite the widespread inclusion of postural correction in therapeutic interventions, there is limited experimental data to support its effectiveness. The intervention for any muscle imbalance is divided into three stages:

1. Restoration of normal length of the muscles
2. Strengthening of the muscles that have become inhibited and weak
3. Establishing optimal motor patterns to secure the best possible protection to the joints and the surrounding soft tissues

Summary

For most individuals, gait and posture are innate characteristics, as much a part of their personality as their smile. Indeed, many people can be recognized in a group by their gait or posture. Normal human gait involves the complex synchronization of the cardiopulmonary and neuromuscular systems. The energy required for gait is largely a factor of the health of the cardiopulmonary systems. The lower kinetic chain is a specialized system designed for human locomotion. Once mastered, gait allows us to move around our environment in an efficient manner and allows the arms and hands to be free for exploration of the environment. Although gait appears to be a simple process consisting of a series of rotations allowing translation of the entire body through space,[89] it is prone to breakdown.

Postural development begins at a very early age. As the infant starts to activate the postural system, skeletal muscles develop according to their predetermined specific uses in various recurrent functions and movement strategies.[86] In a multisegmented organism such as the human body, many postures are adopted throughout the course of a day. Nonneutral alignment, whether maintained statically or performed repetitively, appears to be a key precipitating factor in soft tissue and neurologic pain.[67] This may be the result of an alteration in joint load distribution or in the force transmission of the muscles. This alteration can result in a muscle imbalance.

REVIEW Questions

1. Give three of the major requirements for successful walking.
2. Define the gait cycle.
3. What are the functional tasks associated with normal gait?
4. What are the two periods of the gait cycle?
5. What are the intervals of the stance phase called?
6. What are the four intervals of the swing phase called?
7. What are the three gait parameters that are the most meaningful to measure in the clinic?
8. What are the three primary determinants of gait velocity?
9. What is the average normal cadence in adults without pathology?
10. Where is the center of gravity (COG) of the body located?
11. True or false: During the gait cycle, the COG is displaced both vertically and posteriorly.
12. True or false: During the gait cycle, the thoracic spine and the pelvis rotate in the same direction to enhance stability and balance.
13. Describe the characteristics of a positive Trendelenburg sign.
14. List three effects that a weak tibialis anterior could have on gait.
15. During the normal gait cycle, when do the hamstrings have their maximum activity?
16. A positive Trendelenburg sign results from paralysis of:
    a. Hip flexors
    b. Hip abductors
    c. Hip extensors
    d. Hip adductors
17. You are observing a patient walking. The patient lurches backward during the stance phase. What type of gait is the patient demonstrating?
    a. Wide-based gait
    b. Antalgic gait
    c. Gluteus medius gait
    d. Extensor gait
18. An individual demonstrates a steppage gait pattern during ambulation activities. Steppage gait is characterized by excessive:
    a. Knee and hip extension
    b. Knee and hip flexion
    c. Knee and ankle flexion
    d. Knee and ankle extension
19. Weakness of which muscle can cause a Trendelenburg gait pattern?
20. While observing the gait of a 67-year-old man with arthritis of the left hip, you observe a left lateral trunk lean during stance. Why does the patient present with this gait deviation?
    a. To increase the joint compression force of the involved hip by moving the weight toward it
    b. To decrease the joint compression force by moving the weight toward the involved hip
    c. To bring the line of gravity closer to the involved hip joint
    d. Because his right leg is shorter
21. You observe a patient demonstrating a significant posterior trunk lean at initial contact. Which is the most likely muscle that you will need to focus on during the exercise session in order to minimize this gait deviation?

22. A patient who has had a recent fracture of the right tibia and fibula has developed foot drop of the right foot during gait. Which nerve is causing this loss of motor function?

23. You are observing a patient with excessive subtalar pronation in standing. What other postural adaptations are you likely to notice at the tibia, femur, and pelvis?

24. Which abnormal posture is characterized by an increase in the lumbosacral angle, an increase in lumbar lordosis, and an increase in the anterior pelvic tilt and hip flexion?

25. Which abnormal posture is characterized by a shifting of the entire pelvic segment anteriorly, resulting in relative hip extension, and a shifting of the thoracic segment posteriorly, resulting in a relative flexion of the thorax on the upper lumbar spine?

26. A patient presents with a flat low back posture. Which muscle imbalances would you expect to be associated with this posture?

References

1. Mann RA, Hagy JL, White V, et al: The initiation of gait. J Bone Joint Surg 61A:232–239, 1979

2. Luttgens K, Hamilton N: Locomotion: Solid surface, in Luttgens K, Hamilton N (eds): Kinesiology: Scientific Basis of Human Motion (ed 9). Dubuque, IA, McGraw-Hill, 1997, pp 519–549

3. Donatelli R, Wilkes R: Lower kinetic chain and human gait. J Back Musculoskel Rehabil 2:1–11, 1992

4. Luttgens K, Hamilton N: The center of gravity and stability, in Luttgens K, Hamilton N (eds): Kinesiology: Scientific Basis of Human Motion (ed 9). Dubuque, IA, McGraw-Hill, 1997, pp 415–442

5. Epler M: Gait, in Richardson JK, Iglarsh ZA (eds): Clinical Orthopaedic Physical Therapy. Philadelphia, WB Saunders, 1994, pp 602–625

6. Perry J: Stride analysis, in Perry J (ed): Gait Analysis: Normal and Pathological Function. Thorofare, NJ, Slack, 1992, pp 431–441

7. Perry J: Gait Analysis: Normal and Pathological Function. Thorofare, NJ, Slack, 1992

8. Rogers MM: Dynamic foot mechanics. J Orthop Sports Phys Ther 21:306–316, 1995

9. Gage JR, Deluca PA, Renshaw TS: Gait analysis: Principles and applications with emphasis on its use with cerebral palsy. Inst Course Lect 45:491–507, 1996

10. Levine D, Whittle M: Gait Analysis: The Lower Extremities. La Crosse, WI, Orthopaedic Section, American Physical Therapy Association, 1992

11. Scranton PE, Jr., Rutkowski R, Brown TD: Support phase kinematics of the foot, in Bateman JE, Trott AW (eds): The Foot and Ankle. New York, BC Decker, 1980, pp 195–205

12. Mann RA, Hagy J: Biomechanics of walking, running, and sprinting. Am J Sports Med 8:345–350, 1980

13. Perry J: Gait cycle, in Perry J (ed): Gait Analysis: Normal and Pathological Function. Thorofare, NJ, Slack, 1992, pp 3–7

14. Mann RA, Moran GT, Dougherty SE: Comparative electromyography of the lower extremity in jogging, running and sprinting. Am J Sports Med 14:501–510, 1986

15. Arsenault AB, Winter DA, Marteniuk RG: Is there a "normal" profile of EMG activity in gait? Med Biol Eng Comput 24:337–343, 1986

16. Berchuck M, Andriacchi TP, Bach BR, et al: Gait adaptations by patients who have a deficient anterior cruciate ligament. J Bone Joint Surg 72A:871–877, 1990

17. Boeing DD: Evaluation of a clinical method of gait analysis. Phys Ther 57:795–798, 1977

18. Dillon P, Updyke W, Allen W: Gait analysis with reference to chondromalacia patellae. J Orthop Sports Phys Ther 5:127–131, 1983

19. Giannini S, Catani F, Benedetti MG, et al: Terminology, parameterization and normalization in gait analysis, in Giannini S, Catani F, Benedetti MG, et al (eds): Gait Analysis: Methodologies and Clinical Applications. Washington, DC, IOS Press, 1994, pp 65–88

20. Hunt GC, Brocato RS: Gait and foot pathomechanics, in Hunt GC (ed): Physical Therapy of the Foot and Ankle. Edinburgh, Churchill Livingstone, 1988, pp 39–57

21. Krebs DE, Robbins CE, Lavine L, et al: Hip biomechanics during gait. J Orthop Sports Phys Ther 28:51–59, 1998

22. Murray MP: Gait as a total pattern of movement. Am J Phys Med 46:290, 1967

23. Oberg T, Karsznia A, Oberg K: Basic gait parameters: Reference data for normal subjects, 10–79 years of age. J Rehabil Res Dev 30:210–223, 1993

24. Richardson JK, Iglarsh ZA: Gait, in Richardson JK, Iglarsh ZA (eds): Clinical Orthopaedic Physical Therapy. Philadelphia, Saunders, 1994, pp 602–625

25. Saunders JBD, Inman VT, Eberhart HD: The major determinants in normal and pathological gait. J Bone Joint Surg Am 35:543–558, 1953

26. Whitehouse PA, Knight LA, Di Nicolantonio F, et al: Heterogeneity of chemosensitivity of colorectal adenocarcinoma determined by a modified ex vivo ATP-tumor chemosensitivity assay (ATP-TCA). Anticancer Drugs 14:369–375, 2003

27. Oatis CA: Role of the hip in posture and gait, in Echternach J (ed): Clinics in Physical Therapy: Physical Therapy of the Hip. New York, Churchill Livingstone, 1983, pp 165–179

28. Perry J: The hip, in Perry J (ed): Gait Analysis: Normal and Pathological Function. Thorofare, NJ, Slack, 1992, pp 111–129

29. Dee R: Normal and abnormal gait in the pediatric patient, in Dee R, Hurst LC, Gruber MA, et al (eds): Principles of Orthopaedic Practice (ed 2). New York, McGraw-Hill, 1997, pp 685–692

30. Baker R, Dreyfuss P, Mercer S, et al: Cervical transforaminal injection of corticosteroids into a radicular artery: A possible mechanism for spinal cord injury. Pain 103:211–5, 2003

31. Hoyt DF, Taylor CF: Gait and the energetics of locomotion in horses. Nature 292:239–240, 1981

32. Larish DD, Martin PE, Mungiole M: Characteristic patterns of gait in the healthy old. Ann N Y Acad Sciences 515:18–32, 1987
33. Martin PE, Rothstein DE, Larish DD: Effects of age and physical activity status on the speed-aerobic demand relationship of walking. J Appl Physiol 73:200–206, 1992
34. Waters RL, Hislop HJ, Perry J, et al: Comparative cost of walking in young and old adults. J Orthop Res 1:73–76, 1983
35. Allen W, Seals DR, Hurley BF, et al: Lactate threshold and distance running performance in young and older endurance athletes. J Appl Physiol 58:1281–1284, 1985
36. Trappe SW, Costill DL, Vukovich MD, et al: Aging among elite distance runners: A 22-year longitudinal study. J Appl Physiol 80:285–290, 1996
37. Wells CL, Boorman MA, Riggs DM: Effect of age and menopausal status on cardiorespiratory fitness in masters women runners. Med Sci Sports Exerc 24:1147–1154, 1992
38. Lange GW, Hintermeister RA, Schlegel T, et al: Electromyographic and kinematic analysis of graded treadmill walking and the implications for knee rehabilitation. J Orthop Sports Phys Ther 23:294–301, 1996
39. Molen NH, Rozendal RH, Boon W: Fundamental characteristics of human gait in relation to sex and location. Proceedings of the Koninklijke Nederlandse Akademie van Wetenschappen—Series C. Biomed Sci 45:215–223, 1972
40. Finley FR, Cody KA: Locomotive characteristics of urban pedestrians. Arch Phys Med Rehabil 51:423–426, 1970
41. Sato H, Ishizu K: Gait patterns of Japanese pedestrians. J Hum Ergol (Tokyo) 19:13–22, 1990
42. Richard R, Weber J, Mejjad O, et al: Spatiotemporal gait parameters measured using the Bessou gait analyzer in 79 healthy subjects: Influence of age, stature, and gender. Rev Rhum Engl Ed 62:105–114, 1995
43. Corrigan J, Moore D, Stephens M: The effect of heel height on forefoot loading. Foot Ankle 11:418–422, 1991
44. Foti T, Davids JR, Bagley A: A biomechanical analysis of gait during pregnancy. J Bone Joint Surg 82A:625–632, 2000
45. Shkuratova N, Morris ME, Huxham F: Effects of age on balance control during walking. Arch Phys Med Rehabil 85:582–588, 2004
46. Perry J: Pelvis and trunk pathological gait, in Perry J (ed): Gait Analysis: Normal and Pathological Function. Thorofare, NJ, Slack, 1992, pp 265–279
47. Rengachary SS: Gait and station; examination of coordination, in Wilkins RH, Rengachary SS (eds): Neurosurgery (ed 2). New York, McGraw-Hill, 1996, pp 133–137
48. Eyring EJ, Murray W: The effect of joint position on the pressure of intra-articular effusion. J Bone Joint Surg 47A:313–322, 1965
49. Morag E, Hurwitz DE, Andriacchi TP, et al: Abnormalities in muscle function during gait in relation to the level of lumbar disc herniation. Spine 25:829–833, 2000
50. Bauer DM, Finch DC, McGough KP, et al: A comparative analysis of several crutch length estimation techniques. Phys Ther 71:294–300, 1991
51. Joyce BM, Kirby RL: Canes, crutches and walkers. Am Fam Phys 43:535–542, 1991
52. Deaver GG: What every physician should know about the teaching of crutch walking. JAMA 142:470–472, 1950
53. Baxter ML, Allington RO, Koepke GH: Weight-distribution variables in the use of crutches and canes. Phys Ther 49:360–365, 1969
54. Jebsen RH: Use and abuse of ambulation aids. JAMA 199:5–10, 1967
55. Kumar R, Roe MC, Scremin OU: Methods for estimating the proper length of a cane. Arch Phys Med Rehabil 76:1173–1175, 1995
56. Li S, Armstrong CW, Cipriani D: Three-point gait crutch walking: Variability in ground reaction force during weight bearing. Arch Phys Med Rehab 82:86–92, 2001
57. Kendall FP, McCreary EK, Provance PG: Muscles: Testing and Function. Baltimore, Williams & Wilkins, 1993
58. Turner M: Posture and pain. Phys Ther 37:294, 1957
59. Ayub E: Posture and the upper quarter, in Donatelli RA (ed): Physical Therapy of the Shoulder (ed 2). New York, Churchill Livingstone, 1991, pp 81–90
60. Greenfield B, Catlin P, Coats P, et al: Posture in patients with shoulder overuse injuries and healthy individuals. J Orthop Sports Phys Ther 21:287–295, 1995
61. Jackson-Manfield P, Neumann DA: Structure and function of the vertebral column, in Jackson-Manfield P, Neumann DA (eds): Essentials of Kinesiology for the Physical Therapist Assistant. St Louis, Mosby Elsevier, 2009, pp 177–225
62. Putz-Anderson V: Cumulative Trauma Disorders: A Manual for Musculoskeletal Diseases of the Upper Limbs. Bristol, PA, Taylor & Francis, 1988
63. Neumann DA: Axial skeleton: Osteology and arthrology, in Neumann DA (ed): Kinesiology of the Musculoskeletal System: Foundations for Physical Rehabilitation. St Louis, Mosby, 2002, pp 251–310
64. Jull GA, Janda V: Muscle and motor control in low back pain, in Twomey LT, Taylor JR (eds): Physical Therapy of the Low Back: Clinics in Physical Therapy. New York, Churchill Livingstone, 1987, pp 258–278
65. Janda V: Muscles and motor control in cervicogenic disorders: Assessment and management, in Grant R (ed): Physical Therapy of the Cervical and Thoracic Spine. New York, Churchill Livingstone, 1994, pp 195–216
66. Janda V: Muscle strength in relation to muscle length, pain and muscle imbalance, in Harms-Ringdahl K (ed): Muscle Strength. New York, Churchill Livingstone, 1993, pp 83–91
67. Keller K, Corbett J, Nichols D: Repetitive strain injury in computer keyboard users: Pathomechanics and treatment principles in individual and group intervention. J Hand Ther 11:9–26, 1998
68. Kiser DM: Physiological and biomechanical factors for understanding repetitive motion injuries. Semin Occup Med 2:11–17, 1987
69. Greenfield B: Upper quarter evaluation: Structural relationships and interindependence, in Donatelli R, Wooden M (eds): Orthopedic Physical Therapy. New York, Churchill Livingstone, 1989, pp 43–58
70. Smith A: Upper limb disorders—Time to relax? Physiotherapy 82:31–38, 1996
71. Wilder DG, Pope MH, Frymoyer JW: The biomechanics of lumbar disc herniation and the effect of overload and instability. J Spinal Disord 1:16, 1988
72. Sahrmann SA: Diagnosis and Treatment of Movement Impairment Syndromes. St Louis, Mosby, 2001

73. Babyar SR: Excessive scapular motion in individuals recovering from painful and stiff shoulders: Causes and treatment strategies. Phys Ther 76:226–247, 1996

74. Tardieu C, Tabary JC, Tardieu G, et al: Adaptation of sarcomere numbers to the length imposed on muscle, in Guba F, Marechal G, Takacs O (eds): Mechanism of Muscle Adaptation to Functional Requirements. Elmsford, NY, Pergamon Press, 1981, pp 99–114

75. Seidel-Cobb D, Cantu R: Myofascial treatment, in Donatelli RA (ed): Physical Therapy of the Shoulder (ed 3). New York, Churchill Livingstone, 1997, pp 383–401

76. Darnell MW: A proposed chronology of events for forward head posture. J Craniomandib Prac 1:49–54, 1983

77. Hamilton N, Luttgens K: The standing posture, in Hamilton N, Luttgens K (eds): Kinesiology: Scientific Basis of Human Motion (ed 10). New York, McGraw-Hill, 2002, pp 399–411

78. Magee DJ: Assessment of posture, in Magee DJ (ed): Orthopedic Physical Assessment. Philadelphia, WB Saunders, 2002, pp 873–903

79. Horak FB, Earhart GM, Dietz V: Postural responses to combinations of head and body displacements: Vestibular-somatosensory interactions. Exp Brain Res 141:410–414, 2001

80. Hahn ME, Lee HJ, Chou LS: Increased muscular challenge in older adults during obstructed gait. Gait Posture 22:356–361, 2005

81. Lord SR, Clark RD, Webster IW: Postural stability and associated physiological factors in a population of aged persons. J Gerontol 46:M69–M76, 1991

82. Berg G, Hammar M, Moller-Nielsen J, et al: Low back pain during pregnancy. Obstet Gynecol 71:71–75, 1988

83. Bullock JE, Jull GA, Bullock MI: The relationship of low back pain to postural changes during pregnancy. Aust J Physiother 33:10–17, 1987

84. Franklin ME, Conner-Kerr T: An analysis of posture and back pain in the first and third trimesters of pregnancy. J Orthop Sports Phys Ther 28:133–138, 1998

85. Orloff HA, Rapp CM: The effects of load carriage on spinal curvature and posture. Spine 29:1325–1329, 2004

86. Morris C, Chaitow L, Janda V: Functional examination for low back syndromes, in Morris C (ed): Low Back Syndromes: Integrated Clinical Management. New York, McGraw-Hill, 2006, pp 333–416

87. Kisner C, Colby LA: The spine and posture: Structure, function, postural impairments, and management guidelines, in Kisner C, Colby LA (eds): Therapeutic Exercise. Foundations and Techniques (ed 5). Philadelphia, FA Davis, 2002, pp 383–406

88. Cailliet R: Low Back Pain Syndrome (ed 4). Philadelphia, FA Davis, 1991, pp 263–268

89. Inman VT, Ralston HJ, Todd F: Human Walking. Baltimore, Williams & Wilkins, 1981

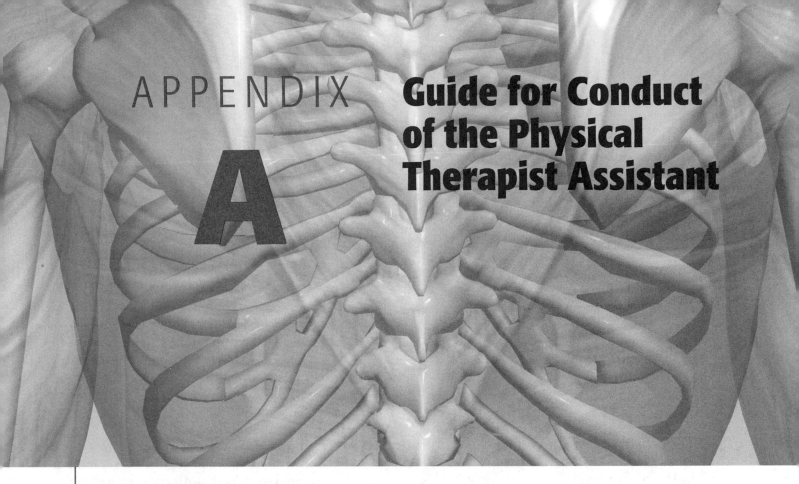

Guide for Conduct of the Physical Therapist Assistant

A

A. Purpose

This Guide for Conduct of the Physical Therapist Assistant (Guide) is intended to serve physical therapist assistants in interpreting The Standards of Ethical Conduct for a Physical Therapist Assistant (Standards) of the American Physical Therapy Association (APTA). The Guide provides guidelines by which physical therapist assistants may determine the propriety of their conduct. It also is intended to guide the development of physical therapist assistant students. The Standards and Guide apply to all physical therapist assistants. These guides are subject to change as the dynamics of the profession change and as new patterns of health-care delivery are developed and accepted by the professional community and the public. This Guide is subject to monitoring and timely revision by the Ethics and Judicial Committee of the Association.

B. Interpreting Standards

The interpretations expressed in this Guide reflect the opinions, decisions, and advice of the Ethics and Judicial Committee. These interpretations are intended to guide a physical therapist assistant in applying general ethical principles to specific situations. They should not be considered inclusive of all situations at a physical therapist assistant may encounter.

Standard 1

1. A physical therapist assistant shall respect the rights and dignity of all individuals and shall provide compassionate care.
   a. Attitude of a physical therapist assistant.
   1. A physical therapist assistant shall recognize, respect, and respond to individual and cultural difference with compassion and sensitivity.
   2. A physical therapist assistant shall be guided at all times by concern for the physical and psychological welfare of patients/clients.
   3. A physical therapist assistant shall not harass, abuse, or discriminate against others.

Standard 2

1. A physical therapist assistant shall act in a trustworthy manner towards patients/clients.
   a. Trustworthiness.
   1. A physical therapist assistant shall always place the patient's/client's interest(s) above those of the physical therapist assistant. Working in the patients/client's best interests requires sensitivity to the patient's/client's vulnerability and an effective working relationship between a physical therapist and a physical therapist assistant.
   2. A physical therapist assistant shall not exploit any aspect of the physical therapist assistant—patient/client relationship.
   3. A physical therapist assistant shall clearly identify him/herself as a physical therapist assistant to patients/clients.
   4. A physical therapist assistant shall conduct him/herself in a manner that supports the physical therapist–patient/client relationship.
   5. A physical therapist assistant shall not engage in any sexual relationship or activity, whether consensual or nonconsensual, with any patient/client entrusted to his/her care.
   6. A physical therapist assistant shall not invite, accept, or offer gifts or other considerations that affect or give an appearance of affecting his/her provision of physical therapy interventions.

b. Exploitation of patients.
   1. A physical therapist assistant shall not participate in any arrangements in which patients/clients are exploited. Such arrangements include situations where referring sources enhance their personal incomes by referring to or recommending physical therapy services.

c. Truthfulness.
   1. A physical therapist assistant shall not make statements that he/she knows or should know are false, deceptive, fraudulent, or misleading.
   2. Although it cannot be considered unethical for a physical therapist assistant to own or have a financial interest in the production, sale, or distribution of products/services, he/she must act in accordance with law and make full disclosure of his/her interest to patients/clients.

d. Confidential information.
   1. Information relating to the patient/client is confidential and shall not be communicated to a third party not involved in that patient's/client's care without the prior consent of the patient/client, subject to applicable law.
   2. A physical therapist assistant shall refer all requests for release of confidential information to the supervising physical therapist.

Standard 3

1. A physical therapist assistant shall provide selected physical therapy interventions only under the supervision and direction of a physical therapist.
   a. Supervisory relationship.
   1. A physical therapist assistant shall provide interventions only under the supervision and direction of a physical therapist.
   2. A physical therapist assistant shall provide only those interventions that have been selected by the physical therapist.
   3. A physical therapist assistant shall not provide any interventions that are outside his/her education, training, experience, or skill, and shall notify the responsible physical therapist of his/her inability to carry out the intervention.

4. A physical therapist assistant may modify specific interventions within the plan of care established by the physical therapist in response to changes in the patient's/client's status.

5. A physical therapist assistant shall not perform examinations and evaluations, determine diagnoses and prognoses, or establish or change a plan of care.

6. Consistent with a physical therapist assistant's education, training, knowledge, and experience, he/she may respond to the patient's/client's inquiries regarding interventions that are within the established plan of care.

7. A physical therapist assistant shall have regular and ongoing communication with a physical therapist regarding the patient's/client's status.

Standard 4

1. A physical therapist assistant shall comply with laws and regulations governing physical therapy.
   a. Supervision.
      1. A physical therapist assistant shall know and comply with applicable law. Regardless of the content of any law, a physical therapist assistant shall provide services only under the supervision and direction of a physical therapist.
   b. Representation.
      1. A physical therapist assistant shall not hold him/herself out as a physical therapist.

Standard 5

1. A physical therapist assistant shall achieve and maintain competence in the provision of selected physical therapy interventions.
   a. Competence.
      1. A physical therapist assistant shall provide interventions consistent with his/her level of education, training, experience, and skill.
   b. Self-assessment.
      1. A physical therapist assistant shall engage in self-assessment in order to maintain competence.

   c. Development.
      1. A physical therapist assistant shall participate in educational activities that enhance his/her basic knowledge and skills.

Standard 6

1. A physical therapist assistant shall make judgments that are commensurate with their educational and legal qualifications as a physical therapist assistant.
   a. Patient safety.
      1. A physical therapist assistant shall discontinue immediately any intervention(s) that, in his/her judgment, may be harmful to the patient/client and shall discuss his/her concerns with the physical therapist.
      2. A physical therapist assistant shall not provide any interventions that are outside his/her education, training, experience, or skill and shall notify the responsible physical therapist of his/her inability to carry out the intervention.
      3. A physical therapist assistant shall not perform interventions while his/her ability to do so safely is impaired.
   b. Judgments of patient/client status.
      1. If in a judgment of the physical therapist assistant, there is a change in the patient/client status he/she shall report this to the responsible physical therapist.
   c. Gifts and other considerations.
      1. A physical therapist assistant shall not invite, accept, or offer gifts, monetary incentives, or other consideration that affect or give an appearance of affecting his/her provision of physical therapy interventions.

Standard 7

1. A physical therapist assistant shall protect the public and the confession from unethical, incompetent, and illegal acts.
   a. Consumer protection.
      1. A physical therapist assistant shall report any conduct that appears to be unethical or illegal.

b. Organizational employment.

1. A physical therapist assistant shall inform his/her employer(s) and/or appropriate physical therapist of any employer practice that causes him or her to be in conflict with the Standards of Ethical Conduct of the Physical Therapist Assistant.

2. A physical therapist assistant shall not engage in any activity that puts him or her in conflict with the Standards of Ethical Conduct for the Physical Therapist Assistant, regardless of directives from a physical therapist or employer.

From Guide to physical therapist practice: Phys Ther 81:S13–S95, 2001. Courtesy of the American Physical Therapist Association.

B

American Physical Therapy Association's Documentation Guidelines

- The documentation must be consistent with the APTA's Standards of Practice.
- All documentation must be legible and use medically approved abbreviations or symbols.
- All documentation must be written in black or blue ink, and the mistakes must be crossed out with a single line through the error, initialed and dated by the PTA.
- Each intervention session must be documented. The patient's name and identification number must be on each page of the documentation record.
- Informed consent for the interventions must be signed by a competent adult. If the adult is not competent, the consent must be signed by the patient/client's legal guardian. If the patient is a minor, the consent must be signed by the parent or an appointed guardian.
- Each document must be dated and signed by the PT/PTA using the first and the last name and the professional designation; professional license number may be included but can be optional.
- All communications with other healthcare providers or healthcare professionals must be recorded.
- The PTA students' notes should be cosigned by the PTA (clinical instructor) or by the PT (clinical instructor).
- Non-licensed personnel notes should be cosigned by the PT.

Data from American Physical Therapy Association: APTA's documentation guidelines. http://www.apta.org; and Dreeben O: Introduction to physical therapy for physical therapist assistants. Sudbury, MA, Jones and Bartlett Publishers, 2007

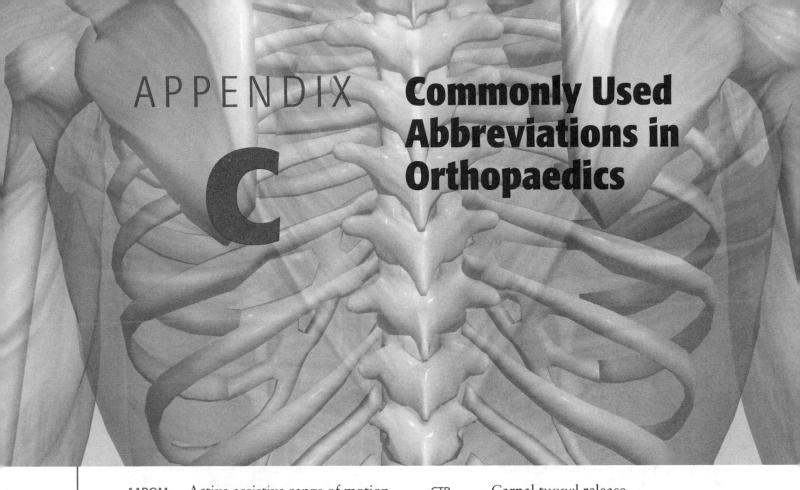

AAROM	Active assistive range of motion	CTR	Carpal tunnel release
abd	Abduction	d/c	Discontinued or discharged
add	Adduction	DDD	Degenerative disk disease
ACL	Anterior cruciate ligament	DF	Dorsiflexion
ADL	Activities of daily living	DIP	Distal interphalangeal
ad lib	As desired	DJD	Degenerative joint disease
AE	Above elbow	DOB	Date of birth
AFO	Ankle foot orthosis	DOE	Dyspnea on exertion
AK	Above knee	DTR	Deep tendon reflexes
amb	Ambulation	DVT	Deep vein thrombosis
ANS	Autonomic nervous system	Dx	Diagnosis
A-P	Anterior-posterior	EMG	Electromyography
AROM	Active range of motion	ER	External rotation or emergency room
ASIS	Anterior superior iliac spine		
BE	Below elbow	E-stim	Electrical stimulation
bid	Twice a day	ex	Exercise
BK	Below knee	ext	Extension
BP	Blood pressure	FES	Functional electrical stimulation
bpm	Beats per minute	Flex	Flexion
CC	Chief complaint	FWB	Full weight bearing
CGA	Contact guard assist	Fx	Fracture
c/o	Complains of	HEP	Home exercise program
CPM	Continuous passive motion	HNP	Herniated nucleus pulposus
CR	Contract-relax	HP	Hot pack
CTLSO	Cervical-thoracic-lumbar-sacral orthosis	HR	Heart rate or hold-relax
		Hx	History

ICU	Intensive care unit	PROM	Passive range of motion
Ind	Independent	PWB	Partial weight bearing
IR	Internal rotation	qid	Four times a day
JRA	Juvenile rheumatoid arthritis	RA	Rheumatoid arthritis
Jt	Joint	r/o	Rule out
KAFO	Knee-ankle-foot orthosis	ROM	Range of motion
LBP	Low back pain	RTC	Rotator cuff
LCL	Lateral collateral ligament	Rx	Treatment
LE	Lower extremity	SCI	Spinal cord injury
LOB	Loss of balance	SLR	Straight leg raise
LTG	Long-term goal	SOB	Short of breath
MCL	Medial collateral ligament	STG	Short-term goal
MCP	Metacarpophalangeal	TBI	Traumatic brain injury
MMT	Manual muscle test	TDWB	Touch down weight bearing
MVA	Motor vehicle accident	TENS	Transcutaneous electrical nerve stimulation
N/A	Not applicable		
NWB	Non–weight-bearing	THA	Total hip arthroplasty
OOB	Out of bed	tid	Three times a day
OP	Outpatient	TKA	Total knee arthroplasty
OR	Operating room	TKE	Terminal knee extension
ORIF	Open reduction and internal fixation	TMJ	Temporomandibular joint
OT	Occupational therapy	TTWB	Toe touch weight bearing
PCL	Posterior cruciate ligament	Tx	Traction
PF	Plantarflexion	UE	Upper extremity
PIP	Proximal interphalangeal	US	Ultrasound
PMH	Past medical history	WB	Weight bearing
PNF	Proprioceptive neuromuscular facilitation	WBAT	Weight bearing as tolerated
		WFL	Within functional limits
Post op	Postoperative	WNL	Within normal limits
PRE	Progressive resistive exercises	y/o	Year(s) old
Prn	As needed		

Common Laboratory Values

Test	Related Physiology	Reference Range Example
Arterial P_{O_2}	Reflects the dissolved oxygen level based on the pressure it exerts on the bloodstream	80–100 mm Hg
Arterial P_{CO_2}	Reflects the dissolved carbon dioxide level based on the pressure it exerts on the bloodstream	36–44 mm Hg
Arterial pH	Reflects the free hydrogen ion concentration; collectively this test and the arterial P_{O_2} and arterial P_{CO_2} tests help reveal the acid–base status and how well oxygen is being delivered to the body	7.35–7.45
Oxygen saturation	Usually a bedside technique (pulse oximetry) to indicate the level of oxygen transport	95–100 percent
Creatine phospho-kinase (CPK)	An enzyme found predominantly in the heart, brain, and skeletal muscle that aids in protein catabolism; can be separated into subunits or isoenzymes, each derived from a specific tissue: • CPK-BB = brain • CPK-MB = cardiac • CPK-MM = skeletal muscle	Total CPK: Less than 30
Lactate dehydroge-nase (LDH)	Present in all body tissues and abundant in red blood cells and acts as a marker for hemolysis; isoenzymes are LDH 1–5	105–333 IU/L (international units per liter)

(continued)

Test	Related Physiology	Reference Range Example
Alkaline phosphate	An enzyme associated with bone metabolism/calcification and lipid transport	Adults: 13–39 IU/L Infants through adolescents: Up to 104 IU/L
Sodium (Na)	Major extracellular cation: serves to regulate serum osmolality, fluid, and acid–base balance; maintains transmembrane electric potential for neuromuscular functioning	136–145 mmol/L
Potassium (K)	Major intracellular cation: maintains normal hydration and osmotic pressure	3.5–5.5 mmol/L
Chloride (Cl)	Extracellular anion: maintains electrical neutrality of extracellular fluid	96–106 mmol/L
Carbon dioxide	Reflects body's ability to control pH; important in bicarbonate–carbonic acid blood buffer system	24–30 mmol/L
Anion gap (sodium minus the sum of chloride and carbon dioxide)	Calculated value helpful in evaluating metabolic acidosis	3–11 mmol/L
Calcium (Ca)	Important for the transmission of nerve impulses and muscle contractility; cofactor in enzyme reactions and blood coagulation	8.5–10.8 mg/dL; inversely related to phosphorus level
Phosphorus (PO_4)	Integral to the structure of nucleic acids, in adenosine triphosphate energy transfer, and in phospholipid function; phosphate helps to regulate calcium levels, metabolism, base balance, and bone metabolism	2.6–4.5 mg/dL; inversely related to calcium level
Blood urea nitrogen (BUN)	Measures renal function and protein intake, and amino acid metabolism in the liver produces urea as waste; urea is filtered by the kidney with the portion passively reabsorbed being measured in the plasma	Adult range: 8–22 mg/dL
Creatinine	A measure of renal function; muscle creatine degradation produces creatinine, which in turn is excreted by the kidneys	Adult range: 0.7–1.4 mg/dL
BUN/creatinine ratio	Assessment of kidney and liver function	Adult range: 6–25 mg/dL
Alanine aminotransferase (ALT)	Enzyme released in cytolysis and necrosis of liver cells	1–21 units/L
Aspartate aminotransferase (AST)	Enzyme released in cytolysis and necrosis of liver cells; also in heart and skeletal muscle tissues	7–27 units/L
Alkaline phosphatase (ALP)	Enzyme released in cytolysis and necrosis of liver cells; also in bone	13–39 units/L
γ-Glutamyltransferase	Enzyme released in cytolysis and necrosis of liver cells; also in kidney tissue	5–38 units/L
Albumin	Index of liver synthetic capacity	3.5–5.0 g/dL
Bilirubin, total	Bilirubin is the predominant pigment in bile, and the major metabolite of hemoglobin	0.2–1.0 mg/dL; direct: 0–0.2 mg/dL; indirect: 0.2–1.0 mg/dL
Ammonium	Liver converts ammonium from blood to urea	12–55 μmol/L

Test	Related Physiology	Reference Range Example
WBC count	Measures mature and immature WBCs in 1 μL of whole blood and is used in conjunction with WBC differential; produced in bone marrow, WBCs provide defense against foreign agents/organisms	4000–10,000 WBCs/μL
WBC differential	Visual or computer observation and count of different types of WBCs with differentiation of white blood cell types by relative percentages; cell types usually seen (in descending order): • Neutrophils (PMN) • Lymphocytes • Monocytes • Eosinophils • Basophils	All components totaled equal 100 percent
Segmented neutrophils	Phagocytizes	~37–77 percent
Band neutrophils	Phagocytizes; less mature neutrophils	~0–11 percent
Lymphocytes	B cells produce immunoglobulins; T cells provide regulatory and effector functions in immunity	~10–44 percent
Monocytes	Phagocytize and contribute to cellular and humoral immunity in association with T lymphocytes	~2–10 percent
Eosinophils	Also function as phagocytes, somewhat less effectively than neutrophils	~0–7 percent
Basophils	Also function as phagocytes; synthesize and store histamine	~0–2 percent
Red blood cell (RBC)/ erythrocyte count	Measures the number of RBCs in 1 μL of blood; produced in bone marrow, RBCs carry oxygen to tissues	4.2–6.2×106 μL
Hemoglobin	Reflects the concentration of hemoglobin in blood	12–16 g/dL (values of 8–10 g/dL typically result in decreased exercise tolerance, increased fatigue, and tachycardia, a condition that may contraindicate aggressive therapeutic measures, including strength and endurance training)
Hematocrit	Measure of the ratio of packed red blood cells to whole blood; by dividing the hematocrit level by three, one can approximate the hemoglobin level	36–54 percent (approximately three times hemoglobin)
Mean cell (corpuscular) volume (MCV)	Measure of average size of RBCs—the ratio of hematocrit to red blood cell count	80–100 fL
Mean cell hemoglobin concentration (MCHC)	Indicates the average concentration of hemoglobin to hematocrit, and measures the percentage of hemoglobin in 100 mL of blood	32–36 g/dL; cannot exceed 37 g/dL

(continued)

Test	Related Physiology	Reference Range Example
Mean cell hemoglobin (MCH)	Indicates average weight of hemoglobin per RBC	32 to 36 g/dl, or between 4.9–5.5 mmol/L
RBC distribution width	Standard deviation of MCV; measure of degree of uniformity in the size of RBCs	11.7–14.2 percent
Erythrocyte sedimentation rate (ESR)	Nonspecific indicator of inflammation or tissue damage	0–20 mm/1 hr
Platelet count	Reflects potential to address injury to vessel walls, thus regulating homeostasis	140,000–450,000 μL

Data from Wall LJ: Laboratory tests and values, in Boissonnault WG (ed): Primary Care for the Physical Therapist: Examination and Triage. St Louis, Elsevier Saunders, 2005, pp 348–367; and Lotspeich-Steinger CA, Stiene-Martin AE, Koepke JA: Clinical Hematology; Principles, Procedures, Correlations. Philadelphia, JB Lippincott, 1992

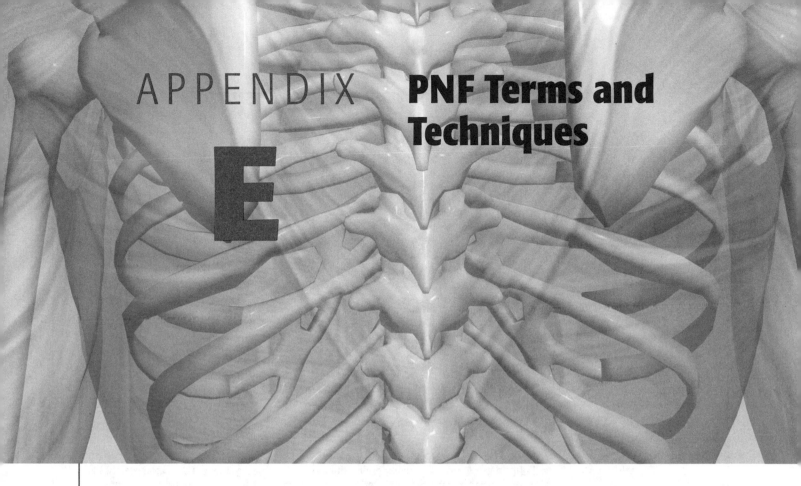

Technique	Description
Irradiation (overflow)	The spread of energy from the prime agonist to complementary agonists and antagonists within a pattern. Can occur from proximal to distal muscle groups, distal to proximal, upper trunk to lower trunk (and vice versa), and from one extremity to another. Weaker muscle groups benefit from the irradiation they gain while working in synergy with stronger, more normal partners. Irradiation is stimulated by the clinician through the use of resistance.
Manual and maximal resistance	In PNF, the direction, quality, and quantity of resistance are adjusted to prompt a smooth and coordinated response, whether for stability (i.e., holds), or for ease, smoothness, and pace of movement. The resistance should be at an appropriate level to prompt proper irradiation and facilitate function, and should be no greater than the resistance that allows full ROM to occur.
Verbal cueing	Effective verbal cues coordinate the clinician's efforts with the patient's.
Approximation and traction	Joint compression stimulates afferent nerve endings, and encourages extensor muscles and stabilizing patterns (co-contraction), thereby inhibiting abnormal tone and enhancing stabilization of the proximal segment. Compression techniques can be used to prepare a joint for weight bearing. Joint traction provides a stretch stimulus and enhances movement by elongating the adjacent muscles. Traction techniques are commonly used in the presence of pain to inhibit excessive compression and facilitation of flexor muscles and mobilizing patterns. May also be used to help decrease spasticity.

(continued)

Technique	Description
Stretch	Stretch is frequently performed at the starting position of the pattern or movement to promote reflexive activity that is facilitating to the desired action. The resulting reflex activation is then synchronized with volitional effort through verbal cues.
Timing	Describes the sequencing of movement. Timing for emphasis suggests that, to facilitate and enhance muscular response, the clinician can intentionally interrupt the normal timing sequence at specific points in the ROM to the more powerful muscle groups to obtain "overflow" to weaker muscle groups. Can be performed within a limb (ipsilateral from one muscle group to another) or using overflow from one limb to contralateral limb, or trunk to limb. Typically combined with repeated contractions to the weak components, or superimposed upon normal timing in a distal to proximal sequence. Indications include weakness and incoordination.
Combination of isotonics (formerly referred to as agonist reversals)	A slow isotonic, shortening contraction through the range followed by an eccentric, lengthening contraction using the same muscle groups. Indications include weak postural muscles and inability to eccentrically control body weight during movement transitions (e.g., sitting down).
Stabilizing reversals (formerly referred to as alternating isometrics)	Isometric holding is facilitated first on one side of the joint, followed by alternate holding of the antagonist muscle groups. Can be applied in any direction (anterior-posterior, medial-lateral, diagonal). Indications include instability in weight bearing and holding, poor antigravity control, weakness, and ataxia.
Contract-relax (CR)	A relaxation technique usually performed at a point of limited range of motion in the agonist pattern: isotonic movement in rotation is performed followed by an isometric hold of the range-limiting muscles in the antagonist pattern against slowly increasing resistance, then voluntary relaxation, and active contraction in the newly gained range of the agonist pattern. The patient is then asked to contract the muscle(s) to be stretched (agonists). The clinician resists this contraction except for the rotary component. The patient is then asked to relax and the clinician moves the joint further into the desired range. Indications include spasticity and limitations in range of motion caused by muscle adaptive shortening. Although primarily used as a stretching technique, due to the isometric contractions involved, some strengthening does occur.
Hold-relax (HR)	A similar technique in principle to contract-relax, except that when the patient contracts, the clinician allows no motion (including rotation) to occur. Following the isometric contraction the patient's own contraction causes the desired movement to occur. Typically used as a relaxation technique in the acutely injured patient because it tends to be less aggressive than the contract-relax technique.
Replication (formerly referred to as hold-relax-active motion)	An isometric contraction performed in the mid to shortened range followed by a voluntary relaxation and passive movement into the lengthened range, and resistance to an isotonic contraction through the range. May be used with patients who have an inability to initiate movement, hypotonia, weakness, or marked imbalances between antagonists.
Manual contact	A deep but painless pressure is applied through the clinician's contact to stimulate a muscle, tendon, and/or joint afferents.
Maximal resistance	Resistance is applied to stronger muscles to obtain overflow to weaker muscles. Indications include weakness and muscle imbalances.
Quick stretch	A motion applied suddenly stimulates the tendon receptors, resulting in a facilitation of motor recruitment and thus more force.
Reinforcement	The coordinated use of the major muscle groups, or other body parts, to produce a desired movement pattern. Often used to increase the stability of the proximal segments.

Technique	Description
Repeated contractions (RC)	A unidirectional technique that involves repeated isotonic contractions induced by quick stretch and that is enhanced by resistance performed to the range or part of range at the point of weakness. Indications include weakness, incoordination, muscle imbalances, and lack of endurance. Facilitation of the agonist and relaxation of the antagonist.
Reversals of antagonists	Many functional tasks involve reversing movement patterns that task body balance and postural stability. For example, the reciprocal activity of the limbs in the swing phase of walking compared with the stance phase. To facilitate static and dynamic postural balance, reciprocal movement of the antagonistic groups are facilitated with static (isometric) or dynamic (isotonic) contractions
Dynamic reversals of antagonists (formerly referred to as slow reversal)	The technique of dynamic reversals enhances reciprocal or reversing motions. Dynamic (isotonic) contractions of antagonistic movements are facilitated reciprocally in a range appropriate to the goal of the exercise. Indications include inability to reverse directions, muscle imbalances, weakness, incoordination, and instability.
Rhythmic initiation (RI)	Unidirectional or bidirectional voluntary relaxation followed by passive movement through increasing range of motion, followed by active-assisted contractions progressing to light tracking resistance to isotonic contractions.Indications include spasticity, rigidity, inability to initiate movement, motor learning deficits, and communication deficits.
Rhythmic stabilization (RS)	The application of alternating isometric contractions of the agonist and antagonist muscles to stimulate movement of the agonist, develop stability, and relax the antagonist. Indications include instability in weight bearing and holding, poor antigravity control, weakness, and ataxia. May also be used to decrease limitations in range of motion caused by adaptive muscle shortening and painful muscle splinting.
Stabilizing reversals	Alternating resistance is applied to an agonist-antagonist pair while seeking a maximal dynamic (isotonic) contraction. The technique is similar in many ways to rhythmic stabilization, but it can also be used when the patient is unable to perform a true static (isometric) contraction.
Rhythmic rotation	Voluntary relaxation combined with slow, passive, rhythmic rotation of the body or body part around a longitudinal axis and passive movement into newly gained range. Active holding in the new range then is stressed. Indications include hypertonia with limitations in functional range of motion.
Resisted progression (RP)	A stretch and tracking resistance is applied in order to facilitate progression in walking, creeping, kneel-walking, or movement transitions. Indications include impaired strength, timing, motor control, and endurance.

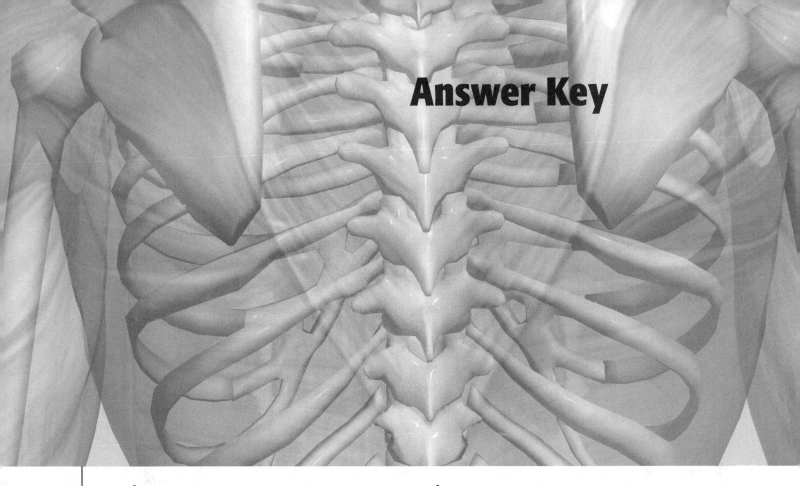

Answer Key

Chapter 1

1. b
2. b
3. b
4. a
5. c
6. b
7. d
8. c
9. d
10. c
11. Subjective, objective, assessment, and plan
12. False
13. True
14. c
15. b
16. a
17. a
18. a
19. a
20. a

Chapter 2

1. True
2. Hyaline cartilage, elastic cartilage, and fibrocartilage
3. False; loose CT
4. True
5. d
6. Hyaline
7. 206
8. True
9. Diaphysis
10. Epiphyseal plate
11. Smooth, skeletal, and cardiac
12. Endomysium
13. Slow twitch, type I fibers
14. To attach muscle to bone
15. True
16. Any four of the following: provide support, enhance leverage, protect vital structures, provide attachments for both tendons and ligaments, and store minerals, particularly calcium

17. d
18. d
19. c
20. d
21. c
22. a
23. a
24. a
25. a

Chapter 3

1. d
2. c
3. a
4. b
5. b
6. C1–C4
7. C5–T1
8. The spinal accessory nerve (XI) and the vagus nerve (X)
9. Spinal accessory
10. Posterior
11. Coracobrachialis, brachialis, and biceps brachii
12. Deep fibular (peroneal) nerve
13. Radial nerve
14. Median nerve
15. Median nerve
16. Ulnar nerve
17. Supraspinatus and infraspinatus
18. Long thoracic nerve
19. Thoracodorsal nerve
20. Gluteus medius and minimus, tensor fascia lata
21. C7
22. Wrist extensors
23. c
24. Median nerve
25. a
26. d
27. e
28. b
29. Flexor pollicis longus and pronator quadratus
30. c
31. d
32. d
33. d
34. a
35. d

Chapter 4

1. True
2. Sagittal, frontal, transverse
3. d
4. c
5. c
6. a
7. Proximal
8. Open-chain
9. Opposite direction
10. c

Chapter 5

1. Inflammatory phase, proliferative phase, and remodeling phase
2. Tendinitis is a microscopic tear at the muscle-tendon junction. Tendinosis usually results from a degenerative process.
3. Inflammatory phase, reparative (callus) phase, and remodeling phase
4. The law describes the ability of bone to adapt by changing size, shape, and structure depending on the mechanical stresses applied to the bone.
5. Any three of the following: the rotator cuff of the shoulder (i.e., supraspinatus, bicipital tendons), insertion of the wrist extensors (i.e., lateral epicondylitis, tennis elbow) and flexors (i.e., medial epicondylitis) at the elbow, patellar and popliteal tendons and iliotibial band at the knee, insertion of the posterior tibial tendon in the leg (i.e., shin splints), and the Achilles tendon at the heel
6. A sprain is an acute injury to the ligament, whereas a strain is an injury to the muscle.
7. d
8. d
9. d
10. c

Chapter 6

1. Three
2. Grade III
3. Grade I
4. Soft tissue approximation

5. Traumatic hyperemia, pain relief, and decreasing scar tissue
6. Effleurage
7. Tapotement
8. Myofascial release techniques

Chapter 7

1. c
2. 165–175°F (73.9–79.4°C)
3. b
4. Ultrasound
5. amps
6. b
7. c
8. d
9. c
10. d
11. a
12. b
13. b
14. a
15. a
16. c
17. b
18. d

Chapter 8

1. Phosphagen and glycolysis
2. Adenosine triphosphate (ATP)
3. The energy expenditure required for sitting quietly, talking on the phone, or reading a book
4. Essential and storage
5. 18.5–24.9
6. Open
7. Static and dynamic
8. False

Chapter 9

1. Range of motion and elongation of muscle
2. Plastic and elastic deformation
3. To reduce contractures, to improve motion, and to minimize risk of soft tissue injury
4. False
5. False
6. True

7. Passive ROM → Active assisted ROM → Active ROM
8. False
9. True
10. Static, cyclic, ballistic, and proprioceptive neuromuscular facilitation stretching

Chapter 10

1. Isometric contraction
2. Eccentric
3. Eccentric
4. Extensibility, elasticity, irritability, and the ability to develop tension
5. False
6. The strength gains are developed at a specific point in the range of motion and not throughout the range; not all of a muscle's fibers are activated.
7. b
8. Type/mode of exercise, intensity, duration, and frequency
9. b
10. c
11. b
12. b
13. c

Chapter 11

1. Proprioception and the mechanoreceptor system
2. Poor coordination, decreased range of motion, weakness, and compromised perception
3. True
4. Automatic postural reactions
5. Somatosensory, visual, and vestibular systems
6. Kinesthesia
7. Ankle, hip, and stepping strategies
8. Balance testing procedures
9. Sitting
10. True

Chapter 12

1. Cervical, thoracic, lumbar, sacral, and coccygeal
2. The lordosis of the cervical and lumbar spine
3. The vertebral bodies and intervertebral disks

4. 24 pairs
5. The neutral zone
6. True

Chapter 13

1. The uncinate processes are considered to be a guiding mechanism for flexion and extension in the cervical spine and to resist posterior translation as well as some degree of side bending.
2. Rectus capitis lateralis
3. Ipsilateral side bending and contralateral rotation of the head and neck
4. Axis
5. Horizontal
6. Extension
7. Frontal
8. True
9. True
10. True
11. The lateral pterygoid and digastric muscles
12. The temporalis, masseter, and medial pterygoid muscles
13. The masseter and temporalis muscles on the right, and the medial and lateral pterygoid muscles on the left
14. The mouth is closed so that the lips touch but the teeth do not, and the tongue is resting gently on the hard palate.
15. Decreased ipsilateral opening and lateral deviation to the involved side

Chapter 14

1. Rotation
2. Diaphragm
3. Upper
4. Erector spinae and hip flexors
5. True
6. True
7. True
8. True
9. Round back
10. A forward and downward projecting sternum

Chapter 15

1. Nucleus pulposus
2. Sagittal
3. Flexion

4. False
5. Anterior spondylolisthesis
6. True
7. False
8. Bending forward in a flexed posture and lifting
9. True
10. True
11. a

Chapter 16

1. Sternoclavicular, acromioclavicular, glenohumeral, and scapulothoracic
2. The acromioclavicular ligament and the coracoclavicular ligament
3. Supination of the forearm
4. Infraspinatus, teres minor, and posterior deltoid
5. d
6. d
7. c
8. A shoulder dislocation is a true separation between the head of the humerus and the glenoid. A shoulder separation involves a disruption of the acromioclavicular joint.
9. d
10. c
11. The sternoclavicular joint
12. Supraspinatus, infraspinatus, teres minor, and pectoralis major
13. The acromioclavicular joint
14. Radial nerve damage
15. c
16. a
17. d
18. a
19. a
20. a

Chapter 17

1. Elbow extension and forearm supination
2. 70 degrees of elbow flexion and 10 degrees of forearm supination
3. 70 degrees of elbow flexion and 35 degrees of forearm supination
4. Elbow extension
5. One
6. Approximately 15 degrees
7. Brachioradialis and biceps brachii

8. Humerus
9. Lateral
10. True
11. a
12. a
13. a

Chapter 18

1. The complex consists of the central fibrocartilage articular disk, palmar and dorsal radioulnar ligament, ulnar collateral ligament, and a sheath from the extensor carpi ulnaris. It attaches to the ulna board of the radius and the distal ulna.
2. A fracture of the radius and the ulna
3. The scaphoid
4. Avascular necrosis
5. MCP flexion and IP extension
6. The distal interphalangeal joints
7. a
8. b
9. c
10. Lateral cord
11. d
12. d
13. a
14. a
15. a

Chapter 19

1. In the direction of hip extension, adduction, and internal rotation
2. Extension
3. Extension, internal rotation, abduction
4. Three
5. Anteriorly
6. Sartorius and rectus femoris
7. b
8. a
9. a
10. c
11. d
12. a

Chapter 20

1. Sartorius, gracilis, and semitendinosis
2. Popliteus

3. The medial meniscus
4. To prevent posterior displacement of the tibia on the femur
5. Hamstrings
6. 12- to 18-year-old females
7. Vastus medialis obliquus
8. c
9. a
10. c
11. b
12. a
13. a
14. d
15. a

Chapter 21

1. a
2. Maximum dorsiflexion
3. The anterior talofibular ligament
4. The calcaneus bone and the talus
5. The plantar calcaneonavicular ligament
6. d
7. a
8. b
9. c
10. b
11. a
12. a
13. a
14. c
15. b

Chapter 22

1. 3–4 months
2. 5–6 months
3. 8–9 months
4. 12 months
5. b
6. a
7. b
8. d
9. c
10. a
11. c
12. c
13. d

Chapter 23

1. Gerontology
2. Weight-bearing joints
3. b
4. b
5. c
6. d
7. c
8. d
9. The onset of chronic, insidious memory loss that is slowly progressive
10. A durable power of attorney for health care and a living will
11. Informed consent
12. a
13. a
14. a

Chapter 24

1. c
2. Kegel exercises
3. Relaxin
4. True
5. True
6. A lateral separation of greater than two fingertip widths of the two bellies of the rectus abdominis at the linea alba (or linea nigra, in pregnancy) that can occur during pregnancy or delivery
7. False
8. Overflow incontinence
9. A mechanical insufficiency that arises in an area when lymph collectors sustain functional and structural damage resulting in the accumulation of hydrophilic proteins in the tissues
10. True
11. a

Chapter 25

1. Support of body mass by the lower extremities, production of locomotor rhythm, and dynamic balance control of the moving body
2. The interval of time between any of the repetitive events of walking

3. Weight acceptance, single limb support, and swing limb advancement
4. Stance and swing
5. Initial contact, loading response, midstance, and terminal stance
6. Preswing, initial swing, midswing, and terminal swing
7. Gait velocity, stride length, and cadence
8. The repetition rate (cadence), physical conditioning, and the length of the person's stride
9. 113 steps/min
10. Approximately midline in the frontal plane and slightly anterior to the second sacral vertebra in the sagittal plane
11. False
12. False
13. A positive Trendelenburg sign is indicated when the pelvis lists toward the non–weight-bearing side during single limb support.
14. Foot slap immediately after initial contact, foot drop during swing, excessive hip and knee flexion during swing
15. During the end of the swing phase
16. b
17. d
18. b
19. Gluteus medius
20. c
21. Gluteus maximus
22. Deep fibular (peroneal)
23. Tibial, femoral, and pelvic internal rotation
24. The lordotic posture
25. The slouched posture
26. Stretched and weak lumbar extensor and possibly hip flexor muscles

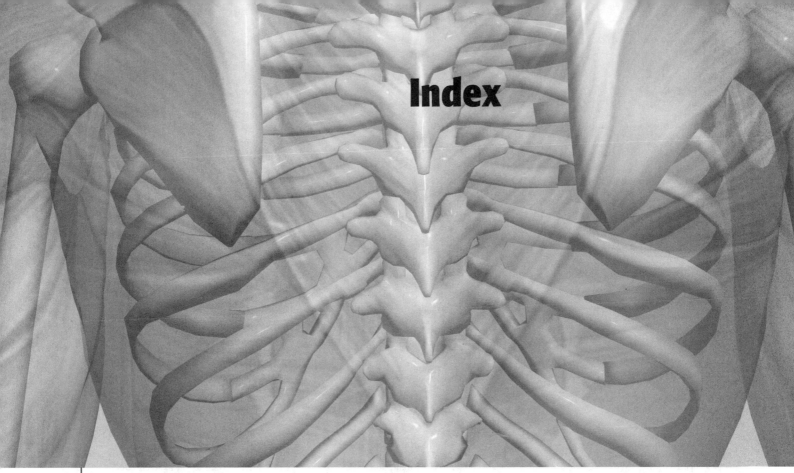

Index

Proximal, 108
Proximal femoral osteotomy, 505
Proximal interphalangeal (PIP) joint, 136, 442, 462
Proximal phalanges, 438
Proximal radioulnar joint, 119, 120, 408–412
Proximal tibiofibular joint, 563
Pseudoclaudication, 344
Pseudomyostatic contracture, 121
Psoas major, 54, 478, 480
Psoas minor, 318, 478
Psychological abuse, screen for, 9
PT or PTA student, role of, 7
PT/OT aide, role of, 7
Pterygoids, 79
Ptosis, 90
Pubic rami fracture, 499
Pubic symphysis, 647
Pubis bone, 317–319, 478, 499
Pubococcygeal muscle, 652
Pubofemoral ligament, 44, 482–483
Puborectalis, 652–653
Pudendal plexus, 85
Pulled elbow, 622
Pulley exercises, 397
Pulling force, 110
Pulmonary embolism, 146
Pulp-to-pulp pinch, 445
Pulse, electrotherapeutic modalities, 189, 192
Pupils, 87
Push-ups, 375
Pyramidalis, 318
Pyrexia, 17
Pyrophosphate arthropathy, 143–144

Q
Q-angle, 520–521
Quad canes, 673
Quadrant mobilizations, hip joint, 507–508
Quadratus femoris
 anatomy, 478, 480, 482
 nerves, 85
 sacroiliac joint, 318
Quadratus lumborum, 318
Quadratus plantae, 87, 562
Quadriceps angle, 520–521
Quadriceps femoris
 knee joint complex, 517–518
 nerves, 86
 strains, 495–496
Quadriceps gait, 672
Quadriceps tendon, 520–521
Quadriceps tendonitis, 544–545
Quadruped stabilization exercise, 304
Questions, 12
Quick stretch, PNF terms, 702
Quinolone, 29

R
Radial artery, 438, 439
Radial collateral ligament
 elbow complex, 43
 wrist, 439
Radial deviation of the carpometacarpal block, 138, 140
Radial deviation, wrist movement, 446
Radial nerves
 elbow complex, 413
 fractures, 143
 injury findings in upper extremity, 92
 upper quadrant, 81, 84
 wrist and forearm, 442
Radiation treatments, stress fractures, 143–144
Radiation, energy from, 175
Radiculopathy, 80, 283, 284–285
Radiocarpal joint
 anatomy, 438–439
 capsular patterns of restriction, 65

close-packed position, 119
 joint mobilizations, 469–470
 manual modalities, 157
 open-packed position, 120
 wrist and hand articulations, 446
Radiohumeral joint
 close-packed position, 119
 open-packed position, 120
 pulled elbow, 622
Radiology, conventional (plain film), 33
Radionucleotide scanning, 34
Radioulnar glide, 430–431
Radioulnar joint, 157, 165
Radius, 43, 425–426, 438–439, 462–466. See also Elbow complex; Wrist
Rami communicantes, 78
Randomized clinical trials, 27
Randomized controlled trials, 26
Range of motion (ROM)
 active range of motion, 57, 61
 ankle and foot, 568–569, 571
 cervical spine, 269, 278, 279
 elbow complex, 415
 exercise, indications and contraindications, 220, 221
 fractures, 146
 glenohumeral joint, 362
 goniometry, 56–61
 hip joint, 487
 improving, 220–222
 joint kinematics, 120–122
 knee joint complex, 514, 522, 525, 540
 lower quarter scanning examination, 100
 lumbar spine, 326
 neurologic exam, 98
 passive range of motion, 61–63
 plan of care, 5
 recording, 63–64
 rheumatoid arthritis and, 141
 shoulder complex, 356, 371, 372, 374–376
 soft tissue injury, exercises for, 133
 therapeutic exercise, 213–214
 total shoulder replacement arthroplasty, 394–395
 vertebral column, 262, 264
 wrist and hand, 450–451, 465
Reach test, 98
Reagan's test, 448
Receptive aphasia, 91
Reciprocal inhibition, 169, 223
Rectilinear motion, 109
Rectus abdominis, 318, 347
Rectus capitis anterior, 81, 270
Rectus capitis lateralis, 81, 271
Rectus capitis posterior major, 271, 290
Rectus capitis posterior minor, 290
Rectus femoris
 anatomy, 478, 480
 force couples, 111
 function of, 56
 knee joint complex, 516, 517
 muscle fiber types, 54
 myotendinous junction tears, 42
 sacroiliac joint, 318
 stretches, 488, 506, 543
Red blood cells, laboratory values, 699
Red flags, 21
Referred pain, 20, 137–138
Reflexes
 autogenic inhibition, 77
 balance, movement strategies, 250–251
 ligamentomuscular reflex, 250
 nervous system and, 89
 pathological, 96
 reflex neurovascular dystrophy, 468–469
 reflex sympathetic dystrophy, 468–469
 testing, 100, 101
Refusal of treatment, 638

Rehabilitation team, members of, 6–7
Rehabilitative modalities, overview, 11–12
Reinforcement, PNF terms, 702
Relafen, 29
Relaxation
 biofeedback, 197
 muscles, 52
 postisometric, 223–224
Remodeling
 bone healing, 144–146
 osteoporosis, 141
 soft tissue injury, 134–135
Renal disease, stress fractures, 143–144
Renal failure, 30
Rent test, shoulder complex, 366
Reparative phase, bone healing, 144
Repeated contractions, PNF terms, 703
Repetition maximum (RM), 237–239
Repetitions, defined, 230
Repetitive joint use
 carpal tunnel syndrome, 95, 454
 iliotibial band friction syndrome, 497–498
 secondary osteoarthritis, 137–138
Replication, defined, 702
Research, evidence-based practice, 26–27
Resistance
 electrical, 191–192
 manual muscle testing, 66
 Ohm's law, 192
 PNF terms, 701
 types of, 235–237
Resisted cervical rotation test, 99
Resisted elbow extension test, 100
Resisted elbow flexion test, 99
Resisted finger adduction test, 99
Resisted hip flexion, 101
Resisted knee extension, 101
Resisted progression, PNF terms, 703
Resisted shoulder abduction test, 99
Resisted shoulder elevation test, 99
Resisted shoulder external rotation test, 99
Resisted thumb extension test, 100
Resisted walking, 526–527
Resisted wrist extension test, 99
Resisted wrist flexion test, 100
Resistive exercises, 133–134
Resistive testing, 98, 100
Respiration, 18, 87, 299
Rest
 exercise intervals, 214
 soft tissue injury, 131
 strength training, 237
Resting energy metabolism, 209
Resting position, 119
Resting potential, defined, 190
Restricted scapulothoracic motion, 396
Reticular fibers, 40
Retraction movement, shoulder complex, 355, 356, 363–365
Retroversion, hip joint, 485
Return to neutral, cervical exercise, 277
Revascularization phase, bone healing, 144
Reversals of antagonists, PNF terms, 703
Reverse curl-up, 335
Reversibility principle, 215
Rheobase, electrotherapeutic modalities, 192
Rheumatoid arthritis (RA), 138, 140–141, 143–144
Rhombencephalon (hindbrain), 75
Rhomboid muscle
 function and innervation, 359
 glenohumeral joint movement, 358
 scapular stabilizer exercises, 280–281
 shape of, 54
 shoulder complex anatomy, 356, 360
 shoulder movement, 363–365
Rhomboideus major muscle, 360
Rhythmic initiation, PNF terms, 703
Rhythmic rotation, PNF terms, 703

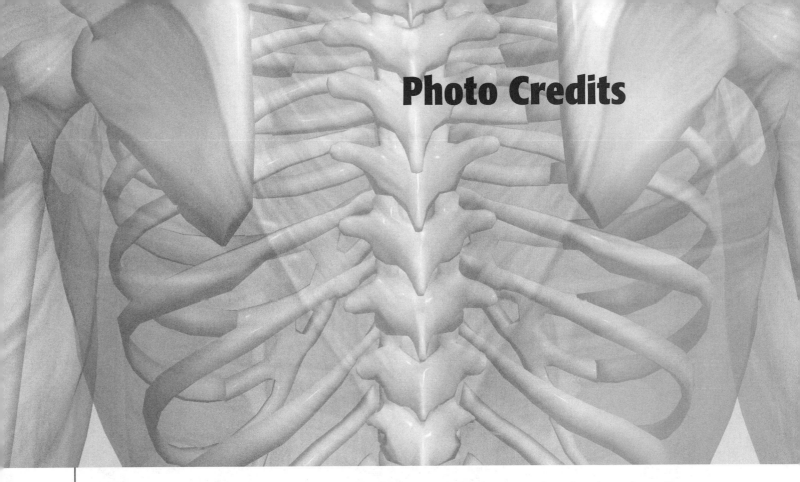

Photo Credits

All chapter and section openers © Patrick Hermans/ShutterStock, Inc.

4-2 Courtesy of Thomas Henderson; 10-1 Used with permission of Biodex Medical Systems; 11-15 Used with permission of Fitter International, Inc.; 14-19 © SPL/Photo Researchers, Inc.; 14-20 © Dr. M.A. Ansary/Photo Researchers, Inc.; 14-22 © Dr. P. Marazzi/Photo Researchers, Inc.; 14-23 © Michael English, M.D./Custom Medical Stock Photo; 15-5 Courtesy of Nikita Vizniak, Professional Health Systems; 15-15A Courtesy of Dr. Robert Burgess, Huggins Back Bay Rehabilitation; 15-15B Courtesy of Dr. Robert Burgess, Huggins Back Bay Rehabilitation; 15-76 © Living Art Enterprises, LLC/Photo Researchers, Inc.; 18-44 Courtesy of Kevin G. Shea, MD, Intermountain Orthopaedics, Boise, Idaho; 19-29 Courtesy of Erik Dalton, Freedom From Pain Institute®; 19-30 Courtesy of DePuy Orthopaedics, Inc. Used with permission; 20-30 © SIU BioMed/Custom Medical Stock Photo; 21-7A © Photos.com; 21-35A © Medical-on-Line/Alamy; 21-35B © Princess Margaret Rose Orthopaedic Hospital/Photo Researchers, Inc.; 22-3 © SIU/Visuals Unlimited, Inc.; 22-4 © Wellcome Images/Custom Medical Stock Photo; 22-14 © Dr. P. Marazzi/Photo Researchers, Inc.

Unless otherwise indicated, all photographs and illustrations are under copyright of Jones & Bartlett Learning or have been provided by the author.